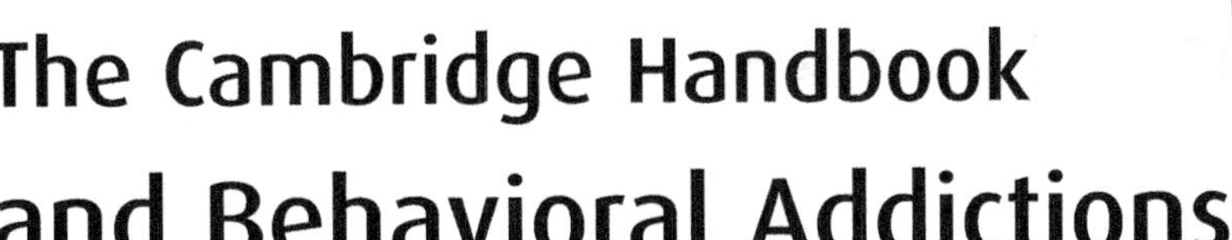

The Cambridge Handbook of Substance and Behavioral Addictions

Edited by

Steve Sussman
University of Southern California

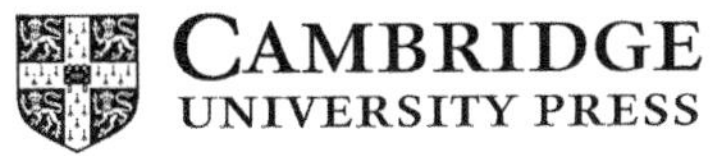

CAMBRIDGE
UNIVERSITY PRESS

University Printing House, Cambridge CB2 8BS, United Kingdom

One Liberty Plaza, 20th Floor, New York, NY 10006, USA

477 Williamstown Road, Port Melbourne, VIC 3207, Australia

314–321, 3rd Floor, Plot 3, Splendor Forum, Jasola District Centre, New Delhi – 110025, India

79 Anson Road, #06–04/06, Singapore 079906

Cambridge University Press is part of the University of Cambridge.

It furthers the University's mission by disseminating knowledge in the pursuit of education, learning, and research at the highest international levels of excellence.

www.cambridge.org
Information on this title: www.cambridge.org/9781108427166
DOI: 10.1017/9781108632591

First published 2020

Printed in the United Kingdom by TJ International Ltd, Padstow Cornwall

A catalogue record for this publication is available from the British Library.

Library of Congress Cataloging-in-Publication Data
Names: Sussman, Steven Yale, editor.
Title: The Cambridge handbook of substance and behavioral addictions / edited by Steve Sussman, University of Southern California.
Description: Cambridge, United Kingdom ; New York, NY : Cambridge University Press, 2020. | Series: Cambridge handbooks in psychology | Includes bibliographical references and index.
Identifiers: LCCN 2020009197 (print) | LCCN 2020009198 (ebook) | ISBN 9781108427166 (hardback) | ISBN 9781108447850 (paperback) | ISBN 9781108632591 (epub)
Subjects: LCSH: Substance abuse. | Substance abuse–Treatment. | Substance abuse–Psychological aspects. | Compulsive behavior.
Classification: LCC RC564 .C29 2020 (print) | LCC RC564 (ebook) | DDC 362.29–dc23
LC record available at https://lccn.loc.gov/2020009197
LC ebook record available at https://lccn.loc.gov/2020009198

ISBN 978-1-108-42716-6 Hardback
ISBN 978-1-108-44785-0 Paperback

The Cambridge Handbook of Substance and Behavioral Addictions

Written by leaders in the addictions field, 100 authors from six countries, this handbook offers a guide to the breadth and depth of addiction processes. Through a detailed explanation of appetitive motivation, incentive sensitization, reward deficiency, and behavioral economics, it provides readers with the necessary conceptual underpinnings to fully grasp this area. Both clinical and research methods are clearly mapped out alongside an outline of their strengths and weaknesses, giving the reader the tools needed to help guide their research and practice aims. The etiology of addiction at various levels of analysis is discussed, including neurobiology, cognition, culture, and environment, which simultaneously lays out the foundations and high-level discourse to serve both novice and expert researchers and clinicians. The volume also explores the prevention and treatment of addictions including alcohol, tobacco, other drugs, food, gambling, sex, work, shopping, the internet, and several seldom-investigated behaviors (e.g., love, tanning, exercise). This practical advice is accompanied with suggestions for future research.

Steve Sussman is Professor of Preventive Medicine, Psychology, and Social Work at University of Southern California, USA. With over 500 publications to his name, he is editor of the journal *Evaluation & the Health Professions* and author of *Substance and Behavioral Addictions: Concepts, Causes, and Cures (2017).*

Contents

Part V Ongoing and Future Research Directions

Figures

Tables

Contributors

Michael Amlung, PhD McMaster University, Hamilton, Ontario, Canada

Fiza Arshad, MS McMaster University, Hamilton, Ontario, Canada

Henri-Jean Aubin, MD, PhD Paris-Sud University, Paris, France

Rajendra D. Badgaiyan, MD cahn School of Medicine, Mount Sinai, New York, NY, USA; University of Texas Medical Center, San Antonio, TX, USA

Sampada Badgaiyan, MD Geneus Health, San Antonio, TX, USA

Iris M. Balodis, PhD McMaster University, Hamilton, Ontario, Canada

David Baron, DO Wright State University, Dayton, OH, USA

Hannah M. Baumgartner, MS University of Michigan, Ann Arbor, MI, USA

Antoine Bechara, PhD University of Southern California, Los Angeles, CA, USA

Mariel S. Bello, MA University of Southern California, Los Angeles, CA, USA

Kent C. Berridge, PhD University of Michigan, Ann Arbor, MI, USA

David S. Black, PhD, MPH University of Southern California, Los Angeles, CA, USA

Donald W. Black, MD University of Iowa, Iowa City, IA, USA

Carlos Blanco, MD, PhD National Institute on Drug Abuse, National Institutes of Health, US Department of Health and Human Services, Bethesda, MD, USA (Foreword)

Austin W. Blum, MD, JD The University of Chicago, Chicago, IL, USA

Kenneth Blum, PhD, DHL Western University Health Sciences, Pomona, CA, USA; Wright University, Dayton, OH, USA; University of Vermont, Burlington, VT, USA

Ricky N. Bluthenthal, PhD University of Southern California, Los Angeles, CA, USA

Maria Bolshakova, BS University of Southern California, Los Angeles, CA, USA

Brent Boyett, DMD, DO Pathway Healthcare, LLC, Birmingham, AL, USA

Eric R. Braverman, MD Path Foundation, New York, NY, USA

Kyle S. Burger, PhD, MPH, RD University of North Carolina at Chapel Hill, Chapel Hill, NC, USA

Nina C. Christie, MA University of Southern California, Los Angeles, CA, USA

Wilson M. Compton, MD, MPE National Institute on Drug Abuse, National Institutes of Health, US Department of Health and Human Services, Bethesda, MD, USA (Foreword)

Ornella Corazza, PhD University of Hertfordshire, Hatfield, Great Britain

Caroline Davis, PhD York University, Toronto, Ontario, Canada

Zsolt Demetrovics, DSc, PhD ELTE Eötvös Loránd University, Budapest, Hungary

Jeffrey L. Derevensky, PhD McGill University, Montreal, Quebec, Canada

Bernard William Downs, BS Victory Nutrition International, Lederach, PA, USA

Danielle Symons Downs, PhD The Pennsylvania State University, University Park, PA, USA

Walter G. Dyer, BS, BA University of Southern California, Los Angeles, CA, USA

Drew Edwards, PhD Lakeview Health, Jacksonville, FL, USA

D. Rose Ewald, MPH University of North Carolina at Greensboro, Greensboro, NC, USA

Helen Fisher, PhD The Kinsey Institute, Bloomington, IN, USA

Charlotte M. Freeland, BS Wesleyan University, Middletown, CT, USA

Artur Galimov, MD University of Southern California, Los Angeles, CA, USA

Ashley N. Gearhardt, PhD University of Michigan, Ann Arbor, MI, USA

Brett W. Gelino, BS University of Kansas, Lawrence, KS, USA

Shane N. Glackin, PhD University of Exeter, Exeter, Great Britain

Mark S. Gold, MD Washington University, St. Louis, MO, USA

Nicholas I. Goldenson, PhD JUUL Labs, Inc., San Francisco, CA, USA

Marjorie C. Gondré-Lewis, PhD Howard University College of Medicine, Washington, DC, USA

Jon E. Grant, JD, MD, MPH The University of Chicago, Chicago, IL, USA

Mark D. Griffiths, PhD Nottingham Trent University, Nottingham, Great Britain

Timothy J. Grigsby, PhD The University of Texas at San Antonio, San Antonio, TX, USA

Joshua B. Grubbs, PhD Bowling Green State University, Bowling Green, OH, USA

Heather A. Hausenblas, PhD Jacksonville University, Jacksonville, FL, USA

Mary Hauser, MA Dominion Diagnostics, North Kingston, Rhode Island, USA

Beth R. Hoffman, PhD California State University, Los Angeles, CA, USA

David P. Jarmolowicz, PhD University of Kansas, Lawrence, KS, USA

Máté Kapitány-Fövény, PhD Semmelweis University, Budapest, Hungary; Nyírő Gyula National Institute of Psychiatry and Addictions, Budapest, Hungary

Afton Kechter, MS University of Southern California, Los Angeles, CA, USA

Shane W. Kraus, PhD University of Nevada at Las Vegas, Las Vegas, NV, USA

Daria J. Kuss, PhD Nottingham Trent University, Nottingham, Great Britain

Anna Yu Lee, BS Claremont Graduate University, Claremont, CA, USA

Adam M. Leventhal, PhD University of Southern California, Los Angeles, CA, USA

Lisa Lott, PhD Geneus Health, San Antonio, TX, USA

James MacKillop, PhD McMaster University, Hamilton, Ontario, Canada

Derek T. Y. Mann, PhD Jacksonville University, Jacksonville, FL, USA

Shanna Marrinan, PhD University of Hertfordshire, Hatfield, Great Britain

Ashley E. Mason, PhD University of California at San Francisco, San Francisco, CA, USA

Darren Mays, PhD, MPH Georgetown University Medical Center and Lombardi Comprehensive Cancer Center, Washington, DC, USA

Thomas McLaughlin, MD Center for Psychiatric Medicine, Lawrence, MA, USA

Kimberly A. Miller, PhD University of Southern California, Los Angeles, CA, USA

Edward J. Modestino, PhD Curry College, Milton, MA, USA

Mark Moran, MD Geneus Health, San Antonio, TX, USA

Vanessa Morris, BA McMaster University, Hamilton, Ontario, Canada

Erin E. Naffziger, MS University of Michigan, Ann Arbor, MI, USA

Gideon P. Naudé, MA University of Kansas, Lawrence, KS, USA

Jeffrey J. Olney, PhD University of Michigan, Ann Arbor, MI, USA

Muhsin Michael Orsini, EdD University of North Carolina at Greensboro, Greensboro, NC, USA

Sheila Pakdaman, MS University of Southern California, Los Angeles, CA, USA

James Russell Pike, MBA Claremont Graduate University, Claremont, CA, USA

Arwen Podesta, MD Tulane University School of Medicine, New Orleans, LA, USA

Jessica Valdez Ponce, MS Geneus Health, San Antonio, TX, USA

Halley M. Pontes, PhD University of Tasmania, Hobart, Australia

Marc N. Potenza, MD, PhD Yale University, New Haven, CT, USA

Cristina Quinones, PhD, CPsychol Open University, Milton Keynes, Buckinghamshire, Great Britain

Derek D. Reed, PhD, BCBA-D University of Kansas, Lawrence, KS, USA

Rory C. Reid, PhD University of California at Los Angeles, Los Angeles, CA, USA

Mike J. F. Robinson, PhD Wesleyan University, Middletown, CT, USA

Alphonse Kenison Roy III, MD, DFASAM, DLFAPA Tulane University School of Medicine, New Orleans, LA, USA

Jennifer R. Sadler, BA University of North Carolina at Chapel Hill, Chapel Hill, NC, USA

Lawrence M. Scheier, PhD LARS Research Institute, Scottsdale, AZ, USA; Prevention Strategies, LLC, Greensboro, Greensboro, NC, USA

Emma. T. Schiestl, MS University of Michigan, Ann Arbor, MI, USA

Tadd D. Schneider, BS University of Kansas, Lawrence, KS, USA

Erica M. Schulte, PhD University of Pennsylvania, Philadelphia, PA, USA

Grace E. Shearrer, PhD University of North Carolina at Chapel Hill, Chapel Hill, NC, USA

Thomas A. Simpatico, MD University of Vermont, Burlington, VT, USA

Kelsey A. Simpson, MA University of Southern California, Los Angeles, CA, USA

David Siwicki, MD Geneus Health, San Antonio, TX, USA

A. Benjamin Srivastava, MD Columbia University, New York, NY, USA

Alan W. Stacy, PhD Claremont Graduate University, Claremont, CA, USA

Bruce Steinberg, PhD Curry College, Milton, MA, USA

Robert W. Strack, PhD University of North Carolina at Greensboro, Greensboro, NC, USA

Steve Sussman, PhD, FAAHB, FAPA, FSPR University of Southern California, Los Angeles, CA, USA

Panayotis K. Thanos, PhD Research Institute on Addictions, University at Buffalo, Buffalo, NY, USA

Jennifer B. Unger, PhD University of Southern California, Los Angeles, CA, USA

Anthony G. Vaccaro, MRes University of Southern California, Los Angeles, CA, USA

Shelley M. Warlow, PhD University of California, San Diego, CA, USA

Daniel H. Willick, PhD, JD Law Offices of Daniel H. Willick, Westlake Village, CA, USA

Foreword

What are the Boundaries of Addictions?

Wilson M. Compton, MD, MPE, and Carlos Blanco, MD, PhD

In addition to substances, a large variety of inherently rewarding behaviors can produce a syndrome with the features of addiction, including severe impairments and consequences, loss of control over the behavior, and excessive salience of the behavior. Individuals who engage in those inherently rewarding behaviors have availed themselves of numerous mutual support programs (twelve-step and others) to ameliorate their symptoms, not only for substance problems but also for nonsubstance issues (Sussman, 2017), suggesting the severity of impairments that persons with nonsubstance addictive syndromes may experience. Furthermore, publication of the DSM-5 (APA, 2013; Hasin et al., 2013) has rekindled interest in defining what an addictive disorder truly is. However, the precise nature of addictive disorders cannot be always exactly delineated, and official nomenclatures only cover a few of the possible behaviors that clinicians and the overall population may consider an addictive disorder in need of prevention or treatment (APA, 2013; Blanco et al., 2008; WHO, 2018).

The boundaries for addictive disorders have been a source of clinical and research inquiry and uncertainty for decades, and the nature of these boundaries exists across a number of dimensions. One source of uncertainty rests within each particular condition. For instance, within each substance addiction, the boundaries between minimal use, misuse, heavy use, problematic use, and addiction are fuzzy. Most research suggests that the disorders exist along a continuum (much like blood pressure) but whether this includes frequency of use of a substance in addition to the number and intensity of symptoms of addiction has remained uncertain (Compton et al., 2009; Dawson, Compton & Grant, 2010; Saha et al., 2010). This same issue may apply to nonsubstance addictive behaviors.

A second area of uncertainty is whether the substance-related disorders are truly separate disorders or represent the expression of an underlying general propensity. Genetic epidemiology research on this question suggests both pathways are found – genetic factors that relate to a general "substance use disorder" propensity as well as genetic risk for specific disorders (Kendler et al., 2003; Tsuang et al., 1998), with additional work suggesting that genetic risks may be distinguished for licit versus illicit substances (Kendler, Myers & Prescott, 2007). Finding an even broader general factor, genetic epidemiology research also suggests an "externalizing spectrum" of disorders (with an underlying antisocial behavior latent trait) that may include substance use addictions and multiple nonsubstance-related disorders (e.g., Krueger et al., 2005; Witkiewitz et al., 2013).

Disclaimer The views expressed in this publication represent the views of the authors and do not necessarily represent the views of the National Institute on Drug Abuse, the National Institutes of Health or the US Department of Health and Human Services.

The third, related, area of uncertainty is whether similar appearing behaviors related to nonsubstance activities are part of a single addictive phenotype. That is, whether other behaviors that share similar symptoms as the substance addictions are part of a single underlying "addiction phenotype" or represent distinct entities. Certainly, individuals struggle to cope with a broad range of compulsive behaviors that share many features with substance addictions. However, are they components of a single dimension, multiple separate dimensions, or some hybrid of these two possibilities? Just as differences and similarities of substance addictions can be studied, research can be used to explore the unique and shared features of substance and nonsubstance addiction phenotypes.

This new *Handbook* explores these important topics in depth and provides an innovative focus on both substance and nonsubstance addictions. Authors include the leaders in the behavioral addiction arena who provide a summary of the breadth of potential behaviors that may be part of the overall addiction phenotype, and explore both the common and unique features of these behaviors. By bringing together this information across a broad range of conditions, this unique *Handbook* provides a wealth of source material to help shape the field of addiction science.

Overall, evidence (including much of the work included in this *Handbook*) suggests considerable, though incomplete, overlap among the substance and nonsubstance conditions. Symptoms of nonsubstance behaviors have been associated with other findings expected to precede, cooccur with, or be the consequences of, an addictive disorder, and the existence of multiple antecedent, concurrent, and consequent correlates supports the validity of behavioral addictions as both related and distinct entities (Franco et al., 2019). That is, for most, but not all, the patterns of risk factors, comorbidity, and outcomes indicate both shared and unique features.

For example, evidence for being part of a common addictive phenotype varies by behavior. The evidence is compelling for gambling disorder, but less so for others. For conditions such as obesity and obsessive-compulsive disorder (OCD), even with repetitive behaviors involved, the link to addictive disorders is much less clear. Gambling disorder (or addiction) shares many risk factors, overlaps extensively in patterns of comorbidity, and shares phenotypic symptom expression with substance addictions. By contrast, overeating, obesity, and substance use addictions appear to share many phenotypic characteristics and underlying neurocircuitry (Volkow et al., 2013) but overlap little in terms of comorbidity (Pickering et al., 2007) and obesity does not appear to fit well in an addictive latent factor (Blanco et al., 2015). In addition, it has been shown that substance addictions share some features with OCD, particularly repetitive, poorly controlled, stereotyped behaviors, which may be mediated by a shared, underlying compulsivity factor (Figee et al., 2016). In addition, negative reinforcement is important in

OCD and may play a key role in later stages of addiction (Koob, 2015). Yet, a key distinction between OCD and addictive disorders is that, while performing the rituals may help relieve distress and thus generate negative reinforcement, OCD does not have the positive reward inherent in the onset of addictive disorders. Such overlaps and differences within overall similarly expressed behaviors are a stark reminder that the boundaries between substance and nonsubstance addictions (and with nonaddictive disorders) need additional research.

What are the implications of this *Handbook*? Most obviously, there are consistent patterns that many practitioners and the public label as "addictions." Such terminology may support treatment-seeking by those who seek relief from distress and dysfunction. Further, even when such terminology does not fully represent the underlying etiology adequately, it may allow for development of interventions and policies that improve patient outcomes and overall public health.

In addition, phenotypic heterogeneity, both within a single behavioral addiction subtype and across different addictions, indicates the involvement of more than one neurobiological pathway for all of these conditions, with multiple causes of the dysfunctions that underlie symptoms. For example, genetic predisposition, childhood maltreatment, or recent stressful events alone or in combination can all affect executive function (Blanco, Compton & Lopez, 2018). Disturbances in executive function can be important in the etiology of multiple addiction phenotypes, and possible integrative models have been proposed (e.g., Blanco et al., 2014; Sussman, 2017). However, a mechanistic understanding is needed of the interplay of risk factors within an individual that may lead to the development of disturbances in executive function (and a likely complex extension to addictive disorders and psychiatric disorders more generally). Such research on these and other neurobiologicial pathways may inform "precision epidemiology," as part of the future of precision medicine and precision public health, thus guiding prevention at the individual and community level (Blanco et al., 2016, 2018; Clayton & Collins, 2014; Collins & Varmus, 2015; Desmond-Hellman, 2016; Kendler, Gardner & Prescott, 2006).

To address these complex issues, integrated science across disciplines is needed. For instance, although epidemiology and neuroscience are often viewed as separate disciplines, there is a growing consensus for the need to better integrate these disciplines. Neuroscience can help uncover the mechanisms underlying population-based findings, whereas epidemiological methods, including use of representative samples, can help generalize the insights generated by neuroscience. In addition, large-scale longitudinal studies would benefit from including information from additional sources, such as use of healthcare services (e.g., prescription information). The ability to combine high-quality diagnostic data (and possibly environmental and biological variables) with service outcomes would generate unprecedented opportunities to advance research and practice. One key example of this type of research is the Adolescent Brain Cognitive Development (ABCD) study (Lisdahl et al., 2018). This landmark project has successfully completed baseline neuropsychiatric, developmental, and neuroimaging assessments of 11,875 children aged nine to ten. The study is currently conducting follow up of these youth and their families with plans to evaluate them repeatedly over the ensuing decade to examine trajectories of normal and pathological conditions (Casey et al., 2018). As such, the ABCD study is poised to address just the sort of questions that remain about the development and overlap of substance and nonsubstance addictions.

A complex but important topic will be the conceptualization of the comorbidity of behavioral addictions (with substance addictions and other psychiatric disorders) and the implications for understanding causal mechanisms, measurement, and treatment. Research is also needed to link epidemiological findings to clinical and basic neuroscience. Are the brain pathways associated with different diagnostic criteria the same in behavioral addictions as in substance addictions? Such work will help to determine the overall validity and significance of behavioral addictions.

As we continue to delineate different levels of description and explanation of what a substance use disorder or (more broadly) an addictive disorder is, there are exciting opportunities for nosological research, precision epidemiology, neurobiology, and intervention development. Iteratively answering those questions should help advance science and, more importantly, improve the health of individuals with a variety of addictive phenotypes.

REFERENCES

American Psychiatric Association [APA] (2013). *Diagnostic and Statistical Manual of Mental Disorders* (5th edition) (DSM-5). Washington, DC: American Psychiatric Publishing.

Blanco, C., Compton, W. M. & Grant, B. F. (2016). Toward precision epidemiology. *JAMA Psychiatry*, **73**(10), 1008–1009.

Blanco, C., Compton, W. M. & Lopez, M. F. (2018). What is an addictive disorder? *JAMA Psychiatry*, **75**(3), 229–230.

Blanco, C., García-Anaya, M., Wall, M., et al. (2015). Should pathological gambling and obesity be considered addictive disorders? A factor analytic study in a nationally representative sample. *Drug and Alcohol Dependence*, **150**, 129–134.

Blanco, C., Ogburn, E., Pérez de Los Cobos, J., et al. (2008). DSM-IV criteria-based clinical subtypes of cannabis use disorders: results from the National Epidemiological Survey on Alcohol and Related Conditions (NESARC). *Drug and Alcohol Dependence*, **96**(1–2), 136–144.

Blanco, C., Rafful, C., Wall, M. M., et al. (2014). Towards a comprehensive developmental model of cannabis use disorders. *Addiction*, **109**(2), 284–294.

Casey, B. J., Cannonier, T., Conley, M. I., et al. (2018). The Adolescent Brain Cognitive Development (ABCD) study: imaging acquisition across 21 sites. *Developmental Cognitive Neuroscience*, **32**, 43–54.

Clayton, J. A. & Collins, F. C. (2014). NIH to balance sex in cell and animal studies. *Nature*, **509**, 282–283.

Collins, F. S. & Varmus, H. (2015). A new initiative on precision medicine. *New England Journal of Medicine*, **372**(9), 793–795.

Compton, W. M., Saha, T. D., Conway, K. P. & Grant, B. F. (2009). The role of cannabis use within a dimensional approach to cannabis use disorders. *Drug and Alcohol Dependence*, **100**(3), 221–227.

Dawson, D. A., Compton, W. M. & Grant, B. F. (2010). Frequency of 5+/4+ drinks as a screener for drug use and drug use disorders. *Journal of Studies on Alcohol and Drugs*, **71**(5), 751–760.

Desmond-Hellmann, S. (2016). Progress lies in precision. *Science*, **353**(6301), 731.

Figee, M., Pattij, T., Willuhn, I., et al. (2016). Compulsivity in obsessive-compulsive disorder and addictions. *European Neuropsychopharmacology*, **26**(5), 856–868.

Franco, S., Olfson, M., Wall, M. M., et al. (2019). Shared and specific associations of substance use disorders on adverse outcomes: a national prospective study. *Drug and Alcohol Dependence*, **201**, 212–219.

Hasin, D. S., O'Brien, C. P., Auriacombe, M., et al. (2013). DSM-5 criteria for substance use disorders: recommendations and rationale. *American Journal of Psychiatry*, **170**(8), 834–851.

Kendler, K. S., Gardner, C. O. & Prescott, C. A. (2006). Toward a comprehensive developmental model for major depression in men. *American Journal of Psychiatry*, **163**(1), 115–124.

Kendler, K. S., Jacobson, K. C., Prescott, C. A. & Neale, M. C. (2003). Specificity of genetic and environmental risk factors for use and abuse/dependence of cannabis, cocaine, hallucinogens, sedatives, stimulants, and opiates in male twins. *American Journal of Psychiatry*, **160**(4), 687–695.

Kendler, K. S., Myers, J. & Prescott, C. A. (2007). Specificity of genetic and environmental risk factors for symptoms of cannabis, cocaine, alcohol, caffeine, and nicotine dependence. *Archives of General Psychiatry*, **64**(11), 1313–1320.

Koob, G. F. (2015). The dark side of emotion: the addiction perspective. *European Journal of Pharmacology*, **753**, 73–87.

Krueger, R. F., Markon, K. E., Patrick, C. J. & Iacono, W. G. (2005). Externalizing psychopathology in adulthood: a dimensional-spectrum conceptualization and its implications for DSM-V. *Journal of Abnormal Psychology*, **114**(4), 537–550.

Lisdahl, K. M., Sher, K. J., Conway, K. P., et al. (2018). Adolescent brain cognitive development (ABCD) study: overview of substance use assessment methods. *Developmental Cognitive Neuroscience*, **32**, 80–96.

Pickering, R. P., Grant, B. F., Chou, S. P. & Compton, W. M. (2007). Are overweight, obesity, and extreme obesity associated with psychopathology? Results from the national epidemiologic survey on alcohol and related conditions. *Journal of Clinical Psychiatry*, **68** (7), 998–1009.

Saha, T. D., Compton, W. M., Pulay, A. J., et al. (2010). Dimensionality of DSM-IV nicotine dependence in a national sample: an item response theory application. *Drug and Alcohol Dependence*, **108**, 21–28.

Sussman, S. (2017). *Substance and Behavioral Addictions: Concepts, Causes, and Cures*. Cambridge, UK: Cambridge University Press.

Tsuang, M. T., Lyons, M. J., Meyer, J. M., et al. (1998). Co-occurrence of abuse of different drugs in men: The role of drug-specific and shared vulnerabilities. *Archives of General Psychiatry*, **55**(11), 967–972.

Volkow, N. D., Wang, G. J., Tomasi, D. & Baler, R. D. (2013). Obesity and addiction: neurobiological overlaps. *Obesity Reviews*, **14**(1), 2–18.

Witkiewitz, K., King, K., McMahon, R. J., et al. (2013). Evidence for a multi-dimensional latent structural model of externalizing disorders. *Journal of Abnormal Child Psychology*, **41**(2), 223–237.

World Health Organization [WHO] (2018). *ICD-11 for Mortality and Morbidity Statistics (ICD-11 MMS)*. Geneva, Switzerland: WHO (https://icd.who.int/)

Preface

The testimonials of countless persons attest to the existence of any number of behaviors that manifest themselves addictively, begetting numerous twelve-step programs and mutual support chatrooms (Sussman, 2017). Conversely, research in its cautious tone, acknowledges the likely existence of a variety of substance and behavioral addictions – but does not yet officially confirm their existence except for gambling (APA, 2013) and, very recently, online and offline gaming disorder (WHO, 2018). Official recognition is derived from the consensus of individuals, who agree or disagree for any number of reasons to include use of a substance or excessive engagement in a behavior as being an addiction.

There are several barriers to achieving a comprehensive understanding of the breadth of addictive behaviors. First, consensus on what is an addiction is not established across all decision makers, and some behaviors have been referred to as impulse control disorders instead of or prior to later being identified as an addiction (e.g., with problem gambling). Also, there may be disagreement regarding the importance of suffering negative consequences for an addiction to be considered in existence (the "positive" addiction). However, this *Handbook* takes the stance that extensive involvement in an activity that causes no problems might be better considered a "passion" rather than an addiction. Arguably, there are common features which may reflect a general understanding of addiction. These features include some type of neurobiological effect reflecting recurrent involvement with a behavior (perhaps subjectively experienced as improved affect, arousal, or cognition), followed by preoccupation with the addictive behavior, loss of control, and experience of undesired, negative consequences (see Sussman & Pakdaman, 2020). The World Health Organization includes these features explicitly in its current definition (WHO, 2018).

Second, given that there is reasonable consensus on what defines an "addiction," some researchers have set up research demands that many addictive behaviors do not yet meet. For example, some professionals desire that there be well-defined criteria specific to an addiction that have been studied in general population samples, along with neurobiological evidence, that the addictive behavior exists – beyond the subjective reports of the sufferer (Sussman, 2017). Some researchers desire that behavioral addictions should emulate drug addictions in topography and neurobiological responses. Some researchers wonder whether some behaviors are impulsive or compulsive disorders rather than addictions (see Blum & Grant, 2020). When one considers the current status of neurobiological knowledge (or lack thereof) regarding even currently recognized addictions (see Burger, Shearrer & Sadler, 2020; Christie & Bechara, 2020; Vaccaro & Potenza, 2020), one may begin to assert that subjective experience and common criteria are the best sources of information available – which do permit examination of addictions as a quantitative phenomenon that can apply to many types of behavior.

Finally, there are practical concerns. Some professionals take a rather skeptical stance and warn that admitting the existence of any number of addictive behaviors would lead to the drying up of precious insurance coverage. So, an addiction arguably may need to demonstrate excessive costs to self and others prior to being labeled as a problematic or "true" addiction. Several addictions that might cause problems to self may not cause tremendous social problems, such as work, shopping, or exercise addictions – although at the extremes anything is possible. For example, consider the social costs incurred by that shopaholic who experiences incredible debt within a family or steals from the workplace to pay off loans.

There is a shallow quality to a conceptual understanding of addictions when one takes a focus on substances, though substance addictions do tend to harm self and others quite unambiguously with recurrent engagement. Unfortunately, substance addictions may get confounded with physiological tolerance and withdrawal which, for many persons, is irritating but not a life-long difficulty. For example, someone taking medication as prescribed may find themselves suffering from withdrawal symptoms when they stop taking the medication. Even though they suffer withdrawal symptoms, it does not well-describe the loss of control or preoccupation aspects of addiction – it is just a painful inconvenience until the (nonvulnerable) person can get through a neurobiological readjustment. Only some people may find it practically impossible to quit substance use, or some other addictive behavior, suggesting that vulnerability, along with living in difficult life contexts, plays a role (e.g., see Blum et al., 2020; Sussman & Pakdaman, 2020).

While perhaps not having a substance addiction problem, there are persons that cause havoc to themselves and families through participation in gambling, gaming, or other behavior addictions. There is no physiological withdrawal due to the intake of exogenous ligands (drugs), though endogenous ligand turnover (naturally occurring neurotransmission) may indeed have become dependent on participation in these behaviors (Sussman, 2017). That is, one's neurobiology is flexible; it "learns" to respond and adapt to behavioral signals. Humans think, and associational memory may impact one in all sorts of ways, including the creation of behavioral addictions (see Stacy, Pike & Lee, 2020). It is reasonable to assert that there are many types of behaviors that can become addictive. It is most feasible that addiction is a problem of life-style and associational memory, which interface with neurobiological processes associated with obtaining appetitive effects. That is, addiction probably reflects an appetitive motivation neurobiological system gone awry; may be recurrent or periodic; may be severe or not; may appear normative or deviant; and is likely to be very distressful only at some point (Sussman, Rozgonjuk & Eijnden, 2017).

This *Handbook*

The purpose of this thirty-four-chapter volume is to summarize and advance work on substance and behavioral addictions as described in multiple disciplines including psychology, sociology, social work, ecology, economics, preventive medicine, neurobiology, neuroscience, law, philosophy, and psychiatry. This text will be a rather useful resource that can assist in graduate-level teaching, research, prevention, and treatment of the addictions broadly defined. There are no handbooks of this scope and length in existence on the topic. Given the fact that addictions broadly defined is a rapidly growing research arena, the time is ripe for such a novel work.

This edited text is designed primarily for graduate students, researchers, and practitioners interested in the breadth and depth of addiction processes to better understand conceptual underpinnings, etiology, prevention, and treatment. Courses might include those for chemical dependence counselors in advanced training, health promotion, health education, health behavior research, public health, social work, and health psychology. It is being written at a level that anyone who has completed college general education requirements might be able to appreciate the text. Still, those with an advanced education may be better able to appreciate several concepts presented (e.g., aspects of neurotransmission, appetitive effects, behavioral economics theorems). The text presents multiple addictions, several of which are not currently recognized as such by the DSM-5 (due to need for additional research support, though acknowledged as potential addictions). The reach of this text is to multiple addictions. We consider eleven focal addictions (Sussman 2017): tobacco, alcohol, other drugs, food, gambling, internet [gaming], love, sex, exercise, shopping, and workaholism. Tanning was added as a twelfth type (see Miller & Mays, 2020).

Each of the thirty-four chapters provides an overview of the topic, citing the most current and credible research. These chapters are grouped within five parts (sections). Part I of the *Handbook* grapples with concepts of addiction in four chapters, being careful to encompass both substance (drugs, food) and behavioral addictions. Three of among the most impactful models of addiction are presented, including a general appetitive needs framework, behavioral economics, and sensitization of incentive salience. Finally, a presentation of philosophical issues in the addictions is presented, to help guide future conceptualizations or integrations of concepts.

Part II of the *Handbook* presents five chapters on clinical and research methods used to tap addictions. These include human neuroimaging, human laboratory paradigms, behavioral economics assessment, clinical assessment instruments, and qualitative assessment of addiction.

Part III of the *Handbook* explores the etiology of the addictions at various levels of analysis. These five chapters examine neurobiology of substance addictions, neurobiology of behavioral addictions, multiple memory systems and addiction, cultural influences on behavioral addictions, and the built environment and policy factors that place persons at risk for addiction.

Part IV of the *Handbook* explores prevention and treatment of the addictions. Separate chapters exist for the prevention and treatment of drug addictions, because much more research has been completed on these. The nine chapters in this section examine the prevention and treatment of: alcohol, tobacco, and other drugs (ATOD) [as two chapters], food addiction, gambling disorders, sex addiction, love addiction, shopping addiction, work addiction, and internet addiction and gaming disorder.

Finally, Part V of the *Handbook* explores ongoing and future research directions. Eleven chapters are in this section. The first chapter in this section (Chapter 24) discusses Precision Behavioral Management techniques to alter dopaminergic function and lessen the vulnerability to addiction, with relevance to the opiate crisis. The next chapter presents novel psychoactive substances and implications for prevention and treatment. This is followed by a chapter on the assessment and treatment of impaired professionals. Chapter 27 is on feedback models to assist in gambling control. The debate on food versus eating addictions is presented in Chapter 28. Next, the measurement, prevention, and treatment of exercise addiction is presented, with a lens on future research directions. Then, tanning addiction is presented as Chapter 30. It oftentimes is not treated as a focal addiction, but its prevalence is surprisingly high. The debate on the overlap among compulsions, impulsions, and addiction composes Chapter 31. Next, emotion-related therapy is discussed for its implications for the remediation of addictive disorders. Chapter 33 discusses the use of mindfulness in prevention and treatment of the addictions. The final chapter explores ethical and legal issues in addiction research and practice.

This text provides a rather comprehensive and novel presentation and should help spur on research and practice in new directions. It is hoped that this *Handbook* will catapult the arena of substance and behavioral addictions.

REFERENCES

American Psychiatric Association (2013). *Diagnostic and Statistical Manual of Mental Disorders*, (5th edition). Washington, DC: American Psychiatric Association Publishing.

Blum, A. W. & Grant, J. E. (2020). Considering the overlap and nonoverlap of compulsivity, impulsivity, and addiction. In S. Sussman (Ed.) *The Cambridge Handbook of Substance and Behavioral Addictions*. Cambridge, UK: Cambridge University Press, pp. 373–385.

Blum, K., et al. (2020). Precision behavioral management (PBM): A novel genetically guided therapy to combat reward deficiency syndrome (RDS) relevant to the opiate crisis. In S. Sussman (Ed.) *The Cambridge Handbook of Substance and Behavioral Addictions*. Cambridge, UK: Cambridge University Press, pp. 297–306.

Burger, K. S., Shearrer, G. E. & Sadler, J. R. (2020). Human neurobiological approaches to hedonically motivated behaviors. In S. Sussman (Ed.) *The Cambridge Handbook of Substance and Behavioral Addictions*. Cambridge, UK: Cambridge University Press, pp. 53–61.

Christie, N. & Bechara, A. (2020). Neurobiology of substance addictions. In S. Sussman (Ed.) *The Cambridge Handbook of Substance and Behavioral Addictions*. Cambridge, UK: Cambridge University Press, pp. 121–135.

Miller, K. A. & Mays, D. (2020). Tanning as an addiction: The state of the research and implications for intervention. In S. Sussman (Ed.) *The Cambridge Handbook of Substance and Behavioral Addictions*. Cambridge, UK: Cambridge University Press, pp. 362–372.

Stacy, A. W., Pike, J. & Lee, A. Y. (2020). Multiple memory systems, addiction, and health habits: New routes for translational science. In S. Sussman (Ed.) *The Cambridge Handbook of Substance and Behavioral Addictions*. Cambridge, UK: Cambridge University Press, pp. 152–170.

Sussman, S. (2017). *Substance and Behavioral Addictions: Concepts, Causes, and Cures*. Cambridge, UK: Cambridge University Press.

Sussman, S. & Pakdaman, S. (2020). Appetitive needs and addiction. In S. Sussman (Ed.) *The Cambridge Handbook of Substance and*

Behavioral Addictions. Cambridge, UK: Cambridge University Press, pp. 3–11.

Sussman, S., Rozgonjuk, D. & van den Eijnden, R. (2017). Substance and behavioral addictions may share a similar underlying process of dysregulation. *Addiction*, **112**, 1717–1718.

Vaccaro, A. G. & Potenza, M. N. (2020). Neurobiological foundations of behavioral addictions. In S. Sussman (Ed.) *The Cambridge Handbook of Substance and Behavioral Addictions*. Cambridge, UK: Cambridge University Press, pp. 136–151.

World Health Organization (WHO) (2018). *ICD-11 for Mortality and Morbidity Statistics (ICD-11 MMS)*. Geneva, Switzerland: WHO (https://icd.who.int/)

Acknowledgements

I would like to thank Steven Acera and Emily Watton of Cambridge University Press, and Beverley Lawrence, for helping me bring this text to print. Their editorial efforts and support are greatly appreciated. I would also like to thank Ellen Galstyan, Leah Meza, and Sheila Pakdaman for their administrative assistance. I would also like to thank the ninety-nine coauthors of this *Handboo*k that created this cohesive and comprehensive volume. We all hope that this text will help boost an understanding of the depth and breadth of addiction, assert for new research directions, and provide solutions within the arena. Finally, I thank Rotchana, Tina, Evelyn, Evan, and Max for their collective family support that helped balance out the bad days and charge up the good days.

Part I

Concepts of Addiction

1 Appetitive Needs and Addiction

Steven Sussman, PhD, FAAHB, FAPA, FSPR, and Sheila Pakdaman, MS

Introduction

The word "addiction" originates from the Latin word "*addictio*", which means to be indebted to or, more colloquially, to be enslaved by (e.g., Mahoney, 2018; Sussman, 2017). Over time, addiction has come to refer to a pathological preoccupation with, and loss of control over, substance use and other behaviors, related to dysregulated activation of the neurobiological motivation–reward system (e.g., Kalivas & Volkow, 2005; Nathan, Conrad & Skinstad, 2016; WHO, 2018). Sussman and Sussman (2011) asserted that addiction involves five distinct components: (a) existence of subjective appetitive needs, (b) repeated attempts at satiation of these needs through engagement in specific behaviors (achieving subjectively experienced "appetitive effects"), (c) preoccupation with obtaining appetitive effects via the associated behavior, (d) loss of control over time spent engaged in the appetitive effect-related behavior, and (e) undesired or negative consequences resulting from continued engagement in the behavior (such as failure to meet work, familial, and social obligations; suffering physical injury or emotional turmoil). As will be described in this chapter, it is theorized that addictive phenomena operate, in part, through learned alteration of appetitive mechanisms involving a misleading, temporary subjective sense of neurobiological fitness (e.g., Sussman, 2017). Unfortunately, the behaviors involved disable the individual over time (Kalivas & Volkow, 2005). The focus of this chapter is to achieve a better understanding of addiction from the perspective of dysregulation of appetitive behaviors.

Appetitive Needs

Over a period of 100 years, evolutionary biologists, ethologists, psychiatrists, motivation psychologists, and neuroscientists have described "appetitive needs" (i.e., roughly synonymous with human instincts, motives, or drives). Appetitive needs have been asserted to be universal among human beings and may support the fulfillment of important survival maintenance functions (Richards, 2018). Early theorists suggested that humans experience innate and secondarily acquired appetitive needs. These needs are invoked by interoceptive (e.g., hunger pangs) and environmental (e.g., sight or smell of food) stimuli that guide behavior toward rewarding outcomes which satiate those needs (e.g., Buss, 2015; Craig, 1917; Darwin, 1871; Kalivas & Volkow, 2005; Lashley, 1938; Maslow, 1954; McDougall, 1932; Murray, 1938; Richards, 2018; Ryan & Deci, 2000). Primary appetitive needs related to survival include hunger, thirst, sleep, and reproduction. In addition, many other primary or secondarily acquired appetitive needs have been suggested, including desires to: (a) increase sociability (be part of a human "herd," relatedness); (b) love and be loved (affection, sexual love, parental love, self- and other nurturance); (c) submit to a social order (be submissive for protection); (d) procure a meaningful position within the human herd (leadership, dominance, competence, power, self-assertion); (e) play and imitate (learn); (f) explore and obtain new resources (curiosity, autonomy); and (g) possess (covet, hoard) things (see Alcoholics Anonymous, 1976; Angell, 1906; Baumeister & Leary, 1995; Buss, 2015; Loonis, Apter & Sztulman, 2000; Maslow, 1943; McClelland, 1961; McDougall, 1932 [eighteen basic needs or instincts are suggested]; Murray, 1938 [twenty manifest needs are suggested]; Ryan & Deci, 2000). More recent evolutionary theories of human behavior have asserted that subjective experience of adaptation attributes such as survival ability and reproductive fitness are reflected biologically in the operations of the mesolimbic dopaminergic system (probably the endpoint of, or nested within, a cascade of other neurobiological systems [e.g., glutaminergic, opioid, serotonergic]; Blum et al., 1996; Kalivas & Volkow, 2005).

Attempts at Classification of Appetitive Needs

A consensus on a systematic typology of appetitive needs does not presently exist. Most mentions of specific types of appetitive needs have been a mere listing (e.g., McDougall, 1932; Murray, 1938), with much overlap across lists. Still, it may be helpful to consider an example of how appetitive needs have been classified prior to tackling an appetitive needs perspective of addiction. A few definitional systems of appetitive needs (motives) have been proposed, perhaps most prominently being Maslow's hierarchy (1943; 1996). Maslow inferred the existence of dimensions of lower-order to higher-order needs (motives, drives). Basic, primitive, "deficiency needs" include physiological (food, water, sleep, sex), safety (personal, financial, well-being), and love/belonging and esteem (respect). Higher-order drive dimensions include self-actualization (being the most one can be) and transcendence (altruism and spirituality).

Some researchers have critiqued the notion of higher-order motives as being culturally nongeneralizable. For example, Hofstede (1984) suggested that higher-order motives are not applicable to collectivistic cultures, which may not emphasize self-actualization as a goal. The general concept of appetitive needs and satiation of those needs, however, appears operative across cultures. For example, Tay and Diener (2011) examined the association between the fulfillment of needs and subjective well-being across 123 countries. Subjective need fulfillment was associated with reports of well-being across world regions. Other research on the relations of appetitive needs with mental and social health indicators is ongoing and includes such topics as appetitive motivation and negative emotion reactivity (Hankin, Wetter & Flory, 2012), aggression reactivity (Beaver et al., 2008), behavioral activation (Jackson & Smillie, 2004; of exploration-related motives), social affiliation/insecurity (Gable, 2006), cognition (Aarts, van Holstein & Cools, 2011), and addiction (Haylett, Stephenson & Lefever, 2004; MacLaren & Best, 2010; Sussman, 2012, 2017).

Both purportedly "innate" and "learned" motives have been studied (e.g., McClelland, 1961, 1987; the achievement motive). Learned motives (needs) may develop through an initial association with innate motives (e.g., Lang & Bradley, 2013). A few studies have even tied study of appetitive needs to substance use. For example, McClelland and colleagues (1972) found evidence that heavy male alcohol drinking was at least partly a function of attempting to satisfy a motive of personalized power (McClelland et al., 1972; also see recent qualitative work by Eng & Woodside, 2012). One may speculate that individuals learn to associate and experience achievement of power within the social herd through engagement in various behaviors, which could include addictive behaviors – such as drinking alcohol. The fact that people learn to adapt to interoceptive stimuli (craving) and environmental stimuli (e.g., colorful advertisements for alcohol) through modification of their behavioral repertoire – to hasten the experience of satiation – is at the very heart of the appetitive needs notion of addiction.

Momentary Dysregulation of Appetitive Effects

Overconsumption of highly processed food, alcohol, and drugs, and overindulgence in other behaviors (e.g., gaming or gambling marathons, shopping sprees, work binges) are common behaviors. Anecdotally, it is well known that in the United States people tend to eat to excess on Thanksgiving in November and tend to drink alcohol to excess on New Year's Eve, suggesting momentary dysregulation of appetitive function. Many activities that facilitate addiction-like behavior are widely promoted and encouraged in modern society (Brown, 2014), such as directions to distribution points (e.g., casino locations, fast food restaurants, nightclubs; Sussman et al., 2011) and information provided by the mass media (e.g., alcohol commercials) that facilitate experimentation with potentially addictive objects, directed by "acquired drives" (Bejerot, 1972), which may come to supplant other activities.

While overindulgence in a variety of behaviors would appear to mimic addictive disorders, such a pattern of behavior generally occurs on rare occasions, tends to be condoned or tolerated within social contexts, and seldom leads to noticeable negative consequences. There are at least four situations or contexts in which excessive behaviors may be condoned, tolerated, or possibly ritualized. First, there are celebratory occasions, such as certain holidays (e.g., New Years Eve), the birth of a child, or marriage-related parties, within which excessive alcohol consumption may be condoned. An infamous example, the night-before bachelor/bachelorette parties are known for overindulgence in the USA. (Note movies such as *The Hangover*, 2009, distributed by Warner Brothers Pictures.) Second, when traumatic events lead one to feel very sad (such as the death of a loved one), some cultures may consider overindulgence (e.g., of alcohol) acceptable (e.g., a New Orleans funeral). Other events (e.g., loss of a job) may lead to temporary overindulgence (e.g., of alcohol), which might be tolerated but probably not condoned. Third, exploration (e.g., with drugs), or "expanding one's mind," during emerging adulthood appears to be tolerated, condoned, and possibly ritualized in the USA (Sussman & Arnett, 2014). For example, college groups like fraternities and sororities may foster substance use as "rites of passage" to adulthood. Finally, there are intra-individual cognitive misperceptions, sometimes promoted by the mass media, which may direct addictive behavior temporarily (Childress et al., 1999; Sussman, 2017). For example, one may believe – perhaps after viewing a movie – that the addictive behavior will help one to be more creative, sophisticated, less bored, or a more critical thinker.

In summary, many behaviors may serve an appetitive function but do not qualify as an addictive, negatively consequential behavior. Engagement in the behavior, temporarily excessive, may not lead to long-lasting functional dysregulation (e.g., overeating at holiday time). Possibly, any appetitive-related behavior might be viewed on a spectrum, from normal to excessive to uncontrolled. If excessive behavior recurs, at some point negative outcomes may result that expert consensus might label as an addiction. That is, excessive, repetitive appetitive behavior may quality as an addiction when it becomes repetitively negatively consequential (Ekhtiari et al., 2016; Orford, 2001; Potenza et al., 2012).

Appetitive Needs and Satiation: Crossing Over to Become an Addiction

In many circumstances, satiation of appetitive needs serves highly adaptive functions. For example, one needs to eat food to live. If one does not obtain food, one will likely crave food and feel as if one will die without eating. (Eventually one will lose his or her appetite – and die.) Conversely, after completing a meal, one may feel satiated (full, satisfied), while bodily cells repair themselves and the individual continues to thrive. As a second example, if one does not feel part of a social herd, one may crave company and possibly even experience phenomena such as "cabin fever" (e.g., restlessness, isolation, boredom; Rosenblatt, Anderson & Johnson, 1984). Conversely, after receiving social supports such as companionship, one may feel satiated (at peace; e.g., Cohen, 1988).

However, an illusory satiation of appetitive needs *via* a learned behavior may develop and become maladaptive ("addiction"). That is, one may experience satiation of a need that does not actually accomplish an adaptive goal. For example, if one suffers from alcoholism, one may feel the need to drink alcohol to live (and possibly achieve a sense of impact on the world or personal power; Eng & Woodside, 2012). If one does not obtain alcohol, one may crave alcohol and feel *as if* one will suffer or die without drinking. (This sort of craving can occur without the experience of acute withdrawal symptoms, or after such symptoms subside.) Once one begins to drink again, one may experience a sense of fulfillment of the appetitive need, at least for a brief period.

One important aspect of an appetitive needs notion of addiction is that, at least temporarily, the individual feels *as if* an appetitive need is resolved by engaging in the behavior; that is, some period may transpire within which cravings/urges are not operative (Foddy & Savulescu, 2010a, 2010b; Hirschman, 1992; Marks, 1990; Orford, 2001; Pearson & Little, 1969). The appetitive need may become reevoked, of course, given renewed exposure to addiction-related cues (Colagiuri & Lovibond, 2015).

Sussman (2017) speculated that satiation is subjectively experienced in at least three ways. First, one may feel an optimal level of pleasure (law of effect). If a person is not feeling good, he/she may engage in certain behaviors to feel better. Second, one may experience an optimal level of arousal. If the person feels over- or under-aroused, the person may modify his/her behavior to obtain a more optimal level of arousal. Finally, one may experience an optimal level of thought activity. If a person is over- or under-thinking, the person may modify his or her mental activity to obtain a more optimal level (exploratory thinking or quieting down thinking).

Ryan and Deci (2000) also refer to the experience of satisfying appetitive needs, in their Self-Determination Theory. They suggest that physiological or psychological needs may be innate, are "energizing states," and include needs for a sense of competence, autonomy, and relatedness. Satisfaction of these needs may be experienced as an ongoing sense of integrity and well-being, self-esteem, self-actualization, or "eudaimonia" (Ryan & Deci, 2000; Ryan & Frederick, 1997). While much more work is needed to objectify the neurobiological constituents of satiation, one may agree that such a state exists, that it is a desired subjective state of being that indicates termination of craving or dissatisfaction, and that is operative temporarily (perhaps even quite briefly) in the case of addictive behavior (Sussman, 2017).

The environmental context discussed later in this chapter as lifestyle "pulls" (seductions) and "pushes" (stresses) may facilitate opportunity for ongoing, recurrent engagement in the addictive behavior and repeated appetitive need-satiation cycles. Through repeated engagement, attentional processes may become increasingly focused on engagement in the addictive behavior. Consequently, the addictive behavior may become highly reliably associated with subjective, temporary fulfillment of an appetitive need. Repeated appetitive need-behavior-satiation cycles may become strongly associated in one's implicit (spontaneous and automatic) memory (e.g., Stacy & Ames, 2001; Wiers et al., 2007). Through repeated exposure, behaviors (e.g., drinking alcohol) associated with appetitive needs (e.g., self-nurturance, personal power) may achieve a relatively high reward value, and become "wanted" (see Warlow et al., 2020, Chapter 3 of *Handbook*). Implicit memory associations, created through experience, may affect which behaviors become relatively more salient for subjectively obtaining specific types of appetitive effects (see Stacy, Pike & Lee, 2020, Chapter 12 of *Handbook*).

Attempts at Classification of Appetitive Needs as Addictive Behaviors

In recent work, appetitive motives have been investigated as a means of differentiating addictive behaviors. Initial work carried out in the 1980s to the early 2000s considered appetitive motives as positive outcome expectancies (see discussion in Wiers et al., 2007), and classified addiction approach motives (primarily alcohol) simply as being either one of positive reinforcement (leading to positive effects) or negative reinforcement (alleviating negative effects). Later, work with the PROMIS questionnaire (Haylett et al., 2004; MacLaren & Best, 2010; PROMIS Clinics, 2018) led researchers to posit at least two general factors, or behavior types, associated with different specific addictive behaviors: "hedonist" types (illegal drugs, tobacco, prescription drugs, gambling, compulsive sex, alcohol, and caffeine) and "nurturant" types (compulsive helping, work, relationships, shopping, eating behaviors, and exercise). Hedonist-type addictive behavior appears to focus on immediate pleasure, whereas nurturant-type addictive behavior appears to focus on personal fulfillment. Haylett et al. (2004) also found some support for dominant and submissive-related factors, possibly nested within hedonist and nurturant factors.

Other literature also has focused on addictions as reflecting fight (e.g., dominance, power) or flight (e.g., retreat into fantasy, submission) motives (Blum et al., 2012; Goeders, 2004; Haylett et al., 2004; Newlin, 2002; Rawson & Condon, 2007; Sunderworth & Milkman, 1991), related to limbic system-based reward and stimulation of the hypothalamic-pituitary-adrenal (HPA) axis (also see Koob & LeMoal, 2001, 2008). Limbic system-associated reward that motivates behaviors to satiate appetitive needs essential to survival is also that system from which drug cravings originate (see Warlow et al., 2020, Chapter 3 of *Handbook*).

Five Appetitive Motive Combinations of Addictions: A Speculative Typology

Sussman (2012, 2017) grouped addictive behaviors into a five appetitive motive combination typology, derived from different logically appearing two-motive combinations of the four previously investigated motives (Haylett et al., 2004): pleasure, self-nurturance, dominance, and submission (withdrawal). (Dominance and submissiveness can't logically occur together.) First, one could withdraw (submission, flight) and feel pleasure. Arousal reduction/sedation might be among subjective effects reported (e.g., opiate drug use). Second, one could dominate and feel pleasure. Subjective effects might include the experience of peak moments or arousal enhancement (e.g., a sex addict who engages in sexual acts that he/she paid for; also, maybe alcohol use). Third, one could achieve self-nurturance and pleasure, subjectively feeling very deeply satisfied at least momentarily (e.g., a food addict after completing a meal). Fourth, one could dominate and feel self-nurturance/self-contained (e.g., a workaholic in action). Finally, one could withdraw and feel self-nurturance (e.g., one who is addicted to engagement in cognitive fantasy or to a spiritual obsession).

Associational Memory-Appetitive System Relations Model (AMASR)

The Associational Memory-Appetitive Systems Relations (AMASR) Model intends to describe how appetitive motives may become excessive, atypically elicited, or misdirected, as an explanation of the addictions. The AMASR Model is depicted in Figure 1.1 below (also see an earlier version of the model in Sussman, 2017). The appetitive needs component has been presented, above. The other components of the AMASR model are described next, and include vulnerability (e.g., genetics), lifestyle, associative learning, and associative memory for alternative behaviors, which act together to lead an individual to addictive (or nonaddictive) appetitive-related behavior.

Vulnerability

It is acknowledged that addictions (e.g., alcohol use) have a substantial genetic component (e.g., up to 50 percent of alcohol use disorders are accounted for by genetics; see Verhulst, Neale & Kendler, 2015). The AMASR model embraces theories which assert that manipulation and dysregulation of one's appetitive needs is partially a function of genetic expression. Individuals with a genetic predisposition to substance or behavioral addictions may have a different physiological reaction when engaging in certain behaviors.

Most addiction researchers appear to attribute appetitive motivation function to the mesolimbic dopaminergic system (Kalivas & Volkow, 2005). This system may be subject to "hijacking" by learned behaviors over time. That is, strong subjective associations may be created between learned behaviors with specific appetitive need attributes (Bejerot, 1972; Blum et al., 2012; Kalivas & Volkow, 2005; Newlin, 2002). The neurochemistry of an individual can potentially create an inclination toward maladaptive appetitive learning and functioning (Laricchiuta & Petrosini, 2014; Panksepp & Moskal, 2008; Wahlstrom, White & Luciana, 2010).

There are at least two competing theories regarding what underlies appetitive system vulnerability: reward deficiency (Blum et al., 2011,

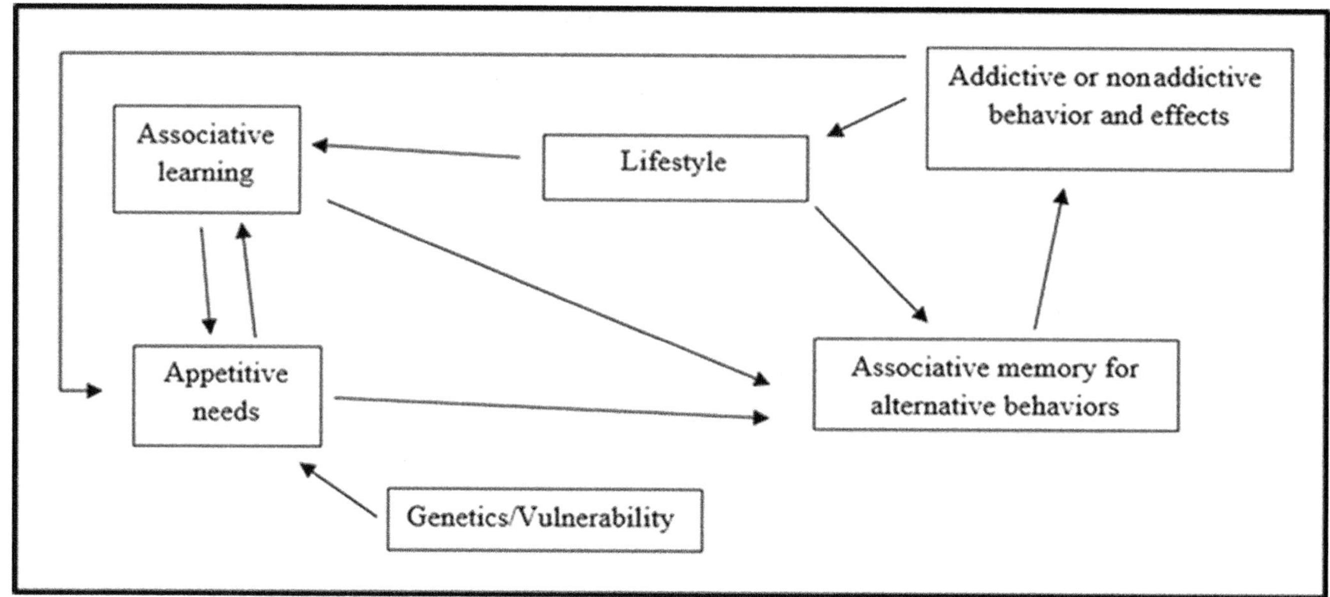

Figure 1.1 AMASR model

2012; see also Blum et al., 2020) versus reward over-reactivity (Berridge, 2017; see Warlow et al., 2020). First, it is possible that dopaminergic gene polymorphisms may be associated with subjective reports of dissatisfaction, anhedonia, or what has been coined as the "reward deficiency syndrome (RDS)" (Blum et al., 2011). The DRD2 gene, which is associated with pleasure or novelty, has been referred to as the "reward gene" (Downs et al., 2009). This gene and the taql A1 allele have been associated with a variety of behavioral disorders such as addiction (Blum et al., 2011; see Blum et al., 2020; Vandenbergh et al., 2007). Extensive behavioral activation may be needed to fulfil appetitive desires in certain individuals; moderation may gradually fail to guide behavior.

Other researchers have argued that maybe mesolimbic suppression is a consequence of engaging in an addictive behavior, rather than a causal factor (Berridge, 2017). Possibly, mesolimbic hyperreactivity to addictive object cues and imagery underlies vulnerability to addiction. Some people may be particularly susceptible to developing a brain response of incentive-sensitization, showing a stronger and quicker response than others to appetitive cues, and this vulnerability may be fundamentally important (Berridge, 2017; Olney et al., 2018). The genetic mechanisms are not yet clear within this perspective.

Certainly, there are yet other possible mechanisms of dysregulation, including – one may speculate – the irregular release of mesolimbic dopamine, or lability of dopamine release, as well as the previous hypo- versus hyperrelease perspectives. In common across these perspectives is atypical mesolimbic dopaminergic responses (as part of a cascade of neurotransmission pathways involving various neurotransmitters). Yet, there are some inconsistencies in current studies regarding addiction-specific neurotransmission pathways (see Vaccaro & Potenza, 2020), and personality factors and brain regions may differ as a function of type of addiction (e.g., see Walther, Morganstern & Hanewinkel, 2012; Zilberman et al., 2019). While assertions regarding specific facets of vulnerability are tentative, the importance of neurobiological vulnerability should not be overlooked. Future research certainly will examine these competing perspectives of mesolimbic dopaminergic vulnerability, as well as potential interactions involving multiple pathways.

Regardless of vulnerability pathway, growth, change, development, adaptation, and phasing take place in every stage of life and alter genetic mapping of appetitive needs. The interface between one's genetics, development, and adaptation with social and physical environmental cues (epigenetics and associative learning) further delineates the potential for addiction (Nestler & Landsman, 2001). For example, prolonged periods of stress, particularly at a young age, may lead to disruption in brain reward cascade functioning (Alexander, 2012; Blum et al., 2011; Fishbein, 2000). Such disruption, in turn, may increase one's susceptibility to addictive behavioral rewards.

Lifestyle

Addictions also may reflect a problem of lifestyle (Sussman, Lisha & Griffiths, 2011). The social and physical environmental settings that one traverses impact what information one learns and how one thinks and may facilitate which behaviors one may select to perform. Daily life events include social "pulls" (seductions) and "pushes" (stresses, social influence) which could potentially facilitate addiction. Regarding the pulls, neurobiological-socio-cultural theories of ill-health note that, as a community settles in one area for a generation, and easily fulfills needs for food, shelter, and protection, sedentary habits may accumulate (Fave, Massimini & Bassi, 2011, p. 25). There may arise a competition between cultural and biological fitness. It is possible that persons may engage in behaviors to help them feel *as if* they are grappling to satiate biological appetitive needs (Newlin, 2002), in a modern societal context which does not provide the arena for application of adaptive physiologic or psychological work to satiate those needs (Blum et al., 2012; Sussman, 2017). From an evolutionary perspective, previous motives of engaging in extensive "work" to satisfy an appetitive motive (e.g., hunting for food, growing one's own food, carefully planning meals, or cooking one's own food) may now be satisfied too easily and quickly (buying a quick meal), also consuming "products" that facilitate "rush" effects (e.g., processed, fatty, or sugary foods), leading to repeated cycles of attempting to satiate the motive with diminishing success (Blum et al., 2012; Hill, 2013; Koob & LeMoal, 2001, 2008; Robinson & Berridge, 2000; Sussman, Reynaud, Aubin & Leventhal, 2011).

For example, there are certain fast-food, drive-thru hamburger restaurants where car drivers may line up for blocks to purchase and consume the food. The experience may constitute an exciting event, involving a social setting and conversation among customers within their cars, and culminating in the ingestion of a 2,000 calorie meal in the United States (e.g., http://calorielab.com/news/2011/03/10/2000-calories-at-in-n-out/; accessed January 15th, 2018), which may permit experiences of both food and adventure satiation (i.e., self-nurturance, pleasure, social herd submission and relatedness motives). Numerous documentaries have been produced exposing the seductive lures of the food, gambling, tobacco, alcohol, and pharmaceutical industries (Courtwright, 2019; McDaniel et al., 2008; Myles, 2014; Sussman, 2017) in enticing engagement in potentially harmful behaviors.

Hill (2013) described several evolutionary theories of addiction, one of which is the *mismatch hypothesis*. Simply put, this social pull notion suggests that triggers in modern civilization (e.g., availability of recreational drugs) may seduce brain reward pathways that had developed through biological evolution to respond promptly to environmental inputs. Subsequent neurobiological adaptations then lead to dysregulation of function over time. It is in this way that one's appetitive functioning may begin to become dysregulated (sometimes rather quickly).

Regarding the social pushes, some authors suggest that modern societies such as the USA are captured by an out-of-control state of expectations conducive to experimentation with addictive behaviors (e.g., Alexander, 2012; Brown, 2014). Emphasis is placed on quick-paced accomplishment-oriented behavior, along with the breaking of extended social cooperative links, and chronic adversity, which may induce some individuals to look for quick ways to relax or distract themselves (Al'Absi, 2007; Sinha, 2008; Sussman, 2017). Certain individuals adapt well to a technologically enhanced, time-pressured lifestyle; others do not. Stress effects may activate the hypothalamic–pituitary–adrenal axis (HPA axis), which can be dampened through activation of the mesolimbic dopaminergic system (Koob & LeMoal, 2001, 2008; Sinha, 2008).

There are many types of lifestyle pushes (i.e., pressures, stressors). Lifestyle stressors which may facilitate coping by engaging in addictive behaviors include experiences of social demands, economic struggles, negative life events (e.g., relationship breakups, violent events), and ethnic/racial discrimination (Jacobs, 1986; Sinha, 2008). Possibly, up to 50 percent of society does not adapt well to the pulls and pushes of modern lifestyles, and some of the resulting patterns of compensatory behavior may become dysregulated (Bechara, 2005; Griffiths & Larkin, 2004; Hatterer, 1982; Holden, 2001; Kourosh, Harrington & Adinoff, 2010; Marks, 1990; Orford, 2001; Sussman, 2017; Sussman, Lisha & Griffiths, 2011).

Associative Learning

Through associative learning and cued adaptive or maladaptive behavioral performance, appetitive needs come to be subjectively evoked and satiated (e.g., Cartoni, Balleine & Baldassarre, 2016). Associational learning and memory have been considered in several recent models of addictive behaviors. One recent "implicit cognition" theory is that addictive behaviors develop as a function of implicit associations between participation in the addictive *behavior* (e.g., smoking cigarettes), *cues* to the addictive behavior (e.g., pipes for smoking, settings, locations), and subjective *outcomes* (physiological or social reward) associated with participating in the addictive behavior (see Stacy et al., 2020). Some individuals may not, through deliberate cognition, recognize that their decisional processes are being influenced by maladaptive reward cues. That is, if implicit cognition-associated cues and outcomes are not channeled through deliberate processes (e.g., introspective self-reflection or causal attribution), then one may behave in concordance with what pops to mind, possibly leading to a maladaptive, addictive chain of behavior.

Wiers et al. (2007) proposed that appetitive motivation is controlled through a dual process of deliberate, conscious, executive, regulatory cognition interacting with relatively automatic, implicit processes, in response to addiction-related cues. He and his colleagues note that adolescence is a particularly vulnerable period for the development of addictions. First, executive inhibitory processes are still developing in adolescence. Second, adolescents may not recognize that engagement in addictive behaviors is a problem. Sussman and Arnett (2014) likewise noted that emerging adulthood is a developmental period in which various addiction-related behaviors are sometimes even promoted by modern society ("sowing the wild oats"). Third, executive cognitive functions may become compromised by engagement in the addictive behavior (e.g., alcohol, marijuana, or tobacco-related impairment of executive cognitive function). Wiers and colleagues (2007) asserted that ability to inhibit or redirect attention or goals (executive functions) and the motivation to do so (expectancies) are the key factors that determine whether an addictive course of action is pursued. These factors are impacted by implicit cognitive processes (e.g., automatic associations among cues, outcomes, and behaviors), individual differences in sensitization effects (craving; also see Warlow and colleagues, 2020), associated stimuli (e.g., negative mood), and social context.

Repeated appetitive need-satiation cycles that become associated with a myriad of cues may become firmly encoded in implicit memory. Over time, partly as a result of relatively automatic prompting by multiple cues, one may experience excessive thoughts and desires to perform a behavior. In turn, excessive time may be spent planning and engaging in the behavior and possibly recovering from its effects (e.g., from "hangovers"). Less time may be spent on other activities, despite potentially diminishing appetitive effects (Sussman & Sussman, 2011). When one considers or "thinks through" (executive cognition) negative consequences resulting from (previous) engagement in the addictive behavior, one may sense or recognize being preoccupied with that addictive behavior.

Difficulty in refraining from an addictive behavior despite attempting to do so may be central to a loss of control aspect of addiction (see Heather, 1998, on "akrasia"; also see Stacy et al., 2020). Attentional narrowing, impulsiveness, along with specific addictive behavior-directed short-term planning (see Stacy et al., 2020), and lack of attention to long-term planning, may all be related to the pattern of addiction-related loss of control (Sussman & Sussman, 2011).

Incomplete memory access appears to be a common feature of substance and behavioral addictions. According to Campbell (2003), the "cognitive impairment" associated with an addiction emerges only when a specific addiction associated with harmful consequences produces a simultaneous positive emotional response. Attentional narrowing minimizes or negates the memory of the negative effects or consequences of previous addictive behavior experiences (or access to aversive memory). Phenomenologically, because of these memory effects, recovering addicts with "sober time" (and who no longer suffer from a cognitive narrowing) may look back at their active addiction days as being fraught with disordered, illogical, fragmented, destructive, and nonsensical thought (Hirschman, 1992).

Associative Memory for Alternative Behaviors

Through vicarious and in-vivo exposure, an addictive behavior may become familiar and be more likely to be recognized as a potential behavioral option. A child who grows up with parents who were engaged in an addictive behavior may be relatively likely to tie appetitive needs fulfillment to an addiction-related lifestyle through vicarious learning (Sussman, 2017). Through participation in an addictive behavior, one may spend less time with others who do not enjoy or approve of the addictive behavior, and one may differentially socialize with similar others who also engage in the addictive behavior (Akers et al., 1979). Through cumulative experience with the addictive behavior, associative memory for alternative behaviors may diminish while number cues that signal anticipation of engaging in the addictive behavior may increase ("vicariance"; Loonis et al., 2000). One becomes more entrenched in the addiction (Sussman, 2017).

Summary

One's neurobiological vulnerability (e.g., genetics), appetitive needs, lifestyle inputs (pulls and pushes), and associative learning (including relative salience of alternative behaviors) impact what behaviors may come to mind in the course of daily life. The elements and potential interactions among constituents of the AMASR Model are depicted in Figure 1.1. Consideration of types of motives is not currently included in the model. At the present time, it is not known for certain if specific appetitive motives are relatively likely to become associated with particular addictive behaviors, or if the same motives might operate for various addictive behaviors. Much more research is needed.

Human Development Contributions to Addictive Behaviors

There are many behaviors that could be experienced as appetitive and become addictive. Some popular behaviors include: tobacco, alcohol, and other drug misuse; binge overeating/food addiction; shopping; electronic media use (e.g., internet use, online gaming); love and sex; workaholism; exercise; and gambling (Sussman, Lisha & Griffiths, 2011). Involvement in different addictions may vary over the course of human development. That is, it is feasible that the development of different types of addictions within the same person may occur over the lifespan. It is possible that the same person may suffer from multiple addictions, longitudinally. Environmental contexts may direct which addictions are accessible to vulnerable persons at different levels of development. Persons as young as three years of age may suffer from television addiction (Sussman & Moran, 2013) though there is little research on this topic. However, anecdotally, parents have observed the consequences of turning off the television on their young children (e.g., the children may become irritable and show difficulties focusing attention), which suggest addiction. Persons as young as eight years of age may become addicted to caffeine (Collins et al., 1997; Sussman & Ames, 2008). They may use caffeine to help regulate their emotions, level of arousal, or cognitive activity, and they may suffer withdrawal symptoms when they are not using caffeine. There is only one study on this topic (i.e., Collins et al., 1997). Additionally, this study found that relatively high and frequent intake of caffeine was predictive of other addictions later on in life (tobacco, alcohol). Persons as young as eleven or twelve years of age may become addicted to cigarette smoking and progress to other drugs when they are maybe fourteen to fifteen years old (e.g., Kandel, 1990). Beginning in the older teen years, people may become addicted to other behaviors (e.g., sex addiction; Sussman, 2007). A person may give up a previous addiction and acquire a new one – or a person may simply add new addictions to their repertoire (i.e., the addiction spectrum may "fan out").

Behaviors That May Not Be Intrinsically Addictive?

There are two parameters of behavior that may not be addictive. First, there may be behaviors, or aspects of behavior, that are unlikely to elicit an appetitive state. Thinking out loud, deliberately focusing one's attention, and self-reflection are not likely to be associated with seeking nurturance, joy, sedation, or arousal, per se; that is, with addictive manifestations of appetitive behaviors (Sussman, Reynaud, Aubin & Leventhal, 2011). Second, the topography of a behavior that is addictive often involves a rapid change in subjective state (a "rush"), whereas behavior that is not addictive may involve a much slower tempo. Gardening, for example, is not addictive for most people because it often involves a slow tempo and patience (Griffiths, 2005). Sleep certainly seems to serve important recuperative functions, but one may be unlikely to become addicted to sleeping.

Furthermore, executive functions or slow-paced behavior may not be aspects of behavior that are likely to become satiated. Consideration of specific goals to be achieved, that necessitate engagement in attentional focus or step-by-step action, certainly may lead one to feel a sense of accomplishment with planning activities, such as completing a gardening sequence. However, this is likely not the same thing as satiating an appetitive motive. Upon ending a period of gardening, one may feel satisfied with the day's work but with a realization that more development of the garden can be completed – and gardening is an ongoing process, which needs to be maintained. Gardening likely does not result in a quick rush or sense of appetitive satiation. Going off to sleep, on the other hand, is an example of an appetitive behavior that can be satiated. However, the fact that sleep does not involve a rapid change in state may underlie its likely nonaddictive status.

Conclusions

Appetitive needs are instinctually embodied in every human being from birth. For over 100 years researchers have been exploring the parameters of human appetitive needs (e.g., Craig, 1917); however, a consensual taxonomy of such needs does not exist yet. A dysregulation of appetitive function, which involves inputs of neurobiological vulnerability, lifestyle factors, and associational memory, is asserted in this chapter as underlying the development of addictive behaviors. If the AMASR Model is applicable, many types of motivation-related behaviors can become addictive (Sussman, Rozgonjuk & Eijnden, 2017). Overindulgence may be condoned under certain conditions (e.g., celebratory), objects of addiction may vary over time (e.g., smartphones were invented in 1992, and their use recently has become problematic), and excessive behavior falls along a continuum which, at some point, comes to be viewed as a negative consequential addiction (Orford, 2001).

Everyday life demands may impact individual decisions and contribute to the development of an addiction. Cooccurrence of addictions may exist, and different addictions may have different appetitive effects across individuals. Research is needed to explore a taxonomy of appetitive needs and how different needs may transform into certain addictive behaviors. There is still much be learned about the role of appetitive needs in the addictive process.

REFERENCES

Aarts, E., van Holstein, M. & Cools, R. (2011). Striatal dopamine and the interface between motivation and cognition. *Frontiers in Psychology*, **2**, 163.

Akers, R. L., Krohn, M. D., Lanza-Kaduce, L. & Radosevich, M. (1979). Social learning and deviant behavior: a specific test of a general theory. *American Sociological Review*, **44**, 636–655.

Al'Absi, M. (Ed., 2007). *Stress and Addiction: Biological and Psychological Mechanisms*. New York, NY: Elsevier/ Academic Press.

Alcoholics Anonymous (1976). *Alcoholics Anonymous*. New York: Alcoholics Anonymous World Services.

Alexander, B. K. (2012). Addiction: The urgent need for a paradigm shift. *Substance Use & Misuse*, **47**, 1475–1482.

Angell, J. R. (1906). The important human instincts. In J. R. Angell (Ed.), *Psychology: An Introductory Study of the Structure and Function of Human Consciousness* (3rd edition). New York: Henry Holt and Company, pp. 294–309.

Baumeister, R. F. & Leary, M. R. (1995). The need to belong: desire for interpersonal attachments as a fundamental human motivation. *Psychological Bulletin*, **117**, 497–529.

Beaver, J. D., Lawrence, A. D., Passamonti, L. & Calder, A. J. (2008). Appetitive motivation predicts the neural response to facial signals of aggression. *Journal of Neuroscience*, **28**, 2719–2725.

Bechara, A. (2005). Decision making, impulse control and loss of willpower to resist drugs: a neurocognitive perspective. *Nature Neuroscience*, **8**, 1458–1463.

Bejerot, N. (1972). A theory of addiction as an artificially induced drive. *American Journal of Psychiatry*, **128**, 842–846.

Berridge, K. C. (2017). Is addiction a brain disease? *Neuroethics*, **10**, 29–33.

Blum, K., et al. (2020). Precision behavioral management (PBM): A novel genetically guided therapy to combat reward deficiency syndrome (RDS) relevant to the opiate crisis. In S. Sussman (Ed.) *The Cambridge Handbook of Substance and Behavioral Addictions*. Cambridge, UK: Cambridge University Press, pp. 297–306.

Blum, K., Chen, A. L., Giordano, J., et al. (2012). The addicted brain: all roads lead to dopamine. *Journal of Psychoactive Drugs*, **44**, 134–143.

Blum, K., Chen, A. L. C., Oscar-Berman, M., et al. (2011). Generational association studies of dopaminergic genes in Reward Deficiency Syndrome (RDS) Subjects: selecting appropriate phenotypes for reward dependence behaviors. *International Journal of Environmental Research and Public Health*, **8**, 4425–4459.

Blum, K., Cull, J. G., Braverman, E. R. & Comings, D. E. (1996). Reward deficiency syndrome. *American Psychologist*, **84**, 132–145.

Brown, S. (2014). *Speed: Facing Our Addiction to Fast and Faster – And Overcoming Our Fear of Slowing Down*. New York, NY: Berkley Books.

Buss, D. (Ed., 2015). *The Handbook of Evolutionary Psychology* (2nd edition). Hoboken, NJ: John Wiley & Sons, Inc.

Campbell, W. G. (2003). Addiction: a disease of volition caused by a cognitive impairment. *Canadian Journal of Psychiatry*, **48**, 669–674.

Cartoni, E., Balleine, B. & Baldassarre, G. (2016). Appetitive Pavlovian-instrumental transfer: a review. *Neuroscience & Biobehavioral Reviews*, **71**, 829–848.

Childress, A. R., Mozley, P. D., McElgin, W., et al. (1999). Limbic activation during cue-induced cocaine craving. *American Journal of Psychiatry*, **156**, 11–18.

Cohen, S. (1988). Psychosocial models of the role of social support in the etiology of physical disease. *Health Psychology*, **7**, 269–297.

Colagiuri, B. & Lovibond, P. F. (2015). How food cues can enhance and inhibit motivation to obtain and consume food. *Appetite*, **84**, 79–87.

Collins, L. M., Graham, J. W., Rousculp, S. S. & Hansen, W. B. (1997). Heavy caffeine use and the beginning of the substance use onset process. In K. Bryant, M. Windle & S. West (Eds.), *The Science of Prevention: Methodological Advances from Alcohol and Substance Abuse Research*. Washington, DC: American Psychological Association, pp. 79–99.

Courtwright, D. T. (2019). *The Age of Addiction: How Bad Habits Became Big Business*. Cambridge, MA: Belnap Press-An Imprint of Harvard University Press.

Craig, W. (1917). Appetites and aversions as constituents of instincts. *Proceedings of the National Academy of Sciences of the United States of America*, **3**(12), 685–688.

Darwin, C. (1871). *The Descent of Man and Selection in Relation to Sex*. London: Murray.

Downs, B. W., Chen, A. L. C., Chen, T. J. H., et al. (2009). Nutrigenomic targeting of carbohydrate craving behavior: Can we manage obesity and aberrant craving behaviors with neurochemical pathway manipulation by Immunological Compatible Substances (nutrients) using a Genetic Positioning System (GPS) Map? *Medical Hypotheses*, **73**, 427–434.

Ekhtiari, H., Nasseri, P., Yavari, F., Mokri, A. & Monterosso, J. (2016) Neuroscience of drug craving for addiction medicine: from circuits to therapies. *Journal of Progress in Brain Research*, **223**, 115–141.

Eng, S. & Woodside, A. G. (2012). Configural analysis of the drinking man: fuzzy-set qualitative comparative analyses. *Addictive Behaviors*, **37**, 541–543.

Fave, A. D., Massimini, F. & Bassi, M. (2011). *Psychological Selection and Optimal Experience across Cultures: Social Empowerment through Personal Growth, Cross Cultural Advancements in Positive Psychology, 2*. New York, NY: Springer.

Fishbein, D. H. (2000). The importance of neurobiological research to the prevention of psychopathology. *Prevention Science*, **1**, 89–106.

Foddy, B. & Savulescu, J. (2010a). A liberal account of addiction. *Philosophy, Psychiatry, & Psychology*, **17**, 1–22.

Foddy, B. & Savulescu, J. (2010b). Relating addiction to disease, disability, autonomy, and the good life. *Philosophy, Psychiatry, & Psychology*, **17**, 35–42.

Gable, R. S. (2006). The toxicity of recreational drugs. *Scientific American*, **94**, 206–208.

Goeders, N. E. (2004). Stress, motivation, and drug addiction. *Current Directions in Psychological Science*, **13**, 33–35.

Griffiths, M. D. (2005). A "components" model of addiction within a biopsychosocial framework. *Journal of Substance Use*, **10**, 191–197.

Griffiths, M. S. & Larkin, M. (2004). Conceptualizing addiction: The case for a "complex systems" account. *Addiction Research and Theory*, **12**, 99–102.

Hankin, B. L., Wetter, E. K. & Flory, K. (2012). Appetitive motivation and negative emotion reactivity among remitted depressed youth. *Journal of Clinical Child and Adolescent Psychology*, **41**, 611–620.

Hatterer, L. J. (1982). The addictive process. *Psychiatric Quarterly*, **54**, 149–156.

Haylett, S. A., Stephenson, G. M. & Lefever, R. M. H. (2004). Covariation in addictive behaviors: A study of addictive orientations using the shorter PROMIS Questionnaire. *Addictive Behaviors*, **29**, 61–71.

Heather, N. (1998). A conceptual framework for explaining drug addiction. *Journal of Psychopharmacology*, **12**, 3–7.

Hill, E. M. (2013). An evolutionary perspective on addiction. In P. Miller (Ed.), *Principles of Addiction (Volume 1)*. New York: Elsevier Inc., pp. 41–50 (chapter 4).

Hirschman, E. C. (1992). The consciousness of addiction: toward a general theory of compulsive consumption. *Journal of Consumer Research*, **19**, 155–179.

Hofstede, G. (1984). The cultural relativity of the quality of life concept. *Academy of Management Review*, **9**, 389–398.

Holden, C. (2001). "Behavioral" addictions: do they exist? *Science*, **294**, 980–982.

Jacobs, D. F. (1986). A general theory of addictions: a new theoretical model. *Journal of Gambling Behavior*, **2**, 15–31.

Jackson, C. J. & Smillie, L. D. (2004). Appetitive motivation predicts the majority of personality and an ability measure: a comparison of BAS measures and a re-evaluation of the importance of RST. *Personality and Individual Differences*, **36**, 1627–1636.

Kalivas, P. W. & Volkow, N. D. (2005). The neural basis of addiction: a pathology of motivation and choice. *American Journal of Psychiatry*, **162**, 1403–1413.

Kandel, D. B. (1990). Parenting styles, drug use, and children's adjustment in families of young adults. *Journal of Marriage and the Family*, **52**, 183–196.

Koob, G. F. & LeMoal, M. (2001). Drug addiction, dysregulation of reward, and allostasis. *Neuropsychopharmacology*, **24**, 97–129.

Koob, G. F. & LeMoal, M. (2008). Neurobiological mechanisms for opponent motivational processes in addiction. *Philosophical Transactions of the Royal Society B: Biological Sciences*, **363**, 3113–3123.

Kourosh, A. S., Harrington, C. R. & Adinoff, B. (2010). Tanning as a behavioral addiction. *The American Journal of Drug and Alcohol Abuse*, **36**, 284–290.

Lang, P. J. & Bradley, M. M. (2013). Appetitive and defensive motivation: goal-directed or goal-determined? *Emotion Review: Journal of International Society for Research on Emotion*, **5**, 230–234.

Laricchiuta, D. & Petrosini, L. (2014). Individual differences in response to positive and negative stimuli: endocannabinoid-based insight on approach and avoidance behaviors. *Frontiers in Systems Neuroscience*, **8** (238), 22 pages.

Lashley, K. S. (1938). Experimental analysis of instinctive behavior. *Psychological Review*, **45**, 445–471.

Loonis, E., Apter, M. J. & Sztulman, H. (2000). Addiction as a function of action system properties. *Addictive Behaviors*, **25** (3), 477–481.

MacLaren, V. V. & Best, L. A. (2010). Multiple addictive behaviors in young adults: student norms for the shorter PROMIS scale. *Addictive Behaviors*, **35**, 252–255.

Mahoney, K. D. (2018). http://latin-dictionary.net/definition/822/addictio-addictionis; accessed October 10th, 2018. Latdict Group.

Marks, I. (1990). Behaviour (non-chemical) addictions. *British Journal of Addiction*, **85**, 1389–1394.

Maslow, A. H. (1943). A theory of human motivation. *Psychological Review*, **50**, 370–396.

Maslow, A. H. (1954). *Instinct Theory Reexamined: Motivation and Personality*. New York: Harper & Row.

Maslow, A. H. (1996). Critique of self-actualization theory. In: E. Hoffman (Ed.), *Future Visions: The Unpublished Papers of Abraham Maslow*. Sage Publications, Inc., pp. 26–32.

McClelland, D. C. (1961). *The Achieving Society*. New York: NY: Free Press.

McClelland, D. C. (1987). *Human Motivation*. Cambridge, Great Britain: Cambridge University Press.

McClelland, D. C., Davis, W. N., Kalin, R. & Wanner, E. (1972). *The Drinking Man: Alcohol and Human Motivation*. New York, NY: Free Press.

McDaniel, P. A., Intinarelli, G. & Malone R. E. (2008). Tobacco industry issues management organizations: creating a global corporate network to undermine public health. *Globalization and Health: Biomed Central*, **4** (2), 18 pages.

McDougall, W. (1932). *The Energies of Men: A Study of the Fundamentals of Dynamic Psychology*. London, Great Britain: Methuen.

Murray, H. A. (1938). *Explorations in Personality*. New York, NY: Oxford University Press.

Myles, I. A. (2014). Fast food fever: reviewing the impacts of Western diet on immunity. *Nutrition Journal: Biomed Central*, **13** (61), 17 pages.

Nathan, P. E., Conrad, M. & Skinstad, A. H. (2016). History of the concept of addiction. *Annual Review of Clinical Psychology*, **12**, 29–51.

Nestler, E. J. & Landsman, D. (2001). Learning about addiction from the genome. *Nature*, **409**, 834–835.

Newlin, D. B. (2002). The self-perceived survival ability and reproductive fitness (SPFit) theory of substance use disorders. *Addiction*, **97**, 427–445.

Olney, J. J., Warlow, S. M., Naffziger, E. E. & Berridge, K. C. (2018). Current perspectives on incentive salience and applications to clinical disorders. *Current Opinion in Behavioral Science*, **22**, 59–69.

Orford, J. (2001). Addiction as excessive appetite. *Addiction*, **96**, 15–31.

Panksepp, J. & Moskal, J. (2008). Dopamine and SEEKING: Subcortical "reward" systems and appetitive urges. In: A. J. Elliot (Ed.), *Handbook of Approach and Avoidance Motivation*. New York: Taylor & Francis Group, pp. 67–87 (chapter 5).

Pearson, M. M. & Little, R. B. (1969). The addictive process in unusual addictions: a further elaboration of etiology. *American Journal of Psychiatry*, **125**, 1166–1171.

Potenza, M. N., Hong, K. I. A., Lacadie, C. M., et al. (2012). Neural correlates of stress-induced and cue-induced drug craving: influences of sex and cocaine dependence. *American Journal of Psychiatry*, **169**, 406–414.

PROMIS Clinics (2018). www.s-p-q.com; accessed October 31st, 2018.

Rawson, R. A. & Condon, T. P. (2007). Why do we need an Addiction supplement focused on methamphetamine? *Addiction*, **102** (Supplement 1), 1–4.

Richards, R. J. (2018). Instinct. In J. Vonk and T. Shackelford (Eds.), *Encyclopedia of Animal Cognition and Behavior*. New York: Springer International Publishing.

Robinson, T. E. & Berridge, K. C. (2000). The psychology and neurobiology of addiction: an incentive-sensitization view. *Addiction*, **95**, 91–117.

Rosenblatt, P. C., Anderson, R. M. & Johnson, P. A. (1984). The meaning of "cabin fever." *The Journal of Social Psychology*, **123**, 43–53.

Ryan, R. M. & Deci, E. L. (2000). Self-determination theory and the facilitation of intrinsic motivation, social development, and well-being. *American Psychologist*, **55**, 68–78.

Ryan, R. M. & Frederick, C. M. (1997). On energy, personality, and health: subjective vitality as a dynamic reflection of well-being. *Journal of Personality*, **65**, 529–565.

Sinha, R. (2008). Chronic stress, drug use, and vulnerability to addiction. *Annals of the New York Academy of Sciences*, **114**, 105–130.

Stacy, A. W. & Ames, S. L. (2001). Implicit cognition theory in drug use and driving under the influence interventions. In S. Sussman (Ed.), *Handbook of Program Development in Health Behavior Research and Practice*. Sage, pp. 107–130.

Stacy, A. W., Pike, J. & Lee, A. Y. (2020). Multiple memory systems, addiction, and health habits: New routes for translational science. In S. Sussman (Ed.) *The Cambridge Handbook of Substance and Behavioral Addictions*. Cambridge, UK: Cambridge University Press, pp. 152–170.

Sunderwirth, S. G. & Milkman, H. (1991). Behavioral and neurochemical commonalities in addiction. *Contemporary Family Therapy*, **13**, 421–433.

Sussman, S. (2007). Sexual addiction among teens: A review. *Sexual Addiction & Compulsivity: The Journal of Treatment and Prevention*, **14**, 257–278.

Sussman, S. (2012). Steve Sussman on Matilda Hellman's "Mind the Gap!" Failure in understanding key dimensions of an addicted drug user's life: addictive Effects. *Substance Use & Misuse*, **47**, 1661–1665.

Sussman, S. (2017). *Substance and Behavioral Addictions: Concepts, Causes, and Cures*. Cambridge, Great Britain: Cambridge University Press.

Sussman, S. Y. & Ames, S. L. (2008). *Drug Abuse: Concepts, Prevention, and Cessation*. Cambridge, Great Britain: Cambridge University Press.

Sussman, S. & Arnett, J. (2014). Emerging adulthood: Developmental period facilitative of the addictions. *Evaluation & the Health Professions*, **37**, 147–155.

Sussman, S. & Moran, M. B. (2013). Hidden addiction: Television. *Journal of Behavioral Addictions*, **2**, 125–132.

Sussman, S. & Sussman, A. N. (2011). Considering the definition of addiction. *International Journal of Environmental Research and Public Health*, **8**, 4025–4038.

Sussman, S., Leventhal, A., Bluthenthal, R. N., Freimuth, M., Forster, M. & Ames, S. L. (2011). A framework for the specificity of addictions. *International Journal of Environmental Research and Public Health*, **8**, 3399–3415.

Sussman, S., Lisha, N. & Griffiths, M. (2011). Prevalence of the addictions: a problem of the majority or the minority? *Evaluation & the Health Professions*, **34**, 3–56.

Sussman, S., Reynaud, M., Aubin, H. J. & Leventhal, A. M. (2011). Drug addiction, love, and the Higher Power. *Evaluation & the Health Professions*, **34**, 362–370.

Sussman, S., Rozgonjuk, D. & van den Eijnden, R. (2017). Substance and behavioral addictions may share a similar underlying process of dysregulation. *Addiction*, **112**, 1717–1718.

Tay, L. & Diener, E. (2011). Needs and subjective well-being around the world. *Journal of Personality and Social Psychology*, **101**, 354–365.

Vaccaro, A. G. & Potenza, M. N. (2020). Neurobiological foundations of behavioral addictions. In S. Sussman (Ed.) *The Cambridge Handbook of Substance and Behavioral Addictions*. Cambridge, UK: Cambridge University Press, pp. 136–151.

Vandenbergh, D. J., O'Connor, R. J., Grang, M. D., et al. (2007) Dopamine receptor genes (DRD2, DRD3, DRD4) and gene-gene interactions associated with smoking-related behaviors. *Addiction Biology*, **12**, 106–116.

Verhulst, B., Neale, M. C. & Kendler, K. S. (2015). The heritability of alcohol use disorders: a meta-analysis of twin and adoption studies. *Psychological Medicine*, **45**, 1061–1072.

Wahlstrom, D., White, T. & Luciana, M. (2010). Neurobehavioral evidence for changes in dopamine system activity during adolescence. *Neuroscience Biobehavior Review*, **34**, 631–648.

Walther, B., Morgenstern, M. & Hanewinkel, R. (2012). Co-occurrence of addictive behaviors: personality factors related to substance use, gambling and computer gaming. *European Addiction Research*, **18**, 167–174.

Warlow, S. M., et al. (2020). Chapter 3 of the current *Handbook*.

Wiers, R. W., Bartholow, B. D., Wildenberg, E. v.d., et al. (2007). Automatic and controlled processes and the development of addictive behaviors in adolescents: a review and a model. *Pharmacology Biochemistry and Behavior*, **86** (2), 263–283.

World Health Organization [WHO] (2018). *ICD-11 for Mortality and Morbidity Statistics (ICD-11 MMS)*. Geneva, Switzerland: WHO (https://icd.who.int/).

Zilberman, N., Lavidor, M., Yadid, G. & Rassovsky, Y. (2019). Qualitative review and quantitative effect size meta-analyses in brain regions identified by cue-reactivity addiction studies. *Neuropsychology*, **33**, 319–334.

2 Behavioral Economics and Addictive Disorders

David P. Jarmolowicz, PhD, and Tadd D. Schneider, BS

Introduction

Addicted individuals often behave in ways that perplex those around them. They put their lives at risk. For example, they use substances that carry a substantial risk of accidental overdose. In 2016 over 70,000 individuals died from drug overdose – over 50,000 of those deaths being from opioids (NIDA, 2017). They put their health at risk. For example, addicted individuals have an elevated rate of sexually transmitted infections (Dembo et al., 2009) and many addicted individuals fail to obtain sufficient nutritional intake (Cowan & Devine, 2012, 2013). Moreover, they put their future at risk. For example, substance abusers are disproportionally unemployed (see Holtyn, DeFulio & Silverman, 2015, for a discussion). Taken together, one may ask, "Why would any rational person do this to themselves?."

There is danger, however, in assuming that people will behave rationally. Prior to the great recession of 2008, the macroeconomic models guiding fiscal policy assumed rationality. In the wake of the crash, President Obama, and Alan Greenspan – the head of the Federal Reserve – noted that current economic models had failed in practice. On a personal level, even the most trustworthy of persons finds it difficult to follow-through on commitments, even ones made in rational best interest. An extreme case of this is found in addicted individuals, out of control, promising to seek treatment but continuing to use instead.[1]

Given the persistent observation that individuals frequently fail to behave in their rational best interests, a science focused on understanding these deviations in rationality has taken hold. Specifically, *behavioral economics* – often defined as the systematic evaluation of choice under conditions of constraint (Bickel & Vuchinich, 2000) – neither assumes nor typically observes rational choice. Instead, behavior economics researchers find that people are hypersensitive to even the smallest delays, are hyposensitive to diminishing odds, and tend to overvalue specific – often harmful – commodities. Notably, although these tendencies are observed in most individuals, they tend to be exaggerated in individuals suffering from substance dependence (Bickel et al., 2011a, 2012a) and other health maladies (Bickel et al., 2012d; Epstein et al., 2010; Jarmolowicz et al., 2016c), including obesity (Epstein et al., 2010), eating disorders (Ritschel et al., 2015), and even pathological gambling (Dixon, Marley & Jacobs, 2003). These tendencies, their measurement, the neurobiology that drives them, and their relevance to addictive disorders are described below.

[1] Although this is a typically seen cycle, there are other routes to recovery that are seen in around one-third of those with substance use disorders. Some addicts age out, or naturally progress out of use disorders on their own through declining valuation of the drug of choice. Others have been known to spontaneously recover without the help of an intervention or assistance (Sobell, Ellingstad & Sobell, 2000).

Delay Discounting

Delay discounting (DD) is the devaluation of a reward as a product of the delay to its receipt (Bickel & Marsch, 2001; Rachlin, 2006). When choosing between a smaller yet sooner (SS) or larger yet later (LL) reward, DD reflects the relative value of these two options. Typically, there is a systematic decrease in the value of a LL reward as the delay to its receipt increases. While this general relation is seen, independent of the size of the delayed reward, prior studies (Green et al., 2014; Kirby, Petry & Bickel, 1999) have found a magnitude effect, wherein individual's discounting rates decrease as the size of the LL reward increases.

When measuring DD rates, the steepness of the slope is reflected by the rate of discounting (Green & Myerson, 2004, 2013). Under typical conditions, passing on the SS and opting for a LL payout is thought to reflect self-control. By contrast, the tendency to opt for the SS in lieu of the LL reward is thought to reflect impulsivity. Choosing the SS reward, however, is not always maladaptive. While choosing the smaller sooner reward can be seen as a negative trait when used as the default choice, not taking advantage of available resources can also be maladaptive when future events (e.g., having to go on a trip to a new location) could prevent the delivery of the delayed reward.

Despite notable empirical consistency, debate continues on the behavioral and/or neurobiological processes driving DD (Loewenstein, 1988; Madden & Bickel, 2009). As such, DD definitions differ in focus, with many focusing on impulsive choice (Bickel & Marsch, 2001), whereas others focus on the ability to value delayed rewards (Bickel et al., 2012c; Bickel & Yi, 2008; Jarmolowicz et al., 2013). These differing foci may obscure the basic nature of DD as reflecting the interaction of at least two behavioral processes (i.e., inhibiting a prepotent response and valuing delayed rewards) subserved by distinct neurobiological processes (Bickel et al., 2007, 2012c).

Of note, individuals' choices are not always consistent across time (Ainslie & Herrnstein, 1981). For example, one hallmark of addiction is the failure of addicted individuals to follow through with choices made at one timepoint at a later time. For example, one may state a desire to go to the gym after work then discuss plans that morning – yet change his/her mind as happy hour approaches. This switch, often called a "preference reversal," is often distressing to those that care about these individuals. These preference reversals, however, are not restricted to addicted individuals. For example, one may express a desire to forgo dessert at the beginning of a meal yet change one's mind and ask for cake as the meal winds down. This does not mean that the individual was lying at the beginning of dinner. Instead, one's choices were inconsistent across two timepoints: (1) at the beginning of the meal, both the dessert and improved health are delayed outcomes versus (2) at the end of the meal the dessert is an immediate outcome, whereas the improved health associated with forgoing the cake is a delayed outcome. At timepoint 1, both the cake and health were devalued because they were both delayed outcomes. At timepoint 2, only the health outcomes were delayed – with their devaluation leaving them unable to compete with the immediate rewards associated with the cake. In terms of DD, this demonstrates a preference reversal toward the SS option which is associated with risky choice behaviors. The behavioral economic models used to describe DD (below) account for these preference reversals in ways that rational choice models cannot (Ainslie & Herrnstein, 1981; Green & Estle, 2003; Green et al., 1981; Monterosso & Ainslie, 2007; Yi, Matusiewicz & Tyson, 2016).

Discounting rates are often stable over time (Kirby, 2009; Takahashi et al., 2007), but can also change as a function of certain conditions, drugs or environmental influences (Koffarnus et al., 2013). Moreover, these DD rates typically differ by individual (Bickel et al., 2012d). As such, some have posited that DD may reflect a personality trait (Odum, 2011). However, although DD rates don't change much over time, response patterns are sensitive to different environments and circumstances. People with substance use disorders have been shown to discount their substance of choice at higher rates than money (Bickel et al., 2012d) while those without substance use disorders have been shown to change discounting rates with acute administration of alcohol (Reynolds, Richards & de Wit, 2006). Effects on discounting have also been seen in those withdrawing from substance use (Ashare & Hawk, 2012) as well as improvements seen with physical activity (Sofis, Carrillo & Jarmolowicz, 2016). As such there is debate as to whether DD should be seen as a behavioral tendency rather than a fixed measure or trait (Dallery & Raiff, 2007; Odum, 2011) or as relatively consistent over time, while exhibiting developmental and experiential changes (Romer, 2010).

Measurement

Delay discounting can be measured in many ways (see Reed et al., 2020). One common approach is the monetary choice questionnaire developed by Kirby and colleagues (Kirby & Marakovic, 1996; Kirby et al., 1999). The Monetary-choice Questionnaire is a fixed set of binary choices ("would you rather have?") juxtaposing smaller immediate rewards against larger rewards to be delivered after a delay. Using this approach, twenty-one to twenty-seven predetermined questions are used to determine discounting rates for small, medium, and large rewards. This commonly used approach has good temporal stability (Kirby, 2009) and predictive validity. Alternatively, DD is often assessed using an adjusting amount procedure wherein the size of a larger delayed reward (e.g., $1,000 in one week) is kept constant while the size of an immediate reward is adjusted until the point at which the subject is indifferent between the two is determined (i.e., $875 today is worth $1,000 a week from now). These indifference points are determined across a range of delays (often presented in ascending order), and the data are analyzed using nonlinear regression (see below). The steeper the curve, the higher the discounting rate, which is often seen as reflective of the degree of impulsivity (Bickel & Marsch, 2001) or executive function (Bickel et al., 2012c).[2] Although the exact algorithms used to adjust the magnitude of the immediate reward vary (Du, Green & Myerson, 2002; Richards et al., 1999), all adjusting amount procedures follow this general logic.

A newer and quicker version of the discounting procedure being used is the five-trial adjusting delay procedure (Koffarnus & Bickel, 2014). When using this updated technique, participants make a total of five choices between smaller/immediately available rewards, and larger/delayed rewards. After each choice the delay to the larger reward is titrated (increased if larger reward had been chosen, decreased if smaller reward had been chosen) with the overall outcome of the five trials being identification of the delay at which the delayed reward loses half of its value (which is used to calculate the discounting rate). This task shortens the task time and give similar results to the adjusting amount tasks previously used (Du et al., 2002; Richards et al., 1999). In the previous versions of DD tasks, participants would answer a slew of questions about the same delay or amount. However, in the five-trial version, the choices are titrated at a higher rate (e.g., sliding the scale multiple spots, instead of only one spot in previous tasks). The resulting indifference points are statistically similar yet reach the endpoint in a much faster time.

Delay discounting involves measuring successive trials at different delays to find multiple indifference points that can then be plotted to see the overall discounting curve for a particular commodity. The steeper the curve, the higher the discounting rate, and the more likely the correlation with maladaptive behaviors such as drug and alcohol addictions, or behavioral addictions. To quantify DD, there are multiple formulas, or variations on formulas, that may be used. The *exponential model*, which arose from standard economic theories (Samuelson, 1937), factors in the additional risk that comes with each additional delay. The smaller-sooner is considered safe because the delayed event implies risk that the reinforcer may not be delivered. The *hyperbolic model* (Mazur, 1987), which comes out of experimental psychology, addresses the choice between two reinforcement values. Each unit of delay results in a proportionally decreasing reduction of the subjective value of the delayed reward. As such, hyperbolic formulas predict rapid devaluation at shorter delays followed by lesser devaluation at longer delays, as seen in DD data. Hyperbolic modeling of DD rates: Mazur (1987) hyperbolic formula,

$$V = \frac{A}{1 + kD}, \tag{2.1}$$

which describes how the value (V) of some amount (A) of a reward decreases at a given rate (k) as a product of the delay (D) to its receipt. The steepness of DD (i.e., k) is typically taken as a direct measure of impulsivity (Bickel & Marsch, 2001) or executive dysfunction (Bickel et al., 2012c; Jarmolowicz et al., 2013). Subsequent iterations of these hyperbolic models have added a scaling parameter (s). For example, Myerson and Green (1995) account for nonlinear perception/scaling of delays by placing a scaling parameter on the entire denominator,

$$V = \frac{A}{(1 + kD)^s} \tag{2.2}$$

fits to the model tend to be superior (Green & Myerson, 2004; McKerchar et al., 2009) to the unscaled hyperbolic model (Mazur, 1987) even when accounting for the additional free parameter in the model (Franck et al., 2015). By contrast, Rachlin (2006) has developed an alternative hyperboloid model,

$$V = \frac{A}{1 + kD^s} \tag{2.3}$$

which focuses exclusively on the subject's scaling of delays. This model tends to have goodness of fits that are superior to both prior discounting models (Franck et al., 2015).

To check for goodness of fit, measures of R^2 or root mean squared error (RMSE) measures are used. These metrics quantify how much better than a straight line through the mean a model performs (R^2), or

[2] When controlling for socioeconomic status.

how far the average datapoint is from the fitted line (RMSE). An alternative approach to summarizing DD data is calculating area under the curve (Myerson, Green & Warusawitharana, 2001). This technique is model free and can be used as an alternative to other methods or paired with other methods to find the best fit to evaluate different fits and outcomes measured by utilizing the different approaches.

Neurobiology of Delay Discounting

When studying relations between DD rates and addiction, the neuroanatomical area most often emphasized is the limbic system, or reward pathway in the brain. More specifically, researchers tend to focus on the ventral striatum (VS) or, even more particularly, the nucleus accumbens (NA). Neuroimaging studies suggest that neuronal responding in the limbic system (reward system), is activated more from the subjective values of the reinforcers rather than objective properties (Miedl, Peters & Buchel, 2012a). For example, a hobby such as coin collecting may be of great subjective value over its objective value, possibly lending itself to become an addiction. Discounting is associated with self-regulation, impulse-control, delay of gratification, and intertemporal choice (Manuck et al., 2003). Elevated reaction of the VS has been associated with steep discounting, and addiction outcomes have been linked to dysregulation of the VS (Kalivas & Volkow, 2005).

Activity in the VS increases in response to both the anticipation and the receipt of reinforcers including primary (e.g., food) and secondary (e.g., money) reinforcers (O'Doherty, 2004). Individual differences may be seen in a preference for smaller-sooner versus larger-later rewards due to the magnitude of activity in the VS, which shows an immediate response to rewards (Hariri, 2009). Through the use of BOLD fMRI, individual differences in DD can be predicted by the activity in the VS (Hariri et al., 2006). Specifically, individual differences in DD correlate positively with the level of VS activation, in response to positive and negative feedback, but also with differential reward-related VS activation in response to positive and/or negative rewards (Hariri, 2009). Dopaminergic drugs, concentrations of neurotransmitters, and brain lesions have also been reported to modulate discounting of delayed rewards (Takahashi, 2006). Dopaminergic midbrain activity after near-misses positively correlates with gambling severity (Miedl et al., 2012a).

Delay Discounting and Clinical Phenomena

Obtaining the high, or eliminating withdrawal symptoms, makes the SS rewards associated with drug consumption more immediately appealing than the LL reward of abstinence, health and having more money or resources. When a person chooses abstinence, one is choosing the LL reward. The challenge is that there are many opportunities for SS rewards along the road to this LL goal. Higher discounting rates have been shown in individuals dependent on opioids (Kirby et al., 1999; Madden et al., 1997), that abuse alcohol (Bickel et al., 2012b; Bjork et al., 2004; Petry, 2001a), cocaine (Coffey et al., 2003; Heil et al., 2006), and cigarette smokers (Bickel, Odum & Madden, 1999; Bickel et al., 2008, 2012b; Odum & Baumann, 2007).[3] Moreover, higher rates of impulsive choice put individuals at higher risk for addictive disorders such as pathological gambling (Dixon et al., 2003). Importantly, the presence of both gambling and substance use problems result in an additive effect on DD (Petry, 2001b; Petry & Casarella, 1999). That is, gamblers, with and without substance abuse issues, have been compared on delay-discounting tasks, and it was seen that higher DD rates correlated with substance abuse problems (Addiction Severity Index, McLellan et al., 1985) and impulsivity (Eysenck Impulsivity Scale, Eysenck & Eysenck, 1978). When quantified using Mazur's (1987) equation, heroin addicts discount money more steeply than controls (0.220 compared to 0.027, respectively), and they discount heroin at an even much higher rate (4.170) (Madden et al., 1997).

Importantly, rates of DD are highly predictive. For example, premorbid DD rates predict individuals' initiation of substance abuse (Audrain-McGovern et al., 2009). Moreover, baseline DD rates predict patients' outcomes of substance abuse treatments (Sheffer et al., 2012, 2014; Washio et al., 2011). As a result, DD rates have increasingly been viewed as a treatment target (Koffarnus et al., 2013). For example, Bickel et al. (2011b) found that exposing patients to a four-to-fifteen-week course of working memory training decreased DD rates in treatment seeking stimulant users. Promising work in preclinical models suggest that DD rates can be decreased by providing explicit and prolonged exposure to delayed rewards. Black and Rosen (2011) found that a money management course resulted in lower than untreated discounting rate in cocaine users. Morrison et al. (2014) found that mindfulness training decreased DD rates in college students. Lastly, Sofis et al. (2016) found that a seven-week exercise program decreased discounting rates in a community sample. While the exact mechanism underlying this improvement is still being researched, the impact on the executive system shows improved functioning that helps to override the reward system in future valuations of reinforcement. This area of research is still in its infancy and, as such, more research is needed to parse out the specific underlying mechanism at play.

Probability Discounting

Delay, however, is not the only variable that impacts choice. Risk is often also considered when individuals make choices. For example, if one is investing for their future, the likelihood of any given investment paying out is often crucial. The old proverb states, "a bird in the hand is worth two in the bush." This, of course, implicitly indicates that organisms often make tradeoffs between the size and certainty of a given reward. As was the case with DD (described above), these sorts of tradeoffs are systematic (i.e., willing to accept less as the certainty of the risky reward decreases) and highly individual. The concept of probability discounting (PD) mirrors that of DD. Specifically, just as DD describes the systematic devaluation of a choice alternative as the delay increases, PD describes the systematic devaluation of a choice alternative as that alternative's reward becomes increasingly improbable. Put simply, each person has a differing tolerance for risk.

Probability discounting provides a lens through which individuals' patterns of tradeoffs between smaller-certain and probabilistic-yet-larger rewards can be examined. Specifically, much like as was seen with DD, individuals' choices between smaller and certain rewards are compared to those for larger and probabilistic rewards across a wide parametric space to determine the smallest certain reward that individuals will accept in lieu of larger rewards across a wide range of probabilities of receipt.

[3] Although drug users typically discount rewards at higher rates than controls, this relation does not appear to hold with marijuana users (Johnson et al., 2010).

Measurement

There are a number of ways to assess PD (Rachlin, Raineri & Cross, 1991). The most common is to compare individuals' choices between a larger reward that will be delivered with some degree of probability (e.g., 50 percent chance of receiving $1,000) and a smaller certain reward. The size of the smaller certain reward is then titrated until the participant is equally likely to choose either reward. This approach is considered a titrating amount procedure. As with DD, the indifference points (i.e., size of the smaller certain award that is subjectively equivalent to the larger yet probabilistic reward) are collected at a range of probabilities, and nonlinear regression is used to describe a larger choice pattern.

Although many mathematical formulas have been used to describe PD, many behavioral economists posit that these data are theoretically, and empirically best fit by hyperbolic (Rachlin, 2006; Rachlin et al., 1991) or hyperbolic-like (Green & Myerson, 2004; Myerson & Green, 1995) formulas. The most basic of these formulas (Rachlin et al., 1991) is a straightforward modification of Mazur's (1987) *hyperbolic function*,

$$V = \frac{A}{1 + h\theta}, \tag{2.4}$$

which describes how the subjective value (V) of a given amount (A) of a commodity decreases at an individualized rate (h) as the odds against ($\theta = 1 - p/p$; p = probability) receiving that reward decrease. Being hyperbolic in form, this formula accounts for the sharp initial decline in subjective value followed by the slow devaluation as poor odds get worse that is typically seen in the data. These fits are improved both theoretically and empirically by the addition of an additional free parameter (s) in Rachlin's (2006) refined equation

$$V = \frac{A}{1 + h\theta^{s}}, \tag{2.5}$$

and Myerson and Green's (1995) hyperboloid formula

$$V = \frac{A}{(1 + h\theta)^{s}}, \tag{2.6}$$

In both of these refined equations, the s parameter accounts for the nonlinear scaling of probabilities. One might note that this scaling is more straight forwards in Rachlin's (2006) equation than Myerson and Green's (1995). The scaling parameter (s) is a nonlinear scaling used to represent the dispersion of the probabilistic distribution. This means that the higher the scaling parameter, the more spread out the data. The scaling parameter can be understood as a similar process to log transformed data. Whereby using a scaling parameter helps to bring the dispersion closer together. In doing so, the model fits are improved, yet the interpretation of the fitted parameters becomes more complicated. Specifically, because these hyperboloid equations include a second fitted parameter, the discounting rate no longer is the sole descriptor of the shape of the curve. Instead, an interaction between the h and s equations describes these choice patterns. As such, statistical analysis of the discounting rate alone does not describe the observed patterns in the data.

Neurobiology of Probability Discounting

Despite the similarities between delay and probability discounting, these two behavioral processes are distinguishable at the neurobiological level. In rats, lesions of the orbitofrontal cortex (OFC) disrupt PD but not DD, whereas the converse is true for lesions of the ventral hippocampus (VHC). Moreover, nucleus accumbens (NAc) lesions have been found to decrease rats' sensitivity to delayed rewards (i.e., flattened the DD function) but have not been found to impact rats' sensitivity to probabilistic rewards (Abela & Chudasama, 2013). Apparently, the basic brain circuitry recruited for these distinct performances are distinct, even in preclinical models.

Although the exact neurobiological structures differ in clinical and preclinical research, patterns of neurobiological differences are also seen in humans. For example, when using fMRI to examine neural correlates of performance on delay and probability discounting in pathological gamblers versus controls, Miedl et al. (2012a) found that PD was associated with activation in the left intraparietal sulcus and ventrial striatum (VS), whereas activation during the DD tasks were associated with activation of the left lateral parietal cortex, right posterior cortex, left medial prefrontal cortex and VS. These findings mirrored those from prior work in nonclinical populations (Peters & Buchel, 2009). When comparing neural activation during PD tasks between clinical samples and controls, the results are varied, yet robust. For example, when comparing individuals with Internet Gaming Disorder (IGD) to controls, researchers have found that IGD subject have less activation in the inferior frontal gyrus and precentral gyrus than controls (Lin et al., 2015).

Probability and Clinical Phenomena

As with DD, there is a growing body of evidence suggesting that PD is directly related to a number of important clinical phenomena. For example, despite prior studies failing to find differences in rates of PD between smokers and nonsmokers, Reynolds et al. (2004) found that cigarette smokers PD rates were higher than those of nonsmokers. These inconsistent findings are echoed in those of a study by Yi, Chase and Bickel (2007). Specifically, Yi et al. found that smokers and nonsmokers did not have statistically significant differences in PD rates, yet indifference points for high probabilities were much lower in smokers, despite their being no discernable differences in indifference points at lower probabilities. That is, even at high percentages, smokers discounted the potential larger reward and took the smaller yet certain reward. Smokers showed sensitivity to the probabilistic reward earlier than nonsmokers and as such preferred the sure thing. In all, the findings with smokers are promising, yet the effect seems to be less robust than the well demonstrated relation between DD and smoking (Bickel et al., 1999).

Probability discounting may be more suited to assessing important differences in other clinically significant populations. For example, on face value, one would expect problematic gamblers to be insensitive to increasingly poor odds – which is what the research has shown. Specifically, Holt, Green and Myerson (2003) conducted a study wherein they compared PD in gambling versus nongambling college students. PD rates were lower in the gamblers, suggesting that they were not as highly impacted by the increased odds against winning (i.e., they were risk seeking). These findings were consistent with those of Madden, Petry and Johnson (2009), who found lower than control rates of PD in a sample of patients that met the DSM-IV criteria for pathological gambling. This relation between PD rate and gambling has been replicated in additional studies (Miedl, Peters & Buchel, 2012b), yet there is no consistent relation between PD rate and the severity of one's gambling problem. Relatedly, individuals suffering from Internet Gaming Disorder tend to discount probabilistic rewards at lower rates than controls (Lin et al., 2015). Moreover, although researchers have failed to find relations between DD and psychopathy, psychopaths tended to be more risk taking than controls on a PD task (Takahashi et al., 2014).

Probability discounting may even be uniquely related to important health maintenance behaviors. Notably, researchers (Bruce et al., 2016) asked multiple sclerosis patients that typically did (n = 38) or did not (n = 38) take their medications the likelihood of taking medications that had various probabilities of preventing a worsening of their symptoms (seven values; 5%–95%) yet carried various risks of side effects (three values; 10%–90%). Patients' choices across probable efficacy were well described by Equation 2.6 above, and systematically decreased as the probability of side effects increased. Importantly, these likelihoods of taking medications were systematically lower in the patients that seldom took their medications, and among those typically nonadherent patients PD based on medication effectiveness was higher. Moreover, follow-up regression analyses found that these discounting rates were uniquely able to predict adherence status. Follow-up analyses based on those data used forecasting techniques to determine the rate of side effects that would be needed to spur typically nonadherent individuals to take their medications (Jarmolowicz et al., 2016b). Unfortunately, the rates required are lower than is feasible in the medication development process, suggesting that behavioral interventions may be needed to increase adherence. Consistent with the decreasing likelihood of taking medications as the probability of side effects increased, patients have also reported a decreased likelihood of taking medications as the severity of side effects that they were risking increased (Jarmolowicz et al., 2017). The culmination of these findings has been the development of a *3-D probability discounting model*,

$$V = \frac{U}{(1 + h_{se}\theta_{se}{}^{s_{se}}) * (1 + h_e\theta_e{}^{s_e})}, \tag{2.7}$$

which describes how the value of a medication (V) decreases as the odd against it working ($\theta_e = \frac{p}{1-p}; p =$ percent efficacy) increases and the odds of experiencing side effects ($\theta_{se} = \frac{1-p}{p}; p =$ probability of side effects) increases, with this effect being modulated by their discounting of treatment based on the side effects (h_{se}) and/or decreased efficacy (h_e) and their weighting of side effects (s_{se}) and/or efficacy (s_e). This model not only adequately described choice data across three different side effect severities (Jarmolowicz et al., 2018) but also served as a significant predictor of MS knowledge, adherence determination, and adherence (Bruce et al., 2018).

Demand

A third major area of behavioral economic research has focused on subjects' willingness to sacrifice more resources, such as time, effort, money, etc., to obtain their substance of abuse (Hursh, 1980, 1984, 1991). Borrowing concepts from the microeconomic literature (Watson & Holman, 1977), these studies typically examine real or hypothetical consumption across a range of drug prices – with the overall patterns of consumption being described by demand curves. These behavioral economic concepts have provided great insight into the valuation of drugs of abuse, and other rewards.

Own Price Elasticity

One important consistency is that as the price to obtain a unit of reward increases, people will typically defend (i.e., maintain) consumption across a range of small price increases, yet will precipitously decrease their consumption as the prices increase further. Along the prices wherein consumption is defended, demand is said to be inelastic. Technically speaking, this inelastic demand means that, for each unit of price increase, consumption decreases by less than one unit (i.e., the slope is greater than –1). As prices continue to increase, consumption begins to decrease by more than one unit per unit of cost (i.e., the slope becomes less than –1), and demand is said to become elastic. The rate at which elasticity changes is often quantified as "alpha" (α; described below), and the price at which demand switches from inelastic to elastic is called "*p-max*" (described below).

These predictable patterns of consumption are echoed by a similarly predictable pattern of expenditure. Specifically, as prices increase through the inelastic portion of the demand curve, expenditure to defend this level of consumption systematically increases. This expenditure, however, precipitously decreases after *p-max*, eventually reaching 0. The price at which consumption/output is driven to zero is the breakpoint. The maximum spent at any price is called "*o-max,*" which often occurs at *p-max*.

Cross-Price Elasticity

Commodities are seldom consumed in a vacuum. Instead, commodities are typically concurrently available. If this concurrent availability of commodities has no impact on consumption, commodities are said to be *independents*. Behavioral economists, however, are often interested in the interactions between commodities, collectively referred to as "cross-price elasticity." For example, consumption of any given commodity is often tied to the cost of other concurrently available commodities. These interactions can often explain a lot about the sort of choices that subjects are likely to make when faced with these trade-offs outside of the laboratory environment.

Some commodities are so closely tied that anything that decreases the consumption of one of the commodities would certainly impact the consumption of the other. For example, some people only smoke cigarettes when they drink alcohol. Thus, if they stopped drinking, they would stop smoking as well. In behavioral economics, these sorts of relations are tested by determining if the consumption of a given commodity (e.g., cigarettes) decreases as increases in the cost of a related commodity (e.g., alcohol) drives its consumption downward. If this relation exists, the items are said to be *complements*. This complementary relation, however, may not be symmetrical. For example, although increases in the price of alcohol may drive down consumption of both alcohol and cigarettes in this example, it is unlikely that increases in the price of cigarettes would have much impact on alcohol consumption. Thus, in this scenario, alcohol and cigarettes are "asymmetrical complements."

By contrast, consumption of other commodities tends to be inversely related. For example, if market pressures were to precipitously increase the cost of red wine, many consumers would increase their consumption of white wine. As with the complements relation described above, behavioral economics researchers would typically test this possibility by keeping the cost of one commodity (e.g., white wine) constant as consumption of the other commodity (e.g., red wine) was suppressed by increasing its price. If consumption of the cost consistent commodity (e.g., white wine) were to increase as a result of this manipulation, the commodities would be said to be *substitutes*.

Measurement

Behavioral economic demand can be analyzed in a wide variety of ways. As with delay and PD, the research tradition has its roots in preclinical models. Specifically, observing regularities in responding from operant conditioning experiments with rats, pigeons, and monkeys that were consistent with microeconomic theory, Hursh (1980) outlined important contributions that a behavioral economic viewpoint could make to the experimental analysis of reward behavior. These included the concepts of own and cross-price elasticity, as well as noting consistently elevated consumption when animals received all of their food during their daily experimental sessions ("closed economy") relative to when the reinforcer that they were working for (i.e., food) was available outside of session. To study these issues, Hursh et al. (1988) developed a general framework wherein rewards were delivered for a set cost (i.e., a fixed number of responses), which escalated across 24-hour sessions. The primary dependent variable was consumption (i.e., the number of rewards earned) at each unit price (i.e., cost/benefit ratio; number of responses per reward), with the overall pattern of responding being well-described via nonlinear regression using the formula

$$\ln Q = \ln L + b \ln p - aP, \tag{2.8}$$

which describes how consumption (Q) changes as a function of price (P), the predicted consumption at the lowest price (L), as a product of the initial slope of the function (b), and acceleration in slope (a).

As the experimental tradition transitioned to the study of human clinical populations, many changes to the overall assessment paradigm became evident. For example, session durations remained relatively long (e.g., three hours), yet the economy - out of necessity - shifted from closed to open. For example, Shahan et al. (1999) had smokers (n = 12) who had abstained from smoking for six hours prior to their three-hour sessions of pull plungers to obtain the opportunity to take three puffs from an experimental cigarette. In some conditions, the cigarettes contained nicotine, in others they did not. Within each condition, the number of plunger pulls to obtain the puffs increased through a set progression (i.e., 2, 100, 300, 1,000, 3,000, 6,000, and 12,000 pulls), which increased across days until the subject stopped earning puffs. Although this procedure was technically an open economy, the data from this procedure were highly consistent with those collected with preclinical models responding in closed economies. As a result, subsequent clinical studies seldom (cf., Greenwald & Hursh, 2006) have used the closed economies so prevalent in the preclinical research (Bickel & Madden, 1999a, 1999b, 1999c; Johnson & Bickel, 2003, 2006; Madden & Bickel, 1999; Madden, Bickel & Jacobs, 2000; Shahan et al., 1999, 2001; Shahan, Odum & Bickel, 2000).

Three hours per day for several consecutive days, however, is beyond the monetary and time investment that many researchers are willing to undertake. Not surprisingly, briefer questionnaire-based measures have since been developed (Jacobs & Bickel, 1999; Murphy & MacKillop, 2006), refined, and widely disseminated (MacKillop et al., 2012; Madden & Kalman, 2010). These highly flexible analogs - often referred to as purchase tasks - have allowed for the rapid assessment of patients' demand for commodities ranging from alcohol (MacKillop & Murphy, 2007; MacKillop et al., 2009, 2010) and cigarettes (MacKillop & Tidey, 2011; MacKillop et al., 2008, 2012) to more specialized commodities such as access to indoor tanning (Reed et al., 2016) and sex (Jarmolowicz et al., 2016a). These measures are stable over time (Acuff & Murphy, 2017; Few et al., 2012; Grace, Kivell & Laugesen, 2015), yet sensitive enough to change when circumstances change (MacKillop et al., 2010; Madden & Kalman, 2010). As such, demand curve measures are thought to reflect the current hedonic value of a given reward.

As the research moved from preclinical models in the laboratory to patients in the clinic, the analytic methods changed. To describe the demand curve in a single fitted parameter - akin to what has allowed DD research to thrive - a single parameter exponential model (Hursh & Silberberg, 2008)

$$\log Q = \log Q_0 + k(e^{-\propto (Q_0 * c)} - 1) \tag{2.9}$$

has been developed. In this equation, Q represents consumption with Q_0 as baseline consumption or maximum demand, c is cost or effort required, and k is the scaling parameter for consumption. This model replaces the dual slope (Hursh et al., 1988) model of Equation 2.8 with a single slope (i.e., free parameter) facilitating the investigation of individual differences in demand. Taking this trend a step further, the prevalence of zero values (i.e., prices at which patients say they would not purchase the good) has risen dramatically as researchers moved from presenting individualized sequences of prices which cease when the organism stops consuming the reinforcer to presenting patients with a questionnaire that has a fixed set of questions designed to extend beyond the prices at which patients will consume the reward. These zero consumption values are problematic for Equation 2.9, because zero cannot be log transformed. As a result, an exponentiated version of Equation 2.9 has been developed (Koffarnus et al., 2015) so that researchers do not need to remove the zero values from consideration.

Neurobiology of Demand

Research on the intercorrelates of demand is markedly underdeveloped. In fact, only one known study has tested the neurocorrelates of demand and the essential value of reinforcers (Mackillop et al., 2014). As such, discussion of the neurobiology of demand is speculative, but built upon decades of neuropsychological research.

Considerations of the essential value of a reinforcer are nearly synonymous with the dense body of literature on *hedonic reward valuation*. Thereby it is proposed that neural considerations of demand can be informed by existing neuroeconomic research on hedonic reward valuation. Extant research on hedonic reward valuation clearly indicates that the orbitofrontal cortex plays a role in modulating the effects of reinforcement (see the review by Kringelbach, 2005). Strong hedonic preferences emerging from the valuation system could overpower cost-benefit analyses and opportunity cost considerations regarding consumption of the reward in the executive processing system. Indeed, researchers have found that the orbitofrontal cortex (OFC) is implicated in reward valuation and expectancies in both human and nonhuman animals (Jones et al., 2012; Schoenbaum & Esber, 2010). One might note that the OFC is also implicated in discounting (e.g., Jo et al., 2013), suggesting some overlap in these mechanisms in a Competing Neurobehavioral Decision System (CNDS). The CNDS is a spectral measure of the competing systems of the limbic system (reward system) versus the frontal region (executive system). This dual system analysis of behavior looks at the competing systems of the evolutionarily older limbic and paralimbic system that drives reward processing and the executive system or prefrontal region that influences tolerance to delay and future planning and valuation. Given the OFC connection to the nucleus accumbens, researchers have associated the OFC with the modulation of responses emerging from the limbic system associated with drug valuation and addiction (Porrino & Lyons, 2000; Volkow & Fowler, 2000). MacKillop and colleagues (2014) asked participants to make decisions to drink by using a hypothetical purchase task during an event-related fMRI protocol. High levels of frontostriatal region activation was seen on trials wherein the participants' level of anticipated consumption began to decrease dramatically.

Demand and Clinical Phenomena

Like delay and probability discounting, demand is relevant to a number of clinical issues. A primary characteristic of addiction is that addicted individuals overvalue the commodity they are addicted to – relative to other commodities. For example, Johnson and Bickel (2006) found that cigarette smokers continued to pull response plungers for cigarette puffs at higher costs (i.e., number of pulls) than they were willing to emit for money. This lower level of demand elasticity was found despite the participants higher valuation of money at lower costs. Similarly, MacKillop et al. (2008) found that that college-aged smokers with greater levels of nicotine dependence had less elastic demand for cigarettes than college-aged smokers with minimal nicotine dependence. These findings suggest that patients' relative lack of elasticity of demand may apply generally for commodities with which they feel addicted.

With demand reflecting individuals' struggle with addictive commodities, it may be an important treatment marker. For example, Madden and Kalman (2010) found that patients using bupropion for smoking cessation had a greater decrease in demand for cigarettes – as evidenced by their responding on a purchase task – than patients that received a placebo. Similarly, Green and Ray (2018) found that the maximum amount that patients indicated being willing to spend (i.e., *o-max*) was lower in patients using varenicline than those using placebo during a quit attempt. Moreover, Murphy et al. (2017) found that NRT and varenicline similarly decreased demand for cigarettes on quit day and that the breakpoint on their purchase task predicted abstinence on quit day, whereas their change in demand intensity (i.e., amount they would consume if cigarettes were free) and breakpoint from intake (i.e., *X* days prior to quit day) to quit day predicted one and three months abstinence, respectively. Lastly, MacKillop et al. (2016) found that demand curve measures (i.e., elasticity, *o-max*, *p-max*) predicted abstinence during a contingent vouchers treatment. In voucher contingency programs, sometimes also called contingency management programs, participants are compensated for compliance to treatment rules, which are usually measured by adherence to behavior and clean urine analysis testing.

Conclusions

There is not a compelling reason to believe that individuals tend to respond in rational ways. In fact, decades of behavioral economic research suggest that people tend to operate in a number of irrational ways. Fortunately, the behavioral economics of addiction arena developed a number of simple ways of determining the degree to which individuals' behavior is likely to deviate from rationality. These data reflect one's disordered valuation of problematic commodities such as drugs or other addictions, predict irrational behavior, and – importantly – predict success when undergoing treatments to improve behavior. With a growing understanding of the base behavioral and neurobiological processes which drive addictive behavior, there is hope that clinical researchers can leverage these insights to improve human health.

REFERENCES

Abela, A. R. & Chudasama, Y. (2013). Dissociable contributions of the ventral hippocampus and orbitofrontal cortex to decision-making with a delayed or uncertain outcome. *European Journal of Neuroscience*, **37**, 640–647.

Acuff, S. F. & Murphy, J. G. (2017). Further examination of the temporal stability of alcohol demand. *Behavioural Processes*, **141**, 33–41.

Ainslie, G. & Herrnstein, R. J. (1981). Preference reversal and delayed reinforcement. *Animal Learning and Behavior*, **9**(4), 476–482.

Ashare, R. L. & Hawk, L. W., Jr. (2012). Effects of smoking abstinence on impulsive behavior among smokers high and low in ADHD-like symptoms. *Psychopharmacology*, **219**(2), 537–547.

Audrain-McGovern, J., Rodriguez, D., Epstein, L. H., et al. (2009). Does delay discounting play an etiological role in smoking or is it a consequence of smoking? *Drug and Alcohol Dependence*, **103**(3), 99–106. doi:10.1016/j.drugalcdep.2008.12.019

Bickel, W. K. & Madden, G. J. (1999a). The behavioral economics of smoking. In F. J. Chaloupka, M. Grossman, W. K. Bickel & H. Saffer (Eds.), *The Economic Analysis of Substance Use and Abuse: An Integration of Econometric and Behavioral Economic Research*. Chicago: University of Chicago Press, pp. 31–61.

Bickel, W. K. & Madden, G. J. (1999b). A comparison of measures of relative reinforcing efficacy and behavioral economics: Cigarettes and money in smokers. *Behavioural Pharmacology*, **10**(6-7), 627–637.

Bickel, W. K. & Madden, G. J. (1999c). Similar consumption and responding across single and multiple sources of drug. *Journal of the Experimental Analysis of Behavior*, **72**(3), 299–316.

Bickel, W. K. & Marsch, L. A. (2001). Toward a behavioral economic understanding of drug dependence: Delay discounting processes. *Addiction*, **96**(1), 73–86. doi:10.1046/j.1360-0443.2001.961736.x

Bickel, W. K. & Vuchinich, R. E. (2000). *Reframing Health Behavior Change with Behavioral Economics*. Mahwah, NJ: Lawrence Erlbaum Associates Publishers.

Bickel, W. K. & Yi, R. (2008). Temporal discounting as a measure of executive function: Insights from the competing neuro-behavioral decision system hypothesis of addiction. In D. Houser & K. McCabe (Eds.), *Neuroeconomics: Advances in Health Services Research (Volume 20)*. Bingley, UK: Emerald Group Publishing, pp. 289–309.

Bickel, W. K., Jarmolowicz, D. P., MacKillop, J., et al. (2012a). The behavioral economics of reinforcement pathologies. In H. J. Shaffer (Ed.), *Addiction Syndrome Handbook*. Washington, DC: American Psychological Association.

Bickel, W. K., Jarmolowicz, D. P., Mueller, E. T., et al. (2012b). Altruism in time: Social temporal discounting differentiates smokers from problem drinkers. *Psychopharmacology*, **224**(1), 109–120. doi:10.1007/s00213-012-2745-6

Bickel, W. K., Jarmolowicz, D. P., Mueller, E. T. & Gatchalian, K. M. (2011a). The behavioral economics and neuroeconomics of reinforcer pathologies: Implications for etiology and treatment of addiction. *Current Psychiatry Reports*, **13**(5), 406–415. doi:10.1007/s11920-011-0215-1

Bickel, W. K., Jarmolowicz, D. P., Mueller, E. T., Gatchalian, K. M. & McClure, S. M. (2012c). Are executive function and impulsivity antipodes? A conceptual reconstruction with special reference to addiction. *Psychopharmacology*, **221**(3), 361–387.

Bickel, W. K., Jarmolowicz, D. P., Mueller, E. T., Koffarnus, M. N. & Gatchalian, K. M. (2012d). Excessive discounting of delayed reinforcers as a trans-disease process contributing to addiction and other disease-related vulnerabilities: Emerging evidence. *Pharmacology and Therapeutics* **134**(3), 287-297. doi:10.1016/j.pharmthera.2012.02.004

Bickel, W. K., Miller, M. L., Yi, R., et al. (2007). Behavioral and neuroeconomics of drug addiction: Competing neural systems and temporal discounting processes. *Drug and Alcohol Dependence*, **90S**, S85–S91. doi:10.1016/j.drugalcdep.2006.09.016

Bickel, W. K., Odum, A. L. & Madden, G. J. (1999). Impulsivity and cigarette smoking: Delay discounting in current, never, and ex-smokers. *Psychopharmacology*, **146**(4), 447–454. doi:10.1007/PL00005490

Bickel, W. K., Yi, R., Kowal, B. P. & Gatchalian, K. M. (2008). Cigarette smokers discount past and future rewards symmetrically and more than controls: Is discounting a measure of impulsivity? *Drug and Alcohol Dependence*, **96** (3), 256–262. doi:10.1016/j.drugalcdep.2008.03.009

Bickel, W. K., Yi, R., Landes, R. D., Hill, P. F. & Baxter, C. (2011b). Remember the future: Working memory training decreases delay discounting among stimulant addicts. *Biological Psychiatry*, **69**(3), 260–265. doi:10.1016/j.biopsych.2010.08.017

Bjork, J. M., Hommer, D. W., Grant, S. J. & Danube, C. (2004). Impulsivity in abstinent alcohol-dependent patients: Relation to control subjects and type 1 /type 2 like traits. *Alcohol*, **34**(2-3), 133–150.

Black, A. C. & Rosen, M. I. (2011). A money management-based substance use treatment increases valuation of future rewards. *Addictive Behaviors*, **36**(1-2), 125–128. doi:10.1016/j.addbeh.2010.08.014

Bruce, J. M., Bruce, A. S., Catley, D., et al. (2016). Being kind to your future self: Probability discounting of health decision-making. *Annals of Behavioral Medicine*, **50**, 297–309.

Bruce, J. M., Jarmolowicz, D. P., Lynch, S., et al. (2018). How patients with multiple sclerosis weigh treatment risks and benefits. *Health Psychology*, **37**, 680–690.

Coffey, S. F., Gudleski, G. D., Saladin, M. E. & Brady, K. T. (2003). Impulsivity and rapid discounting of delayed hypothetical rewards in cocaine-dependent individuals. *Experimental and Clinical Psychopharmacology*, **11**(1), 18–25.

Cowan, J. A. & Devine, C. M. (2012). Process evaluation of an environmental and educational nutrition intervention in residential drug-treatment facilities. *Public Health Nutrition*, **15**, 1159–1167.

Cowan, J. A. & Devine, C. M. (2013). Diet and body composition outcomes of an environmental and educational intervention among men in treatment for substance addiction. *Journal of Nutrition Education and Behavior*, **45**, 154–158.

Dallery, J. & Raiff, B. R. (2007). Delay discounting predicts cigarette smoking in a laboratory model of abstinence reinforcement. *Psychopharmacology*, **190**, 485–496.

Dembo, R., Belenko, S., Childs, K. & Wareham, J. (2009). Drug use and sexually transmitted diseases among female and male arrested youths. *Journal of Behavioral Medicine*, **32**, 129–141.

Dixon, M. R., Marley, J. & Jacobs, E. A. (2003). Delay discounting by pathological gamblers. *Journal of Applied Behavior Analysis*, **36**(4), 449–458.

Du, W., Green, L. & Myerson, J. (2002). Cross-cultural comparisons of discounting delayed and probabilistic rewards. *The Psychological Record*, **52**, 479–492.

Epstein, L. H., Salvy, S. J., Carr, K. A., Dearing, K. K. & Bickel, W. K. (2010). Food reinforcement, delay discounting and obesity. *Physiology and Behavior*, **100**(5), 438–445. doi:10.1016/j.physbeh.2010.04.029

Eysenck, S. B. G. & Eysenck, H. J. (1978). Impulsiveness and venturesomeness: Their position in a dimensional system of personality description. *Psychological Reports*, **43**, 1247–1255.

Few, L. R., Acker, J., Murphy, J. G. & MacKillop, J. (2012). Temporal stability of a cigarette purchase task. *Nicotine and Tobacco Research*, **14**, 761–765.

Franck, C. T., Koffarnus, M. N., House, L. L. & Bickel, W. K. (2015). Accurate characterization of delay discounting: A multiple model approach using approximate Bayesian model selection and a unified discounting measure. *Journal of the Experimental Analysis of Behavior*, **103**, 218–233.

Grace, R. C., Kivell, B. M. & Laugesen, M. (2015). Assessing the temporal stability of a cigarette purchase task after an excise tax increase for factory-made and roll-your-own smokers. *Nicotine & Tobacco Research: Official Journal of the Society for Research on Nicotine and Tobacco*, **17**, 1393–1396.

Green, L. & Estle, S. J. (2003). Preference reversals with food and water reinforcers in rats. *Journal of the Experimental Analysis of Behavior*, **79**(2), 233–242. doi:10.1901/jeab.2003.79-233

Green, L. & Myerson, J. (2004). A discounting framework for choice with delayed and probabilistic rewards. *Psychological Bulletin*, **130**(5), 769–792.

Green, L. & Myerson, J. (2013). How many impulsivities? A discounting perspective. *Journal of the Experimental Analysis of Behavior*, **99**, 3–13.

Green, L., Fisher, E. B., Perlow, S. & Sherman, L. (1981). Preference reversal and self-control: Choice as a function of reward amount and delay. *Behaviour Analysis Letters*, **1**(1), 43–51.

Green, L., Myerson, J., Oliveira, L. & Chang, S. E. (2014). Discounting of delayed and probabilistic losses over a wide range of amounts. *Journal of the Experimental Analysis of Behavior*, **101**, 186–200.

Green, R. & Ray, L. A. (2018). Effects of varenicline on subjective craving and relative reinforcing value of cigarettes. *Drug and Alcohol Dependence*, **188**, 53–59.

Greenwald, M. K. & Hursh, S. R. (2006). Behavioral economic analysis of opioid consumption in heroin-dependent individuals: Effects of unit price and pre-session drug supply. *Drug and Alcohol Dependence*, **85**(1), 35–48. doi:Doi 10.1016/J.Drugalcdep.2006.03.007

Hariri, A. (2009). The neurobiology of individual differences in complex behavioral traits. *Annual Review of Neuroscience*, **32**, 225–247.

Hariri, A. R., Brown, S. M., Williamson, D. E., et al. (2006). Preference for immediate over delayed rewards is associated with magnitude of ventral striatal activity. *Journal of Neuroscience*, **26**(51), 13213–13217.

Heil, S. H., Johnson, M. W., Higgins, S. T. & Bickel, W. K. (2006). Delay discounting in currently using and currently abstinent cocaine-dependent outpatients and non-drug-using matched controls. *Addictive Behaviors*, **31**(7), 1290–1294.

Holt, D. D., Green, L. & Myerson, J. (2003). Is discounting impulsive? Evidence from temporal and probability discounting in gambling and non-gambling college students. *Behavioural Processes*, **64**(3), 355–367. doi:10.1016/S0376-6357(03)00141-4

Holtyn, A. F., DeFulio, A. & Silverman, K. (2015). Academic skills of chronically unemployed drug-addicted adults. *Journal of Vocational Rehabilitation*, **42**, 67–74.

Hursh, S. R. (1980). Economic concepts for the analysis of behavior. *Journal of the Experimental Analysis of Behavior*, **34**(2), 219–238.

Hursh, S. R. (1984). Behavioral economics. *Journal of the Experimental Analysis of Behavior*, **42**(3), 435–452.

Hursh, S. R. (1991). Behavioral economics of drug self-administration and drug abuse policy. *Journal of the Experimental Analysis of Behavior*, **56**(2), 377–393. doi:10.1901/jeab.1991.56-377

Hursh, S. R. & Silberberg, A. (2008). Economic demand and essential value. *Psychological Review*, **115**(1), 186–198. doi:2008-00265-008 [pii] 10.1037/0033-295X.115.1.186

Hursh, S. R., Raslear, T. G., Shurtleff, D., Bauman, R. & Simmons, L. (1988). A cost-benefit analysis of demand for food. *Journal of the Experimental Analysis of Behavior*, **50**(3), 419–440. doi:10.1901/jeab.1988.50-419

Jacobs, E. A. & Bickel, W. K. (1999). Modeling drug consumption in the clinic via simulation procedures: Demand for heroin and cigarettes in opioid-dependent outpatients. *Journal of Experimental and Clinical Psychopharmacology*, **7**(4), 412–426.

Jarmolowicz, D. P., Bruce, A. S., Glusman, M., et al. (2017). On how patients with multiple sclerosis weigh side effect severity and treatment efficacy when making treatment decisions. *Experimental and Clinical Psychopharmacology*, **25**, 479–484.

Jarmolowicz, D. P., Lemley, S. M., Mateos, A. & Sofis, M. J. (2016a). A multiple-stimulus-without-replacement assessment for sexual partners: Purchase task validation. *Journal of Applied Behavior Analysis*, **48**(3), 723–729.

Jarmolowicz, D. P., Mueller, E. T., Koffarnus, M. N., et al. (2013). Executive dysfunction in addiction. In J. MacKillop & H. de Wit (Eds.), *The Wiley-Blackwell Handbook of Addiction Psychopharmacology*. Oxford: Wiley-Blackwell.

Jarmolowicz, D. P., Reed, D. D., Bruce, A. S., et al. (2016b). Using EP50 to forecast treatment adherence in individuals with multiple sclerosis. *Behavioural Processes*, **132**, 94–99.

Jarmolowicz, D. P., Reed, D. D., Bruce, A. S., et al. (2018). Modeling effects of side-effect probability, side effect severity, and medication efficacy on patients with multiple sclerosis medication choice. *Experimental and Clinical Psychopharmacology*, **26**(6), 599.

Jarmolowicz, D. P., Reed, D. D., DiGennaro Reed, F. D. & Bickel, W. K. (2016c). The behaviroal and neuroeconomics of reinforcer pathologies: Implications for manigerial and health decision making. *Managerial and Decision Economics*, **37**, 274–293. doi:10.1002/mde.2716

Jo, S., Kim, K. U., Lee, D. & Jung, M. W. (2013). Effect of orbitofrontal cortex lesions on temporal discounting in rats. *Behavioural Brain Research*, **245**, 22–28. doi:10.1016/j.bbr.2013.02.014

Johnson, M. W. & Bickel, W. K. (2003). The behavioral economics of cigarette smoking: The concurrent presence of a substitute and an independent reinforcer. *Behavioral Pharmacology*, **14**(2), 137–144.

Johnson, M. W. & Bickel, W. K. (2006). Replacing relative reinforcing efficacy with behavioral economic demand curves. *Journal of the Experimental Analysis of Behavior*, **85** (1), 73–93.

Johnson, M. W., Bickel, W. K., Baker, F., et al. (2010). Delay discounting in current and former marijuana-dependent individuals. *Experimental and Clinical Psychopharmacology*, **18**(1), 99–107.

Jones, J. L., Esber, G. R., McDannald, M. A., et al. (2012). Orbitofrontal cortex supports behavior and learning using inferred but not cached values. *Science*, **338**(6109), 953-956. doi:10.1126/science.1227489

Kalivas, P. W. & Volkow, N. D. (2005). The neural basis of addiction: A pathology of motivation and choice. *The American Journal of Psychiatry*, **162**(8), 1403–1413.

Kirby, K. N. (2009). One-year temporal stability of delay-discount rates. *Psychonomic Bulletin and Review*, **16**(3), 457–462. doi: 10.3758/Pbr.16.3.457

Kirby, K. N. & Marakovic, N. N. (1996). Delay-discounting probabilistic rewards: rates decrease as amounts increase. *Psychonomic Bulletin and Review*, **33**, 100–104.

Kirby, K. N., Petry, N. M. & Bickel, W. K. (1999). Heroin addicts have higher discount rates for delayed rewards than non-drug using controls. *Journal of Experimental Psychology: General*, **128**(1), 78–87.

Koffarnus, M. N. & Bickel, W. K. (2014). A 5-trial adjusting delay discounting task: Accurate discount rates in less than one minute. *Experimental and clinical psychopharmacology*, **22**, 222–228.

Koffarnus, M. N., Franck, C. T., Stein, J. S. & Bickel, W. K. (2015). A modified exponential behavioral economic demand model to better describe consumption data. *Experimental and Clinical Psychopharmacology*, **23**, 504–512.

Koffarnus, M. N., Jarmolowicz, D. P., Mueller, E. T. & Bickel, W. K. (2013). Changing discounting in light of the competing neurobehavioral decision systems theory *Journal of the Experimental Analysis of Behavior*, **99**(1), 32–57.

Kringelbach, M. L. (2005). The orbitofrontal cortex: Linking reward to hedonic experience. *Nature Reviews Neuroscience*, **6**, 691–702.

Lin, X., Zhou, H., Dong, G. & Du, X. (2015). Impaired risk evaluation in people with Internet gaming disorder: fMRI evidence from a probability discounting task. *Progress in Neuro-Psychopharmacology and Biological Psychiatry*, **56**, 142–148.

Loewenstein, G. F. (1988). Frames of the mind in intertemporal choice. *Management Science*, **34**(2), 200–214.

MacKillop, J. & Murphy, J. G. (2007). A behavioral economic measure of demand for alcohol predicts brief intervention outcomes. *Drug and Alcohol Dependence*, **89**(2-3), 227–233.

MacKillop, J. & Tidey, J. W. (2011). Cigarette demand and delayed reward discounting in nicotine-dependent individuals with schizophrenia and controls: An initial study. *Psychopharmacology*, **216**(1), 91–99.

Mackillop, J., Amlung, M. T., Acker, J., et al. (2014). The neuroeconomics of alcohol demand: An initial investigation of the neural correlates of alcohol cost-benefit decision making in heavy drinking men. *Neuropsychopharmacology*. doi:10.1038/npp.2014.47

MacKillop, J., Few, L. R., Murphy, J. G., et al. (2012). High-resolution behaviroal economic analysis of cigarette demand to inform tax policy. *Addiction*, **107**(12), 2191–2200.

MacKillop, J., Murphy, C. M., Martin, R. A., et al. (2016). Predictive validity of a cigarette purchase task in a randomized controlled trial of contingent vouchers for smoking in individuals with substance use disorders. *Nicotine & Tobacco Research: Official Journal of the Society for Research on Nicotine and Tobacco*, **18**, 531–537.

MacKillop, J., Murphy, J. G., Ray, L. A., et al. (2008). Further validation of a cigarette purchase task for assessing the relative reinforcing efficacy of nicotine in college smokers. *Experimental and Clinical Psychopharmacology*, **16**(1), 57–65. doi:10.1037/1064-1297.16.1.57

MacKillop, J., Murphy, J. G., Tidey, J. W., et al. (2009). Latent structure of facets of alcohol reinforcement from a behavioral economic demand curve. *Psychopharmacology*, **203**(1), 33–40.

MacKillop, J., O'Hagen, S., Lisman, S. A., et al. (2010). Behavioral economic analysis of cue-elicited craving for alcohol. *Addiction*, **105**(9), 1599–1607. doi:10.1111/j.1360-0443.2010.03004.x

Madden, G. J. & Bickel, W. K. (1999). Abstinence and price effects on demand for cigarettes: A behavioral-economic analysis. *Addiction*, **94**(4), 577–588.

Madden, G. J. & Bickel, W. K. (2009). *Impulsivity: The Behavioral and Neurological Science of Discounting*. Washington, DC: APA.

Madden, G. J. & Kalman, D. (2010). Effects of bupropion on simulated demand for cigarettes and the subjective effects of smoking. *Nicotine and Tobacco Research*, **12**, 416–422.

Madden, G. J., Bickel, W. K. & Jacobs, E. A. (2000). Three predictions of the economic concept of unit price in a choice context. *Journal of the Experimental Analysis of Behavior*, **73**(1), 45–64.

Madden, G. J., Petry, N. M., Badger, G. J. & Bickel, W. K. (1997). Impulsive and self-control choices in opioid-dependent patients and non-drug-using control participants: Drug and monetary rewards. *Experimental and Clinical Psychopharmacology*, **5**(3), 256–262.

Madden, G. J., Petry, N. M. & Johnson, P. S. (2009). Pathological gamblers discount probabilistic rewards less steeply than matched controls. *Experimental and Clinical Psychopharmacology*, **17**(5), 283–290. doi:10.1037/a0016806

Manuck, S. B., Flory, J. D., Muldoon, M. F. & Ferrell, R. E. (2003). A neurobiology of intertemporal choice. In G. Loewenstein, D. Read & R. Baumeister (Eds.), *Time and Decision: Economic and Psychological Perspectives on Intertemporal Choice*. New York: Russell Sage Foundation, pp. 139–172.

Mazur, J. E. (1987). An adjusting procedure for studying delayed reinforcement. In M. L. Commons, J. E. Mazur, J. A. Nevin & H. Rachlin (Eds.), *Quantitative Analysis of Behavior (Volume 5)*. Hillsdale, NJ: Erlbaum, pp. 55–73.

McKerchar, T. L., Green, L., Myerson, J., et al. (2009). A comparison of four models of delay discounting in humans. *Behavioural Processes*, **81**(2), 256–259. doi:10.1016/j.beproc.2008.12.017

McLellan, A. T., Luborsky, L., Cacciola, J., et al. (1985). New data from the Addiction Severity Index: Reliability and validity in three centers. *Journal of Nervous and Mental Disorders*, **173** (7), 412–423.

Miedl, S. F., Peters, J. & Buchel, C. (2012a). Altered neural reward representations in pathological gamblers revealed by delay and probability discounting. *Archives of General Psychiatry*, **69**(2), 177–186.

Miedl, S. F., Peters, J. & Buchel, C. (2012b). Altered neural reward representations in pathological gamblers revealed by delay and probability discounting. *JAMA Psychiatry*, **69**, 177–186.

Monterosso, J. & Ainslie, G. (2007). The behavioral economics of will in recovery from addiction. *Drug and Alcohol Dependence*, **90** (Supplement 1), S100–111. doi:10.1016/j.drugalcdep.2006.09.004

Morrison, K. L., Madden, G. J., Odum, A. L., Friedel, J. E. & Twohig, M. P. (2014). Altering impulsive decision making with an acceptance-based procedure. *Behavior Therapy*, **45**, 630–639.

Murphy, C. M., MacKillop, J., Martin, R. A., et al. (2017). Effects of varenicline versus transdermal nicotine replacement therapy on cigarette demand on quit day in individuals with substance use disorders. *Psychopharmacology*, **234**, 2443–2452.

Murphy, J. G. & MacKillop, J. (2006). Relative reinforcing efficacy of alcohol among college student drinkers. *Experimental and Clinical Psychopharmacology*, **14**(2), 219–227. doi:10.1037/1064-1297.14.2.219

Myerson, J. & Green, L. (1995). Discounting of delayed rewards: Models of individual choice. *Journal of the Experimental Analysis of Behavior*, **64**(3), 263–276.

Myerson, J., Green, L. & Warusawitharana, M. (2001). Area under the curve as a measure of discounting. *Journal of the Experimental Analysis of Behavior*, **76**(2), 235–243. doi: 10.1901/jeab.2001.76-235

NIDA. (2017). Overdose death rates. Retrieved from www.drugabuse.gov/related-topics/trends-statistics/overdose-death-rates

O'Doherty, J. P. (2004). Reward representations and reward-related learning in the human brain: insights from neuroimaging. *Current Opinion in Neurobiology*, **14**, 769–776.

Odum, A. L. (2011). Delay discounting: Trait variable? *Behavioral Processes*, **87**, 1–9.

Odum, A. L. & Baumann, A. A. (2007). Cigarette smokers show steeper discounting of both food and cigarettes than money. *Drug and Alcohol Dependence*, **91**(2–3), 293–296.

Peters, J. & Buchel, C. (2009). Overlapping and distinct neural systems code for subjective value during intertemporal and risky decision making. *The Journal of Neuroscience*, **29**, 15727–15734.

Petry, N. M. (2001a). Delay discounting of money and alcohol in actively using alcoholics, currently abstinent alcoholics, and controls. *Psychopharmacology*, **154**(3), 243–250.

Petry, N. M. (2001b). Pathological gamblers, with and without substance use disorders, discount delayed rewards at high rates. *Journal of Abnormal Psychology*, **110**(3), 482–487.

Petry, N. M. & Casarella, R. (1999). Excessive discounting of delayed rewards in substance abusers with gambling problems. *Drug and Alcohol Dependence*, **56**(1), 25–32.

Porrino, L. J. & Lyons, D. (2000). Orbital and medial prefrontal cortex and psychostimulant abuse: studies in animal models. *Cerebral Cortex*, **10**(3), 326–333.

Rachlin, H. (2006). Notes on discounting. *Journal of the Experimental Analysis of Behavior*, **85**(3), 425–435. doi: 10.1901/jeab.2006.85-05

Rachlin, H., Raineri, A. & Cross, D. (1991). Subjective probability and delay. *Journal of the Experimental Analysis of Behavior*, **55**(2), 233–244. doi: 10.1901/jeab.1991.55-233

Reed, D. D., Kaplan, B. A., Becirevic, A., Roma, P. G. & Hursh, S. R. (2016). Toward quantifying the abuse liability of ultraviolet tanning: A behavioral economic approach to tanning addiction. *Journal of the Experimental Analysis of Behavior*, **106**, 93–106.

Reed, D. D., Naudé, G. P. Gelino, B. W. & Amlung, M. (2020). Behavioral economic considerations of novel addictions and nonaddictive behavior: Research and analytic methods. In S. Sussman (Ed.) *The Cambridge Handbook of Substance and Behavioral Addictions*. Cambridge, UK: Cambridge University Press, pp. 73–86.

Reynolds, B., Richards, J. B., Horn, K. & Karraker, K. (2004). Delay discounting and probability discounting as related to cigarette smoking status in adults. *Behavioral Processes*, **30**(65), 35–42. doi:10.1016/S0376-6357(03)00109-8

Reynolds, B., Richards, J. B. & de Witt, H. (2006). Acute-alcohol effects on the Experiential Discounting Task (EDT) and a question-based measure of delay discounting. *Pharmacology, Biochemistry, and Behavior*, **83**(2), 194–202.

Richards, J. B., Zhang, L., Mitchell, S. H. & de Wit, H. (1999). Delay or probability discounting in a model of impulsive behavior: Effect of alcohol. *Journal of the Experimental Analysis of Behavior*, **71**(2), 121–143.

Ritschel, F., King, J. A., Geisler, D., et al. (2015). Temporal delay discounting in acutely ill and weight-recovered patients with anorexia nervosa. *Psychological Medicine*, **45**(6), 1229–1239.

Romer, D. (2010). Adolescent risk taking, impulsivity, and brain development:

Implications for prevention. *Developmental Psychobiology*, **52**, 263–276.

Samuelson, P. (1937). A note on measurement of utility. *The Review of Economic Studies*, **4**, 155–161.

Schoenbaum, G. & Esber, G. R. (2010). How do you (estimate you will) like them apples? Integration as a defining trait of orbitofrontal function. *Current Opinion in Neurobiology*, **20** (2), 205–211. doi:10.1016/j.conb.2010.01.009

Shahan, T. A., Bickel, W. K., Badger, G. J. & Giordano, L. A. (2001). Sensitivity of nicotine-containing and de-nicotinized cigarette consumption to alternative non-drug reinforcement: A behavioral economic analysis. *Behavioral Pharmacology*, **12**(4), 277–284.

Shahan, T. A., Bickel, W. K., Madden, G. J. & Badger, G. J. (1999). Comparing the reinforcing efficacy of nicotine containing and de-nicotinized cigarettes: A behavioral economics analysis. *Psychopharmacology*, **147**(2), 210–216.

Shahan, T. A., Odum, A. L. & Bickel, W. K. (2000). Nicotine gum as a substitute for cigarettes: A behavioral economics analysis. *Behavioral Pharmacology*, **11**(1), 71–76.

Sheffer, C. E., Christensen, D. R., Landes, R. D., et al. (2014). Delay discountin rates: A strong prognastic indicator of smoking relapse. *Addictive Behaviors*, **39**, 1682–1689.

Sheffer, C. E., MacKillop, J., McGeary, J., et al. (2012). Delay discounting, locus of control, and cognitive impulsiveness independently predict tobacco dependence treatment outcomes in a highly dependent, lower socioeconomic group of smokers. *American Journal on Addictions*, **21**(3), 221–232.

Sofis, M. J., Carrillo, A. & Jarmolowicz, D. P. (2016). Maintained physical activity induced changes in delay discounting. *Behavioral Modification*. doi:10.1177/0145445516685047

Sobell, L. C., Ellingstad, T. P. & Sobell, M. B. (2000). Natural recovery from alcohol and drug problems: Methodological review of the research with suggestions for future directions. *Addiction*, **95**(5), 749–764.

Takahashi, T. (2006). Time-estimation error following Weber–Fechner law may explain subadditive time-discounting. *Medical Hypotheses*, pp. 1372–1374.

Takahashi, T., Furukawa, A., Miyakawa, T., Maesato, H. & Higuchi, S. (2007). Two-month stability of hyperbolic discount rates for delayed monetary gains in abstinent inpatient alcoholics. *Neuroendocrinology Letters*, **28**(2), 131–136.

Takahashi, T., Takahashi, H., Nishinaka, H., Makino, T. & Fukui, H. (2014). Neuroeconomics of psychopathy: Risk taking in probability discounting of gain and loss predicts psychopathy. *Neuroendocrinology Letters*, **35**, 510–517.

Volkow, N. D. & Fowler, J. S. (2000). Addiction, a disease of compulsion and drive: Involvement of the orbitofrontal cortex. *Cerebral Cortex*, **10**(3), 318–325. doi:10.1093/cercor/10.3.318

Washio, Y., Higgins, S. T., Heil, S. H., et al. (2011). Delay discounting is associated with treatment response among cocaine-dependent outpatients. *Experimental and Clinical Psychopharmacology*. doi:10.1037/a0023617

Watson, D. S. & Holman, M. A. (1977). *Price Theory and Its Uses* (4th edition.). Boston: Houghton Mifflin.

Yi, R., Chase, W. D. & Bickel, W. K. (2007). Probability discounting among cigarette smokers and nonsmokers: Molecular analysis discerns group differences. *Behavioural Pharmacology*, **18**(7), 633–639. doi:10.1097/FBP.0b013e3282effbd3 [doi]:00008877-200711000-00006 [pii]

Yi, R., Matusiewicz, A. K. & Tyson, A. (2016). Delay discounting and preference reversals by cigarette smokers. *The Psychological Record*, **66**, 235–242.

3 Sensitization of Incentive Salience and the Transition to Addiction

Shelley M. Warlow, PhD, Hannah M. Baumgartner, MS, Charlotte M. Freeland*, BS, Erin E. Naffziger*, MS, Jeffrey J. Olney*, PhD, Kent C. Berridge, PhD, and Mike J. F. Robinson, PhD, *authorship shared equally

Introduction

Most people have at one time in their lives indulged in drugs or other incentives with known addictive properties. This includes legal and illicit drugs such as alcohol, nicotine, cocaine or heroin, or behaviors such as gambling, shopping or indoor tanning (Petit et al., 2014; also see Derevensky, 2020; Galimov & Black, 2020; Miller & Mays, 2020; also see Sussman & Bolshakova, 2020). Yet for most individuals such behavior is largely recreational or done with moderation, and it is balanced by other life pursuits. For some people, however, the consumption of these rewards can escalate and lead to a dominant compulsive behavior, focused heavily on obtaining and consuming a given reward. This pattern of misuse can develop into addiction, hallmarks of which include compulsive use despite negative consequences, and persistent pursuit and escalated consumption often triggered by intense cravings. Drug cravings originate from the same brain reward systems that have evolved to encourage seeking out natural rewards crucial to survival (Sussman, Rozgonjuk & van den Eijnden, 2017). In drug addiction, these reward 'wanting' systems may be sensitized, and thus become hijacked to narrowly focus on taking drugs as an addictive target (Robinson & Berridge, 1993). The result is reward 'wanting' systems hyperreactive to drugs and their cues, especially after specific patterns of drug use among at-risk individuals. Similar hijacking of brain 'wanting' systems may also occur in especially susceptible individuals in other addictions. The neural adaptations underlying the sensitization of brain reward systems have been shown to be extremely long-lasting, and independent of the brain systems responsible for the pleasure or 'liking' associated with many of these rewards. As a result, exposure to drugs and their cues, even after years of abstinence, can trigger bouts of intense desire and craving for the drug that may lead to relapse. As such, addiction is a chronic relapsing disorder characterized by excessive 'wanting' for the drug and its cues, even in the absence of corresponding changes in 'liking.'

'Wanting' and 'Liking'

The brain is responsible for generating motivation for rewards, such as food, sex, and social relationships. This motivation for reward can be further parsed into three distinct psychological components, that each serve their own independent function, consisting of liking, wanting, and learning (Berridge & Robinson, 2003). Specifically, a reward is usually both liked and wanted, and often has been learned about, to help guide future behavior. In most situations, liking, wanting, and learning seamlessly function together to influence motivation. For example, when one thinks about what they want to eat for dinner, pleasurable meals that have been eaten in the past are instantly recalled. In this way, 'liking' and 'wanting' naturally act in tandem to generate motivation to seek out and obtain the rewards that produce pleasure. However, each of these functions is attributed to distinct but overlapping brain mechanisms. Separable brain systems permit the possibility that these components can diverge under certain conditions. Whereas people typically 'want' what they 'like,' and 'like' what they 'want,' after mesolimbic sensitization a person can at times develop excessive motivation for rewards known to evoke only moderate amounts of expected pleasure. In some cases, this might even generate excessive craving for rewards which have in the past been repeatedly paired with unpleasant consequences. Such is the case in the transition from recreational drug use to addiction, and a similar process may operate with behavioral addictions as well.

Addiction can cause an individual to perform irrational behavior when compulsively seeking drugs, with only limited insight into the origin of their behavior. This is because both 'wanting' and 'liking' do not necessarily have to be consciously experienced to influence behavior. For instance, subliminally presented pictures of happy faces can increase incentive motivation and make thirsty participants drink more of a sweet beverage and highly rate it, without those thirsty participants reporting any changes in conscious feelings (Winkielman, Berridge & Wilbarger, 2005). Similarly with drug rewards, 'wanting' and 'liking' can occur below consciousness. For example, recovering cocaine addicts have been described to consistently choose a very low dose of cocaine over an injection of saline, despite reporting no more subjective feelings of pleasure than with saline, no cardiovascular responses, and indicating that they thought they were sampling both options equally (Fischman & Foltin, 1992). Furthermore, presenting cocaine addicts with brief (33 ms) images of drug-related stimuli (e.g., a pipe) or sexual stimuli, that are masked by the longer presentation of another subsequent image to prevent conscious perception, activates similar reward brain circuitry and causes an enhancement of that brain's reactivity to a later, consciously-seen drug stimulus (Childress et al., 2008). Thus, drug craving ('wanting'), can often be generated unconsciously, only reaching at times the level of conscious awareness. As such, we refer to 'wanting' as incentive salience and 'liking' as hedonic impact in quotations to distinguish those objective psychological processes, which can occur either unconsciously or consciously, from subjective feelings of wanting and liking that are necessarily conscious.

Pleasure 'Liking' as a Distinct Psychological Component

Pleasure is more than a property of a physical reward stimulus – it is actively generated by the brain as one of the components of an experienced reward (Berridge, 2009; Dai, Brendl & Ariely, 2010; Litt, Khan & Shiv, 2010). 'Liking' refers to the objective hedonic impact, measurable in affective reactions, derived from a pleasant reward. Although rewards such as food, drink, or sex comprise multiple sensory properties that elicit pleasurable reactions, 'liking' is a distinct psychological component that goes beyond the mere sensory qualities of a reward. The sensory properties of a reward such as the sweetness of ice cream can remain constant, yet the pleasurable sensation associated with the reward itself may be dramatically reduced, if the flavor was previously paired with the nausea of visceral sickness (Berridge et al., 2010; Garcia et al., 1985; Rozin, 2000). Conversely, the bitter taste of beer or coffee can become not only desired but also positively enjoyed for many people, when repeatedly paired with the pharmacological properties of alcohol and caffeine. Furthermore, sudden changes in internal physiological state can produce a dynamic shift in hedonic tone known as "alliesthesia" (Cabanac, 1971). And whereas hunger can make foods more 'liked' (Cabanac, 1971; Cabanac & Lafrance, 1990; Kaplan, Roitman & Grill, 2000), satiation can dampen the pleasure elicited by chocolate, even in self-proclaimed "chocoholics" (Lemmens et al., 2009; Small et al., 2001).

'Liking' as an affective response to hedonic stimuli can be measured in behavior and physiology even in the absence of subjective liking. Orofacial hedonic reactions to sweet versus bitter tastes were first measured in human infants by Jacob Steiner (Steiner, 1973), and subsequently extended to rats in the taste reactivity test (Grill & Norgren, 1978), which measures orofacial reactions elicited in response to different tastes. These include objective patterns of hedonic reactions such as lip licking and rhythmic tongue protrusions in response to 'liked' tastes such as sweet sugars, and negative gapes and headshakes in response to 'disliked' tastes such as bitter quinine. These reactions are highly conserved and homologous across species including humans, rats and apes (Berridge & Kringelbach, 2008; Steiner et al., 2001). Importantly, these hedonic orofacial reactions to pleasantness are separable from just sweet or bitter sensations and track the hedonic impact of the taste rather than its sensory properties. For example, a once 'liked' sweet taste that elicits tongue protrusion 'liking' reactions, can become 'disliked,' causing gaping 'disliking' reactions when paired with sickness (Delamater & McNamara, 1986; Itoga, Berridge & Aldridge, 2016; Parker, 2014). Subjective ratings of pleasure and pain can be difficult to compare across individuals, if they have different experiences leading to different standards by which they evaluate an affective stimulus (Bartoshuk, 2014). For example, those with limited experience of extreme pain may rate a given stimulus as more painful than someone who has previously experienced severely painful events. On the other hand, a limiting feature of orofacial affective reactions is that the measure is restricted to taste pleasures. However, evidence suggests there is extensive overlap in the brain circuitry that is responsive to different types of pleasures (e.g., food, sex, or music pleasures) (Cacioppo et al., 2012; Georgiadis & Kringelbach 2012; Salimpoor et al., 2011; Xu et al., 2011), opening a possibility that orofacial affective reactions to taste pleasure can be used as a means of providing insight into brain mechanisms of pleasure more generally.

Neuroanatomy of 'Liking': Hedonic Hotspots

Where in the brain is pleasure generated? Using the taste reactivity test that measures changes in hedonic orofacial reactions in response to passively infused tastes, researchers in the Berridge laboratory have identified small cubic-millimeter-sized zones in which neurochemicals such as opioids, endocannabinoids, and orexin, but not dopamine, can enhance 'liking' reactions to the hedonic impact of sweetness pleasure. These small zones, located in distinct sites within larger brain structures, are called hedonic hotspots because of their unique capacity to cause hedonic enhancements of sweetness pleasure (Berridge & Robinson, 2003; Smith & Berridge, 2007). Thus far, identified hedonic hotspots include subregions, such as the the rostrodorsal quadrant of the medial shell of nucleus accumbens (Castro & Berridge, 2014; Castro, Terry & Berridge, 2016; Peciña & Berridge, 2000, 2005), the posterior half of ventral pallidum (whose hotspot is crucial for 'liking') (Cromwell & Berridge, 1993; Ho & Berridge, 2013; Smith & Berridge, 2005), cortical subregions such as medial orbitofrontal cortex and posterior insula (Castro & Berridge, 2017; Georgiadis & Kringelbach, 2012), and the parabrachial nucleus of the brainstem pons (Söderpalm and Berridge, 2000) (Figure 3.1a). These hedonic hotspots seem to function as a cooperative network that requires a unanimous vote to engender a 'liking' response. While stimulation of just one hotspot will typically recruit others, pharmacologically inhibiting activity in one hot spot will prevent an enhancement of 'liking' from opioid stimulation in one of the other hotspots (Castro & Berridge, 2017; Smith & Berridge, 2007).

'Wanting' and the Attribution of Incentive Salience

While 'liking' refers to the pleasure derived from rewards, 'wanting' refers to incentive salience, a specific motivation process underlying the desire to obtain and seek out those rewards. This "motivational desire" given to a reward can be conferred to learned cues and objects associated with that reward (Bindra, 1978), transforming them also into "wanted" incentives. Reward-related cues have the powerful ability to trigger bursts of motivation and reward seeking, mediated by mesolimbic circuitry involving dopamine and other neurotransmitters in nucleus accumbens (Holmes, Marchand & Coutureau, 2010; Peciña & Berridge, 2013). For example, the enticing smell of freshly baked cookies or the aroma of freshly brewed coffee can elicit consumption even in the absence of any need. However, in cases of pathological motivation, such as addiction, cues can become powerful enough to trigger intense cravings for rewards that may not even be consciously wanted or may have adverse consequences. Even an addict who has been able to abstain for many years may encounter a drug-related cue such as a physical location where purchases of an illicit drug had occurred, drug paraphernalia, or smell the odor of an alcoholic drink, which then causes intense cravings that become hard to ignore, possibly resulting in relapse.

By being paired with a particular reward and its outcome, cues become imbued with incentive salience, making them attractive targets of attention and desire (Hickey & Peelen, 2015). For example, virtual reality environments with casino-related cues evoke a significant urge to gamble in recreational gamblers, and this craving increases significantly when participants transition from the practice environment to the gambling environment (Giroux et al., 2013; Park et al., 2015). "Wanted" reward-related cues attract approach behavior and invigorate actions. Experimentally, the attribution of incentive salience to cues can be measured using a variety of tests. Pavlovian sign-tracking or autoshaping assesses how attractive the cue has become by examining whether an animal will sniff, nibble, or even bite inedible objects such as a protruding metal lever because it has been previously paired with a reward (Brown & Jenkins, 1968; DiFeliceantonio & Berridge, 2012;

Mahler & Berridge, 2012; Uslaner et al., 2006). Whether the cue has become a valued and desired object on its own is sometimes measured in animals by using the conditioned reinforcement test (Robbins, 1976), asking whether the animal will work to gain the cue. Similarly, the ability of the reward-paired cue to trigger bursts of more intense motivation to seek the reward itself can be established using Pavlovian-to-Instrumental Transfer (PIT), a measure of cue-triggered bursts of increased 'wanting' to obtain the unconditioned reward (Ostlund et al., 2014; Zhou et al., 2012; Peciña & Berridge, 2013). For example, PIT studies in animal models have demonstrated that the mere presence of cues associated with various drugs of abuse (i.e., ethanol or cocaine) can drive intense bursts of seeking behaviors for those particular drugs through a Pavlovian motivational process such as incentive salience (Corbit & Janak, 2007; LeBlanc, Ostlund & Maidment, 2012). These well-established behavioral paradigms have offered a valuable tool for investigating the brain mechanisms involved in generating 'wanting' for either rewards themselves or for reward-paired cues, and for modeling transition to addiction and relapse by assessing the invigorating effects of reward cues.

The ability of reward-related cues to invigorate 'wanting' is dependent on two major components, the reward cue's predictive value and incentive value. The predictive value of a cue is essentially pure learning: on how well it predicts the presence of reward. Yet prediction by itself does not necessarily imbue the cue with incentive value (Anselme & Robinson, 2013; Berridge, 2012; Robinson & Flagel, 2009). Only when the cue also carries incentive value does it become powerfully able to motivate reward seeking. The attribution of incentive value to a cue by an individual can be measured in Pavlovian autoshaping. In autoshaping, the presentation of a discrete, localizable cue that predicts reward delivery triggers powerful attraction and interaction with the cue itself in some animals, known as "sign-trackers." Sign-trackers assign incentive value to the reward predictive cue and are thus attracted to and engage with the lever cue. In contrast, "goal-trackers" assign only predictive value to the same cue, and instead are drawn to the location where the reward will be delivered (Robinson et al., 2014a). Such individual differences in sensitivity to reward-related cues indicate that sign-trackers and goal-trackers process motivationally salient stimuli in different ways. For example, a lever cue has the powerful ability to become an attractive motivational target in sign-trackers, spurring much higher levels of reward/drug seeking, even despite adverse consequences (e.g., a foot shock) than goal-trackers (Saunders & Robinson, 2010, 2011). By contrast, contextual cues have greater influence on directing motivated behavior in goal-trackers (Boakes et al., 1978; Flagel & Robinson, 2017; Flagel, Akil & Robinson, 2009; Robinson & Flagel, 2009). These reward-related cues illicit large increases in dopamine release from the nucleus accumbens in sign-trackers, which are absent in goal-trackers (Flagel et al., 2011). In this way, sign-trackers seem to be especially sensitive to the motivational power of reward-related cues, which may relate to addiction vulnerability. Indeed, several lines of research have shown that sign-trackers show a greater propensity to undergo psychomotor sensitization to cocaine with repeated treatment (Flagel et al., 2008), exhibit more intense cue-triggered relapse behavior (Saunders & Robinson, 2010) and are more prone to impulsive behavior (Lovic et al., 2011), another behavioral trait associated with addiction (Robinson et al., 2014a).

This distinction between predictive and incentive value of reward cues can be further exemplified by modulating the strength of the predictive value. For example, reward uncertainty, in which the cue predicts delivery of the reward only 50 percent of the time, degrades a cue's predictive value, and yet increases the amount to which that cue is attributed with incentive value (Anselme & Robinson, 2013; Robinson et al., 2015b). Similarly, incentive value of a cue can persist even when the cue's predictive value has declined by changing reward contingencies to omit the delivery of rewards when the lever is pressed. Evidence shows that although rats learn to stop pressing the lever, they continue to show appetitive approach behaviors toward that lever, at the same rate as another group who never experienced the change in predictive value. This would indicate that the cue (the lever) has acquired incentive value, able to motivate actions such as sniffing and biting, which persist beyond the cue's predictive ability (Chang & Smith, 2016; Hellberg, Levit & Robinson, 2018). As such, there is a clear distinction between predictive and incentive value that a cue acquires, with the latter being most important for intensifying 'wanting.' This is of particular interest to addiction, since the incentive salience value attributed to a cue can determine its ability to trigger bouts of craving and drug-seeking.

However, it is important to note that the intensity of 'wanting' triggered by a predictive cue not only depends on the cue's incentive value, but also the current dopamine-related brain state of the individual (Berridge & Robinson, 2016; Zhang et al., 2009). The motivation triggered by a reward-related cue can be exponentially increased in the moment by current brain dopamine levels. Physiological states such as stress, relevant appetites, intoxication or excitement (Anselme, 2016; Robinson & Berridge, 2013; Sinha, 2013) which heighten dopaminergic brain reactivity state, can combine with the cue's presentation to raise the intensity of triggered bursts of 'wanting.' This mirrors real-world situations of addictive relapse, where an abstinent addict can successfully resist a cue multiple times without succumbing to relapse, but subsequently upon a single presentation of that cue under conditions of higher stress or excitement, can suddenly heighten the incentive value and drug 'wanting' triggered by that cue to a point where temptation is overwhelming and results in relapse. This heightened 'wanting' in situations of stress, for example, can be further exacerbated by short-circuiting of executive function, particularly in prefrontal cortical projections to striatum (Garcia-Keller et al., 2013; Kalivas, Volkow & Seamans, 2005). Thus incentive salience is thought to integrate two separate factors – current neurobiological state plus a cue's incentive value, which are integrated together to determine the level of 'wanting' triggered at that moment by the cue (Berridge, 2012).

Brain Generators of 'Wanting'

'Wanting' generators in the brain are much more robust and diffuse than those brain mechanisms generating 'liking.' 'Wanting' includes dopaminergic (and opioid, glutamate and other) systems across mesocorticolimbic structures. Dopamine neurons residing in the midbrain ventral tegmental area send projections and release dopamine in limbic structures such as the nucleus accumbens and prefrontal cortex, interacting with other structures such as the amygdala, ventral pallidum, and lateral hypothalamus to enhance motivation for rewards (both natural and drug rewards) and reward-paired cues (Cameron, Wightman & Carelli, 2014; Castro, Cole & Berridge, 2015) (Figure 3.1a). In laboratory experiments, stimulations of these structures (for example, by infusing a dopamine agonist, or by optogenetic stimulation of neurons) can increase 'wanting' to consume rewards, as well as enhance cue-triggered reward seeking and approach of reward cues, and the same has also been shown with the infusion of opioid agonists such as DAMGO

(Castro & Berridge, 2014; DiFeliceantonio & Berridge, 2012; Mahler & Berridge, 2012; Peciña & Berridge, 2013; Smith & Berridge, 2005; Smith, Berridge & Aldridge, 2011). In contrast, drugs that block dopamine transmission, such as the dopamine antagonist pimozide, or treatments (i.e., 6-OHDA) that destroy over 99 percent of mesolimbic and neostriatal dopamine afferents, disrupt 'wanting' – animals lack the motivation to feed themselves and display life-threatening aphagia and adipsia (Berridge, Venier & Robinson, 1989). In humans, drugs that block dopamine function completely fail to reduce the subjective ratings of pleasure people give to an addictive drug, such as amphetamine, cocaine or methamphetamine, yet diminish craving to take more drug (Brauer & de Wit, 1997; Leyton et al., 2007; Wachtel, Ortengren & de Wit, 2002), and diminish cue-induced craving (Berger et al., 1996). Similarly, studies in which dopamine transmission was decreased by interfering with dopamine synthesis (acute phenylalanine/tyrosine depletion; APTD) show that the subjective pleasure ratings and mood altering effects of a wide range of abused substances, such as alcohol (Barrett et al., 2008; Leyton et al., 2000), tobacco (Casey et al., 2006; Munafò, Zetterler & Clark, 2007), amphetamine (Leyton et al., 2007), and cocaine (Leyton et al., 2005), remain intact, while subjective ratings of drug 'wanting' and cocaine-induced confidence are reduced (Leyton et al., 2005). In contrast, application of a drug that blocks opioid function impacts both 'wanting' and 'liking' due to opioids' role in both processes, particularly in areas such as the nucleus accumbens shell (Castro & Berridge, 2014; Shin et al., 2010; Smith & Berridge, 2007).

Natural rewards such as food, water, and sex all generate pleasure, while also triggering the release of mesolimbic dopamine and coactivating the 'wanting' system (Hernandez & Hoebel, 1988; Pfaus et al., 1990). In drug, food, and gambling addictions, there exists evidence of hypersensitive 'wanting' systems taking incentive salience attribution to maladaptive levels, often with very little change in pleasure responding (Robinson & Berridge, 2008; Robinson et al., 2015b; Rømer Thomsen et al., 2014).

Sensitized 'Wanting' in Incentive Sensitization Theory

While mesocorticolimbic brain structures evolved to generate 'wanting' for natural rewards crucial to survival, they are especially heavily activated by modern drugs of abuse, hyperpalatable foods, and rewarded behaviors such as gambling. Activation of 'wanting' circuitry by these rewarding stimuli or incentive cues related to them, involves surges of dopamine release. Over time, drugs can induce particular neural changes called sensitization in mesolimbic circuitry, which once formed may be extremely long lasting (Evans et al., 2006; Paulson, Camp & Robinson, 1991; Robinson & Becker, 1986). Conceivably behavioral addictions may involve similar meoscorticolimbic changes through repetition and alteration of endogenous ligands in particularly susceptible individuals. Sensitization causes mesocorticolimbic activation to become increasingly sensitive to those particular rewards and their related cues, such that higher levels of dopamine are released and greater neural responses are evoked in target structures when cues are encountered. This is especially true in a subset of individuals partaking in particular binge/purge patterns of drug use or behaviors, such as episodic/binge gambling (Cowlishaw et al., 2018), who may be particularly vulnerable to sensitization due to their genes, steroid hormones, previous stress experiences, etc. (Kawa, Bentzley & Robinson, 2016; Rougé-Pont et al., 1993; Piazza et al., 1989, 2000). In sensitized individuals, presentation of the reward or reward-related cue causes an enhanced release of dopamine among mesocorticolimbic brain structures responsible for generating reward 'wanting.' Further, the magnitude of incentive salience evoked by a cue can be augmented even further by current states of intoxication or stress (Berridge, 2012). Thus, being primed with drug consumption, stress or emotional excitement states, and then encountering incentive cues, can cause intense cravings for the drug/behavior and heightened motivation to seek out that particular drug or engage in that particular behavior. For many individuals with addiction, this desire can become overwhelming and undeniable enough to cause relapse.

The notion that drug-induced sensitization among brain mesolimbic structures renders them hyperreactive to the addict's drug of choice and its cues is the basis for the Incentive Sensitization theory of addiction first proposed by Robinson and Berridge (Robinson & Berridge, 1993). This hyperreactivity caused by drugs or drug-paired cues triggers an increase in cravings for that particular drug of abuse, and results in patterns of excessive drug use. In individuals recovering from drug abuse, these cravings can become so overwhelmingly tempting (especially in times of stress or excitement) as to result in relapse (Figure 3.1b).

Over the years there has been a substantial amount of evidence accumulated to support this theory. For example, drugs of abuse cause anatomical and morphological sensitization (i.e., increased dendritic spines and amount of dendrites capable of responding to drug) in mesolimbic brain structures, and this morphological sensitization can result in behavioral sensitization to that drug (Robinson & Kolb, 2004; Singer et al., 2009; Steketee & Kalivas, 2011; Wolf, 2010). Furthermore, history and pattern of drug use play a key role in sensitized dopaminergic response to drugs of abuse or their paired cues (Robinson & Becker, 1986). For example, sensitization especially occurs in cases of drug binges and patterns of intermittency (Kalivas & Stewart, 1991; Kawa et al., 2016; Robinson & Becker, 1986). As a result, addicts show heightened mesolimbic activation in response to drugs (Boileau et al., 2007; Cox et al., 2009). Similar neuroplasticity has been observed in nondrug addictions. Several studies reviewed by Zeeb and colleagues found that compared to healthy controls, individuals with gambling disorder exhibited an average of 50 percent more dopamine release in the ventral striatum and midbrain and increased locomotion in response to a challenge dose of amphetamine (Zeeb et al., 2017). Mesolimbic sensitization has also been observed in rats exposed to a junk-food diet. For example, rats fed a junk-food diet for one month showed cross-sensitization to amphetamine-induced locomotion and downregulation of striatal dopamine D2 receptor mRNA. This morphological sensitization likely resulted in behavioral sensitization, as rats that developed obesity following exposure to junk-food diet showed increased willingness to gain access to a sucrose cue, but without increased hedonic impact ('liking') of sucrose (Robinson et al., 2015b; Zeeb et al., 2017).

Not only does a sensitized mesolimbic structure become hyperreactive to the drug of choice itself, but it also becomes hyperreactive to drug-related cues and contexts that have been paired with drug-taking. For example, a heightened brain response in limbic circuitry is triggered by reward-related cues after sensitization (Tindell et al., 2005) and drug paraphernalia in human addicts (Cox et al., 2009; Kühn & Gallinat, 2011; Leyton & Vezina, 2013; Vezina & Leyton, 2009). Furthermore, cue reactivity in mesolimbic ventral striatum correlates with years of cocaine use such that the more years of use, the greater the brain activation (Prisciandaro et al., 2014). Additionally, time-dependent increases in cue-induced craving have been observed in methamphetamine addicts

(a)

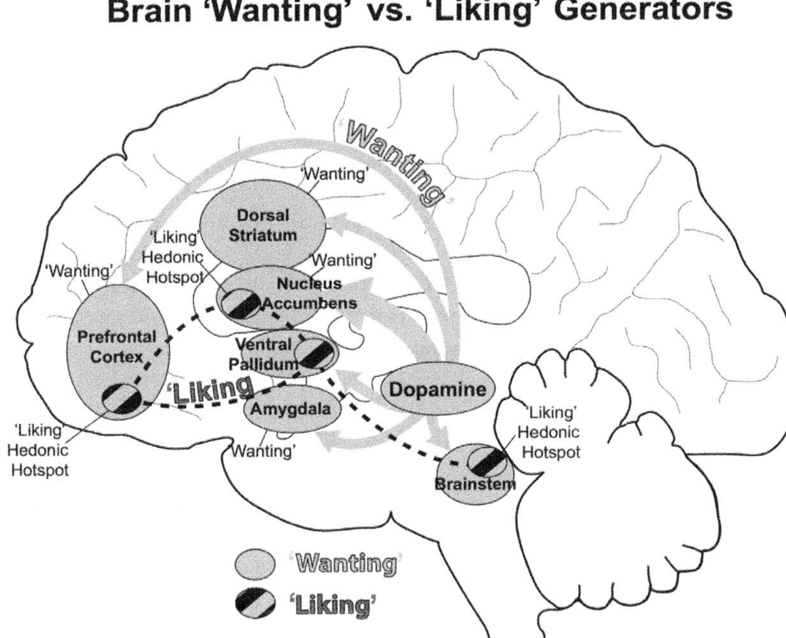

Figure 3.1a Brain 'Wanting' vs. 'Liking' Generators.
Modified from (Berridge and Robinson, 2016) and (Robinson and Berridge, 1993) 'Wanting' is mediated by robust brain systems, including dopamine (a brain neurochemical produced in midbrain; light grey solid arrows), which is released onto various limbic and cortical structures (light grey ovals). By contrast 'liking' is produced in smaller, more restricted zones within the same limbic and cortical structures, and these zones are referred to as 'liking' hedonic hotspots (black and grey diagonal striped ovals). As such, 'liking' and 'wanting' brain systems may overlap, but are capable of being dissociated from one another

(b)

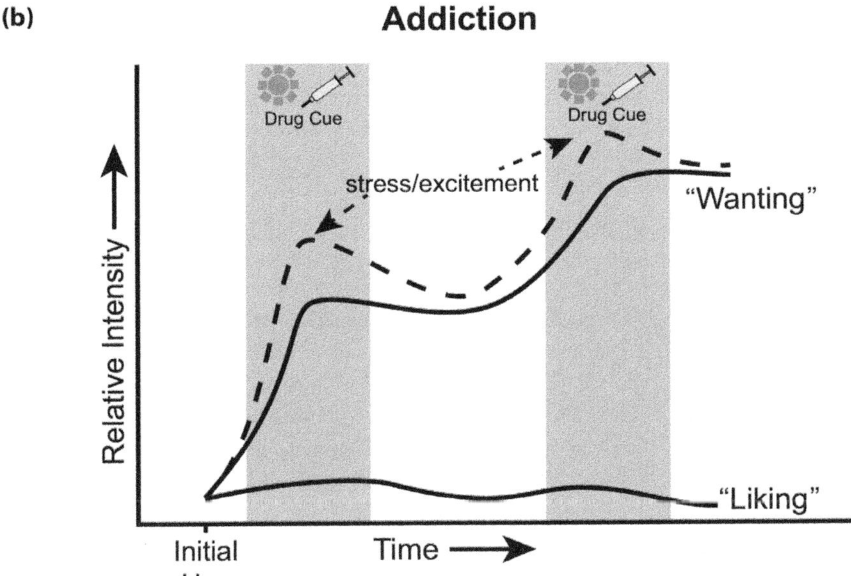

Figure 3.1b Addiction.
Incentive sensitization theory proposes after drug exposure, reactivity of brain 'wanting' systems related to drug-seeking increases over time, while 'liking', or the pleasure derived from taking drugs, stays relatively the same or even decreases. Sensitized 'wanting' systems are not just continuously hyperactive, but are instead hyper-reactive to drug cues and contexts, and this hyperreactivity is pronounced during times of stress or excitement (dotted line). Drug cues and contexts cause peaks of 'wanting' or drug craving (potentiated by stress or excitement) that render an individual vulnerable to relapse.

(Wang et al., 2013) as well as in alcoholics (P. Li et al., 2015), and these time-dependent increases in cue-induced craving (also referred to as incubation) are dependent on mesolimbic structures such as the central amygdala (Lu et al., 2005, 2007; X. Li et al., 2015) and nucleus accumbens (Xi et al., 2013). A study of recovering cocaine addicts showed that those who reported sensitization of other drug-related effects, such as paranoid psychosis, were also more likely to relapse (Bartlett et al., 1997). This suggests that sensitization of drug effects is linked to the risk of relapse, even when sensitization simultaneously increases the intensity and occurrence of adverse effects of the drug, such as drug-induced paranoia. This body of evidence suggests a possible reason for how drug craving increases over time to a point where an addict's drug of choice is almost impossible to ignore, and where motivation to obtain that reward, even after withdrawal or other noxious effects subside, is so high that relapse becomes a recurrent problem.

Focusing of 'Wanting'

Incentive sensitization theory also hinges on the idea that mesolimbic sensitization occurs in a common neural network that is responsible for the attribution of incentive salience to all addictive rewards (e.g., drugs, food, gambling). Sensitization of 'wanting' systems in the brain may therefore increase reactivity to a number of other drugs and rewards, a phenomenon known as "cross-sensitization." Cross-sensitization, in the context of drug use, refers to a situation when sensitization to one drug will produce a sensitized response to other drugs (such as from heroin to cocaine, or the converse). In cases of cross-sensitization of 'wanting,' an individual, as a result of excessively consuming one drug, is rendered hyperresponsive to the motivational effects of other drugs, including ones that may have never been previously consumed. A study by Horger and colleagues found that, when rats were given nine daily injections of amphetamine or nicotine, they acquired a cocaine self-administration habit much more quickly than control animals, thus indicating that prior exposure to either amphetamine or nicotine sensitized the pretreated rats to the incentive motivation effects of cocaine (Casey et al., 2006; Horger, Giles & Schenk, 1992; Munafò et al., 2007). Similarly, a study by Cunningham and colleagues found that rats who were given intra-accumbens treatment of certain opiates (such as morphine) later proved to be sensitized to the behavioral effects of amphetamine (Cunningham & Kelley, 1992; Leyton et al. 2007). Cross-sensitization and resulting hyperresponsivity of dopaminergic systems also occurs between drugs of abuse and some natural rewards, such as sugar (Avena & Hoebel, 2003) and between drugs of abuse and stress (at both behavioral and physiological levels) (Cruz et al., 2011; Garcia-Keller et al., 2013; Piazza et al., 1990). This latter finding highlights the important role that stress may play in relapse, whereby stressful life events can act as powerful triggers of cravings, and a history of stressful life events may even predispose a person to drug or other behavioral addiction. Cross-sensitization of dopaminergic systems from gambling has also been seen in humans, indicating some especially vulnerable individuals may develop mesocorticolimbic sensitization even without taking drugs. Boileau and colleagues found that problem gamblers have increased dopamine release in response to amphetamine and in response to gambling-related cues, compared with healthy controls (Boileau et al., 2014). These examples of cross-sensitization support the idea that an underlying sensitization of neural circuitry may be common to all addictive drugs and other addictive behaviors.

However, if sensitization appears to promote dopaminergic activity, then why aren't addicts addicted to all drugs of abuse, even across reward types such as gambling, food, or sex? There are a few possible explanations for this. First, a degree of comorbidity does exist between various addictions, where human drug addicts 'want' several different drugs, may be hypersexual, and are prone to other compulsions (Benotsch, Kalichman & Kelly, 1999; Leeman & Potenza, 2012; Washton & Stone-Washton, 1993). However, incentive-sensitization may become quite focused on one particular reward target and not generalize to other rewards. Evidence from our lab and others shows that the narrow focusing of 'wanting' to one particular target in addiction may involve dopamine-circuitry interactions with the amygdala (DiFeliceantonio & Berridge, 2012; Koob & Volkow, 2010; Mahler & Berridge, 2012; Robinson, Warlow & Berridge, 2014b; Venniro, Caprioli & Shaham, 2016; Warlow, Robinson & Berridge, 2017). For example, optogenetic stimulation of the central amygdala caused paired drug or food rewards to become almost compulsively preferred, and that persisted despite adverse consequences (paired footshock) or greater alternative rewards. This strong preference was not due to an intrinsic rewarding effect of the laser stimulation itself, nor did stimulation affect how much the reward was 'liked' (Robinson et al., 2014b; Tom et al., 2019; Warlow et al., 2017). These findings implicate a role for amygdala-related circuitry in focusing incentive salience toward particular learned targets that generates compulsive-like seeking of that reward target.

Sensitized 'wanting' is also focused temporally to particular moments in time. Rather than creating an overall hyperactive dopaminergic state, implying that those brain areas are always driving intense 'wanting,' incentive sensitization creates a hyperreactive response to discrete, localized stimuli at particular times when they are encountered. Incentive sensitization theory posits that it is the hyperreactivity to rewards and their cues that triggers intense motivation and cravings leading to relapse – not any baseline hyperactivity or constant drive in these brain mesolimbic structures.

Dopamine as 'Wanting,' not 'Liking'

It was once popularly thought that dopamine mediates the pleasure of rewards. However, a majority of the traditional experimental designs that gave rise to that idea by their nature confounded measures of pleasure with motivation. For instance, blocking or depleting dopamine levels in the brains of rats renders them unwilling to eat, which was initially interpreted as them not deriving pleasure from food. However, beginning with early studies using the taste reactivity test, which more specifically separated 'liking' from 'wanting' because it doesn't rely on the rat's willingness to eat, a different dopamine story has emerged. First, the early animal studies showed that dopamine is not necessary for 'liking,' as 6-OHDA lesions of nearly all nigrostriatal and mesolimbic dopamine neurons leave 'liking' responses intact (Berridge & Robinson, 1998; Berridge et al., 1989). Second, elevations in dopamine signaling fail to enhance 'liking,' though do increase 'wanting' as shown through increased reward consumption and cue-triggered reward seeking (Peciña & Berridge, 2013; Peciña et al., 2003). Further, electrode stimulation of the lateral hypothalamus enhances 'wanting' and actually causes a decrease in 'liking' (Berridge & Valenstein, 1991). Third, human studies starting around 2000 began to further support the role of dopamine in mediating 'wanting,' as deep brain stimulation in the nucleus accumbens produces feelings of desire but not feelings of experienced pleasure (Schlaepfer et al., 2008), whereas pharmacological dopamine disruption reduces subjective 'wanting' ratings for drugs without reducing subjective 'liking' ratings (Boileau et al., 2007; Brauer & de Wit, 1997; Evans & Lees, 2004; Leyton et al., 2002; O'Sullivan et al., 2011). Furthermore, dopamine depletion in Parkinson's disease preserves normal hedonic ratings to sweet tastes despite earlier views that the disease produces anhedonia (Sienkiewicz-Jarosz et al., 2013). Finally, in the most recent decade, it's become clear that some Parkinson's patients who receive direct-receptor dopamine agonist treatments show an abnormal increase in addictive-type 'wanting' that may result in compulsive hypersexuality, gambling, shopping or other addictive behaviors (Bostwick et al., 2009; Delpont et al., 2017; Vela et al., 2016; Voon et al., 2017; Warren et al., 2017). Altogether, these studies suggest that dopamine does not play a role in 'liking,' but instead is necessary and sufficient for 'wanting.'

Mesolimbic Suppression versus Sensitization in Addiction

Yet, despite the evidence for dopamine-related sensitization above, some studies have actually reported suppression or down-regulation of brain dopamine D2 receptor levels or a blunted release of dopamine in addiction. This has led to an alternative "reward-deficiency" view that addiction arises because of too little brain dopamine, and drugs are sought to restore dopamine to baseline levels. The reward deficiency theory posits that individuals who have naturally low functioning dopamine self-medicate by taking drugs of abuse, suggesting that low dopamine is the cause for drug-seeking and the development of addiction. The reward deficiency theory also seems to presume either that dopamine still mediates the 'liking' for drugs and other rewards (so that low dopamine reduces pleasure to produce "reward deficiency") (see Blum et al., 2020), or that lowered D2 receptors specifically remove an antimotivation "brake" (that normally opposes motivation for rewards mediated by D1 receptors, leading to imbalance in accumbens/striatal circuitry) (Volkow, Koob & McLellan, 2016). This is in stark contrast to the incentive sensitization view of addiction, that suggests that dopamine function is increased in addiction, producing hyperreactivity in accumbens/striatal circuitry and higher cue-triggered 'wanting,' and that D2 downregulation in addicts is mostly a consequence rather than the cause of drug-taking. There are several possibilities that may address this discrepancy. First, suppressed brain dopamine among addicts is typically observed in response to the actual drug, not drug cues (Volkow et al., 2016). Second, suppression of D2 receptors or dopamine responses isn't always present, and opposite sensitization has instead been reported in several studies in response to abused drugs (Boileau et al., 2016; Evans et al., 2006; Prisciandaro et al., 2014). The difference between observing suppressions versus sensitization may heavily depend on the setting in which neural activity is being measured. For example, test situations (i.e., MRI machines within hospital and lab settings) are different from real-life settings in which drugs are generally taken (e.g., at home or in social settings) (Leyton & Vezina 2013). Artificial medical settings may be more likely to report neural suppressions, because dopamine-related sensitization is known to appear specifically in drug-taking situations but to be masked in situations where drugs have never been taken (Browman, Badiani & Robinson, 1998; Crombag et al., 2000, 2001). When effort is taken to make the drug cues and contexts more realistic, sensitized activations have been suggested to be more likely to be found (Leyton & Vezina, 2013). Additionally, instances of observed mesolimbic dopamine suppression (i.e., receptor downregulation occurring during drug use) are restricted to PET measures of radioactive drug binding to the dopamine D2 receptor. Lower D2 binding could also result from higher levels of endogenous or drug-stimulated dopamine that occupies more D2 receptors and leaves fewer available to bind to radioactive drug, and could be downregulated in addicts as a compensatory tolerance consequence resulting from high dopamine stimulation of receptors during heavy drug consumption (Berridge & Robinson, 2016). In the short term, tolerance can often mask neural sensitization even when both occur simultaneously in parallel, as long as drugs are still being taken. Some recent evidence has suggested that downregulation of dopamine D2 receptors may actually facilitate drug-induced behavioral sensitization (Kai et al., 2015). But, in the longer run, many tolerance-related mesolimbic suppressions are temporary and fade shortly after drug discontinuation, whereas sensitization processes are long lasting and grow over time, even long after drug-taking has ceased (Paulson & Robinson, 1995). In rats, sensitization has been reported to persist for up to a year after drugs were discontinued (Paulson et al., 1991), while monkeys still display a sensitized response to amphetamine even two years posttreatment (Castner & Goldman-Rakic, 1999).

Emergence of neural sensitization causes increased vulnerability to relapse after being drug-abstinent for over a month, a phenomenon referred to as incubation of drug craving (Pickens et al., 2011). This incubation of drug craving can only be explained by sensitization mechanisms rather than neural suppressions of reward-deficiency. Finally, the reward deficiency theory of addiction cannot fully explain why dopamine stimulation (either pharmacologically in animal models, or via direct D2-receptor agonist medications combined with L-Dopa medication in Parkinson's patients) actually increases drug-seeking and triggers the emergence of new compulsive motivations to pursue drugs, gambling, shopping, and sex (Callesen et al., 2013; Friedman & Chang, 2013; Ondo & Lai, 2008; Politis et al., 2013), which cease as soon as dopamine-stimulating medication is discontinued.

Support for Incentive Sensitization in Drug Addiction

In support of incentive sensitization theory, mesolimbic hyperreactivity to drugs of abuse has been well documented. For example, repeated amphetamine administration in both humans and rodents causes sensitization to reward cues in limbic areas such as the amygdala, ventral pallidum, and nucleus accumbens (O'Daly et al., 2014; Tindell et al., 2005; Wyvell & Berridge, 2001), and this sensitization involves an increase in dopamine release (Evans et al., 2006; Kalivas & Duffy, 1990; Thomas, Kalivas & Shaham, 2008). Similarly, repeated cocaine administration induces long-lasting sensitization of the mesolimbic dopamine system (Calipari et al., 2013; Pascoli, Turiault & Lüscher, 2011). Animal studies have also shown elevated dopamine levels (Carlson & Drew Stevens, 2006; McBride, 2002), increased dopamine receptor expression and sensitivity (Tournier et al., 2016), and enhanced synaptic strength (Saal et al., 2003; Stuber et al., 2008) in reward-related brain regions following repeated exposure to such drugs as alcohol, marijuana, or nicotine. Further, those changes and increased dopamine release causes heightened responses and attribution of incentive salience to reward cues (Ostlund et al., 2014; Tindell et al., 2005). Indeed, in humans a direct link between the amount of time using cocaine to the intensity of their mesolimbic response to cocaine-related cues has been demonstrated (Prisciandaro et al., 2014). Heightened incentive-salience attributed to drug cues may explain why sensitized people addicted to crack cocaine have been seen to "chase ghosts," where individuals compulsively search for small white specks on the ground, even when they know that they are probably only small bits of sugar or pebbles (Rosse et al., 1993, 1994). Animal models have further demonstrated that this drug-induced sensitization chronically heightens dopamine release, increases susceptibility to drug cues, and causes increases in 'wanting' (Peciña et al., 2003; Wyvell and Berridge, 2000, 2001). Further, this increased 'wanting' has been shown to produce a narrow focus onto one particular reward, even when equivalent alternatives are available (DiFeliceantonio & Berridge, 2012; Mahler & Berridge, 2009; Robinson, Warlow & Berridge, 2014b; Warlow et al., 2017). In line with this narrowing of cue salience, human studies have shown the heightened response to drug cues and heightened dopamine release is directly related to reports of drug 'wanting' (Boileau et al., 2016; Evans et al., 2006).

Individuals with a history of extensive alcohol, marijuana, and/or nicotine use also exhibit heightened activity in various reward-related regions in response to drug or drug-related cues, whereas casual users or nonusers do not exhibit hyperreactivity to such stimuli (Charboneau et al., 2013; Claus et al., 2011; Cousijn et al., 2013; Filbey et al., 2009; Ihssen et al., 2011; Kühn & Gallinat, 2011; Metrik et al., 2016; Myrick et al., 2004; Tapert et al., 2003). Furthermore, activity in these regions has been shown to be directly correlated with self-reported craving (Charboneau et al., 2013; Myrick et al., 2004; Tapert et al., 2003), the individual's drug use habits (i.e. frequency of use) (Tapert et al., 2003), and duration of dependence (Claus et al., 2011; Filbey et al., 2009). As a whole, these findings demonstrate that abuse of such substances is characterized by hyperreactive limbic-related brain structures. This heightened activity is not observed in casual users and/or nonusers and often corresponds with the severity of abuse. Thus, incentive sensitization likely can be attributed to neurobiological changes in the mesolimbic dopamine pathway that leaves the individual primed to respond to drugs and drug-related cues.

Incentive Sensitization in Behavioral Addictions

Gambling

Pathological gambling is inarguably a growing public health concern, with societal costs estimated to exceed $5 billion per year in the United States alone (Gerstein et al., 1999), and rates steadily increasing over the past few decades (Nowak & Aloe, 2014; Petry & Blanco, 2013). Gambling disorder shares many characteristics with substance disorders, including the inability to cut down on gambling, continued gambling despite adverse consequences such as loss of money or job, and cravings for gambling (Potenza, 2008). In gambling addiction, gambling-related cues also seem to take on increased incentive salience, where they become motivational stimuli that can drive behavior. One of the hallmarks of gambling, and indeed of most games, is the presence of uncertainty (Costikyan, 2013). Studies in rats suggest that uncertainty pertaining to the probability and magnitude of the reward outcome can cause attribution of additional incentive salience to reward-related cues (Anselme & Robinson, 2013; Hellberg et al., 2018; Robinson et al., 2014b, 2015a). This finding is paradoxical from the point of view that reward prediction determines motivation, since reward uncertainty degrades the predictive value of a cue, yet appears to enhance a cue's incentive value (Zhang et al., 2009). Uncertainty of reward also produces a greater dopaminergic response (Fiorillo, Tobler & Schultz, 2003), promotes risk-seeking behavior (Fiorillo, 2011), and can induce behavioral cross-sensitization in animals, as measured by an increased locomotor response to and greater motivation to self-administer amphetamine (Mascia et al., 2019; Singer, Scott-Railton & Veniza, 2012; Zack et al., 2014). In line with the hypothesis that reward uncertainty can enhance incentive salience, problem gamblers exhibit a strong attentional bias toward gambling-related cues (Brevers et al., 2014a;, 2014b). Similarly, dopamine release is increased in problem gamblers (van Holst et al., 2012), the magnitude of increase is correlated to the severity of problem gambling (Joutsa et al., 2012), and pathological gamblers show increased dopamine-synthesis capacity in areas such as the ventral striatum (van Holst et al., 2018). In conjunction with the finding that problem gamblers also report lower euphoria than control participants in response to an amphetamine challenge (Mick et al., 2014), this suggests that there may be a dissociation between 'wanting' and 'liking' in compulsive gambling similar to drug addiction.

Food Addiction

Features of incentive sensitization also have been reported in putative cases of food addiction (Gearhardt et al., 2009, 2011). Although food addiction remains a controversial disorder, there are important neural correlates to food cues overlapping with those to drug cues in drug addiction (Davis & Carter, 2009; Finlayson, 2017; Gearhardt et al., 2011; Kelley & Berridge, 2002; Volkow et al., 2012). Indeed, cross-sensitization between drugs of abuse and long-term access to junk-food diets has been reported in rodent studies (Robinson et al., 2015b; Oginsky et al., 2016a, 2016b). In humans, higher cue-triggered ratings of food 'wanting' were reported in participants who completed a questionnaire in a cue-rich, simulated fast-food restaurant compared to those in a standard lab setting (despite no differences in baseline hunger or any change in meal 'liking') (Joyner, Kim & Gearhardt, 2017). Applied to a clinical population, individuals with binge-eating disorder (BED) are reported to show significant attentional biases to food cues, illustrating the capability for food cues themselves to become more attractive and "wanted" in that condition (Deluchi et al., 2017; Popien et al., 2015; Schmidt et al., 2016; Schmitz et al., 2014; Sperling et al., 2017).

Future Research

Recently, research has begun increasingly to focus on individual differences in cue sensitivity and attentional bias. For example, recent research has suggested that excessive attentional bias and incentive salience attributed to reward-related cues, as seen in sign-tracking, is associated with higher rates of relapse, obesity and food craving, along with cravings and urges to gamble (Goudriaan et al., 2010; van Holst et al., 2012; Versace et al., 2016). The ability to determine individual differences in cue reactivity may provide insight into those who are at greatest risk for incentive sensitization, and who ultimately bear the greatest risk of developing addiction. Correspondingly, treatments that may reduce someone's heightened attentional bias toward addiction-related cues could provide a respite from craving and reduce the risk of relapse. Recent findings examining the use of transcranial magnetic stimulation (TMS) in cocaine users has been shown to reduce craving (Terraneo et al., 2016), and could provide similar benefits to individuals suffering from food addictions or behavioral addictions such as gambling.

Similarly, a crucial factor in need of more research is sex differences in incentive salience attribution, and as a result sex differences in addiction vulnerability. Some key differences include the fact that, in cases of alcohol, illicit drugs, and gambling, women who are vulnerable to addiction tend to escalate their use to the point of addiction more rapidly than do men in several studies (Barker & Taylor, 2019; Becker, 2016; Doran, 2014; Fattore et al., 2014; however, see Keyes et al., 2010). Laboratory experiments have demonstrated that female rats more rapidly acquire drug self-administration and are more motivated to earn drugs (i.e., cocaine). Furthermore, this enhancement of motivation may be caused by circulating ovarian hormones such as estradiol and its interaction with mesolimbic dopamine transmission (Becker & Hu, 2008; Hu & Becker, 2008). In addition to a more rapid escalation of use, women who are abstinent also report greater cue-induced craving leading to relapse (Fox et al., 2013), making treatment outcomes more dire. Thus, future research that addresses incentive sensitization mechanisms underlying other addictions (gambling, etc.) with particular emphasis on sex differences could contribute greatly to the field.

Conclusions

In summary, 'wanting' and 'liking' are produced by separable brain mechanisms, with intense 'wanting' being more robust and diffusely generated and tied to dopamine-related systems, whereas intense 'liking' or pleasure is functionally fragile, mediated only by other neurotransmitters, and needs unanimity among various multiple hedonic hotspots. The incentive-sensitization theory of addiction originally proposed that 'wanting' brain systems, including mesocorticolimbic dopamine, become sensitized with repeated drug use, rendering them hyperreactive to drug-paired cues. By contrast, 'liking' systems (independent of dopamine) remain relatively unchanged in addiction, or may even decline, and at any rate do not strongly sensitize. Dissociation of 'liking' and 'wanting' brain systems help explain how drugs become "wanted" more and more, while not necessarily being 'liked' at the same level. This selective sensitization of 'wanting' independent of 'liking' produces hyperreactivity of mesocorticolimbic systems to drug cues causing higher pulses of dopamine release and impact on target structures. These pulses of 'wanting' can be further exacerbated by some current neurobiological states (stress or excitement), to cause more intense peaks of drug craving and seeking, which can lead to relapse even long after withdrawal symptoms fade. Research over the past few decades continues to support these incentive sensitization features in drug addiction, and there is mounting evidence that incentive sensitization also extends to some other behavioral addictions, such as compulsive gambling and food addiction. Developing better treatments able to target sensitized brain 'wanting' systems and attenuation of craving may be helpful in eventually reducing addiction.

REFERENCES

Anselme, P. (2016). Motivational control of sign-tracking behaviour: a theoretical framework. *Neuroscience and Biobehavioral Reviews*, **65**, 1–20.

Anselme, P. & Robinson, M. J. F. (2013). What motivates gambling behavior? Insight into dopamine's role. *Frontiers in Behavioral Neuroscience*, **7**, 182.

Avena, N. M. & Hoebel, B. G. (2003). Amphetamine-sensitized rats show sugar-induced hyperactivity (cross-sensitization) and sugar hyperphagia. *Pharmacology, Biochemistry, and Behavior*, **74**(3), 635–639.

Barker, J. M. & Taylor, J. R. (2019). Sex differences in incentive motivation and the relationship to the development and maintenance of alcohol use disorders. *Physiology & Behavior*, **203**, 91–99.

Barrett, S. P., Pihl, R. O., Benkelfat, C., et al. (2008). The role of dopamine in alcohol self-administration in humans: individual differences. *European Neuropsychopharmacology*, **18**(6), 439–447.

Bartlett, E., Hallin, A., Chapman, B. & Angrist, B. (1997). Selective sensitization to the psychosis-inducing effects of cocaine: a possible marker for addiction relapse vulnerability? *Neuropsychopharmacology*, **16** (1), 77–82.

Bartoshuk, L. (2014). The measurement of pleasure and pain. *Perspectives on Psychological Science: A Journal of the Association for Psychological Science*, **9**(1), 91–93.

Becker, J. B. (2016). Sex differences in addiction. *Dialogues in Clinical Neuroscience*, **18**(4), 395–402.

Becker, J. B. & Hu, M. (2008). Sex differences in drug abuse. *Frontiers in Neuroendocrinology*, **29**(1), 36–47.

Benotsch, E. G., Kalichman, S. C. & Kelly, J. A. (1999). Sexual compulsivity and substance use in HIV-seropositive men who have sex with men: prevalence and predictors of high-risk behaviors. *Addictive Behaviors*, **24**(6), 857–868.

Berger, S. P., Hall, S., Mickalian, J. D., et al. (1996). Haloperidol antagonism of cue-elicited cocaine craving. *The Lancet*, **347** (9000), 504–508.

Berridge, K. C. (2012). From prediction error to incentive salience: mesolimbic computation of reward motivation. *The European Journal of Neuroscience*, **35**(7), 1124–1143.

Berridge, K. C. (2009). "liking" and "wanting" food rewards: brain substrates and roles in eating disorders. *Physiology & Behavior*, **97**(5), 537–550.

Berridge, K. C. & Kringelbach, M. L. (2008). Affective neuroscience of pleasure: reward in humans and animals. *Psychopharmacology*, **199**(3), 457–480.

Berridge, K. C. & Robinson, T. E. (2016). Liking, wanting, and the incentive-sensitization theory of addiction. *The American Psychologist*, **71**(8), 670–679.

Berridge, K. C. & Robinson, T. E. (2003). Parsing reward. *Trends in Neurosciences*, **26**(9), 507–513.

Berridge, K. C. & Robinson, T. E. (1998). What is the role of dopamine in reward: hedonic impact, reward learning, or incentive salience? Brain Research. *Brain Research Reviews*, **28**(3), 309–369.

Berridge, K. C. & Valenstein, E. S. (1991). What psychological process mediates feeding evoked by electrical stimulation of the lateral hypothalamus? *Behavioral Neuroscience*, **105** (1), 3–14.

Berridge, K. C., Ho, C.-Y., Richard, J. M. DiFeliceantonio, A. G. (2010). The tempted brain eats: pleasure and desire circuits in obesity and eating disorders. *Brain Research*, **1350**, 43–64.

Berridge, K. C., Venier, I. L. & Robinson, T. E. (1989). Taste reactivity analysis of 6-hydroxydopamine-induced aphagia: implications for arousal and anhedonia hypotheses of dopamine function. *Behavioral Neuroscience*, **103**(1), 36–45.

Bindra, D. (1978). How adaptive behavior is produced: a perceptual-motivational alternative to response reinforcements. *Behavioral and Brain Sciences*, **1**(01), 41.

Blum, K., et al. (2020). Chapter 24 of the *Handbook*.

Boakes, R. A., Poli, M., Lockwood, M. J. & Goodall, G. (1978). A study of misbehavior: token reinforcement in the rat. *Journal of the*

Experimental Analysis of Behavior, **29**(1), 115–134.

Boileau, I., Dagher, A., Leyton, M., et al. (2007). Conditioned dopamine release in humans: a positron emission tomography [11C]raclopride study with amphetamine. *The Journal of Neuroscience*, **27**(15), 3998–4003.

Boileau, I., Payer, D., Chugani, B., et al. (2014). In vivo evidence for greater amphetamine-induced dopamine release in pathological gambling: a positron emission tomography study with [(11)C]-(+)-PHNO. *Molecular Psychiatry*, **19**(12), 1305–1313.

Boileau, I., Payer, D., Rusjan, P. M., et al. (2016). Heightened dopaminergic response to amphetamine at the D3 dopamine receptor in methamphetamine users. *Neuropsychopharmacology*, **41**(13), 2994–3002.

Bostwick, J. M., Hecksel, K. A., Stevens, S. R., Bower, J. H. & Ahlskog, J. E. (2009). Frequency of new-onset pathologic compulsive gambling or hypersexuality after drug treatment of idiopathic Parkinson disease. *Mayo Clinic Proceedings*, **84**(4), 310–316.

Brauer, L. H. & de Wit, H. (1997). High dose pimozide does not block amphetamine-induced euphoria in normal volunteers. *Pharmacology, Biochemistry, and Behavior*, **56**(2), 265–272.

Brevers, D., Cleeremans, A., Bechara, A., et al. (2014a). Impaired metacognitive capacities in individuals with problem gambling. *Journal of Gambling Studies*, **30**(1), 141–152.

Brevers, D., Koritzky, G., Bechara, A. & Noël, X. (2014b). Cognitive processes underlying impaired decision-making under uncertainty in gambling disorder. *Addictive Behaviors*, **39** (10), 1533–1536.

Browman, K. E., Badiani, A. & Robinson, T. E. (1998). Modulatory effect of environmental stimuli on the susceptibility to amphetamine sensitization: a dose-effect study in rats. *The Journal of Pharmacology and Experimental Therapeutics*, **287**(3), 1007–1014.

Brown, P. L. & Jenkins, H. M. (1968). Auto-shaping of the pigeon's key-peck. *Journal of the Experimental Analysis of Behavior*, **11**(1), 1–8.

Cabanac, M. (1971). Physiological role of pleasure. *Science*, **173**(4002), 1103–1107.

Cabanac, M. & Lafrance, L. (1990). Postingestive alliesthesia: the rat tells the same story. *Physiology & Behavior*, **47**(3), 539–543.

Cacioppo, S., Bianchi-Demicheli, F., Frum, C., Pfaus, J. G. & Lewis, J. W. (2012). The common neural bases between sexual desire and love: a multilevel kernel density fMRI analysis. *The Journal of Sexual Medicine*, **9**(4), 1048–1054.

Calipari, E. S., Ferris, M. J., Zimmer, B. A., Roberts, D. C. S. & Jones, S. R. (2013). Temporal pattern of cocaine intake determines tolerance vs sensitization of cocaine effects at the dopamine transporter. *Neuropsychopharmacology*, **38**(12), 2385–2392.

Callesen, M. B., Scheel-Krüger, J., Kringelbach, M. L. & Møller, A. (2013). A systematic review of impulse control disorders in Parkinson's disease. *Journal of Parkinson's Disease*, **3**(2), 105–138.

Cameron, C. M., Wightman, R. M. & Carelli, R. M. (2014). Dynamics of rapid dopamine release in the nucleus accumbens during goal-directed behaviors for cocaine versus natural rewards. *Neuropharmacology*, **86**, 319–328.

Carlson, J. N. & Drew Stevens, K. (2006). Individual differences in ethanol self-administration following withdrawal are associated with asymmetric changes in dopamine and serotonin in the medial prefrontal cortex and amygdala. *Alcoholism, Clinical and Experimental Research*, **30**(10), 1678–1692.

Casey, K. F., Benkelfat, C., Young, S. N. & Leyton, M. (2006). Lack of effect of acute dopamine precursor depletion in nicotine-dependent smokers. *European Neuropsychopharmacology*, **16**(7), 512–520.

Castner, S. A. & Goldman-Rakic, P. S. (1999). Long-lasting psychotomimetic consequences of repeated low-dose amphetamine exposure in rhesus monkeys. *Neuropsychopharmacology*, **20**(1), 10–28.

Castro, D. C. & Berridge, K. C. (2014). Opioid hedonic hotspot in nucleus accumbens shell: mu, delta, and kappa maps for enhancement of sweetness "liking" and "wanting." *The Journal of Neuroscience*, **34** (12), 4239–4250.

Castro, D. C. & Berridge, K. C. (2017). Opioid and orexin hedonic hotspots in rat orbitofrontal cortex and insula. *Proceedings of the National Academy of Sciences of the United States of America*, **114**(43), E9125–E9134.

Castro, D. C., Cole, S. L. & Berridge, K. C. (2015). Lateral hypothalamus, nucleus accumbens, and ventral pallidum roles in eating and hunger: interactions between homeostatic and reward circuitry. *Frontiers in Systems Neuroscience*, **9**, 90.

Castro, D. C., Terry, R. A. & Berridge, K. C. 2016. Orexin in rostral hotspot of nucleus accumbens enhances sucrose "liking" and intake but scopolamine in caudal shell shifts "liking" toward "disgust" and "fear." *Neuropsychopharmacology*, **41**(8), 2101–2111.

Chang, S. E. & Smith, K. S. (2016). An omission procedure reorganizes the microstructure of sign-tracking while preserving incentive salience. *Learning & Memory*, **23**(4), 151–155.

Charboneau, E. J., Dietrich, M. S., Park, S., et al. (2013). Cannabis cue-induced brain activation correlates with drug craving in limbic and visual salience regions: preliminary results. *Psychiatry Research*, **214**(2), 122–131.

Childress, A. R., Ehrman, R. N., Wang, Z., et al. (2008). Prelude to passion: limbic activation by "unseen" drug and sexual cues. *PLos ONE*, **3**(1), e1506.

Claus, E. D., Ewing, S. W. F., Filbey, F. M., Sabbineni, A. & Hutchison, K. E. (2011). Identifying neurobiological phenotypes associated with alcohol use disorder severity. *Neuropsychopharmacology*, **36**(10), 2086–2096.

Corbit, L. H. & Janak, P. H. (2007). Ethanol-associated cues produce general pavlovian-instrumental transfer. *Alcoholism, Clinical and Experimental Research*, **31**(5), 766–774.

Costikyan, G. (2013). *Uncertainty in Games*. MIT Press.

Cousijn, J., Goudriaan, A. E., Ridderinkhof, K. R., et al. (2013). Neural responses associated with cue-reactivity in frequent cannabis users. *Addiction Biology*, **18**(3), 570–580.

Cowlishaw, S., Nespoli, E., Jebadurai, J. K., Smith, N. & Bowden-Jones, H. (2018). Episodic and binge gambling: an exploration and preliminary quantitative study. *Journal of Gambling Studies*, **34**(1), 85–99.

Cox, S. M. L., Benkelfat, C., Dagher, A., et al. (2009). Striatal dopamine responses to intranasal cocaine self-administration in humans. *Biological Psychiatry*, **65**(10), 846–850.

Crombag, H. S., Badiani, A., Chan, J., et al. (2001). The ability of environmental context to facilitate psychomotor sensitization to amphetamine can be dissociated from its effect on acute drug responsiveness and on conditioned responding. *Neuropsychopharmacology*, **24**(6), 680–690.

Crombag, H. S., Badiani, A., Maren, S. & Robinson, T. E. (2000). The role of contextual versus discrete drug-associated cues in promoting the induction of psychomotor sensitization to intravenous amphetamine. *Behavioural Brain Research*, **116**(1), 1–22.

Cromwell, H. C. & Berridge, K. C. (1993). Where does damage lead to enhanced food aversion: the ventral pallidum/substantia innominata or lateral hypothalamus? *Brain Research*, **624**(1–2), 1–10.

Cruz, F. C., Quadros, I. M., Hogenelst, K., Planeta, C. S. & Miczek, K. A. (2011). Social defeat stress in rats: escalation of cocaine and "speedball" binge self-administration, but not heroin. *Psychopharmacology*, **215**(1), 165–175.

Cunningham, S. T. & Kelley, A. E. (1992). Opiate infusion into nucleus accumbens: contrasting effects on motor activity and responding for conditioned reward. *Brain Research*, **588**(1), 104–114.

Dai, X., Brendl, C. M. & Ariely, D. 2010. Wanting, liking, and preference construction. *Emotion*, **10**(3), 324–334.

Davis, C. & Carter, J. C. (2009). Compulsive overeating as an addiction disorder. A review of theory and evidence. *Appetite*, **53**(1), 1–8.

Delamater, R. J. & McNamara, J. R. (1986). The social impact of assertiveness. Research findings and clinical implications. *Behavior Modification*, **10**(2), 139–158.

Delpont, B., Lhommée, E., Klinger, H., et al. (2017). Psychostimulant effect of dopaminergic treatment and addictions in Parkinson's disease. *Movement Disorders*, **32** (11), 1566–1573.

Deluchi, M., Costa, F. S., Friedman, R., Gonçalves, R. & Bizarro, L. (2017). Attentional bias to unhealthy food in individuals with severe obesity and binge eating. *Appetite*, **108**, 471–476.

Derevensky, J. L. (2020). The prevention and treatment of gambling disorders: some art, some science. In S. Sussman (Ed.) *The Cambridge Handbook of Substance and Behavioral Addictions*. Cambridge, UK: Cambridge University Press, pp. 241–253.

DiFeliceantonio, A. G. & Berridge, K. C. (2012). Which cue to "want"? Opioid stimulation of central amygdala makes goal-trackers show stronger goal-tracking, just as sign-trackers show stronger sign-tracking. *Behavioural Brain Research*, **230**(2), 399–408.

Doran, N. (2014). Sex differences in smoking cue reactivity: craving, negative affect, and preference for immediate smoking. *The American Journal on Addictions*, **23**(3), 211–217.

Evans, A. H. & Lees, A. J. (2004). Dopamine dysregulation syndrome in Parkinson's disease. *Current Opinion in Neurology*, **17**(4), 393–398.

Evans, A. H., Pavese, N., Lawrence, A. D., et al. (2006). Compulsive drug use linked to sensitized ventral striatal dopamine transmission. *Annals of Neurology*, **59**(5), 852–858.

Fattore, L., Melis, M., Fadda, P. & Fratta, W. (2014). Sex differences in addictive disorders. *Frontiers in Neuroendocrinology*, **35**(3), 272–284.

Filbey, F. M., Schacht, J. P., Myers, U. S., Chavez, R. S. & Hutchison, K. E. (2009). Marijuana craving in the brain. *Proceedings of the National Academy of Sciences of the United States of America*, **106**(31), 13016–13021.

Finlayson, G. (2017). Food addiction and obesity: unnecessary medicalization of hedonic overeating. *Nature Reviews Endocrinology*, **13**(8), 493–498.

Fiorillo, C. D. (2011). Transient activation of midbrain dopamine neurons by reward risk. *Neuroscience*, **197**, 162–171.

Fiorillo, C. D., Tobler, P. N. & Schultz, W. (2003). Discrete coding of reward probability and uncertainty by dopamine neurons. *Science*. **299**(5614), 1898–1902.

Fischman, M. W. & Foltin, R. W. (1992). Self-administration of cocaine by humans: a laboratory perspective. *Ciba Foundation Symposium*, **166**, 165–173; discussion 173.

Flagel, S. B. & Robinson, T. E. (2017). Neurobiological basis of individual variation in stimulus-reward learning. *Current Opinion in Behavioral Sciences*, **13**, 178–185.

Flagel, S. B., Akil, H. & Robinson, T. E. (2009). Individual differences in the attribution of incentive salience to reward-related cues: Implications for addiction. *Neuropharmacology*, **56** (Supplement 1), 139–148.

Flagel, S. B., Clark, J. J., Robinson, T. E., et al. (2011). A selective role for dopamine in stimulus-reward learning. *Nature*, **469**(7328), 53–57.

Flagel, S. B., Watson, S. J., Akil, H. & Robinson, T. E. (2008). Individual differences in the attribution of incentive salience to a reward-related cue: influence on cocaine sensitization. *Behavioural Brain Research*, **186** (1), 48–56.

Fox, H. C., Sofuoglu, M., Morgan, P. T., Tuit, K. L. & Sinha, R. (2013). The effects of exogenous progesterone on drug craving and stress arousal in cocaine dependence: impact of gender and cue type. *Psychoneuroendocrinology*, **38**(9), 1532–1544.

Friedman, J. H. & Chang, V. (2013). Crack cocaine use due to dopamine agonist therapy in Parkinson disease. *Neurology*, **80**(24), 2269–2270.

Galimov, A. & Black, D. W. (2020). Prevention and treatment of compulsive buying disorder. In S. Sussman (Ed.) *The Cambridge Handbook of Substance and Behavioral Addictions*. Cambridge, UK: Cambridge University Press, pp. 271–279.

Garcia, J., Lasiter, P. S., Bermudez-Rattoni, F. & Deems, D. A. (1985). A general theory of aversion learning. *Annals of the New York Academy of Sciences*, **443**, 8–21.

Garcia-Keller, C., Martinez, S. A., Esparza, M. A., et al. (2013). Cross-sensitization between cocaine and acute restraint stress is associated with sensitized dopamine but not glutamate release in the nucleus accumbens. *The European Journal of Neuroscience*, **37**(6), 982–995.

Gearhardt, A. N., Corbin, W. R. & Brownell, K. D. (2009). Food addiction: an examination of the diagnostic criteria for dependence. *Journal of Addiction Medicine*, **3**(1), 1–7.

Gearhardt, A. N., Yokum, S., Orr, P. T., et al. (2011). Neural correlates of food addiction. *Archives of General Psychiatry*, **68**(8), 808–816.

Georgiadis, J. R. & Kringelbach, M. L. (2012). The human sexual response cycle: brain imaging evidence linking sex to other pleasures. *Progress in Neurobiology*, **98**(1), 49–81.

Gerstein, D., Hoffmann, J., Larison, C., et al. 1999. *Gambling impact and behavior study*. Report to the National Gambling Impact Study Commission. National Opinion Research Center at the University of Chicago, Chicago.

Giroux, I., Faucher-Gravel, A., St-Hilaire, A., Boudreault, C., Jacques, C. & Bouchard, S. (2013). Gambling exposure in virtual reality and modification of urge to gamble. *Cyberpsychology, Behavior and Social Networking*, **16**(3), 224–231.

Goudriaan, A. E., de Ruiter, M. B., van den Brink, W., Oosterlaan, J. & Veltman, D. J. (2010). Brain activation patterns associated with cue reactivity and craving in abstinent problem gamblers, heavy smokers and healthy controls: an fMRI study. *Addiction Biology*, **15**(4), 491–503.

Grill, H. J. & Norgren, R. (1978). The taste reactivity test. I. Mimetic responses to gustatory stimuli in neurologically normal rats. *Brain Research*, **143**(2), 263–279.

Hellberg, S. N., Levit, J. D. & Robinson, M. J. F. (2018). Under the influence: Effects of adolescent ethanol exposure and anxiety on motivation for uncertain gambling-like cues in male and female rats. *Behavioural Brain Research*, **337**, 17–33.

Hernandez, L. & Hoebel, B. G. (1988). Feeding and hypothalamic stimulation increase dopamine turnover in the accumbens. *Physiology & Behavior*, **44**(4–5), 599–606.

Hickey, C. & Peelen, M. V. (2015). Neural mechanisms of incentive salience in naturalistic human vision. *Neuron*, **85**(3), 512–518.

Ho, C.-Y. & Berridge, K. C. (2013). An orexin hotspot in ventral pallidum amplifies hedonic "liking" for sweetness. *Neuropsychopharmacology*, **38**(9), 1655–1664.

Holmes, N. M., Marchand, A. R. & Coutureau, E. (2010). Pavlovian to instrumental transfer: a neurobehavioural perspective. *Neuroscience and Biobehavioral Reviews*, **34**(8), 1277–1295.

Holst, van, R. J., Sescousse, G., Janssen, L. K., et al. (2018). Increased striatal dopamine synthesis capacity in gambling addiction. *Biological Psychiatry*, **83**(12), 1036–1043.

Holst, van, R. J., Veltman, D. J., van den Brink, W. & Goudriaan, A. E. (2012). Right on cue? Striatal reactivity in problem gamblers. *Biological Psychiatry*, **72**(10), e23–24.

Horger, B. A., Giles, M. K. & Schenk, S. (1992). Preexposure to amphetamine and nicotine predisposes rats to self-administer a low dose of cocaine. *Psychopharmacology*, **107**(2–3), 271–276.

Hu, M. & Becker, J. B. (2008). Acquisition of cocaine self-administration in ovariectomized female rats: effect of estradiol dose or chronic estradiol administration. *Drug and Alcohol Dependence*, **94**(1–3), 56–62.

Ihssen, N., Cox, W. M., Wiggett, A., Fadardi, J. S. & Linden, D. E. J. (2011). Differentiating heavy from light drinkers by neural responses to visual alcohol cues and other motivational stimuli. *Cerebral Cortex*, **21**(6), 1408–1415.

Itoga, C. A., Berridge, K. C. & Aldridge, J. W. (2016). Ventral pallidal coding of a learned taste aversion. *Behavioural Brain Research*, **300**, 175–183.

Joutsa, J., Johansson, J., Niemelä, S., et al. (2012). Mesolimbic dopamine release is linked to symptom severity in pathological gambling. *Neuroimage*, **60**(4), 1992–1999.

Joyner, M. A., Kim, S. & Gearhardt, A. N. (2017). Investigating an incentive-sensitization model of eating behavior: Impact of a simulated fast-food laboratory. *Clinical Psychological Science*, p. 216770261771882.

Kai, N., Nishizawa, K., Tsutsui, Y., Ueda, S. & Kobayashi, K. (2015). Differential roles of dopamine D1 and D2 receptor-containing neurons of the nucleus accumbens shell in behavioral sensitization. *Journal of Neurochemistry*, **135**(6), 1232–1241.

Kalivas, P. W. & Duffy, P. (1990). Effect of acute and daily cocaine treatment on extracellular dopamine in the nucleus accumbens. *Synapse*, **5**(1), 48–58.

Kalivas, P. W. & Stewart, J. (1991). Dopamine transmission in the initiation and expression of drug- and stress-induced sensitization of motor activity. Brain Research. *Brain Research Reviews*, **16**(3), 223–244.

Kalivas, P. W., Volkow, N. & Seamans, J. (2005). Unmanageable motivation in addiction: a pathology in prefrontal-accumbens glutamate transmission. *Neuron*, **45**(5), 647–650.

Kaplan, J. M., Roitman, M. & Grill, H. J. (2000). Food deprivation does not potentiate glucose taste reactivity responses of chronic decerebrate rats. *Brain Research*, **870**(1–2), 102–108.

Kawa, A. B., Bentzley, B. S. & Robinson, T. E. (2016). Less is more: prolonged intermittent access cocaine self-administration produces incentive-sensitization and addiction-like behavior. *Psychopharmacology*, **233**(19–20), 3587–3602.

Kelley, A. E. & Berridge, K. C. (2002). The neuroscience of natural rewards: relevance to addictive drugs. *The Journal of Neuroscience*, **22**(9), 3306–3311.

Keyes, K. M., Martins, S. S., Blanco, C. & Hasin, D. S. (2010). Telescoping and gender differences in alcohol dependence: new evidence from two national surveys. *The American Journal of Psychiatry*, **167**(8), 969–976.

Koob, G. F. & Volkow, N. D. (2010). Neurocircuitry of addiction. *Neuropsychopharmacology*, **35**(1), 217–238.

Kühn, S. & Gallinat, J. (2011). Common biology of craving across legal and illegal drugs – a quantitative meta-analysis of cue-reactivity brain response. *The European Journal of Neuroscience*, **33**(7), 1318–1326.

LeBlanc, K. H., Ostlund, S. B. & Maidment, N. T. (2012). Pavlovian-to-instrumental transfer in cocaine seeking rats. *Behavioral Neuroscience*, **126**(5), 681–689.

Leeman, R. F. & Potenza, M. N. (2012). Similarities and differences between pathological gambling and substance use disorders: a focus on impulsivity and compulsivity. *Psychopharmacology*, **219**(2), 469–490.

Lemmens, S. G. T., Schoffelen, P. F. M., Wouters, L., et al. (2009). Eating what you like induces a stronger decrease of "wanting" to eat. *Physiology & Behavior*, **98**(3), 318–325.

Leyton, M. & Vezina, P. (2013). Striatal ups and downs: their roles in vulnerability to addictions in humans. *Neuroscience and Biobehavioral Reviews*, 37(9 Pt A), 1999–2014.

Leyton, M., Boileau, I., Benkelfat, C., et al. (2002). Amphetamine-induced increases in extracellular dopamine, drug wanting, and novelty seeking: a PET/[11C]raclopride study in healthy men. *Neuropsychopharmacology*, **27**(6), 1027–1035.

Leyton, M., Casey, K. F., Delaney, J. S., Kolivakis, T. & Benkelfat, C. (2005). Cocaine craving, euphoria, and self-administration: a preliminary study of the effect of catecholamine precursor depletion. *Behavioral Neuroscience*, **119**(6), 1619–1627.

Leyton, M., aan het Rot, M., Booij, L., et al. (2007). Mood-elevating effects of d-amphetamine and incentive salience: the effect of acute dopamine precursor depletion. *Journal of Psychiatry & Neuroscience*, **32**(2), 129–136.

Leyton, M., Young, S. N., Blier, P., et al. (2000). Acute tyrosine depletion and alcohol ingestion in healthy women. *Alcoholism, Clinical and Experimental Research*, **24**(4), 459–464.

Li, P., Wu, P., Xin, X., et al. (2015). Incubation of alcohol craving during abstinence in patients with alcohol dependence. *Addiction Biology*, **20**(3), 513–522.

Li, X., Zeric, T., Kambhampati, S., Bossert, J. M. & Shaham, Y. (2015). The central amygdala nucleus is critical for incubation of methamphetamine craving. *Neuropsychopharmacology*, **40**(5), 1297–1306.

Litt, A., Khan, U. & Shiv, B. (2010). Lusting while loathing: parallel counterdriving of wanting and liking. *Psychological Science*, **21**(1), 118–125.

Lovic, V., Saunders, B. T., Yager, L. M. & Robinson, T. E. (2011). Rats prone to attribute incentive salience to reward cues are also prone to impulsive action. *Behavioural Brain Research*, **223**(2), 255–261.

Lu, L., Hope, B. T., Dempsey, J., et al. (2005). Central amygdala ERK signaling pathway is critical to incubation of cocaine craving. *Nature Neuroscience*, **8**(2), 212–219.

Lu, L., Uejima, J. L., Gray, S. M., Bossert, J .M. & Shaham, Y. (2007). Systemic and central amygdala injections of the mGluR(2/3) agonist LY379268 attenuate the expression of incubation of cocaine craving. *Biological Psychiatry*, **61**(5), 591–598.

Mahler, S. V. & Berridge, K. C. (2009). Which cue to "want?" Central amygdala opioid activation enhances and focuses incentive salience on a prepotent reward cue. *The Journal of Neuroscience*, **29**(20), 6500–6513.

Mahler, S. V. & Berridge, K. C. (2012). What and when to "want?" Amygdala-based focusing of incentive salience upon sugar and sex. *Psychopharmacology*, **221**(3), 407–426.

Mascia, P., Neugebauer, N. M., Brown, J., et al. (2019). Exposure to conditions of uncertainty promotes the pursuit of amphetamine. *Neuropsychopharmacology*, **44**(2), 274–280.

McBride, W. J. (2002). Central nucleus of the amygdala and the effects of alcohol and alcohol-drinking behavior in rodents. *Pharmacology, Biochemistry, and Behavior*, **71**(3), 509–515.

Metrik, J., Aston, E. R., Kahler, C. W., et al. (2016). Cue-elicited increases in incentive salience for marijuana: craving, demand, and attentional bias. *Drug and Alcohol Dependence*, **167**, 82–88.

Mick, I., Myers, J., Stokes, P. R. A., et al. (2014). Amphetamine induced endogenous opioid release in the human brain detected with [^{11}C]carfentanil PET: replication in an independent cohort. *The International Journal of Neuropsychopharmacology*, **17**(12), 2069–2074.

Miller, K. A. & Mays, D. (2020). Tanning as an addiction: The state of the research and implications for intervention. In S. Sussman (Ed.) *The Cambridge Handbook of Substance and Behavioral Addictions*. Cambridge, UK: Cambridge University Press, pp. 362–372.

Munafò, M. R., Zetteler, J. I. & Clark, T. G. (2007). Personality and smoking status: a meta-analysis. *Nicotine & Tobacco Research*, **9**(3), 405–413.

Myrick, H., Anton, R. F., Li, X., et al. (2004). Differential brain activity in alcoholics and social drinkers to alcohol cues: relationship to craving. *Neuropsychopharmacology*, **29**(2), 393–402.

Nowak, D. E. & Aloe, A. M. (2014). The prevalence of pathological gambling among college students: a meta-analytic synthesis, 2005–2013. *Journal of Gambling Studies*, **30**(4), 819–843.

O'Daly, O. G., Joyce, D., Tracy, D. K., et al. (2014). Amphetamine sensitization alters reward processing in the human striatum and amygdala. *PLos ONE*, **9**(4), e93955.

Oginsky, M. F., Goforth, P. B., Nobile, C. W., Lopez-Santiago, L. F. & Ferrario, C. R. (2016a). Eating "junk-food" produces rapid and long-lasting increases in nac cp-ampa receptors: implications for enhanced cue-induced motivation and food addiction. *Neuropsychopharmacology*, **41**(13), 2977–2986.

Oginsky, M. F., Maust, J. D., Corthell, J. T. & Ferrario, C. R. (2016b). Enhanced cocaine-induced locomotor sensitization and intrinsic excitability of NAc medium spiny neurons in adult but not in adolescent rats susceptible to diet-induced obesity. *Psychopharmacology*, **233**(5), 773–784.

Ondo, W. G. & Lai, D. (2008). Predictors of impulsivity and reward seeking behavior with dopamine agonists. *Parkinsonism & Related Disorders*, **14**(1), 28–32.

Ostlund, S. B., LeBlanc, K. H., Kosheleff, A. R., Wassum, K. M. & Maidment, N. T. (2014). Phasic mesolimbic dopamine signaling encodes the facilitation of incentive motivation produced by repeated cocaine exposure. *Neuropsychopharmacology*, **39**(10), 2441–2449.

O'Sullivan, S. S., Wu, K., Politis, M., et al. (2011). Cue-induced striatal dopamine release in Parkinson's disease-associated impulsive-compulsive behaviours. *Brain: A Journal of Neurology*, **134**(Part 4), 969–978.

Park, C.-B., Park, S. M., Gwak, A. R., et al. (2015). The effect of repeated exposure to virtual gambling cues on the urge to gamble. *Addictive Behaviors*, **41**, 61–64.

Parker, L. A. (2014). Conditioned flavor avoidance and conditioned gaping: rat models of conditioned nausea. *European Journal of Pharmacology*, **722**, 122–133.

Pascoli, V., Turiault, M. & Lüscher, C. (2011). Reversal of cocaine-evoked synaptic potentiation resets drug-induced adaptive behaviour. *Nature*, **481**(7379), 71–75.

Paulson, P. E. & Robinson, T. E. (1995). Amphetamine-induced time-dependent sensitization of dopamine neurotransmission in the dorsal and ventral striatum: a microdialysis study in behaving rats. *Synapse*, **19**(1), 56–65.

Paulson, P. E., Camp, D. M. & Robinson, T. E. (1991). Time course of transient behavioral depression and persistent behavioral sensitization in relation to regional brain monoamine concentrations during amphetamine withdrawal in rats. *Psychopharmacology*, **103**(4), 480–492.

Peciña, S. & Berridge, K. C. (2000). Opioid site in nucleus accumbens shell mediates eating and hedonic "liking" for food: map based on microinjection Fos plumes. *Brain Research*, **863**(1–2), 71–86.

Peciña, S. & Berridge, K. C. (2005). Hedonic hot spot in nucleus accumbens shell: where do mu-opioids cause increased hedonic impact of sweetness? *The Journal of Neuroscience*, **25**(50), 11777–11786.

Peciña, S. & Berridge, K. C. (2013). Dopamine or opioid stimulation of nucleus accumbens similarly amplify cue-triggered "wanting" for reward: entire core and medial shell mapped as substrates for PIT enhancement. *The European Journal of Neuroscience*, **37**(9), 1529–1540.

Peciña, S., Cagniard, B., Berridge, K. C., Aldridge, J. W. & Zhuang, X. (2003). Hyperdopaminergic mutant mice have higher "wanting" but not "liking" for sweet rewards. *The Journal of Neuroscience*, **23**(28), 9395–9402.

Petit, A., Lejoyeux, M., Reynaud, M. & Karila, L. (2014). Excessive indoor tanning as a behavioral addiction: a literature review. *Current Pharmaceutical Design*, **20**(25), 4070–4075.

Petry, N. M. & Blanco, C. (2013). National gambling experiences in the United States: will history repeat itself? *Addiction*, **108**(6), 1032–1037.

Pfaus, J. G., Damsma, G., Nomikos, G. G., et al. (1990). Sexual behavior enhances central dopamine transmission in the male rat. *Brain Research*, **530**(2), 345–348.

Piazza, P. V., Deminière, J. M., Le Moal, M. & Simon, H. (1989). Factors that predict individual vulnerability to amphetamine self-administration. *Science*, **245**(4925), 1511–1513.

Piazza, P. V., Deminiere, J. M., Le Moal, M. & Simon, H. (1990). Stress- and pharmacologically-induced behavioral sensitization increases vulnerability to acquisition of amphetamine self-administration. *Brain Research*, **514**(1), 22–26.

Piazza, P. V., Deroche-Gamonent, V., Rouge-Pont, F. & Le Moal, M. (2000). Vertical shifts in self-administration dose-response functions predict a drug-vulnerable phenotype predisposed to addiction. *The Journal of Neuroscience*, **20**(11), 4226–4232.

Pickens, C. L., Airavaara, M., Theberge, F., et al. (2011). Neurobiology of the incubation of drug craving. *Trends in Neurosciences*, **34** (8), 411–420.

Politis, M., Loane, C., Wu, K., et al. (2013). Neural response to visual sexual cues in dopamine treatment-linked hypersexuality in Parkinson's disease. *Brain: A Journal of Neurology*, **136**(Part 2), 400–411.

Popien, A., Frayn, M., von Ranson, K. M. & Sears, C. R. (2015). Eye gaze tracking reveals heightened attention to food in adults with binge eating when viewing images of real-world scenes. *Appetite*, **91**, 233–240.

Potenza, M. N. (2008). The neurobiology of pathological gambling and drug addiction: an overview and new findings. *Philosophical Transactions of the Royal Society of London B: Biological Sciences*, **363**(1507), 3181–3189.

Prisciandaro, J. J., Joseph, J. E., Myrick, H., et al. (2014). The relationship between years of cocaine use and brain activation to cocaine and response inhibition cues. *Addiction*, **109** (12), 2062–2070.

Robbins, T. W. (1976). Relationship between reward-enhancing and stereotypical effects of psychomotor stimulant drugs. *Nature*, **264** (5581), 57–59.

Robinson, M. J. F. & Berridge, K. C. (2013). Instant transformation of learned repulsion into motivational "wanting." *Current Biology*, **23**(4), 282–289.

Robinson, M. J. F., Anselme, P., Fischer, A. M. & Berridge, K. C. (2014a). Initial uncertainty in Pavlovian reward prediction persistently elevates incentive salience and extends sign-tracking to normally unattractive cues. *Behavioural Brain Research*, **266**, 119–130.

Robinson, M. J. F., Anselme, P., Suchomel, K. & Berridge, K. C. (2015a). Amphetamine-induced sensitization and reward uncertainty similarly enhance incentive salience for conditioned cues. *Behavioral Neuroscience*, **129**(4), 502–511.

Robinson, M. J. F., Burghardt, P. R., Patterson, C. M., et al. (2015b). Individual differences in cue-induced motivation and striatal systems in rats susceptible to diet-induced obesity. *Neuropsychopharmacology*, **40**(9), 2113–2123.

Robinson, M. J. F., Warlow, S. M. & Berridge, K. C. (2014b). Optogenetic excitation of central amygdala amplifies and narrows incentive motivation to pursue one reward above another. *The Journal of Neuroscience*, **34**(50), 16567–16580.

Robinson, T. E. & Becker, J. B. (1986). Enduring changes in brain and behavior produced by chronic amphetamine administration: a review and evaluation of animal models of amphetamine psychosis. *Brain Research*, **396** (2), 157–198.

Robinson, T. E. & Berridge, K. C. (1993). The neural basis of drug craving: an incentive-sensitization theory of addiction. *Brain Research. Brain Research Reviews*, **18**(3), 247–291.

Robinson, T. E. & Berridge, K. C. (2008). Review. The incentive sensitization theory of addiction: some current issues. *Philosophical Transactions of the Royal Society of London. Series B, Biological Sciences*, **363**(1507), 3137–3146.

Robinson, T. E. & Flagel, S. B. (2009). Dissociating the predictive and incentive motivational properties of reward-related cues through the study of individual differences. *Biological Psychiatry*, **65**(10), 869–873.

Robinson, T. E. & Kolb, B. (2004). Structural plasticity associated with exposure to drugs of abuse. *Neuropharmacology*, **47** (Supplement 1), 33–46.

Rømer Thomsen, K., Fjorback, L. O., Møller, A. & Lou, H. C. (2014). Applying incentive sensitization models to behavioral addiction. *Neuroscience and Biobehavioral Reviews*, **45**, 343–349.

Rosse, R. B., Fay-McCarthy, M., Collins, J. P., Alim, T. N. & Deutsch, S. I. (1994). The relationship between cocaine-induced paranoia and compulsive foraging: a preliminary report. *Addiction*, **89**(9), 1097–1104.

Rosse, R. B., Fay-McCarthy, M., Collins, J. P., et al. (1993). Transient compulsive foraging behavior associated with crack cocaine use. *The American Journal of Psychiatry*, **150**(1), 155–156.

Rougé-Pont, F., Piazza, P. V., Kharouby, M., Le Moal, M. & Simon, H. (1993). Higher and longer stress-induced increase in dopamine concentrations in the nucleus accumbens of animals predisposed to amphetamine self-administration. A microdialysis study. *Brain Research*, **602**(1), 169–174.

Rozin, E. (2000). The flavor principle: comment on use of the concept by Pliner and Stallberg-White (2000). *Appetite*, **34**(2), 224; discussion 225–226.

Saal, D., Dong, Y., Bonci, A. & Malenka, R. C. (2003). Drugs of abuse and stress trigger a common synaptic adaptation in dopamine neurons. *Neuron*, **37**(4), 577–582.

Salimpoor, V. N., Benovoy, M., Larcher, K., Dagher, A. & Zatorre, R. J. (2011). Anatomically distinct dopamine release during anticipation and experience of peak emotion to music. *Nature Neuroscience*, **14**(2), 257–262.

Saunders, B. T. & Robinson, T. E. (2010). A cocaine cue acts as an incentive stimulus in some but not others: implications for addiction. *Biological Psychiatry*, **67**(8), 730–736.

Saunders, B. T. & Robinson, T. E. (2011). Individual variation in the motivational properties of cocaine. *Neuropsychopharmacology*, **36**(8), 1668–1676.

Schlaepfer, T. E., Cohen, M. X., Frick, C., et al. (2008). Deep brain stimulation to reward circuitry alleviates anhedonia in refractory major depression. *Neuropsychopharmacology*, **33**(2), 368–377.

Schmidt, R., Lüthold, P., Kittel, R., Tetzlaff, A. & Hilbert, A. (2016). Visual attentional bias for food in adolescents with binge-eating disorder. *Journal of Psychiatric Research*, **80**, 22–29.

Schmitz, F., Naumann, E., Trentowska, M. & Svaldi, J. (2014). Attentional bias for food cues in binge eating disorder. *Appetite*, **80**, 70–80.

Shin, A. C., Pistell, P. J., Phifer, C. B. and Berthoud, H. R. (2010). Reversible suppression of food reward behavior by chronic mu-opioid receptor antagonism in the nucleus accumbens. *Neuroscience*, **170**(2), 580–588.

Sienkiewicz-Jarosz, H., Scinska, A., Swiecicki, L., et al. (2013). Sweet liking in patients with Parkinson's disease. *Journal of the Neurological Sciences*, **329**(1–2), 17–22.

Singer, B. F., Scott-Railton, J. & Vezina, P. (2012). Unpredictable saccharin reinforcement enhances locomotor responding to amphetamine. *Behavioural Brain Research*, **226**(1), 340–344.

Singer, B. F., Tanabe, L. M., Gorny, G., et al. (2009). Amphetamine-induced changes in dendritic morphology in rat forebrain correspond to associative drug conditioning rather than nonassociative drug sensitization. *Biological Psychiatry*, **65**(10), 835–840.

Sinha, R. (2013). The clinical neurobiology of drug craving. *Current Opinion in Neurobiology*, **23**(4), 649–654.

Small, D. M., Zatorre, R. J., Dagher, A., Evans, A. C. & Jones-Gotman, M. (2001). Changes in brain activity related to eating chocolate: from pleasure to aversion. *Brain: A Journal of Neurology*, **124**(Pt 9), 1720–1733.

Smith, K. S. & Berridge, K. C. (2007). Opioid limbic circuit for reward: interaction between hedonic hotspots of nucleus accumbens and ventral pallidum. *The Journal of Neuroscience*, **27**(7), 1594–1605.

Smith, K. S. & Berridge, K. C. (2005). The ventral pallidum and hedonic reward: neurochemical maps of sucrose "liking" and food intake. *The Journal of Neuroscience*, **25** (38), 8637–8649.

Smith, K. S., Berridge, K. C. & Aldridge, J. W. (2011). Disentangling pleasure from incentive salience and learning signals in brain reward circuitry. *Proceedings of the National Academy of Sciences of the United States of America*, **108** (27), E255–264.

Söderpalm, A. H. & Berridge, K. C. (2000). The hedonic impact and intake of food are increased by midazolam microinjection in the parabrachial nucleus. *Brain Research*, **877**(2), 288–297.

Sperling, I., Baldofski, S., Lüthold, P. & Hilbert, A. (2017). Cognitive food processing in binge-eating disorder: an eye-tracking study. *Nutrients*, **9**(8), 903.

Steiner, J. E. (1973). The gustofacial response: observation on normal and anencephalic newborn infants. *Symposium on Oral Sensation and Perception*, **4**, 254–278.

Steiner, J. E., Glaser, D., Hawilo, M. E. & Berridge, K. C. (2001). Comparative expression of hedonic impact: affective reactions to taste by human infants and other primates. *Neuroscience and Biobehavioral Reviews*, **25**(1), 53–74.

Steketee, J. D. & Kalivas, P. W. (2011). Drug wanting: behavioral sensitization and relapse to drug-seeking behavior. *Pharmacological Reviews*, **63**(2), 348–365.

Stuber, G. D., Hopf, F. W., Hahn, J., et al. (2008). Voluntary ethanol intake enhances excitatory synaptic strength in the ventral tegmental area. *Alcoholism, Clinical and Experimental Research*, **32**(10), 1714–1720.

Sussman, S. & Bolshakova, M. (2020). Treatment of alcohol, tobacco, and other drug (ATOD) misuse. In S. Sussman (Ed.) *The Cambridge Handbook of Substance and Behavioral Addictions*. Cambridge, UK: Cambridge University Press, pp. 215–229.

Sussman, S., Rozgonjuk, D. & van den Eijnden, R. J. J. M. (2017). Substance and behavioral addictions may share a similar underlying process of dysregulation. *Addiction*, **112**(10), 1717–1718.

Tapert, S. F., Cheung, E. H., Brown, G. G., et al. (2003). Neural response to alcohol stimuli in adolescents with alcohol use disorder. *Archives of General Psychiatry*, **60**(7), 727–735.

Terraneo, A., Leggio, L., Saladini, M., et al. (2016). Transcranial magnetic stimulation of dorsolateral prefrontal cortex reduces cocaine use: A pilot study. *European Neuropsychopharmacology*, **26**(1), 37–44.

Thomas, M. J., Kalivas, P. W. & Shaham, Y. (2008). Neuroplasticity in the mesolimbic dopamine system and cocaine addiction.

British Journal of Pharmacology, **154**(2), 327–342.

Tindell, A. J., Berridge, K. C., Zhang, J., Peciña, S. & Aldridge, J. W. (2005). Ventral pallidal neurons code incentive motivation: amplification by mesolimbic sensitization and amphetamine. *The European Journal of Neuroscience*, **22**(10), 2617–2634.

Tom, R. L., Ahuja, A., Maniates, H., Freeland, C. M. & Robinson, M. J. F. (2019). Optogenetic activation of the central amygdala generates addiction-like preference for reward. *The European Journal of Neuroscience*, **50**(3), 2086–2100.

Tournier, B. B., Tsartsalis, S., Dimiziani, A., Millet, P. & Ginovart, N. (2016). Time-dependent effects of repeated THC treatment on dopamine D2/3 receptor-mediated signalling in midbrain and striatum. *Behavioural Brain Research*, **311**, 322–329.

Uslaner, J. M., Acerbo, M. J., Jones, S. A. & Robinson, T. E. (2006). The attribution of incentive salience to a stimulus that signals an intravenous injection of cocaine. *Behavioural Brain Research*, **169**(2), 320–324.

Vela, L., Martínez Castrillo, J. C., García Ruiz, P., et al. (2016). The high prevalence of impulse control behaviors in patients with early-onset Parkinson's disease: a cross-sectional multicenter study. *Journal of the Neurological Sciences*, **368**, 150–154.

Venniro, M., Caprioli, D. & Shaham, Y. (2016). Animal models of drug relapse and craving: From drug priming-induced reinstatement to incubation of craving after voluntary abstinence. *Progress in Brain Research*, **224**, 25–52.

Versace, F., Kypriotakis, G., Basen-Engquist, K. & Schembre, S. M. (2016). Heterogeneity in brain reactivity to pleasant and food cues: evidence of sign-tracking in humans. *Social Cognitive and Affective Neuroscience*, **11**(4), 604–611.

Vezina, P. & Leyton, M. (2009). Conditioned cues and the expression of stimulant sensitization in animals and humans. *Neuropharmacology*, **56** (Supplement 1), 160–168.

Volkow, N. D., Koob, G. F. & McLellan, A. T. (2016). Neurobiologic advances from the brain disease model of addiction. *The New England Journal of Medicine*, **374**(4), 363–371.

Volkow, N. D., Wang, G. J., Fowler, J. S., Tomasi, D. & Baler, R. (2012). Food and drug reward: overlapping circuits in human obesity and addiction. *Current Topics in Behavioral Neurosciences*, **11**, 1–24.

Voon, V., Napier, T. C., Frank, M. J., et al. (2017). Impulse control disorders and levodopa-induced dyskinesias in Parkinson's disease: an update. *Lancet Neurology*, **16**(3), 238–250.

Wachtel, S. R., Ortengren, A. & de Wit, H. (2002). The effects of acute haloperidol or risperidone on subjective responses to methamphetamine in healthy volunteers. *Drug and Alcohol Dependence*, **68**(1), 23–33.

Wang, G., Shi, J., Chen, N., et al. (2013). Effects of length of abstinence on decision-making and craving in methamphetamine abusers. *PLos ONE*, **8**(7), e68791.

Warlow, S. M., Robinson, M. J. F. & Berridge, K. C. (2017). Optogenetic central amygdala stimulation intensifies and narrows motivation for cocaine. *The Journal of Neuroscience*, **37**(35), 8330–8348.

Warren, N., O'Gorman, C., Lehn, A. & Siskind, D. (2017). Dopamine dysregulation syndrome in Parkinson's disease: a systematic review of published cases. *Journal of Neurology, Neurosurgery, and Psychiatry*, **88**(12), 1060–1064.

Washton, A. M. & Stone-Washton, N. (1993). Outpatient treatment of cocaine and crack addiction: a clinical perspective. *NIDA Research Monograph*, **135**, 15–30.

Winkielman, P., Berridge, K. C. & Wilbarger, J. L. (2005). Unconscious affective reactions to masked happy versus angry faces influence consumption behavior and judgments of value. *Personality and Social Psychology Bulletin*, **31**(1), 121–135.

Wolf, M. E. (2010). The Bermuda Triangle of cocaine-induced neuroadaptations. *Trends in Neurosciences*, **33**(9), 391–398.

Wyvell, C. L. & Berridge, K. C. (2000). Intra-accumbens amphetamine increases the conditioned incentive salience of sucrose reward: enhancement of reward "wanting" without enhanced "liking" or response reinforcement. *The Journal of Neuroscience*, **20**(21), 8122–8130.

Wyvell, C. L. & Berridge, K. C. (2001). Incentive sensitization by previous amphetamine exposure: increased cue-triggered "wanting" for sucrose reward. *The Journal of Neuroscience*, **21**(19), 7831–7840.

Xi, Z.-X., Li, X., Li, J., et al. (2013). Blockade of dopamine D3 receptors in the nucleus accumbens and central amygdala inhibits incubation of cocaine craving in rats. *Addiction Biology*, **18**(4), 665–677.

Xu, X., Aron, A., Brown, L., et al. (2011). Reward and motivation systems: a brain mapping study of early-stage intense romantic love in Chinese participants. *Human Brain Mapping*, **32**(2), 249–257.

Zack, M., Featherstone, R. E., Mathewson, S. & Fletcher, P. J. (2014). Chronic exposure to a gambling-like schedule of reward predictive stimuli can promote sensitization to amphetamine in rats. *Frontiers in Behavioral Neuroscience*, **8**, 36.

Zeeb, F. D., Li, Z., Fisher, D. C., Zack, M. H. & Fletcher, P. J. (2017). Uncertainty exposure causes behavioural sensitization and increases risky decision-making in male rats: toward modelling gambling disorder. *Journal of Psychiatry & Neuroscience*, **42**(6), 404–413.

Zhang, J., Berridge, K. C., Tindell, A. J., Smith, K. S. & Aldridge, J. W. (2009). A neural computational model of incentive salience. *PLoS Computational Biology*, **5**(7), e1000437.

Zhou, L., Smith, R. J., Do, P. H., Aston-Jones, G. & See, R. E. (2012). Repeated orexin 1 receptor antagonism effects on cocaine seeking in rats. *Neuropharmacology*, **63**(7), 1201–1207.

4 Philosophical Issues in the Addictions

Shane N. Glackin, PhD

Introduction

As this *Handbook* demonstrates, the phenomenon of addiction straddles a dizzying number of fields of enquiry; even at a very coarse disciplinary grain, it throws up biomedical, neurological, pharmacological, clinical, social, legal, political, and moral issues, among numerous others. So it is no surprise that the multitude of disciplinary perspectives, methodologies, terminologies, and research programs, all working at cross-purposes, should generate conceptual misunderstandings and disputes.

Philosophy is, of course, dedicated as a field of study to the analysis and clarification of such conceptual quandaries, and many of the particular issues that have arisen in the course of the interdisciplinary study of addiction over the past few decades will be extremely familiar to ethicists, metaphysicians, and philosophers of science. Philosophers may address these problems directly; philosophical attention to them can also be hugely beneficial to researchers in the range of other "stakeholder" disciplines by increasing the conceptual consistency and rigor of the insights they produce into the nature, treatment, and prevention of addiction. Furthermore, philosophical analysis can help to integrate different disciplinary approaches to addiction together, by elaborating the range of possible metaphysical relations between various levels of causation and epistemic relations between levels of explanation, as well as by analyzing the relations between their distinctive frameworks and definitions – facilitating, in effect, intertheoretical translation.

I begin this chapter by summarizing the historical views of the major philosophers who have discussed or described addiction, whether explicitly or in arguments clearly pertaining to it, as well as those who, according to others, seem to have suffered from it. I then turn to the literature of the past few decades, in which addiction has become a specific topic of interest for philosophers. It would be beyond the scope of this chapter (not to mention deeply tedious for the nonspecialist) to provide a comprehensive review of this literature. Instead, I will focus on four current debates about the concept of addiction, each of which clearly invites philosophical analysis. The first concerns the scope of the concept, and whether it should be restricted to substance abuse, or expanded to cover, for example, sexual, gambling, or other behavioral, compulsions. The second is the ongoing tension between biomedical accounts of addiction, focussing on physiological and neural mechanisms and effects, and accounts which focus on social patterns of addiction, for which they in turn seek social-level explanations. A third concerns the question of whether addiction should be regarded as a disease or not, while the fourth concerns the agency of addicts, and the degree to which they can be regarded as being in control of, and responsible for, their actions, or powerless to overcome their compulsions.

I will deal with these controversies in turn over the following five sections. Each links to important ongoing debates in the wider philosophical literature; I summarize those debates and the major positions within them, before showing their relevance for the understanding of addiction and examining some of the ways that philosophers of addiction have in recent decades applied them. Of course, there is a considerable amount of overlap between these issues; the metaphysical question whether addictions form a "natural kind," for instance, hinges in significant part on whether they possess some causal mechanism in common, which in turn pertains to both the debate over whether addiction is caused primarily by social or biomedical phenomena, and the debate about compulsion, free will, and the moral responsibility of the addict for her actions. Nevertheless, the issues have frequently been unduly conflated too; the question whether addiction is a "brain disease," for instance, is often regarded as settling whether or not addicts are morally responsible. Separating the issues out as far as possible in this way will allow us to gain maximum conceptual clarity, and the connections can be noted in passing.

Addiction and the Ancients

The history of Western philosophy was memorably characterized by Whitehead as "an extended series of footnotes to Plato" (1929), and, certainly, a historical overview of any philosophical topic must start with the Ancient Greeks. Addictive substances were certainly known to the Greeks; Hesiod records the cultivation of poppies for their somniferous juice, *opion*, which was recommended by such pioneering physicians as Hippocrates and Galen, while alcohol – wine in particular – was of sufficient cultural prominence to have its own God in the person of Dionysos. Intoxication seems to have had religious significance too, and the famous Oracle is now widely supposed to have made her prophecies under the influence of a natural gas vent near the temple at Delphi.

The Greeks were undoubtedly familiar with alcoholism and the abuse of opiates, too; both Hippocrates and Galen, again, identified the causes and symptoms of *delirium tremens* (Leibowitz, 1967). The philosophers in particular will have been well-acquainted; Aristotle's most famous pupil Alexander the Great was legendary for his drunken escapades and enthusiastic consumption of opium, and he may have hastened his own mysterious early death by his prodigious over-indulgence. Moreover, the "Symposia" described by Plato, in which Socrates and others typically developed and expounded their philosophical views, were lengthy after-dinner boozing sessions not at all similar to the genteel modern staples of the academic calendar that bear their name. And, as Bruce Alexander has pointed out (2008, p. 318), Socrates does seem in Plato's *Republic* to be describing something strongly akin to the

Acknowledgements The author is grateful to Jonathan Davies, Hannah Farimond, Hannah Galvin, Joel Krueger, Celia Morgan, Tom Roberts, and Steve Sussman, as well as to the participants in the British Academy/Leverhulme Trust-funded workshop on "Philosophy and the Interdisciplinary Study of Addiction" at the University of Exeter in February 2019, for their helpful discussion of these and related issues.

stereotype of addiction in his discussion of "master passions," which may compel a man to expend:

> whatever income he has . . . and next of course he'll start borrowing and drawing on capital . . . when he comes to the end of his father's and mother's resources. . . he'll start by burgling a house or holding someone up at night, and go on to clean out a temple. Meanwhile [his] older beliefs about honour and dishonour, which he was brought up to accept as right, will be overcome by others once held in restraint but now free to become the bodyguard of his master passion. . . His passion tyrannizes over him, a despot without restraint or law.
>
> (2003, 573d–575a)

Yet it is not clear that the Greeks had any distinct concept of addiction, or that addiction in its modern sense was a significant problem in Greek society. At any rate, in the surviving writings of the Greek philosophers we find no explicit discussions of addicts or addictive behavior.

What we do find, nevertheless, are discussions of concepts which have shaped our understanding of addiction and moral responsibility ever since. In Plato's dialogue *Protagoras*, Socrates declares that it is impossible for us to act in ways that we know we shouldn't. "No one," he states, "who either knows or believes that there is another possible course of action, better than the one he is following, will ever continue on his present course" (2009, 358b-c). Like many philosophers' pronouncements, this seems straightforwardly false on first consideration; I know perfectly well that I should finish my overdue draft of this chapter rather than going to the pub for the evening, yet against my better judgement I go to the pub anyway. But is this really "against my better judgement"? Certainly, I would *prefer* to go to the pub; whatever I tell the volume's editor, there is a clear sense in which this seems the better option to me, which is why I do it.

Aristotle's solution to this puzzle is to draw a distinction between our reason and our appetites. If our moral education and development has proceeded properly, reason and the appetites will be aligned; we naturally want what is good for ourselves and others to have. This is, indeed, the mark of the *eudaimon*; the "happy," "excellent," or "flourishing" person who serves as the moral exemplar in Aristotle's system. But if our moral development has not been fully or properly formed, and we have failed to achieve *eudaimonia*, our animal passions may be out of kilter with our reasons. In this case, very few of us will be so thoroughly corrupt or depraved that we cannot see the right course of action at all; more likely we will recognize what is best but fail to desire it as we should. Aristotle calls this condition *akrasia* or "weakness of the will" (literally, "incontinence"); although we know what we ought to do, our appetites point us to a different course of action, and we lack the strength of will to overcome them. Moral education consists in large part of developing the strength of will to resist our appetites, until they have been realigned and acting rightly becomes "second nature" to us (2004, Bk VII).

In addition to our everyday failings – missing deadlines, skipping gym sessions, having a second biscuit during a coffee break – *akrasia* has been widely thought to illuminate the moral situation of addicts. We don't suppose that addicts are unaware that their actions are wrong; yet nor do we judge those actions in the same way as we would if they were carried out by a nonaddict. Addiction, on this view, is properly regarded as a derangement of the appetites; the addict is not a moral monster or ignoramus, but simply someone whose appetitive desires are too uncommonly strong for them to overcome and observe the same moral standards as the rest of us.

This line of reasoning was taken to its extreme – as philosophers are wont to do – by the Stoics, who taught that *all* desire was at odds with the virtuous life, which could be reached only by serene acceptance of one's lot. However, for our purposes the most notable thing about the Stoic school is not the analgesic undertone of this doctrine, but one of its prominent members; the Roman emperor Marcus Aurelius, who appears to have been the first significant philosopher who was himself an addict. Administered opium by his physician Galen, Marcus' seemingly bottomless appetite for the drug was recorded in Galen's notes, and remarked upon by his contemporaries, with his withdrawal symptoms at one point conspicuously affecting the course of a military campaign (Africa, 1961; Trancas, Borja Santos & Patrício, 2004).

Marcus was not the last philosopher of antiquity to succumb to addiction. The great Persian philosopher and physician Ibn Sina (Avicenna), perhaps the greatest intellect of the Islamic world, prescribed himself enemas of opium poppy and celery seeds for the treatment of severe colic, and is reported to have died following an overdose, perhaps deliberately administered by larcenous slaves. Sina's death was also attributed by some observers to his compulsive sexual appetites, perhaps indicating an addiction that embraced both substance and behavior.

By some distance the most remarkable such figure, however, is St. Augustine of Hippo. More than any other, the figure who marks the intellectual transition between the Greco-Roman and the Christian worlds, Augustine is perhaps best known for his *Confessions*; a text that is often regarded as the first autobiography. In it, he recounts the trauma of being forced by his mother to abandon the mother of his child – his beloved partner of eleven years – in favor of a more politically auspicious marriage, and the years of compulsive promiscuity he was plunged into as a result, before adopting chastity following a religious conversion.

Augustine seems to have had trouble controlling his sexual impulses from a young age, his teenage promiscuity having been a source of concern to his alcoholic mother and amusement to his philandering father. At sixteen, he recounts, "the madness of lust. . . took complete control of me, and I surrendered wholly to it" (2002, 24:2.2; cf. James, 1987; Soble, 2002, p. 561). To Carthage then he came as a student, as T. S. Eliot wrote, "burning burning burning burning" (1922). For several years in the great city he gave himself over to his desires, until the formation of his exclusive relationship with the mother of his child, itself a "mere bargain of lustful love" (Augustine, 2002, 52:4.2; Soble, 2002, p. 555).

He seems to have behaved stably for the duration of that relationship, until it was broken by his mother's ambition and an arranged marriage. However, his bethrothed would not be of age to marry for another two years, during which time – now a professor in Milan – he threw himself headlong back into promiscuity. Augustine describes in excruciating detail his inability to moderate his sexual appetites; no middle ground was possible for him between a state of complete abstinence and one of being completely "given over" – literally, *ad-dicted* – to his obsession (Alexander, 2008, pp. 27–28; Bowers, 1990, p. 112). He describes, in terms that would become familiar over the following centuries, the sense of being inescapably compelled by his addiction:

> The enemy held my will captive; therefore he kept me, chained down and bound. For out of a rebellious will lust had sprung; and lust pampered had become custom; and custom indulged had become necessity. These were the links of the chain; this was the bondage in which I was bound, and that new will which was already born in me, freely to serve you, wholly to enjoy you, God, the only true joy, was not yet able to subdue my former willfulness, strengthened by the wantonness of years. So did my two wills, one new, the other old, one spiritual, the other carnal, fight within me, and by their discord undo my soul.
>
> (2002, 8.5–11)

He recounts more and yet more reckless behavior in pursuit of his addiction, rising to the coyly described extreme of a sexual encounter during Holy Mass, a debasement which he believed "deserved death as its reward" (2002, 3.3). Though he feels the pull of Christianity strongly, he resists it because "(t)he plain truth is that I thought I should be impossibly miserable if I had to forego the embraces of a woman" (2002, 100–101; 6.11). Augustine is tormented, divided by his desire for sex, and his desire to be free of it. *Lord, make me chaste,* he famously prayed . . . *but not yet.*

If so many of the classic themes of addiction are already present in Augustine's story – family history and coaddiction, social and geographic dislocation, guilt and self-loathing, doubt in one's free will, even the suspicion of moralising exaggeration – it ends with another: spontaneous remission. In the terms of a much later vocabulary of addiction, he embraced a higher power, abandoning his Manichaean beliefs, breaking his engagement, and converting to Christianity. He renounced sex, was ordained a bishop, and devoted his energies to writing. The Lord had seen fit, finally, to make Augustine chaste.

Classifying Addiction

When we talk about "addiction," it is not always clear how wide the term's scope is intended to be. Is alcoholism the same *sort* of thing, in some relevant sense, as addiction to crack cocaine, or the habitual abuse of prescription opioids? Most controversially, are addictions of this putative sort – addictions to *substances* – relevantly similar to what are frequently regarded as "addictions" to certain sorts of *behavior,* such as gambling or sexual activity? And how closely do the classifications of these phenomena suggested by science correspond to the everyday or "folk" use of the term "addiction"?

In philosophers' terminology, what we are asking here is whether or not the addictions – or some subset of them – form a "natural kind"; whether, that is, such groupings of conditions reflect real distinctions and similarities in nature, or are simply artefacts of our human interests and classificatory practices (Bird & Tobin, 2018). These poles delimit a whole spectrum of positions in the debate; very broadly speaking, we call those closer to the first "realist," and those closer to the second "nominalist."

But to be more precise, we should distinguish two further broad families of position. "*Naturalists*" believe, as realists do, that good classifications "carve nature at the joints" like good butchers, in Plato's famous image (2005, 265e); the distinctions posited by our best conceptual schemes correspond to genuine, objective distinctions in the nature of the things classified. But naturalists are not thereby committed to the view that the kinds or categories posited by those schemes thereby "really" exist as abstract objects. So, the *realist* positions are a metaphysically ambitious subset of the naturalist ones. That is to say, what nominalists deny is not naturalism, the view that our classifications are rooted in and reflect natural distinctions, but realism, the view that the groupings thus classified exist abstractly. The view properly opposed to naturalism is "*conventionalism*" which holds, in its various strengths, that our classifications fail to reflect genuine distinctions in nature either because such distinctions are unknowable to us (weak conventionalism) or because no such distinctions exist (strong conventionalism). Again, the conventionalist positions are a subset of the nominalist ones; it is possible to be both a naturalist and a nominalist. Of course, one may adopt different views of different classificatory schemes; to regard, for example, positional distinctions between soccer-players – is Mohamed Salah a winger or a wide-lying striker? – as useful but essentially arbitrary does not commit one to taking a similar view about the chemical elements.

There are a variety of reasons for supposing that "natural kinds" exist; conversely, each of these imposes conditions on what can count as a natural kind. The most influential such view is that natural kinds support inductive inferences; familiarity with some members of the kind allows us to make relevant predictions about the others, owing to their natural similarities, while in turn it is frequently the ability to make such inductive judgements reliably that alerts us to the existence of relevant similarities. This is the view advanced by W. V. Quine, perhaps the central figure in post-World War II US philosophy; we begin with a good evolved ability to discern similarities, since "creatures inveterately wrong in their inductions have a pathetic but praiseworthy tendency to die before reproducing their kind" (1969, p. 126). However, the inductions made possible by this "folk-psychological" ability allow us to develop natural science, which goes on to inductively refine and supersede our folk classifications by revealing deeper and more significant levels of similarity, producing progressively better candidates for natural kindhood.

This view is notably liberal, since any natural property will permit inductive inferences to be drawn and so count as supporting a natural kind. Moreover, as Peter Godfrey-Smith observes, some inductive inferences do not rest on shared properties or natural kinds at all; thus, electoral polling requires only that the sample be sufficiently large and drawn at random (2011). So this may be a necessary condition for kindhood, but is not a sufficient one.

A more robust, and discriminating, variant appeals to the *clustering* of such properties. In a multidimensional graph representing all the objects in the world by dots, Ruth Millikan points out, taking each of their properties as corresponding to a dimension, "all but very small areas of the graph will remain empty" and "where not empty the graph would contain mostly clumps of dots that were in close proximity along multiple dimensions, closely clustered in . . . property space. There would be a clump that was all the rabbits, say, and another that was all the Gothic cathedrals, . . . and so forth, and there would be, for the most part, very sizable empty areas surrounding each of these clusters in most dimensions" (2017, p. 12). A great number of these clusters, Millikan speculates, will exist for historical reasons; they are formed because objects are typically created by copying other existent objects in some way. More generally, in Richard Boyd's formulation, such clusters will be supported by "homeostatic" mechanisms which in some way cause the properties in the cluster to associate with each other, thereby making divergent individuals comparatively unlikely to arise or persist. *Homeostatic property clusters* are thus self-regulating, and support much more robust, informative inductions; from some individual's membership in the cluster, we may infer a great deal more about its properties beyond merely the visible ones which lead us to classify it (Boyd, 1991, 1999).

An alternative approach is to require that natural kinds support *laws of nature,* rather than inductive inferences. Thus, the fact that some class of items always and everywhere behaves in a particular way is explained by the members of that class possessing the relevant properties. However, this approach seems of limited use in the biological and social sciences, which it is now widely agreed contain no exceptionless, nontrivial generalizations of this sort (see e.g., Sterelny & Griffiths, 1999, p. 366).

A similar problem seems to afflict inductive accounts. The theory of natural selection requires that there be considerable variation within any biological grouping, so there is likely to be no property that all members of the kind possess, over which inductive inferences may be drawn. Cluster-based accounts can go some way to addressing this concern, since kind-membership is determined not by possession of any particular property, but only of subsets of the clustered properties. But even these accounts have trouble grounding inductive inferences over species that display significant polymorphism; much of what we might infer from observing Great Danes will not extend to Beagles, or Chihuahuas. Nor will it do to simply locate our kinds at a different level, such as breeds, since polymorphisms seem to cross-cut any such divisions; we can learn even less about male angler-fish by observing female ones.

One solution to this conundrum begins by taking seriously Millikan's idea that the clustering of properties in biological kinds is the result of the historical processes which formed them. What unites the members of such kinds is not some (disjunctive) set of properties they possess, but their common history. Seeing kinds as historical in this way allows us to focus on several important features they possess. One of these is the fact that their members' characteristic features are not inevitable, but can change over time; famously, the typical peppered moth became much darker as the Industrial Revolution took hold of England, lightening again when pollution reduced. Likewise, criminalizing – or legalizing – a drug of addiction can radically alter the social profile of the addicted population.

So, classifying a case as belonging to a kind does not, on this view, fix its properties. On the contrary, as Ian Hacking (1995) has argued, what the criminalization/legalization case shows is that human kinds tend to be "interactive" rather than natural; any act of classification itself produces "looping" feedback effects which alter the profile of the classified kind. To identify any group by some distinctive features its members possess does not thereby bring it into existence – the features, of necessity, already exist – but it does provide its members and those around them with a new way to understand their lives. When "alcoholism" was first identified as a kind, in other words, those with drinking problems found themselves in a new conceptual world. Likewise, once we conceptualize problem gambling as an "addiction" – as Gamblers Anonymous has long done, officially followed only since 2013 by the American Psychiatric Association – we can expect such gamblers to be treated, and to regard themselves, in a similar way to alcoholics and chain-smokers; and, for better or worse, to behave (and perhaps to respond to therapy) accordingly. And this may alter those features by which we initially picked out the group beyond recognition. As Scott Vrecko (2010, pp. 40–41; *cf.* Foddy & Savulescu, 2010a, p. 11) points out, members of the kind "addict" were identified in the mid-twentieth century by withdrawal symptoms. Yet as our understanding of the same group has deepened and expanded, and as the group itself has responded, this has become an inessential characteristic of the kind; we recognize many addictions with no such symptoms, and cases of physical dependence on drugs like Prozac, which sometimes are not considered addictions at all. Similarly, the way we recognize afflicted groups can – through the provision of clean needles, access to therapeutic resources, etc. – have transformative effects on the overall health profile typical of their members, including particularly the incidence of comorbidity with other medical issues. Demanding that social welfare and healthcare recipients pass drug-tests before accessing resources, or labeling them as morally corrupted, conversely, may have a similarly profound, but negative, effect on health and well-being.

What we are seeing here is the idea that classifications are extremely contingent, perhaps radically so. According to Nelson Goodman (1978), this is not just a feature of the human sciences, but of classification generally. The world does not come prepackaged into categories; if kinds are historical entities, then they must have beginnings and, in principle, ends. For any given set of data, multiple classificatory schemes of equivalent accuracy are available, and the choice between them is typically made on grounds of convenience. Classification is not then a matter of identifying or discovering the "correct" natural kinds already existing in the world, but of "making" a conceptual world by identifying and selecting relevant kinds for our purposes.

Hacking and Goodman are therefore both pluralists and nominalists about kinds – they think there are a myriad of equally accurate potential classificatory systems, none of them uniquely "real," and the choice as to which is appropriate is determined by the purposes to which we wish to put them – but they are not conventionalists. The natural properties that form the basis of classification are genuine, for all that they may be altered by the act of classifying. It is just in respect of those properties that such kinds do prove themselves useful for our purposes; the projects of "worldmaking" (Goodman, 1978) and "making up people" (Hacking, 1986) are constrained by reality.

How much, then, rests on the kinds in question existing "abstractly"? Perhaps not a lot (Glackin, 2012). Hacking himself describes his view as a "dynamic nominalism," but grants that one might just as well regard the same position as a "*dialectical realism*, preoccupied by the interactions between what there is (and what comes into being) and our conceptions of it" (2004, p. 2). And certainly it is open to realists, too, to reject the idea that there is a single, uniquely correct schema for the classification of kinds in nature. One can choose, instead, to adopt a realist stance toward kinds across the board, or "promiscuously." John Dupré (1995) argues that there are countless ways of classifying the world into real, abstract kinds, all equally legitimate for some theoretical or inductive purpose or other. This *promiscuous realism* is not a conventionalist or nominalist view; it holds that genuine natural features of the world differentiate the members of natural kinds from nonmembers, and denies that the mere multiplicity of such groupings gives us any reason for modesty about their metaphysical status. Better to take our folk and scientific classifications at face value; when we say that groupings exist, we mean that they exist, whether we are talking about "living things that are vertebrates" or "living things that are kosher." We may be concerned with either, depending on whether the natural features we are interested in have to do with physiology or religious law. The mere fact that two phenomena are kind-mates, then, doesn't necessarily tell us much more about their similarities; what matters is whether the shared features which underpin the kind are useful for diagnostic, etiological, therapeutic, or other uses.

So much for the theory, let's have the pay-off; what use is all of this metaphysical musing for the study of addiction? A key dispute concerning the terms of addiction research in recent decades has been the question whether, when we talk about "addiction," we are dealing with one sort of thing, or many. Likewise within more narrowly grained categories; are "substance addictions" or "drug addictions," for instance, one kind of phenomenon, or many? What is at stake in these debates is the question of similarity between ostensibly different cases, and the inductive generalizations that can be drawn over them as a result.

The answers to these questions matter because if cases are indeed relevantly similar – if they are part of the same natural kind – then we can profitably understand and treat them in similar ways. If the neurobiological phenomena characteristic of alcoholics resemble those of sex addicts, say, then pharmaceutical or behavioral interventions that are effective for one group may be similarly beneficial for the other.

And our understanding of the moral situation of alcoholics – the degree to which they are or are not "responsible for their actions" – may likewise clarify our attitudes toward those who engage compulsively in sexual behavior.

The relevance of natural kinds is double-edged, then; if they are to be useful, they should rest on underlying similarities between different cases, and they should in turn justify treating those different cases similarly. We can illustrate this with some concrete examples.

The American Psychiatric Association's current *Diagnostic and Statistical Manual of Mental Disorders* ("DSM-5") groups disorders according to outward phenomena involving "clinically significant disturbances of cognition, emotion or behavior," rather than the underlying biological or neurological dysfunctions that they reflect (APA, 2013; Murphy, 2017). This prioritizes diagnostic reliability over diagnostic validity; it is concerned with categories that clinicians can identify consistently, rather than categories which "really exist" (Hempel, 1994). Accordingly, it defines a category of "Gambling Disorder" (previously "Pathological Gambling"), where the patient indulges in gambling of a sort and to a degree that causes significant problems for his or her life (e.g., Criterion 2; "Is restless or irritable when attempting to cut down or stop gambling": Criterion 8; "Has jeopardized or lost a significant relationship, job, or educational or career opportunity because of gambling"). But critics have charged that this overlooks the key explanatory fact about such gamblers; despite the very different outward manifestation, their neurology is strikingly similar to those of drug addicts. Those diagnosed with Gambling Disorder typically "exhibit classic patterns of addictive behavior as a result of a specific kind of dysfunction in their dopaminergic reward system and consequent neuroadaptation impairing frontal control circuits," and critics therefore recommend "replacing the behaviorally derived concept of PG with the neuroscientifically anchored concept of addictive gambling" (Ross et al., 2012, p. 200).

This reflects more practical concerns than a philosopher's taste for taxonomic precision. First, the DSM-5 criteria provide at best a fuzzy basis for demarcating genuinely addicted gamblers from those who merely gamble habitually or excessively (Ross et al., 2012, p. 201*ff.*; Murphy, 2017; see also Sinnott-Armstrong & Pickard, 2013, Griffiths, 2013). Despite the outward similarities in their defining behavior, it is crucial for the purposes of understanding and treating both groups to recognize that their brains work in fundamentally different ways. A classification combining them is likely to be profoundly misleading on both scores; it therefore provides a poor basis for inductive generalizations, if comprehension and treatment are our aims. Conversely, recognizing gambling addiction as part of a broader natural kind, "addiction," adds to our understanding both of pathological gamblers and of other substance and behavioral addictions. Most strikingly, from 1998 onwards it began to be recognized that the opiate antagonist Naltrexone and other anticraving medications, widely used in treating alcoholism and heroin addiction, were effective in reducing the compulsion of addicts to gamble (Vrecko, 2010, pp. 42–43). These drugs act upon the endorphin and dopamine systems; that is to say, they have similar therapeutic effects in drug addicts and gambling addicts (as well as sex addiction, eating disorders, and kleptomania) because of similarities in the brain chemistry of these groups that a purely behavioral view of their conditions could not have predicted. Note again, too, how induction and classification support each other here. We posit kinds because we recognize underlying similarities among the members which will support inductive generalization; and it is the success of those generalizations that persuades us that the members are indeed similar and the kind genuine, leading us to discover further useful similarities (though see the methodological reservations expressed in Vrecko, 2010, pp. 43–45).

Similar issues arise at every level of analysis and classification. Thus, Jeremy Pober (2013) argues that substance addictions do not themselves form a natural kind, since not all such "addicts" do share the relevant brain chemistry. Cannabis addiction, he argues, does not affect Dopamine type-2/type-3 receptor availability in the way that addiction to other legal and illegal substances seems to; the relevant sort of neuroadaptation doesn't occur (2013, pp. 128–129). Nor does it share several other neural mechanisms that have been posited as the basis of addiction. So addiction – whether confined to substances of abuse or expanded to include behavioral compulsions – does not look like a natural kind; inductions drawn over the group will not be reliable for cannabis addicts. This is not to claim that cannabis addiction is illusory; Pober suggests splitting the kind into "S-addiction" and "T-addiction." But it suggests that interventions effective in one type of case may not translate to other types, and that the degree of autonomy one sort of addict displays may not reflect the moral capacity we can ascribe to others. Alternatively, we might find that our generalisations do hold up; in that case, the dissimilar properties Pober identifies will not have been the ones supporting the natural kind of addiction after all.

There is a further wrinkle in our talk of kinds and induction. Human kinds, according to Hacking, are interactive; they "loop," and alter over time. But chemical kinds, for the most part, do not. An addict is a social being, who responds to being classified as an addict by altering his or her behavior in various ways, some predictable and some not. But an addict is also, if defined neurochemically or pharmacologically rather than socially or behaviorally, a complex amalgam of biochemical reactions and processes, which are not similarly responsive to our taxonomic processes. So addicts are plausibly members of multiple kinds at once; at any rate, there are multiple levels of causation which affect them, not all of which are similarly dynamic, or responsive to the same things. An addict's underlying pharmacology may not loop at all, and there's an interesting and important question how much can loop without it; how much it thereby constrains kind-behavior.

Addiction and Levels of Causation

This raises another vexed question in the literature: is addiction a social phenomenon, or a biomedical or chemical one? In some sense, clearly, it seems to be both; addicts are, like all of us, both social and biochemical beings. But is one level of causation and explanation dominant over the other? Might one perhaps be epiphenomenal, just a causally inert companion of the other? Or do both work independently but in tandem, both contributing in crucial ways to the addicted person's behavior? I'll try to avoid getting involved in the scientific and empirical (and often philosophical) debate about which view of the relation is *right* here; rather, I'll summarize some of the conceptual apparatus that philosophers have developed to analyze questions of this sort, and how it may bear on our understanding of addiction.

One of the defining tasks of philosophy, particularly as it has been understood in the English-speaking world since the end of the nineteenth century, has been the analysis of how different vocabularies, apparently concerned with the same subjects, are related (Brandom, 2008, chapter 1). How can we understand talk about modality – how the world *could be* or *must be* – in terms of our familiar talk about how it actually *is*? What is the relation between brain events, like the firing of C-fibers, and mental events, like the feeling of pain? What place have moral and other *reasons* for action in the picture of the world and ourselves revealed to us by natural science? And how exactly do the theories that make up our sciences depend on the observational data our senses accrue? The question of whether addiction is primarily social or pharmacological in nature seems to have this character. Indeed, it has close affinities with the second and third of the puzzles above; the mind–body problem and the problem of morality, respectively.

A first candidate relation for this sort of puzzle would be *reduction*. That is, the vocabulary and any rules in one level of analysis might be straightforwardly translatable into those of the other or shown to be their logical consequence (Nagel, 1961). In this case, everything that can be said about social and behavioral addiction-related phenomena might have its correlate at the more fundamental neuropharmacological level, where all causal and explanatory interest resides. But this surely cannot be the case, and the view does not seem to have been advanced seriously in the literature. Looping phenomena would seem to be inexplicable on this view, as would the fact that – despite the similarities in brain chemistry – alcoholics cannot simply substitute gambling for drink, nor smokers relieve their cravings with theft or cocaine. And we would have no way to understand the persistent comparative prevalence of addictions in certain demographic groups rather than others. Instead, figures like Leshner have contended that although addiction is a neurochemical condition, it is one "for which the social contexts in which it has both developed and is expressed are critically important" (1997, p. 46).

More unusually, something like a reductive relation might be plausible in the other direction. On this view, all the interesting causal and explanatory work would be done at the social and behavioral levels. There are associated neurological phenomena, of course, because that is simply how our minds and brains work, but their significance and pervasiveness have been overstated by researchers wedded to an overly materialist worldview. Something like this position is often suggested by writers employing the rhetoric of a "myth" of addiction (Davies, 1997; Hammersley & Reid, 2002); researchers, policy-makers, and the public have been systematically misled by the idea that addictive behavior is an inevitable consequence of neurochemistry, rather than a complex of social and behavioral phenomena. Bruce Alexander, in his seminal work on the concept of addiction, distinguishes a spurious "restrictive" concept involving chemical compulsion – "a relic of 19th century temperance doctrine that penetrated the 20th century dressed up as medical or scientific knowledge [whose] origins are neither medical nor scientific and [which] does not mesh well with contemporary knowledge" (Alexander & Schweighofer, 1988, p. 159) – from the true, broader concept, a multivalent behavioral category caused throughout history by recurrent patterns of social dislocation (Alexander, 2008).

Hanna Pickard is a philosopher who seems to hold a view of this sort too, albeit rather more nuanced than this simple taxonomy suggests. Data suggest that there are overwhelmingly two classes of addicts, she argues; those with underlying psychiatric disorders and those whose addiction "peak(s) in adolescence and early adulthood and then . . . (resolve) permanently, without clinical intervention, by the late twenties or early thirties" (2012, pp. 40–41). This in turn shows that addiction is not a "chronic, relapsing neurobiological disease . . . characterised by compulsive use" (2012, p. 41; I consider the conceptually separate question of whether addiction is a disease in a section below) as the common image suggests; for the second group, it is neither chronic nor relapsing, whereas for the first group it is neurobiological, but not a disease of compulsion. Rather, for those suffering from comorbid psychiatric disorders, it is used "purposively: to alleviate severe psychological distress. Consumption is a chosen means to desired ends. If the ends are no longer as pressing, or alternative ways of achieving them are available, it is possible to choose differently: Use is not compulsive" (2012, p. 42). Building on the previous vocabulary: the class of "addicts" comprises two discrete natural kinds, on this view, one of which is defined behaviorally with no distinctive neurochemical characteristics, while the other has neurological characteristics which are not distinctive to addiction, and is again defined by the behavioral response of self-medication.

Reductive views imply that one apparent level of causation can, in principle, be dispensed with entirely, or at least regarded merely as a useful shorthand. If we want to acknowledge genuine causal influences at multiple levels, some other relation is necessary. One candidate, which has generated immense quantities of discussion among philosophers while seeming entirely unknown to the rest of the world, is that of *supervenience* (Kim, 1984; McLaughlin & Bennett, 2018). A set of properties supervenes upon another just in case the first set of properties cannot change without a change in the second. Consider the property *brittle*. Panes of glass can be brittle – hard but easily broken – as can fingernails, decorative ironwork, etc. Brittleness in each of these is a matter of having a certain molecular microstructure. But brittleness does not reduce to having such a microstructure; it is realized by decidedly different microstructures in each case. The property of brittleness is thus multiply realisable; but however it is realized in a given case, it cannot change unless the microstructure changes. Any pane with the relevant microstructure will be brittle. This provides another possibility; the behavioral phenomena of addiction may supervene upon the associated facts about brain chemistry. This will allow a correspondence between neurochemical facts and behavioral ones, which still permits each a significant measure of causal autonomy.

A similar candidate relation, which has been widely discussed in recent years, is *grounding* (Bliss & Trogdon, 2016). Metaphysical grounding, unlike supervenience, is *directional*. Supervenience is concerned only with modal covariance; A-properties cannot change without changes in B-properties. Grounding is concerned with the existence of properties, or objects, or facts, "in virtue of" more fundamental ones. On this view, behavioral phenomena such as compulsion are explained by neurochemical phenomena; they happen as they do *owing to* what occurs in the dopamine and endorphin systems. This reflects a shift from a "flat" ontology, where all properties are equally basic, to an "ordered" one, in which some exist or obtain in virtue of others doing so (Schaffer, 2009, pp. 354–356). The neurochemical facts are "more basic," metaphysically speaking, than the behavioral ones; but the behavioral ones are nevertheless causally efficacious as well. In this case there will be a behavioral kind *because* there is a neurochemical kind.

Grounding also seems particularly suited to the analysis of social kinds; according to the schema outlined in a recent book by Brian Epstein (2015), social facts can hold in virtue of – be grounded by – some more basic underlying facts just in case a convention known as a "frame principle" exists establishing that grounding relation. And the facts establishing that convention are termed its "anchors." So, for instance, a certain piece of paper ("Billy the dollar bill") is legal tender; this social fact is grounded by the fact that Billy is printed in a certain way by the Bureau of Engraving and Printing. And it is grounded by this fact because the framing principle that all such papers printed by the BEP are legal tender is anchored by further facts about the operative statues, acts of Congress, and so forth. Likewise, various social facts about addiction might be grounded by neurochemical facts about the brains of addicts because of framing principles themselves anchored by further facts about the law, social deprivation, genetic susceptibility, the availability of addictive substances, and so forth (Glackin, 2019). This approach allows us to describe and analyze a reticulated, multilayered range of cross-cutting causal relations between different, causally autonomous, kinds and their associated facts.

In such an intricate causal scenario, however, philosophical worries about ontological priority may add an unnecessary extra level of complexity. What matters from the point of view of both research and therapy in addiction is causal efficacy; which phenomena are doing which work. So, a less unwieldy way to capture this same intricacy is to follow the heuristic principle that Philip Kitcher terms "causal democracy" (2003). Developed initially to help analyze the complicated patterns of causal interaction between genes and environment in biological development, the principle holds that such questions cannot be satisfactorily answered by aprioristic metaphysical or methodological assumptions, but only by careful and patient case-by-case empirical research, which gives every causal factor its due. Causal democracy does not hold that all factors are equally important, or of equal metaphysical standing; it espouses equality of opportunities rather than of outcomes (Griffiths, 2016, p. 74; Stotz & Griffiths, 2016, p. 148), demanding only that "if the effect E is the product of factors in set S, then, for any $C \in S$, it is legitimate to investigate the dependence of E on C when the other factors in S are allowed to vary" (Kitcher, 2003, p. 290). Let a thousand research programmes bloom, in other words; and let all eschew "the usual preference for overly simple, often monocausal explanations," at least until inquiries are concluded (Griffiths, 2016, p. 76).

Addiction as Disease

One persistent question in the literature concerns whether or not addiction is, or should be regarded as, a brain disease (e.g., Alexander, 2008; Foddy & Savulescu, 2010a; Leshner, 1997; Levy, 2013). But this question appears to conflate two others; whether or not it is principally neurochemical, a condition of the brain, and whether or not it is a disease. The first of these was dealt with in the previous section, albeit to no firm conclusion; I consider the second, which has not been much considered in the literature (notable exceptions are Foddy [2010] and Segal [2013]), here.

To know whether or not addiction is a disease, one thing we need to know is what it *means* for something to be a disease. There are three principal accounts of disease in the philosophical literature, plus an additional one which we should consider in this context. These can be subdivided into "*naturalist*" theories, which regard disease as a value-free, objective concept, and "*normativist*" ones, which regard it as inherently evaluative, so that it is an intrinsically bad thing for one to have a disease, even if – as when a very minor complaint such as bone-spurs prevents one from being conscripted and losing one's life at war – it is on the whole beneficial.

The most influential account of disease, and certainly the most discussed, is the Biostatistical Theory of Disease (BST) first advanced by Christopher Boorse (1975, 1977). Boorse's theory is a naturalistic one; its criteria purport to be value-free, and to appeal only to entities and quantities that can be observed and measured by the methods of the natural sciences. According to Boorse, disease can be defined as the absence of health, where health is regarded as statistical normality of function. Function here is defined "causally"; an organ or trait's function is whatever contribution it typically makes (according to the "species design") to the body's overall operation. Now, merely taking a statistical average across the whole population will produce some unwelcome results. For instance, almost all males will have higher levels of testosterone, and almost all females less, than the statistical norm. Likewise, since heart-rate drops steadily as one ages, the population mean will not produce a useful figure for young or old people. Accordingly, Boorse takes the relevant statistical norm to be that displayed in a *reference class*, or an age-group of a sex of a species.

There have been numerous objections to, and defenses of, the BST, which I will not attempt to summarize here. Our question is: does addiction, by the BST standard, count as a disease? It seems likely to; it represents in all age-groups a departure from normal functioning in several respects which are usually profoundly deleterious for the addict. It shortens life and impairs life-chances, it greatly increases the risk of several other diseases, and it represents in itself a severe impairment in the person's functional ability to make and act on rational choices. One worry we might have concerns the relativizing of the standard to the reference class; if almost all members of a demographic group smoke or drink alcohol to excess, does that addiction thereby cease to count as a disease? Boorse accounts for such "universal disorders," however, by appealing again to the species design. In some cases, he writes – dental caries and arteriosclerosis, for example – the entire reference class may have its functional ability limited by comparison to the species design because of environmental influences (Boorse, 1977, p. 567). So addiction will count as an impairment of normal functioning either relevant to the reference class's statistical norm or, failing that, for the class as a whole in an adverse environment.

One objection is worth mentioning here, however, since it directly concerns addicted populations. As Elselijn Kingma has pointed out (2007), the liver function of alcoholics, or the lung function of smokers, will differ from that of the wider population in just the same way that the body-fat percentages of males and females, or the heart-rates of the elderly, will. We account for the latter cases by relativizing to a reference class, and saying that someone has a normal body fat percentage *for a male*, or that so-and-so's heart-rate is in the normal range *for someone of her age*. Why not say in the same way: Nigel's liver functions well *for an alcoholic*? The answer seems straightforward; alcoholism is a disease, whereas being male or female, or elderly, is not. But remember that the reference classes were to be used to give us an objective, value-free account of what disease is; they cannot, on pain of circularity, themselves be based on our intuitive sense of which conditions do and do not count as diseases.

The main alternative biomedical account of disease is properly speaking a normativist account, though it is sometimes regarded as a hybrid one, having both a normativist and a naturalist element. The Harmful Dysfunction Theory (HDT), developed by Jerome Wakefield (e.g., Wakefield, 1992), combines the judgements that a condition represents a dysfunction (naturalist) that is harmful for the patient (normativist). "Dysfunction" here is understood in a different sense from the BST; Wakefield appeals to the "etiological" or "selected effect" function developed by Ruth Millikan (1989). On this view, the function of a trait or organ is whatever it has evolved to do; specifically, whatever task its precursors having performed in the bodies of the organism's ancestors helps to explain its current presence and configuration. A disease, in turn, will be where any trait or organ does not function in the way it has evolved to do, and this failure negatively impacts its owner.

Does addiction qualify on this score? It is controversial on both counts. Certainly, most addictions are harmful, though the addict may not always think so at the time (see below). But is an addiction *intrinsically* harmful – is a harmful effect a necessary condition of addiction? It certainly seems conceptually possible for some addictions to be benign, or even beneficial. That, at any rate, is what I tell myself about my morning coffee. Indeed, *all* addictions arguably are functional; they do something positive for the addict, and then do something negative to the addict. So unless harmful to the individual, addiction will not count as a disease on Wakefield's view. Many will find counterintuitive, though, the idea that the same neurochemical response to the same substance may in one circumstance be a disease, and, in another, not.

Does addiction represent a dysfunction in Wakefield's and Millikan's evolutionary sense? Perhaps. However, a number of studies have suggested that addiction is evolutionarily significant; that humans and psychoactive plants may have coevolved, or that humans have developed specific adaptations (e.g., for metabolizing alcohol; Durrant et al., 2009). This raises the possibility that addictive behavior may be functional; it may reflect an evolved response to adverse social environments. This conjecture is *extremely* speculative. But if it is true, we cannot use the HDT to classify addiction as a disease however harmful it may be, as it would then represent the system functioning in the way it was designed to (Levy, 2013).

What is the alternative to a biomedical account of disease? It, too, may be better regarded as a social kind rather than a natural kind. After all, even if there is some natural property that asthma, fractured scaphoids, prostate cancer, and myopia possess in common, it is far from clear that such a property is anything like what we have in mind when we class them together. Rather, we think of those with such conditions as having suffered a *misfortune* of some kind, as being in a bodily state that is *disvalued* in certain ways, of *experiencing* their body in a disrupted fashion, or as being the proper objects of *medicalized* practices in our society (e.g., Engelhart, 1976; Glackin, 2010, 2019; Nordenfelt, 2018). Such views are termed social constructivist (or social constructionist); they assume that the diseases are a kind constructed on the basis of a certain sort of social status which its members share. Moreover, insofar as there are underlying physiological similarities between cases of disease, this is because the classification reflects a social effort to *direct the attention* of the medical profession to the treatment of those physiological features.

On this view, the disease status of addiction will hang on social attitudes to addicts and their status. And this may be a double-edged sword. One of the things we typically intend by calling something a disease is to entitle those afflicted by it to a certain moral status; we devote resources to their treatment or protection, and excuse the inconvenience their condition causes for others as beyond their control. But this "social justice" aspect of the disease concept, which seems to be conspicuous in many of its invocations by addiction researchers, is not on offer from a social constructionist account of disease. That is to say, the constructionist takes the relevant evaluative attitudes to precede the classification rather than to follow from it, so the classification cannot be used to justify holding those attitudes (Kukla, 2014). Moreover, the status of disease may itself be regarded as stigmatizing, or to reflect stigmatizing social attitudes. We can usefully compare the history of homosexuality's classification here; its declassification as a psychiatric disorder was both a major step in destigmatizing it, and a reflection of large-scale change in stigmatizing social attitudes toward gay people. On the other hand, its *initial* classification as a psychiatric disorder, prior to which it had been regarded as merely immoral, licentious behavior, was similarly hailed as a move against stigmatization and a reflection of newly enlightened social attitudes. So it is plausible that addiction might follow the same moral trajectory over time, depending on the progress of the debates summarized in the next section.

One final theory of disease is worth considering here, not least for its connection to the issues of free will and choice, which the next section discusses, though it does not command a significant following among serious contemporary philosophers of medicine (though Pickard [2009] is a sympathetic reinterpretation by an important philosopher of addiction). The Hungarian "anti-"psychiatrist Thomas Szasz, following the nineteenth-century doctrine of Rudolf Virchow, held that the "gold standard" for disease was the presence of lesion, or damage to physical tissue (Szasz, 1960; Virchow, 1860). Szasz, a radical libertarian politically, meant this not as a vague metaphor, but as a very specific one; he abhorred the proliferation of "fiat money" not backed by gold reserves (Szasz, 2006). In analogous fashion, Szasz decried the false currency – the "myth" – of mental illness; since the mind is not the kind of thing which can have lesions, he argued, it is not the kind of thing which can become ill. "Mental illness" is not therefore a medical category at all, but rather a pretext for the use of medical institutions to repress behavior that society finds disgusting, inconvenient, or otherwise unacceptable. This is not to say that there cannot be brain diseases; the brain can have lesions the way any other physical organ can. So insofar as addiction is a distinct neurochemical kind, it may count as a disease. But insofar as it is social and behavioral, it is merely a "problem of living." The addict is somebody who makes choices to behave in particular ways, for his or her own reasons. The behavior is distinctive insofar as it displays a high degree of inelasticity (Foddy, 2010, p. 27); the addict continues acting on the same preferences, even when the costs of doing so are very considerable. But this is simply unusual economic activity, which the rest of us may disapprove of, but have no legitimate basis to restrict. To smuggle our moral attitudes under cover of a medical – and thus implicitly scientific or objective – classification would according to this perspective be to act both unjustly and in patently bad faith.

Addiction and Moral Agency

This brings us on, finally, to the issue where philosophers may have the most obvious contribution to make to debates over addiction; the problems it raises regarding morality, responsibility, and free will. Addicts regularly perform actions that, in isolation, would elicit unequivocal moral condemnation. And the fact of addiction is almost universally taken to qualify our attitudes toward the perpetrators in at least some regard; heartbreaking, degrading scenarios, and the sequences of events which bring them about, become "tragic," rather than "evil," failures of society and its support systems rather than failures uniquely attributable to the particular individuals involved. This can be double-edged; treating addicts as thereby lacking in moral agency may mitigate their wrongdoing, but often at the cost of regarding them as less than fully human, as less than full participants in a moral society in which we are accountable to others for our actions.

As is often the case in philosophy, a good place to start is to revisit the discussions of 2,000 years ago, since the question of *akrasia* continues to loom large over contemporary discussions, particularly since its revival in recent decades by R. M. Hare (1952, 1963) and Donald Davidson (1970, 1982); for a particular application of Davidson's argument to addiction, see Heather and Segal (2013, 2015). One very plausible reason for the "orthodox conception" of addicts as acting under compulsion, and unable to control their urges, is what might be called "common-sense" Socratism (Pickard, 2018). If a person knows their action will have unacceptable consequences, we suppose, and can avoid doing it, then they will avoid doing it. Ergo, the reasoning goes, since addicts are surely aware of the negative consequences of their actions, it follows that they must lack self-control. And if somebody is not in control of their actions, they cannot be responsible for them.

But absolving addicts of *any* responsibility in this way strikes most people as both morally and factually wrong. Various scientific studies have cast doubt upon the idea that addicts are lacking in the neurological capacity for self-control, while only minimal personal acquaintance or sociological study is necessary to debunk the image of addicts as automatons driven only by amoral compulsion; and we know that many addicts do succeed in quitting without intervention. So it cannot simply be the case that addicts are, per se, unable to control their actions. We must suppose, then, either that they are akratic - being aware of the wrongness of actions but failing to refrain from them accordingly - or that they are in some way unaware of the actions' wrongness. Of course, this simply demarcates three extreme limits of the debate; most views of addiction will hold some combination of them, in more-or-less qualified form.

While it is commonly assumed, there is surprisingly little explicit defense of the "common-sense" view in the literature. Perhaps this should not be surprising; nobody gains tenure by arguing for what everyone already knows. So the majority of critical opinion inevitably runs against the popular stereotype, the pantomime character of *The Addict* (Pickard, 2016, p. 454). Nevertheless, the contrast in this regard with major philosophical writers of earlier generations (e.g., James, 1890) is striking.

One observation about addiction worth taking seriously, then, is that the substance or behavior of choice *really may seem genuinely beneficial* to the addict. That is, we take the Socratic inference - if acting freely, people will act as it seems to them for the best - seriously, but perform a *modus ponens* rather than a *modus tollens* over it; we don't reject the idea that they are acting freely, but that they are failing to act in the way that - all things considered - seems to them best. Bruce Alexander (2008) points to persistent patterns of social dislocation that have, across geography and history, been accompanied by widespread phenomena of addiction. And his seminal experiments on rats appear to support the view that addictive behavior is heavily contingent on an impoverished environment (Alexander et al., 1981). Similarly, Hanna Pickard claims, the majority of addicts who are not afflicted by comorbid psychiatric disorder appear to recover permanently from the condition without intervention as they reach their late twenties or early thirties (Pickard & Pearce, 2014, pp. 166–167). Those who are so afflicted, moreover, are principally using the substances they do as "a way of coping with psychological distress" (p. 170). So the strong preferences displayed by addicts simply reflect the fact that substance abuse - or gambling, or promiscuous sexuality - seems to them the best response to their current circumstances; when circumstances improve, they cease to prefer that sort of response. Bennett Foddy and Julian Savulescu accordingly give a strikingly simple "liberal" account of addiction; "an addiction is a strong appetite" (2010b, p. 35; see also Foddy & Savulescu, 2010a, pp. 14–15).

What are the implications of this view for the moral responsibility of addicts for their actions? It might seem, at first glance, to give them full responsibility; if they are not under compulsion, then they are in control of their actions, and can be held accountable for their choices, and their failure to assess the best course of action. But the causal antecedents of addiction are not under an individual's control; the addict cannot reasonably be blamed for experiencing psychiatric disorder or social dislocation, and so for finding themselves in a situation where the best course of action seems as it does. This raises a problem, which philosophers have termed "Moral Luck" (Nagel, 1979; Williams, 1976); it is widely assumed that we are morally assessible only to the extent that what we are morally assessed for depends on factors under our control, yet it also frequently seems *correct* to morally assess us for things that are out of our control. Thomas Nagel distinguished four kinds of luck that might bear on moral assessment: resultant luck, or "luck in the way one's actions and projects turn out"; circumstantial luck, or "the luck involved in "the kind of problems and situations one faces"; causal luck, or "luck in how one is determined by antecedent circumstances"; and constitutive luck, or the luck involved in one's having the "inclinations, capacities and temperament" that one does (Nagel, 1979, p. 28). The last three of these seem clearly pertinent to the moral position of addicts. According to Nagel, the problem exposes a general issue with the possibility of moral assessment:

> The area of genuine agency, and therefore of legitimate moral judgment, seems to shrink under this scrutiny to an extensionless point . . . in a sense the problem has no solution, because something in the idea of agency is incompatible with actions being events, or people being things. But as the external determinants of what someone has done are gradually exposed, in their effect on consequences, character, and choice itself, it becomes gradually clear that actions are events and people things. Eventually nothing remains which can be ascribed to the responsible self, and we are left with nothing but a portion of the larger sequence of events, which can be deplored or celebrated, but not blamed or praised.
>
> (Nagel, 1979, pp. 35–37)

Various attempts have been made to resolve this problem. Pickard (2017), for one, outlines a framework for "responsibility without blame" allowing genuine moral agency to be acknowledged while nevertheless refraining from hostile or stigmatizing attitudes toward the affected individuals; though she confesses to initially having "no idea how this stance was so much as conceptually possible" (p. 174), Pickard describes in detail its functioning in a therapeutic community where she worked. And while the theoretical details require a great deal of further elaboration within the philosophy of action literature, philosophers should be wary in the extreme about dismissing from the couch as a-priori conceptually impossible what practitioners observe in the field.

Another possible resolution, advanced by Chandra Sripada (2018), concerns the ubiquitous phenomenon of *fallibility*. All complex human activity, he notes, however expert the practitioner, carries a nonzero possibility of failure due to error; even Homer nods, as the saying goes. The recovering addict typically faces a constant stream of drug-directed desires, each of which *individually* requires significant cognitive effort to overcome; their *cumulative* effect is therefore to significantly raise the probability of a failure of self-control. Thus, Sripada argues, it can be simultaneously true that each individual drug-directed desire is fully resistible by the addict as a free moral agent, and that the addict's overall ability to resist eventually succumbing to those desires and relapsing is greatly diminished.

So, there is a seeming tension between acknowledging the freedom of agency addicts possess, mitigating the actions they nevertheless take, and attributing to them a full understanding of those actions' consequences. The Aristotelian solution, of invoking *akrasia*, is a tempting one. According to Neil Levy, the neurological evidence suggests a version of this thesis; addicts' judgement may *shift* temporarily to make the pursuit of addictive preferences seem temporarily to be the best course of action, even if at other times they would not endorse those decisions. Again, he argues, this may also explain the phenomena of addicts "maturing out" or of ceasing to act compulsively when removed to a significantly different environment (as with many of the heroin-using US servicemen who returned from Vietnam in the early 1970s); the "judgement-shift" is a response to particular environmental circumstances (Levy, 2011; see also Ainslie, 2000). Richard Holton presents a slightly different understanding of *akrasia* as a mismatch between *values* and *desires*; the addict is somebody who exhibits "an almost complete disconnection between judging an outcome good and wanting it, or, conversely, between judging it bad and not wanting it" (2009, p. 109; see also Holton, 1999).

Lubomira Radoilska's rival account counters that the Holton analysis "is best understood as an unsuccessful attempt to tackle akrasia… a secondary failure of intentional agency which follows from and is partly explained by the primary failure that it tries to redress" (2013, p. xi). On Radoilska's view, true akratic action is successful insofar as it brings something intended about, but fails insofar as it is wrongly aimed, and thus both intends and brings about something other than what the agent truly values. This suggests, in classic Aristotelian fashion, that addiction reflects a failure of *development*; moral actors who have matured in the species-appropriate way will not experience this sort of mismatch between their intentions and their "true" aims. But those who have not reached this point successfully, and so display "evaluative immaturity," can even find themselves acting akratically when the behavior in question is "devoid of pleasure. Paradoxically, this is what accounts for the sense of compulsion typically associated with addiction," but not with my blown deadline, or skipped workout (p. xi).

According to Gideon Yaffe, Holton and others wrongly interpret what neuroscientific data are available in characterizing addicts in this way. Like Levy, he takes it to show that addicts, "at the time of action, value what they choose." And this, he argues, shows that "addiction influences what people do intentionally by working through, rather than against, the valuing system" (Yaffe, 2013, p. 194). In turn, he takes this to show that the moral situation of addicts is not dissimilar to that of victims of duress, who "find themselves valuing criminal conduct more than they value refraining from such conduct. And like those under duress, and unlike those with such values who are not under duress, addicts have the values they have thanks to the fact that they bear burdens that are not, themselves, reflective of morally or legally objectionable attitudes on their parts" (p. 195). But addiction is *not*, says Yaffe, a form of duress, wherein "(i)t is not that they cannot comply; it is, rather, that they cannot be expected to bear the burdens of withdrawal that compliance would lead them to suffer" (2011, p. 116). If this is indeed the way that duress-based accounts work, as most of the literature has assumed (e.g., Husak, 1999; Morse, 2000; Watson, 1999), then they seem unlikely to be successful; only a small number of the range of conditions widely regarded as addictions involve anything like withdrawal symptoms, which are consequently no longer widely appealed to – as we have seen – in characterizing addictions. Moreover, it is not empirically clear that withdrawal-avoidance does play any significant motivational role in addicts' reasoning.

But while this corresponds to the classical legal doctrine of duress, there is another view, which may avoid these problems and has not been widely discussed in the addiction literature. In an influential article, Patrick Atiyah (1982) argued that the classical doctrine did not well characterize the emerging case-law on *economic* duress. A better view than the idea that the agent's will was "overborne" in duress cases, he argued, was to recognize that while the agent had been presented a genuine choice, it was not the choice facing most agents, but one between evils. The problem with contracts entered into under duress is therefore not that the agent has not consented, but that she has been wrongfully faced with a set of choices in which the usual reasons not to behave in some particular way have been superseded. A duress-based account of addiction along these lines would thus acknowledge the patient's freedom of action but recognize that the "motivational space" she inhabits is radically different from that familiar to most people.

This brings such accounts into close proximity with a rich philosophical literature on the possibility of mutually inaccessible and incomprehensible ways of experiencing and inhabiting the world. Some philosophers have dismissed the very possibility as incoherent; according to Donald Davidson (1974), the description of such radically different "conceptual schemes" is self-defeating, since we could only recognize and assert their existence in the event that we could, after all, comprehend them. (To see the force of this objection, consider the commonly cited problem with Internet "listicles" with titles such as "20 words in foreign languages that can't be translated into English"; by explaining the terms to the (anglophone) reader the author has, precisely, translated them, thereby contradicting his premise). But countless others have found this a fruitful way of understanding various phenomena. One of these was Ludwig Wittgenstein, whose influential notion of "forms of life" organized and made internally comprehensible by their characteristic "language games" (Wittgenstein, 1953) has been usefully applied by Peg O'Connor – herself a recovering alcoholic – to the lived world of addiction, and its contrast with that of sobriety:

> In many ways, I think active alcoholics have a form of life different from that of recovered alcoholics, as well as from that of non-alcoholics. The world we all share is the same in important respects. But in some deep ways, the lived world and its meanings are radically different. Consider some differences between people with long-term sobriety and those who are actively alcoholic, or even newly entering a recovery program. An unrecovered alcoholic often can't even understand the alcoholic who says, "Your life will be better without alcohol. You will like yourself more. You will have more friends and a lot more fun." To the unrecovered, people in recovery can seem preachy and sanctimonious. Early on, no matter how many times and in how many ways a long-timer says this, what the unrecovered person hears is more like, "Blah, blah, serenity. Blah, blah, blah, serenity," as a great Gary Larson cartoon reminds us.
>
> Non-alcoholics can't fathom alcoholics, those of us who would risk our livelihoods, families, and whatever else we hold near and dear in order to drink. We can offer huge chains of reasoning that make sense to us, and to other alcoholics. But to non-alcoholics, unless they've been enlisted in enabling us, we can seem to be beyond logic and sanity.
>
> (Morris, 2011)

A very recent trend in the philosophical literature, which provides another useful way to think about these issues, concerns the nature of "transformative experiences." Beginning with L. A. Paul's analysis of the experience of pregnancy (Paul, 2015a), this work concerns a certain class of experiences which by their nature cannot be the subjects of rational decision-making. This is because they are both epistemically and personally *transformative*; that is, they change our points of view, including our core preferences, and the only way to know what they are like is to have them ourselves (Paul, 2015b). Becoming a parent, according to Paul, is something that alters one's core preferences in a way that – as they never seem to tire of telling us – only someone who has experienced it can understand. And this means that the decision to become a parent or not cannot be evaluated rationally, since one cannot, prior to the decision, access the preferences or values that would motivate one after the decision, and therefore justify it. Addiction, as O'Connor describes it, or on the model of the second form of duress we considered, may be a transformative experience of this sort; the motivational structure of the addict's world may be fundamentally inaccessible to those who are not addicted, and that of somebody recovering similarly barred to the addict. And this would explain the difficulty we commonly have in knowing how to morally assess the actions of addicts; we know perfectly well how these actions would be assessed if performed by somebody whose "motivational space" is comprehensible to us, but we also know that that of the addict is not.

Conclusions

Just as the study of addiction spans a huge number of academic disciplines, its philosophical study embraces a great many of philosophy's subdisciplines. We have considered debates here in normative and applied ethics, the philosophy of action, metaphysics, philosophy of medicine, philosophy of psychiatry, epistemology, philosophy of biology, philosophy of medicine, and jurisprudence; no doubt a more comprehensive overview would add more to the list. This reflects the rich, cross-cutting intellectual interest of addiction as a topic of philosophical study.

It also reflects the wide-ranging and versatile toolkit which philosophers have, over the centuries, developed for the analysis of such phenomena. This conceptual apparatus is not proprietary; it represents a public resource available to investigators across all the myriad fields gathered together in this *Handbook*, and many more beside. As the various social and life sciences tell us more about addiction, philosophers will continue to be on hand to interpret and analyze the results, clarifying the issues and – perhaps – thereby suggesting further avenues for future research. Intellectually interesting though the philosophical study of addiction may be in its own right, a subdiscipline where philosophers of addiction spoke only to each other would be an arid and pointless one; the true value of the work described in this chapter lies in its potential to enable dialogue and collaboration between and across disciplines.

REFERENCES

Africa, T. W. (1961). The opium addiction of Marcus Aurelius. *Journal of the History of Ideas*, **22**, 97–102.

Ainslie, G. (2000). A research-based theory of addictive motivation. *Law and Philosophy*, **19**, 77–115.

Alexander, B. K. (2008). *The Globalization of Addiction: A Study in the Poverty of the Spirit.* Oxford: Oxford University Press.

Alexander, B. K., Beyerstein, B. L., Hadaway, P. F. & Coambs, R. B. (1981). Effect of early and later colony housing on oral ingestion of morphine in rats. *Pharmacology Biochemistry & Behavior*, **15**, 571–576.

Alexander, B. K. & Schweighofer, A .R. F. (1988). Defining "addiction." *Canadian Psychology/Psychologie Canadienne*, **29**, 151–162.

American Psychiatric Association. (2013). *Diagnostic and Statistical Manual of Mental Disorders* (5th edition). Arlington, VA: American Psychiatric Publishing.

Aristotle. (2004). *The Nicomachean Ethics (Penguin Classics Edition)*, trans. J. A. K. Thomson. London: Penguin.

Atiyah, P. S. (1982). Economic duress and the overborne will. *Law Quarterly Review*, **98**, 197.

St. Augustine (2002). *Confessions (Penguin Classics Edition)*, trans. R. S. Pine-Coffin. London: Penguin.

Bird, A. & Tobin, E. (2018). Natural kinds. In E. N. Zalta (Ed.), *The Stanford Encyclopedia of Philosophy* (Spring 2018 Edition). https://plato.stanford.edu/archives/spr2018/entries/natural-kinds/

Bliss, R. & Trogdon, K. (2016). Metaphysical grounding. In E. N. Zalta (Ed.), *The Stanford Encyclopedia of Philosophy* (Winter 2016 Edition). https://plato.stanford.edu/archives/win2016/entries/grounding/

Boorse, C. (1975). On the distinction between disease and illness. *Philosophy and Public Affairs*, **5**, 49–68.

Boorse, C. (1977). Health as a theoretical concept. *Philosophy of Science*, **44**, 542–573.

Bowers, J. M. (1990). Augustine as addict: Sex and texts in the *Confessions*. *Exemplaria*, **2**, 403–448.

Boyd, R. (1991). Realism, anti-foundationalism and the enthusiasm for natural kinds. *Philosophical Studies*, **61**, 127–148.

Boyd, R. (1999). Homeostasis, species, and higher taxa. In R. Wilson (Ed.), *Species: New Interdisciplinary Essays*. Cambridge: MIT Press, pp. 141–186.

Brandom, R. B. (2008). *Between Saying and Doing: Towards and Analytic Pragmatism.* Oxford: Oxford University Press.

Davidson, D. C. (1970). How is weakness of the will possible? In D. C. Davidson (1980) *Essays on Actions and Events*. Oxford: Clarendon Press, pp. 21–42.

Davidson, D. C. (1974). On the very idea of a conceptual scheme. *Proceedings and Addresses of the American Philosophical Association*, **47**, 5–20.

Davidson, D. C. (1982). Paradoxes of irrationality. In D. C. Davidson (2004) *Problems of Rationality*. Oxford: Clarendon Press, pp. 169–187.

Davies, J. B. (1997). *The Myth of Addiction* (2nd edition). Amsterdam: Harwood Academic Publishers.

Dupré, J. (1995). *The Disorder of Things: Metaphysical Foundations of the Disunity of Science.* Cambridge MA: Harvard University Press.

Durrant, R., Adamson, S., Todd, F. & Sellman, D. (2009). Drug use and addiction: Evolutionary perspective. *Australian and New Zealand Journal of Psychiatry*, **43**, 1049–1056.

Eliot, T. S. (1922). *The Waste Land.* New York: Horace Liveright.

Engelhart, H. T. (1976). Ideology and etiology. *Journal of Medicine and Philosophy*, **1**, 256–268.

Epstein, B. (2015). *The Ant Trap: Rebuilding the Foundations of the Social Sciences.* Oxford: Oxford University Press.

Foddy, B. (2010). Addiction and its sciences – philosophy. *Addiction*, **106**, 25–31.

Foddy, B. & Savulescu, J. (2010a). A liberal account of addiction. *Philosophy, Psychiatry, & Psychology*, **17**, 1–22.

Foddy, B. & Savulescu, J. (2010b). Relating addiction to disease, disability, autonomy, and the good life. *Philosophy, Psychiatry, & Psychology*, **17**, 35–42.

Glackin, S. N. (2010). Tolerance and illness: The politics of medical and psychiatric classification. *Journal of Medicine and Philosophy*, **35**, 449–465.

Glackin, S. N. (2012). Kind-making, objectivity, and political neutrality; the case of Solastalgia. *Studies in History and Philosophy of Biological and Biomedical Sciences*, **43**, 209–218.

Glackin, S. N. (2019). Grounded disease: The biological and the social in medicine. *The Philosophical Quarterly*, **69**, 258–276.

Godfrey-Smith, P. (2011). Induction, samples, and kinds. In J. K. Campbell, M. O'Rourke & M. H. Slater (Eds.), *Carving Nature at Its Joints: Natural Kinds in Metaphysics and Science*. Cambridge: MIT Press, pp. 33-52.

Goodman, N. (1978). *Ways of Worldmaking*. Indianapolis: Hackett.

Griffiths, M. D. (2013). Is loss of control always a consequence of addiction? *Frontiers in Psychiatry*, **4**, 36.

Griffiths, P. E. (2016). Proximate and ultimate information in biology. In J. Pfeifer & M. Couch (Eds.), *The Philosophy of Philip Kitcher*. Oxford: Oxford University Press, pp. 74-93.

Hacking, I. (1986). Making up people. In T. Heller, M. Sosna & D. Wellberry (Eds.), *Reconstructing Individualism*. Stanford CA: Stanford University Press, pp. 222-236.

Hacking, I. (1995). The looping effects of human kinds. In D. Sperber & A. Premark (Eds.), *Causal Cognition*. Oxford: Clarendon Press, pp. 351-394.

Hacking, I. (2004). *Historical Ontology*. Cambridge, MA and London: Harvard University Press.

Hammersley, R. & Reid, M. (2002). Why the pervasive addiction myth is still believed. *Addiction Research & Theory*, **10**, 7-30.

Hare, R. M. (1952). *The Language of Morals*. Oxford: Clarendon Press.

Hare, R. M. (1963). *Freedom and Reason*. Oxford: Clarendon Press.

Heather, N. & Segal, G. (2013). Understanding addiction: Donald Davidson and the problem of akrasia. *Addiction Research & Theory*, **21**, 445-452.

Heather, N. & Segal, G. (2015). Is addiction a myth? Donald Davidson's solution to the problem of akrasia says not. *The International Journal of Alcohol and Drug Research*, **4**, 77-83.

Hempel, C. G. (1994). Fundamentals of taxonomy. In J. S. Sadler, O. P. Wiggins & M. A. Schwartz (Eds.), *Philosophical Perspectives on Psychiatric Diagnostic Classification*. Baltimore: Johns Hopkins University Press, pp. 315-331.

Holton, R. (1999). Intention and weakness of will. *Journal of Philosophy*, **96**, 241-262.

Holton, R. (2009). *Willing, Wanting, Waiting*. Oxford: Oxford University Press.

Husak, D. (1999). Addiction and criminal liability. *Law and Philosophy*, **18**, 655-684.

James, F. A. III (1987). Augustine's sex-life change: From profligate to celibate. *Christian History*, 15.

James, W. (1890). *Principles of Psychology*. New York: Henry Holt.

Kim, J. (1984). Concepts of supervenience. *Philosophy and Phenomenological Research*, **45**, 153-176.

Kingma, E. (2007). What is it to be healthy? *Analysis*, **67**, 128-133.

Kitcher, P. (2003). Battling the undead: How (and how not) to resist genetic determinism. In *In Mendel's Mirror: Philosophical Reflections on Biology*. Oxford: Oxford University Press, pp. 283-300.

Kukla, R. (2014). Medicalization, "normal function," and the definition of health. In J. D. Arras, E. Fenton & R. Kukla (Eds.), *The Routledge Companion to Bioethics*. London: Routledge.

Leibowitz, J. O. (1967). Studies in the history of alcoholism II: Acute alcoholism in Ancient Greek and Roman medicine. *British Journal of Addiction to Alcohol and Other Drugs*, **62**, 83-86.

Leshner, A. I. (1997). Addiction is a brain disease, and it matters. *Science*, **278**, 45-47.

Levy, N. (2011). Addiction, responsibility, and ego depletion. In J. Poland & G. Graham (Eds.), *Addiction and Responsibility*. Cambridge, MA: MIT Press, pp. 89-111.

Levy, N. (2013). Addiction is not a brain disease (and it matters). *Frontiers in Psychiatry*, **4**, 24. In J. Poland & G. Graham (Eds.), *Addiction and Responsibility*. Cambridge, MA: MIT Press, pp. 89-111.

McLaughlin, B. & Bennett, K. (2018). Supervenience. In E. N. Zalta (Ed.), *The Stanford Encyclopedia of Philosophy* (Spring 2018 Edition). https://plato.stanford.edu/archives/spr2018/entries/supervenience/

Millikan, R. G. (1989). In defense of proper functions. *Philosophy of Science*, **56**, 288-302.

Millikan, R. G. (2017). *Beyond Concepts: Unicepts, Language, and Natural Information*. Oxford: Oxford University Press.

Morris, T. (2011). Interview with a Philosopher: Aristotle and Wittgenstein walk into a bar - Philosophy and addiction. *Huffington Post*. 10/12/2011. www.huffingtonpost.com/tom-morris/philosophy-and-addiction_b_999933.html

Morse, S. (2000). Hooked on hype: Addiction and responsibility. *Law and Philosophy*, **19**, 3-49.

Murphy, D. (2017). Philosophy of psychiatry. In E. N. Zalta (Ed.), *The Stanford Encyclopedia of Philosophy* (Spring 2017 Edition). https://plato.stanford.edu/archives/spr2017/entries/psychiatry/

Nagel, E. (1961). *The Structure of Science*. London: Routledge and Kegan Paul.

Nagel, T. (1979). Moral luck. In *Mortal Questions*. Cambridge: Cambridge University Press, pp. 24-38.

Nordenfelt, L. (2018). Functions and health: Towards a praxis-oriented conception of health. *Biological Theory*, **13**, 10-16.

Paul, L. A. (2015a). What you can't expect when you're expecting. *Res Philosophica*, **92**, 1-23.

Paul, L. A. (2015b). *Transformative Experience*. Oxford: Oxford University Press.

Pickard, H. (2009) Mental illness is indeed a myth. In L. Bortolotti & M. Broome (Eds.), *Psychiatry as Cognitive Science: Philosophical Perspectives*. Oxford: Oxford University Press, pp. 83-101.

Pickard, H. (2012). The purpose in chronic addiction. *AJOB Neuroscience*, **3**, 40-49.

Pickard, H. (2016). Addiction. In K. Timpe, M Griffith & N. Levy (Eds.), *The Routledge Companion to Free Will*. London: Routledge, pp. 454-468.

Pickard, H. (2017). Responsibility without blame for addiction. *Neuroethics*, **10**, 169-180.

Pickard, H. (2018). The puzzle of addiction. In H. Pickard & S. H. Ahmed (Eds.), *The Routledge Handbook of Philosophy and Science of Addiction*. London: Routledge.

Pickard, H. & Pearce, S. (2014). Addiction in context: Philosophical lessons from a personality disorder clinic. In N. Levy (Ed.), *Addiction and Self-Control: Perspectives from Philosophy, Psychology, and Neuroscience*. Oxford: Oxford University Press, pp. 165-189.

Plato (2003). *The Republic (Penguin Classics Edition)*, trans. H. D. P. Lee. London: Penguin.

Plato (2005). *Phaedrus (Penguin Classics Edition)*, trans. C. Rowe. London: Penguin.

Plato (2009). *Protagoras (Oxford World's Classics)*, trans. C .C. W. Taylor. Oxford: Oxford University Press.

Pober, J. M. (2013). Addiction is not a natural kind. *Frontiers in Psychiatry*, **4**, 123.

Quine, W. V. (1969). Natural kinds. *Ontological Relativity & Other Essays*. New York: Columbia Press.

Radoilska, L. (2013). *Addiction and Weakness of Will*. Oxford: Oxford University Press.

Ross, D. Sharp, C., Vuchinich, R. E. & Spurrett, D. E. (2012). *Midbrain Mutiny: The Picoeconomics and Neuroeconomics of Disordered Gambling: Economic Theory and Cognitive Science*. Cambridge, MA: MIT Press.

Schaffer, J. (2009). On what grounds what. In D. Manley, D. J. Chalmers & R. Wasserman (Eds.), *Metametaphysics: New Essays on the Foundations of Ontology*. Oxford: Oxford University Press, pp. 347-383.

Segal, G. (2013). Alcoholism, disease, and insanity. *Philosophy, Psychiatry, & Psychology*, **20**, 297-315.

Sinnott-Armstrong, W. & Pickard, H. (2013). What is addiction? In K. W. M. Fulford, M. Davies, R. T. Gipps, G. Graham, J. Z. Sadler, G. Stanghellini & T. Thornton (Eds.), *The Oxford*

Handbook of Philosophy and Psychiatry. Oxford: Oxford University Press, pp. 851–864.

Soble, A. G. (2002). Correcting some misconceptions about St. Augustine's sex life. *Journal of the History of Sexuality,* **11**, 545–569.

Sripada, C. S. (2018), Addiction and fallibility. *Journal of Philosophy,* **115**, 569–587.

Sterelny, K. & Griffiths, P. E. (1999). *Sex and Death: An Introduction to Philosophy of Biology.* Chicago: University of Chicago Press.

Stotz, K. & Griffiths, P. E. (2016). A niche for the genome. *Biology and Philosophy,* **31**, 143–157.

Szasz, T. (1960). The myth of mental illness. *American Psychologist,* **15**, 113–118.

Szasz, T. (2006). Defining disease: The Gold Standard of Disease versus the Fiat Standard of Diagnosis. *The Independent Review,* **10**, 325–336.

Trancas, B., Borja Santos, N. & Patrício, L.D. (2004). O Uso do Ópio na Sociedade Romana e a Dependência do *Princeps* Marco Aurélio. *Acta Médica Portuguesa,* **21**, 581–590.

Virchow, R. (1860). *Cellular Pathology as based upon Physiological and Pathological Histology.* London: John Churchill.

Vrecko, S. (2010). "Civilizing Technologies" and the control of deviance. *BioSocieties,* **5**, 36–51.

Wakefield, J. C. (1992). The concept of mental disorder: On the boundary between biological facts and social values. *American Psychologist,* **47**, 373–388.

Watson, G. (1999). Excusing addiction. *Law and Philosophy,* **18**, 589–619.

Williams, B. A. O. (1976). Moral luck. *Proceedings of the Aristotelian Society,* Supplementary volumes, **50**, 115–135.

Whitehead, A. N. (1929). *Process and Reality: An Essay in Cosmology. Gifford Lectures Delivered in the University of Edinburgh During the Session 1927–1928.* Cambridge: Cambridge University Press.

Wittgenstein, L. (1953). *Philosophical Investigations.* Oxford: Blackwell.

Yaffe, G. (2011). Lowering the bar for addicts. In J. Poland & G. Graham (Eds.), *Addiction and Responsibility.* Cambridge, MA: MIT Press, pp. 113–138.

Yaffe, G. (2013). Are addicts akratic? Interpreting the neuroscience of reward. In N. Levy (Ed.), *Addiction and Self-Control: Perspectives from Philosophy, Psychology, and Neuroscience.* Oxford: Oxford University Press, pp. 190–213.

Part II

Clinical and Research Methods in the Addictions

5 Human Neurobiological Approaches to Hedonically Motivated Behaviors

Kyle S. Burger, PhD, MPH, RD, Grace E. Shearrer, PhD, and Jennifer R. Sadler, BA

Introduction

The goal of this chapter is to provide the reader with a concrete understanding of the neuroimaging techniques used for evaluating hedonically motivated behaviors, such as addictions, primarily focusing on aspects of functional magnetic resonance imaging (fMRI) data. Here, we present an overview of general study designs and neuroimaging methods, including discussion of each methods' strengths and weaknesses. This chapter also describes the application of various study designs to addiction research and opportunities to improve the field. The chapter concludes with a discussion of neurobehavioral theories of addiction and how they are assessed using neuroimaging techniques.

Overarching Study Designs: Strengths and Limitations

After determining a research question and defining a-priori hypotheses, research design is the critical determinant of the type of inferences one can draw from a neuroimaging study. Before delving into the variety of neuroimaging approaches discussed throughout this chapter, it is pertinent to briefly discuss how basic study designs can be applied in neurobiological research.

Cross-Sectional, Between-Group Designs

Cross-sectional research designs typically comprise multiple groups with no temporal component. Since participants are evaluated at a single moment of time, this design tests for existing differences between groups or conditions rather than changes following intervention or treatment. The cross-sectional design can measure differences among a group of people on specific characteristics, such as correlating drug use frequency with a health outcome. Also, this design can measure differences between groups of people defined by specific characteristics, such as comparing a health outcome between a group of drug users versus a group of nonusers.

To date, the majority of neuroimaging-based studies are cross-sectional. Neuroimaging techniques can be expensive and invasive, so cross-sectional study designs are often used to minimize the number of measurements an individual must complete. Valuable information can be gained in these designs, yet the limitations are considerable. Typically, due to the cost, sample sizes are small, which can increase the likelihood of an unknown third variable confounding the observed results. Moreover, the within-subject test-retest reliability, or temporal satiability, of neuroimaging techniques has been questioned in recent discussions of neuroimaging research (e.g., Haller & Bartsch, 2009). If neuroimaging results lack temporal stability, taking a "snapshot" of brain response over a single imaging session may produce highly variable results that do not generalize to responses that occur when participants are not being observed. For example: is brain response during exposure to alcohol cues while in a brain imaging scan similar to a response seen in the "real world" or is it more representative of the individuals state at the time of the scan? With a single timepoint, it is challenging to answer this question.

Cohort/Longitudinal Designs

Cohort/longitudinal study designs are, typically, conducted over a period of time, involving a group of individuals selected from a larger population. The sample is recruited to be representative of the population of interest for that study. The population of interest may have a wide breadth (e.g., college students) or be focused on variables of interest (e.g., young adults with parents that have a history of a substance use). Typically, cohort studies test for how sample characteristics at baseline predict the emergence of an outcomes of interest (prospective), or how current characteristics relate to an event/exposure that occurred in the past (retrospective).

Relative to cross-sectional designs, there are few neuroimaging cohort studies in the literature. However, the *brain-as-predictor* approach, particularly in longitudinal cohort studies, is becoming increasingly popular (Berkman and Falk, 2013). In the *brain-as-predictor* approach in longitudinal research, the cohort completes a baseline neuroimaging assessment, and then behavioral outcomes are measured over a follow-up period that extends beyond the initial study session. Neuroimaging data can then be used to understand and predict behavior measured at follow-up. While the *brain-as-predictor* approach does not necessary require a longitudinal study design, it is best utilized in these designs. Similar to cross-sectional studies, sample sizes for longitudinal/cohort studies are typically small. This can be a particular concern, as participants will drop out of the study over time. With a smaller sample sizes, this loss to follow-up can reduce the power of the experiment and, in worse-case scenarios, bias the outcomes. Therefore, longitudinal/cohort studies must recruit a larger sample, assuming some participants will be lost to follow-up.

Experimental/Quasi-Experimental Designs

Experimental designs, such as a randomized controlled trials (RCT), are studies where participants are randomly assigned to an experimental condition or control condition. Experimental designs should be used when three criteria of a relationship between an independent variable (cause) and outcome (effect) are met: (1) there is observational evidence that the cause precedes effect (called temporal precedence); (2) there is consistency in the causal relationship (the cause will always lead to the same effect); and (3) the magnitude of the correlation between cause and effect is large. These three criteria are suggestive of a causal relationship, so an experimental study design can be applied to test causality. The classic experimental design randomly assigns individuals or subjects to an experimental group and a control group. The independent variable is administered to the experimental group as a "treatment" and is not given to the control group. Both groups are measured on the same outcome before and after treatment or placebo. Quasi-experimental designs have treatments and outcome measures, but do not use random assignment. Without randomization, quasi-experiments provide less support for inferences of causality. There are typically two types of quasi-experiments: (1) those that lack a control group or lack a pretest on the outcome of interest (e.g., multiple baseline designs) and (2) those that use control groups and pretests but lack random assignment. Most commonly, quasi-experimental designs are used when it is unethical to randomly assign individuals to treatment or control groups. For example, it would be unethical to randomly assign individuals to take a life-saving medication or a placebo medication.

The greatest strength of an experimental design is that individuals can serve as their own control, since measurement is taken before and after experimental manipulation. However, for neuroimaging research, using this "self-as-control" approach can inflate error, due to low test-retest reliability of the neuroimaging measurements as previously discussed. In experimental designs, this can be compounded by an order effect, where the experience of being scanned in the preintervention session influences the data systematically when compared to the second scanning session, since participants have experience with the measurement at the second session. This is particularly troublesome in MRI and PET environments, where the scanning environment may induce more stress at the first session (i.e., unfamiliar large machine, unfamiliar loud noises, apprehension about task performance). This stress diminishes with subsequent scanning and familiarity with the scanning environment or task. Given these challenges, few neuroimaging-based studies use experimental/quasi-experimental designs (e.g., Benedict et al., 2012; Burger, 2017). Careful planning when designing these experiments can address some of the issues e.g., scanning control groups, mock scanning), nevertheless consideration of the unique vulnerabilities to bias when using neurobiological approaches in experiments is warranted.

Neuroimaging Techniques

In this section, we discuss the various neuroimaging approaches used to provide insight into human brain response in addiction research (Blum et al., 1996; Volkow et al., 2009; Wang et al., 2004). This discussion primary focuses on functional magnetic resonance imaging (fMRI) and its comparison to other brain assessment techniques. We also describe many of the design considerations needed for a robust fMRI experiment, the strengths and weakness of fMRI, and opportunities to improve the field.

Functional Magnetic Resonance Imaging

Over the past 20 years, fMRI has been the most common method to experimentally assess human brain function, in particular addiction, psychiatric, and eating-related research (Babbs et al., 2013; Benedict et al., 2012; Berridge, 2012; Crockford et al., 2005; Dawe & Loxton, 2004; Wang et al., 2004). Functional MRI measures localized changes in metabolic activity (the uptake and release of oxygen due to metabolic needs of the surrounding tissue) that reflect neural action called the blood oxygen level dependent (BOLD) response. BOLD response is considered a proxy for brain activity. Activity firing neurons require more oxygen via increased local blood. As such, the oxyhemoglobin (oxygen-rich) concentration increases and the deoxyhemoglobin concentration decreases in the region where neuronal activation occurs. Oxyhemoglobin and deoyhemoglobin have differential magnetic properties (diamagnetic and paramagnetic respectively).

The MRI measures BOLD response by applying a radiofrequency pulse to all atoms in its magnetic field (B0; for fMRI this is the strength of the magnet used, usually between 1.5 T and 7 T (tesla) units), then measuring the magnetic signal that is emitted as the atoms realign ("relax" or "dephase") to the magnetic field. Changes in the ratio of oxyhemoglobin to deoxyhemoglobin manifest as alterations to the magnetic signal. This allows fMRI to detect regional brain activity in regions where change from oxygenated to deoxygenated blood is the strongest. Physiologically, this change is greater in active tissues. For example, the muscles of someone running produce a greater BOLD response than the muscles of someone sitting, as running requires an increase in oxygen supply to the leg muscles. Similarly, firing neurons require more oxygen than those at rest due to high metabolic activity. While it is well-established that increased blood flow relates to neural firing, the exact mechanism is not fully understood, though it is likely caused by increased uptake of glutamate in astrocytes (star-shaped glial cells of the central nervous system). Functional MRI *evoked* paradigms expose the brain to stimuli and ideally excite specific parts of the brain invoking a BOLD response. For example, a person pushing a button in their right hand with their eyes closed should have a greater BOLD response in their left motor cortex, as that part of the brain is required for the button push. At the same time, activity in the occipital cortex will not increase because participants are not receiving visual stimuli. Further, because the brain is constantly working, BOLD responses can also be assessed during rest (resting state fMRI; rsfMRI), which provide information about basal brain activity independent of specific stimuli.

In health-related cognitive research, functional images are typically collected using echo planar imaging (EPI). This approach has been frequently used in drug addiction, smoking, gambling, and disordered eating (Frank et al., 2012; Goldstein et al., 2009; Goudiraan et al., 2010; Potenza et al., 2003). EPIs acquire slices of brain images, repeatedly, every few seconds, to then reconstruct whole brain images over time. Consider slicing a loaf of bread into hundreds of slices, and then reconstructing these slices to form the same loaf of bread; this is what EPI does with brain activity. During one scan session, hundreds of EPI images are acquired, allowing for the statistical power to detect a ~2 percent to 3 percent change in BOLD signal associated with response to stimuli. As these assessments can last up to an hour or beyond, the session is typically broken down into "runs" that are considerably shorter. This allows for the participants to relax momentarily between runs to reduce fatigue, and provide feedback to the researcher over the intercom. A common repetition time (TR) is two seconds (2 s). This time refers to the amount of time it will take to obtain a whole brain image in three dimensions (3D). As mentioned, the individual whole brain image is acquired in slices. Across various studies, these slices can be different thicknesses, have intentional gaps, and can be assessed in different orders (e.g., interleaved, ascending, descending). Owing to their rapid acquisition, EPI images are of average quality and prone to various types of artifacts, including head movement, irregularities in the magnetic field, and scanner drift over time. To account for these problems, techniques for fMRI acquisition are rapidly advancing. For example, some techniques that were commonplace around five years ago are considered outdated or less preferable today. With these rapid changes in the "gold-standard" for fMRI methods, researchers must be as clear as possible when reporting fMRI techniques in publications, allowing for the reader to truly understand the parameters of the experiment. Outlined below are a few critical choice points in fMRI acquisition that should be considered when designing an imaging study and be reported on in publications (Haller & Bartsch, 2009; Poldrack et al., 2008).

- Scanner attributes, such as the magnetic field strength, given in tesla (T) and the scanner manufacturer and product name, e.g., Siemens TIM/Trio.
- The Rx (head) coil, e.g., a twelve-channel phased-array coil, a sixteen-leg birdcage coil. In the case of a custom head coil, a detailed description should be used.
- The pulse sequence type (gradient/spin echo EPI/spiral).
- The field of view, the distance over which an MR image is acquired typically presented in mm.
- The slice order, for example *interleaved*, descending, ascending, any interslice gap (in mm), slice thickness and the orientation.
- The TE (echo time), the time from the center of the radio-frequency pulse to the center of the echo.
- The TR, the repetition time of the sequence.
- The flip angle, the amount of rotation the net magnetization experiences during the RF pulse; typically presented in degrees.
- The number of acquisitions per run, the total number of runs, total number of stimuli (if applicable) and the total time in the scanner.

Resting-State fMRI

Resting-state fMRI (rsfMRI) assesses intrinsic activity while the brain is "resting." During data collection, participants typically are asked to remain still with their eyes open, allow their mind to wander, avoid thinking about specific daily tasks or list making, and to fixate on a fixation cross displayed on a screen. Response in resting-state fMRI is often examined in the context of connectivity. Resting-state connectivity is commonly quantified by measuring the synchronization of low-frequency BOLD fluctuations across pairs of brain regions of interest (ROIs). This is done by using correlation coefficients, or can be derived via data-driven techniques such as Independent Components Analyses (ICA). Regions that show temporal connectivity are described as "functionally connected" (e.g., Koob & Volkow, 2010; Liu et al., 2009) Functional connections can be transformed into networks of connectivity. The topology of these networks can be described or compares across groups of subjects.

Structural Magnetic Resonance Imaging (sMRI)

Unlike the above-mentioned research methods, structural magnetic resonance imaging (sMRI) images the anatomy of the brain. The identification of structural phenotypes and alterations in the brain has become increasingly important in the study of addiction and psychiatric diseases (Goldstein & Volkow, 2011; Koehler et al., 2015). Similar to the process of assessing BOLD response during an fMRI, structural MRI differentiates between tissues by the rate at which protons in the tissues return to their equilibrium state after excitation from a RF pulse. Tissues that contain more fat, specifically white matter, show a different rate of return than tissues containing more water, like gray matter. This allows the sMRI to differentiate between the two types of tissues. In sMRI, there are two commonly used image types, T1- and T2-weighted images. A T1-weighted image measures the time for spinning protons to realign with the external magnetic field (the field strength of the magnet, usually 1.5 T to 7 T; spin-lattice relaxation), which is assessed by changing the TR. A T2-weighted image is a measure of the time for protons to decay in the transverse plane (spin–spin relaxation; imagine the time a tether ball takes to spin all the around a pole where the pole is the magnetic field and the ball is the spinning proton; this is essentially spin–spin relaxation), which is done by changing the TE. Typically, T1-weighted images are produced by using short TE and TR times, relative to the longer TE and TR times associated with T2-weighted images.

A T1-weighted image can be used to assess aspects of the cerebral cortex and differentiate between gray and white matter. In contrast, a T2-weighted image is useful for assessing inflammation, because it produces a better image of fluid in the brain. It is easy to differentiate between T1- and T2-weighted images as the cerebral spinal fluid (CSF) is very bright on T2-weighted images, though different sequences and suppression techniques can be applied that alter the brightness of structures. Structural MRI images can be used to identify causes of cognitive impairment, and have become key in understanding underlying structural correlates of aberrant behavioral patterns, such as addiction. The typical analytic approaches used with sMRI are: voxel-based morphometry (VBM), a technique that allows investigation of specific differences in brain anatomy, such as gray matter or white matter volume or density, and cortical thickness, an approach that focuses on estimating the thickness of grey matter on the cerebral cortex. These analytic approaches are discussed in detail later in this chapter.

Positron-Emission Tomography (PET) Imaging

Positron-emission tomography (PET) is a functional imaging approach used to directly observe metabolic processes within the brain, for example in the context of addiction (Fowler et al., 1998; Martinez et al., 2009; Volkow et al., 2001; Wilcox et al., 2010). Unlike fMRI, PET is a direct measure of neuronal function. It directly assesses cerebral blood flow (CBF) and receptor binding. This is accomplished by administering a radioactive tracer (positron-emitting radionuclide) that is taken up by blood cells. Blood flow, marked by the tracer, is then detected by pairs of gamma rays administered in the PET scanner. Similar to fMRI, a 3D image of tracer concentration in the brain can be constructed with computer analyses. This 3D image is used to assess a variable of interest, such as dopamine-receptor binding. Recent advances in PET imaging have allowed for simultaneous fMRI BOLD assessment and PET CBF, capitalizing on the strengths of both techniques.

Electroencephalogram (EEG) / Magnetoencephalography (MEG)

An electroencephalogram (EEG) is a noninvasive technique that records electrical patterns (brain waves) in the brain. These patterns represent regional brain function. During an EEG, small electrodes are attached to the participant's head. The electrodes detect brain waves, then the EEG machine amplifies the signal, and records the signal in a wave pattern on graph paper or a computer screen. EEG is limited, measuring subcortical activity. Similar to EEG, magnetoencephalography (MEG) is a functional neuroimaging method that assesses brain activity via recording magnetic fields produced by electrical currents. This noninvasive technique uses sensitive magnetometers that are placed around the head. Arrays of superconducting quantum interference devices (SQUIDs) are a common type of magnetometer. Similar to EEG, MEG is used to test basic research questions about cognitive brain processes. In particular, MEG is used to localize regions affected by stimuli or regions that drive a behavior. It also is used as an etiological tool to determine the function of various parts of the brain, and response to neurofeedback. An example of neurofeedback includes a task where participants who are in recovery from a substance use disorder are instructed to inhibit cravings as they view images of drug paraphernalia while undergoing an MEG scan. The MEG can provide real-time feedback by measuring response in the prefrontal cortex, and showing participants a "progress bar" that increases as they exert cognitive control, as measured by an increase in prefrontal response. This can be applied in a clinical setting to strengthen the effectiveness of interventions, as well as in an experimental setting to measure brain activity.

Both EEG and MEG measure electricity generated by brain function, but do not assess thoughts or feelings, per se. More accurately, they assess physiological correlates that are associated with affective or arousal states, physiological differences between groups, or brain patterning during the performance of behaviors. Of note, unlike transcranial magnetic stimulation (TMS), EEG and MEG do not send any electricity into the brain to manipulate brain function. Clinically, these measures are most often used to determine the type and origin of seizures, but also are used heavily in research. The noninvasive nature, relative ease of use, and the low cost of assessment make these approaches attractive for research; however, these two methods can only assess activity occurring in the cortex.

Comparison of Functional Neurological Measurement Techniques

There are several distinct advantages to fMRI relative to other approaches for neurological assessment. Unlike positron-emission tomography (PET), fMRI is performed in standard MRI scanners and does not require radioactive contrast agents, allowing for a less-invasive assessment and the ability to study young adults and children. Because fMRI does not use a radioactive tracer, repeated assessments can be completed without concern of frequent exposure to radioactive materials. Unlike electroencephalogram (EEG) imaging and magnetoencephalography (MEG) imaging, which only assess cortical activity, and PET imaging, which targets specific receptors, fMRI involves whole brain coverage. Functional MRI also is highly flexible in the type of experimental conditions it allows. Response to sound, visual cues, taste, smell, and touch all are used with fMRI.

Despite these advantages, fMRI does have notable drawbacks. The spatial and temporal resolution, or the spatial clarity of the images and how quickly it can assess repeated images, is lacking. Functional MRI has a spatial resolution of approximately one millimeter (1 mm), which is inferior in clarity relative to other imaging techniques. More importantly, fMRI measures a proxy of cerebral blood flow (CBF), not CBF or receptor binding itself. Unlike EEG/MEG, BOLD response lags behind the underlying neuronal events by seconds, due to slow vascular response. Thus, to assess time-dependent response to a stimulus, BOLD response must be mapped onto a standard function for hemodynamic response. As such, fMRI is considered to be lackluster for studying fast, dynamic spread of neuronal activations across brain areas. When using a 3 T magnet for fMRI measurement, a trade-off between the temporal resolution and its spatial resolution exists. The introduction of stronger magnetic field magnets, e.g., 7 T, allows for increased spatial resolution and/or increased temporal resolution. However, these advances in technology also come at a cost, specifically, the impact of head motion. Head motion can greatly influence the quality of fMRI images, because it registers as false BOLD activity. Head motion acts as a confounder. Increasing the spatial resolution of a scan from $2 \times 2 \times 2$ mm to $1 \times 1 \times 1$ mm can inflate the impact of small, involuntary movements. Moreover, increasing the temporal resolution by increasing frequency at which images are acquired can also inflate in the negative impact of motion. With higher temporal resolution, movement "spikes" in BOLD response will span across multiple slices, resulting in more false responses in the 3D images. Multiple techniques can be implemented to counteract the impact of motion during acquisition. For example, Prospective Acquisition CorrEction (PACE), is a technique that adjusts the slice position and orientation, as well as regrids residual volume to volume motion in real-time during data acquisition. Postacquisition, motion correction is applied during preprocessing of fMRI data by identifying and deweighting individual scans/runs within which motion spikes occurred. Also, during preprocessing, measures of motion are regressed out of data to reduce confounding effects. Sometimes even elimination of participants is used to prevent the undue effects of motion; however, each of these adjustments changes the data and reduces the accuracy of results. The elimination of scans/runs/subjects due to motion also contributes to the most pervasive issue in fMRI research, inadequate power. Beyond adding more subjects or increasing the number of scans performed on any given subject, careful design of the paradigm (type and sequence of stimuli exposure) is the best way to maximize the efficacy of the signal from each participant while avoiding excessive motion.

fMRI Paradigm Design and Stimuli

The fMRI paradigms frequently use visual, auditory, gustatory, or other stimuli to induce one or more cognitive states during a scan. Evoked paradigms (block and event-related, as discussed below) present multiple conditions to *evoke* a response. For example, researchers might use a two-condition paradigm to test hypotheses about brain response to drug images. One condition is the variable of interest (e.g., images of drugs), while the other is the control condition (e.g., images of tools). A direct contrast of the conditions is completed.

One key component of the paradigm design is the impact of the "baseline" exposure. Frequently, the baseline is a fixation cross on a visual screen, or no stimuli. Depending on the analytic approach and the contrast of interest, an accurate representation of baseline activity can be very important. Beyond the baseline activity, there are a number of "rules of thumb" about the required number of events, or instances that a single stimulus or set of stimuli are presented, to see a reliable response. Power analysis tools and fMRI design optimization programs are currently the best approach to determine the required number of events and how to order events within the paradigm. Below are brief descriptions of typical fMRI paradigms.

Block fMRI Designs. In a block design, the events are arranged to present the experimental and control conditions, with each block typically being often 10–15 s in length, but occasionally longer. During a block, the participant experiences the stimuli for an extended period. For example, in a visual experiment, a participant may be asked to examine a piece of art projected on a screen for a 30 s block. After the block, the participant often will see a "null" image, such as a cross-hair for a small period of time (5 s), before starting the next block of looking at art. The block design is optimal for detecting activation, because its long exposure allows response reflecting actual blood flow to be captured. Additionally, a block design is needed for dynamic functional connectivity analyses and other emerging dynamic analytic techniques because it best captures change over time. The duration of the stimuli exposure spans acquisition of multiple images, so in a block design the number of stimuli presented can be less than event-related designs to adequately model the BOLD signal.

Event-Related fMRI Designs. Event-related designs are better suited to characterize the strength and timing of BOLD in response to a stimulus. In the event-related designs, stimuli and/or task related events (both experimental and control) can be very brief and occur between nonconstant interstimuli-intervals via jitters. A jitter is similar to the null image described above but, rather than lasting a fixed period, the jitter is variable in how long it occurs. Commonly, the mean jitter is recommended to last one-third of the total event time. Therefore, if an event lasts 9 s, the mean jitter will be 3 s. An individual jitter in this example could be 2 s or 5 s, as long as the mean across the paradigm is 3 s. In event-related designs, a longer baseline is important as it allows the BOLD response to return more fully to the baseline before the onset of the next event (the jitter is included in this time). Unlike block designs, the duration of the stimuli exposure in event-related designs can be a little as a fraction of a second. Also, compared to a block design, more events are required to effectively model the BOLD signal in event related designs.

Passive and Behaviorally Active fMRI Paradigms. In addition to the type of stimuli presentation (block or event related), fMRI paradigms can be either passive or behaviorally active. During passive paradigms, the participant simply observes/receives the stimuli. For example, a participant viewing images of alcohol, rewarding/aversive images, receiving puffs of air, or administration of a cold object all constitute passive paradigms. Conversely, behaviorally active paradigms require the participant to interact in real time while being exposed to, or in response to, the stimuli presented. Typically, behaviorally active fMRI paradigms are adapted from tasks that are performed outside of the scanner to meet the timing/stimuli requirements of an fMRI paradigm. An example of a behaviorally active task is a stop signal task, in which the participant is told to press a button when they see an object on the screen, but to withhold a button press if they see a second object. This task requires the participant to actively engage with the paradigm while in the magnet. More in-depth examples of both passive and behavioral paradigms follow.

Sample Passive fMRI Paradigm. In one example, researchers would like to assess the neural responses to substance-related cues, so they employ a basic visual cue fMRI paradigm. In the task, participants view the visual cues on a head-coil-mirror system in the fMRI scanner. The paradigm includes substance-related cues subdivided into six categories related to: (1) beer, (2) wine, (3) hard liquor, (4) cannabinoids, (5) stimulants, and (6) depressants. Also included is a series of control stimuli that would consist of objects used for arts and crafts (paint brush, clay). There are twenty events of interest presented per category, resulting in 120 events of drug stimuli and forty events of control images, totalling 160 events. Images are presented in a hybrid block and event related design. Each image presented for 6 s followed by a 2–4 s jitter, during which a fixation cross appears, representing one event. All images in a category are presented together, represented a block of similar stimuli. The order of the blocks is randomized to prevent prediction of stimuli and decrease boredom. These stimuli are presented in two runs, and the stimuli blocks are counterbalanced across participants to protect against order effects by runs. The analyses evaluate BOLD response to drug cues by contrasting response during presentation of drug images versus response during presentation of the control images.

Sample Behaviorally Active fMRI Paradigms. As a first example, researchers would like to assess the neural responses during decision processes of an immediate versus delayed reward, so they perform a delay discounting task. Specifically, the task assesses the BOLD response to the magnitude and delay of a future reward. On any given trial, subjects choose between (1) an immediate reward, which always offers a reward magnitude of \$10.00 at a delay of 0 days and (2) a future reward that varies over seven amounts (\$10.00, \$10.50, \$11.00, \$13.00, \$15.00, \$20.00, and \$25.00) and six delays (0, 7, 30, 60, 90, and 180 days). During the task, the first screen presents the immediate option for 2 s. Next, the magnitude of the future option is presented for 2 s, followed by the delay of the future option displayed for another 2 s. The next screen prompts participants to choose between the immediate or future option with the appearance of left and right arrows (2 s), which corresponds the right or left button to be pressed on a button box. A 2–6 s jitter occurs between each trial with presentation of a fixation cross. One run includes 42 trial types, such that every combination of payout magnitude and delay is presented once. Stimuli are presented in two runs, yielding a total of 84 trials. In the analysis, there are nine events of interest according to a 3×3 factorial design with payout magnitude and delay as factors: low (\$10.00, \$10.50), medium (\$11.00, \$13.00, \$15.00), and high (\$20.00, \$20.00) amount $\times$ low (0, 7 days), medium (30, 60 days), and long delays (90, 180 days).

As a second example, researchers want to examine brain response during simple cognitive reappraisal techniques for reducing hyper-responsivity of reward circuitry and increasing inhibitory region activation in response to drug cues. In this paradigm, participants attempt to manipulate their cognitive state during the scan in a craving suppression paradigm. At the start of each trial, a drug cue is shown, and one of the following instructions is presented above the picture: (1) "use," (2) "health benefits of not using," (3) "health costs of using " (4) "appearance benefits of not using," and (5) "appearance costs of using." Participants are instructed to look at the image and think about it in the manner instructed by the text. On half of the trials, participants rate how much they want to use the drug using a button box after the image and instruction are shown. A 1–4 s jitter is be presented between each picture and rating scale, during which the screen shows a cross-hair. Before scanning, the participants are familiarized with the fMRI paradigm through practice on a desktop computer, during which they receive training in use of the reappraisal strategies. Stimuli are presented in a randomized order across four counter-balanced runs. This paradigm allows for researchers to directly measure brain response during use of various strategies to elicit mental effort to not consume the drug. Similar approaches have been used for other health-related research (Boswell et al., 2018; Buhle et al., 2014; Zhao et al., 2012).

fMRI Processing and Analysis

The analysis of fMRI data is challenging. To go from raw data to the finished product requires the use of complex techniques for acquisition, image processing, and statistical modeling. The end-product of fMRI analysis is generally a statistical map showing which brain regions responded to the condition of interest contrasted against baseline. Results are then interpreted to suggest a particular cognitive or psychological process. There are several software packages available to complete fMRI data analysis that have been debated since the beginning of research focused fMRI (Morgan et al., 2007). Overall, the packages have very similar functions, but there are small differences, some of which are noted below.

The "pipeline" for fMRI data analyses includes a number of steps prior to the formation of statistical maps and analytic testing. One of the main goals of preprocessing is to minimize the impact of noise on the data. Because the BOLD contrast is small (<1 percent in many studies of higher cognitive processes), simply averaging images over the experimental and control conditions and then subtracting control response from experimental response is inadequate to reliably determine differences. Instead, noise will compete with true signal, and render false positives and negatives in the results. Noise comes from sources within the subject: head motion, cardiac and respiratory noise, and variations in brain metabolism, or from the scanner itself. Occasionally, noise can be larger than the signal of interest, so fMRI analyses use relative contrasts (experimental condition versus control condition) in analyses to detect the signal. These contrast tests result in a statistical activation map that represents the probability that the brain states significantly differ. The statistical test for a BOLD response can use a general linear model (GLM; Chen et al., 2013), cross-correlation with modeled regressors, or data-driven approaches (e.g., independent components analysis [ICA]). Similar to standard statistics, fMRI statistical models include the experimental test as well as "nuisance regressors" of no interest, such as signal drift, and head motion parameters.

After data acquisition preprocessing is required for all fMRI analyses. The steps in preprocessing typically include the following.

- Brain extraction: removal of the skull and other nonbrain head matter images ("skull stripping").
- Motion correction: the center slice is chosen as a reference, all other slices are aligned to this center slice, and the amount of alignment is measured in terms of motion in the *x*, *y*, and *z* directions. This generally is a good way to measure and account for motion, unless the center slice is very different than the rest of the scan. For example, the participant moved right at the center moment, but did not move the rest of the scan. In that case a different reference scan can be used. In general, motion correct provides six parameters than can then be used to regress out motion in the images. This can be done though the general linear model used to set up contrasts. Generally, the derivatives of the motion regressors are also included.
- Bias field (B0) correction: this corrects for inhomogeneity in the magnetic field. This requires the acquisition of field maps. In general, two field-map images are acquired, the field map and a magnitude image. Of note, the magnitude image must be skull stripped. Depending on the software used, one may additionally need to know magnet parameters like the echo-planar imaging (EPI) echo spacing, TE (echo time), and unwarp direction. Also, researchers may need to specify the percent signal loss, which represents at what threshold the signal loss in the EPI is too great for registration to get a good match between the EPI data and reference image. The field map parameters are highly depended on the type of scanner used (Siemens, GE, Philips). Special attention should be paid to what type of scanner was used to acquire the field maps when preprocessing.
- Spatial smoothing: spatial smoothing generally uses a Gaussian (normally distributed) filter with full width half maximum to reduce noise in the fMRI data, slice by slice, in millimeters. This is generally performed by averaging activity in a voxel (volumetric pixel: the 3D unit used in data analysis) with neighboring voxels. The goal of spatial smoothing is to reduce the signal-to-noise ratio. In practice, this is optimal when the area of activation is larger than the smoothing parameter. Therefore, if one is interested in a small region (for example, the nucleus accumbens), a smaller smoothing threshold should be used. Care should be taken when determining how much spatial smoothing, as it may inflate functional connectivity measurements.
- Temporal filtering: temporal filtering uses a Gaussian-weighted straight line to remove frequency artefacts. The efficacy of the temporal filter is related to TR, therefore, if the TR is too high, filtering will only remove so much noise. In general, only highpass filtering is used, meaning that only a high-frequency signal "passes." This removes low-frequency artefacts such as heartbeat, respiration, and low-frequency oscillations (equipment noise). Lowpass filtering is possible, in which high-frequency signals are removed. Care should be taken with lowpass filtering, as it can reduce a signal of interest. In general, it is not widely used. When performing resting state analyses, care should be taken in considering an appropriate highpass filter as, by definition, resting-state frequencies are lower than task-based frequencies. A highpass filter that is too aggressive could potentially remove all resting-state frequencies.
- Slice timing correction: this accounts for the fact that although researchers consider the 4D BOLD image to be taken at a single timepoint, each slice is acquired at a slightly different time.
- Prewhitening: because the 4D image is acquired over time, each voxel is temporally correlated; this is sometimes referred to as intrinsic smoothness. In essence, a voxel is more likely to be active due to time rather than due to the experimental condition. This is particularly problematic if the task is time sensitive. Without correcting for the autocorrection in the data, conclusions can be inaccurate or invalid. During prewhitening, a statistical adjustment is applied to remove autocorrelation in fMRI data. It is particularly important for nonblock-related designs, where the correlation cannot be shaped or "colored." Jittering-event-related designs additionally reduce some autocorrelation. Depending on the software used, different statistical processes are used to account for the autocorrelation in the data. Regardless of software used, prewhitening or some form of autocorrelation correction should be used for designs with greater than 50 timepoints.
- Framewise displacement: framewise displacement refers to the change in rotation and displacement frame, per TR. This is an additional motion-correction measure. TRs with large framewise displacement can be censored or regressed out of the model like the motion correction, above. In general, the threshold for framewise displacement should be chosen based on the task or resting state.
- DVARS: the derivative of the time-course, or root mean squared variance over voxels, is an index of the rate of change in BOLD signal per frame of data, or a measure of difference of signal intensity. The use of DVARS is still being established, since there is no consensus on what difference in intensity is a cut-off for a spike, but can, within a sample, indicate possible outliers.

Debate regarding the "best" steps for preprocessing, the ideal order of steps, and the program/approach for preprocessing is ongoing and constant. As such, careful research and discussion with experts in the field is recommended before preprocessing data.

Structural MRI Processing and Analyses

Similar to fMRI, the end result of structural MRI analysis is a statistical map. However, rather than mapping the BOLD response, structural MRI aims to measure variations in tissue concentrations. Meaningful differences in tissue concentrations may be related to cognitive or psychological processes. Overall, analysis of sMRI data is more straightforward. Again, the main concern is noise reduction. Structural MRI preprocessing aims to minimize noise and improve signal differentiation between tissues. Most structural preprocessing includes the following.

- Brain extraction: need to remove the dura, eyes, and any neck images that may be present. Failure to properly skull strip can result in inflated volumetric data.
- Intensity nonuniformity: owing to B0 inhomogeneity some areas may appear artificially bright or dark. A field map can estimate the bias field and a correction can be applied. Errors in tissue intensity can lead to segmentation failures.
- Spatial normalization: all brains are slightly different. However, to perform statistical analysis and make comparisons, brains need to conform to the same shape. To do this, each individual brain needs to be fitted to a standard space. Generally, this requires two steps. First, a 12° affine transformation is completed to match overall position and size of the subject brain to the template (parallel spacing is preserved); second, a nonlinear transformation to "warp" the subject brain to the template is done, aligning the sulci and other structures. A note on templates: generally, standard templates are available (MNI, Talairach); if studying a specific population (infants, elderly, a disease state) a custom template is preferable.
- Segmentation: the purpose of this step is to define what is gray matter, white matter, and cerebral spinal fluid (CSF). This can be done using prior probability maps (maps in which the gray and white matter are known), mixed-model cluster analysis, or a combination of both. A partial-volume model is also possible using software like FSL's FAST, in which each the proportion of a tissue type is estimated per voxel.
- Modulation: because each brain is registered to a template brain, the process of "warping" the brain using nonlinear registration may induce volume changes. To correct for potential volume changes, Jacobian modulation is used to multiply the normalized tissue by its volume before and after warping.
- Smoothing: voxels are averaged with neighboring voxels, usually using an isotropic Gaussian kernel. The process of smoothing overall improves the signal-to-noise ratio and, in the process, the data become more normally distributed. Additionally, a certain amount of smoothing can compensate for imperfect registration. Care should be taken though, as too much smoothing will result in a loss of specificity in the brain.

At this point the structural data should be ready for statistical analysis. Based on the research question, a variety of methods exist to assess localized brain volumes and cortical thickness.

Voxel-Based Morphometry (VBM) Structural Analysis

Voxel-based morphometry (VBM) detects variations in regional concentrations of tissues while correcting for global brain-shape differences. Both FSL and SPM software investigates voxel-wise differences in the tissue of choice (gray or white matter) through parametric mapping. Voxel differences can be computed between hemispheres, between two or more groups, over time, to a case study, or a clinical variable. As with fMRI, a general linear model is created to assess differences in voxel intensity. Nuisance regressors can be also be added to the model; for instance, age, sex, and global brain volume (total intercranial volume). Keep in mind that potential covariates may contribute to uniformly larger or smaller brains that have the same proportion of white or gray matter; therefore, they need to be modeled to account for equally distributed differences. As with any statistical test, multiple comparisons can become an issue. Permutation testing with VBM results is possible by using FSL's RANDOMISE tool to correct for potential false positives.

Cortical-Thickness Structural Analysis

If one was to stretch and iron an adult human brain it would result in a cortical sheet about 2.5 ft^3 in area and about 3 mm thick. The thickness of the human cortex is not uniform throughout the brain, and has been shown to change with certain pathologies and age. Tissue segmentation is critical for determining cortical thickness, as it is defined as the measure between the pial matter (gray matter boundary) and the white matter boundary.

Freesurfer is an excellent tool for cortical-thickness estimation. The automatic segmentation uses information from known intensity profiles, nearest neighbor, and probability based on voxel location to assess if the voxel is white or gray matter. Control points can be added manually to improve the hard segmentation; however, the utility in doing so is subject to debate. A finite-element model is then constructed, made up of thousands of triangles that form vertices where they meet. Each vertex has a value and label in *xyz* space. The white-matter surface is created from T1 gradients and has a smoothness constraint. Pial surface "grows" from the white-matter surface, meaning that is follows both the white-matter surface and T1 gradients. Therefore, if the boundaries in the pial look poor, it may be due to poor boundaries in the white-matter surface and can be corrected with control points. Cortical thickness can be calculated as the difference between the white-matter and pial surfaces at each vertex. Finally, statistics can be performed by using a general linear model to assess differences in cortical thickness for the whole brain between subjects or correlated to behavioral or psychological variables. The output generally is a surface map of the cortex with "clusters" of significantly thick or thin areas.

Pitfalls of Neuroimaging Approaches

The reproducibility of scientific results has come under increasing scrutiny in recent years (Haller & Bartch, 2009; Vul & Pashler, 2012; Woo, Krishnan & Wager, 2014). As a result, a more-focused evaluation considers whether some common research practices can be problematic, and where these issues contribute to high rates of false findings in the scientific literature. This is particularly relevant to neuroimaging as a number of concerns become increasing unveiled during the maturation of the field. These factors include: researchers drawing inappropriate inferences from their results, general study design that may inadvertently introduce bias, low statistical power, and flexibility in data-collection approaches and analytic methods.

Inferences Drawn from Brain Imaging Studies

Interpretation results from neuroimaging studies can be challenging. The foremost error in the literature presently concerns the inferences drawn for the presented brain data. Typically, the inference drawn from (functional) neuroimaging studies is that, when a specific cognitive process occurs, a particular brain area is active and, thus, that region is responsible for that cognitive process. The underlying issue here is one of forward versus reverse inference; specifically, regarding affirming the consequent. The issues arise when there is an induction entailing reasoning backwards from the observed brain activity to a particular cognitive process not directly tested, but with which it is associated. A simple example of how this issue may arise is the thought exercise of: "I ate a lot of pizza, therefore I am full" and "I am full therefore I ate a lot of pizza." Clearly, the latter could be accurate, but fails to address alternative possibilities (e.g., other foods).

In the case of neuroimaging, forward inference is the question of what brain activity/region is associated with a given experimental condition/ cognitive function, ultimately giving information about brain functioning. While this is a rational way to interpret brain functioning, it may lead to inappropriate interpretations. Conversely, reverse inference is the question of what cognitive process/behavior, etc., is occurring given the brain activity. In essence, this is interpreting "backwards" from brain activity. Typically, the overarching goal is to infer something about unmeasured internal mental processes; yet, inferring reverse inference can lead the field in a poor direction. For example, if a "reward brain region" was active during presentation of drug cues, the researcher might report "drug cues causes reward," following this logic further, "If brain region X lights up, that means addiction, region Y means smoking cigarettes," and so on. Clearly these are inaccurate conclusions and they may also influence the research that others conduct, wasting large amounts of time and funding while researchers examine questions that do not meaningfully lead the field forward.

Low Statistical Power and Multiple Comparisons

Low power not only reduces the likelihood of finding a true result if it exists, but also raises the likelihood that any positive result is false, as well as causing substantial inflation of observed positive effect sizes (Lieberman & Cunningham, 2009; Yarkoni, 2009). When possible, all sample sizes should be justified by an a-priori power analysis. However, one must be cautious in extrapolating from effect sizes estimated from small studies, because they are almost certainly inflated. When previous data are not available to support a power analysis, one can instead identify the sample size that would support finding the minimum effect size that would be theoretically informative. The use of heuristic sample size guidelines (for example, that are based on sample sizes used in previously published studies) is likely to result in a misuse of resources, either by collecting too many or (more likely) too few subjects.

The most common approach to neuroimaging analysis involves mass univariate testing, in which a separate hypothesis test is performed for each voxel. In such an approach, the false positive rate will be inflated if there is no correction for multiple tests. The problem of multiplicity in neuroimaging analysis was recognized very early, and the past twenty-five years have seen the development of now well-established and validated methods for correction of family-wise error rate (FEW) and false discovery rate (FDR) in neuroimaging data. However, recent work has suggested that even some very well-established inferential methods (specifically, ones that are based on the spatial extent of activations) can produce inflated Type I error rates in certain settings. There is an ongoing debate between neuroimaging researchers who feel that conventional approaches to multiple comparison correction are too lax and allow too many false positives, and those who feel that thresholds are too conservative, and risk missing most of the interesting effects.

As the complexity of a software program increases, the likelihood of undiscovered bugs quickly reaches certainty. Errors are more likely to be discovered when a code has a larger user base, and larger projects are more likely to follow better software-development practices. Researchers should learn and implement good programming practices, including the judicious use of software testing and validation. Validation methodologies (such as comparing with another existing implementation or using simulated data) should be clearly defined.

Conclusions

Ultimately, the goal of human neuroimaging is to examine the relation between brain functioning and cognitive states, behaviors, and disease states. Each of the approaches discussed can provide a highly valuable insight the etiology of disorders associated with hedonically motive behaviors, including substance and behavioral addictions. It is noteworthy that a use of single-brain-imaging methodology in isolation to study aspects of addiction is relatively insufficient to understand the neural underpinnings and heterogeneity of addiction disorders. Further, each methodology provides a balance of strengths and weakness (e.g., fMRI is less invasive than PET; however, PET specifically tests receptor binding). Results from neuroimaging studies can also be misinterpreted and/or overly sensationalized. Researchers engaging in performing these studies should pay particular attention to their chosen method and make efforts to be as transparent as possible in data acquisition and statistical methods. The advent of human neuroimaging in the past 20 years has ushered in the availability to study the human brain in vivo, providing insight to the understanding of neurobiological approaches processes associated with addiction and addictive-type behaviors that previously could only be studied in "proxy" animal models. As the field of addiction research advances, there will be an increased need for cross-species research, each maximizing their relative strengths. Human imaging is a key approach in that future. Ideally, these approaches and subsequent insights will provide the foundation for more effective treatment and prevention programs.

REFERENCES

Babbs, R. K., Sun, X., Felsted, J., et al. (2013). Decreased caudate response to milkshake is associated with higher body mass index and greater impulsivity. *Physiology & Behavior*, **121**, 103–111.

Benedict, C., Brooks, S. J., O'Daly, O. G., et al. (2012). Acute sleep deprivation enhances the brain's response to hedonic food stimuli: an fMRI study. *Journal of Clinical Endocrinology and Metabolism*, **97**(3), E443–447. doi: 10.1210/jc.2011-2759

Berkman, E. T. & Falk, E. B. (2013). Beyond brain mapping using neural measures to predict real-world outcomes. *Current*

Directions in Psychological Science, **22**(1), 45–50.

Berridge, K. C. (2012). From prediction error to incentive salience: mesolimbic computation of reward motivation. *European Journal of Neuroscience*, **35**(7), 1124–1143. doi: 10.1111/j.1460-9568.2012.07990.x

Blum, K., Cull, J. G., Braverman, E. R. & Comings, D. E. (1996). Reward deficiency syndrome. *American Scientist*, **84**(2), 132–145.

Boswell, R. G., Sun, W., Suzuki, S. & Kober, H. (2018). Training in cognitive strategies reduces eating and improves food choice. *Proceedings of the National Academy of Sciences*, **115**(48), E11238–E11247.

Buhle, J. T., Silvers, J. A., Wager, T. D., et al. (2014). Cognitive reappraisal of emotion: a meta-analysis of human neuroimaging studies. *Cerebral Cortex*, **24**(11), 2981–2990.

Burger, K. S. (2017). Frontostriatal and behavioral adaptations to daily sugar-sweetened beverage intake: a randomized controlled trial. *The American Journal of Clinical Nutrition*, **105**(3), 555–563. doi: 10.3945/ajcn.116.140145

Chen, G., Saad, Z. S., Britton, J. C., Pine, D. S. & Cox, R. W. (2013). Linear mixed-effects modeling approach to fMRI group analysis. *Neuroimage*, **73**, 176–190.

Crockford, D. N., Goodyear, B., Edwards, J., et al. (2005). Cue-induced brain activity in pathological gamblers. *Biological Psychiatry*, **58**(10), 787–795.

Dawe, S. & Loxton, N. J. (2004). The role of impulsivity in the development of substance use and eating disorders. *Neuroscience and Biobehavioral Reviews*, **28**(3), 343–351. doi: 10.1016/j.neubiorev.2004.03.007

Fowler, J. S., Volkow, N. D., Ding, Y. S., et al. (1998). PET and the study of drug action in the human brain. *Pharmaceutical News*, **5**, 11–16.

Frank, G. K. W., Reynolds, J. R., Shott, M. E., et al. (2012). Anorexia nervosa and obesity are associated with opposite brain reward response. *Neuropsychopharmacology*, **37**(9), 2031–2046.

Goldstein, R. Z. & Volkow, N. D. (2011). Dysfunction of the prefrontal cortex in addiction: neuroimaging findings and clinical implications. *Nature Reviews Neuroscience*, **12**(11), 652.

Goldstein, R. Z., Tomasi, D., Alia-Klein, N., et al. (2009). Dopaminergic response to drug words in cocaine addiction. *Journal of Neuroscience*, **29**(18), 6001–6006.

Goudriaan, A. E., et al. (2010). Brain activation patterns associated with cue reactivity and craving in abstinent problem gamblers, heavy smokers and healthy controls: an fMRI study. *Addiction Biology*, **15**(4), 491–503.

Haller, S. & Bartsch, A. J. (2009). Pitfalls in fMRI. *European Radiology*, **19**(11), 2689–2706.

Koehler, S., Hasselmann, E., Wüstenberg, T., et al. (2015). Higher volume of ventral striatum and right prefrontal cortex in pathological gambling. *Brain Structure and Function*, **220**(1), 469–477. doi: 10.1007/s00429-013-0668-6

Koob, G. F. & Volkow, N. D. (2010). Neurocircuitry of addiction. *Neuropsychopharmacology*, **35**(1), 217–238. doi: http://dx.doi.org/10.1038/npp.2009.110

Lieberman, M. D. & Cunningham, W. A. (2009). Type I and Type II error concerns in fMRI research: re-balancing the scale. *Social Cognitive and Affective Neuroscience*, **4**(4), 423–428.

Liu, J., Liang, J., Qin, W., et al. (2009). Dysfunctional connectivity patterns in chronic heroin users: an fMRI study. *Neuroscience Letters*, **460**(1), 72–77. doi: 10.1016/j.neulet.2009.05.038

Martinez, D., Slifstein, M., Narendran, R., et al. (2009). Dopamine D1 receptors in cocaine dependence measured with PET and the choice to self-administer cocaine. *Neuropsychopharmacology*, **34**(7), 1774.

Morgan, V. L., Dawant, B. M., Li, Y. & Pickens, D. R. (2007). Comparison of fMRI statistical software packages and strategies for analysis of images containing random and stimulus-correlated motion. *Computerized Medical Imaging and Graphics*, **31**(6), 436–446.

Poldrack, R. A., Fletcher, P. C., Henson, R. N., et al. (2008). Guidelines for reporting an fMRI study. *Neuroimage*, **40**(2), 409–414.

Potenza, M. N., Steinberg, M. A., Skudlarski, P., et al. (2003). Gambling urges in pathological gambling: a functional magnetic resonance imaging study. *Archives of General Psychiatry*, **60**(8), 828–836. doi: 10.1001/archpsyc.60.8.828

Volkow, N., Chang, L., Wang, G. J., et al. (2001). Low level of brain dopamine D2 receptors in methamphetamine abusers: association with metabolism in the orbitofrontal cortex. *American Journal of Psychiatry*, **158**(12), 2015–2021.

Volkow, N. D., Fowler, J. S., Wang, G. J., et al. (2009). Imaging dopamine's role in drug abuse and addiction. *Neuropharmacology*, **56**, 3–8.

Vul, E. & Pashler, H. (2012). Voodoo and circularity errors. *Neuroimage*, **62**(2), 945–948.

Wang, G.-J., Volkow, N. D., Thanos, P. K. & Fowler, J. S. (2004). Similarity between obesity and drug addiction as assessed by neurofunctional imaging: a concept review. *Journal of Addictive Diseases*, **23**(3), 39–53.

Wilcox, C. E., Braskie, M. N., Kluth, J. T. & Jagust, W. J. (2010). Overeating behavior and striatal Dopamine with 6-[1 8 F]-Fluoro-L-m-Tyrosine PET. *Journal of Obesity*, **2010**, 909348.

Woo, C. W., Krishnan, A. & Wager, T. D. (2014). Cluster-extent based thresholding in fMRI analyses: pitfalls and recommendations. *Neuroimage*, **91**, 412–419.

Yarkoni, T. (2009). Big correlations in little studies: Inflated fMRI correlations reflect low statistical power – Commentary on Vul et al. (2009). *Perspectives on Psychological Science*, **4**(3), 294–298.

Zhao, L. Y., Tian, J., Wang, W., et al. (2012). The role of dorsal anterior cingulate cortex in the regulation of craving by reappraisal in smokers. *PLoS ONE*, 7(8) e43598.

6 Human Laboratory Paradigms in Addictions Research

Vanessa Morris, BA, Fiza Arshad, MS, Iris M. Balodis, PhD, Derek D. Reed, PhD, BCBA-D, James MacKillop, PhD, and Michael Amlung, PhD

Introduction

Addictive disorders continue to be a substantial public health problem. According to data from the World Health Organization (WHO), the number of people using illicit drugs between 2006 and 2015 increased by 38 million (World Health Organization, 2015). Of this, an estimated 12 million people were using drugs intravenously, and an estimated 1.65 million were infected by HIV as a result. Moreover, the WHO found that in 2012 alcohol consumption contributed to 6 percent of deaths worldwide (World Health Organization, 2015). The economic burden of alcohol and drug use is also substantial. The National Institute on Drug Abuse (NIDA) estimated that misuse of tobacco, alcohol, and illicit drugs costs in excess of $740 billion annually, including costs related to crime, lost productivity, and health care (National Institute on Drug Abuse, 2017). Behavioral addictions are also relatively common and associated with numerous negative consequences (e.g., see Sussman, 2017). As examples, meta-analysis of over 160 studies on problem gambling found that in the past year, 2.8 percent of people met criteria for gambling disorder, and 3.8 percent of people had a lifetime prevalence of problem gambling (Shaffer, Hall & Bilt, 1999). With regards to food addictions, it has been estimated that more than 5 percent of the population suffers from food addiction and that it is more than twice as likely to affect women than men (Pedram et al., 2013). Finally, an estimated 3 percent of online gamers experience symptoms of Internet Gaming Disorder (Ferguson, Coulson & Barnett, 2011) and an estimated 0.3 percent to 0.5 percent of the population struggles with exercise addiction (Mónok et al., 2012).

Taken together, these high rates of substance and behavioral addictions and their associated consequences underscore the need for additional research to identify the causes of addiction, and to develop more effective treatment and prevention programs. As such, the need for additional research studies and paradigms, especially in the realm of behavioral addictions, are essential to ameliorating the current climate of addictive disorders and their associated damage. Human laboratory research is well-suited to address this need by providing a range of cost-effective options with respect to study designs and the use of validated tasks and assessment measures.

Cues Exposure Paradigms

Background and Practical Aspects

The basic principle of a cue exposure paradigm is presentation of stimuli or cues associated with one or more addictive behaviors and examining an individual's psychological, behavioral, or physiological responses to those cues. The use of cue exposure is based on a foundation of classical conditioning (Pavlov & Anrep, 2003). Within the cue exposure paradigm, cues that are previously associated with engaging in addictive behaviors elicit subjective (e.g., craving, anxiety, pleasure), physiological (e.g., increase heart rate, salivation), and behavioral responses (e.g., drug seeking behavior). The cues act as powerful conditioned stimuli (CS) evoking a conditioned response (CR) in the individual. For example, an intravenous drug user may begin to associate a syringe with the rewarding/euphoric effects of the drug. The individual may come to associate the syringe with the subjective high so much so that eventually simply being visually exposed to the syringe evokes similar physiological responses and cravings for the high provided by the drug. In the case of behavioral addictions, for example gambling, poker chips, playing cards, or slot machines may be presented to the participant to elicit subjective, behavioral, or physiological responses.

Regardless of the type of addictive behavior being examined, most cue exposure protocols follow a similar procedure (e.g., MacKillop et al., 2012). Participants are typically asked to interact with one or more cues according to instructions provided in a script that is read aloud by a researcher. Responses to addiction-related cues are commonly compared to responses to a neutral cue condition (i.e., alcohol versus water cues). In this scenario, cue reactivity is reflected in the difference in responses to the active/experimental cue and the neutral cue. Importantly, the order of cue presentation is often not counterbalanced, with neutral cues presented first followed by the active addiction-related cues. This is because of well-established carryover effects when the active cues are presented first (MacKillop et al., 2012).

The cues used are often designed to engage multiple senses and vary in the extent to which the cues are imaginal versus physically present (see Table 6.1, top). At one end of the spectrum, imaginal cues involve participants mentally envisioning situations related to engaging in addictive behaviors. This often involves a guided imagery script that attempts to standardize the experience across participants in the study. At the other end of the spectrum are in-vivo and virtual-reality protocols that are designed to be highly immersive and realistic. These types of exposures have a number of ethical limitations that must be considered (see below). In between, visual and audio cues are commonly used to balance the realistic nature of the cues without necessarily having a physical object or stimulus present. Examples of representative visual cues are presented in Figure 6.1.

Measurement of cue reactivity during cue exposure paradigms also spans a continuum (Table 6.1, bottom). Ideally, studies should combine assessment types to capture the multifaceted nature of cue-evoked responses. For example, subjective measures of craving or desire could be paired with physiological measures such as heart rate or skin conductance. Behavioral measures such as latency to take a sip of alcohol or

Table 6.1 Common cue presentation and assessment modalities for cue exposure paradigms

Mode of cue presentation	Example
Imaginal	Ask the participant to imagine they are at a bar ordering their preferred alcoholic beverage
Photographic	Show the participants high-quality photographs related to smoking, such as cigarettes, lighters, ash trays, cigarette brand logos
Audio	Have the participant listen to a recording of casino sounds and description of a row of slot machines
Video	Have the participant watch a video of a person preparing heroin for intravenous injection
In vivo	Pouring a full glass of a person's preferred alcoholic beverage in a simulated bar laboratory environment and asking them to hold and smell the drink
Virtual Reality	Use a head-mounted virtual reality setup to immerse the person in a gambling environment such as a casino or horse track
Assessment modality	**Example**
Self-report	Craving scales, subjective affect, etc.
Neruocognitive measures	Response inhibition, attention bias, impulsivity, risk taking, behavioral economic demand, etc.
Behavioral	Drinking latency, approach/avoidance behaviors, eye tracking, etc.
Physiological	Heart rate, blood pressure, skin conductance, salivary cortisol, etc.
Neuroimaging techniques	Functional magnetic resonance imaging, electroencephalography, etc.

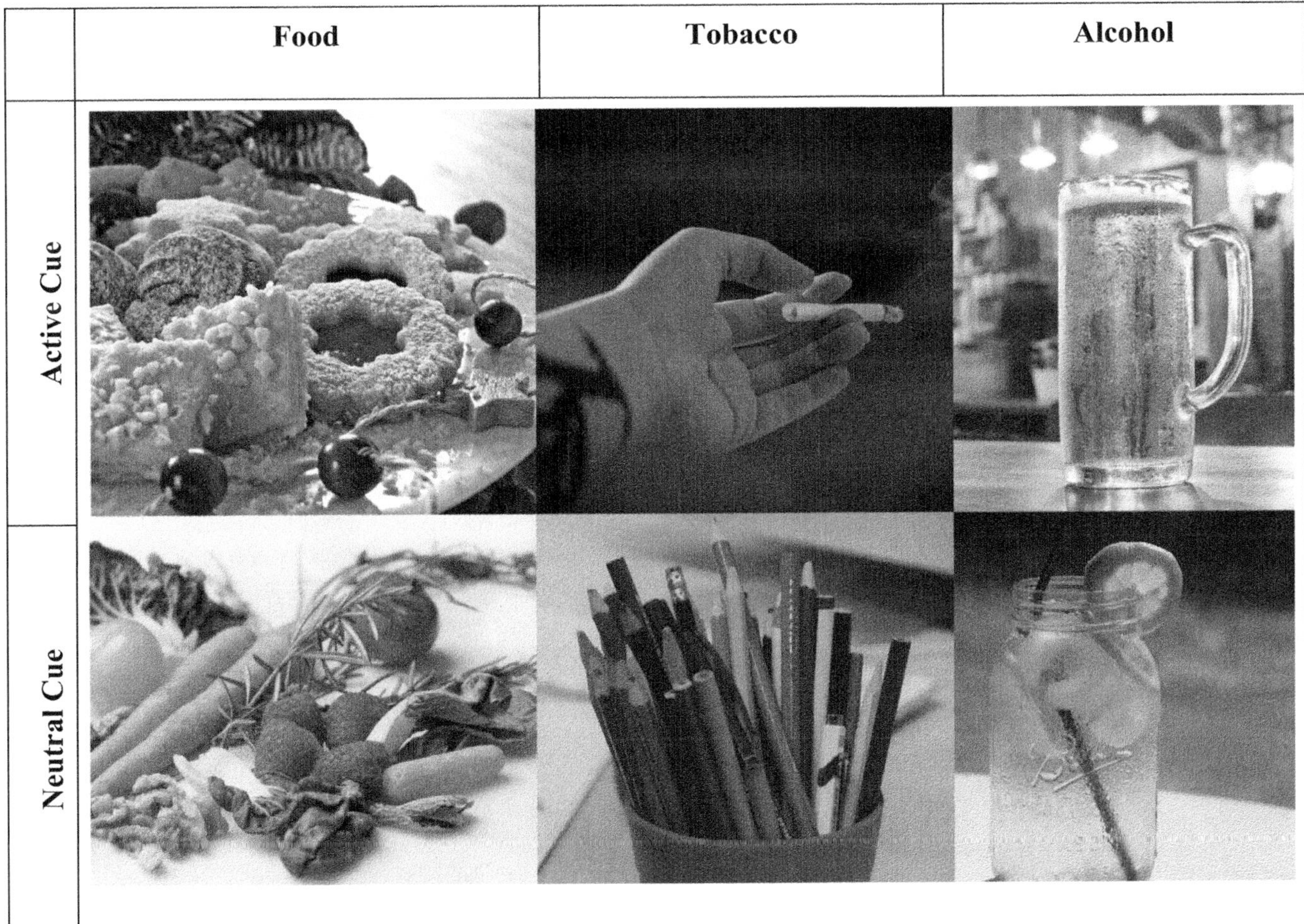

Figure 6.1 Representative photographic cues used in cue exposure paradigms

a puff of a cigarette can also be collected to provide objective measures of approach motivation. A relatively recent addition to the cue reactivity assessment repertoire includes behavioral economic demand measures. These measures assess hypothetical consumption of a substance at different levels of price and provide a measure of reinforcing value of the substance (see Jarmolowicz & Schneider, 2020; Reed et al., 2020). Initial research has shown that behavioral economic demand measures are sensitive to acute effects of addictive cues, including alcohol, tobacco, cannabis, among others (MacKillop et al., 2010, 2012; Metrik et al., 2016). Finally, neuroimaging techniques have been extensively used to examine the neural correlates of cue-elicited craving. While this technology poses unique challenges (e.g., being inside an MRI scanner), researchers have developed creative ways to provide multimodal cues during brain imaging scans. This includes standardized photo cue sets (e.g., Pulido et al., 2010) and taste cues (e.g., Filbey et al., 2007, 2008).

Ethical Considerations

Although relatively limited in terms of ethical concerns, cue exposure paradigms still have several important aspects that need to be considered, especially with regard to which groups are being studied and the types of cues being used. The majority of human laboratory studies on addictive disorders recruit participants who are either substance naive, currently using or misusing addictive substances, or in recovery from substance use disorders. Most ethical issues arise when studies seek to recruit participants who are currently in recovery. Even though a participant may have given informed consent to participate in the study, there remains the concern that being exposed to cues and stimuli associated with substance use may "trigger" the participant or encourage them to abandon their recovery. In fact, The National Advisory Guidelines state that "subjects who have achieved a sustained period of abstinence while living in the community should not be included as subjects in research involving alcohol administration" (Enoch et al., 2009).

While studying individuals in recovery is scientifically important, care must be exercised when selecting cues. For example, presenting in-vivo alcohol beverage cues in a simulated bar laboratory may be too powerful for someone in recovery. This is not to say that such research cannot be done; however, special attention should be paid to ensuring that participants are not actively craving the substance or at an increased likelihood of relapse immediately following the session. Other types of cues that are less immersive may be better suited for this population. As well, the amount of time in recovery should be considered with extreme caution. For example, one study found that even after twelve months of intensive inpatient treatment, participants with opioid-use disorder still experienced an increase in craving, feelings of depression, and anger in response to drug-related stimuli (Franken et al., 1999).

Cue exposure paradigms with participants in recovery should also include clinical safeguards, such as conducting the study in a safe and controlled environment, establishing rapport with the participant and providing a clear explanation of the study, checking-in with the participant throughout the study to assess any possible discomfort, and having personnel who are specifically trained in managing acute distress and cravings (Dolinsky & Babor, 1997).

On the other side of the spectrum, cue reactivity paradigms may recruit participants who are either substance naive or who are able to use substances moderately without any symptoms of addiction. Studying this population, or using this group as control participants, may provide important insights about why some people develop substance use disorder while others do not. Researchers may examine whether these groups display different behavioral or physiological responses to the cues and stimuli presented.

Potential Limitations

Aside from the ethical considerations and the need to critically evaluate the population of interest, cue exposure paradigms remain one of the most commonly used methods of studying human evoked responses in a laboratory setting. Before adopting a cue exposure protocol for a research study, it is critical to consider potential limitations of these approaches.

An important limitation of cue reactivity paradigms is ecological validity of the cues used, or the extent to which the cues are realistic of real-world situations. In-vivo and virtual-reality cues are highly immersive and may have increased ecological validity compared to pictorial or imagery-based cues. There is also no guarantee that all participants will be affected by the cues chosen; there may be "nonreactors," or the cue simply may not be salient to a portion of participants (Avants et al., 1995). Participants may show reduced responses because they are aware that they do not have actual access to the substances (Powell, 2006). Finally, the laboratory environment itself may impact response. Cues presented in the controlled laboratory settings may not be as stimulating as in a naturalistic setting. As with all laboratory studies, it is often difficult to elicit a typical response given that participant is not in a typical substance use environment; in fact, some authors argue that the environment is more important than the cue itself (MacKillop & Lisman, 2008). That is, the addictive behavior environment may provide a whole constellation of cues, which may be more salient than one or two cues in an otherwise novel environment.

Another potential limitation of cue exposure paradigms is related to the type of assessments used. Self-report assessments may be subject to systematic bias or demand characteristics if participants are aware of the purpose of the exposure. In addition, assessment of craving based solely on self-report has been criticized in the literature, particularly for single item measures of craving (Sayette et al., 2000). An ideal approach is to combine self-report subjective reports with arguably more objective measures such as physiological arousal or behavioral performance. Objective measures provide data irrespective of mood, demand characteristics, personality, and various other factors that can discredit subjective measures. Moreover, these assessments of physiological responses can be reassessed across time points to examine whether a participant is becoming more or less sensitive to the presented cues.

Future Directions

The majority of cue exposure studies have focused on substance use, including an extensive body of research on alcohol, tobacco, and drug cue reactivity (for meta-analyses of this literature, see Carter & Tiffany, 1999; Kuhn & Gallinat, 2011; Norberg et al., 2016). By comparison, the literature on behavioral additions and cue exposure paradigms is rather small (Sussman, 2017). One explanation for the relative lack of studies on cue reactivity in these disorders is the relative recency of their emergence in mainstream addictions research, including their inclusion in more recent editions of the DSM (APA, 2013). As attention on behavioral addictions increases, it is expected that research focusing on the role of cue reactivity in these disorders will become more prevalent. Nevertheless, several excellent examples of cue exposure paradigms have been developed for behavioral addictions. Food-related addictions are the most common (Ferrer-García et al., 2017; Maxwell, LOxton & Hennegan, 2017), followed by gambling (Balodis et al., 2012; Clark et al., 2016; Kushner et al., 2007; Park et al., 2015; Symes & Nicki, 1997), whereas behavioral addictions such as shopping, tanning, video gaming, and exercise are relatively understudied. Ferrer-García and colleagues examined the use of virtual-reality cue exposure in a group of forty eating-disorder patients who had been resistant to their initial structured cognitive-behavioral treatment (CBT) program. Results demonstrated that the use of virtual-reality cue exposure therapy had a significantly positive effect for the clinical group in behavioral features, attitude, anxiety, food craving, and abstinence rates (Ferrer-García et al., 2017).

In a gambling study, Park and colleagues used virtual-reality cue exposure to examine whether the effect of repeated gambling cues affected one's urge to gamble. The study consisted of twelve recreational gamblers who were exposed to five virtual casino environments with various casino type cues. Results demonstrated that all virtual environments and casino type cues produced increased craving and urge to gamble in the sample (Park et al., 2015).

Although cue exposure protocols have an extensive history in addictions research, several methodological and theoretical questions remain to be examined, including: improving ecological validity, establishing a clear link between elicited response and relapse, examining subtypes of participants (e.g., sex differences, nonreactors), and expanding the use of cue exposure paradigms in the context of behavioral addictions.

The most notable future direction for cue exposure paradigms would be to improve the ecological validity of the exposure itself. From a research standpoint, performing cue exposure paradigms within a laboratory setting provides researchers with the most control over the experiment and the setting; however, when one compares the laboratory setting to a real-world drug use or gambling environment, questions arise about the generalizability of the results. With regards to treatment, some authors argue that cue exposures performed in a lab or treatment setting are impractical based on the notion that cues do not generalize well to typical situations outside the laboratory (MacKillop & Lisman, 2008; Niaura, 2002; Niaura et al., 1999). Importantly, though, some studies have found that responses to cues in the lab setting do not significantly differ from those in real-life situations (Amlung et al., 2011).

Another aspect of cue exposure paradigms that needs additional study is determining the link between subjective and objective (i.e., behavioral, physiological) responses following a cue exposure and subsequent consumption or relapse. This topic has been actively debated by leading craving and cue reactivity researchers (Drummond et al., 2000). Indeed, there is limited research demonstrating a link between relapse risk and self-reported craving in response to presented cues (Abrams et al., 1988; Niaura et al., 1989). Moreover, objective responses such as heart rate, have produced inconsistent results in response to cues (Avants et al., 1995; Sayette et al., 2000; Sterling et al., 2004).

Lastly, there are a limited number of articles that have focused on individual differences in cue reactivity. First, gender differences may play an important role in cue reactivity (Niaura et al., 1989; Saladin et al., 2012). Saladin and colleagues have demonstrated that women experience greater stress, craving, and arousal in response to stressful script cues, as well as showing marginally greater levels of stress, craving and arousal in response to smoking cues (Saladin et al., 2012). Second, previous studies have identified a group of individuals termed "nonreactors" (i.e., the presented stimulus does not elicit any response) (Avants et al., 1995; Szegedi et al., 2000) Some may argue that this group of people may be less addicted than those who do exhibit a response, or that the nonreactors may only elicit a response when in a specific mood or frame of mind (Avants et al., 1995); however, this remains an empirical question that requires additional research. Lastly, the genetic underpinnings of cue reactivity remain to be completely characterized, despite some promising research on the topic such as the finding that the *SLC6A4* gene may play a role in cue-induced alcohol cravings and may have an association to heavy drinking (Ait-Daoud et al., 2012). Moreover, research examining cannabis dependence has found that carriers of the *CNR1* G allele and *FAAH* C/C genotype seem to experience enhanced neural response in reward areas of the brain in response to cannabis related cues (Filbey et al., 2009).

Stress Induction Paradigms

Background and Practical Aspects

An adaptive response to stress is important for the survival of the organism. The origin of a stressor can be biological, physical, or psychological, with the latter as one of the most common forms of stress experienced by humans in the modern-day world. Biological stressors include toxins, viruses, bacteria, or drugs, such as *Streptococcus pneumoniae*, Human Immunodeficiency Virus or cocaine. Physical stressors induce stress by placing physical demands on the body, such as through exercise. Psychological stressors include psychosocial stressors, such as social or emotional stressors.

Importantly, stress leads to increased vulnerability for health-related problems (DeLongis, Folkman & Lazarus, 1988), including addiction (Goeders, 2003). The relationship between stress and addiction can be bidirectional; chronic stress may promote substance use and in turn, substance use may alter stress responsivity through its effects on the body's stress systems, including the Hypothalamic-Pituitary-Adrenal (HPA) (Goeders, 2003; Sinha, 2008) and Sympathetic-Adrenal-Medullary (SAM) axes (Fosnocht & Briand, 2016). Both the HPA and SAM axes appear dsyregulated in populations with substance use disorders (Koob, 1999; Koob & Kreek, 2007). There is also some evidence for stress effects in the pathophysiology of behavioral addictions, such as Gambling Disorder (GD), the first nonsubstance-based addiction in the *Diagnostic and Statistical Manual of Mental Disorders* (DSM-5; APA, 2013). For example, there is evidence that gambling increases cortisol levels and heart rate in recreational gamblers (Meyer et al., 2000). In problem gamblers, gambling activity also raises norepinephrine and dopamine levels (Meyer et al., 2004), both of which act on the brain's reward and motivational pathways (Sinha, 2008), including neural regions involved in regulating stress responsivity (Arnsten, 2009; Radley, Arias & Sawchenko, 2006). Early-life stressors may lead to dissociation between executive function and reward processing pathways, which may then increase propensity toward risk-taking behaviors and reduced impulse control, potentially prompting substance use and risky behaviors (Watt et al., 2017).

While stress plays a key role in addiction, studying stress effects in a controlled laboratory setting can be difficult. Though stress can be measured using self-report methods, physical and psychological stress induction protocols in the laboratory permit direct investigation of acute stress effects and stress reactivity. Several validated stress induction protocols have been developed to produce psychophysiological responses similar to real-world stressful events, including the Trier Social Stress Test (TSST), the Guided-Imagery Script Paradigm (GISP), the Cold Pressor Test (CPT), and the Socially Evaluated Cold Pressor Test (SECPT) (Kirschbaum, Pirke & Hellhammer, 1993; Miller et al., 1987; Schwabe, Haddad & Schachinger, 2008). While the CPT is a physical stress induction procedure, the TSST and GISP are psychological stressors, and the SECPT combines the two. Although both physical and psychological stressors activate the HPA axis, there are stressor-type dependent nuances in its response pattern (McRae et al., 2006; Singh et al., 1999). When compared to the CPT, TSST-induced cortisol and adrenocorticotropic hormone (ACTH) levels are significantly higher; in addition, the former biomarker takes longer to decline (McRae et al., 2006). However, the combination of the two, as is the case with SECPT, leads to significant increases in levels of cortisol when compared to the CPT (Schwabe et al., 2008). Other physical stress induction procedures, such as the high-intensity exercise test, lead to significant differences in levels of ACTH in high responders to stress when compared to low responders, but the TSST does not (Singh et al., 1999). Therefore, both physical and psychological stressors have differential effects, and the choice to include one over the other depends on the research question and related methodological considerations. Here, we discuss the TSST and the Guided-Imagery Script Paradigm, two ecologically valid stressors that are used to probe acute stress effects on human neurobiology and behavior.

Kirschbaum and colleagues (Kirschbaum et al., 1993) developed the Trier Social Stress Test (TSST) as a standardized protocol to induce psychological stress under controlled laboratory conditions. The TSST is a reliable and validated measure that potentiates the experience of socio-evaluative threat and uncontrollability (Dickerson & Kemeny, 2004; Gruenewald et al., 2004). The TSST procedure (Kirschbaum et al., 1993) involves three different stressor phases: (1) speech preparation (ten minutes), (2) speech task (five minutes), and (3) mental arithmetic (five minutes). In the protocol, a participant first enters a room where three panel members are seated; the individual is introduced to the panel members who maintain serious and neutral expressions. The participant is asked to prepare a speech on why they would be a good job candidate and informed that they have ten minutes to prepare the speech. Anticipatory anxiety is increased by introducing panel members as experts in the field and telling them that the speech will be recorded for later analysis. During the speech, panel members maintain a neutral face and provide little feedback. If a participant stops their speech early, the panel chairperson lets them know: "You have X minutes left." Following long pauses, panel members may ask prompting questions, such as: "What personality characteristics do you think would be good for the job?" to extend the speech portion to the full five minutes. Following the speech, participants are asked to perform mental arithmetic in front of the panel for another five minutes. This consists of subtracting prime numbers from other larger numbers (e.g., "Subtract 13 from 1022, as quickly and as accurately as possible."). The combination of public speaking and cognitive components in the TSST increases subjective reports of stress, but also psychophysiological measures of arousal and increased levels of stress hormones (Kirschbaum et al., 1993).

Similar to the TSST, the Guided-Imagery Script Paradigm is a stress induction tool for psychological stress. However, in contrast to the TSST, the guided-imagery procedure involves personalized scripts based on individual stressors unique to each participant. The procedure is adapted from Miller and colleagues (Miller et al., 1987) who demonstrated how emotional imagery can produce greater physiological activity and heightened intrinsic emotion-specific responses. This paradigm begins with a participant meeting for a script-development session with a trained researcher in which they complete a scene-development questionnaire identifying stressful and neutral relaxing situations from the past year. Stressful situations often include fighting with loved ones, breakups, performing badly at work/school or finding out about the death of a loved one. Neutral situations often consist of watching TV or reading at home, or going for a relaxing walk. The details from the script development session are then used by the researcher to develop an imagery script, which is subsequently recorded and played back to the participant at a later date when they are in the laboratory or undergoing neuroimaging. These scripts can produce increases in subjective ratings of craving and anxiety, but can also produce increases in stress hormones as well as cardiovascular measures (Sinha et al., 2003).

Ethical Considerations

The primary ethical consideration when implementing a stress-induction protocol is the potential for serious adverse reactions during or after the procedure. While the goal of the TSST or guided-imagery protocol is to increase psychosocial stress, researchers should exercise caution that the responses are not excessively distressing for participants. For instance, acute stress from these manipulations could potentially induce excessive anxiety or even a panic attack in participants who have a history of anxiety disorders. For this reason, participants with a history of anxiety disorders are often excluded from research studies using these paradigms.

Another important ethical concern related to guided-imagery protocols is the content of the imagery script. Researchers should be careful to select life events that have high potential to elicit stress responses, but not be excessively traumatic. For example, certain life events such as physical abuse, sexual assault, death of a loved one, or other traumas would likely not be appropriate for most stress-induction paradigms because of the potential for an adverse reaction. Similar to the concerns above, individuals with a history of trauma or posttraumatic stress disorder may need to be excluded from stress induction protocols to reduce the risk of serious adverse reactions to the manipulation.

Potential Limitations

Two notable potential limitations of stress induction paradigms include differential stress responses between men and women and individual differences in cortisol responses. In the first case, sex-specific considerations for the TSST are observed with respect to cortisol reactivity and hormonal status (Kirschbaum et al., 1999; Kudielka et al., 2004; Phan et al., 2017); for example, females in their luteal phase show higher cortisol responses than women on oral contraceptives or those in the follicular phase (Kirschbaum et al., 1999). In addition, females and males also show differences in cortisol recovery (Chen et al., 2017; Phan et al., 2017). Females demonstrate a flatter recovery curve (Phan et al., 2017), whereas males show a steeper linear cortisol decrease (Chen et al., 2017). A steep decrease reflects faster recovery after a stressor in men, while a flatter curve shows the opposite, and may have negative health consequences in women. This is seen in work investigating the health-related implications of diurnal cortisol slope; for example, in lung cancer patients, a flatter cortisol rhythm and a higher slope is related to an early mortality rate (Sephton et al., 2013). Therefore, the investigation of cortisol reactivity and reactivity curves is important as it has implications for accurately profiling differential states of stress responsivity. These sex-related differences are therefore important to consider when accurately reflecting the cortisol response; combining across genders may produce equivocal findings, therefore data analyses should explore potentially unique sex-related stress profiles. Further, the study of sex-related fluctuations may reveal interactions with androgenic or estrogenic hormones. For example, Phan and colleagues (2017) found both testosterone and dehydroepiandosterone predict levels of cortisol, showing potential coupling between the HPA and Hypothalamic–Pituitary–Gonadal axes.

A recent meta-analysis highlighted a variety of factors influencing cortisol responsiveness, including sensitivity to differences in sampling protocol, pre-TSST acclimation and activities, speech and arithmetic components, panel gender composition, and the time of the day (Goodman, Janson & Wolf, 2017). For example, morning TSST sessions lead to lower cortisol reactivity than those in the afternoon, likely related to higher levels of this hormone earlier in the day (Balodis, Wynne-Edwards & Olmstead, 2010), and after awakening, which is known as the cortisol awakening response (CAR) (Pruessner et al., 1997). Both the CAR and levels of cortisol are sensitive to circadian rhythm and physiological dysregulations, so alterations in sleep–wake timings or health complications can affect these variables. For example, an elevated CAR is seen in problem gamblers as compared to recreational gamblers (Wohl et al., 2008). Additionally, the length of time individuals spend in the lab prior to the TSST is important: both cortisol and alpha-amylase are elevated when the participants first arrive at the lab (Balodis et al., 2010; Goodman et al., 2017) and participants spending more time in the lab (i.e., sixteen to thirty minutes) have a higher cortisol response to a stressor (Goodman et al., 2017), demonstrating the importance of establishing a clear biomarker baseline prior to the TSST. During the mental math phase, there is some evidence for different numbers leading to higher cortisol reactivity (Phan et al., 2017) and introducing a social evaluative component including loss framing (i.e., loss of compensation for failure to improve performance) can produce a sharper cortisol rise and steeper decline during recovery (Goodman et al., 2017). There is also evidence that a mixed-gender panel produces greater cortisol reactivity than an all-female panel (Van Hedger, Bershad & de Wit, 2017). Other considerations include the ingestion of caffeine or nicotine both of which may alter stress reactivity either through their acute drug or withdrawal effects (Van Hedger et al., 2017).

Future Directions

Further research in stress responses is important in behavioral addictions, particularly in Gambling Disorder, which include multiple subgroups with potentially different pathways and mechanisms underlying this disorder (Kirschbaum & Hellhammer, 1994; Laudat et al., 1988; Loo et al., 2010). Given the important role of stress in the facilitation, maintenance, and relapse of addiction, more research is needed to effectively investigate stress reactivity in these populations as well as its influence on risky behaviors.

Both the TSST and Guided-Imagery Script Paradigm are effective laboratory paradigms to systematically induce psychological stress. While stress is unpleasant and associated with negative effects, the level of distress experienced in the laboratory from these paradigms is not more than an individual might experience in their everyday life. Aside from obesity research, very few studies using the Guided-Imagery Script Paradigm have been conducted in populations beyond substance use disorders. Future studies will provide more information on similarities and differences in stress and urge behaviors across substance-based and nonsubstance-based addictions. Understanding stress responses is of great importance as stress-induced craving remains a strong predictor of relapse in substance use disorders, and likely operates with behavioral addictions as well.

Self-Administration and Acute Challenge Paradigms

Background and Practical Aspects

These two paradigms were developed to investigate substance addictions (though some examples in this section suggest that they may be used to examine some behavioral addictions). Self-administration and acute challenge paradigms both involve participants consuming substances in a laboratory setting. Protocols in this domain provide a unique opportunity to examine consummatory behavior along with the acute effects of addictive substances in controlled laboratory settings that ensure the safety of participants. The central feature of *self-administration* paradigms is that the participants consume as much of the commodity as they want (often up to a predetermined maximum) at their own pace, thereby providing a measure of the total amount consumed and the rate at which it is administered. For example, participants in a food addiction study may be given free access to a "buffet" of snack foods and healthy foods over a set amount of time (e.g., Goldman et al., 2011). Self-administration paradigms allow researchers to investigate motivation for substances through use of operant responding paradigms. For example, someone who is willing to press a button 500 times to receive a portion of a substance would presumably have a higher motivation for the substance than someone who is only willing to press the button fifty times for the same amount. Additional motivation aspects that can be examined in addition to amount are speed, force, duration, mood, and, in some situations, money.

Acute challenge studies, on the other hand, typically involve participants consuming a specific amount of a substance or partaking in a behavior for a specific amount of time that is determined in advance by the research staff. For example, participants may consume a preset amount of an alcoholic beverage that is measured to raise their blood alcohol level to a target point, or they may ask participants to shop until they've spent a specific amount of money (e.g., potentially relevant to shopping addiction). In contrast to self-administration protocols, acute challenge studies are ideally suited to examine effects of a fixed amount of a substance or time spent engaging in behavior that is equated across participants. In other words, in acute challenge studies, the challenge is the manipulation and not the outcome (as is typically the case with self-administration protocols). The focus is largely on the effects or impact of the presence of the substance or behavior and not necessarily the motivational factors that influence how much a person will consume or how hard they are willing to work to obtain the substance or engage in the behavior.

These protocols necessarily have unique requirements related to environment and participant safety. Self-administration paradigms can be conducted in laboratory settings, inpatient clinical settings, as well as outpatient and community settings. Inpatient settings typically allow for more flexible scheduling time, along with complete control of conditions and consequences. Moreover, inpatient settings may allow for study sessions to be conducted in multiple, shorter sessions that extend over numerous days. Outpatient and community settings are typically time-limited, and require long study sessions, sometimes multiple hours in duration. Moreover, conducting self-administration paradigms in community settings is often much less controlled and, in some cases, less safe if proper ethical and security precautions are not in place.

Along with the setting come the necessary and associated costs, resources, task choice, possible number of participants, types of substances administered, and mode of administration. The use of inpatient settings can often be less costly and resource intensive, safe for substance administration, and unrestricted in the tasks being administered. However, the number of participants may be lower and recruitment time may take longer based on intake and discharge within the hospital. Outpatient and community settings may require traveling to various settings in the community to collect data and recruit participants; this will inevitably increase the required resources for the study. In addition, these various outpatient and community settings may introduce unforeseen confounds (such as variations in social-community contexts) and may not allow for proper task administration. A benefit of the outpatient and community setting, however, is the ability to constantly recruit new, diverse participants from an ever-changing domain. Outpatient and community settings, although less controlled, may also benefit the study by allowing participants to interact with typical environments (i.e., shopping malls, casinos, buffets), which improves the ecological validity and allows researchers to study participants in their typical use environments.

Ethical Considerations

Self-administration paradigms carry many ethical questions that need to be considered. The most prominent ethical issue to consider when conducting a self-administration study is selecting the most appropriate sample for the study. There are some obvious groups that are inappropriate for a self-administration study (e.g., pregnant women, children). However, it is also ethically questionable to administer alcohol or other substances to individuals who are currently in treatment or in recovery (NIAAA, 2005) owing to concerns about prompting relapse. Individuals who have never used substances (e.g., substance naïve) should also not be administered alcohol or drugs. In this case, NIAAA guidelines state that the first exposure to alcohol is associated with an unknown level of risk because researchers cannot predict with certainty who is at risk for later development of alcohol-related problems (NIAAA, 2005). In the realm of behavioral addictions, self-administration paradigms are often easier, and less ethically concerning (i.e., food, gambling, video games); however, there are a few cases in which the amounts used or consumed need to be carefully monitored. For example, there is growing evidence for the overuse of tanning beds in what may be termed "tanning addiction" (see Miller & Mays, 2020). Use of tanning beds for self-administration research provides an excellent way to study tanning addiction, yet researchers need to carefully consider the amount of time they are allowing participants to engage in the activity, given that tanning beds have been deemed carcinogenic (Mogensen & Jemec, 2010).

An additional ethical consideration for self-administration paradigms is supplying medically safe and legal substances. Researchers must carefully consider the legality of the substance (e.g., cannabis or other drug self-administration paradigms may be prohibited by law), the amount that will be administered or the maximum amount that a participant can receive. In the case of alcohol, for example, NIAAA guidelines recommend that the dose administered not exceed an amount that the participant has consumed at least occasionally in the last year (NIAAA, 2005). Additionally, for ad-libitum self-administration protocols in which participants are able to drink freely, care must be exercised to limit the maximum amount of alcohol available that is often dosed to reach a target maximum blood alcohol level. In the case of persons with substance use disorders, appropriate dosing can create a problem with regard to ecological validity, given that most severe users consume quantities that may be medically unsafe for a research study.

In the case of nondrug substance or behavioral addictions, the risk of ad-libitum self-administration protocols is often less risky but should still be considered carefully depending on the behavior. For example, in extreme cases, overeating an immense amount of food (a nondrug substance addiction) can cause health complications, shopping or gambling addictively with personal money can lead to financial trouble, excessive video gaming can lead to self-neglect, and an extreme amount of time using tanning beds can lead to health concerns (Miller & Mays, 2020). Although behavioral addictions can often be considered less dangerous given that dangerous amounts of alcohol and drugs are not being consumed, precautions still need to be implemented given that any substance or behavior taken in excess can be dangerous.

Potential Limitations

When implemented properly and following appropriate safety guidelines, self-administration and acute challenge protocols are powerful tools to examine acute effects of addictive substances, motivation, and consummatory behavior. However, the self-administration paradigm also has a number of potential limitations. Most commonly, research studies using self-administration are conducted in laboratory settings. Although this allows for greater control and standardization on the part of the researcher, it is often difficult for participants to view a research laboratory as a real-world situation for substance use. This raises the question of whether the lab is an ideal location to conduct the self-administration protocols. In contrast, if researchers were to choose a more realistic environment in the community, the amount of experimental control is dramatically reduced and additional safety concerns come into play. Real-world testing also could potentially increase the number of distractions that can affect responses during the protocol.

Another potential challenge is identifying an appropriate control condition for self-administration or acute challenge studies. This includes the use of placebo substances, such as a nonalcoholic beverage. Although researchers have developed methods to create realistic placebo substances (e.g., floating a small amount of alcohol on the top of a nonalcoholic mixer to mimic the taste and olfactory properties of alcohol), placebo manipulations are not universally effective (Testa et al., 2006).

A final limitation of self-administration studies relates to the substantially increased requirements for ensuring participant and staff safety. If the study is administering a psychoactive substance, the risk of adverse reactions or other unexpected responses is greater. This is especially true for alcohol studies, where participants may become sick or uncomfortable after consuming alcohol in the laboratory. Additional safeguards must be put in place to ensure that participants are continuously monitored (e.g., via a closed-circuit camera system or a two-way mirror). Finally, safety is also critical at the end of the session because participants who have consumed alcohol or other substances may still be experiencing intoxicating effects that could impair cognition or behavior. For this reason, researchers involved in alcohol studies are encouraged to keep participants in the laboratory until blood alcohol levels fall below 0.02–0.04 percent. Researchers should also carefully consider any transportation restrictions following the study and, where possible, participants should be encouraged not to drive themselves home from the study.

Future Directions

The literature on self-administration paradigms for nondrug substance addictions or behavioral addictions is quite limited, partly because many behavioral addictions are still being identified and classified in the DSM. In addition, the studies that have been conducted using self-administration paradigms often have small sample sizes, rely entirely on self-report questionnaires, or lack adequate ecological validity.

With regard to food addictions, Epstein and colleagues have conducted many studies examining the reinforcing value of food in samples such as infants, children and women (Epstein et al., 2010). These studies have used paradigms such as computer choice tasks (Epstein et al., 2010), an online grocery store with altered prices based on nutritional value (Epstein et al., 2015), and food purchase tasks (Epstein et al., 2006). In the future, many of these paradigms could be modified and applied to various forms of food addiction and disordered eating.

On the topic of problem gambling, some impressive work has been produced by Dixon and colleagues (Dixon et al., 2013a, 2013b, 2014, 2017; Templeton et al., 2014). This group has conducted several studies in which problem gamblers are provided with slot machines to use while their skin conductance, behavior, and force applied on the buttons are recorded (Dixon et al., 2017). Although this work focuses largely on cognitive variables and participants' responses to wins, losses and near-misses, many of their paradigms could lend themselves nicely to future studies on problem gambling from a behavioral addictions standpoint.

A small sample of studies on other behavioral addictions such as shopping (Hartston, 2012; Rose & Dhandayudham, 2014), video gaming (Vadlin, Åslund & Nilsson, 2015), exercise (Márquez & De la Vega, 2015; Weinstein & Weinstein, 2014), and tanning (Becirevic et al., 2017; Reed, 2015), have been conducted; however, the literature on these topics in conjunction with self-administration paradigms is still relatively limited and in need of development.

Conclusions

As behavioral addictions continue to be identified and classified in the DSM, increased research on the etiological factors that contribute to these disorders will also be necessary. This chapter has reviewed various paradigms and methods that can be used to study addictive disorders among humans in laboratory settings. Moreover, this chapter has touched on each method's practical aspects, ethical considerations, limitations, and areas for future work.

Ultimately, the paradigm selected for a given study should be driven by the specific research question and hypotheses, available resources, location, study population, as well as any other relevant details of the study. An advantage to human laboratory paradigms in general is the high level of experimental control that they provide, but this can sometimes come at the cost of reduced ecological validity. Therefore, the advantages and disadvantages of laboratory paradigms should be weighed carefully during the design of new research studies.

A general conclusion that can be drawn from this overview is that application of validated laboratory paradigms to the study of behavioral addictions is relatively limited to date. Therefore, expanded research on behavioral addictions is an important priority for the future. Through this, researchers will continue to add to the scientific literature on these disorders, while also identifying gaps and developing novel methods for conducting the human laboratory paradigms in various behavioral addictions. Expanding knowledge, adapting methods, and identifying areas for development are fundamental aspects needed not only for behavioral addictions, but for addictions research as a whole.

REFERENCES

Abrams, D. B., Monti, P. M., Carey, K. B., Pinto, R. P. & Jacobus, S. I. (1988). Reactivity to smoking cues and relapse: Two studies of discriminant validity. *Behaviour Research and Therapy*, **26**(3), 225–233. doi:10.1016/0005-7967(88)90003-4

Ait-Daoud, N., Seneviratne, C., Smith, J. B., et al. (2012). Preliminary evidence for cue-induced alcohol craving modulated by serotonin transporter gene polymorphism rs1042173. *Frontiers in Psychiatry*, **3**. doi:10.3389/fpsyt.2012.00006

American Psychiatric Association (2013). *Diagnostic and Statistical Manual of Mental Disorders* (5th edition). Washington, DC: American Psychiatric Association Publishing.

Amlung, M. T., Acker, J., Stojek, M. K., Murphy, J. G. & MacKillop, J. (2011). Is talk "cheap"? An initial investigation of the equivalence of alcohol purchase task performance for hypothetical and actual rewards. *Alcoholism: Clinical and Experimental Research*, **36**(4), 716–724. doi:10.1111/j.1530-0277.2011.01656.x

Arnsten, A. F. T. (2009). Stress signalling pathways that impair prefrontal cortex structure and function. *Nature Reviews Neuroscience*, **10**(6), 410–422. https://doi.org/10.1038/nrn2648

Avants, S., Margolin, A., Kosten, T. R. & Cooney, N. L. (1995). Differences between responders and nonresponders to cocaine cues in the laboratory. *Addictive Behaviors*, **20**(2), 215–224. doi:10.1016/0306-4603(94)00066-2

Balodis, I. M., Wynne-Edwards, K. E. & Olmstead, M. C. (2010). The other side of the curve: Examining the relationship between pre-stressor physiological responses and stress reactivity. *Psychoneuroendocrinology*, **35**(9), 1363–1373. https://doi.org/10.1016/j.psyneuen.2010.03.011

Balodis, I. M., Kober, H., Worhunsky, P. D., et al. (2012). Diminished frontostriatal activity during processing of monetary rewards and losses in pathological gambling. *Biological Psychiatry*, **71**(8), 749–757.

Becirevic, A., Reed, D. D., Amlung, M., et al. (2017). An initial study of behavioral addiction symptom severity and demand for indoor tanning. *Experimental and Clinical Psychopharmacology*, **25**(5), 346–352. doi:10.1037/pha0000146

Carter, B. L. & Tiffany, S. T. (1999). Meta-analysis of cue-reactivity in addiction research. *Addiction*, **94**(3), 327–340. doi:10.1046/j.1360-0443.1999.9433273.x

Chen, X., Gianferante, D., Hanlin, L., et al. (2017). HPA-axis and inflammatory reactivity to acute stress is related with basal HPA-axis activity. *Psychoneuroendocrinology*, **78**, 168–176. https://doi.org/10.1016/j.psyneuen.2017.01.035

Clark, G. I., Rock, A. J., Mckeith, C. F. & Coventry, W. L. (2016). Cue-reactive rationality, visual imagery and volitional control predict cue-reactive urge to gamble in poker-machine gamblers. *Journal of Gambling Studies*, **33**(3), 807–823. doi:10.1007/s10899-016-9650-6

DeLongis, A. Folkman, S. & Lazarus, R. S. (1988). The impact of daily stress on health and mood: Psychological and social resources as mediators. *Journal of Personality and Social Psychology*, **54**(3), 486–495. https://doi.org/10.1037/0022-3514.54.3.486

Dickerson, S. S. & Kemeny, M. E. (2004). Acute stressors and cortisol responses: A theoretical integration and synthesis of laboratory research. *Psychological Bulletin*, **130**(3), 355–391. https://doi.org/10.1037/0033-2909.130.3.355

Dixon, M. J., Harrigan, K. A., Santesso, D. L., et al. (2013a). The impact of sound in modern multiline video slot machine play. *Journal of Gambling Studies*, **30**(4), 913–929. doi:10.1007/s10899-013-9391-8

Dixon, M. J., Collins, K., Harrigan, K. A., Graydon, C. & Fugelsang, J. A. (2013b). Using sound to unmask losses disguised as wins in multiline slot machines. *Journal of Gambling Studies*, **31**(1), 183–196. doi:10.1007/s10899-013-9411-8

Dixon, M. J., Graydon, C., Harrigan, K. A., et al. (2014). The allure of multi-line games in modern slot machines. *Addiction*, **109**(11), 1920–1928. doi:10.1111/add.12675

Dixon, M. J., Larche, C. J., Stange, M., Graydon, C. & Fugelsang, J. A. (2017). Near-misses and stop buttons in slot machine play: An investigation of how they affect players, and may foster erroneous cognitions. *Journal of Gambling Studies*, **34**(1), 161–180. doi:10.1007/s10899-017-9699-x

Dolinsky, Z. S. & Babor, T. F. (1997). Ethical, scientific and clinical issues in ethanol administration research involving alcoholics as human subjects. *Addiction*, **92**, 1087–1097.

Drummond, D. C., et al. (2000). Craving research: Future directions. *Addiction*, **95** (8s2), 247–255. doi:10.1046/j.1360-0443.95.8s2.13.x

Enoch, M.-A., et al. (2009). Ethical considerations for administering alcohol or alcohol cues to treatment-seeking alcoholics in a research setting: Can the benefits to society outweigh the risks to the individual? *Alcoholism: Clinical and Experimental Research*, **33**(9), 1508–1512. doi:10.1111/j.1530-0277.2009.00988.x

Epstein, L. H., Handley, E. A., Dearing, K. K., et al. (2006). Purchases of food in youth. Influence of price and income. *Psychological Science*, **17**(1), 82–89. doi:10.1111/j.1467-9280.2005.01668.x

Epstein, L. H., Salvy, S. J., Carr, K. A., Dearing, K. K. & Bickel, W. K. (2010). Food reinforcement, delay discounting and obesity. *Physiology & Behavior*, **100**(5), 438–445. doi:10.1016/j.physbeh.2010.04.029

Epstein, L. H., Finkelstein, E., Raynor, H., et al. (2015). Experimental analysis of the effect of taxes and subsides on calories purchased in an on-line supermarket. *Appetite*, **95**, 245–251. doi:10.1016/j.appet.2015.06.020

Ferguson, C. J., Coulson, M. & Barnett, J. (2011). A meta-analysis of pathological gaming prevalence and comorbidity with mental health, academic and social problems. *Journal of Psychiatric Research*, **45**(12), 1573–1578. doi:10.1016/j.jpsychires.2011.09.005

Ferrer-García, M., Gutiérrez-Maldonado, J., Pla-Sanjuanelo, J., et al. (2017). A randomised controlled comparison of second-level treatment approaches for treatment-resistant adults with bulimia nervosa and binge eating disorder: Assessing the benefits of virtual reality cue exposure therapy. *European Eating Disorders Review*, **25**(6), 479–490. doi:10.1002/erv.2538

Filbey, F. M., Claus, E., Audette, A. R., et al. (2007). Exposure to the taste of alcohol elicits activation of the mesocorticolimbic neurocircuitry. *Neuropsychopharmacology*, **33** (6), 1391–1401. doi:10.1038/sj.npp.1301513

Filbey, F. M., Ray, L., Smolen, A., et al. (2008). Differential neural response to alcohol priming and alcohol taste cues is associated with DRD4 VNTR and OPRM1 genotypes. *Alcoholism: Clinical and Experimental Research*, **32**(7), 1113–1123. doi:10.1111/j.1530-0277.2008.00692.x

Filbey, F. M., Schacht, J. P., Myers, U. S., Chavez, R. S. & Hutchison, K. E. (2009). Individual and additive effects of the CNR1 and FAAH genes on brain response to marijuana cues. *Neuropsychopharmacology*, **35**(4), 967–975. doi:10.1038/npp.2009.200

Fosnocht, A. Q. & Briand, L. A. (2016). Substance use modulates stress reactivity. *Behavioral and Physiological Outcomes*, **166**, 32–42. https://doi.org/10.1126/science.1249098.Sleep

Franken, I. H. a., et al. (1999). Cue reactivity and effects of cue exposure in abstinent posttreatment drug users. *Journal of Substance Abuse Treatment*, **16**(1), 81–85. doi:10.1016/s0740-5472(98)00004-x

Goeders, N. E. (2003). The impact of stress on addiction. *European Neuropsychopharmacology*, **13**(6), 435–441. https://doi.org/10.1016/j.euroneuro.2003.08.004

Goldman, R. L., Borckardt, J. J., Frohman, H. A., et al. (2011). Prefrontal cortex transcranial direct current stimulation (tDCS) temporarily reduces food cravings and increases the self-reported ability to resist food in adults with frequent food craving. *Appetite*, **56**(3), 741–746. doi:10.1016/j.appet.2011.02.013

Goodman, W. K., Janson, J. & Wolf, J. M. (2017). Meta-analytical assessment of the effects of protocol variations on cortisol responses to the Trier Social Stress Test. *Psychoneuroendocrinology*, **80**, 26–35. https://doi.org/10.1016/j.psyneuen.2017.02.030

Gruenewald, T. L., Kemeny, M. E., Aziz, N. & Fahey, J. L. (2004). Acute threat to the social self: Shame, social self-esteem, and cortisol activity. *Psychosomatic Medicine*, **66**(6), 915–924. https://doi.org/10.1097/01.psy.0000143639.61693.ef

Hartston, H. (2012). The case for compulsive shopping as an addiction. *Journal of Psychoactive Drugs*, **44**(1), 64–67. doi:10.1080/02791072.2012.660110

Jarmolowicz, D. P. & Schneider, T. D. (2020). Behavioral economics and addictive disorders. In S. Sussman (Ed.) *The Cambridge Handbook of Substance and Behavioral Addictions*, Cambridge, UK: Cambridge University Press, 12–22.

Kirschbaum, C., Pirke, K.-M. & Hellhammer, D. H. (1993). The "Trier Social Stress Test" – A tool for investigating psychobiological stress responses in a laboratory setting. *Neuropsychobiology*, **28**, 76–81.

Kirschbaum, C. & Hellhammer, D. H. (1994). Review: Salivary cortisol in psychoneuroendocrine research: Recent developments and applications. *Psychoneuroendocrinology*, **19**(4), 313–333.

Kirschbaum, C., Kudielka, B. M., Gaab, J., Schommer, N. C. & Hellhammer, D. H. (1999). Impact of gender, menstrual cycle phase, and oral contraceptives on the activity of the hypothalamus-pituitary-adrenal axis. *Psychosomatic Medicine*, **61**(2), 154–162. https://doi.org/10.1097/00006842-199903000-00006

Koob, G. F. (1999). Corticotopin-releasing factor, norephinephrine, and stress. *Stress: The International Journal on the Biology of Stress*, **1800**, 47–59. https://doi.org/10.1016/j.bbagen.2009.07.018

Koob, G. & Kreek, M. J. (2007). Stress, dysregulation of drug reward pathways, and the transition to drug dependence. *American Journal of Psychiatry*, **164**(8), 1149–1159. https://doi.org/10.1176/appi.ajp.2007.05030503

Kudielka, B. M., Buske-Kirschbaum, A., Hellhammer, D. H. & Kirschbaum, C. (2004). HPA axis responses to laboratory psychosocial stress in healthy elderly adults, younger adults, and children: Impact of age and gender. *Psychoneuroendocrinology*, **29**(1), 83–98. https://doi.org/10.1016/S0306-4530(02)00146-4

Kuhn, S. & Gallinat, J. (2011). Common biology of craving across legal and illegal drugs – A quantitative meta-analysis of cue-reactivity brain response. *European Journal of Neuroscience*, **33**(7), 1318–1326. doi:10.1111/j.1460-9568.2010.07590.x

Kushner, M. G., Abrams, K., Donahue, C., et al. (2007). Urge to gamble in problem gamblers exposed to a casino environment. *Journal of Gambling Studies*, **23**(2), 121–132. doi:10.1007/s10899-006-9050-4

Laudat, M. H., Cerdas, S., Fournier, C., et al. (1988). Salivary cortisol measurement: A practical approach to assess pituitary-adrenal function. *Journal of Clinical Endocrinology and Metabolism*, **66**(2), 343–348. https://doi.org/10.1210/jcem-66-2-343

Loo, J. A., Yan, W., Ramachandran, P. & Wong, D. T. (2010). Comparative human salivary and plasma proteomes. *Journal of Dental Research*, **89**(10), 1016–1023. https://doi.org/10.1177/0022034510380414

MacKillop, J. & Lisman, S. A. (2008). Effects of a context shift and multiple context extinction on reactivity to alcohol cues. *Experimental and Clinical Psychopharmacology*, **16**(4), 322–331. doi:10.1037/a0012686

MacKillop, J., et al. (2010).Behavioral economic analysis of cue-elicited craving for alcohol. *Addiction*, **105**(9), 1599–1607. doi:10.1111/j.1360-0443.2010.03004.x

MacKillop, J., et al. (2012). Behavioral economic analysis of withdrawal- and cue-elicited craving for tobacco: An initial investigation. *Nicotine & Tobacco Research*, **14**(12), 1426–1434., doi:10.1093/ntr/nts006

Maxwell, A. L., Loxton, N. J. & Hennegan, J. M. (2017). Exposure to food cues moderates the indirect effect of reward sensitivity and external eating via implicit eating expectancies. *Appetite*, **111**, 135–141. doi:10.1016/j.appet.2016.12.037

Márquez, S. & De la Vega, R. (2015). [Exercise addiction: An emergent behavioral disorder]. *Nutricion Hospitalaria*, **31**(6). doi:10.3305/nh.2015.31.6.8934

McRae, A. L., Saladin, M. E., Brady, K. T., et al. (2006). Stress reactivity: Biological and subjective responses to the cold pressor and Trier Social stressors. *Human Psychopharmacology*, **21**(August), 377–385. https://doi.org/10.1002/hup.778

Metrik, J., et al. (2016). Cue-elicited increases in incentive salience for marijuana: Craving, demand, and attentional bias. *Drug and Alcohol Dependence*, **167**, 82–88. doi:10.1016/j.drugalcdep.2016.07.027

Meyer, G., Hauffa, B. P., Schedlowski, M., et al. S. (2000). Casino gambling increases heart rate and salivary cortisol in regular gamblers. *Biological Psychiatry*, **48**(9), 948–953. https://doi.org/10.1016/S0006-3223(00)00888-X

Meyer, G., Schwertfeger, J., Exton, M. S., et al. (2004). Neuroendocrine response to casino gambling in problem gamblers. *Psychoneuroendocrinology*, **29**(10), 1272–1280. https://doi.org/10.1016/j.psyneuen.2004.03.005

Miller, G. A., Levin, D. N., Kozak, M. J., et al. (1987). Individual differences in imagery and the psychophysiology of emotion. *Cognition and Emotion*, **1**(4), 367–390. https://doi.org/10.1080/02699938708408058

Miller, K. A. & Mays, D. (2020). Tanning as an addiction: The state of the research and implications for intervention. In S. Sussman (Ed.) *The Cambridge Handbook of Substance and Behavioral Addictions*. Cambridge, UK: Cambridge University Press, pp. 362–372.

Mónok, K., Berczik, K., Urbán, R., et al. (2012). Psychometric properties and concurrent validity of two exercise addiction measures: A population wide study. *Psychology of Sport and Exercise*, **13**(6), 739–746. doi:10.1016/j.psychsport.2012.06.003

Mogensen, M. & Jemec, G. B. (2010). The potential carcinogenic risk of tanning beds: clinical guidelines and patient safety advice. *Cancer Management and Research*, **2**, 277–282.

National Institute on Drug Abuse [NIDA] (2017). *Trends & Statistics*. NIDA, 24 April 2017. www.drugabuse.gov/related-topics/trends-statistics

NIAAA. (2005). *National Advisory Council on Alcohol Abuse and Alcoholism – Recommended Council Guidelines on Ethyl Alcohol Administration in Human Experimentation*. Retrieved from www.niaaa.nih.gov/Resources/ResearchResources/Pages/job22.aspx

Niaura, R., Abrams, D., Demuth, B., Pinto, R. & Monti, P. (1989). Responses to smoking-related stimuli and early relapse to smoking. *Addictive Behaviors*, **14**(4), 419–428. doi:10.1016/0306-4603(89)90029-4

Niaura, R., Abrams, D. B., Shadel, W. G., et al. (1999). Cue exposure treatment for smoking relapse prevention: A controlled clinical trial. *Addiction*, **94**(5), 685–695. doi:10.1046/j.1360-0443.1999.9456856.x

Niaura, R. (2002). Does "unlearning" ever really occur: Comment on Conklin & Tiffany. *Addiction*, **97**(3), 357. doi:10.1046/j.1360-0443.2002.0055a.x

Norberg, M. M., et al. (2016). Craving cannabis: A meta-analysis of self-report and psychophysiological cue-reactivity studies. *Addiction*, **111**(11), 1923–1934. doi:10.1111/add.13472

Park, C., Park, S. M., Gwak, A. R., et al. (2015). The effect of repeated exposure to virtual gambling cues on the urge to gamble. *Addictive Behaviors*, **41**, 61–64. doi:10.1016/j.addbeh.2014.09.027

Pavlov, I. P. & Anrep, G. V. (2003). *Conditioned Reflexes*. Mineola, NY: Dover Publications.

Pedram, P., Wadden, D., Amini, P., et al. (2013). Food addiction: Its prevalence and significant association with obesity in the general population. *PLoS ONE*, **8**(9). doi:10.1371/journal.pone.0074832

Phan, J. M., Schneider, E., Peres, J., et al. (2017). Social evaluative threat with verbal performance feedback alters neuroendocrine response to stress. *Hormones and Behavior*, **96**(September), 104–115. https://doi.org/10.1016/j.yhbeh.2017.09.007

Powell, J. (2006). Conditioned responses to drug-related stimuli: Is context crucial. *Addiction*, **90**(8), 1089–1095. doi:10.1046/j.1360-0443.1995.90810897.x

Pruessner, J. C., Wolf, O. T., Hellhammer, D. H., et al. (1997). Free cortisol levels after awakening: A reliable biological marker for the assessment of adrenocortical activity. *Life Sciences*, **61**(26), 2539–2549.

Pulido, C., Brown, S. A., Cummins, K., Paulus, M. P. & Tapert, S. F. (2010). Alcohol cue reactivity task development. *Addictive Behaviors*, **35**(2), 84–90. doi:10.1016/j.addbeh.2009.09.006

Radley, J. J., Arias, C. M. & Sawchenko, P. E. (2006). Regional differentiation of the medial prefrontal cortex in regulating adaptive responses to acute emotional stress. *The Journal of Neuroscience: The Official Journal of the Society for Neuroscience*, **26**(50), 12967–12976. https://doi.org/10.1523/JNEUROSCI.4297-06.2006

Reed, D. D. (2015). Ultra-violet indoor tanning addiction: A reinforcer pathology interpretation. *Addictive Behaviors*, **41**, 247–251. doi:10.1016/j.addbeh.2014.10.026

Reed, D. D, Naudé, G. P., Gelino, B. W. & Amlung, M. (2020). Behavioral economic considerations of novel addictions and nonaddictive behavior: Research and analytic methods. In S. Sussman (Ed.) *The Cambridge Handbook of Substance and Behavioral Addictions*, Cambridge, UK: Cambridge University Press, pp. 73–86.

Rose, S. & Dhandayudham, A. (2014). Towards an understanding of Internet-based problem shopping behaviour: The concept of online shopping addiction and its proposed predictors. *Journal of Behavioral Addictions*, 3(2), 83–89. doi:10.1556/jba.3.2014.003

Saladin, M. E., Gray, K. M., Carpenter, M. J., et al. (2012). Gender differences in craving and cue reactivity to smoking and negative affect/stress cues. *The American Journal on Addictions*, **21**(3), 210–220. doi:10.1111/j.1521-0391.2012.00232.x

Sayette, M. A., Shiffman, S., Tiffany, S. T., et al. (2000). The measurement of drug craving. *Addiction*, **95**(8s2), 189–210. doi:10.1046/j.1360-0443.95.8s2.8.x

Schwabe, L., Haddad, L. & Schachinger, H. (2008). HPA axis activation by a socially evaluated cold-pressor test. *Psychoneuroendocrinology*, **33**(6), 890–895. https://doi.org/10.1016/j.psyneuen.2008.03.001

Sephton, S. E., Lush, E., Dedert, E. A., et al. (2013). Diurnal cortisol rhythm as a predictor of lung cancer survival. *Brain, Behavior, and Immunity*, **30**(Supplement), S163–S170. https://doi.org/10.1016/j.bbi.2012.07.019

Shaffer, H. J., Hall, M. N. & Bilt, J. V. (1999). Estimating the prevalence of disordered gambling behavior in the United States and

Canada: A research synthesis. *American Journal of Public Health*, **89**(9), 1369–1376. doi:10.2105/ajph.89.9.1369

Singh, A., Petrides, J. S., Gold, P. W., Chrousos, G. P. & Deuster, P. A. (1999). Differential hypothalamic-pituitary-adrenal axis reactivity to psychological and physical stress. *The Journal of Clinical Endocrinology & Metabolism*, **84**(6), 1944–1948.

Sinha, R. (2008). Chronic stress, drug use, and vulnerability to addiction. *Annals of the New York Academy of Sciences*, **1141**, 105–130. https://doi.org/10.1196/annals.1441.030 .Chronic

Sinha, R., Talih, M., Malison, R., et al. (2003). Hypothalamic-pituitary-adrenal axis and sympatho-adreno-medullary responses during stress-induced and drug cue-induced cocaine craving states. *Psychopharmacology*, **170**(1), 62–72. https://doi.org/10.1007/ s00213-003-1525-8

Sterling, R. C., Dean, J., Weinstein, S. P., Murphy, J. & Gottheil, E. (2004). Gender differences in cue exposure reactivity and 9-month outcome. *Journal of Substance Abuse Treatment*, **27**(1), 39–44. doi:10.1016/ j.jsat.2004.03.008

Sussman, S. Y. (2017). *Substance and Behavioral Addictions: Concepts, Causes, and Cures.* Cambridge, United Kingdom: Cambridge University Press.

Symes, B. A. & Nicki, R. M. (1997). a preliminary consideration of cue-exposure, response-prevention treatment for pathological gambling behaviour: Two case studies. *Journal of Gambling Studies*, **13**(2), 145–157. https://doi.org/10.1023/ A:1024951301959

Szegedi, A., Lörch, B., Scheurich, A., et al. (2000). Cue exposure in alcohol dependent patients: preliminary evidence for different types of cue reactivity. *Journal of Neural Transmission*, **107**(6), 721–730. doi:10.1007/ s007020070073

Templeton, J. A., Dixon, M. J., Harrigan, K. A. & Fugelsang, J. A. (2014). Upping the reinforcement rate by playing the maximum lines in multi-line slot machine play. *Journal of Gambling Studies*, **31**(3), 949–964. doi:10.1007/s10899-014-9446-5

Testa, M., et al. (2006). Understanding alcohol expectancy effects: Revisiting the placebo condition. *Alcoholism: Clinical and Experimental Research*, 30(2), 339–348. doi:10.1111/j.1530-0277.2006.00039.x

Vadlin, S., Åslund, C. & Nilsson, K. W. (2015). Development and content validity of a screening instrument for gaming addiction in adolescents: The Gaming Addiction Identification Test (GAIT). *Scandinavian Journal of Psychology*, **56**(4), 458–466. doi:10.1111/sjop.12196

Van Hedger, K., Bershad, A. K. & de Wit, H. (2017). Pharmacological challenge studies with acute psychosocial stress. *Psychoneuroendocrinology*, **85**(August), 123–133. https://doi.org/10.1016/j.psyneuen .2017.08.020

Watt, M. J., Weber, M. A., Davies, S. R. & Forster, G. L. (2017). Impact of juvenile chronic stress on adult cortico-accumbal function: Implications for cognition and addiction. *Progress in Neuro-Psychopharmacology and Biological Psychiatry*, **79**(June), 136–154. https://doi.org/ 10.1016/j.pnpbp.2017.06.015

Weinstein, A. & Weinstein, Y. (2014). Exercise addiction - Diagnosis, bio-psychological mechanisms and treatment issues. *Current Pharmaceutical Design*, **20**(25), 4062–4069. doi:10.2174/13816128113199990614

Wohl, M. J. A., Matheson, K., Young, M. M. & Anisman, H. (2008). Cortisol rise following awakening among problem gamblers: Dissociation from comorbid symptoms of depression and impulsivity. *Journal of Gambling Studies*, **24**(1), 79–90. https://doi.org/10.1007/s10899-007-9080-6

World Health Organization. (2015, December). Health in 2015: From MDGs to SDGs. Retrieved March 02, 2018, from www.who.int/ gho/publications/mdgs-sdgs/en/

7 Behavioral Economic Considerations of Novel Addictions and Nonaddictive Behavior: Research and Analytic Methods

Derek D. Reed, PhD, BCBA-D, Gideon P. Naudé, MA, Brett W. Gelino, BS, and Michael Amlung, PhD

Introduction

Since the inception of behavioral pharmacology, addiction researchers have sought to explain substance use and issues of dependence via hedonic mechanisms (Bickel et al., 2014; Hursh & Silberberg, 2008). Early behavioral pharmacologists conceptualized substance use within Skinnerian (operant) behaviorism (Skinner, 1953, 1961), wherein the rewarding properties of substances reinforced substance-related behavior, such as consumption and actions associated with accessing those substances for consumption (Branch, 2006; Comer et al., 2010). In this perspective, consumption of a drug reward reinforces drug-seeking and associated consummatory behavior, potentially leading to a cycle of abuse.

Concurrent with advances in behavioral pharmacology was the development of hedonic scaling to quantify reinforcer efficacy (Herrnstein, 1971). It is no surprise, then, that early applications of behavioral pharmacology sought to produce precise quantification of relative reinforcer efficacy (Griffiths, Brady & Bradford, 1979). A specific example of this approach is the progressive-ratio analysis proposed by Hodos in 1961 (Hodos, 1961). In this progressive-ratio approach, animals earn consummatory access to a reinforcer upon completion of a specified number of responses (i.e., a ratio schedule). Completion of the ratio requirement renders two outcomes (Jarmolowicz & Lattal, 2010): (1) consummatory access to the reward and (2) an increase in the next ratio requirement. For example, in the seminal Hodos study, rats first earned access to sweetened condensed milk by completing two lever presses. After consuming the milk, the next ratio requirement was four lever presses; each earned access increased the ratio requirement by two lever presses. Progressive ratios increased upon each earned access to milk, resulting in suppressed reinforcer access at larger ratio values. Thus, rewards with higher hedonic value will maintain responding across larger ratio values, relative to rewards with lower hedonic value. In this approach, the last-completed ratio is considered the breakpoint in the progressive-ratio arrangement. Higher breakpoint values are thereby indicative of stronger relative reinforcing efficacy.

Since Hodos' (1961) conceptualization of breakpoint as a marker of hedonic scaling, behavioral pharmacologists have used this metric and its offshoots to describe various facets of drug valuation in self-administration studies, such as the effects of deprivation, abuse liability, and impacts of contextual manipulations on drug-seeking (Bradshaw & Killeen, 2012; Stafford, LeSage & Glowa, 1998). The success the breakpoint approach in the behavioral pharmacology literature underscored the importance of response-reward relations when drug access is constrained in some parametric approach. Reinforcer constraint occurs when some contingency is placed on drug consumption – dimensions of constraint include effort, delay, unit price, and reinforcement schedule variations. This interplay of constraint and consumption emulates economic pressures, which serves as the foundation for behavioral economic approaches to quantifying relative reinforcing efficacy of rewards – substance-related or otherwise (Hursh, 1980, 1984, 1993).

As described in Chapter 2 (Jarmolowicz & Schneider, 2020), behavioral economics is the intersection of microeconomics and behavioral psychology. The subdiscipline of behavioral economics has proven especially advantageous to addiction fields given its ability to model economic pressures on reward attainment, simulating drug-seeking responses in real-world markets (Bickel, Degrandpre & Higgins, 1993; Jarmolowicz, Reed & Bickel, 2015). Two major themes have evolved from this behavioral economic tradition: (1) delay discounting and (2) operant demand. Delay discounting describes the devaluation of reward value as a function of consummatory delay (Madden & Bickel, 2010), while demand describes an organisms' operant defense of baseline drug consumption amidst increasing constraints (Reed, Kaplan & Becirevic, 2015) (see Figure 7.1). Because of the robust degree to which discounting and demand describe addiction-related phenomena, a novel reinforcement pathologies model of addiction has emerged (Bickel et al., 2011, 2014), providing unique behavioral economic insights into addiction profiles.

The reinforcement pathologies model of addiction posits that clinical issues of substance use and dependence arise when there is a confluence of excessive (a) preference for immediate consumption of a reward and (b) persistence in demand for a reward relative to other substitutable commodities/rewards (Bickel et al., 2014). While the explicit formulation of the reinforcement pathologies model is relatively new, discounting and demand have been independently applied to addiction topics over the past several decades. Specific areas of discounting and demand research include a range of both substance-related problems such as nicotine dependence (MacKillop & Tidey, 2011), alcohol use (Lemley et al., 2016), stimulant dependence (Greenwald & Hursh, 2006), and marijuana use (Collins et al., 2014), as well as behavioral addictions such as gambling (Madden, Petry & Johnson, 2009), indoor tanning (Reed, 2015), sexual acts (Johnson & Bruner, 2012), and technology dependence (Saville et al., 2010).

The rise and success of applying behavioral economics to areas of addiction is due in no small part to the pragmatic nature of discounting and demand research approaches (Hursh et al., 2013). Discounting and demand analyses provide unique behavioral insights to addiction in several ways. First, behavioral economic procedures simulate real-world market pressures associated with accessing addictive rewards. Second, the metrics rendered from behavioral economic procedures yield precise

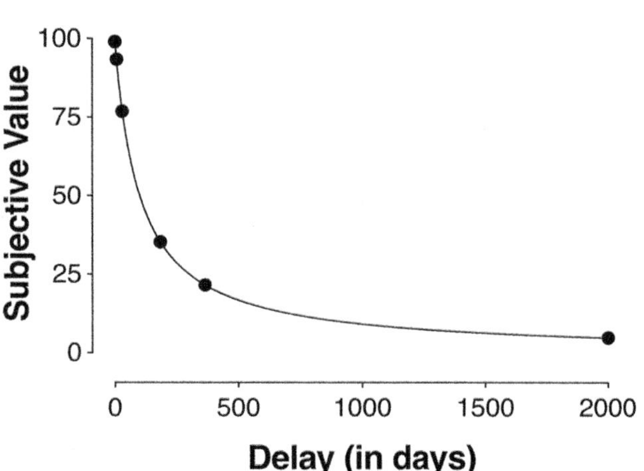

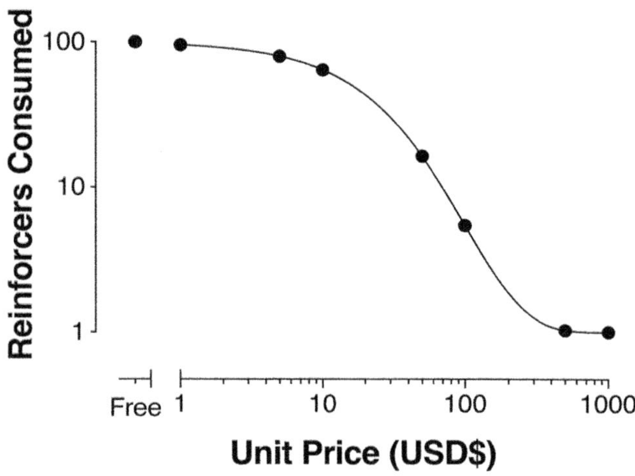

Figure 7.1 Graphical examples of delay discounting (left panel) and operant demand (right panel; note use of log scales)

quantification of various facets of addictive behavior; such metrics describe novel aspects of addiction profiles. Third, behavioral economic metrics can be translated to real-world variables with substantial social validity, such as effective pricing of drugs, delays associated with differing levels of reinforcer efficacy, and expected behavioral output associated with differing levels of consumption at differing constraint values – each of these variables directly inform policy and intervention considerations (Hursh & Roma, 2013).

The purpose of this chapter is to detail both human and nonhuman assays associated with quantifying the behavioral economics of addiction. Toward this end, we describe the historical foundations and evolution of behavioral economic methodology in the addiction literature. Following discussion of methods aimed at rendering behavioral economic data, we present the various models and approaches associated with behavioral economic metrics and the unique insights such metrics provide in an understanding of addiction.

History of Intertemporal Reward Valuation in Behavioral Economics

Nonhuman Intertemporal Choice

Mazur's (1987) adjusting delay procedure was among the first methods to directly measure discounting (see Lea [1976], Navarick & Fantino [1972], and Rachlin & Green [1972] for other work on intertemporal choice). In Mazur's experimental preparation, White Carneaux pigeons allocated pecking responses to keys producing either a small amount of food after a fixed delay or a larger amount after delays adjusting up or down based on the subject's previous response. Consistent preference for the smaller amount on the first block of trials resulted in a shorter delay to the larger option in the subsequent block, while preference for the larger delayed option lengthened the delay to that option. After reaching stable responding, the mean adjusted delay for each trial block served as the indifference point (i.e., the subject chose the fixed and adjusting options with equal frequency; Richards et al., 1997). Contrary to economic models of intertemporal choice that propose constant-rate reductions in reinforcer value as a function of delay (e.g., Samuelson, 1937), discounting in these experiments approximated the shape of a hyperbola, aligning with earlier behavioral economic accounts of intertemporal choice (Chung & Herrnstein, 1967; Rachlin & Green, 1972; Ainslie, 1975).

An alternate and extensively used method of measuring discounting in nonhumans is the procedure pioneered by Evenden and Ryan (1996), which provides a parametric comparison of sensitivity to magnitude and delay to reinforcement on operant responding. As mentioned elsewhere (Madden & Bickel, 2010), this procedure produces an ideal baseline for pharmacological and neurological experimentation after stable responding occurs across days. In the original experiments, twenty-four male Sprague-Dawley rats chose between immediate and delayed alternatives (e.g., a single food pellet now versus five pellets in ten seconds). Sessions began with a pair of forced-choice trials, with each alternative presented singularly as a means of exposing subjects to the contingencies of the preparation. In the subsequent six trials, choosing the immediate alternative produced a single pellet and initiated the programmed delay followed by a variable-length inter-trial interval (ITI). If the subject chose the delayed alternative, it experienced the same programmed delay followed simultaneously by the larger reinforcer and ITI. Time to the delayed alternative increased in systematic increments from 0.5 to 60 seconds across the seven remaining trial blocks.

In a variation of Mazur's (1987) adjusting delay procedure, Richards et al. (1997) assessed discounting in eight Sprague-Dawley rats using a novel adjusting *amount* method. Like Mazur's approach, this task featured a fixed (i.e., delayed) alternative (100 μl of water) and an adjusting alternative. If the subject chose the fixed option, the *amount* of the adjusting option increased by 10 percent on the subsequent trial, while choosing the adjusting option resulted in a 10 percent decrease in its amount on the next trial. Delay intervals associated with the fixed alternative were 0, 2, 4, 8, and 16 seconds and remained constant throughout each session. The amount of the adjusting alternative began between 71 μl (high amount) and 35 μl (low amount) and alternated across repeated assessments of each delay. Discount functions obtained aligned with those reported by Mazur (1987) and subsequent research suggests close correspondence between adjusting amount and adjusting delay procedures (Green et al., 2007).

Intertemporal Choice in Humans

In the early 1960s, Walter Mischel began his seminal investigations on self-control and delay of gratification in young children. Recruiting participants with a modal age of four years from Stanford University's Bing Nursery School and neighboring communities, Mischel initially assessed preference for pairs of reinforcers at varying delays and magnitudes. Given their curiosity about children's behavior during the delays to the larger (or more preferred) reinforcer(s), Mischel & Ebbesen (1970) initiated a long-running series of *experiential* delay of gratification experiments involving real reinforcers and real delays. These experiments featured a two-option choice paradigm: receive a smaller (or less-preferred) reinforcer immediately, or tolerate a delay to receive a larger (or more-preferred) reinforcer. Prior to leaving the room, the experimenter informed the child that emitting a specific operant (e.g., sounding a bell) at any point prior to end of the delay would result in receipt of the less-preferred (or smaller quantity) reinforcer(s). Longitudinal data from participants in these experiments revealed clear and robust differences between those who did and did not select the smaller more immediate reinforcer (Mischel, Ebbesen & Raskoff Zeiss, 1972; Mischel, Shoda & Peake, 1988; Mischel, Shoda & Rodriguez, 1989). In particular, the children who withstood the fifteen- to-twenty-minute waiting period – when followed up as adolescents – rated their social and cognitive behaviors higher, demonstrated better scores on college entrance exams, had lower body-mass indexes, were rated by parents and caregivers as exhibiting better self-control, and were more tolerant of frustrating environmental conditions than those who chose the immediately available reinforcer. In later adolescence, these same participants produced higher Scholastic Aptitude Test (SAT) scores and, as adults, reported greater job and marital satisfaction (Shoda, Mischel & Peake, 1990).

Development of Hypothetical Discounting Tasks

The first hypothetical discounting assessment was developed by Rachlin, Raineri and Cross (1991) using an undergraduate sample (N = 80). Seated across the table from an experimenter, participants indicated their preference for one of two hypothetical monetary options presented on index cards. Half the participants made choices between immediate and delayed outcomes while the other half experienced an analogous condition with outcomes framed as guaranteed or probabilistic. In the delay condition, the larger delayed alternative remained constant at $1,000 while the immediate alternative either increased from $1 or decreased from $1,000 in increments of $4 to $50 (half of the participants began at $1 and the other half at $1,000). Each participant experienced the increasing and decreasing sequences across seven delays (one month, six months, one year, five years, ten years, twenty-five years, and fifty years). Those assigned to the probability group experienced the same increasing and decreasing sequences, instead choosing between an amount to be paid for sure, or the chance of receiving $1,000 at seven probabilities (0.95, 0.9, 0.7, 0.5, 0.3, 0.1, and 0.05). Participants were said to have switched to the initially dispreferred alternative after making two consecutive choices of that alternative. Calculating the mean of the amounts just prior to and after the switch produced points of equivalence between the competing amounts, and the mean of these points in the increasing and decreasing sequences of each block produced indifference points. The authors fit the single-parameter hyperbolic equation (Mazur, 1987), $V = A/(1+kD)$, to the median indifference points generated in the delay condition, where V provides a description of how an outcome (A) loses value as a function of delay (D) to receipt, and k is a free parameter representing rate of discounting. The authors applied a variant of the hyperbolic model to the indifference points generated in the probability condition. In this model, h takes the place of k, and Θ, the odds against receipt of the larger amount, replaces D. Here, $\Theta = (1/p) - 1$, with p representing the probability of the outcome occurring. It is important to note the relation between the k and h parameters: k values in the high range suggest outcome devaluation as a function of delay, whereas high h values suggest an aversion to risk (i.e., devaluation as a function of uncertainty; Gray et al., 2016). Rachlin's approach can be administered in person by an experimenter, or on a computer. While the task has the benefit of assessing a relatively large range of immediate values, the drawback lies in the time cost relative to the procedures described below.

Monetary Choice Questionnaire

The Monetary Choice Questionnaire (MCQ; Kirby & Maraković, 1996) features a fixed sequence of twenty-one dichotomous choices between immediate and larger delayed options across small, medium, and large magnitudes of the delayed alternative. Kirby, Petry and Bickel (1999) developed a twenty-seven-item version several years later and this will be the focus of the present discussion, although the logic of the twenty-one- and twenty-seven-item assessments are essentially the same. Values of the delayed alternative are grouped into small ($25, $30, and $35), medium ($50, $55, and $60), and large ($75, $80, and $85) magnitudes, resulting in nine logarithmically spaced k values at each grouping. This tool has been extensively validated and has demonstrated utility in both clinical and research settings. Indeed, the MCQ is presently one of the most widely used contemporary human discounting assessments (Kaplan et al., 2016; MacKillop & Tidey, 2011). Scoring the MCQ has since been simplified by the development of automated scoring calculators (see Gray et al., 2016; Kaplan et al., 2016), which yield discounting rates across each magnitude as well as a consistency metric. A consistency score reflects the proportion of each participant's responses that align with the assigned k value as defined by the MCQ. Low consistency scores may suggest task inattention or haphazard responding. Toward this end, scores below 75 percent should be examined and *considered* for exclusion (Kaplan et al., 2016; cf. Gray et al., 2016).

Probability Discounting Questionnaire

The Probability Discounting Questionnaire (PDQ; Madden, Petry & Johnson, 2009) is a thirty-item assessment consisting of three ten-item blocks and it shares similarities with the MCQ to the extent that each consist of preconfigured choices and yield discounting rates across three magnitude groupings ($20 for sure or $80 at 10–83 percent chance.; $40 for sure or $100 at 18–91 percent chance; and $40 for sure or $60 at 40–97 percent chance). Producing a consistency score for each block of the PDQ follows the same logic as for the MCQ and is the sum of the number of certain choices prior to the proposed h value and the number of risky choices occurring at and after that h value, divided by the total number of choices in the block. Because the level of risk across choices on the PDQ clearly decreases (i.e., is not randomized), alternating between certain and risky options beyond the initial switch may suggest haphazard responding or task inattention. Accordingly, consistency scores <80 percent on any of the three blocks should be considered for possible removal (Gray et al., 2016).

Adjusting Amount

Du, Green and Myerson (2002) developed a variant of Richards and colleagues' (1997, 1999) titration procedure and, similar to other adjusting methods, operates as a function of each participant's choice pattern. Like Rachlin et al. (1991), the authors assessed delay and probability discounting across seven delays, selecting instead the following time blocks: one month, three months, nine months, two years, five years, ten years, and twenty years. The probability condition featured the same odds of receiving the reward used in Rachlin et al. (1991). Participants made six choices at each delay or probability across \$200 and \$10,000 magnitudes of the delayed/probabilistic alternative. The adjusting (i.e., immediate/guaranteed) alternative began at half the value of the fixed (delayed/probabilistic) alternative and, on the second trial, either increased or decreased by 50 percent of its initial value, depending on whether the participant chose the fixed or adjusting option, respectively. For the remaining trials, the adjusting option increased or decreased by 50 percent of the previous adjustment until the sixth choice, at which point the procedure repeated on the next delay (or probability) block. As in the Rachlin et al. task, the researchers obtained an indifference point at each delay or probability by determining the midpoint between the last chosen and unchosen immediate (or guaranteed) options. The seven resulting indifference points, like those generated by the Rachlin et al. task, can be fit with the hyperbolic equation (Mazur, 1987), or a hyperboloid variant that contains the additional free parameter *s*, which represents psychophysical scaling of delay and/or reward magnitude (see Myerson & Green, 1995; Rachlin, 2006). The authors, however, advise against a comparison of discount rates when using the hyperboloid equations, given the interaction between *k* (or *h*) and *s* parameters (Du et al., 2002; Myerson, Green & Warusawitharana, 2001).

Five-Trial Adjusting Delay

Koffarnus and Bickel (2014) developed an efficient method of measuring delay discounting involving just five choices that can be completed in approximately thirty to forty seconds. In this task the immediate and delayed amounts are fixed (e.g., \$500 and \$1,000), while delays to the larger option adjust up or down based on the participants responses. A benefit of this task is the ability to assess nonmonetary commodities, since tasks in which the amount fluctuates (e.g., Du, Green & Myerson, 2002; Richards et al., 1999) may present participants with awkward fractional commodities (e.g., 0.85 of a refrigerator). This task measures well against more established discounting procedures (e.g., Du et al., 2002) and, in addition to a *k* value, provides the effective delay-50 (ED_{50}) metric, which represents the delay at which the value of an outcome has lost 50 percent of its initial value.

Common Measures of Discounting

Discounting procedures that yield indifference points across blocks of delays (e.g., Du et al., 2002; Rachlin et al., 1991) are amenable to fitting nonlinear functions that describe the decrease in subjective value of an outcome as a function of delay (*k* parameter) or probability (*h* parameter). Mazur's (1987) hyperbolic equation or one of several variants described earlier can be fit to the obtained indifference points using a number of statistical packages (e.g., GraphPad Prism; SPSS; R). The resultant R^2 metric provides an estimate of the variance in the discounting function accounted for by the equation; common practice is to fit to the median indifference points generated by the dataset (rather than the means) to minimize the influence of outliers.[1] Because *k* and *h* values tend to follow nonnormal distributions (i.e., are positively skewed), performing log or natural log (ln) transformations will facilitate parametric statistical comparisons across groups and/or conditions. Again, it is important to note that discounting equations containing more than one free parameter (e.g., the psychophysical scalar in hyperboloid variants) preclude any direct comparison of the *k* (or *h*) values across participants due to the interaction between parameters.

Yoon and Higgins (2008) adapted the ED_{50} metric used to describe drug action in pharmacological research as a novel method to characterize discounting. In pharmacology, ED_{50} is the *dose* associated with a 50 percent reduction in the maximum drug effect (Ross & Kenakin, 2001). The authors opted to retain the name ED_{50}, referring instead to the effective *delay* rather than effective dose. Calculating ED_{50} is accomplished by substituting $A/2$ for V in Mazur's (1987) hyperbolic equation and, in so doing, this identifies the specific delay at which the value of an outcome is equal to 50 percent of its initial amount. Conveniently, as the authors point out, ED_{50} is equivalent to $1/k$ as derived by the hyperbolic equation. The related EP_{50} (Jarmolowicz et al., 2016) is the *probability* at which an outcome decreases to 50 percent of its initial value. A minor alteration of Rachlin et al.'s (1991) single parameter equation renders $E\Theta_{50}$ equivalent to $1/h$, and EP_{50} equivalent to $1/(E\Theta_{50}+1)$. This measure is useful when measuring decisions between guaranteed and uncertain outcomes (e.g., medication adherence with varying chances of side effects).

Several alternative methods of measuring discounting provide an atheoretical (i.e., model-free) account of the impact of delay or uncertainty on the subjective value of an outcome. One approach involves simply calculating the number or proportion of delayed or probabilistic choices across the discounting assessment. This method is a particularly suitable substitute for the *k* value when using the MCQ, given the strong correspondence between these metrics (Myerson, Baumann & Green, 2014). Another model-free approach involves calculating the total area under the empirical discounting function (i.e., indifference points), resulting in a value known as area-under-the-curve (AUC; Myerson et al., 2001). As is the case when fitting a nonlinear function, this method can only be directly applied to discounting assessments that produce indifference points across blocks of delays or probabilities. Calculating AUC for an empirical discounting function involves converting each delay (or odds-against occurrence) into a proportion of the longest delay (or lowest odds-against occurrence), while converting each indifference point into a proportion of the undiscounted amount. These proportions

[1] Several methods for identifying nonsystematic and outlier responding can be applied to discounting data (e.g., the algorithm developed by Johnson & Bickel (2008); removing participants whose proportion of immediate choices result in *z*-scores or a median absolute deviation outside of a decided cut-off criterion). There is, however, no consensus on how to best handle nonsystematic responding on discounting assessments.

then serve as the x (delay or odds-against) and y (subjective value) coordinates. The distance between each normalized indifference point and the x-axis (which can be represented by hypothetical vertical lines) creates a succession of trapezoids, each of which can be explained mathematically as $(x_2 - x_1)\,[(y_1 + y_2)/2]$. Here, x_1 and x_2 represent sequential delays (or decreasing odds-against), and y_1 and y_2 are the obtained indifference points associated with those values. The authors note that, for the first trapezoid, the x_1 and y_1 values are set at 0.0 and 1.0, respectively (Myerson et al., 2001, p. 240). Summing the calculated areas of each trapezoid yields the total area under the empirical discounting function, with proportions further below 1.0 indicative of steeper discounting. Two recent variants of AUC incorporate $\log_{10}$ and ordinal transformations of the delays to account for nonlinear scaling of time intervals (or probability) and the consequently disproportionate contribution of successive delays (or odds against occurrence) to the total AUC (see Borges et al., 2016).

Novel Discounting Applications

Research on discounting has provided important information about unsafe sexual behavior in vulnerable populations including at-risk youth (Dariotis & Johnson, 2015), individuals with alcohol-use disorder (Jarmolowicz, Bickel & Gatchalian, 2013; Johnson et al., 2017), opioid-dependent women (Herrmann et al., 2014), and cocaine users (Jarmolowicz et al., 2014). Johnson and Bruner (2012) presented a sample of cocaine-dependent individuals with a novel hypothetical discounting task, involving decisions between an immediate unprotected sexual encounter and a delayed sexual encounter where a condom was available. Participants made choices across four conditions: (1) a hypothetical partner least likely to have a sexually transmitted infection, (2) most likely to have a sexually transmitted infection, (3) most attractive, and (4) least attractive. Results indicated that risky sexual decisions are strongly mediated by delays to protected sex.

College-age individuals generally spend upwards of five hours a day on the internet or engaging with a smartphone (Cheever et al., 2014; Junco & Cotten, 2012; Roberts, Petnji Yaya & Manolis, 2014) and there is growing evidence that chronic smartphone and internet use may be markers of a behavioral addiction (Kwon et al., 2013; O'Donnel & Epstein, 2019). Reed et al. (2016a) validated and extended a discounting task developed by Atchley and Warden (2012) to assess the effect of delays on the value of unlocking a received text message. Participants read a vignette explaining that their cellular-phone provider has instituted a new plan whereby subscribers must pay a fee to immediately open text messages or may open the messages for free after a delay. Fees for immediately unlocking the text message feature were \$0.50 and \$5.00, and both were assessed across delays ranging from one minute to twenty-four hours. The discounting task effectively captured a magnitude effect between the \$0.50 and \$5.00 conditions and differentiated chronic text-messaging users and less-frequent users.

Other novel research has examined discounting of "erotic stimuli" (Lawyer, 2008), food (Epstein et al., 2010; Odum, Baumann & Remington, 2006), marijuana and alcohol (Strickland, Lile & Stoops, 2017), cigarettes (Bickel, Odum & Madden, 1999), and internet use in college students (Saville et al., 2010). In sum, discounting provides useful tools to better understand neuroeconomic and contextual factors that exert influence on decision making.

History of Operant Demand Assessment in Behavioral Economics

Nonhuman Operant Demand

As operant approaches to behavioral pharmacology became increasingly popular in the literature (see Leslie, 2003), researchers began examining the effects of drug administration on rates of responding under differing levels of reinforcement constraint, typically in the form of simple reinforcement schedules. Organisms' rates of responding across differing "costs" of reinforcement under differing drugs and doses provided an objective measure of abuse liability. Common across these early operant behavioral pharmacology assays was a parametric evaluation of reinforcement costs (e.g., a range of fixed ratio or variable interval requirements). To understand drug effects, however, nondrug operant baselines were necessary to serve as a comparison for operant responding under the influence of drug administration. In a classic study by Catania and Reynolds (1968), researchers conducted a series of six experiments examining pigeons' key-pecking across differing reinforcement constraints (e.g., variable and fixed interval schedules, omission of reinforcement following long intervals). These experiments illustrated the orderly parametric effects of reinforcement cost on responding, providing other researchers a baseline against which drug discrimination and administration studies could be compared.

In the late 1970s and early 1980s, Dr. Steven Hursh (at the time, a behavioral pharmacologist and scientist at Walter Reed Institute of Research) began summarizing the known literature on the effects reinforcement costs and constraints on operant responding. In a seminal review paper (1980), Hursh outlined the many ways in which operant responding under differing constraints conformed to basic principles of microeconomics (e.g., Law of Demand, economy types). Hursh subsequently proposed the field of behavioral economics as a novel means of understanding operant phenomena (1984). For example, Hursh noted that the precipitous decrease in operant behavior across increasing fixed ratio responses in Felton and Lyon's (1966) study of pigeons resembled demand curves from the economic literature.

As behavioral pharmacologists became acquainted with the behavioral economic framework, operant demand emerged as the gold standard in operant assessment of drug abuse liability. For example, Winger et al. (2002) examined drug self-administration across differing unit prices and doses of ketamine, phencyclidine, and dizocilpine in rhesus monkeys. Within drugs, the doses yielded equivalent demand elasticities. However, in a reanalysis of the data, Hursh (2014) illustrated that ketamine featured the strongest levels of demand, while dizocilipine featured the lowest. These demand levels were perfectly rank-order correlated with the drugs' time to peak effect, offering novel insight into how drug metabolization and effect timing interact with the organism's demand. These analyses serve as prototypic examples of nonhuman operant demand assays' insights into drug rewards.

Human Operant Demand

Given the success of the behavioral economic approach to behavioral pharmacology in the nonhuman literature, behavioral pharmacologists began extending these demand assays to human drug self-administration in the 1980s (see Griffiths, Bigelow & Henningfield (1980) for a review of this translational work). This human drug demand work was specifically pioneered by Dr. Warren Bickel and Dr. Steven

Higgins, who were interested in identifying humans' valuation of drug reinforcers to design novel behavioral interventions. In early extensions to human behavioral pharmacology, Bickel and colleagues (1990, 1991) offered human participants the opportunity to earn puffs of preferred cigarettes contingent on meeting schedule requirements by pulling levers in a laboratory. Their results rendered demand curves similar to the example in the right panel of Figure 7.1, directly replicating the general function observed in highly controlled nonhuman work.

Following Bickel and colleagues' seminal work outlining their success in translating nonhuman demand findings to human samples (see also Bickel, DeGrandpre & Higgins, 1993; DeGrandpre et al., 1992, 1993), other behavioral scientists began using their procedures to answer similar issues regarding human drug abuse liability. For example, Greenwald and Hursh (2006) offered heroin-dependent research participants the option between money or hydromorphone, both at escalating "costs" in the form of working on a computer task. Participant choices were aggregated to create demand curves.

Careful consideration of the aforementioned human demand studies reveals a number of procedural limitations. First, drug administration requires intense institutional oversight and safety precautions. Second, procurement of the drug rewards requires significant financial resources. Third, rendering a demand curve requires repeated assessment across a range of drugs costs, often necessitating scores of hours of participant time with data collection taking weeks or months for each individual participant. For these reasons, actual drug administration in human operant demand work is infeasible for many laboratories and investigators. Advances in simulated demand assays in the form of hypothetical purchase tasks circumvents these concerns while still returning valid responses that conform to behavioral economic expectations. The remainder of this section focuses exclusively on purchase task methods.

Development of the Hypothetical Purchase Task

By the end of the 1990s, researchers had begun to place a greater emphasis on the utility of behavioral economic methods as a framework to better understand illicit drug use. Published findings proposing a relation between operant demand indices and reinforcing efficacy underscored the application of human operant methodology to facets of addiction (see Bickel & Madden, 1999). However, because the difficulties of a translational behavioral economic study of human respondents proved troublesome in many respects (e.g., concerns surrounding the administration of potentially addictive drugs to rehabilitation-seeking users), research teams moved to develop a survey-type measure capable of producing operant demand indices expected from laboratory work without the significant time investment or ethical concerns of traditional methods. The literature highlighted in this section embodies the general advancement of purchase task methodology; for a more comprehensive review of purchase task literature, see Kaplan et al. (2018) and Reed et al. (2020).

The first instance of the hypothetical purchase task (HPT) was presented by Petry and Bickel (1998) as a simplified assessment of decision making by drug users – one that circumvents the concerns associated with preceding human operant substance abuse work while still drawing upon principles from the behavioral economic laboratory. Forty (n = 25 male) self-reported substance users were granted a balance of hypothetical currency and asked to make decisions regarding the purchasing and consumption of illicit drugs (e.g., heroin, Valium) under changing stipulations; price constraints were framed as per unit (e.g., *per bag* of heroin; *per pill* of Valium) and presented in a random order to more closely approximate the instability of real-world price fluctuation. Prior to responding, a context for decision making was established by a vignette that described a hypothetical scenario and imposed restrictions on purchasing and substance use (e.g., "You may buy any drugs you'd like with this money, and there are no consequences to using these drugs"; "You cannot purchase more drugs, or any other drugs except those you choose below"; p. 323).

Hypothetical purchases demonstrated the characteristic positive deceleration with increasing price expected from laboratory progressive-ratio assessments. Regarding the continued application of simulation studies to general behavioral economic investigation, such a replication of laboratory findings was a necessary precedent. Researchers concluded in favor of the potential viability of simulation tasks to describe these economic relations, given the extension of laboratory findings embodied by purchase task responding. Interestingly, respondents reported that the contrived nature of the task (e.g., the limitations imposed by the vignette) aided in establishing relations to real-world events and thus may have aided in generating more authentic responding.

In a replication of this initial success, Jacobs and Bickel (1999) used a hypothetical purchase task to assess the previously described relations between behavioral economic indices (e.g., breakpoint, elasticity) and measures of reinforcer efficacy in a sample of cigarette and opioid users. Simplification of the simulation task via the removal of hypothetical money in favor of participants' verbal reporting of purchases permitted a more rapid task administration and completion as compared to the previous installation. The task instructed seventeen respondents to report hypothetical purchases of cigarettes and heroin at unit prices (i.e., *per cigarette* and *per bag*, respectively) ranging from $0.01 (free) to $1,120, with and without the competing commodity made concurrently available; an included vignette was used to stimulate more authentic task responding.

Responses again demonstrated features of operant demand expected in laboratory studies (e.g., positive deceleration at increasing price). This successful modeling of behavioral economic demand for target commodities extended the early success of the purchase task, with notable differences in methodology. Researchers did not present respondents with mock currency, but instead asked them to report hypothetical purchasing under *imagined* usage constraints (e.g., respondents were informed that all "purchased" units of a commodity were for personal consumption within the set temporal restriction). This modification reportedly resulted in less costly data acquisition but may have inflated respondent purchasing. Differences notwithstanding, a replicated success of purchase tasks bolstered confidence in the utility of these simulations for assessing reinforcer efficacy.

The early success of the purchase task brought to light the growing need for investigation to better understand the limitations necessarily imposed by a simulation-type assessment to generate responding representative of that occurring under natural contingencies. Several extensions followed (e.g., Petry, 2000, 2001a, 2001b; see also Petry & Bickel, 1999) and served as replications of the efficiency and value of purchase task application, yet throughout these works the role of the vignette remained largely unmodulated. Work seeking to narrow constraints and create a more valid context through which purchasing decisions are made was a logical next step for purchase task methodology.

Alcohol Purchase Task

As purchase tasks continued to grow in popularity, their applicability for more nuanced use – facilitated by vignette modifications – became increasingly evident with the work of Murphy and MacKillop (2006). In their study, researchers demonstrated use of a novel purchase task (i.e., the alcohol purchase task; APT) to assess the reinforcing efficacy of alcohol in a sample of undergraduate students. Researchers drew from earlier efforts in their development of a vignette to constrain hypothetical purchases; limitations on the size and type of purchased alcoholic beverages, the setting of proposed alcohol intake, and the use of purchased beverages (i.e., drinks could be consumed only by the respondent within the specified timeframe) narrowed the possibility of inflated responding. In addition, researchers heeded the advice of Jacobs and Bickel (1999) to include budgetary constraints – participants were asked to imagine their current financial situation when making their purchasing decisions. Fourteen price points ranging from $0 (free) to $9 served as discrete, within-subject assessments of demand for alcoholic beverages. Model-derived behavioral economic indices demonstrated conceptual consistency with previously validated clinical scales of alcohol use (i.e., Daily Drinking Questionnaire; Collins, Parks & Marlatt, 1985), in that self-identified *heavy drinkers* (n = 189) demonstrated greater demand for alcohol at zero-cost as compared to *light drinkers,* as well as more persistent demand for alcohol in the face of increasing price. Despite promising initial findings, researchers acknowledged limitations to their design, notably the focus on undergraduate students as the sole sample of interest, the novel vignette design, which may not represent the natural contingencies of alcohol consumption for all respondents, and a limited range of prices, which resulted in a small subset of respondents that did not report a break in consumption.

Work by Murphy et al. (2009) advanced the APT on several fronts. The goal of the work was to build added support for the application of a purchase task to measure demand for alcohol by again demonstrating the relation between indices generated via task responding and aspects of reinforcer efficacy as measured by established clinical scales (e.g., twenty-eight-day Timeline Follow-Back interview (Sobell & Sobell, 1973, 1992); Young Adult Alcohol Problems Screening Test (Hurlbut & Sher, 1992). A refined vignette more extensively framed responding (e.g., clarification on nonalcoholic drug use) and specified a new location for purchases (i.e., the respondent is now attending a party, as opposed to the previously assumed bar setting). Results confirmed the proposed relations between indices, supporting the use of the APT as a measure of reinforcing efficacy of alcohol.

As a critical next step for the utility of the APT and, broadly, HPTs, Amlung et al. (2012) assessed the degree to which alcohol consumption reported on the APT is representative of behavior observed in natural settings and under relevant contingencies. Forty-one respondents completed purchase tasks in a "neutral" lab environment, during which time researchers recorded reported and simulated (i.e., using tangible mock currency) purchases of alcoholic beverages. Subsequent validation took place in a cue-primed bar environment wherein respondents were presented with a quantity of drinks corresponding to self-reported purchases at a randomly selected price-point. Responding was assessed for consistency between real and hypothetical purchases, and for consistency between reported and actual consumption (essential given the vignette-specified purchase–consumption relation). Analysis indicated acceptable validity for the use of the APT; examination of predictive validity suggested the simulation task is indeed tapping a behavioral construct similar to that observed in a typical setting.

As a final exemplary contribution to the APT literature, Yurasek et al. (2013) presented several modifications to the standard APT format in their investigatory comparison of APT responding in self-identified tobacco users and nonusers. In contrast to previous work, the employed APT featured a price structure extended to include seventeen prices ranging from $0 (free) to $20. The vignette was also modified to reflect the absence of *next day responsibilities*, in that respondents were asked to imagine a scenario in which no obligations were scheduled on the day following the proposed alcohol consumption. Obtained alcohol demand metrics adequately predicted consumption values collected via clinical measures (e.g., DDQ) and, as such, lend support for the use of this most recent vignette adaptation as a standard for APT methodology.

Cigarette Purchase Task

In the same year that Murphy and MacKillop (2006) proposed their novel application of purchase tasks, Field et al. (2006) presented an extension to the measurement of operant demand for cigarettes. More specifically, researchers were interested in replicating the findings of an earlier study (i.e., Madden & Bickel, 1999) that revealed a potential sensitivity of behavioral economic measures to periods of smoking abstinence in regular cigarette smokers. This foundational version of a cigarette purchase task (CPT) instructed participants to imagine a fixed budget and to report their allocation of weekly disposable income (e.g., after vignette-indicated necessary costs) to various common daily expenses (e.g., food, travel, leisure activities) when faced with an increasing price *per pack* of cigarettes; prices served as discrete assessments of reinforcing efficacy and ranged from £3 to £7 in whole unit increments. Broadly, task responding demonstrated positive deceleration of purchasing with respect to increasing cost, as well as several other relevant features of laboratory assessment. Reported cigarette purchasing did not appear to be impacted by periods of smoking abstinence, although participants exhibited a willingness to reduce spending in other, often more essential domains of daily living (e.g., clothing, household goods) in order to compensate for increasing cigarette prices.

A subsequent version of the CPT proposed by MacKillop et al. (2008) employed a methodology drawing more heavily upon components of previously established HPTs (e.g., Jacobs & Bickel, 1999). The primary aim was to assess the ability of the proposed CPT to identify individuals with an elevated risk for nicotine dependence; toward this end, respondents completed the Fagerström Test of Nicotine Dependence (Fagerström, 1978; Heatherton et al., 1991) as a comparator for convergent validity. A vignette constrained purchasing in a fashion similar to natural contingencies – all purchasing decisions should be characteristic of those occurring during a typical day and should draw from a budget representative of the individual's ongoing financial status. Respondents received further instructions to assume no access to potential substitutes (e.g., nicotine replacement therapies), and that any purchased product was to be consumed within a twenty-four-hour period. Nineteen *per cigarette* prices, ranging from $0 (free) to $1,120 and presented in ascending order, assessed demand in the face of changing cost stipulations. Indices generated by CPT responding demonstrated a significant relation to nicotine-related variables (i.e., nicotine dependence) and successfully discriminated between individuals of varying self-reported nicotine dependence, thereby lending further support for CPT administration.

Murphy et al. (2011) sought to extend this demonstrated validity to use with an adolescent population. One-hundred and thirty-eight adolescent smokers completed a modified CPT; relative to the version employed by MacKillop et al. (2008), the range of prices was expanded to include twenty-six values ranging from $0 (free) to $1,120 *per cigarette.* Respondents also completed clinically relevant measures of nicotine use that had been previously validated for use with adolescent populations. As with previous work focused in adult populations, CPT responding demonstrated significant relations to indices of nicotine use and thus illustrated an alternative approach to examining nicotine use in adolescents.

Few et al. (2012) evaluated the temporal stability of indices generated via application of the CPT by examining consistency of task responding when completed at two instances separated by a one-week delay. To "smooth" price gaps and create a high-resolution view of cigarette demand, the task assessed *per cigarette* purchases at seventy-three prices ranging from $0 (free) to $10. Responding on the task demonstrated strong test–retest reliability, while indices generated from each instance of measurement demonstrated a strong relation to indices of self-reported nicotine use as collected on the Fagerström Test of Nicotine Dependence (Heatherton et al., 1991). As such, data support the use of the purchase task for the measurement of cigarette demand across time.

Novel Hypothetical Purchase Task Applications

The continued success of purchase task methodology in evaluating and describing operant demand for drugs of abuse has inspired numerous extensions examining commodities that fall outside the typical purview of behavioral economic investigation. Advancing both the understanding of purchase task utility and the relative demand for these commodities, novel examinations have greatly contributed to the present viability of hypothetical purchase tasks as a jack-of-all-trades assessment. The first representation of these outside-the-box applications, Epstein, Dearing and Roba (2010) examined demand for preferred snack food using a nineteen-price hypothetical purchase task; *per portion* pricing ranged from $0 (free) to $1,120 and was assessed in an ascending fashion. Twenty-four (n = 12 identified as obese; i.e., having a BMI of at least 30 kg/m^2) individuals completed the task under constraints typical of previous purchase tasks (e.g., these products are for your consumption *only*). Responding revealed similarities to preceding laboratory food assessments, leading researchers to conclude in favor of the use of a simulation task to more quickly determine reinforcing efficacy of various snack foods.

Similarly, Pope et al. (2010) used an extension of the hypothetical purchase task to evaluate demand for anabolic-androgenic steroids (AAS) in a sample of forty-two men, all having used AAS at least once. Owing to the unorthodox nature of AAS use (i.e., individuals must maintain regular use for up to twelve weeks at a time), the standard vignette constraints were modified such that purchases were for planned, long-term use. Respondents thus indicated *per 10 ml bottle* purchases at prices ranging from £1 to £987 with the goal of stockpiling the commodity. Individuals identified as having a potential dependence also demonstrated significantly greater demand, illustrating the robust applicability of purchase task methodology to situations necessitating adaptability. These and the following studies represent a synopsis of the wide-ranging use of HPTs in recent behavioral economic literature.

Marijuana Purchase Task

The marijuana purchase task (MPT) was first used by Collins et al. (2014) as a rapid evaluation of the reinforcing efficacy of cannabis in a sample of fifty-nine regular users. Respondents reported hypothetical *per joint* purchases at sixteen prices ranging from $0 (free) to $160. Constraints were largely typical of previous work (e.g., consumption within an allotted period of time) but contained additional information relevant to purchases of the novel commodity (e.g., specification of marijuana quality). Responses on the task were significantly related to self-reported rates of commodity ingestion, providing some initial support for the use of the MPT as a brief measure of operant demand for marijuana.

Subsequent applications of the MPT sought to extend demonstrations of validity via relations between responding and other measures of marijuana abuse liability. Aston et al. (2015) examined responding of 104 self-reported marijuana users on a twenty-two-price installation of the MPT. Results confirmed previous findings, in that demand metrics significantly predicted risk for substance dependence. Similarly, Aston, Metrik and MacKillop (2015) recruited ninety-nine self-reported frequent marijuana users to report hypothetical *per puff* purchases at twenty-two price-points ranging from $0 (free) to $10. Again, task responding demonstrated significant relations to variables relevant to cannabis use (e.g., dependence symptoms). Further extensions of the MPT have employed a variety of aims, including the demonstration of cue-elicited demand for marijuana (Metrik et al., 2016), the importance of perceived product quality for demand (Vincent et al., 2017), and the presence of a latent factor structure (i.e., "persistence" and "amplitude"; Aston et al., 2017) — all support use of the MPT for describing the reinforcing efficacy of cannabis.

Cocaine Purchase Task

In their novel presentation of a cocaine purchase task, Bruner and Johnson (2014) reported hypothetical purchases of eighty-six self-identified cocaine-dependent individuals residing in a metropolitan location. Respondents could purchase *nickel bags* of crack rock or *vials* of powdered cocaine at fifteen prices ranging from $0.01 to $1,000, presented in an ascending fashion. Strickland et al. (2016), too, examined purchasing of rock or powered cocaine, adding a specified weight of 0.1 grams per unit. Forty verified (i.e., via urinalysis) cocaine users reported purchases for their preferred form of the commodity at sixteen per-unit prices ranging from $0 (free) to $1,000. Strickland, Reynolds & Stoops (2016) applied a similar price structure and vignette to evaluate cocaine demand in a sample of forty-four self-identified active cocaine users. In all exhibitions, cocaine demand metrics served as adequate predictors of reported cocaine use.

Tanning Purchase Task

Taking a step away from the typical frame of substance abuse, Reed et al. (2016b) examined the utility of a hypothetical purchase task to evaluate operant demand for ultraviolet (UV) indoor tanning. A sample of 102 undergraduate females completed the novel tanning purchase task (TPT), indicating their subjective *likelihood* of signing up for a month of unlimited tanning at a variety of costs. Commodity *base price* was stated to be $30, and respondents were instructed to indicate purchasing intentions when presented with fifteen different *tax prices*, ranging from $0 (no tax) to $60, added to the base price. Those identified by clinically-relevant measures as being at greater risk for tanning abuse concurrently demonstrated a significantly elevated demand for tanning services.

More recent TPT applications have evaluated the effects of a varied price structure and purchasing method (i.e., number of tanning sessions purchased in a month). Becirevic et al. (2017) examined the predictive ability of this updated TPT to predict scores on a validated, clinical measure of UV indoor tanning abuse liability. Metrics of demand exhibited by differing risk classification groups showed significant differences, where those at the highest risk for tanning abuse also maintained purchases at higher costs. Becirevic, Reed and Amlung (2017) used the same purchasing guidelines and price structure to assess the ability of cues to modulate demand and, subsequently, reported purchases. Self-identified regular tanners exposed to cues associated with indoor tanning exhibited elevated demand as compared to those exposed to neutral cues, providing support for the sensitivity of the TPT to differences in setting events, and highlighting a potential risk for relapse (i.e., cue-elicited cravings) in the treatment of tanning dependence.

Gambling Purchase Task

To evaluate the prevalence and reinforcing efficacy of gambling-type behavior, Weinstock et al. (2016) developed a gambling purchase task (GPT) that assesses monthly gambling session entries as a factor of varying cover charges. Seventy-three respondents reported the number of times they would gamble in a month if cover charges were set at each of eighteen prices, ranging from $0 (free) to $50 *per entry*. Demand metrics were then compared to responding on a clinical assessment of lifetime gambling use; individuals flagged as having, or being at risk for, a gambling-use disorder also demonstrated – on average – greater demand for gambling and more willingness to pay expensive cover fees for access to gambling.

Pornography Purchase Task

In light of growing concerns surrounding pornography use, Mulhauser, Short and Weinstock (2018) developed a pornography purchase task (PPT) for use in assessing reinforcing efficacy of the content. A sample of 369 individuals was recruited via an online crowdsourcing service and instructed to make decisions regarding access of pornographic material. Notably, respondents were asked to imagine that their only means of accessing pornography was through a website with a daily access fee, although no specific definition of pornography was provided. Participants reported the *number of days* in a thirty-day span they would purchase access to the site. Twenty-nine entry costs ranging from $0 (free) to $500 served to evaluate defense of baseline consumption. Evaluation of task responding suggested adequate test-retest reliability and construct validity, and thus suggests the PPT may embody a viable approach for evaluating demand for pornography.

Internet Purchase Task

Broadbent and Dakki (2015) demonstrated the utility of a hypothetical purchase task to measure operant demand for internet use. Given the absence of preceding work examining the reinforcing efficacy of internet exposure and the growing concern surrounding excessive internet use, the internet purchase task (IPT) examined willingness to pay for internet access in a sample of 253 undergraduate students. Respondents were instructed to make *per hour* purchases of internet access in an imagined air travel scenario, in turn limiting purchases to a maximum of five hours (i.e., travel duration) and preventing other availability of internet services. The presented *per hour* price sequence contained thirteen values ranging from $0 (free) to $25. Task responding demonstrated predictive validity with respect to self-reported rates of daily internet use, as well as significant differences for those identified by relevant validated scales as being at risk for problematic use.

Other Applications of HPTs

A growing segment of what continues to prove itself a robust body of literature, hypothetical purchase task studies have shown applicability to a range of measures within (e.g., Pickover et al., 2016) and beyond the realm of addiction. As of the writing of this chapter, purchase tasks have been used to assess travel habits (Reed et al., 2014), sexual partner preference (Jarmolowicz et al., 2016), willingness to work (Henley et al., 2016), and use of reusable shopping bags (Kaplan, Gelino & Reed, 2018). As the use of these tasks progresses, validation and thorough evaluation of task responding will likely continue to support the use of the method as a gold-standard for measuring operant demand.

Conclusions

Behavioral economics provides novel insights into consumer behavior. When applied to addiction and behavioral addictions, behavioral economic principles offer many meaningful metrics to understand motivations to consume or behave. Discounting provides specific insight into how future and/or uncertain outcomes become devalued, often leading to risky present-focused behaviors that could lead to dependence problems or addictive behaviors. Likewise, the notion of demand operationalizes motivational aspects of consumption by translating microeconomic principles to understand organisms' willingness to defend access to potentially addictive substances or behaviors. Organisms with strong and persistent demand are more likely to be treatment-resistant and dependent. Thus, it is no surprise that the confluence of discounting and demand has been proposed as a novel behavioral indicator addiction via *reinforcement pathologies* (Bickel et al., 2011, 2014). Given the relative ease with which discounting or demand measures can be used to measure behavioral tendencies that are robustly related to issues of dependence, addiction professionals should seriously consider adopting such procedures in either clinical or research settings.

REFERENCES

Ainslie, G. (1975). Specious reward: A behavioral theory of impulsiveness and impulse control. *Psychological Bulletin*, **82**(4), 463–496. doi: 10.1037/h0076860

Amlung, M. T., Acker, J., Stojek, M. K., Murphy, J. G. & MacKillop, J. (2012). Is talk "cheap"? An initial investigation of the equivalence of alcohol purchase task performance for hypothetical and actual rewards. *Alcoholism: Clinical and Experimental Research*, **36**(4), 716–724. https://doi.org/10.1111/j.1530-0277.2011.01656.x

Aston, E. R., Farris, S. G., MacKillop, J. & Metrik, J. (2017). Latent factor structure of a behavioral economic marijuana demand curve. *Psychopharmacology*, **234**(16), 2421–2429. https://doi.org/10.1007/s00213-017-4633-6

Aston, E. R., MacKillop, J., Cassidy, R. & Metrik, J. (2015). Initial validation of a marijuana purchase task. *Drug and Alcohol Dependence,* **146**, e212. https://doi.org/10.1016/j.drugalcdep.2014.09.044

Aston, E. R., Metrik, J. & MacKillop, J. (2015). Further validation of a marijuana purchase task. *Drug and Alcohol Dependence,* **152**, 32–38. https://doi.org/10.1016/j.drugalcdep.2015.04.025

Atchley, P. & Warden, A. C. (2012). The need of young adults to text now: Using delay discounting to assess informational choice. *Journal of Applied Research in Memory and Cognition,* **1**(4), 229–234. doi: 10.1016/j.jarmac.2012.09.001

Becirevic, A., Reed, D. D. & Amlung, M. (2017). An initial investigation of the effects of tanning-related cues on demand and craving for indoor tanning. *Psychological Record,* **67** (2), 149–160. https://doi.org/10.1007/s40732-017-0246-z

Becirevic, A., Reed, D. D., Amlung, M., et al. (2017). An initial study of behavioral addiction symptom severity and demand for indoor tanning. *Experimental and Clinical Psychopharmacology,* **25**(5), 346–352. https://doi.org/10.1037/pha0000146

Bickel, W. K. & Madden, G. J. (1999). A comparison of measures of relative reinforcing efficacy and behavioral economics: Cigarettes and money in smokers. *Behavioural Pharmacology,* **10**(6–7), 627–637. https://doi.org/10.1097/00008877-199908001-00023

Bickel, W. K., Degrandpre, R. J. & Higgins, S. T. (1993). Behavioral economics: A novel experimental approach to the study of drug dependence. *Drug and Alcohol Dependence,* **33**(2), 173–192. https://doi.org/10.1016/0376-8716(93)90059-Y

Bickel, W. K., DeGrandpre, R. J., Higgins, S. T. & Hughes, J. R. (1990). Behavioral economics of drug self-administration. I. Functional equivalence of response requirement and drug dose. *Life Sciences,* **47**(17), 1501–1510.

Bickel, W. K., DeGrandpre, R. J., Hughes, J. R. & Higgins, S. T. (1991). Behavioral economics of drug self-administration. II. A unit-price analysis of cigarette smoking. *Journal of the Experimental Analysis of Behavior,* **55**(2), 145–154.

Bickel, W. K., Jarmolowicz, D. P., Mueller, E. T. & Gatchalian, K. M. (2011). The behavioral economics and neuroeconomics of reinforcer pathologies: Implications for etiology and treatment of addiction. *Current Psychiatry Reports,* **13**(5), 406–415. https://doi.org/10.1007/s11920-011-0215-1

Bickel, W. K., Johnson, M. W., Koffarnus, M. N., MacKillop, J. & Murphy, J. G. (2014). The behavioral economics of substance use disorders: reinforcement pathologies and their repair. *Annual Review of Clinical Psychology,* **10**, 641–677. https://doi.org/10.1146/annurev-clinpsy-032813-153724

Bickel, W. K., Odum, A. L. & Madden, G. J. (1999). Impulsivity and cigarette smoking: Delay discounting in current, never, and ex-smokers. *Psychopharmacology,* **146**(4), 447–454. doi: 10.1007/PL00005490

Borges, A. M., Kuang, J., Milhorn, H. & Yi, R. (2016). An alternative approach to calculating area-under-the-curve (AUC) in delay discounting research. *Journal of the Experimental Analysis of Behavior,* **106**(2), 145–155. doi: 10.1002/jeab.219

Bradshaw, C. M. & Killeen, P. R. (2012). A theory of behaviour on progressive ratio schedules, with applications in behavioural pharmacology. *Psychopharmacology (Berl),* **222**(4), 549–564. https://doi.org/10.1007/s00213-012-2771-4

Branch, M. N. (2006). How research in behavioral pharmacology informs behavioral science. *Journal of the Experimental Analysis of Behavior,* **85**(3), 407–423. https://doi.org/10.1901/jeab.2006.130-04

Broadbent, J. & Dakki, M. A. (2015). How much is too much to pay for internet access? A behavioral economic analysis of internet use. *Cyberpsychology, Behavior, and Social Networking,* **18**(8), 457–461. https://doi.org/10.1089/cyber.2014.0367

Bruner, N. R. & Johnson, M. W. (2014). Demand curves for hypothetical cocaine in cocaine-dependent individuals. *Psychopharmacology,* **231**(5), 889–897. https://doi.org/10.1007/s00213-013-3312-5

Catania, A. C. & Reynolds, G. S. (1968). A quantitative analysis of the responding maintained by interval schedules of reinforcement. *Journal of the Experimental Analysis of Behavior,* **11**(3S2), 327–383.

Cheever, N. A., Rosen, L. D., Carrier, L. M. & Chavez, A. (2014). Out of sight is not out of mind: The impact of restricting wireless mobile device use on anxiety levels among low, moderate and high users. *Computers in Human Behavior,* **37**, 290–297. doi: 10.1016/j.chb.2014.05.002

Chung, S. & Herrnstein, R. J. (1967). Choice and delay of reinforcement. *Journal of the Experimental Analysis of Behavior,* **10**(1), 67–74. doi: 10.1901/jeab.1967.10-67

Collins, R. L., Parks, G. A. & Marlatt, G. A. (1985). Social determinants of alcohol consumption: The effects of social interaction and model status on the self-administration of alcohol. *Journal of Consulting and Clinical Psychology,* **53**(2), 189–200. https://doi.org/10.1037/0022-006X.53.2.189

Collins, R. L., Vincent, P. C., Yu, J., Liu, L. & Epstein, L. H. (2014). A behavioral economic approach to assessing demand for marijuana. *Experimental and Clinical Psychopharmacology,* **22**(3), 211–221. https://doi.org/10.1037/a0035318

Comer, S. D., Bickel, W. K., Yi, R., et al. (2010). Human behavioral pharmacology, past, present, and future: Symposium presented at the 50th annual meeting of the Behavioral Pharmacology Society. *Behavioural Pharmacology,* **21**(4), 251–277. https://doi.org/10.1097/Fbp.0b013e32833bb9f8

Dariotis, J. K. & Johnson, M. W. (2015). Sexual discounting among high-risk youth ages 18–24: Implications for sexual and substance use risk behaviors. *Experimental and Clinical Psychopharmacology,* **23**(1), 49–58. doi: 10.1037/a0038399

DeGrandpre, R. J., Bickel, W. K., Hughes, J. R. & Higgins, S. T. (1992). Behavioral economics of drug self-administration. *Psychopharmacology,* **108**(1–2), 1–10.

DeGrandpre, R. J., Bickel, W. K., Hughes, J. R., Layng, M. P. & Badger, G. (1993). Unit price as a useful metric in analyzing effects of reinforcer magnitude. *Journal of the Experimental Analysis of Behavior,* **60**(3), 641–666.

Du, W., Green, L. & Myerson, J. (2002). Cross-cultural comparisons of discounting delayed and probabilistic rewards. *The Psychological Record,* **52**(4), 479–492.

Epstein, L. H., Dearing, K. K. & Roba, L. G. (2010). A questionnaire approach to measuring the relative reinforcing efficacy of snack foods. *Eating Behaviors,* **11**(2), 67–73. https://doi.org/10.1016/j.eatbeh.2009.09.006

Epstein, L. H., Salvy, S. J., Carr, K. A., Dearing, K. K. & Bickel, W. K. (2010). Food reinforcement, delay discounting and obesity. *Physiology & Behavior,* **100**(5), 438–445. doi: 10.1016/j.physbeh.2010.04.029

Evenden, J. L. & Ryan, C. N. (1996). The pharmacology of impulsive behaviour in rats: The effects of drugs on response choice with varying delays of reinforcement. *Psychopharmacology,* **128**(2), 161–170. doi: 10.1007/s002130050121

Fagerström, K. O. (1978). Measuring degree of physical dependence to tobacco smoking with reference to individualization of treatment. *Addictive Behaviors,* **3**(3–4), 235–241. https://doi.org/10.1016/0306-4603(78)90024-2

Felton, M. & Lyon, D. O. (1966). The post-reinforcement pause. *Journal of the Experimental Analysis of Behavior,* **9**(2), 131–134.

Few, L. R., Acker, J., Murphy, C. & MacKillop, J. (2012). Temporal stability of a cigarette purchase task. *Nicotine & Tobacco Research,*

14(6), 761–765. https://doi.org/10.1093/ntr/ntr222

Field, M., Santarcangelo, M., Sumnall, H., Goudie, A. & Cole, J. (2006). Delay discounting and the behavioural economics of cigarette purchases in smokers: The effects of nicotine deprivation. *Psychopharmacology*, **186**(2), 255–263. https://doi.org/10.1007/s00213-006-0385-4

Gray, J. C., Amlung, M. T., Palmer, A. A. & MacKillop, J. (2016). Syntax for calculation of discounting indices from the monetary choice questionnaire and probability discounting questionnaire. *Journal of the Experimental Analysis of Behavior*, **106**(2), 156–163. doi: 10.1002/jeab.221

Green, L., Myerson, J., Shah, A. K., Estle, S. J. & Holt, D. D. (2007). Do adjusting-amount and adjusting-delay procedures produce equivalent estimates of subjective value in pigeons? *Journal of the Experimental Analysis of Behavior*, **87**(3), 337–347. doi: 10.1901/jeab.2007.37-06

Greenwald, M. K. & Hursh, S. R. (2006). Behavioral economic analysis of opioid consumption in heroin-dependent individuals: Effects of unit price and pre-session drug supply. *Drug and Alcohol Dependence*, **85**(1), 35–48. https://doi.org/http://dx..org/10.1016/j.drugalcdep.2006.03.007

Griffiths, R. R., Bigelow, G. E. & Henningfield, J. E. (1980). Similarities in animal and human drug-taking behavior. In N. K. Mello (Ed.), *Advances in Substance Abuse (Volume 1)*. Greenwich, CT: JAI Press, pp. 1–90.

Griffiths, R. R., Brady, J. V. & Bradford, L. D. (1979). Predicting the abuse liability of drugs with animal drug self-administration procedures: Psychomotor stimulants and hallucinogens. In T. Thompson & P. B. Dews (Eds.), *Advances in Behavioral Pharmacology (Volume 2)*. New York: Academic Press, pp. 163–208.

Heatherton, T. F., Kozlowski, L. T., Frecker, R. C. & Fagerström, K. O. (1991). The Fagerström test for nicotine dependence: A revision of the Fagerström Tolerance Questionnaire. *British Journal of Addiction*, **86**(9), 1119–1127. https://doi.org/10.1111/j.1360-0443.1991.tb01879.x

Henley, A. J., DiGennaro Reed, F. D., Kaplan, B. A. & Reed, D. D. (2016). Quantifying efficacy of workplace reinforcers: An application of behavioral economic demand to evaluate hypothetical work performance. *Translational Issues in Psychological Science*, **2** (2), 174–183. https://doi.org/10.1037/tps0000068

Herrmann, E. S., Hand, D. J., Johnson, M. W., Badger, G. J. & Heil, S. H. (2014). Examining delay discounting of condom-protected sex among opioid-dependent women and non-drug-using control women. *Drug and Alcohol Dependence*, **144**, 53–60. doi: 10.1016/j.drugalcdep.2014.07.026

Herrnstein, R. J. (1971). Quantitative hedonism. *Journal of Psychiatric Research*, **8**(3–4), 399–412. https://doi.org/Doi 10.1016/0022-3956(71)90033-1

Hodos, W. (1961). Progressive ratio as a measure of reward strength. *Science*, **134** (3483), 943–944. Retrieved from www.ncbi.nlm.nih.gov/pubmed/13714876

Hurlbut, S. C. & Sher, K. J. (1992). Assessing alcohol problems in college students. *Journal of the American College Health Association*, **41** (2), 49–58. https://doi.org/10.1080/07448481.1992.10392818

Hursh, S. R. (1980). Economic concepts for the analysis of behavior. *Journal of the Experimental Analysis of Behavior*, **34**(2), 219–238. https://doi.org/http://dx..org/10.1901/jeab.1980.34-219

Hursh, S. R. (1984). Behavioral economics. *Journal of the Experimental Analysis of Behavior*, **42**(3), 435–452. https://doi.org/http://dx..org/10.1901/jeab.1984.42-435

Hursh, S. R. (1993). Behavioral economics of drug self-administration – An introduction. *Drug and Alcohol Dependence*, **33**(2), 165–172. https://doi.org/10.1016/0376-8716(93)90058-X

Hursh, S. R. (2014). Behavioral economics and analysis of consumption and choice. In F. K. McSweeney & E. S. Murphy (Eds.), *The Wiley Blackwell Handbook of Classical and Operant Conditioning*. West Sussex, UK: John Wiley & Sons, pp. 275–305.

Hursh, S. R. & Roma, P. G. (2013). Behavioral economics and empirical public policy. *Journal of the Experimental Analysis of Behavior*, **99**(1), 98–124. https://doi.org/10.1007/s00213-008-1120-0

Hursh, S. R. & Silberberg, A. (2008). Economic demand and essential value. *Psychological Review*, **115**(1), 186–198. https://doi.org/10.1037/0033-295x115.1.186

Hursh, S. R., Madden, G. J., Spiga, R., DeLeon, I. G. & Francisco, M. T. (2013). *The Translational Utility of Behavioral Economics: The Experimental Analysis of Consumption and Choice*. Washington, DC: American Psychological Association. https://doi.org/http://dx..org/10.1037/13938-008

Jacobs, E. A. & Bickel, W. K. (1999). Modeling drug consumption in the clinic using simulation procedures: Demand for heroin and cigarettes in opioid-dependent outpatients. *Experimental and Clinical Psychopharmacology*, **7**(4), 412–426. https://doi.org/10.1037//1064-1297.7.4.412

Jarmolowicz, D. P. & Lattal, K. A. (2010). On distinguishing progressively increasing response requirements for reinforcement. *The Behavior Analyst*, **33**(1), 119–125.

Jarmolowicz, D. P. & Schneider, T. D. (2020). Behavioral economics and addictive disorders. In S. Sussman (Ed.) *The Cambridge Handbook of Substance and Behavioral Addictions*, Cambridge, UK: Cambridge University Press, pp. 12–22.

Jarmolowicz, D. P., Bickel, W. K. & Gatchalian, K. M. (2013). Alcohol-dependent individuals discount sex at higher rates than controls. *Drug and Alcohol Dependence*, **131**(3), 320–323. doi: 10.1016/j.drugalcdep.2012.12.014

Jarmolowicz, D. P., Landes, R. D., Christensen, D. R., et al. (2014). Discounting of money and sex: Effects of commodity and temporal position in stimulant-dependent men and women. *Addictive Behaviors*, **39**(11), 1652–1657. doi: 10.1016/j.addbeh.2014.04.026

Jarmolowicz, D. P., Lemley, S. M., Mateos, A. & Sofis, M. J. (2016). A multiple-stimulus-without-replacement assessment for sexual partners: Purchase task validation. *Journal of Applied Behavior Analysis*, **49**(3), 723–729. https://doi.org/10.1002/jaba.313

Jarmolowicz, D. P., Reed, D. D. & Bickel, W. K. (2015). Neuroeconomics: Implications for understanding and treating addictive behavior. In S. W. Feldstein Ewing & F. M. Filbey (Eds.), *Neuroimaging and Psychosocial Addiction Treatment: An Integrative Guide for Researchers and Clinicians*. New York, NY: Palgrave Macmillan, pp. 141–157.

Jarmolowicz, D. P., Reed, D. D., Bruce, A. S., et al. (2016). Using EP50 to forecast treatment adherence in individuals with multiple sclerosis. *Behavioural Processes*, **132**, 94–99. doi: 10.1016/j.beproc.2016.09.003

Johnson, M. W. & Bickel, W. K. (2008). An algorithm for identifying nonsystematic delay-discounting data. *Experimental and Clinical Psychopharmacology*, 16(3), 264–274. doi:10.1037/1064-1297.16.3.264

Johnson, M. W. & Bruner, N. R. (2012). The Sexual Discounting Task: HIV risk behavior and the discounting of delayed sexual rewards in cocaine dependence. *Drug and Alcohol Dependence*, **123**(1–3), 15–21. https://doi.org/10.1016/j.drugalcdep.2011.09.032

Johnson, M. W., Herrmann, E. S., Sweeney, M. M., LeComte, R. S. & Johnson, P. S. (2017). Cocaine administration dose-dependently increases sexual desire and decreases condom use likelihood: The role of delay and probability discounting in connecting cocaine with HIV. *Psychopharmacology*, **234**(4), 599–612. doi: 10.1007/s00213-016-4493-5

Junco, R. & Cotten, S. R. (2012). No A 4 U: The relationship between multitasking and academic performance. *Computers & Education*, **59**(2), 505–514. doi: 10.1016/j.compedu.2011.12.023

Kaplan, B. A., Amlung, M., Reed, D. D., et al. (2016). Automating scoring of delay discounting for the 21- and 27-item monetary choice questionnaires. *The Behavior Analyst*, **39**(2), 293–304. doi: 10.1007/s40614-016-0070-9

Kaplan, B. A., Foster, R. N. S., Reed, D. D., et al. (2018). Understanding alcohol motivation using the alcohol purchase task: A methodological systematic review. *Drug and Alcohol Dependence*, **191**, 117–140. https://doi.org/10.1016/J.DRUGALCDEP.2018.06.029

Kaplan, B. A., Gelino, B. W. & Reed, D. D. (2018). A behavioral economic approach to green consumerism: Demand for reusable shopping bags. *Behavior and Social Issues*, **27**, 20–30. https://doi.org/10.5210/bsi.v.27i0.8003

Kirby, K. N. & Maraković, N. N. (1996). Delay-discounting probabilistic rewards: Rates decrease as amounts increase. *Psychonomic Bulletin & Review*, **3**(1), 100–104. doi: 10.3758/BF03210748

Kirby, K. N., Petry, N. M. & Bickel, W. K. (1999). Heroin addicts have higher discount rates for delayed rewards than non-drug-using controls. *Journal of Experimental Psychology: General*, **128**(1), 78–87. doi: 10.1037/0096-3445.128.1.78

Koffarnus, M. N. & Bickel, W. K. (2014). A 5-trial adjusting delay discounting task: Accurate discount rates in less than one minute. *Experimental and Clinical Psychopharmacology*, **22**(3), 222–228. doi: 10.1037/a0035973

Kwon, M., Lee, J., Won, W., et al. (2013). Development and validation of a smartphone addiction scale (SAS). *PLoS ONE*, **8**(2), 7.

Lawyer, S. R. (2008). Probability and delay discounting of erotic stimuli. *Behavioural Processes*, **79**(1), 36–42. doi: 10.1016/j.beproc.2008.04.009

Lea, S. E. (1976). Titration of schedule parameters by pigeons. *Journal of the Experimental Analysis of Behavior*, **25**(1), 43–54. doi: 10.1901/jeab.1976.25-43

Lemley, S. M., Kaplan, B. A., Reed, D. D., Darden, A. C. & Jarmolowicz, D. P. (2016). Reinforcer pathologies: Predicting alcohol related problems in college drinking men and women. *Drug and Alcohol Dependence*, **167**, 57–66. https://doi.org/10.1016/j.drugalcdep.2016.07.025

Leslie, J. C. (2003). A history of reinforcement: The role of reinforcement schedules in behavior pharmacology. *The Behavior Analyst Today*, **4**(1), 98–108. http://dx.doi.org/10.1037/h0100017

MacKillop, J. & Tidey, J. W. (2011). Cigarette demand and delayed reward discounting in nicotine-dependent individuals with schizophrenia and controls: An initial study. *Psychopharmacology*, **216**(1), 91–99. https://doi.org/10.1007/s00213-011-2185-8

MacKillop, J., Murphy, J. G., Ray, L. A., et al. (2008). Further validation of a cigarette purchase task for assessing the relative reinforcing efficacy of nicotine in college smokers. *Experimental and Clinical Psychopharmacology*, **16**(1), 57–65. https://doi.org/10.1037/1064-1297.16.1.57

Madden, G. J. & Bickel, W. K. (1999). Abstinence and price effects on demand for cigarettes: A behavioral-economic analysis. *Addiction*, **94**(4), 577–588. https://doi.org/10.1046/j.1360-0443.1999.94457712.x

Madden, G. J. & Bickel, W. K. (2010). *Impulsivity: The Behavioral and Neurological Science of Discounting* (1st edition). Washington, DC: American Psychological Association.

Madden, G. J., Petry, N. M. & Johnson, P. S. (2009). Pathological gamblers discount probabilistic rewards less steeply than matched controls. *Experimental and Clinical Psychopharmacology*, **17**(5), 283–290. https://doi.org/10.1037/A0016806

Mazur, J. E. (1987). An adjusting procedure for studying delayed reinforcement. In M. L. Commons, J. E. Mazur, J. A. Nevin & H. Rachlin (Eds.), *Quantitative Analysis of Behavior: Volume 5. The Effect of Delay and Intervening Events on Reinforcement Value*. Hillsdale, NJ: Erlbaum, pp. 55–73. Retrieved from https://search.proquest.com/docview/617226485?accountid=14556

Metrik, J., Aston, E. R., Kahler, C. W., et al. (2016). Cue-elicited increases in incentive salience for marijuana: Craving, demand, and attentional bias. *Drug and Alcohol Dependence*, **167**, 82–88. https://doi.org/10.1016/j.drugalcdep.2016.07.027

Mischel, W. & Ebbesen, E. B. (1970). Attention in delay of gratification. *Journal of Personality and Social Psychology*, **16**(2), 329–337. doi: 10.1037/h0029815

Mischel, W., Ebbesen, E. B. & Raskoff Zeiss, A. (1972). Cognitive and attentional mechanisms in delay of gratification. *Journal of Personality and Social Psychology*, **21**(2), 204–218. doi: 10.1037/h0032198

Mischel, W., Shoda, Y. & Peake, P. K. (1988). The nature of adolescent competencies predicted by preschool delay of gratification. *Journal of Personality and Social Psychology*, **54**(4), 687–696. doi: 10.1037/0022-3514.54.4.687

Mischel, W., Shoda, Y. & Rodriguez, M. L. (1989). Delay of gratification in children. *Science*, **244**(4907), 933–938. doi: 10.1126/science.2658056

Mulhauser, K., Short, E. M. & Weinstock, J. (2018). Development and psychometric evaluation of the pornography purchase task. *Addictive Behaviors*, **84**(December 2017), 207–214. https://doi.org/10.1016/j.addbeh.2018.04.016

Murphy, J. G. & MacKillop, J. (2006). Relative reinforcing efficacy of alcohol among college student drinkers. *Experimental and Clinical Psychopharmacology*, **14**(2), 219–227. https://doi.org/10.1037/1064-1297.14.2.219

Murphy, J. G., MacKillop, J., Skidmore, J. R. & Pederson, A. A. (2009). Reliability and validity of a demand curve measure of alcohol reinforcement. *Experimental and Clinical Psychopharmacology*, **17**(6), 396–404. https://doi.org/10.1037/a0017684

Murphy, J. G., MacKillop, J., Tidey, J. W., Brazil, L. A. & Colby, S. M. (2011). Validity of a demand curve measure of nicotine reinforcement with adolescent smokers. *Drug and Alcohol Dependence*, **113**(2–3), 207–214. https://doi.org/10.1016/J.DRUGALCDEP.2010.08.004

Myerson, J. & Green, L. (1995). Discounting of delayed rewards: Models of individual choice. *Journal of the Experimental Analysis of Behavior*, **64**(3), 263–276. doi: 10.1901/jeab.1995.64-263

Myerson, J., Baumann, A. A. & Green, L. (2014). Discounting of delayed rewards: (A) theoretical interpretation of the Kirby questionnaire. *Behavioural Processes*, **107**, 99–105. doi: 10.1016/j.beproc.2014.07.021

Myerson, J., Green, L. & Warusawitharana, M. (2001). Area under the curve as a measure of discounting. *Journal of the Experimental Analysis of Behavior*, **76**(2), 235–243. doi: 10.1901/jeab.2001.76-235

Navarick, D. J. & Fantino, E. (1972). Interresponse time as a factor in choice. *Psychonomic Science*, **27**(1), 4–6. doi: 10.3758/BF03328868

O'Donnell, S. & Epstein, L. H. (2019). Smartphones are more reinforcing than food for students. *Addictive Behaviors*, **90**, 124–133.

Odum, A. L., Baumann, A. A. L. & Rimington, D. D. (2006). Discounting of delayed Hypothetical money and food: Effects of amount. *Behavioural Processes*, **73**(3), 278–284. doi: 10.1016/j.beproc.2006.06.008

Petry, N. M. (2000). Effects of increasing income on polydrug use: A comparison of heroin, cocaine and alcohol abusers. *Addiction*, **95**(5), 705–717. https://doi.org/10.1046/j.1360-0443.2000.9557056.x

Petry, N. M. (2001a). A behavioral economic analysis of polydrug abuse in alcoholics: Asymmetrical substitution of alcohol and cocaine. *Drug and Alcohol Dependence*, **62**(1), 31–39. https://doi.org/10.1016/S0376-8716(00)00157-5

Petry, N. M. (2001b). The effects of housing costs on polydrug abuse patterns: A comparison of heroin, cocaine, and alcohol abusers. *Experimental and Clinical Psychopharmacology*, **9**(1), 47–58. https://doi.org/10.1037/1064-1297.9.1.47

Petry, N. M. & Bickel, W. K. (1998). Polydrug abuse in heroin addicts: A behavioral economic analysis. *Addiction*, **93**(3), 321–335. https://doi.org/10.1046/j.1360-0443.1998.9333212.x

Petry, N. M. & Bickel, W. K. (1999). A behavioral economic analysis of polydrug abuse in heroin addicts. In F. J. Chaloupka, M. Grossman, W. K. Bickel & H. Saffer (Eds.), *The Economic Analysis of Substance Use and Abuse: An Integration of Econometrics and Behavioral Economic Research*. Chicago, IL: University of Chicago Press, pp. 213–250. https://doi.org/10.1046/j.1360-0443.1998.9333212.x

Pickover, A. M., Messina, B. G., Correia, C. J., Garza, K. B. & Murphy, J. G. (2016). A behavioral economic analysis of the nonmedical use of prescription drugs among young adults. *Experimental and Clinical Psychopharmacology*, **24**(1), 38–47. https://doi.org/10.1037/pha0000052

Pope, H. G., Kean, J., Nash, A., et al. (2010). A diagnostic interview module for anabolic-androgenic steroid dependence: Preliminary evidence of reliability and validity. *Experimental and Clinical Psychopharmacology*, **18**(3), 203–213. https://doi.org/10.1037/a0019370

Rachlin, H. (2006). Notes on discounting. *Journal of the Experimental Analysis of Behavior*, **85**(3), 425–435. doi: 10.1901/jeab.2006.85-05

Rachlin, H. & Green, L. (1972). Commitment, choice and self-control. *Journal of the Experimental Analysis of Behavior*, **17**(1), 15–22. doi: 10.1901/jeab.1972.17-15

Rachlin, H., Raineri, A. & Cross, D. (1991). Subjective probability and delay. *Journal of the Experimental Analysis of Behavior*, **55**(2), 233–244. doi: 10.1901/jeab.1991.55-233

Reed, D. D. (2015). Ultra-violet indoor tanning addiction: A reinforcer pathology interpretation. *Addictive Behaviors*, **41**, 247–251. https://doi.org/10.1016/j.addbeh.2014.10.026

Reed, D. D., Becirevic, A., Atchley, P., Kaplan, B. A. & Liese, B. S. (2016a). Validation of a novel delay discounting of text messaging questionnaire. *The Psychological Record*, **66**(2), 253–261. doi: 10.1007/s40732-016-0167-2

Reed, D. D., Kaplan, B. A. & Becirevic, A. (2015). Basic research on the behavioral economics of reinforcer value. In *Autism Service Delivery: Bridging the Gap Between Science and Practice*. Springer Science + Business Media, pp. 279–306. https://doi.org/10.1007/978-1-4939-2656-5_10

Reed, D. D., Kaplan, B. A., Becirevic, A., Roma, P. G. & Hursh, S. R. (2016b). Toward quantifying the abuse liability of ultraviolet tanning: A behavioral economic approach to tanning addiction. *Journal of the Experimental Analysis of Behavior*, **106**(1), 93–106. https://doi.org/10.1002/jeab.216

Reed, D. D., Kaplan, B. A., Roma, P. G. & Hursh, S. R. (2014). Inter-method reliability of progression sizes in a hypothetical purchase task: Implications for empirical public policy. *Psychological Record*, **64**(4), 671–679. https://doi.org/10.1007/s40732-014-0076-1

Reed, D. D., Naudé, G. P., Salzer, A. R., et al. (2020). Behavioral economic measurement of cigarette demand: A descriptive review of published approaches to the Cigarette Purchase Task. *Experimental and Clinical Psychopharmacology*. Advance online publication. doi: 10.1037/pha0000347

Richards, J. B., Mitchell, S. H., de Wit, H. & Seiden, L. S. (1997). Determination of discount functions in rats with an adjusting-amount procedure. *Journal of the Experimental Analysis of Behavior*, **67**(3), 353-366. doi: 10.1901/jeab.1997.67-353

Richards, J. B., Zhang, L., Mitchell, S. H. & de Wit, H. (1999). Delay or probability discounting in a model of impulsive behavior: Effect of alcohol. *Journal of the Experimental Analysis of Behavior*, **71**(2), 121–143. doi: 10.1901/jeab.1999.71-121

Roberts, J. A., Petnji Yaya, L. H. & Manolis, C. (2014). The invisible addiction: Cell-phone activities and addiction among male and female college students. *Journal of Behavioral Addictions*, **3**(4), 254–265. doi: 10.1556/JBA.3.2014.015

Ross, E. & Kenakin, T. (2001). Pharmacodynamics – Mechanisms of drug action and the relationship between drug concentration and effect. In J. G. Hardman & A. J. Gilman (Eds.), *The Pharmacological Basis of Therapeutics* (10th edition). London: McGraw.

Samuelson, P. A. (1937). A note on measurement of utility. *Review of Economic Studies*, **4**, 155–161.

Saville, B. K., Gisbert, A., Kopp, J. & Telesco, C. (2010). Internet addiction and delay discounting in college students. *Psychological Record*, **60**(2), 273–286.

Shoda, Y., Mischel, W. & Peake, P. K. (1990). Predicting adolescent cognitive and self-regulatory competencies from preschool delay of gratification: Identifying diagnostic conditions. *Developmental Psychology*, **26**(6), 978–986. doi: 10.1037/0012-1649.26.6.978

Skinner, B. F. (1953). *Science and Human Behavior*. Macmillan: Oxford.

Skinner, B. F. (1961). What is the experimental analysis of behavior? *Journal of the Experimental Analysis of Behavior*, **9**(3), 213–218. https://doi.org/http://dx.doi.org/10.1037/11324-008

Sobell, L. C. & Sobell, M. B. (1992). Timeline follow-back. In R. Z. Litten & J. P. Allen (Eds.), *Measuring Alcohol Consumption*. Totowa, NJ: Humana Press, pp. 41–72. https://doi.org/10.1007/978-1-4612-0357-5_3

Sobell, M. B. & Sobell, L. C. (1973). Individualized behavior therapy for alcoholics – Republished. *Behavior Therapy*, **4**(1), 49–72. https://doi.org/https://doi.org/10.1016/S0005-7894(73)80074-7

Stafford, D., LeSage, M. G. & Glowa, J. R. (1998). Progressive-ratio schedules of drug delivery in the analysis of drug self-administration: A review. *Psychopharmacology*, **139**(3), 169–184. https://doi.org/10.1007/s002130050702

Strickland, J. C., Lile, J. A. & Stoops, W. W. (2017). Unique prediction of cannabis use severity and behaviors by delay discounting and behavioral economic demand. *Behavioural Processes*, **140**, 33–40. doi: 10.1016/j.beproc.2017.03.017

Strickland, J. C., Lile, J. A., Rush, C. R. & Stoops, W. W. (2016). Comparing exponential and exponentiated models of drug demand in cocaine users. *Experimental and Clinical Psychopharmacology*, **24**(6), 447–455. https://doi.org/10.1037/pha0000096

Strickland, J. C., Reynolds, A. R. & Stoops, W. W. (2016). Regulation of cocaine craving by cognitive strategies in an online sample of cocaine users. *Psychology of Addictive Behaviors*, **30**(5), 607–612. https://doi.org/10.1037/adb0000180

Vincent, P. C., Collins, R. L., Liu, L., et al. (2017). The effects of perceived quality on behavioral economic demand for marijuana: A web-based experiment. *Drug and Alcohol Dependence*, **170**, 174–180. https://doi.org/10.1016/j.drugalcdep.2016.11.013

Weinstock, J., Mulhauser, K., Oremus, E. G. & D'Agostino, A. R. (2016). Demand for gambling: Development and assessment of a gambling purchase task. *International Gambling Studies*, **16**(2), 316–327. https://doi .org/10.1080/14459795.2016.1182570

Winger, G., Hursh, S. R., Casey, K. L. & Woods, J. H. (2002). Relative reinforcing strength of three methyl-d-aspartate antagonists with different onsets of action. *Journal of Pharmacology and Experimental Therapeutics*, **301**(2), 690–697.

Yoon, J. H. & Higgins, S. T. (2008). Turning *k* on its head: Comments on use of an ED50 in delay discounting research. *Drug and Alcohol Dependence*, **95**(1–2), 169–172. doi: 10.1016/ j.drugalcdep.2007.12.011

Yurasek, A. M., Murphy, J. G., Clawson, A. H., Dennhardt, A. A. & MacKillop, J. (2013). Smokers report greater demand for alcohol on a behavioral economic purchase task. *Journal of Studies on Alcohol and Drugs*, **74**(4), 626–34. https://doi.org/http://dx.doi.org/10 .15288/jsad.2013.74.626

8 Substance and Behavioral Addictions Assessment Instruments

Timothy J. Grigsby, PhD

Introduction

Assessment of substance use has a long psychometric and clinical history. On the other hand, behavioral, or nonsubstance, addictions generally lack a diagnostic guide – with the exception of gambling (as discussed below) – leaving clinicians and researchers to develop their own psychometric inventories to assess excessive reward-seeking behaviors (Albrecht, Kirschiner & Grusser, 2007). Instruments designed to assess behavioral addictions commonly tap one of two theoretical frameworks (West & Brown, 2013): substance-like or impulse-control disorder. Scales developed using a substance-dependence model assess constructs such as escalation of behavior, preoccupation with the behavior, loss of control, negative consequences associated with the behavior, craving, tolerance, and withdrawal (see Griffiths, 1996; Sussman & Sussman, 2011). Scales developed using an impulse-control disorder model, on the other hand, while assessing constructs including compulsivity and self-control, also tap emotional detachment (being ego dystonic) and guilt among others (see Brewer & Potenza, 2008; Grant et al., 2014). Researchers studying and advocating for recognition of behavioral addictions tend to align with the substance-like model (Sussman, 2017).

Assessment of problem use, misuse, dependence, or addiction occurs for various reasons (Grigsby et al., 2017). Efficient and systematic measurement of addiction is essential for establishing population estimates – incidence and prevalence – and for developing treatment planning for afflicted individuals. Assessment may be used for screening ("proactive assessment"). For example, professionals may be asked to screen for drug misuse among employment candidates for jobs in which public safety is paramount (e.g., lifeguards, delivery personnel, vehicle drivers, babysitters, or airplane pilots) or researchers might conduct epidemiological assessments to understand population trends of substance use disorders in order to advocate for policies and resources to address "epidemics" of drug use problems afflicting disparate populations (e.g., the opioid crisis). Assessment may also be used as a tool to clarify a presenting medical or social-psychological problem in clinical settings ("reactive assessment"). Here, a medical professional would be asked to "rule out" addiction as a cause of a presenting condition or to determine the severity of a known addictive behavior. Historically, community and population level assessment of addiction has been nearly synonymous to the measurement of negative substance use consequences in individuals or populations (American Psychiatric Association, 2013).

More scales exist to measure addiction to a substance than addiction to food or any nonsubstance, reward producing stimulus (termed "behavioral" or "process" addictions; Sussman, 2017). Of the many excessive reward-seeking behaviors that have been researched, only gambling has received a formal diagnosis in the *Diagnostic and Statistical Manual* (currently in its fifth edition; DSM-5). This is significant as the American Psychiatric Association (APA) previously characterized Pathological Gambling (PG) as persistent and recurrent maladaptive gambling behavior in the DSM-IV and classified it as an "Impulse-Control Disorder Not Elsewhere Classified." In the DSM-5, a formal gambling disorder diagnosis was formed and was reclassified to one of the "Substance-Related and Addictive Disorders" in an effort to clarify the diagnosis and treatment of gambling disorder, to increase its recognition, and to improve research efforts directed to the disorder (Petry et al., 2013). DSM-5 diagnostic criteria for gambling disorder are presented in Table 8.1. While neuroscience and genetics research played an important role in this decision, no other behavioral addiction was included or reclassified. Internet addiction was also considered, but the American Psychiatric Association work group members decided there were insufficient research data for it to be included. Sex addiction was also discussed but not included because the work group found no scientific evidence that "reward circuitry is operative in the same way as in addictive areas" (Reilly & Smith, 2013). This has repercussions on general population and clinical assessment as no diagnostic framework exists to guide the development of survey, screening, or clinical assessments of behavioral addiction.

This chapter reviews frequently used assessments of drug and behavioral addiction and concludes with recommendations for theoretical and transdisciplinary efforts to improve assessment. The assessment approaches reviewed in this chapter include examples of survey measures (e.g., Likert scales, true/false questionnaires), unstructured and structured interviews (e.g., life and behavioral history interviews), subscales of comprehensive psychological inventories, structured ("screener") assessments, and diagnostic inventories. The purpose of *screening* is to determine whether a client needs a more in-depth assessment. The purpose of *assessment* is to gather the detailed information needed for a treatment plan that meets individual needs. Many standardized instruments exist, more than one chapter can cover, but references to additional resources are provided throughout the chapter for further reading.

Drug and Alcohol Addiction

Alcohol, tobacco, and other drug (ATOD) use is most commonly assessed by asking patients or research participants about the quantity of frequency of their ATOD use. Frequency of drug use indicates how often individuals are using a drug. Frequency of use can be measured through self-reports of lifetime estimates of use, yearly estimates of use, monthly use, and/or daily estimates of use. A prominent measure of drug use frequency is the timeline follow-back method (Sobell & Sobell, 1992). This technique requires individuals to recall previous drug use behavior over a specified time period using memorable life events and a personalized calendar to assist with recall, and it has been shown to be a

Table 8.1 Diagnostic criteria for "Gambling Disorder" in the *Diagnostic and Statistical Manual of Mental Disorders*, 5th edition (DSM-5)

A. Persistent and recurrent problematic gambling behavior leading to clinically significant impairment or distress, as indicated by the individual exhibiting four (or more) of the following in a 12-month period:
  a. Needs to gamble with increasing amounts of money in order to achieve the desired excitement.
  b. Is restless or irritable when attempting to cut down or stop gambling.
  c. Has made repeated unsuccessful efforts to control, cut back, or stop gambling.
  d. Is often preoccupied with gambling (e.g., having persistent thoughts of reliving past gambling experiences, handicapping or planning the next venture, thinking of ways to get money with which to gamble).
  e. Often gambles when feeling distressed (e.g., helpless, guilty, anxious, depressed).
  f. After losing money gambling, often returns another day to get even ("chasing" one's losses).
  g. Lies to conceal the extent of involvement with gambling.
  h. Has jeopardized or lost a significant relationship, job, or educational or career opportunity because of gambling.
  i. Relies on others to provide money to relieve desperate financial situations caused by gambling.

B. The gambling behavior is not better explained by a manic episode.
  Specify if:
  Episodic: Meeting diagnostic criteria at more than one time point, with symptoms subsiding between periods of gambling disorder for at least several months.
  Persistent: Experiencing continuous symptoms, to meet diagnostic criteria for multiple years.
  Specify if:
  In early remission: After full criteria for gambling disorder were previously met, none of the criteria for gambling disorder have been met for at least 3 months but for less than 12 months.
  In sustained remission: After full criteria for gambling disorder were previously met, none of the criteria for gambling disorder have been met during a period of 12 months or longer.
  Specify current severity:
  Mild: 4–5 criteria met.
  Moderate: 6–7 criteria met.
  Severe: 8–9 criteria met.

Note: From the American Psychiatric Association, *Diagnostic and Statistical Manual of Mental Disorders*, 5th Edition (2013) (section 312.31).

reliable and valid self-report measure of alcohol and illicit drug use in the general population (Hjorthøj, Hjorthøj & Nordentoft, 2012; Robinson et al., 2014; Sobell & Sobell, 1992). Unfortunately, relying on frequency of drug use as the primary assessment of drug misuse lacks precision, as it is not designed to compare disparate patterns of drug use. For example, consuming one "hit" of methamphetamine can lead to a psychological effect of feeling high for six to twelve hours (Krasnova & Cadet, 2009), whereas generally it would take several servings of standard alcoholic beverages to achieve a similar sense of drug induced euphoria. As such, recent frequency of drug use may differ somewhat due to psychoactive effects of the drug – and is not entirely related to craving. Of course, regular use over longer periods of time (e.g., a year or longer) is commonly accepted as a high use frequency. Quantity of use is more predictive of problems or disruptive drug use and is used to describe problem behaviors such as binge drinking or heavy drinking (see Newcomb & Felix-Ortiz, 1992; Sanchez-Craig et al., 1984). While quantity of use has been most systematically measured in relation to alcohol use, the association of relatively high quantities of use of various illicit drugs with negative consequences (e.g., overdoses, fainting, loss of behavioral control) is well-known.

Survey Measures

More measures exist to assess alcohol and drug addiction with specific substances or poly-substance use than can be discussed in this chapter. For a comprehensive list of available measures, the reader is referred to the University of New Mexico's Center on Alcoholism, Substance Abuse, and Addictions (CASAA) (https://casaa.unm.edu/Instruments; accessed June 17, 2018). The primary feature of commonly employed survey assessments with community samples focus on negative consequences related to substance use such as neglecting responsibilities, blacking out after binge use, and conflict with loved ones.

The original *Rutgers Alcohol Problem Index (RAPI)* (White & Labouvie, 1989) consists of twenty-three items that address consequences of alcohol use related to psychological functioning, delinquency, social relations, family, physical problems, and neuropsychological functioning. Shorter versions of the measure are available (Earlywine, LaBrie & Pederson, 2008) and the measure has been considered a reliable and valid estimate of other drug use consequences (Ginzler et al., 2007). The original measure has been found to correlate highly with DSM-III-R criteria for alcohol use disorders (r = 0.75–0.95; White & Labouvie, 1989), and recent evidence showed it significantly correlates with DSM-IV abuse and dependence criteria (r = 0.31–0.82; Ginzler et al., 2007).

The *Drinker Inventory of Consequences (DrInC)* is a self-administered fifty-item measure of the adverse consequences of alcohol use. Its parallel form, the fifty-item *Inventory of Drug Use Consequences (InDUC)* (Blanchard et al., 2003; Tonigan & Miller, 2002) was designed as a standardized measure of alcohol and other drug use consequences. The measure includes the same five scales as the DrInC measuring (1) impulse control, (2) social responsibility, (3) physical, (4) interpersonal, and (5) intrapersonal consequences. Similar to other drug use consequence scales, this measure excludes topics related to pathological use, dependence symptoms (i.e., craving), and intent to seek treatment. The InDUC has been shown to effectively measure the severity of drug use consequences over time (Tonigan & Miller, 2002). The *Short Inventory of Problems – Alcohol and Drugs (SIP-AD)* and *Short Inventory of Problems – Revised (SIP-R)* are fifteen-item brief scales that demonstrated comparable, albeit weaker internal consistency compared to the original scale consistency (SIP-AD Cronbach's alpha = 0.95; SIP-R Cronbach's alpha = 0.95), good concurrent and discriminant validity that is also sensitive to detect change in negative consequences over time

(Forcehimes et al., 2007; Kiluk et al., 2013; Miller, Tonigan & Longabaugh, 1995). All scales were designed to assess consequences in the previous three months.

The *Alcohol Use Inventory (AUI)* (Horn, Wanberg & Foster, 1990; Littrell, 1991; Rychtarik, Koutsky & Miller, 1998) is a 228-item multiple-choice self-report inventory. It was systematically developed to measure alcohol problems. There are twenty-four subscales with seventeen primary scales characterizing individuals along various dimensions. The dimensions are grouped according to benefits from drinking, drinking styles, drinking consequences, and concerns about, and recognition of, a drinking problem. The primary scale factors include the following: (1) drinking to improve sociability; (2) drinking to improve mental functioning; (3) drinking to manage or change mood; (4) drinking to cope with marital problems; (5) gregarious versus solitary drinking; (6) obsessive-compulsive drinking or constantly thinking about drinking; (7) continuous, sustained drinking; (8) loss of behavior control when drinking; (9) social-role maladaptation; (10) perceptual withdrawal symptoms such as alcohol hallucinosis and delirium tremors; (11) somatic or physical withdrawal (e.g., shakes, hangovers, convulsions); (12) drinking provokes marital problems; (13) quantity of alcohol used; (14) postdrinking worry, fear, and guilt; (15) external support to stop drinking; (16) ready to quit; and (17) recognition of drinking problems.

The AUI primary scales often identify three general profiles of problem drinkers (Rychtarik, Koutsky & Miller, 1998, 1999; Sussman & Ames, 2008). First, there are low-impairment problem drinkers. They are likely to show a later onset of problem drinking and seek treatment as outpatients. They also are likely to be relatively successful in their social and vocational lives. Second, there are medium-impairment drinkers. They are similar to the first type of drinker in that they show relatively good social adjustment. However, they are more likely to report a history of physical, emotional or sexual abuse, and depression. Finally, there are high-impairment drinkers. They show the greatest social and vocational impairments, high levels of previous physical, emotional, or sexual abuse, highest levels of sustained drinking, and highest levels of psychopathology (i.e., depression, anger, or sociopathy).

The *MacAndrew Alcoholism Scale/Revised (MAC/MAC-R)* (MacAndrew, 1965, 1981) is a subscale of the *Minnesota Multiphasic Personality Inventory (MMPI)*, a standardized questionnaire developed by Hathaway and McKinley (1951). This inventory can be used to help rule out possible psychopathology that is important when investigating the causes of maladaptive behaviors. Some profiles characterize alcohol and/or drug abuse as a form of self-medication for depression (e.g., the 24/42 scale). The MAC/MAC-R consists of forty-nine items that differentiate between alcoholic patients and nonalcoholic psychiatric patients (Clopton, 1978, Clopton, Weiner & Davis, 1980, Svanum, Levitt & McAdoo, 1982). The scale also has been found to help identify individuals who are at risk for developing alcohol-related problems (McCourt, Williams & Schneider, 1971). Early work demonstrated that the scale did not effectively differentiate alcohol abusers from other drug abusers (Burke & Markus, 1977) and that the scale should only be used for its intended purpose, but later work has shown it may be useful at as a screening device with cluster B personality disorders (Smith & Hilsenroth, 2001). Additionally, female alcoholics consistently obtain higher scores than males with similar difficulties (Butcher & Owen, 1978), and among general substance users males scored higher than females (Wong & Besett, 1999). Higher scores suggest potential drug abuse but are also suggestive of extraversion, assertiveness, risk-taking, and the possibility of having experienced blackouts and difficulty concentrating. Low scores are suggestive of introversion, conformity, and low self-confidence, as well as being contraindicative of drug abuse. The MAC should be considered a comprehensive assessment section assuming it is administered as part of the MMPI, which is more common than being used as a standalone measure. This is an advantageous approach, as other subscales on the MMPI can help identify other psychological problems that are associated with or underlie drug misuse.

There are several further measures that have been validated and used with community and college student samples, in particular, that are worthy of exploration, including, but not limited to, the *Young Adult Alcohol Problem Screening Test (YAAPST)* (Hurlbut & Sher, 1992); *Marijuana Problem Scale* (Stephens, Roffman & Cutin, 2000); *Young Adult Alcohol Consequences Scale (YAACQ)* (Read et al., 2006); *Risks and Consequences estionnaire (RCQ)* (Stein et al., 2010), and the *Marijuana Consequences Questionnaire (MACQ)* (Simons et al., 2012).

At present, the *Tobacco and Nicotine Consequences Scale (TANCS)* (Grigsby, 2019) is the only scale measuring negative consequences of tobacco and nicotine products although a number of measures assessing nicotine dependence exist. A split-half validation study with a community-based sample of cigarette and e-cigarette users (n = 491) produced a seventeen-item, five-factor solution (psychological consequences, physical consequences, personal/interpersonal consequences, physical dependence, psychological dependence) that showed excellent fit to the data and good internal consistency of α = 0.91 (subscales 0.68–0.90). The scale was correlated with Fagerström Test for Cigarette Dependence (Fagerström, 2011) and Smoking Effects Questionnaire (Rohsenow et al., 2003) providing preliminary support for its validity as a measure of tobacco/nicotine misuse.

Screener and Clinical Interview Assessment Tools

The *Alcohol Use Disorders Identification Test (AUDIT)* is a well-known and rigorously evaluated ten-question test developed by the World Health Organization to determine if alcohol consumption is harmful (Babor et al., 2001; Saunders et al., 1993). The test was designed to be used internationally and was validated in a study using patients from six countries. Questions 1–3 deal with alcohol consumption, 4–6 relate to alcohol dependence, and 7–10 consider alcohol-related negative consequences. A score of 8 or more in men and 7 or more in women indicates a strong likelihood of hazardous or harmful alcohol consumption. A score of 20 or more is suggestive of alcohol dependence. A systematic review of forty-seven studies evaluating the psychometric properties of the original AUDIT (de Meneses-Gaya et al., 2009) demonstrated acceptable internal consistency across ten studies (mean Cronbach's alpha = 0.80) and evidence for construct validity with different factor structures when assessing populations with low versus high alcohol use disorder prevalence. Psychometrics for non-English versions also support its reliability and validity across populations. Meneses-Gaya et al. (2010) assessed the psychometric qualities of the abbreviated versions of the Alcohol Use Disorders Identification Test (AUDIT-3, AUDIT-4, AUDIT-C, AUDIT-PC, AUDIT-QF, FAST, and Five-Shot), comparing them to the ten-item AUDIT and the CAGE in 2 samples of Brazilian adults. The abbreviated versions showed high sensitivity (of 0.78–0.96) and specificity (of 0.74–0.94) indices, with areas under the curve as elevated as those of the AUDIT (0.89 and 0.92 to screen for abuse, and 0.93 and 0.95 in the screening of dependence) and Cronbach's alpha coefficients between 0.83 and 0.94.

The *CAGE questionnaire* (Ewing, 1984) is a self-report screening instrument that uses the mnemonic CAGE to assess problems with alcohol. The four-item instrument assesses attempts to *Cut down* on drinking, *Annoyance* with criticisms of drinking, *Guilt* feelings about drinking, and use of alcohol as a *morning Eye opener.* When someone responds "yes" to two or more questions, that individual is suspected of having alcohol problems. These questions can be adapted for other drug use, as well, by replacing the word *drinking* with *drug use*, and *a morning eye opener* with *the drug to get you started in the morning.* The focus of this questionnaire is on consequences of use related to an individual's response to others' perceptions of his or her use, resultant feelings, and attempts to quit. Attempts to change behavior may or may not come from outside sources (e.g., one's small social group) that, in turn, may cause guilt feelings or cognitively based conflict. Dhalla and Kopec (2007) reviewed the psychometric properties of the CAGE noting it demonstrated high test–retest reliability (0.80–0.95), and adequate correlations (0.48–0.70) with other screening instruments. The authors conclude that the CAGE is a valid tool for detecting alcohol abuse and dependence in medical and surgical inpatients, ambulatory medical patients, and psychiatric inpatients (average sensitivity 0.71, specificity 0.90). However, they caution its use with white women, prenatal women, and college students, based on existing performance with these groups. Furthermore, it is not recommended as an appropriate screening test for less severe forms of drinking than those listed above.

The *RAFFT test* (Relax, Alone, Friends, Family, Trouble) was developed similarly to the CAGE, but as a brief screen specifically for teens and emerging adults. The RAFFT consists of five items (e.g., "Do you drink to relax, to feel better about yourself, or to fit in?" (Riggs & Alario, 1989). Additionally, Knight and colleagues (1999) adapted several questions from the RAFFT, RAPI and DAP to create a brief screening of alcohol and other drug abuse resulting in the nine-item *CRAFFT test* – which was later reduced to six items (Car, Relax, Alone, Forget, Family or friends complain, Trouble) used primarily in adolescent samples. Items address riding in a car driven by someone under the influence, drinking or using to relax, drinking or using alone, forgetting things while drinking or using, family or friends telling one to cut down, and getting into trouble while under the influence. A review by Dhalla, Zumbo and Poole (2011) found that, across studies, sensitivities of the CRAFFT ranged from 0.61 to 1.00 at optimal cut points, and specificities ranged from 0.33 to 0.97. Additionally, the CRAFFT showed modest to adequate internal consistency values ranging from 0.65 to 0.86, and high test–retest reliability. However, the authors note that more studies of the psychometric properties of the CRAFFT need to be carried out to further assess and improve generalizability to other age groups, to further explore possible gender and ethnic differences, and examine the utility of the scale when adapted for different languages and cultures. The items on these assessment tools represent neurobiologically based (drinking to relax), cognitively based (poor decision making, as in riding in a car driven by someone under the influence, forgetting things while drinking or using), and socially based (drinking alone) drug use motivations, as well as socially based consequences of use (family or friends telling one to cut down) and environmentally related consequences (getting into trouble while under the influence).

The *Michigan Alcohol Screening Test (MAST)* is a twenty-five-item questionnaire used to screen for consequences of problem alcohol use and perceptions of alcohol-related problems. This questionnaire was originally developed to place drinkers into early (mild impairment), middle (moderate impairment), and late (severe impairments) stages (or levels of impairment) of alcoholism (Selzer, 1971). This measure can be self-administered and used to identify abnormal drinking by addressing social and behavioral consequences (Selzer, Vinokur & van Rooijin, 1975). The items are designed to describe extreme drinking behaviors and to establish the presence of negative consequences of excessive alcohol consumption. Examples of discriminating items are as follows: Have you ever attended a meeting of Alcoholics Anonymous? Have you ever gone to anyone for help about your drinking? Have you ever been in a hospital because of drinking? A recent psychometric synthesis of 103 MAST publications (Minnich et al., 2018) derived an aggregated internal consistency estimate of 0.84 (Kuder–Richardson Formula 20 [KR-20]), and test–retest correlations at 0.97, 0.94, and 0.95 at one-, three- and seven-day intervals, respectively. Factor structure analyses support a one-factor model using current factor analysis guidelines for fit. At the suggested cut-off score of 5, the percent correctly classified was 80 percent, sensitivity was 0.70, and specificity was 0.71. However, evidence from the weighted analysis of seven studies and 1,343 participants suggested an optimal cut-off score of 8 improved the overall percentage of correct classification to 81 percent, sensitivity of 0.84, and specificity of 0.75. However, more work is needed as authors of some studies did not specify if the unit scoring or weighted scoring method was used in their analyses which could confound this result. Men appear to be more likely to be classified as having a drinking disorder, and future research is needed to determine if gender-based cut-offs improve the accuracy of the scale.

The *Short MAST (SMAST)* and *Brief MAST (BMAST)* are the shortened thirteen-item and ten-item versions that are relatively effective in discriminating alcoholics from nonalcoholics (Pokorny, Miller & Kaplan, 1972; Selzer et al., 1975). Minnich et al.'s (2019) psychometric synthesis of 13 SMAST studies provided a mean internal consistency for the SMAST, using the KR-20 statistic, of 0.77 with higher internal consistency among nonclinical (0.75) compared to clinical (0.67) samples after all studies were weighted and averaged. Two-week test–retest reliability was estimated at r = 0.74 and one study produced a test–retest estimate of r = 0.89. Exploratory factor analysis (EFA) of the scale produced a three-factor solution (help seeking/conflict, not normal, and family discord) across two studies. Across studies, the suggested cut-off score for the SMAST of 3 resulted in a sensitivity of 0.68 and specificity of 0.74, whereas a cut-off score of 4 actually appeared slightly more parsimonious at a sensitivity of 0.70 and specificity of 0.71. The BMAST has been used less frequently with psychometric data from five studies. Comparatively, using the same methodology for the SMAST analysis, the mean internal consistency for the BMAST was 0.73 with higher internal consistency among clinical (0.82) compared to nonclinical samples (0.71). One study reported five-day test–retest reliability of 0.71 and factor structure analyses suggest a two-factor solution of current drinking and drinking consequences dimensions. Across studies, the suggested cut-off score for the BMAST of 6 resulted in a sensitivity of 0.48 and specificity of 0.90 with a percentage correctly classified of 0.80.

Variations of the MAST scale exist to assess alcoholism in veteran (VAST; Magruder-Habib, Harris & Fraker, 1982) and geriatric (SMAST-G; Blow et al., 1998) populations. Additionally, the ten-item *The Drug Abuse Screening Test (DAST)* (Skinner, 1982) was developed as a twenty-eight-item dichotomously scored self-report measure comprised of modified items from the MAST. The DAST can be self-administered as a screener of consequences and problem experiences from drug abuse and dependence, with a cut-off score of 6 generally used to indicate a drug abuse or dependence problem. The scale has demonstrated good internal consistency (α = 0.86–0.94). Research has found the ten-item version (DAST-10) to have comparable reliability in addition to strong criterion validity (r = 0.31–0.39) and construct validity (r = 0.40; Yudko et al., 2007).

The *Subtle Substance Abuse Screening Inventory (SASSI)* is a longer self-report screening measure that is available in separate versions for adults and adolescents (Miller 1985, 1999). The Adult SASSI-3 is a ninety-three-item (ten subscale) survey – with sixty-seven dichotomous and twenty-six Likert items – used to identify individuals who have a high probability of having a substance dependence disorder with an overall accuracy of 93 percent. The Adolescent one-hundred-item (twelve subscale) SASSI-A2 is designed to identify individuals who have a high probability of having a substance use disorder, including both substance abuse and substance dependence, with its decision rules yielding an overall accuracy of 94 percent. The SASSI includes both face valid and subtle items that have no apparent relationship to substance use that has strong reliability (Cronbach's alpha = 0.93). The subtle items are used to identify individuals with alcohol and other drug problems who are unwilling or unable to acknowledge substance misuse or related symptoms. A review of the SASSI (Feldstein & Miller, 2007) found generally lower internal consistency for the SASSI subtle scales in adult samples with high variability, test–retest reliability lower than that reported in the test manuals. Sensitivity was found to be similar to public domain screening instruments, but specificity estimates suggest the SASSI yields a high rate of false positives.

The *Drug and Alcohol Problem (DAP) Quickscreen* consists of thirty yes/no items and discriminates well between high-risk and low-risk users (Schwartz & Wirtz, 1990). This assessment was developed for use by pediatricians to assess adolescents for alcohol and other drug abuse and includes the prototypical item: "Has anyone (friend, parent, teacher, or counselor) ever told you that they believe that you may have a drinking or drug problem?." Results from the psychometric evaluation showed that four items accounted for 70 percent of the variation between high-risk and low-risk users. Further analyses with these four items (Knight et al., 1999) showed poor internal consistency (α = 0.46), which is to be expected as it was not intended as standalone scale.

The *Comprehensive Drinker Profile (CDP)* (Miller & Marlatt, 1984) is a structured interview that collects detailed information on an individual's alcohol consumption history, motivation, behavior, and self-efficacy, and has shown acceptable reliability for regular (consistent) drinking patterns, but may not be optimal for assessing episodic or infrequent, but heavy, drinking sessions (Miller et al., 1992; Miller & Del Boca, 1994). The CDP includes a section related to alcohol-related problems that can be used to assess drug misuse. The measure produces two scores: a score for alcohol abuse symptomology (problems) derived from the Michigan Alcohol Screening Test and an indicator of physical dependency. This interview was originally developed to determine treatment modality for a male inpatient population but has been revised for use in clinical and research applications.

Alexander and Leung's (2004) *Marijuana Screening Inventory (MSI-X)* is a thirty-one-item screening tool evaluated with a court mandated clinical sample (n = 107) in treatment for marijuana related problems. The MSI-X reliability was 0.90 with factor analysis explaining 72.2 percent of the variance deriving nine factors: job and interpersonal interference (five items), frequent pattern of use (five items), internal consequences (five items), external consequences (three items), memory and physical effects (five items), under the influence (two items), use to feel normal with interpersonal costs (three items), sought help for use (two items), and marijuana arrest (one item). These results were consistent with the development and testing of the experimental version of the scale with a community sample (n = 408) that found it to be internally reliable (α = 0.89), with nine factors explaining 65.8 percent of the variance (Alexander, 2003). Receiver operating characteristic analysis determined MSI-X accuracy and cut-off points in relation to four DSM IV-TR diagnostic classifications. The MSI-X obtained the highest probability (0.91) for accuracy in identifying both cannabis dependence and abuse, with a cut-off score of 6 producing maximum sensitivity (0.83) and specificity (0.89). A cut-off score of 3 was associated with (probability 0.90; sensitivity 0.85; specificity 0.81) identifying cannabis abuse only risk, leading the authors to define moderate risk as a score of 3–5. The MSI-X identified 43 percent of lifetime users and 29 percent of past-year users with moderate- to high-risk marijuana patterns in need of comprehensive evaluation. More males (15.9 percent) than females (7.5 percent) scored in the "high-risk" range on the MSI-X. Subsequent work (Alexander & Leung, 2006) found concurrent validity between the MSI-X, Drug Abuse Screening Test (DAST-20), five Substance Abuse Subtle Screening Inventory (SASSI-3) subscales, a Diagnostic Statistical Manual (DSM) IV-TR Guided Marijuana Inventory, and two Addiction Severity Index variables. MSI-X discriminant validity was supported by a lack of correlations with three alcohol measures. Convergent validity, determined by t-test associations between MSI-X total problems with SASSI-3 substance dependence scores, evidenced further support for the $\geq$6 scoring cut-off.

Bashford, Flett and Copeland (2010) developed and tested the sixteen-item *Cannabis Use Problems Identification Test (CUPIT)* among high-risk cannabis users ranging in age from thirteen to sixty-one years old. Two subscales were derived from principal components analysis and scale showed exhibited good to excellent one-week test–retest reliability (0.89–0.99) and internal consistency (0.92, 0.83). The scale is able to discriminate diagnostic subgroups along the severity continuum (non-problematic, risky, problematic use). A cut-off score of 12 produced maximum sensitivity for both currently diagnosable cannabis use disorder and those at risk of meeting diagnostic criteria in the following twelve months. Readers are encouraged to explore other marijuana screeners including the Cannabis Abuse Syndrome Screening Test (CASST; Hannifin, 1990), the Cannabis Use Disorder Identification Test (CUDIT; Adamson & Sellman, 2003), and the Cannabis Abuse Screening Test (CUST; Legleye et al., 2007).

Diagnostic Interviews

The *Substance Dependence Severity Scale (SDSS)*; (Miele et al., 2000) is a clinician-administered structured interview (composed of thirteen items) that was developed to assess severity and frequency of dependence across a range of drugs, based on the DSM-IV diagnostic criteria for substance use disorders. The test–retest, joint rating, and internal consistency reliabilities across alcohol, cocaine, heroin, marijuana, and sedative users are good.

The *Addiction Severity Index (ASI)*, currently in the sixth version (Denis, Cacciola & Alterman, 2013), is a 200-item structured clinical research interview designed to provide information about various areas of an individual's life in which there often exists dysfunction associated with drug abuse. Problem areas assessed include medical, legal, drug abuse, alcohol abuse, employment, family, and psychiatric problems. For each domain, lifetime and past thirty-day time frames remain the primary assessment intervals. Reliability and validity data for past versions of the ASI have been extensively reported (McLellan et al., 1980, 1985; Rounsville et al. 1986). Work by McLellan and colleagues (1985) and subsequent work (Mäkelä, 2004; McDermott et al., 1996) have resulted in a useful strategy for obtaining a composite score based on the sum of several individual questions within specific problem areas. However, the composite scores are not standardized, resulting in skewed scores and different distributions across problem areas. Nonparametric Item Response Theory (NIRT) analyses were performed with ASI-6 recent status items, which resulted in nine summary measures for the ASI-6, called Recent Status Scores (RSSs). There is one summary measure for each of six areas – Medical, Employment/Finances, Alcohol, Drugs, Legal, Psychiatric; and three summary measures derived for the Family/Social area – Family/Social Problems, Family/Social Support, Children Problems. Each RSSs was significantly correlated with its corresponding CS. The Medical, Alcohol, Drug ,and Psychiatric scales all had correlations higher or equal to 0.70. The ASI-6 showed acceptable discriminant and concurrent validity as well.

The *Comprehensive Addiction Severity Index for Adolescents (CASI-A)* was designed to provide an in-depth, comprehensive assessment of the severity of adolescents' addiction and problem consequences. This structured interview is also adapted from the Addiction Severity Index (ASI; McLellan et al., 1980). The CASI-A is composed of ten modules assessing the following: psychological, peer relationships, family history, sexual relationships, physical abuse, significant life changes, use of free time, substance use effects and treatment experiences, leisure activities, educational experiences and plans, legal history, and psychiatric status, including prior treatment experiences (Meyers et al., 1995).

The *Adolescent Drug Abuse Diagnosis (ADAD)* is a comprehensive structured interview consisting of 150 items used to assess substance abuse and other problem areas. The format is adapted from the well-known adult tool, the Addiction Severity Index (ASI; McLellan et al., 1980). This interview produces composite scores rating the severity of problems in nine life areas including: medical, school, work, social relations, family relationships, legal, psychological, and alcohol and drug use (Friedman & Utada, 1989).

The *Adolescent Diagnostic Interview (ADI)* (Winters & Henly, 1993) is a fifteen-minute evaluation used to assess the need for treatment of drug misuse among adolescents. This interview includes the evaluation of various cognitive, interpersonal, and school functioning factors that may contribute to alcohol or drug misuse. The instrument consists of twenty-four items and has shown good inter-rater and test–retest reliability in both clinical and nonclinical adolescent samples.

The Structured Clinical Interview for the Diagnostic Statistical Manual V (SCID-V)

The *Diagnostic and Statistical Manual of Mental Disorders of the American Psychiatric Association (DSM)* is widely used in diagnosing substance use disorder, and is currently in its fifth edition (APA, 2013). The previous version of this manual contains specific criteria sets for substance abuse, dependence, intoxication, and withdrawal applicable across different classes of drugs (APA, 2000). The structured clinical interview was a primary measure of substance abuse and substance dependence disorders, the former pertaining to the exhibition of one or more of the following symptoms due to recurrent use, in the past twelve months: (a) failure to fulfill role obligations, (b) hazardous use (physical danger), (c) legal problems, and (d) social problems. Substance dependence disorder was intended to be a more severe disorder with three or more of the following symptoms, due to recurrent use, in the past twelve months including (a) tolerance, (b) withdrawal (c) using more than intended, (d) desiring, but being unable, to quit or cut down, (e) taking up a lot of time, (f) other activities being neglected or given up, and (g) continued use despite related psychological or physical problems due to use.

The DSM-5 version describes a single "substance use disorder," which is described along a continuum of severity including moderate and severe categories depending on whether one exhibits two to three or four or more of the following symptoms, respectively, due to recurrent use over the past twelve months: (a) using more than intended, (b) desiring, but being unable, to quit or cut down, (c) taking up a lot of time, (d) exhibiting craving, a strong desire to use, (e) failure to fulfill role obligations, (f) continued use despite related social problems, (g) other activities being neglected or given up, (h) hazardous use (physical danger), (i) continued use despite related psychological or physical problems due to use, (j) tolerance, and (k) withdrawal symptoms.

This revision combines the criteria of substance abuse and substance dependence from the previous version to create an overarching diagnosis for substance use disorders. The "problems with law enforcement" symptom has been removed from the list due to cultural factors that make it difficult to apply internationally, according to the APA. The symptom, "exhibiting craving, a strong desire to use" has been added as a criterion to increase consistency with the *International Classification of Diseases* (10th edition) criteria and indirect evidence and rationale that it is central to the diagnosis and treatment of substance use disorder (Hasin et al., 2013).

The *Structured Clinical Interview for the Diagnostic Statistical Manual (SCID)* is a broad-spectrum instrument that adheres to the DSM-5 decision trees for psychiatric diagnosis and encourages multiple paths of exploration, clarification, and clinical decision-making, with specific clarification regarding efforts to decrease or control use, continued use despite problems, specific withdrawal symptoms of a drug, and assessment of comorbidity. This interview is a primary measure of substance use disorders in the field of clinical psychology.

Food Addiction

Gearhardt, Corbin and Brownell (2009) developed the *Yale Food Addiction Scale (YFAS)* to determine whether the diagnostic criteria for substance dependence were present in eating problems. The scale questions fall under specific criteria that resemble the symptoms for substance dependence as stated in the *Diagnostic and Statistical Manual of Mental Disorders IV-R* and operationalized in the *Structured Clinical Interview for DSM-IV Axis I Disorders*.

The *Yale Food Addiction Scale* was developed to identify individuals exhibiting signs of substance dependence when consuming high fat/high sugar foods. This twenty-five-item self-report measure includes mixed-response categories (dichotomous and Likert-type format). A food addiction symptom (e.g., tolerance, withdrawal, loss of control) count can be obtained, which is similar to the criteria for substance dependence of the *DSM-IV-TR* (American Psychiatric Association, 2000). Additionally, two items assess clinically significant impairment or distress from eating. Food addiction can be "diagnosed" when three symptoms and clinically significant impairment or distress are present.

Following the release of the *Diagnostic and Statistical Manual of Mental Disorders* (5th edition; DSM-5), which included significant changes to the substance-related and addictive disorders (SRAD) section, the *Yale Food Addiction Scale 2.0 (YFAS 2.0)* was developed.

Gearhardt, Corbin and Brownell (2016) revised the scale to maintain consistency with the current diagnostic understanding of addiction and to improve the psychometric properties of the original YFAS. In the initial validation sample of 550 participants, 14.6 percent met criteria for food addiction. The YFAS 2.0 is a thirty-five-item measure reflecting the DSM-5 diagnostic criteria for addiction and includes two scoring options: (1) a continuous symptom count that reflects the number of diagnostic criteria met by the participant and (2) a diagnosis of food addiction based on the number of symptoms and clinically significant impairment or distress. The diagnostic scoring option reflects the same criteria of the DSM-5 and provides cut-offs for mild, moderate, and severe forms. The YFAS 2.0 produced a one-factor solution and demonstrated good internal consistency (Kuder–Richardson alpha = 0.90), as well as convergent, discriminant, and incremental validity. Elevated scores on the YFAS 2.0 were associated with higher rates of obesity and more severe pathological eating (e.g., binge eating). The YFAS 2.0 also appeared to capture a related, but unique, construct relative to traditional eating disorders.

The *Binge Eating Scale (BES)* is a sixteen-item questionnaire used to assess the presence of binge-eating behavior indicative of an eating disorder specifically for use with obese individuals. The questions are based upon both behavioral characteristics (e.g., amount of food consumed) and the emotional, cognitive response, guilt, or shame related to binge eating (Gormally et al., 1982). The range of scores is 0–46, with scores of 17 or less indicating nonbingeing, 18–26 indicating moderate bingeing, and scores of 27 or more indicating severe bingeing. Grupski and colleagues (2013) assessed the clinical utility of the BES to predict binge-eating disorder in a sample of patients seeking bariatric surgery. ROC curve analyses identified an optimal BES cut-score of 17, which correctly classified 78 percent of patients with binge-eating disorder. Increasing the cut-off to 27 improved the correct classification statistic, but significantly increased the number of false positives. Additionally, discriminant function analyses revealed that nearly all BES items significantly predicted binge-eating disorder in the sample. Prevalence rates of these food addiction diagnoses according to the YFAS range between approximately 5 percent to 10 percent in nonclinical samples, 15 percent to 25 percent in obese samples, and 30 percent to 50 percent in morbidly obese bariatric patients or obese individuals with binge-eating disorder (Meule & Gearhardt, 2014).

Ruddock and colleagues (2017) questioned the ecological validity of previous food and eating disorder scales using a substance-based model given the limited comparability between food and drug addiction in relation to their neurological, behavioral, and social effects. They developed the *Addiction like-Eating Behavior Scale (AEBS)* to quantify the dimensions of observable behaviors related to eating addiction. Psychometric analyses in a community sample (n = 511) produced a two-factor structure to explain the data. Factor 1 (nine items) consists of items that referred to appetitive drive, whereas factor 2 (six items) consists of items that referred to dietary control practices. Both subscales demonstrated good internal reliability (Factor 1 α = 0.85–0.90; Factor 2 α = 0.83–0.85) and test–retest reliability (Factor 1 r = 0.74, Factor 2 r = 0.74, total scale r = 0.77), and a confirmatory factor analysis confirmed the two-factor scale structure. AEBS scores correlated positively with body mass index (BMI) ($p < 0.001$) and self-report measures of overeating. The AEBS significantly predicted variance in BMI above that accounted for by both the YFAS and BES (p = 0.027). Readers should note that food addiction is closely related to higher current and lifetime BMI, with participants meeting the "food addiction" threshold being obese (BMI $\geq$ 30) on average, but not universally (Gearhardt, Boswell & White, 2014).

Exercise Addiction

Survey Tools

One of the earliest psychometric inventories, the *Obligatory Exercise Questionnaire* (Thompson & Pasman, 1991) is a twenty-item measure with a four-point Likert response where 1 = "never" and 4 = "always." This nonspecific measure of exercise activity includes exercise addiction items such as "When I don't exercise I feel guilty" and "I have had daydreams about exercise." The internal consistency (Cronbach's alpha) was 0.96 and the test–retest reliability was also 0.96. Construct validity was established as it discriminated between exercisers and control subjects (Pasman & Thompson, 1988) and was correlated with behavioral dimensions of obligatory running, where higher scores were correlated with reporting anxiety when unable to run and to run despite injury (Coen & Ogles, 1993).

The *Bodybuilding Dependency Scale* (Smith, Hale & Collins, 1998) was developed specifically to assess compulsive training in bodybuilding and has satisfactory reliability (Smith & Hale, 2005; Smith et al., 1998). It comprises three subscales: (1) social dependence (the need to be in the gym), (2) training dependence (compulsion to train), and (3) mastery dependence (the need to control training), with satisfactory internal consistency for each subscale at 0.76, 0.75, and 0.78, respectively. Administration of the social dependency subscale with the Athletic Identity Measurement Scale and years of training experience led to the correct classification of 92 percent of participants with bodybuilding dependency. The clinical utility of the training and mastery dependence scales were not entirely supported by the initial psychometric analysis.

Bamber and colleagues' (2000) *Exercise Dependence Interview (EXDI)* assesses compulsive exercising behavior and eating disorders. The EXDI gauges excessive engagement in physical activity in the three months prior to the date of assessment, the associated thoughts, and their association with the eating behavior. It also determines the self-appraisal of exercise dependence and exercise habits; however, the psychometric properties have not been reported.

Another measure, the *Commitment to Exercise Scale (CES)* developed by Davis, Brewer and Ratusny (1993), is an eight-item measure that examines the pathological aspects of exercising (e.g., continued training following injury) and compulsory activities (e.g., feeling guilty when exercise is not completed). The CES has a satisfactory level of reliability (Cronbach's alpha = 0.77) and is correlated with frequency of physical activity participation and weight occupation. Finally, the *Exercise Orientation Questionnaire (EOQ)* (Yates et al., 2001) measures attitudes toward exercise and related behaviors. The twenty-seven-item EOQ comprises six factors: (1) self-control, (2) orientation to exercise, (3) self-loathing, (4) weight reduction, (5) competition, and (6) identity. Alpha coefficients for the factors ranged from 0.74 to 0.87, with 0.92 for the total score, suggesting excellent reliability. Good concurrent validity was indicated by significant correlations between EOQ scores and ratings of exercise investment, frequency, and duration. Gender differences were observed, with females scoring higher on the weight reduction subscale whereas males scored higher on identity.

Screeners and Clinical Assessment Tools

Hausenblas and Symons Downs'(2002) *Exercise Dependence Scale* was originally twenty-seven items but later refined to a final scale of twenty-one statements that establishes exercise dependence based on the *Diagnostic and Statistical Manual IV* (DSM-IV, 1994) criteria for substance dependence. The original scale showed excellent reliability (Cronbach's alpha = 0.93) and evidenced concurrent and construct validity. The revised *Exercise Dependence Scale-21 (EDS-21)* responses were measured on a six point Likert scale where 1 = "always" and 6 = "never" such that lower scores reflect more attributes of exercise dependence. Scale components include (a) withdrawal effects, (b) continuance, (c) tolerance, (d) lack of control, (e) reduction in other activities, (f) time, and (g) intention effects. On the EDS-21 measure, individuals scoring 1 or 2 on three or more of the seven components are classified as exercise dependent. Those scoring in the 3–4 range are classified as symptomatic and those scoring in the range of 5–6 are classified as asymptomatic. The internal consistency of the EDS-21 was excellent ($\alpha = 0.95$) and the seven-day test-retest reliability was strong ($r = 0.92$, $p < 0.001$).

The *Exercise Addiction Inventory (EAI)* (Szabo & Griffiths, 2004) was operationalized using the components of behavioral addiction proposed by Griffiths (1996). The scale was developed with the intent of having a short six-item inventory that would be quick and simple to administer. The initial psychometric analysis of the EAI evidenced good internal reliability (Cronbach's alpha = 0.84), content validity, concurrent validity with the OEQ ($r = 0.80$) and the EDS ($r = 0.81$), and construct validity (Szabo & Griffiths, 2004). It should be noted that, among the instruments outlined for exercise addiction, the most popular currently are the EDS and the EAI (due to their brevity and easy scoring). Research has shown that these two instruments yield comparable results (see Berczik et al., 2012).

Gambling Addiction

Survey Tools

An abbreviated form of the thirty-one-item *Canadian Problem Gambling Index*, the *Problem Gambling Severity Index (PGSI)* is a nine-item self-assessment of gambling problems (Ferris & Wynne, 2001). The response choices for each PGSI item are "never," "sometimes," "most of the time," or "almost always," with a total score ranging from 0 to 27. Cut-offs are used to assign gamblers to categories consisting of "nonproblem gamblers" (total = 0), "low-risk" (total = 1–2), "moderate-risk" (total = 3–7), or "problem-gambler" (total > 7). The PGSI has become one of the most commonly referenced assessments for assessing gambling related harms and has been evaluated qualitatively (McCready & Adlaf, 2006) and quantitatively (Currie, Casey & Hodgins, 2010; Orford et al., 2010). One issue with the measure is that that the problem gambler category was the only one that underwent extensive validity testing. Using the initial scoring rules, there was strong evidence for the validity of the nonproblem and problem gambler categories; however, the low-risk and moderate-risk categories showed poor discriminant validity though this was corrected with a small modification to the scoring (Currie et al., 2012).

Screeners and Clinical Assessment Tools

The *Lie-Bet Tool* (Johnson et al., 1997, 1998) is a valid and reliable two-item measure used to rule out pathological gambling behaviors. The Lie-Bet's two questions ("Have you ever had to lie to people important to you about how much you gambled?" and "Have you ever felt the need to bet more and more money?") consistently differentiate between pathological gambling and nonproblem gambling (Johnson et al., 1998) and are useful in screening to determine whether a longer tool (see below) should be used to assess the extent of a gambling problem. The *DSM-5 Screen for Pathological Gambling* is a nine-item yes/no checklist of past year pathological gambling symptoms based on the DSM-5 diagnostic criteria. A total score of 4 or more "yes" responses indicates a likely diagnosis of a gambling disorder, and scores less than 4, but greater than 0, indicates a potential problem or at-risk indicators that may place the respondent in need of future intervention. Similarly, the *NODS-CLiP* is a three-item screening tool that demonstrated excellent sensitivity (96.2 percent) and acceptable specificity (90.2 percent) in a large study of US adults (Toce-Gerstein, Gerstein & Volberg, 2009). Additional psychometric analyses (Volberg, Munck & Petry, 2011) indicate that the items captured 96 percent of the male problem gamblers and 91 percent of the female problem gamblers. The NODS-CLiP captured 100 percent of the Hispanic problem gamblers, 94 percent of the Caucasian problem gamblers, and 87 percent of the African American problem gamblers. Finally, while the screen captured 100 percent of the problem gamblers aged eighteen to twenty-nine, and 97 percent of those aged thirty to forty-four, it captured only 89 percent of the problem gamblers aged forty-five and over. Alternative item combinations captured more than 90 percent of pathological gamblers in the study.

The *Gambling Symptom Assessment Scale (G-SAS)* is a twelve-item self-rated scale designed to assess gambling symptom severity and change during treatment (Kim et al., 2009). In a sample of 207 patients with DSM IV Pathological Gambling Disorder, the G-SAS had a Cronbach's alpha of 0.87 and a one-week test-retest correlation of $r = 0.56$ indicating moderate reliability over time. The G-SAS was compared to the PG-YBOCS on symptom change scores and percent symptom change scores which showed good agreement (0.81 and 0.85, respectively).

The *South Oaks Gambling Screen (SOGS)* is a twenty-item questionnaire based on the DSM-III criteria for pathological gambling (Lesieur & Bloom, 1987) that was initially developed for screening purposes in clinical settings. As the use of the SOGS expanded to other settings and populations, Stinchfield (2002) examined its psychometric properties in a general population sample ($n = 803$) and a gambling treatment sample ($n = 1{,}589$). The SOGS was found to have satisfactory reliability with coefficient alphas of 0.69 and 0.86 in the general population and gambling treatment samples, respectively. The SOGS differentiated between the general population and the gambling treatment sample and by exhibiting high correlations with DSM-IV diagnostic criteria and moderate correlations with other measures of gambling problem severity. The SOGS demonstrated good-to-excellent classification accuracy in the gambling treatment sample but had worse accuracy in the general population sample with a 50 percent false positive rate. The SOGS overestimated the number of pathological gamblers in the general population, as compared to DSM-IV diagnostic criteria. Evidence suggests the SOGS may be more appropriate for use as a screener with clinical or treatment seeking populations, but criticism and subsequent rebuttal that the SOGS overestimates false positives (Gambino & Lesieur, 2006; Ladouceur et al., 2000; Stinchfield, 2002) has been ongoing as its use has declined in the research setting.

This tool was adapted for use with adolescent populations (Winters et al., 1993) as the twelve-item *South Oaks Gambling Screen: Revised for Adolescents (SOGS-RA)*. Initial findings reliably discriminated between participants who gambled regularly and those who did not, and correlated with the amount of money spent on gambling in the past year ($p < 0.01$). Poulin (2002) investigated the SOGS-RA for identifying daily gamblers, at a cut-point of 4, and found that the sensitivity, specificity and percent classified correct were 22, 99, and 95 percent, respectively. Boudreau and Poulin (2007) used ROC curve analyses on the SOGS-RA, and concluded that the recommended cut-point of 4 performed satisfactorily as measured against the proxy gold standards of either needing, or having received, help for gambling. The SOGS-RA was better at identifying true negative cases (i.e., gamblers who indicated they did not need or did not receive help for their gambling) than true positive cases.

Browne, Goodwin and Rockloff's (2018) *Short Gambling Harm Screen (SGHS)* is a ten-item measure developed to detect the presence and degree of harm caused by gambling. Nonzero responses on the SGHS were associated with a large decrease in personal wellbeing, with wellbeing decreasing linearly with the number of harms (i.e., negative consequences of excessive gambling) indicated. Psychometric analyses showed high alpha reliability ($\alpha = 0.93$), strong correlation with the PGSI (Spearman's $r = 0.68$), near perfect correlation with the initial seventy-two-item pool of harms considered for the scale (Spearman's $r = 0.94$), and invariance across gender and age.

The *National Opinion Research Center DSM-IV Screen (NODS) for Gambling Problems* is a thirty-four-item dichotomous [yes/no] questionnaire administered in two phases (Gerstein et al., 1999). First, respondents are screened for lifetime problems, and then are screened for past-year problems only among lifetime items that were endorsed. Using NORC typology and DSM-IV criteria, a gambler who scores 0 points is classified as a Type B gambler ("low-risk gambler"). Scoring 1–2 points is classified as a Type C gambler ("at-risk gambler"), and a gambler who scores 3–4 points is classified as a Type D gambler ("problem gambler"). Finally, scoring 5 or more points classifies gamblers as a Type E gambler ("probable pathological gambler"). Classification can be determined using lifetime or past year responses. Initial psychometric analyses with a clinical sample (Gerstein et al., 1999) found that test-retest reliability in a sample of forty-four gamblers in treatment using a two- to four-week test-retest period was high ($r = 0.99$ lifetime version and 0.98 past year). Thirty-eight of forty individuals (95 percent) receiving problem gambling treatment achieved scores of 5 or greater on the lifetime version, supporting the validity of the classification. Further investigation of the scale by Hodgins (2004) found a three-factor structure from a sample of problem gamblers one year after a brief treatment ($n = 86$). The Cronbach's alpha (α) values for the three factors were 0.75, 0.61, and 0.56, respectively. The NODS total score correlated highly with the SOGS total score ($r = 0.86$, $p < 0.0001$) and showed moderate correlations with gambling behavior (days spent gambling, dollars spent, and dollars spent per day) over the previous six months.

The *Yale-Brown Obsessive-Compulsive Scale – Pathological Gambling (PG-YBOCS)* was developed to measure the severity and change in severity of pathological gambling symptoms. A ten-item clinician-administered questionnaire measures the severity of PG over a recent time interval of one or two weeks. Initial development of the scale (Pallanti et al., 2005) with 337 participants (188 pathological gamblers and 149 healthy controls) produced subscales pertaining to "thoughts/urges" and "behaviors" with good reliability coefficients of 0.94 and 0.93, respectively, and inter-rater reliability ICCs of 0.936 and 0.943, respectively. Test-retest reliability was moderate (ICC range: 0.294–0.556) but statistically significant as was the subscale correlation with the SOGS. The PG-YBOCS, unlike the GSAS and CGI-Improvement scales, was able to significantly discriminate mild from moderate groups (Grant, Odlaug & Chamberlain, 2017). Thus, this scale may be preferable as a measure in clinical trials or for treatment planning and intake.

Additional clinician-administered screening and diagnostic tools for gambling addiction include the *Structured Clinical Interview for Pathological Gambling* (Grant et al., 2004), which assesses the 10 DSM-IV inclusion criteria for pathological gambling and the exclusionary criteria of "not better accounted for by a manic episode," and the *Diagnostic Interview for Gambling Severity*, which is a structured interview of twenty lifetime and past-year symptoms, treatment history, age of onset of gambling, and family and social functioning (Winters, Specker & Stinchfield, 2002). Though beyond the scope of this chapter, readers with an interest in clinical measurement may want to explore the *Inventory of Gambling Situations (IGS)* as a treatment and relapse prevention tool that emphasizes antecedents and triggers for gambling (Weiss & Petry, 2008).

Sex/Love Addiction

There has been considerable debate about how to label a psychological problem defined by a person's inability to control their sexual behavior (Bancroft & Vukadinovic, 2004; Gold & Heftner, 1998; Klein, 2003). This has led to a proliferation of conceptualizations for the phenomena including sexual addiction, compulsive sexual behavior, sexual compulsivity, and sexual impulsivity (Barth & Kinder, 1987; Carnes, 1983; Coleman, 1991; Kalichman & Rompa, 1995). As such, many existing scales have been constructed using a compulsivity model drawing on underlying obsessive-compulsive disorder or a dependence model drawing on a substance use disorder framework describing the behaviors as a traditional form of addiction. The instruments described here commonly assess objective and subjective symptomology of sexual addiction and the negative consequences associated with sex addiction. A more exhaustive list of inventories for assessing sex addiction are available elsewhere (Karila et al., 2014). Additionally, readers with an interest in these measurements are encouraged to read the Hook et al. (2010) review of seventeen instruments created to assess sexual addiction, including self-report rating scales, self-report checklists, and clinician rating scales measuring symptoms of sexual addiction, as well as self-report rating scales measuring consequences associated with sexual addiction.

Survey Tools

The twenty-eight-item *Compulsive Sexual Behavior Inventory (CSBI)* assesses sexual control, past history of sexual abuse, and experience of sexual violence (Coleman et al., 2001) with total scores ranging between 28 and 140, where lower scores are indicative of higher compulsive sexual behavior. Factor analysis resulted in a three-factor solution that appeared to measure Control (thirteen items), Abuse (eight items), and Violence (seven items), with good reliability ($\alpha = 0.96$ for Control, 0.91 for Abuse, and 0.88 for Violence). Internal consistency has consistently rated as good (α = 0.67–0.87) and the one-week test-retest reliability was acceptable ($r = 0.86$). When tested with a Latino MSM (men who have sex with men) sample (Miner et al., 2007) the scale produced a two-factor solution (control and violence), showed good consistency between English and Spanish versions ($r = 0.88$), and had good test-retest reliability in both languages (English, $r = 0.86$; Spanish, $r = 0.93$).

The *Sexual Compulsivity Scale* (Kalichman et al., 1994) is composed of tenitems yielding a total score to measure sexual addiction with total scores ranging from 10 to 40 and a cut-off score of 24 indicating problems of sexual addiction (Benotsch, Kalichman & Kelly, 1999; Parsons et al., 2001). The scale has been extensively evaluated in community samples of heterosexual and homosexual men and women producing alpha values ranging from 0.59 to 0.92, and acceptable test-retest reliability estimates (two-week, $r = 0.95$; three-month, $r = 0.80$). A follow-up factor analysis of the scale produced a two-factor solution representing social disruptiveness and personal discomfort (Kalichman & Cain, 2004), though a subsequent study was unable to produce the same findings (McBride et al., 2008).

Love addiction is considered a process addiction; that is, it pertains to a pattern of recurrent behavior that, at first, results in reports of pleasurable feelings and obsessive thinking, but has not been as well studied as sex addiction (Sussman, 2010). As such, fewer scales have been developed and tested to measure love addiction, but a few notable measures are discussed here briefly. Feeney and Noller (1990) constructed twelve love addiction-type items that were scored from strongly agree (1) to strongly disagree (5) and formed two factors: reliance on partner (e.g., "want us to be together all the time"), and unfulfilled hopes (e.g., "never satisfied with partners"). Hunter, Nitschke and Hogan (1981) developed a twenty-item four-point self-report "Love Scale" (e.g., "Soon after I met my partner, I knew this person was my 'other half' and made my life complete"), which they administered to fifty-eight undergraduates (mean age twenty-eight years) twice during a two-week period and found high test-retest reliability. Similar items are included in the Passionate Love Scale (PLS; Hatfield & Sprecher, 1986). Feeney & Noller's measure, the Love Scale, and the Passionate Love Scale were tested solely with college undergraduate students and have not been replicated with larger community or clinical samples.

Screeners and Clinical Assessment Tools

The original twenty-five-item *Sexual Addiction Screening Test (SAST)* indicated good internal consistency and the ability to discriminate between male sex addicts and male control populations, making it a widely used tool in various settings and programs (Hueppelheuser et al., 1997; Weiss, 2004). Yet, when used with women or homosexual males, the SAST did not perform as well. A specific scale for women (the W-SAST) and homosexual men (G-SAST) were subsequently developed using a similar format with twenty-five items each (see Carnes, Green & Carnes, 2010). Later the *SAST-R (SAST – Revised)* was developed as a single screener that would capture sexual addiction across multiple populations (Carnes et al., 2010). The scale consists of forty-five yes/no "core items" that allow for direct comparison across groups and allows the assessor to measure unique patterns within specific populations of interest. Of note, readers searching for a brief scale might consider the *PATHOS* screener (Preoccupied, Ashamed, Treatment, Hurt others, Out of control, Sad), a six-item brief screen using a subset of items from the original SAST and SAST-R, which has the potential to detect sex addicts in clinical settings (Carnes et al., 2012).

Morgenstern and colleagues' (2004) *Yale-Brown Obsessive-Compulsive Scale – Compulsive Sexual Behavior* is a ten-item clinician-administered scale that has been evaluated with samples of gay and bisexual males in community settings with internal consistency reported between $\alpha = 0.80$ and 0.91. Initial factor analysis has supported a one-factor, unidimensional scale, but this has not been replicated in further research. Additionally, temporal stability of the scale has not been demonstrated.

The *Internet Sex Screening Test* (Delmonico & Miller, 2003) is a twenty-five-item true/false measure with acceptable internal consistency ($\alpha = 0.78$) with subscale α values ranging between 0.51 and 0.86. Total scale scores correlate with the SAST, boredom proneness, low social connectedness, and time spent online in sexual activity. Though not reviewed here, there are numerous measures of cybersex and Internet sex addiction including, but not limited to, the *Cyber-Pornography Use Inventory* (Grubbs et al., 2010), the *Internet Addiction Test – Sex* (Brand et al., 2011; Laier et al., 2013), and the *Online Sexual Experience Questionnaire* (Shaughnessy, Byers & Walsh, 2011). For a more comprehensive review of scales assessing online sexual activities and addictions see Eleuteri et al. (2014).

The *Hypersexual Behavior Consequences Scale (HBCS)* is a structured diagnostic interview with twenty-two items assessed with a five-point Likert Scale (Reid, Garos & Fong, 2012). Internal consistency is good ($\alpha = 0.84$), as was the two-week test-retest reliability ($r = 0.76$). The related nineteen-item *Hypersexual Behavior Inventory (HBI)* was developed by using a sample of male sex addict outpatients. Factor analysis produced a three-factor solution measuring control, consequences, and coping associated with sexual thoughts, feelings and behaviors (Reid, Garos & Carpenter, 2011). Cronbach's alpha scores have been high for the overall scale ($\alpha = 0.95$–0.96) and for the subscales. Two-week test-retest coefficients were also excellent ($r = 0.91$). Preliminary psychometric analyses supported the concurrent and discriminant validity of the scale, and the authors proposed using a preliminary cut-off score of 53 to distinguish clinically elevated scores for men. More work is needed to test this tentative cut-off score.

Work Addiction

To date, only a few instruments have been designed and validated to assess work addiction. Originally, researchers discussed "workaholism," which was described by Oates (1971) as an "addiction to work, the compulsion or uncontrollable need to work incessantly" (p. 11). Further conceptual and empirical work refined the definition of workaholism to describe workaholism as a subtype of heavy work involvement which can be defined in terms of both a time and space dimension (Snir & Harpaz, 2012). Of course, disagreement on the conceptualization of work addiction, or workaholism, continues today. Some have described workaholism as a positive attribute encompassing high work motivation (Scott, Moore & Miceli, 1997), for example, and others have described it as a negative attribute characterized by compulsiveness and overindulgence (Ng, Sorensen & Feldman, 2007; Robinson, 1998). The latter definition has continued to dominate the conceptualization an operationalization of workaholism (Clark et al., 2016) as indicated by the popular measures commonly employed to measure work addiction as discussed below.

The earliest measure of work addiction was Robinson's (1989) *Work Addiction Risk Test (WART)*, a twenty-five-item scale scored on a four-point Likert scale. Like other scales there has been conflict regarding the factor structure of the measure. Originally, Robinson (1989) reported a one-factor solution but later work (Robinson & Post, 1994) reported a five-factor solution of overdoing, self-worth, control-perfection, intimacy, and future reference/mental preoccupation. Further research reported another five-factor solution (Flowers & Robinson, 2002), and one study suggested a second-order factor composed of five first-order factors (Robinson, 2001). Spence and Robbin's (1992) *Workaholism Battery (WorkBAT)* was initially tested with undergraduate students and then revised and administered to a sample of social workers. The twenty-five-item scale was originally described as having three subscales (work involvement, drive, and enjoyment of work). Using cluster analysis, the developers defined several groups of workers. Workaholics, for instance, scored above the average on work involvement and drive but below the average on enjoyment of work, and work enthusiasts scored above the average on work involvement and enjoyment of work and below the average on drive. The most recently developed scale, the *Dutch Work Addiction Scale (DUWAS)* is a shorter ten-item scale of which five items assess working excessively and five items assess working compulsively (Taris, Schaufeli & Verhoeven, 2005). The five items measuring working compulsively were adapted from the WorkBAT (four items) and the WART (one item). Replication of the initial study found the DUWAS has good psychometric properties (Líbano et al., 2010).

Andreassen et al. (2012) compared the WART, WorkBAT, and DUWAS on cross-validation, temporal stability, and their respective factor structures. The measures were given to 661 cross-occupational Norwegian workers, and 368 workers completed the measures again twenty-four to thirty months later. Briefly, temporal stability (test–retest reliability) was good for all measures. The WorkBAT and WART produced a four-factor solution while the DUWAS produced a two-factor solution. Cross-validation was low between the measures, suggesting that the scales may not be measuring the same construct.

The *Workaholism subscale of the Schedule for Non-adaptive and Adaptive Personality (Workaholism-SNAP)* is composed of eighteen items from a 375-item true/false inventory designed to discriminate normal and abnormal personality traits. Thirteen items focus on work and five items are shared with the obsessive–compulsive subscale (Clark et al., 1993, 1996). In a later study (McMillan et al., 2002), the Cronbach alpha was 0.82 (split half $r = 0.82$) and the measure has shown good convergent validity when used with broader populations (Clark et al., 1996).

A final instrument worth a mention was developed by Buelens and Poelmans (2004). The scale was constructed based on the workaholism structure developed by Spence and Robbins (1992). By using a total of twenty items from different scales, including the WorkBAT and the WART, in an explorative factor analysis they found support for a three-factor solution reflecting the three dimensions of Spence and Robbins (1992): enjoyment, work involvement, and feeling driven. Based on these dimensions the scale described eight subtypes of workers (see Buelens & Poelmans, 2004).

Internet Addiction

An exhaustive review of psychometric inventories measuring Internet addiction found forty-five tools used to measure Internet addiction; with seventeen having been evaluated more than once (Laconi, Rodgers & Chabrol, 2014). While psychometric inventories have been developed to address addiction to specific websites such as Facebook (Andreaseen et al., 2012) or Internet gaming (Király, Griffiths & Demetrovics, 2015; Pontes & Griffiths, 2015), this subsection focuses on general Internet addiction scales. Of note, it is expected that more scales assessing Internet gaming addiction will become available following the 2018 announcement that the World Health Organization's International Classification of Diseases (WHO ICD) would include a diagnosis of gaming disorder (active as of June, 2018). The ICD presently defines gaming disorder as a "pattern of gaming behavior ("digital-gaming" or "video-gaming") characterized by impaired control over gaming, increasing priority given to gaming over other activities to the extent that gaming takes precedence over other interests and daily activities, and continuation or escalation of gaming despite the occurrence of negative consequences" (retrieved December 9, 2018, from www.who.int/features/qa/gaming-disorder/en/). Diagnosis of gaming disorder is assessed based on a twelve-month evaluation of impairment in personal, family, social, educational, occupational, or other important areas of functioning (Table 8.2). The scales summarized below are among the most reviewed and widely used scales of general Internet addiction but is not an exhaustive review of all available scales.

Survey Tools

Young's (1998) twenty-item *Internet Addiction Test (IAT)* is the most rigorously evaluated psychometric tool for Internet addiction.

Table 8.2 Diagnostic criteria for Gaming Disorder from DSM-5 and WHO ICD-11

DSM-5	ICD-11
1. Repetitive use of Internet-based games, often with other players, that leads to significant issues with functioning. Five of the following criteria must be met within one year: 1. Preoccupation or obsession with Internet games. 2. Withdrawal symptoms when not playing Internet games. 3. A build-up of tolerance – more time needs to be spent playing the games. 4. The person has tried to stop or curb playing Internet games but has failed to do so. 5. The person has had a loss of interest in other life activities, such as hobbies. 6. A person has had continued overuse of Internet games even with the knowledge of how much they impact a person's life. 7. The person lied to others about his or her Internet game usage. 8. The person uses Internet games to relieve anxiety or guilt – it's a way to escape. 9. The person has lost or put at risk and opportunity or relationship because of Internet games.	*Gaming disorder, predominantly online* Gaming disorder, predominantly online is characterized by a pattern of persistent or recurrent gaming behavior ("digital gaming" or "video-gaming") that is primarily conducted over the internet and is manifested by: (1) impaired control over gaming (e.g., onset, frequency, intensity, duration, termination, context); (2) increasing priority given to gaming to the extent that gaming takes precedence over other life interests and daily activities; and (3) continuation or escalation of gaming despite the occurrence of negative consequences. The behavior pattern is of sufficient severity to result in significant impairment in personal, family, social, educational, occupational or other important areas of functioning. The pattern of gaming behavior may be continuous or episodic and recurrent. The gaming behavior and other features are normally evident over a period of at least 12 months in order for a diagnosis to be assigned, although the required duration may be shortened if all diagnostic requirements are met and symptoms are severe.

Note: From the American Psychiatric Association *Diagnostic and Statistical Manual of Mental Disorders*, 5th Edition (2013) (section III as a "Condition for further study" and not as a formal diagnosis) and ICD-11 diagnostic code 6C51.0.

Psychometric analyses carried out by Widyanto & McMurran (2004) in a sample of eighty-six Internet users revealed that the IAT had six factors – salience, excessive use, neglecting work, anticipation, lack of control, and neglecting social life – with Cronbach's alpha ratings varying between 0.54 and 0.82. The salience and excessive use factors were associated with greater daily and weekly Internet usage, and this psychometric evaluation corroborated previous findings (Brenner, 1997) that younger Internet users tend to have more problems related to work. A shortened twelve-item version of the scale was developed with a two-factor solution – loss of control/time management and craving/social problems – which showed acceptable reliability and validity estimates across several study samples (Pawlikowski, Altstötter-Gleich & Brand, 2013). The scale continues to be widely used in epidemiological and survey-based research, and has been validated in multiple languages.

The *Chen Internet Addiction Scale (CIAS*; Chen et al., 2003) is twenty-six 6-items and has been shown to have cut-offs for screening and diagnostic points (Ko et al., 2005) with evidence suggesting a total score of 58 for screening and 64 for diagnosis of an Internet use disorder. Alpha reliabilities have been high across studies and are strongly correlated with the IADQ and time spent online.

Derived from the earlier *Internet Related Addictive Behavior Inventory* (Brenner, 1997), the *Internet Related Problem Scale (IRPS)* is a twenty-item scale with a ten-point Likert scale (Armstrong, Phillips & Saling, 2000). Across studies, the IRPS was significantly correlated with time spent on the Internet (Armstrong et al., 2000; Widyanto, Griffiths & Brunsden, 2011). The scale has shown acceptable internal consistency (α = 0.88) but has produced different factor structures across studies (Widyanto et al., 2008).

Initially evaluated in a sample of 277 undergraduate students, the *Problematic Internet Use Scale (PIUS)* (Morahan-Martin & Schumacher, 2000) produced a Cronbach's alpha of 0.88 and correlated with time spent online. An adolescent version – the *Problematic Internet Use Scale Adolescents (PIUS-a)* was recently developed (Boubeta et al., 2015). The scale was developed in Spain and adapted to the Spanish cultural context with a brief 11-item tool using the language of young people. It has satisfactory psychometric properties in terms of reliability of the scores (α = 0.82), sensitivity (81 percent), and specificity (82.6 percent). Another scale developed and validated by using college students is Kelly and Gruber's (2010) *Problematic Internet Use Questionnaire (PIUQ)*. A short (six-item) version of the PIUQ called the *PIUQ short form (PIUQ-SF-6)* was developed with a nationally representative adolescent sample (n = 5,005; mean age 16.4 years) and showed an alpha of 0.77 (Demetrovics et al., 2016). Using at-risk latent profile analysis as the gold standard, a cut-off value of 15 (out of a possible score of 30) was established based on sensitivity and specificity analyses.

The *Compulsive Internet Use Scale (CIUS)* is a fourteen-item dichotomously scored scale that has shown good reliability and validity (Meerkerk et al., 2009). The initial psychometric analysis with three large convenience samples showed that the scale displayed strong reliability and validity over time with different samples. Six of seven psychometric evaluation studies have supported a one-factor solution (see Laconi et al., 2014). The scale has been validated in several languages with adolescent and adult populations.

Caplan's (2010) *Generalized Problematic Internet Use Scale-2 (GPIUS-2)* is a fifteen-item scale revised from an earlier version (Caplan, 2002). Unlike the earlier version, the GPIUS-2 does not have a cut-off score but consists of five subscales made up of three items each: preference for online social interaction, mood regulation, cognitive preoccupation, compulsive internet use, and negative outcomes. The overall scale showed good reliability (α = 0.91) with subscale values ranging between 0.82 and 0.87. The revised scale has shown good concurrent validity with the IAT (Barke et al., 2012; Floravanti, Primi & Casale, 2013) in addition to being correlated with time spent online and depression.

The *Korea Internet Addiction Scale (K-Scale)* is a forty-item scale that has been used in several studies carried out in Korea (Kim, 2008; Kim et al., 2002; Lee et al., 2013). Internal consistency has been reported as good to excellent, but other psychometric results could not be identified.

Screeners and Clinical Assessment Tools

The earliest measure of Internet Addiction is Young's (1996) *Internet Addiction Diagnostic Questionnaire (IADQ)*. Different versions of the scale have been used with seven, eight or ten items (Shek, Tang & Lo, 2008). In the original eight-item version, a score of 3–4 identified "at risk" users, while a score of 5 or more discriminated between addicts and nonaddicts, though these cut-offs may not be reliable (Dowling & Quirk, 2009). The scale has demonstrated good split half reliability (Johansson & Götestam, 2004) and correlated with the CIAS and time spent on the Internet.

The *Problematic and Risky Internet Use Screening Scale (PRIUSS)* is an eighteen-item scale with three subscales: Social Impairment, Emotional Impairment, and Risky/Impulsive Internet Use with Cronbach's alpha values between 0.88 and 0.90. Initially validated with college students between the ages of eighteen to twenty-five (Jelenchick et al., 2014), the scale has shown promising content and concurrent validity but requires more evaluation as a clinical tool.

Conclusions

Assessment of addictive behavior is essential in evaluating an individual's treatment needs and in ruling out other potential reasons for aberrant changes in behavior. This chapter provided an overview of the most frequently described and most commonly used measures of substance and nonsubstance (behavioral) addictions. Considering the still nascent state of behavioral addiction pertaining to the areas discussed here (food, exercise, gambling, working, internet, and sex) the statements of statistical quality (e.g., validation and reliability) and selectivity require further investigation by the reader. It is worth noting to the reader that this chapter was not intended to be all inclusive and that readers should continue to explore issues related to the assessment of other addictions not mentioned here, including shopping addiction (Andreassen et al., 2015; Clark & Calleja, 2008; see Galimov & Black, 2020; Sohn & Choi, 2014) and indoor tanning addiction (see Miller & Mays, 2020; Petit et al., 2014) among others.

Characteristics of behavioral addiction was not consistent between or within the assessment of various behaviors mostly based on the theoretical frameworks used to define the addictive process (i.e., substance dependence or impulse-control disorder). Moreover, the lack of replication research with many assessment tools and poor cross-validation with others makes population assessment, screening, and diagnosis difficult. In developing self-report and clinician-administered tools for assessing behavioral addiction, Grüsser, Thalemann and Griffiths (2006) recommend that each individual case should to be examined to ascertain if the suspected behavior evidences addiction or is just excessive (i.e., nonpathological or belonging to other diseases).

The debate continues as to how best classify behavioral "addictions" as either impulse-control disorders or similar to substance dependence. Others have explored the possibility of behavioral addictions as a form of process addiction. Process addiction is similar in concept to behavioral addiction (in fact it is often used interchangeably) but it may emphasize the desires of an individual immersed in the process leading up to the behavior rather than the direct impact of the behavior itself such as a heroin addict becoming nostalgic about "cooking up" their hit, or a gambling addict anticipating the gambling table as the lights of the casino come into view. Northrup and colleagues (2015), for example, questioned the meaning of "Internet Addiction," as the Internet facilitates addictive behaviors but is not the addictive agent. As such, they created the Internet Process Addiction Test to identify the addictive processes resulting from problematic Internet use. One advantage of this approach is that researchers can screen for multiple addictive processes simultaneously.

The inclusion of Gambling Disorder in the "Substance-Related and Addictive Disorders" section of the DSM-5 and the World Health Organization's classification of gaming disorder as a mental health condition recognizes possible commonalities of behavioral and substance-related conditions. While research has begun to identify common underlying neurobiological factors (Robbins & Clark, 2015; Vaccaro & Potenza, 2020), the need for research that cross-validates the assessment of general core components of behavioral and substance-related addictions is needed. Evidence is mounting that supports common features such as craving, withdrawal, and interruptions to daily life being shared across multiple addictions (Grant et al., 2010), but no research has established this empirically. Identifying a common set of indicators reflecting symptoms of dependence and impairment in intrapersonal, behavioral, social, and occupational functioning similar to substance addictions is a necessary next step as research that leads to the understanding of addiction progresses. As such, the construction and validation of comparable measurement instruments across substances and behavioral problems is needed to systematically identify useful treatment targets (Simons et al., 2012) – especially for comorbid substance and behavioral addictions.

In addition, future work is needed to develop measures that assess multiple addictions simultaneously for populations with comorbid substance and behavioral addictions. The motivations for engaging in multiple addictive behaviors are diverse. At times, people may use a less shameful addiction to mask or dismiss another, perhaps more stigmatized, addiction. For example, an individual may deny having a problem with sex addiction and insist that their pattern of sexual problem behaviors only occurs because of their constant intoxication brought on by excessive drinking. In other cases, the drugs or alcohol are used to cope with underlying pain and shame associated with a sex addiction and help the person disengage from the emotional consequences of their actions. In other instances, both addictions may result from continued use of one to intensify the other. For example, when a person engages in risky sexual behaviors under the influence of alcohol or drugs – such as seen in populations engaging in "chemsex" (McCall et al., 2015) – a continued pattern of simultaneously problematic behaviors might develop into addictive patterns of behavior requiring treatment. Multiple addictions require special attention in measurement and treatment as the cooccurring addictions serve to protect one another and ensure that patterns are stable and predictable (Schneider et al., 2005).

The measurement of addiction remains challenging, and the rather nascent exploration of various nonsubstance, behavioral, addictions contributes to the ongoing debate of when behavior becomes pathological, interferes with our "day to day" lives, and requires intervention. In an attempt to clarify what should be considered a behavioral addiction, and to prevent over-pathologizing common behaviors, Kardefelt-Winther and colleagues (2017) propositioned to define it as "repeated behavior leading to significant harm or distress of a functional impairing nature, which is not reduced by the person and persists over a significant period of time." Identifying with precision when substance misuse or rewarding behaviors elicit "significant" impairment that justifies screening or diagnosis, unfortunately tends to be a function of subjective self-judgements, may be context-driven, and involves making qualitative decisions regarding quantitative phenomena (Sussman, 2017). Establishing a systematic and inclusive definition of addiction is a much-needed next step for developing comparable, valid measures of addiction for substance and nonsubstance addictions alike.

REFERENCES

Adamson, S. J. & Sellman, J. D. (2003). A prototype screening instrument for cannabis use disorder: The Cannabis Use Disorders Identification Test (CUDIT) in an alcohol-dependent clinical sample. *Drug and Alcohol Review*, **22**(3), 309–315.

Albrecht, U., Kirschner, N. E. & Grüsser, S. M. (2007). Diagnostic instruments for behavioural addiction: an overview. *GMS Psycho-Social Medicine*, 4.

Alexander, D. (2003). A marijuana screening inventory (experimental version): description and preliminary psychometric properties. *The American Journal of Drug and Alcohol Abuse*, **29**(3), 619–646.

Alexander, D. E. & Leung, P. (2004). The Marijuana Screening Inventory (MSI-X): Reliability, factor structure, and scoring criteria with a clinical sample. *The American Journal of Drug and Alcohol Abuse*, **30**(2), 321–351.

Alexander, D. & Leung, P. (2006). The Marijuana Screening Inventory (MSI-X): Concurrent, convergent and discriminant validity with multiple measures. *The American Journal of Drug and Alcohol Abuse*, **32**(3), 351–378.

American Psychiatric Association. (2000). *Diagnostic Criteria from DSM-IV-TR*. Washington, DC: American Psychiatric Publishing.

American Psychiatric Association. (2013). *Diagnostic and statistical manual of mental disorders (DSM-5®)*. Washington, DC: American Psychiatric Association Publishing.

Andreassen, C. S., Griffiths, M. D., Hetland, J. & Pallesen, S. (2012). Development of a work addiction scale. *Scandinavian Journal of Psychology*, **53**(3), 265–272.

Andreassen, C. S., Griffiths, M. D., Pallesen, S., et al. (2015). The Bergen Shopping Addiction Scale: Reliability and validity of a brief screening test. *Frontiers in Psychology*, **6**. doi: https://doi.org/10.3389/fpsyg.2015.01374.

Andreassen, C. S., Torsheim, T., Brunborg, G. S. & Pallesen, S. (2012). Development of a Facebook addiction scale. *Psychological Reports*, **110**(2), 501–517.

Armstrong, L., Phillips, J. G. & Saling, L. L. (2000). Potential determinants of heavier internet usage. *International Journal of Human-Computer Studies*, **53**(4), 537–550.

Babor, T. F., de la Fuente, J. R., Saunders, J. & Grant, M. (2001). *The Alcohol Use Disorders Identification Test: Guidelines for use in Primary Health Care.* WHO Publication number 89.4, World Health Organization. Accessed November 7, 2018 from http://citeseerx.ist.psu.edu/viewdoc/download?doi=10.1.1.505.4146&rep=rep1&type=pdf

Bamber, D., Cockerill, I. M. & Carroll, D. (2000). The pathological status of exercise dependence. *British Journal of Sports Medicine*, **34**(2), 125–132.

Bancroft, J. & Vukadinovic, Z. (2004). Sexual addiction, sexual compulsivity, sexual impulsivity, or what? Toward a theoretical model. *Journal of Sex Research*, **41**(3), 225–234.

Barke, A., Nyenhuis, N. & Kröner-Herwig, B. (2012). The German version of the internet addiction test: a validation study. *Cyberpsychology, Behavior, and Social Networking*, **15**(10), 534–542.

Barth, R. J. & Kinder, B. N. (1987). The mislabeling of sexual impulsivity. *Journal of Sex & Marital Therapy*, **13**(1), 15–23.

Bashford, J., Flett, R. & Copeland, J. (2010). The Cannabis Use Problems Identification Test (CUPIT): Development, reliability, concurrent and predictive validity among adolescents and adults. *Addiction*, **105**(4), 615–625.

Benotsch, E. G., Kalichman, S. C. & Kelly, J. A. (1999). Sexual compulsivity and substance use in HIV-seropositive men who have sex with men: Prevalence and predictors of high-risk behaviors. *Addictive Behaviors*, **24**(6), 857–868.

Berczik, K., Szabó, A., Griffiths, M. D., et al. (2012). Exercise addiction: Symptoms, diagnosis, epidemiology, and etiology. *Substance Use & Misuse*, **47**(4), 403–417.

Blanchard, K. A., Morgenstern, J., Morgan, T. J., Lobouvie, E. W. & Bux, D. A. (2003). Assessing consequences of substance use: Psychometric properties of the inventory of drug use consequences. *Psychology of Addictive Behaviors*, **17**(4), 328.

Blow, F. C., Gillespie, B. W., Barry, K. L., Mudd, S. A. & Hill, E. M. (1998). Brief screening for alcohol problems in elderly populations using the Short Michigan Alcoholism Screening Test - Geriatric Version (SMAST-G). *Alcoholism: Clinical and Experimental Research*, **22**(3). Paper presented at: Research Society on Alcoholism; June 20–25, 1998; Hilton Head Island, SC.

Boubeta, A. R., Salgado, P. G., Folgar, M. I., Gallego, M. A. & Mallou, J. V. (2015). PIUS-a: Problematic Internet Use Scale in adolescents. Development and psychometric validation. *Adicciones*, 27(1), 27–63.

Boudreau, B. & Poulin, C. (2007). The South Oaks Gambling Screen-revised Adolescent (SOGS-RA) revisited: A cut-point analysis. *Journal of Gambling Studies*, **23**(3), 299–308.

Brand, M., Laier, C., Pawlikowski, M., et al. (2011). Watching pornographic pictures on the Internet: Role of sexual arousal ratings and psychological-psychiatric symptoms for using Internet sex sites excessively. *Cyberpsychology, Behavior, and Social Networking*, **14**(6), 371–377.

Brenner, V. (1997). Psychology of computer use: XLVII. Parameters of Internet use, abuse and addiction: the first 90 days of the Internet Usage Survey. *Psychological Reports*, **80**(3), 879–882.

Brewer, J. A. & Potenza, M. N. (2008). The neurobiology and genetics of impulse control disorders: relationships to drug addictions. *Biochemical Pharmacology*, **75**(1), 63–75.

Browne, M., Goodwin, B. C. & Rockloff, M. J. (2018). Validation of the Short Gambling Harm Screen (SGHS): A tool for assessment of harms from gambling. *Journal of Gambling Studies*, **34**(2), 499–512.

Buelens, M. & Poelmans, S. A. (2004). Enriching the Spence and Robbins' typology of workaholism: Demographic, motivational and organizational correlates. *Journal of Organizational Change Management*, **17**(5), 440–458.

Burke, H. R. & Marcus, R. (1977). MacAndrew MMPI alcoholism scale: Alcoholism and drug addictiveness. *The Journal of Psychology*, **96** (1), 141–148.

Butcher, J. N. & Owen, P. L. (1978). Objective personality inventories: Recent research and some contemporary issues. In *Clinical Diagnosis of Mental Disorders.* Boston, MA: Springer, pp. 475–545.

Caplan, S. E. (2002). Problematic Internet use and psychosocial well-being: Development of a theory-based cognitive–behavioral measurement instrument. *Computers in Human Behavior*, **18**(5), 553–575.

Caplan, S. E. (2010). Theory and measurement of generalized problematic Internet use: A two-step approach. *Computers in Human Behavior*, **26**(5), 1089–1097.

Carnes, P. (1983). *The Sexual Addiction.* Minneapolis, MN: CompCare Publications.

Carnes, P. J., Green, B. A., Merlo, L. J., et al. (2012). PATHOS: A brief screening application for assessing sexual addiction. *Journal of Addiction Medicine*, **6**(1), 29.

Carnes, P., Green, B. & Carnes, S. (2010). The same yet different: Refocusing the Sexual Addiction Screening Test (SAST) to reflect orientation and gender. *Sexual Addiction & Compulsivity*, **17**(1), 7–30.

Chen, S. H., Weng, L. J., Su, Y. J., Wu, H. M. & Yang, P. F. (2003). Development of a Chinese Internet addiction scale and its psychometric study. *Chinese Journal of Psychology*, **45**, 251–266.

Clark, L. A., Livesley, W. J., Schroeder, M. L. & Irish, S. L. (1996). Convergence of two systems for assessing specific traits of personality disorder. *Psychological Assessment*, **8**(3), 294.

Clark, L. A., McEwen, J. L., Collard, L. M. & Hickok, L. G. (1993). Symptoms and traits of personality disorder: Two new methods for their assessment. *Psychological Assessment*, **5**(1), 81–91.

Clark, M. A., Michel, J. S., Zhdanova, L., Pui, S. Y. & Baltes, B. B. (2016). All work and no play? A meta-analytic examination of the correlates and outcomes of workaholism. *Journal of Management*, **42**(7), 1836–1873.

Clark, M. & Calleja, K. (2008). Shopping addiction: A preliminary investigation among Maltese university students. *Addiction Research & Theory*, **16**(6), 633–649.

Clopton, J. R. (1978). Alcoholism and the MMPI. A review. *Journal of Studies on Alcohol*, **39**(9), 1540–1558.

Clopton, J. R., Weiner, R. H. & Davis, H. G. (1980). Use of the MMPI in identification of alcoholic psychiatric patients. *Journal of Consulting and Clinical Psychology*, **48**(3), 416.

Coen, S. P. & Ogles, B. M. (1993). Psychological characteristics of the obligatory runner: A critical examination of the anorexia analogue hypothesis. *Journal of Sport and Exercise Psychology*, **15**(3), 338–354.

Coleman, E. (1991). Compulsive sexual behavior: New concepts and treatments. *Journal of Psychology & Human Sexuality*, **4**(2), 37–52.

Coleman, E., Miner, M., Ohlerking, F. & Raymond, N. (2001). Compulsive Sexual Behavior Inventory: A preliminary study of reliability and validity. *Journal of Sex & Marital Therapy*, **27**(4), 325–332.

Currie, S. R., Casey, D. M. & Hodgins, D. C. (2010). *Improving the Psychometric Properties of the Problem Gambling Severity Index.* Ottawa: Canadian Consortium for Gambling Research.

Currie, S. R., Hodgins, D. C., Casey, D. M., et al. (2012). Examining the predictive validity of low-risk gambling limits with longitudinal data. *Addiction*, **107**(2), 400–406.

Davis, C., Brewer, H. & Ratusny, D. (1993). Behavioral frequency and psychological commitment: Necessary concepts in the study of excessive exercising. *Journal of Behavioral Medicine*, **16**(6), 611–628.

de Meneses-Gaya, C., Zuardi, A. W., Loureiro, S. R. & Crippa, J. A. S. (2009). Alcohol Use Disorders Identification Test (AUDIT): An updated systematic review of psychometric properties. *Psychology & Neuroscience*, **2**(1), 83.

Delmonico, D. & Miller, J. (2003). The Internet Sex Screening Test: A comparison of sexual compulsives versus non-sexual compulsives. *Sexual and Relationship Therapy*, **18**(3), 261–276.

Demetrovics, Z., Király, O., Koronczai, B., et al. (2016). Psychometric properties of the Problematic Internet Use Questionnaire Short-Form (PIUQ-SF-6) in a nationally representative sample of adolescents. *PLoS ONE*, **11**(8), e0159409.

Denis, C. M., Cacciola, J. S. & Alterman, A. I. (2013). Addiction Severity Index (ASI) summary scores: Comparison of the Recent Status Scores of the ASI-6 and the Composite Scores of the ASI-5. *Journal of Substance Abuse Treatment*, **45**(5), 444–450.

Dhalla, S. & Kopec, J. A. (2007). The CAGE questionnaire for alcohol misuse: A review of reliability and validity studies. *Clinical & Investigative Medicine*, **30**(1), 33–41.

Dhalla, S., Zumbo, B. D. & Poole, G. (2011). A review of the psychometric properties of the CRAFFT instrument: 1999–2010. *Current Drug Abuse Reviews*, **4**(1), 57–64.

Dowling, N. A. & Quirk, K. L. (2009). Screening for internet dependence: do the proposed diagnostic criteria differentiate normal from dependent internet use? *CyberPsychology & Behavior*, **12**(1), 21–27.

Earleywine, M., LaBrie, J. W. & Pedersen, E. R. (2008). A brief Rutgers Alcohol Problem Index with less potential for bias. *Addictive Behaviors*, **33**(9), 1249–1253.

Eleuteri, S., Tripodi, F., Petruccelli, I., Rossi, R. & Simonelli, C. (2014). Questionnaires and scales for the evaluation of the online sexual activities: A review of 20 years of research. *Cyberpsychology: Journal of Psychosocial Research on Cyberspace*, **8**(1), article 2. http://dx.doi.org/10.5817/CP2014-1-2

Ewing, J. A. (1984). Detecting alcoholism: the CAGE questionnaire. *JAMA*, **252**(14), 1905–1907.

Fagerström, K. (2011). Determinants of tobacco use and renaming the FTND to the Fagerström Test for Cigarette Dependence. *Nicotine & Tobacco Research*, **14**(1), 75–78.

Feeney, J. A. & Noller, P. (1990). Attachment style as a predictor of adult romantic relationships. *Journal of Personality and Social Psychology*, **58**(2), 281–291.

Feldstein, S. W. & Miller, W. R. (2007). Does subtle screening for substance abuse work? A review of the Substance Abuse Subtle Screening Inventory (SASSI). *Addiction*, **102** (1), 41–50.

Ferris, J. A. & Wynne, H. J. (2001). *The Canadian Problem Gambling Index*. Ottawa, ON: Canadian Centre on Substance Abuse, pp. 1–59.

Fioravanti, G., Primi, C. & Casale, S. (2013). Psychometric evaluation of the generalized problematic internet use scale 2 in an Italian sample. *Cyberpsychology, Behavior, and Social Networking*, **16**(10), 761–766.

Flowers, C. P. & Robinson, B. (2002). A structural and discriminant analysis of the Work Addiction Risk Test. *Educational and Psychological Measurement*, **62**(3), 517–526.

Forcehimes, A. A., Tonigan, J. S., Miller, W. R., Kenna, G. A. & Baer, J. S. (2007). Psychometrics of the drinker inventory of consequences (DrInC). *Addictive Behaviors*, **32**(8), 1699–1704.

Friedman, A. S. & Utada, A. (1989). A method for diagnosing and planning the treatment of adolescent drug abusers (the Adolescent Drug Abuse Diagnosis [ADAD] instrument). *Journal of Drug Education*, **19**(4), 285–312.

Galimov, A. & Black, D. W. (2020). Prevention and treatment of compulsive buying disorder. In S. Sussman (Ed.) The *Cambridge Handbook of Substance and Behavioral Addictions*. Cambridge, UK: Cambridge University Press, pp. 271–279.

Gambino, B. & Lesieur, H. (2006). The south oaks gambling screen (SOGS): A rebuttal to critics. *Journal of Gambling Issues*, **17**, doi: http://dx.doi.org/10.4309/jgi.2006.17.10.

Gearhardt, A. N., Boswell, R. G. & White, M. A. (2014). The association of "food addiction" with disordered eating and body mass index. *Eating Behaviors*, **15**(3), 427–433.

Gearhardt, A. N., Corbin, W. R. & Brownell, K. D. (2009). Preliminary validation of the Yale food addiction scale. *Appetite*, **52**(2), 430–436.

Gearhardt, A. N., Corbin, W. R. & Brownell, K. D. (2016). Development of the Yale Food Addiction Scale Version 2.0. *Psychology of Addictive Behaviors*, **30**(1), 113–121.

Gerstein, D., Hoffmann, J., Larison, C., et al. (1999). *Gambling Impact and Behavior Study*. National Opinion Research Center at the University of Chicago.

Ginzler, J. A., Garrett, S. B., Baer, J. S. & Peterson, P. L. (2007). Measurement of negative consequences of substance use in street youth: An expanded use of the Rutgers Alcohol Problem Index. *Addictive Behaviors*, **32**(7), 1519–1525.

Gold, S. N. & Heffner, C. L. (1998). Sexual addiction: Many conceptions, minimal data. *Clinical Psychology Review*, **18**(3), 367–381.

Gormally, J., Black, S., Daston, S. & Rardin, D. (1982). The assessment of binge eating severity among obese persons. *Addictive Behaviors*, 7(1), 47–55.

Grant, J. E., Atmaca, M., Fineberg, N. A., et al. (2014). Impulse control disorders and "behavioural addictions" in the ICD-11. *World Psychiatry*, **13**(2), 125–127.

Grant, J. E., Odlaug, B. L. & Chamberlain, S. R. (2017). Gambling disorder, DSM-5 criteria and symptom severity. *Comprehensive Psychiatry*, **75**, 1–5.

Grant, J. E., Potenza, M. N., Weinstein, A. & Gorelick, D. A. (2010). Introduction to behavioral addictions. *The American Journal of Drug and Alcohol Abuse*, **36**(5), 233–241.

Grant, J. E., Steinberg, M. A., Kim, S. W., Rounsaville, B. J. & Potenza, M. N. (2004). Preliminary validity and reliability testing of a structured clinical interview for pathological gambling. *Psychiatry Research*, **128**(1), 79–88.

Griffiths, M.D. (1996). Behavioural addiction: An issue for everybody? *Journal of Workplace Learning*, **8**(3), 19–25.

Grigsby, T. J. (2019). Development and psychometric properties of the tobacco and nicotine consequences scale (TANCS) to screen for cigarette and e-cigarette misuse in community settings. *Addictive Behaviors*, **98**, 106058.

Grigsby, T. J., Sussman, S., Chou, C. P. & Ames, S. L. (2017). Assessment of substance misuse. In *Research Methods in the Study of Substance Abuse*. Cham: Springer, pp. 197–233.

Grubbs, J. B., Sessoms, J., Wheeler, D. M. & Volk, F. (2010). The Cyber-Pornography Use Inventory: The development of a new assessment instrument. *Sexual Addiction & Compulsivity*, **17**(2), 106–126.

Grupski, A. E., Hood, M. M., Hall, B. J., et al. (2013). Examining the Binge Eating Scale in screening for binge eating disorder in bariatric surgery candidates. *Obesity Surgery*, **23**(1), 1–6.

Grüsser, S. M., Thalemann, R. & Griffiths, M. D. (2006). Excessive computer game playing: Evidence for addiction and aggression?. *Cyberpsychology & Behavior*, **10**(2), 290–292.

Hannifin, J. (1990). *The cannabis abuse syndrome screening test: a brief report*. Unpublished report. Wellington: Drugs Advisory Committee.

Hasin, D. S., O'Brien, C. P., Auriacombe, M., et al. (2013). DSM-5 criteria for substance use disorders: Recommendations and rationale. *American Journal of Psychiatry*, **170**(8), 834–851.

Hatfield, E. & Sprecher, S. (1986). Measuring passionate love in intimate relationships. *Journal of Adolescence*, **9**(4), 383–410.

Hathaway, S. R. & McKinley, J. C. (1951). *Minnesota Multiphasic Personality Inventory*; Manual, revised.

Hausenblas, H. A. & Symons Downs, D. (2002). Exercise Dependence Scale-21 Manual. Retrieved from www.personal.psu.edu/dsd11/EDS/EDS21Manual.pdf.

Hjorthøj, C. R., Hjorthøj, A. R. & Nordentoft, M. (2012). Validity of timeline follow-back for self-reported use of cannabis and other illicit substances – systematic review and meta-analysis. *Addictive Behaviors*, **37**(3), 225–233.

Hodgins, D. C. (2004). Using the NORC DSM Screen for Gambling Problems as an outcome measure for pathological gambling: Psychometric evaluation. *Addictive Behaviors*, **29**(8), 1685–1690.

Hook, J. N., Hook, J. P., Davis, D. E., Worthington Jr, E. L. & Penberthy, J. K. (2010). Measuring sexual addiction and compulsivity: A critical review of instruments. *Journal of Sex & Marital Therapy*, **36**(3), 227–260.

Horn, J. L., Wanberg, K. W. & Foster, F. M. (1990). *Guide to the Alcohol Use Inventory (AUI)*. Minneapolis, MN: National Computer Systems.

Hueppelsheuser, M., Crawford, P. & George, D. (1997). The link between incest abuse and sexual addiction. *Sexual Addiction & Compulsivity: The Journal of Treatment and Prevention*, **4**(4), 335–355.

Hunter, M. S., Nitschke, C. & Hogan, L. (1981). A scale to measure love addiction. *Psychological Reports*, **48**(2), 582–582.

Hurlbut, S. C. & Sher, K. J. (1992). Assessing alcohol problems in college students. *Journal of American College Health*, **41**(2), 49–58.

Jelenchick, L. A., Eickhoff, J., Christakis, D. A., et al. (2014). The Problematic and Risky Internet Use Screening Scale (PRIUSS) for adolescents and young adults: Scale development and refinement. *Computers in Human Behavior*, **35**, 171–178.

Johansson, A. & Götestam, K. G. (2004). Internet addiction: Characteristics of a questionnaire and prevalence in Norwegian youth (12–18 years). *Scandinavian Journal of Psychology*, **45**(3), 223–229.

Johnson, E. E., Hamer, R. M. & Nora, R. M. (1998). The Lie/Bet Questionnaire for screening pathological gamblers: A follow-up study. *Psychological Reports*, **83**(Supplement 3), 1219–1224.

Johnson, E. E., Hamer, R., Nora, R. M., et al. (1997). The Lie/Bet Questionnaire for screening pathological gamblers. *Psychological Reports*, **80**(1), 83–88.

Kalichman, S. C. & Cain, D. (2004). The relationship between indicators of sexual compulsivity and high risk sexual practices among men and women receiving services from a sexually transmitted infection clinic. *Journal of Sex Research*, **41**(3), 235–241.

Kalichman, S. C. & Rompa, D. (1995). Sexual sensation seeking and sexual compulsivity scales: Validity and predicting HIV risk behavior. *Journal of Personality Assessment*, **65**(3), 586–601.

Kalichman, S. C., Johnson, J. R., Adair, V., et al. (1994). Sexual sensation seeking: Scale development and predicting AIDS-risk behavior among homosexually active men. *Journal of Personality Assessment*, **62**(3), 385–397.

Kardefelt-Winther, D., Heeren, A., Schimmenti, A., et al. (2017). How can we conceptualize behavioural addiction without pathologizing common behaviours? *Addiction*, **112**(10), 1709–1715.

Karila, L., Wéry, A., Weinstein, A., et al. (2014). Sexual addiction or hypersexual disorder: different terms for the same problem? A review of the literature. *Current Pharmaceutical Design*, **20**(25), 4012–4020.

Kelley, K. J. & Gruber, E. M. (2010). Psychometric properties of the problematic internet use questionnaire. *Computers in Human Behavior*, **26**(6), 1838–1845.

Kiluk, B. D., Dreifuss, J. A., Weiss, R. D., Morgenstern, J. & Carroll, K. M. (2013). The Short Inventory of Problems – Revised (SIP-R): Psychometric properties within a large, diverse sample of substance use disorder treatment seekers. *Psychology of Addictive Behaviors*, **27**(1), 307–314.

Kim, C. T., Kim, D. I., Park, J. K. & Lee, S. J. (2002). *A Study on Internet Addiction Counseling and the Development of Prevention Programs*. Seoul: National IT Industrial Promotion Agency.

Kim, J. U. (2008). The effect of a R/T group counseling program on the Internet addiction level and self-esteem of Internet addiction university students. *International Journal of Reality Therapy*, **27**(2), 4–12.

Kim, S. W., Grant, J. E., Potenza, M. N., Blanco, C. & Hollander, E. (2009). The Gambling Symptom Assessment Scale (G-SAS): A reliability and validity study. *Psychiatry Research*, **166**(1), 76–84.

Király, O., Griffiths, M. D. & Demetrovics, Z. (2015). Internet gaming disorder and the DSM-5: Conceptualization, debates, and controversies. *Current Addiction Reports*, **2**(3), 254–262.

Klein, M. (2003). Sex addiction: A dangerous clinical concept. *Siecus Report*, **31**(5), 8–12.

Knight, J. R., Shrier, L. A., Bravender, T. D., et al. (1999). A new brief screen for adolescent substance abuse. *Archives of Pediatrics & Adolescent Medicine*, **153**(6), 591–596.

Ko, C. H., Yen, C. F., Yen, C. N., et al. (2005). Screening for Internet addiction: an empirical study on cut-off points for the Chen Internet Addiction Scale. *The Kaohsiung Journal of Medical Sciences*, **21**(12), 545–551.

Krasnova, I. N. & Cadet, J. L. (2009). Methamphetamine toxicity and messengers of death. *Brain Research Reviews*, **60**(2), 379–407.

Laconi, S., Rodgers, R. F. & Chabrol, H. (2014). The measurement of Internet addiction: A critical review of existing scales and their psychometric properties. *Computers in Human Behavior*, **41**, 190–202.

Ladouceur, R., Bouchard, C., Rhéaume, N., et al. (2000). Is the SOGS an accurate measure of pathological gambling among children, adolescents and adults? *Journal of Gambling Studies*, **16**(1), 1–24.

Laier, C., Pawlikowski, M., Pekal, J., Schulte, F. P. & Brand, M. (2013). Cybersex addiction: Experienced sexual arousal when watching pornography and not real-life sexual contacts makes the difference. *Journal of Behavioral Addictions*, **2**(2), 100–107.

Lee, Y. S., Han, D. H., Kim, S. M. & Renshaw, P. F. (2013). Substance abuse precedes internet addiction. *Addictive Behaviors*, **38**(4), 2022–2025.

Legleye, S., Karila, L., Beck, F. & Reynaud, M. (2007). Validation of the CAST, a general population Cannabis Abuse Screening Test. *Journal of Substance Use*, **12**(4), 233–242.

Lesieur, H. R. & Blume, S. B. (1987). The South Oaks Gambling Screen (SOGS): A new instrument for the identification of pathological gamblers. *American Journal of Psychiatry*, **144**(9), 1184–1188.

Líbano, M. D., Llorens, S., Salanova, M. & Schaufeli, W. (2010). Validity of a brief workaholism scale. *Psicothema*, **22**(1), 143–150.

Littrell, J. (1991). *Understanding and Treating Alcoholism: Biological, Psychological, and Social Aspects of Alcohol Consumption and Abuse (Volume 2)*. Hillsdale, NJ: Lawrence Erlbaum Associates.

MacAndrew, C. (1965). The differentiation of male alcoholic outpatients from nonalcoholic psychiatric outpatients by means of the MMPI. *Quarterly Journal of Studies on Alcohol*, **26**(2), 238–246.

MacAndrew, C. (1981). What the MAC scale tells us about men alcoholics. An interpretive review. *Journal of Studies on Alcohol*, **42**(7), 604–625.

Magruder-Habib, K., Harris, K. E. & Fraker, G. G. (1982). Validation of the Veterans Alcoholism Screening Test. *Journal of Studies on Alcohol*, **43**(9), 910–926.

Mäkelä, K. (2004). Studies of the reliability and validity of the Addiction Severity Index. *Addiction*, **99**(4), 398–410.

McBride, K. R., Reece, M. & Sanders, S. A. (2008). Using the Sexual Compulsivity Scale to predict outcomes of sexual behavior in young adults. *Sexual Addiction & Compulsivity*, **15**(2), 97–115.

McCall, H., Adams, N., Mason, D. & Willis, J. (2015). What is chemsex and why does it matter? *BMJ*, **2015**, e351.

McCourt, W. F., Williams, A. F. & Schneider, L. (1971). Incidence of alcoholism in a state mental hospital population. *Quarterly Journal of Studies on Alcohol*, **32**(4), 1085–1088.

McCready, J. & Adlaf, E. (2006). *Performance and Enhancement of the Canadian Problem Gambling Index (CPGI): Report and Recommendations.* Prepared for Inter-provincial Funding Partners for Research Into Problem Gambling.

McDermott, P. A., Alterman, A. I., Brown, L., et al. (1996). Construct refinement and confirmation for the Addiction Severity Index. *Psychological Assessment*, **8**(2), 182–189.

McLellan, A. T., Luborsky, L., Cacciola, J., et al. (1985). New data from the Addiction Severity Index: Reliability and validity in three centers. *Journal of Nervous and Mental Disease*, **173** (3), 412–423.

McLellan, A. T., Luborsky, L., Woody, G. E. & O'Brien, C. P. (1980). An improved diagnostic evaluation instrument for substance abuse patients. *Journal of Nervous and Mental Disease*, **168**, 26–33.

McMillan, L. H., Brady, E. C., O'Driscoll, M. P. & Marsh, N. V. (2002). A multifaceted validation study of Spence and Robbins'(1992) Workaholism Battery. *Journal of Occupational and Organizational Psychology*, **75**(3), 357–368.

Meerkerk, G. J., Van Den Eijnden, R. J., Vermulst, A. A. & Garretsen, H. F. (2009). The compulsive internet use scale (CIUS): Some psychometric properties. *Cyberpsychology & Behavior*, **12**(1), 1–6.

Meneses-Gaya, C., Zuardi, A. W., Loureiro, S. R., et al. (2010). Is the full version of the AUDIT really necessary? Study of the validity and internal construct of its abbreviated versions. *Alcoholism: Clinical and Experimental Research*, **34**(8), 1417–1424.

Meule, A. & Gearhardt, A. (2014). Food addiction in the light of DSM-5. *Nutrients*, **6** (9), 3653–3671.

Meyers, K., McLellan, A. T., Jaeger, J. L. & Pettinati, H. M. (1995). The development of the Comprehensive Addiction Severity Index for Adolescents (CASI-A): An interview for assessing multiple problems of adolescents. *Journal of Substance Abuse Treatment*, **12**(3), 181–193.

Miele, G. M., Carpenter, K. M., Cockerham, M. S., et al. (2000). Concurrent and predictive validity of the Substance Dependence Severity Scale (SDSS). *Drug and Alcohol Dependence*, **59**(1), 77–88.

Miller, G. A. (1985). *The Substance Abuse Subtle Screening Inventory (SASSI) Manual* (2nd edition). Springville, IN: The SASSI Institute.

Miller, G. A. (1999). *The Substance Abuse Subtle Screening Inventory (SASSI) Manual* (3rd edition). Springville, IN: The SASSI Institute.

Miller, K. A. & Mays, D. (2020). Tanning as an addiction: The state of the research and implications for intervention. In S. Sussman (Ed.) *The Cambridge Handbook of Substance and Behavioral Addictions*, Cambridge, UK: Cambridge University Press, pp. 362–372.

Miller, W. R. & Del Boca, F. K. (1994). Measurement of drinking behavior using the Form 90 family of instruments. *Journal of Studies on Alcohol, Supplement*, **12**, 112–118.

Miller, W. R. & Marlatt, G. A. (1984). *Manual for the Comprehensive Drinker Profile.* Psychological Assessment Resources.

Miller, W. R., Leckman, A. L., Delaney, H. D. & Tinkcom, M. (1992). Long-term follow-up of behavioral self-control training. *Journal of Studies on Alcohol*, **53**(3), 249–261.

Miller, W. R., Tonigan, J. S. & Longabaugh, R. (1995). The drinker inventory of consequences (DrInC). *Project MATCH Monograph Series*, 4.

Miner, M. H., Coleman, E., Center, B. A., Ross, M. & Rosser, B. S. (2007). The compulsive sexual behavior inventory: Psychometric properties. *Archives of Sexual Behavior*, **36**(4), 579–587.

Minnich, A., Erford, B. T., Bardhoshi, G. & Atalay, Z. (2018). Systematic review of the Michigan Alcoholism Screening Test. *Journal of Counseling & Development*, **96**(3), 335–344.

Minnich, A., Erford, B. T., Bardhoshi, G., et al. (2019). Systematic evaluation of psychometric characteristics of the Michigan Alcoholism Screening Test 13-Item Short (SMAST) and 10-Item Brief (BMAST) versions. *Journal of Counseling & Development*, **97**(1), 15–24.

Morahan-Martin, J. & Schumacher, P. (2000). Incidence and correlates of pathological Internet use among college students. *Computers in Human Behavior*, **16**(1), 13–29.

Morgenstern, J., Parsons, J., Muench, F., et al. (2004, May). *Understanding and Treating Compulsive Sexual Behavior.* New York, NY: Paper presented at the American Psychiatric Association Annual Conference.

Newcomb, M. D. & Felix-Ortiz, M. (1992). Multiple protective and risk factors for drug use and abuse: Cross-sectional and prospective findings. *Journal of Personality and Social Psychology*, **63**(2), 280.

Ng, T. W., Sorensen, K. L. & Feldman, D. C. (2007). Dimensions, antecedents, and consequences of workaholism: A conceptual integration and extension. *Journal of Organizational Behavior: The International Journal of Industrial, Occupational and Organizational Psychology and Behavior*, **28**(1), 111–136.

Northrup, J., Lapierre, C., Kirk, J. & Rae, C. (2015). The Internet Process Addiction Test: Screening for addictions to processes facilitated by the Internet. *Behavioral Sciences*, **5**(3), 341–352.

Oates, W. E. (1971). *Confessions of a Workaholic: The Facts about Work Addiction.* New York: World Publishing Company.

Orford, J., Wardle, H., Griffiths, M., Sproston, K. & Erens, B. (2010). PGSI and DSM-IV in the 2007 British Gambling Prevalence Survey: Reliability, item response, factor structure and inter-scale agreement. *International Gambling Studies*, **10**(1), 31–44.

Pallanti, S., DeCaria, C. M., Grant, J. E., Urpe, M. & Hollander, E. (2005). Reliability and validity of the pathological gambling adaptation of the Yale-Brown Obsessive-Compulsive Scale (PG-YBOCS). *Journal of Gambling Studies*, **21**(4), 431–443.

Parsons, T., Bimbi, D., Perry, N. & Halkitis, J. (2001). Sexual compulsivity among gay/bisexual male escorts who advertise on the Internet. *Sexual Addiction & Compulsivity: The Journal of Treatment and Prevention*, **8**(2), 101–112.

Pasman, L. & Thompson, J. K. (1988). Body image and eating disturbance in obligatory runners, obligatory weightlifters, and sedentary individuals. *International Journal of Eating Disorders*, **7**(6), 759–769.

Pawlikowski, M., Altstötter-Gleich, C. & Brand, M. (2013). Validation and psychometric properties of a short version of Young's Internet Addiction Test. *Computers in Human Behavior*, **29**(3), 1212–1223.

Petit, A., Lejoyeux, M., Reynaud, M. & Karila, L. (2014). Excessive indoor tanning as a behavioral addiction: A literature review. *Current Pharmaceutical Design*, **20**(25), 4070–4075.

Petry, N. M., Blanco, C., Stinchfield, R. & Volberg, R. (2013). An empirical evaluation of proposed changes for gambling diagnosis in the DSM-5. *Addiction*, **108**(3), 575–581.

Pokorny, A. D., Miller, B. A. & Kaplan, H. B. (1972). The brief MAST: A shortened version of the Michigan Alcoholism Screening Test. *American Journal of Psychiatry*, **129**(3), 342–345.

Pontes, H. M. & Griffiths, M. D. (2015). Measuring DSM-5 Internet gaming disorder: Development and validation of a short psychometric scale. *Computers in Human Behavior*, **45**, 137–143.

Poulin, C. (2002). An assessment of the validity and reliability of the SOGS-RA. *Journal of Gambling Studies*, **18**(1), 67–93.

Read, J. P., Kahler, C. W., Strong, D. R. & Colder, C. R. (2006). Development and preliminary validation of the young adult alcohol consequences questionnaire. *Journal of Studies on Alcohol*, **67**(1), 169–177.

Reid, R. C., Garos, S. & Carpenter, B. N. (2011). Reliability, validity, and psychometric development of the Hypersexual Behavior Inventory in an outpatient sample of men. *Sexual Addiction & Compulsivity*, **18**(1), 30–51.

Reid, R. C., Garos, S. & Fong, T. (2012). Psychometric development of the hypersexual behavior consequences scale. *Journal of Behavioral Addictions*, **1**(3), 115–122.

Reilly, C. & Smith, N. (2013). The evolving definition of pathological gambling in the DSM-5. *National Center for Responsible Gaming*, **1**, 1–6.

Riggs, S. G. & Alario, A. J. (1989). Adolescent substance abuse. *The Project ADEPT curriculum for primary care physician training*, 27.

Robbins, T. W. & Clark, L. (2015). Behavioral addictions. *Current Opinion in Neurobiology*, **30**, 66–72.

Robinson, B. E. (1989). *Work Addiction: Hidden Legacies of Adult Children*. Deerfield Beach, FL: Health Communications.

Robinson, B. E. (1998). The workaholic family: A clinical perspective. *American Journal of Family Therapy*, **26**(1), 65–75.

Robinson, B. E. (2001). Workaholism and family functioning: A profile of familial relationships, psychological outcomes, and research considerations. *Contemporary Family Therapy*, **23**(1), 123–135.

Robinson, B. E. & Post, P. (1994). Validity of the Work Addiction Risk Test. *Perceptual and Motor Skills*, **78**(1), 337–338.

Robinson, S. M., Sobell, L. C., Sobell, M. B. & Leo, G. I. (2014). Reliability of the Timeline Followback for cocaine, cannabis, and cigarette use. *Psychology of Addictive Behaviors*, **28**(1), 154.

Rohsenow, D. J., Abrams, D. B., Monti, P. M., et al. (2003). The Smoking Effects Questionnaire for adult populations: Development and psychometric properties. *Addictive Behaviors*, **28**(7), 1257–1270.

Rounsaville, B. J., Kosten, T. R., Weissman, M. M. & Kleber, H. D. (1986). Prognostic significance of psychopathology in treated opiate addicts: A 2.5-year follow-up study. *Archives of General Psychiatry*, **43**(8), 739–745.

Ruddock, H. K., Christiansen, P., Halford, J. C. & Hardman, C. A. (2017). The development and validation of the Addiction-like Eating Behaviour Scale. *International Journal of Obesity*, **41**(11), 1710–1717.

Rychtarik, R. G., Koutsky, J. R. & Miller, W. R. (1998). Profiles of the Alcohol Use Inventory: A large sample cluster analysis conducted with split-sample replication rules. *Psychological Assessment*, **10**(2), 107–119.

Rychtarik, R. G., Koutsky, J. R. & Miller, W. R. (1999). Profiles of the Alcohol Use Inventory: Correction to Rychtarik, Koutsky, and Miller (1998). *Psychological Assessment*, **11**(3), 396–402.

Sanchez-Craig, M., Annis, H. M., Bronet, A. R. & MacDonald, K. R. (1984). Random assignment to abstinence and controlled drinking: evaluation of a cognitive-behavioral program for problem drinkers. *Journal of Consulting and Clinical Psychology*, **52**(3), 390–403.

Saunders, J. B., Aasland, O. G., Babor, T. F., De la Fuente, J. R. & Grant, M. (1993). Development of the alcohol use disorders identification test (AUDIT): WHO collaborative project on early detection of persons with harmful alcohol consumption-II. *Addiction*, **88**(6), 791–804.

Schneider, J. P., Sealy, J., Montgomery, J. & Irons, R. R. (2005). Ritualization and reinforcement: Keys to understanding mixed addiction involving sex and drugs. *Sexual Addiction & Compulsivity*, **12**(2–3), 121–148.

Schwartz, R. H. & Wirtz, P. W. (1990). Potential substance abuse: Detection among adolescent patients using the Drug and Alcohol Problem (DAP) Quick Screen, a 30-item questionnaire. *Clinical Pediatrics*, **29**(1), 38–43.

Scott, K. S., Moore, K. S. & Miceli, M. P. (1997). An exploration of the meaning and consequences of workaholism. *Human Relations*, **50**(3), 287–314.

Selzer, M. L. (1971). The Michigan Alcoholism Screening Test: The quest for a new diagnostic instrument. *American Journal of Psychiatry*, **127**(12), 1653–1658.

Selzer, M. L., Vinokur, A. & van Rooijen, L. (1975). A self-administered short Michigan alcoholism screening test (SMAST). *Journal of Studies on Alcohol*, **36**(1), 117–126.

Shaughnessy, K., Byers, E. S. & Walsh, L. (2011). Online sexual activity experience of heterosexual students: Gender similarities and differences. *Archives of Sexual Behavior*, **40**(2), 419–427.

Shek, D. T., Tang, V. M. & Lo, C. Y. (2008). Internet addiction in Chinese adolescents in Hong Kong: assessment, profiles, and psychosocial correlates. *The Scientific World Journal*, **8**, 776–787.

Simons, J. S., Dvorak, R. D., Merrill, J. E. & Read, J. P. (2012). Dimensions and severity of marijuana consequences: Development and validation of the Marijuana Consequences Questionnaire (MACQ). *Addictive Behaviors*, **37**(5), 613–621.

Skinner, H. A. (1982). The drug abuse screening test. *Addictive Behaviors*, **7**(4), 363–371.

Smith, D. K., Hale, B. D. & Collins, D. (1998). Measurement of exercise dependence in bodybuilders. *The Journal of Sports Medicine and Physical Fitness*, **38**(1), 66–74.

Smith, D. & Hale, B. (2005). Exercise-dependence in bodybuilders: Antecedents and reliability of measurement. *Journal of Sports Medicine and Physical Fitness*, **45**(3), 401–408.

Smith, S. R. & Hilsenroth, M. J. (2001). Discriminative validity of the MacAndrew Alcoholism Scale with Cluster B personality disorders. *Journal of Clinical Psychology*, **57** (6), 801–813.

Snir, R. & Harpaz, I. (2012). Beyond workaholism: Towards a general model of heavy work investment. *Human Resource Management Review*, **22**(3), 232–243.

Sobell, L. C. & Sobell, M. B. (1992). Timeline follow-back. In *Measuring Alcohol Consumption*. Totowa, NJ: Humana Press, pp. 41–72.

Sohn, S. H. & Choi, Y. J. (2014). Phases of shopping addiction evidenced by experiences of compulsive buyers. *International Journal of Mental Health and Addiction*, **12**(3), 243–254.

Spence, J. T. & Robbins, A. S. (1992). Workaholism: Definition, measurement, and preliminary results. *Journal of Personality Assessment*, **58**(1), 160–178.

Stein, L. A., Lebeau, R., Clair, M., et al. (2010). Validation of a measure to assess alcohol-and marijuana-related risks and consequences among incarcerated adolescents. *Drug and Alcohol Dependence*, **109**(1–3), 104–113.

Stephens, R. S., Roffman, R. A. & Curtin, L. (2000). Comparison of extended versus brief treatments for marijuana use. *Journal of Consulting and Clinical Psychology*, **68**(5), 898–908.

Stinchfield, R. (2002). Reliability, validity, and classification accuracy of the South Oaks Gambling Screen (SOGS). *Addictive Behaviors*, **27**(1), 1–19.

Sussman, S. (2010). Love addiction: Definition, etiology, treatment. *Sexual Addiction & Compulsivity*, **17**(1), 31–45.

Sussman, S. (2017). *Substance and Behavioral Addictions: Concepts, Causes, and Cures*. Cambridge: Cambridge University Press.

Sussman, S. & Ames, S. L. (2008). *Drug Abuse: Concepts, Prevention, and Cessation*. Cambridge: Cambridge University Press.

Sussman, S. & Sussman, A. N. (2011). Considering the definition of addiction. *International Journal of Environmental and Public Health*, **8**(10), 4025–4038.

Svanum, S., Levitt, E. E. & McAdoo, W. G. (1982). Differentiating male and female alcoholics from psychiatric outpatients: The MacAndrew and Rosenberg alcoholism scales. *Journal of Personality Assessment*, **46**(1), 81–84.

Szabo, A. & Griffiths, M. D. (2004). The exercise addiction inventory: A new brief screening tool. *Addiction Research and Theory*, **12**(5), 489–499.

Taris, T. W., Schaufeli, W. B. & Verhoeven, L. C. (2005). Internal and external validation of the Dutch Work Addiction Risk Test: Implications for jobs and non-work conflict. *Journal of Applied Psychology: An International Review*, **54**, 37–60.

Thompson, J. K. & Pasman, L. (1991). The obligatory exercise questionnaire. *The Behavior Therapist*, **14**, 137.

Toce-Gerstein, M., Gerstein, D. R. & Volberg, R. A. (2009). The NODS-CLiP: A rapid screen for adult pathological and problem gambling. *Journal of Gambling Studies*, **25**(4), 541.

Tonigan, J. S. & Miller, W. R. (2002). The Inventory of Drug Use Consequences (InDUC): Test-retest stability and sensitivity to detect change. *Psychology of Addictive Behaviors*, **16**(2), 165.

Vaccaro, A. G. & Potenza, M. N. (2020). Neurobiological foundations of behavioral addictions. In S. Sussman (Ed.) *The Cambridge Handbook of Substance and Behavioral Addictions*. Cambridge, UK: Cambridge University Press, pp. 136–151.

Volberg, R. A., Munck, I. M. & Petry, N. M. (2011). A quick and simple screening method for pathological and problem gamblers in addiction programs and practices. *The American Journal on Addictions*, **20**(3), 220–227.

Weiss, D. (2004). The prevalence of depression in male sex addicts residing in the United States. *Sexual Addiction & Compulsivity*, **11**(1–2), 57–69.

Weiss, L. M. & Petry, N. M. (2008). Psychometric properties of the inventory of gambling situations with a focus on gender and age differences. *The Journal of Nervous and Mental Disease*, **196**(4), 321–328.

West, R. & Brown, J. (2013). *Theory of Addiction*. Chichester: John Wiley & Sons.

White, H. R. & Labouvie, E. W. (1989). Towards the assessment of adolescent problem drinking. *Journal of Studies on Alcohol*, **50**(1), 30–37.

Widyanto, L. & McMurran, M. (2004). The psychometric properties of the internet addiction test. *Cyberpsychology & Behavior*, **7** (4), 443–450.

Widyanto, L., Griffiths, M. D. & Brunsden, V. (2011). A psychometric comparison of the Internet Addiction Test, the Internet-Related Problem Scale, and self-diagnosis. *Cyberpsychology, Behavior, and Social Networking*, **14**(3), 141–149.

Widyanto, L., Griffiths, M., Brunsden, V. & McMurran, M. (2008). The psychometric properties of the Internet related problem scale: a pilot study. *International Journal of Mental Health and Addiction*, **6**(2), 205–213.

Winters, K. C. & Henly, G. A. (1993). *Adolescent diagnostic interview (ADI): Manual*. Western Psychological Services.

Winters, K. C., Specker, S. & Stinchfield, R. (2002). Measuring pathological gambling with the diagnostic interview for gambling severity (DIGS). In: J. J. Marotta, J. A. Cornelius & W. R. Eadington (Eds.),*The Downside: Problem and Pathological Gambling*. Reno, NV: University of Nevada, pp. 143–148.

Winters, K. C., Stinchfield, R. D. & Fulkerson, J. (1993). Toward the development of an adolescent gambling problem severity scale. *Journal of Gambling Studies*, **9**(1), 63–84.

Wong, J. L. & Besett, T. M. (1999). Sex differences on the MMPI-2 Substance Abuse Scales in psychiatric inpatients. *Psychological Reports*, **84**(2), 582–584.

Yates, A., Edman, J. D., Crago, M. & Crowell, D. (2001). Using an exercise-based instrument to detect signs of an eating disorder. *Psychiatry Research*, **105**(3), 231–241.

Young, K. S. (1996). Internet addiction diagnostic questionnaire (IADQ).

Young, K. S. (1998). Internet addiction: The emergence of a new clinical disorder. *Cyberpsychology & Behavior*, **1**(3), 237–244.

Yudko, E., Lozhkina, O. & Fouts, A. (2007). A comprehensive review of the psychometric properties of the Drug Abuse Screening Test. *Journal of Substance Abuse Treatment*, **32**(2), 189–198.

9 Qualitative Approaches to the Study of Substance and Behavioral Addictions

Kelsey A. Simpson, MA, and Ricky N. Bluthenthal, PhD

Introduction

One of the most difficult challenges facing researchers, practitioners, and social scientists operating in the field of addictions is the decision and application of appropriate research methodologies that depict the uniqueness, complexity, and meaningfulness of human experience. Addiction and addiction science are in some notable measure regarded as social and historical constructs (Reinarman, 2005). This means that the adversarial effects of addictive behaviors, whether pleasurable or problematic, have a fundamentally social basis (Reinarman, 2005). Accordingly, patterns of addictive behaviors, whether it be in drug use and dependency (a substance addiction), or in pathological gambling (a behavioral addiction), have been found to not obey universal laws (though at the extremes of behavior there is much consensus), but to be shaped by the social, environmental, and cultural contexts of their occurrences (Rhodes & Coomber, 2010).

Although contemporary addictions research has been largely dominated by quantitative methodologies, qualitative research has gained increased acceptance in recent years as an investigative tool in understanding how particular constructions of knowledge, practice, and subjectivity come to be taken as real (Miles & Huberman, 1994; Neale, Allen & Coombes, 2005; Orosz, 1997). Qualitative knowledge of substance and behavioral addictions has been part of the human sciences since their institutionalization in the nineteenth century (Agar, 1973; Becker, 1953; Preble & Casey, 1969; Lindesmith, 1947). In fact, qualitative case studies, interviews, and observations have formed the foundation of many theoretical and practice approaches in mental health and psychiatry used today. For example, Sigmund Freud integrated participant observations, descriptions of his own first person experiences, and interviews with his patients to generate theories and constructs regarding psychoanalysis (Gewurtz et al., 2016). Lindesmith's (1947) study on opiate dependence and withdrawal among heroin users has been thought to pioneer the industry of modern qualitative research within this field (Denzin & Lincoln, 2011). Using a combination of case studies and unstructured interviews, Lindesmith developed the idea that the experience of addiction had a social rather than purely physiological basis.

The importance of research methods that produce qualitative knowledge has long been understood, and qualitative practices have been formalized and available in university curricula, scientific associations, conferences, funded research projects, journal publications, education settings, workshops, as well as computer software programs for data management and analysis. Qualitative research paradigms have been found to provide in-depth knowledge of the social, political, and economic environments in which actions, diseases, and policies interact (Denzin & Lincoln, 2011). This chapter contributes to the emerging interest in qualitative research methods by bringing together a number of contemporary contributions on the method, practice, and findings of qualitative research in the field of substance use and behavioral addictions.

What Is Qualitative Research?

Qualitative research refers to a vast and diverse set of methodological views and practices aimed at describing and understanding the social meaning of different phenomena (Miles & Huberman, 1994). Qualitative research has been adopted by a variety of different academic disciplines within the social sciences, and developed as a result of multiple theoretical and historical influences. Although there are varying definitions and interpretations of qualitative approaches, qualitative research methods are generally aimed at gaining a deep understanding of a specific organization or event rather than a surface description of a large sample of a population. It aims to provide an explicit rendering of the structure, order, and broad patterns found among a specific subset of human participants within a social setting.

While quantitative research involves testing predefined, a-priori hypotheses, qualitative research is more exploratory in nature, and emphasizes subjectivity and individual-level perspectives as central to the research process (Denzin & Lincoln, 2011). In the context of construct and theory development, qualitative research utilizes an inductive design framework aimed at developing concepts and theories concerning aspects of the social world based on direct encounters with participants; whereas quantitative research adopts a deductive framework designed to test hypotheses as more or less of the "truth" according to a specific theoretical framework or hypothesis (Rhodes & Moore, 2001).

Qualitative researchers can address broad explanatory concepts using an iterative approach to inquiry focused on the collection of data in natural settings that are sensitive to those being analyzed (Creswell, 2013). The products of qualitative research include descriptions and rich interpretations that depict the depth and complexity of social and cultural phenomena. Qualitative research does not introduce treatments or manipulate variables or impose the researcher's operational definitions of variables on the participants. Rather, it lets the meaning emerge from the participants, to understand how participants derive meaning from their surroundings and how their meaning influences their behaviors.

According to Reinarman (2005), addiction and addiction science are largely social and historical constructions. Such constructions can result from a series of complex social processes that are inherently relational and in which identity is embedded (Reinarman, 2005). Moreover, the idea that addiction resides solely within the individual continues to foster significant limitations in the field of addictions research, treatment, and prevention. Thus, qualitative research spans past an individual, neurobiological level of analysis, and provides additional layers of information regarding the social and relational processes that take place within a certain context (Nichter et al., 2004). This integrative approach considers manifest behaviors, internal and communicative processes, and the social meaning of addiction when describing different addictions populations, and is grounded in the notion that lived realities that people experience are multiple, social, and subjective (Graham et al., 2008). Furthermore, the primary focus of qualitative research within the field of substance and behavioral addictions is to explore and demonstrate how particular social constructions of knowledge, practice, and subjectivity come to be taken as real (Neale et al., 2005).

Qualitative Methods in Addictions Research

Qualitative research is generated using a variety of different methods including but not limited to: ethnography, participant and nonparticipant observation, interviews, focus groups, and participatory action research (PAR). Here we define and discuss these methods, and provide evidence of each from addictions research. Following these sections, we provide a brief summary of each approach and generally understood advantages and disadvantages of each methodology (see Table 9.2).

Ethnography

The most in-depth form of qualitative research is ethnography, which seeks to describe or explain the shared and learned patterns of values, beliefs, behaviors, and language of a group or culture (Rhodes & Coomber, 2010). Ethnographic research is distinct from other forms of qualitative research in its emphasis on learning through direct immersion into the social contexts that are under investigation (Rhodes & Coomber, 2010). According to Nurani (2008), two basic characteristics of ethnography are: (i) the observation takes place in a natural setting and (ii) researchers must understand how an event is perceived and interpreted within the culture-sharing group. Accordingly, ethnographers are thought to be their own research instruments, and are trained to conduct participant observation fieldwork, conduct qualitative interviews, and analyze and record data to systematically describe the socio-cultural processes of a specific lifeway. Agar (1986) noted, "Such work requires an intensive personal involvement, an abandonment of traditional scientific control, an improvisational style to meet situations not of the researcher's making, and an ability to learn from a long series of mistakes." Ideally, the product of ethnographic research is a systematic description and analysis of an individual's or group's culture (e.g., morals, attitudes, values, beliefs, and symbolic meanings) that is oriented by a specific research question or theory.

Ethnographic research has been widely used in the study of drug use patterns and dependency across a variety of different substance using populations (Nichter et al., 2004). In fact, the earliest traditions of ethnographic research can be traced back to Thomas De Quincey's (1822) study on opium users living amongst the poor in London, England. In this, De Quincey illustrated a colorful depiction of the opium experience by describing his personal experiences with drug use as well as the experiences of those around him (De Quincey, 2013). Another renown ethnographic account of substance use that emerged during the same time frame was Engels' study on opium and alcohol users. Engels' findings elucidated how substance use functioned to provide escape for members of the urban poor during the Industrial Revolution (Engels, 2005). These landmark qualitative studies have yielded profound information and frameworks for understanding how drug-use is shaped by complex sets of factors situated within social contexts.

While there are many advantages to using ethnographic research methods, there are several limitations that must be considered. First, the overall effectiveness of data being collected requires the researcher to have a complex understanding of the cultural group and system they are studying. Thus, experience, knowledge, and rapport with study participants can greatly influence the data obtained (Creswell, 2013). Second, the data-collection process is lengthy, and involves an extensive amount of time spent in the field. Third, results are presented in narratives written in a literary fashion that may limit the audience for authors more accustomed to scientific writing approaches. Lastly, there is a possibility that results may be subject to personal and cultural biases bestowed by the researcher (Nichter et al., 2004). Thus, researchers must be able to practise a considerable degree of reflexivity when collecting data and interpreting their results. That is, researchers must convey how their personal background (e.g., work experiences, cultural experiences) may inform their interpretations of the information being studied.

There are two types of observational approaches that might be considered as specific examples of ethnographic methods: participant and nonparticipant observation. Both participant and nonparticipant observations are composed of notes about physical setting, participant demographics, activities, interactions, conversations, and the researcher's own behaviors during the observation.

Participant Observation. Participant observation is a systematic process of collecting information in which researchers observe a given phenomenon in its naturally occurring environment (Creswell, 2013). There are two main types of participant observation that are distinguishable by the role of the inquirer (Creswell, 2013). The first type is known as a "*participant as observer*" observation, which involves observing events or activities from the inside by being directly engaged with the group being observed (Angrosino, 2007). In this process, the researcher freely interacts with the other group members, participates in various activities of the group, acquires the way of life of the observed group or his own, and studies their behavior or other activities not as an outsider but by becoming a member of that group. This methodological approach is commonly exemplified in ethnographic studies.

According to Mason (1996), participant observations are composed of ontological and epistemological perspectives. Ontological perspectives are those that view interactions, actions, and behaviors and the way people interpret them as central to the research process (Mason, 1996). This perspective also allows for the observer to observe interactions that take place in a certain context and enables the conceptualization and observation of the setting itself. Epistemological perspectives suggest that knowledge or evidence of one's social world can be generated by observing or participating in, or experiencing, "natural" or "real life" behaviors. This position is grounded on the premise that these kinds of settings, situations, and interactions reveal data and make it possible for a researcher to be an interpreter or "knower" of such data (Mason, 1996). The rationale for observing behaviors rather than simply asking participants directly or using self-report questionnaires is that what people say they do and what they actually do is often inconsistent. Thus, participant observation grants researchers the ability to develop insight into how a behavior is practiced.

Participant observations are especially useful in the field of addictions research when describing a topic that has been relatively unexplored. For example, Lima-Rodriguez et al. (2015) used participant observation to investigate the way in which addictions develop from the perspective of alcoholics and their families on issues involved with modifying addictive behaviors and seeking rehabilitation. After observing fifty Alcoholics Anonymous (AA) meetings with twenty-five alcoholic patients and fifteen family members, evidence revealed the development of disease behavior in alcoholism to be a complex issue. Moreover, the addiction recovery process was constrained by sociocultural attitudes as well as self-stigma, leading alcoholics and their families to deny the disease, condition of the patient, and help. These findings illuminate (or highlight) the importance of self-help groups and the involvement of health professionals in the rehabilitation and recovery process of addiction populations.

Participant observation has served as a useful methodology in studying pathological gambling across different populations (Mathur, 2009; Saldanha, D'Souza & Madangopal, 2018). For example, in a study documenting the socioeconomic realities of street children in Mumbai, researchers found that games and participation patterns varied according to age (Saldanha et al., 2018). Moreover, younger children tended to participate in short games with small stakes, and older children gambled continuously or until their money ran out (Saldanha et al., 2018). Similarly, Mathur (2009) discovered that the most common modes of entertainment for street children to include gambling, as well as watching films/television, smoking, drinking, and doing other drugs. Thus, gambling provided more of a social reward rather than economic reward for children in India. These empirical investigations based upon observations of gambling within different social and interpersonal contexts elucidate causes that account for the initiation and persistence of gambling as well as some of the social functions gambling serves.

Naturalistic, Nonparticipant Observation. The second form of observation is known as "*nonparticipant*" observation (Creswell, 2013). In this approach, the researcher is an outsider of the group, and makes observations passively from a distance without influencing or participating in group activities. Nonparticipant observations of addiction processes including escalation of use and help-seeking have yielded important findings. For instance, Simmons and colleagues, in a series of papers using nonparticipant observations of heroin using couples, described how environmental, dyadic, and individual factors contributed to continuation (Simmons & Singer, 2006) and escalation of drug use (Simmons, Rajn & McMahon, 2012) as well as to efforts to enter substance use treatment (Simmons, 2006; Simmons & McMahon, 2012). Non-participant observation techniques have also been used to examine gambling addiction (Rossol, 2001), experiences of substance use treatment (Moskalewicz, 2016), and smoking behaviors (Geraghty, 2012).

Challenges of Observational Approaches. There are several challenges associated with conducting participant and nonparticipant observational studies. First, there are issues surrounding the mechanics of observing, such as difficulty taking notes and having to rely on memory, recording quotes accurately, and determining the most important subject/subjects or event/events worthy of being observed. Accordingly, researchers must be trained to be able to recognize situations that are sociologically significant and worth further attention. A second limitation is that sample sizes are usually small due to the researcher's ability to only obtain in-depth information on a small number of people at any given time (Creswell, 2013). This limits the ability to generalize findings to broader populations or communities. A third limitation is that observations are susceptible to observer bias; meaning that people may consciously or subconsciously change the way they behave due to the fact that they're being observed. Therefore, observational accounts of behaviors may inaccurately represent how people truly behave in their natural environments. Finally, ethical issues regarding the collection of informed consent, confidentiality toward participants, and violations of privacy may arise when conducting participant observations. Researchers must act in accordance with ethical guidelines, and take appropriate steps such as seeking permission to conduct on-site research, and conversing with gatekeepers or authority figures to insure their research will provide the least amount of disruption and harm to their community members (Bryman, 2017).

Qualitative Interviews

The interview is considered the most commonly employed qualitative method used in addictions research (Rhodes & Coomber, 2010). There are various types of qualitative interviews. The ones selected depend on the purpose of the inquiry, the characteristics of the sample of interest, and the kind of knowledge sought (Glasser & Strauss, 1967). In this section we define and provide information about *semistructured, in-depth,* and *key informant* interviews.

In general, interviews are best used when:

- The meaning, motivations, and sequalae of behaviors are not well understood
- Follow-up questions are needed to clarify initial responses to structured questions
- Clarification of questions, phrases, or words in the interview are necessary
- Follow-up questions are based on participant's initial responses to questions
- Some respondents may not have sufficient reading skills, or auditory disabilities that would restrict them from auditory recording techniques
- The target population includes individuals who are likely to become inattentive during data collection
- Sensitive information is being collected and the development of personal rapport may increase trust and comfort
- Nonverbal behaviors are used to identify inconsistencies in responses
- There are judgements required for coding procedures.

Semistructured Interviews. Semistructured qualitative interviews consist of a series of close-ended questions, as well as questions that enable more detail, and open-ended responses from study participants. They are typically administered by trained researchers, and facilitated one-on-one and in groups. The inclusion of open-ended questions and training of interviewers to follow relevant topics that may stray from the interview guide fosters the opportunity for identifying new ways of seeing and understanding the research question at hand (Jamshed, 2014). Semistructured interviews are often preceded by participant observation, as well as informal and unstructured interviewing, in order to allow the researchers to develop a keen understanding of the topic(s) of interest necessary for the development of relevant and meaningful semistructured questions. Semi-structured interviews are best used when researchers only have one chance to interview a participant, and several interviewers are sent out into the field to collect data (Bernard & Bernard, 2013). In general, semistructured interviews are administered using a paper-based interview guide that the interviewer follows throughout the interview. Data are typically collected with audio recordings and/or hand-written notes (Jamshed, 2014).

The success and validity of semistructured qualitative interviews in addictions literature rests on their ability to capture a respondent's ideas and opinions about a particular phenomenon. Thus, the product of such interviews is thought to encapsulate the interviewee's true "voice" and perspective (Rhodes & Coomber, 2010). Jones (1985) summarizes this purpose:

> In order to understand other persons' constructions of reality, we would do well to ask them. and to ask them in such a way that they can tell us in their terms (rather than those imposed rigidly and a priori by ourselves) and in a depth which addresses the rich context that is the substance of the meanings.

A few studies have utilized semistructured interviews in the context of food addictions. For example, studies on members of Overeaters Anonymous found participants to describe addiction symptoms using words such as "physically addicted," "hangover," "withdrawal," "craving," and "drug of choice" (Ronel & Libman, 2003; Russell-Mayhew, von Ranson & Masson, 2010). Green, Larkin and Sullivan (2009) also reported similar terminology in a sample of chronic dieters who were asked to describe their weight-loss failures. In a qualitative study designed to explore how obese women with and without binge-eating disorder (BED) conceptualized overeating in comparison to DSM-5 diagnostic criterion, results revealed that food addiction can occur in individuals with and without BED (Curtis & Davis, 2014). Findings from these studies highlight the utility of semistructured interviews in characterizing the nature of food addictions and depicting commonalities between food addicts and other addiction populations. A more detailed understanding of how different subgroups of the general population perceive food addiction may enable more refined measurement of this construct in diagnostic interviews and assessment measures. In addition, interventions may be designed to reflect the language most consistent with participants' conceptualizations of their addiction.

In-Depth Interviews. The in-depth interview is a qualitative data collection technique designed to elicit a vivid picture of the participants' perspective on a research topic. In-depth interviews are typically administered face-to-face and generally involve a smaller number of participants to explore their perspectives on a particular idea, program, or situation. In general, in-depth interviews are exploratory in nature, and focus on elaboration through guided conversation of a few topics of interest. In-depth interviews are often used to provide context to other data by offering a more complete picture of the specific conditions in which a behavior occurred. For example, in a study looking at the relationship between alcoholism and condom use in a sample of eighty-four male drinkers, in-depth interviews revealed that alcohol use alone was not sufficient to explain the occurrence of unprotected sexual behaviors (Schensul et al., 2010). Instead, circumstantial factors including marriage status, peer pressure to have sex, media influence, as well as location (home environment versus being at a brothel) were predictive of risky sexual behaviors (Schensul et al., 2010).

During in-depth interviews, the person being interviewed is considered to be the expert and the interviewer is considered the student (Rhodes & Coomber, 2010). In-depth interviews are facilitated using open and nondirective interviewing techniques that are driven by the desire to absorb as much information as possible from participants. This process requires the researcher to closely engage with participants by actively listening and posing questions to participants' responses in a neutral manner. In-depth interviewing is most effective when there is established trust and rapport built between the researcher and subject.

In-depth interviews have been useful in studying the psychological motivations of online gaming addicts. For example, in a sample of Taiwanese adolescents who spent over forty-eight hours playing online games per week, in-depth interviews revealed a set of four major areas of needs for playing online games including: entertainment and leisure, emotional coping, excitement and challenge seeking, and escape from reality (Wan & Chiou, 2006). Additionally, they found that the functionality of playing games provided subjects with a compensatory channel for dealing with unmet needs or motivations in their real life (Wan & Chiou, 2006). This evidence sheds light regarding the importance of in-depth interviewing in granting researchers the opportunity to uncover underlying cultural interpretations and shared meanings of addictions. Thus, utilization of these methods is very useful to interpret, classify, and better describe the world of addictions through the lens of addicts, themselves. Additionally, information obtained from in-depth interviews is crucial in the development of culturally sensitive intervention methods (Nichter et al., 2004).

Key Informant Interviews. Key informant interviews are qualitative in-depth interviews with people who have an "inside track" regarding experiences of a particular community being studied. The purpose of key informant interviews is to collect information from a wide range of people including but not limited to: community leaders, professionals, and residents who have first-hand knowledge about the community (Nichter et al., 2004). As wide a range of key informants as possible is necessary to avoid bias by obtaining only the perspective of a few individuals or groups. For example, key informants who may be interviewed in a study investigating how drug dealers experience the adverse effects of drug use could include: drug treatment providers and counselors, outreach workers, general health practitioners, and emergency ambulance teams and hospital staff. The overall goal of key informant interviews is to obtain insight on the nature of different issues and recommended solutions. The primary advantage of key informant interviews is to provide researchers with an opportunity to build or strengthen relationships with important community informants and stakeholders. These relationships can aid in the development of culturally appropriate assessment tools, and improve participant retention in research studies.

In a study looking at gambling-related embezzlement in the workplace, key informant interviews were conducted with professionals in security and drug use prevention services, therapists specializing in problem gambling treatment, counselors from gambling support groups, and recovered problem gamblers with histories of embezzlement to illustrate the processual perspective of a typical severe case of gambling embezzlement (Binde, 2016). Altogether, their data suggested that four processes interact systemically in aggravating and perpetuating the onset and maintenance of gambling addiction. These interacting systemic processes behave in a dynamic like a slippery slope that descends deeper and deeper, making it increasingly more challenging for the individual to regain control once he or she has begun. Such a process has a remarkable power to make individuals who differ greatly in terms of their personality and sociodemographic background to become very similar in their experiences and suffering. More generally, this study suggested that a processual perspective in addition to consideration of psychological and environmental factors is important for understanding the severity of problem gambling.

Limitations in Conducting Interviews. There are several limitations to conducting qualitative interviews. First, the process of transcribing is very time-consuming, and transcription software can be costly. Next, the ability to obtain valuable data relies heavily on the interviewer–interviewee relationship. Thus, the overall effectiveness of an interview can be a direct reflection of the interviewer's skillset. Accordingly, qualitative interviewers should be properly trained to build rapport, respond to unexpected behaviors and emotions, and ask appropriate questions that probe participants to divulge the deeper meanings of their experiences. Such training involves patience and skill on the part of the interviewer. Lastly, the process of developing a qualitative interview guide can be lengthy and difficult to perfect (Creswell, 2013). Researchers must dedicate a considerable amount of time to creating good instructions, and correctly phrasing questions to avoid subtle persuasive questions, responses or explanations that may bias the data.

Focus Groups

Focus groups are a data collection method that may also involve tools including: semistructured interviews, responses to visual material, and generating alternative ideas for a treatment program, in group settings (Nichter et al., 2004). Focus groups are led by a highly skilled moderator who can lead a group of generally six to eight individuals and successfully retrieve information from all members in the group. Typically, focus group members are carefully selected from a pool of persons who share similar experiences to facilitate an exchange of opinions on a topic of interest. For example, Li et al. (2015) used focus groups to explore the etiology and correlates of internet addiction/pathological internet use in a sample of Korean university students who identified as internet addicts. This method was employed with the aim of fostering group dialogue in a setting within which participants felt comfortable and safe sharing personal experiences and perspectives. Also, this method was used to tease out the nuances and complexities of collected survey data.

Focus group data is usually recorded using audio and visual recording as well as hand-written note-taking. Like every other research technique having its own merits, focus group discussions elicit intrinsic worth and meaning through the open expression of ideas in participants (Jamshed, 2014). For example, Howard et al. (2002) conducted a study using focus groups to investigate how chemically dependent clients conceptualized the construct of denial and the role it played in individual substance abuse histories. This study design utilized a *grounded theory approach* to qualitative research design in that its primary aim was to reconceptualize the construct of denial based on data from substance-dependent clients themselves (Glaser & Strauss, 1967). Accordingly, investigators sought to develop a comprehensive and integrative theory of denial that reflected modern perspectives on the etiology and treatment of chemical dependency. Three major models of denial emerged from the dataset including: reasons for failing to recognize and/or acknowledge the seriousness of substance dependency problems, stages of awareness of the seriousness of substance using behaviors, and intra- and interpersonal characteristics shared by subjects at each stage (Howard et al., 2002). Findings from this study offered insight into the conceptualization of denial from the perspective of substance-dependent clients.

Limitations of Focus Groups. There are several disadvantages to the use of focus group methodologies. First, there is a possibility that all members in the group may not express their honest and personal opinions about the topics at hand. When dealing with topics that may be sensitive to some people, the implications of self-report may limit the breadth and depth of the data being collected. Next, in comparison to surveys and questionnaires, focus groups require much more time and money to administer and execute. Accordingly, questionnaire guides must be carefully created to ask the right questions that elicit the types of responses that will be most valuable to a research team. Another disadvantage of focus group methodology is the potential for moderator bias to influence the outcome of focus group discussions (Creswell, 2013). Whether it be intentional or unintentional, moderators may inject their personal biases about a particular phenomenon into the participants' exchange of ideas. Such information may lead to inaccurate results. Lastly, focus group discussions generally are audio recorded or video recorded, and transcribed verbatim. This process imposes certain challenges in terms of analysis. For example, it may be difficult to tease out individual voices and determine the speaker, and certain outspoken individuals may dominate focus group discussions. Despite these challenges, focus group methodologies yield rich, in-depth illustrations that clarify the extent to which behaviors, meanings, or events are socially accepted. Additionally, through the direct observation of group dynamics, they reveal how identities, hierarchies, and meanings are negotiated within particular addiction populations.

Participatory Action Research

Action research, sometimes referred to as "participatory action research (PAR)" or "community-based research" or "advocacy research," has been a fairly common method of investigation in qualitative research for the past few decades. Many sources credit the social psychologist known as Kurt Lewin as the originator of action research (Adelman, 1993). According to Lewin, action research is a process that "gives credence to the development of powers of reflective thought, discussion, decision and action by ordinary people participating in collective research on 'private troubles' that they have in common" (Adelman, 1993). Today, action research represents a collaborative framework that provides social scientists with the means to take systematic action in an effort to resolve specific problems in particular communities.

Participatory action research draws upon the paradigms of critical theory and constructivism and encompasses a range of qualitative research methods. It is distinct from other forms of research in that it involves entire communities as members of the research process (Garcia & Gonzalez, 2011). Specifically, it involves community residents and stakeholders, not as passive research subjects answering survey questions, but as active research collaborators. This method is unique in that it views study participants as experts due to their lived experiences related to the research topic, ensuring that relevant issues are being studied. This involves: making suggestions as to what needs to be studied, assisting in establishing trust and rapport, building community connections, and explaining how the findings of a study can be used to benefit that community directly. The overall goal of action research is to influence social change (Gardner, 2004).

Steps in Implementing Community-Based PAR Projects. Although every community is unique and, hence, every PAR project is different, Kelly (2005) identified a series of steps that can be used as a general foundation for developing and implementing a PAR project. These steps are illustrated in Table 9.1.

Community assessment, which almost always is yoked to a community partnership step, provides opportunities for an informal assessment about current local issues and can provide the stimulus for a PAR project. This step generally involves researchers posing initial ideas about a problem and broadening their knowledge through discussions with colleagues at community agencies, local health departments, or other local experts. In Shannon and colleagues' (2007) community-based HIV prevention study on drug-using women working in sex work markets, an

Table 9.1 Steps in the process of conducting participatory action research projects

Step 1	Community assessment as the basis of action
Step 2	Finding community partnerships
Step 3	Resources
Step 4	Ethical approval
Step 5	Planning cycle
Step 6	Acting cycle

initial development of community partnerships was established through informal conversations between health providers, staff, and sex workers at an inner city drop-in center. In 2004, the project investigators approached the drop-in center to perform a needs assessment, which identified a primary issue of concern – a gap in access to services for HIV prevention and harm reduction.

The "resources step" involves the consideration of existing resources available for implementing a PAR project (Kelly, 2005). For example, local churches with a tradition of activism, or local community health organizations tied to previous research projects within the academic community, often provide a good source of volunteers. Next, ethical approval must be obtained by the Institutional Review Board (IRB) to ensure that research subjects are not abused or harmed during the process of the study. This involves the preparation of the official informed consent document and formal documentation of the potential risks and benefits of entering a research study. IRB approval also delineates the agency's responsibility if harm occurs as a result of participation in the research.

The next step in PAR, according to Kelly (2005), is the planning cycle, which involves a balance between presenting ideas developed from a formal community assessment and working with community groups on the creation of priorities or strategies. The focus of activities during this cycle is to identify and hear from a variety of community members to help clarify the program philosophy and the type of programming needed in the target community (Kelly, 2005). Finally, during the acting cycle, community members and researchers collaborate to assess the process of the research and the outcomes of any health promotion efforts. Outcome evaluation documents are produced and the group determines how to share the study results most effectively.

Participatory action research methods have been successfully applied in smoking cessation studies in a variety of communities identified as "high risk" or "hard-to-reach" (Burton, 2004; Tsark, 2001). For example, Burton (2004) addressed the need for smoking cessation services in the Chinese American community in New York City. In this collaboration between professional and community participants, a multimodal intervention was developed composed of awareness campaigns, telephone support, print materials, and neighborhood groups (Burton, 2004). Tsark (2001) employed similar methods among native Hawaiian residents in a community-based PAR initiative to develop culturally/ethnically relevant tools for tobacco cessation. This project resulted in the development of a user-friendly survey tool designed to gather and evaluate data across a variety of different communities and led to the revision of ongoing intervention designs (Tsark, 2001).

More recently, the Students Against Nicotine and Tobacco Addiction (SANTA) project was developed to engage local medical and mental health providers in partnership with students, teachers and administrators to reduce on-campus smoking in the Minneapolis/St, Paul Jobs Corps community (Mendenhall et al., 2011). In this study, researchers sought to better understand the causes of students' smoking behaviors by gathering and evaluating data in a four-phase research design. In Phase 1, researchers distributed campus-wide surveys to determine overall smoking prevalence and causal factors linked to smoking initiation. This resulted in the recognition of stress and boredom as the primary antecedents to smoking behaviors. The project then continued with three additional phases designed to better characterize students' stress and resulted in the integration of stress management and coping skills into ongoing cessation and support interventions (Mendenhall et al., 2011).

In summary, PAR offers a radical alternative to knowledge development as collective, self-reflective inquiry for the purpose of improving a situation or program in a community or marginalized group of individuals (Koch, Selim & Kralik, 2002). It is a methodology that fosters collaboration among participants and researchers and promotes capacity development and capacity building in all who participate.

Limitations of PAR. As with all methodological approaches, there are some challenges involved with conducting PAR research. First, PAR studies do not have a concrete research leader; thus the group involvement and democratic processes may lead to competing research agendas. Additionally, categorizing a group with a shared interest or problem as a "community" does not automatically result in a consensus on what the problem is and how it might best be addressed. Thus, the process by which collecting differing perspectives of a particular problem and need of a community can be lengthy in terms of time and resources. Even selection of community participants may impact or bias what information results. Nonetheless, PAR is a valuable research tool to be considered by any researcher wanting to influence change within a community. Understanding PAR in terms of its design, principles, definitions, and strengths is imperative for scientists.

Qualitative Data Analysis

Qualitative data analysis is the classification and interpretation of linguistic or visual material to make statements about implicit and explicit dimensions and structures of meaning in the data. Meaning-making is most often subjective and refers to the social interpretations of different phenomena. Qualitative data analysis has several primary aims. The first aim often is to formulate or refine concepts and theories (Flick, 2013). As described above, qualitative research has led to some fundamental rethinking regarding the concepts of addiction and withdrawal (Ronel & Libman, 2003; Russell-Mayhew et al., 2010). The second aim generally involves description of a certain condition or situation from the perspective of a specific individual or group of individuals. This method of analysis can focus on the case (individual or group) and its special features, or it can focus on comparing several cases and identifying commonalities and differences. For example, Neale, Nettleton & Pickering's (2014) study highlighted gender similarities and differences in recovery from heroin dependence.

Third, qualitative analyses explore associations between different variables. For example, Dingle, Cruwys and Frings' (2015) study investigated the potential role of social relationships and social identities on pathways leading into and out of addiction in adults undergoing drug and alcohol treatment. Lastly, qualitative analyses help look for explanations of conditions in which differences between variables or groups occurred (Rhodes & Coomber, 2010). For example, Kougiali and colleagues'

Table 9.2 Comparison among qualitative approaches

Method	Advantages	Disadvantages
Ethnography	Can account for the complexity of group behaviors Reveals interrelationships among several dimensions of group interactions Can provide context for which a behavior or event occurred rather than just describe an occurrence Provides a holistic account to the study of cultural systems	Very time consuming Requires the researcher to have a complex understanding of the cultural group and system they are studying Results are subject to personal and cultural biases bestowed by the researcher Narratives are written in a literary fashion, which may limit the audience for authors more accustomed to scientific writing approaches
Participant observation	Flexible and oriented to knowledge discovery Participants are likely to behave normally because they are in their normal environments Can provide a rich source of data including conversations and descriptions of participant's feelings	Often criticized for its subjectivity Sample sizes are usually small due to the researcher's ability to only obtain in-depth information on a small number of people at any given time Observers have difficulty taking notes and often have to rely on memory Data is open to distortion Ethical issues: Privacy may be violated by the researcher Informed consent is not obtained
Focus groups	Lower in cost and more time effective compared to individual interviews Can get faster results from a larger group of people Economically efficient Clarify the extent to which behaviors, meanings, or events are socially accepted Enable exposure to group language that may not emerge in individual interviews Group dynamics can be directly observed, and reveal how identities, hierarchies and meanings are negotiated Participants may be more comfortable disclosing	Data is difficult to analyze A few individuals may take over the interview Participants may be less apt to disclose When dealing with topics that may be sensitive to some people, the implications of self-report may limit the breadth of the interviews Subject to moderator bias
Qualitative interviews	Provides greater breadth and coverage of a topic that spans past what could be determined by observation alone Can allow access to a wider variety of people and situations Interview development is an iterative process that can be amended throughout the research process depending on experiences with interviewees Ideal for when participants are asked information that they may be unlikely to share in a group setting (e.g., substance use)	Relies on the interviewer–interviewee relationship Transcribing often takes a lot of time The phrasing of questions may lead to subtle persuasive questions, responses or explanations Asking appropriate questions and relying on participants to divulge the meaning of their experiences requires patience and skill on the part of the interviewer Analysis and coding procedure is often time consuming
Participatory action research	PAR focuses on problem solving and permits practical outcomes and positive change within a particular group or community The community locus of control leads to the identification of problems that are important to the community, not diagnosed from outside PAR is committed research The commitment of the community of interest enables the research project to access community understanding, knowledge and collective memory	PAR has no concrete research leader; thus the group involvement and democratic processes may lead to competing research agendas Categorizing a group with a shared interest or problem as a "community" does not automatically result in a consensus on what the problem is, and how it might best be addressed PAR can be lengthy in terms of time and resources

(2017) study examined personal and contextual factors that influenced the addiction and recovery processes in active versus recovered substance users.

There are various accepted methods of conducting qualitative data analyses, such as narrative and discourse analysis, grounded theory, analytical induction, iterative categorization, framework analysis, constant comparative method, and deviant cases. While it is impossible to examine each of these here, the following section will briefly define and discuss three of the primary methodological approaches in addictions research: narrative and discourse analysis, grounded theory analysis, and thematic analysis.

Narrative and Discourse Analysis

Narrative and discourse analysis utilizes a variety of analytic practices involving the collection of stories about individuals' lived and told experiences (Rhodes & Coomber, 2010). Narrative and discourse researchers analyze *narratives* or spoken texts describing accounts of events, actions, or series of events/actions that are temporally connected (Czarniawska, 2004). Narrative stories are gathered from interviews, observations, documents, and group conversations, and emerge from the interaction or dialogue of the researcher and the participant(s). According to Gergen and Gergen (1983), "it is not single events which dictate the shape of a life story, but the life story as a whole – its overall narrative form – which assigns meaning to single events." Furthermore, narrative and discourse analyses are thought of as holistic documentations of meaning that make sense of different events and the cross-time trajectories of which they are evaluated (Gergen & Gergen, 1983).

In contrast to other qualitative analysis procedures, which seek to break data apart into many subsections, researchers in narrative and discourse analysis are wary of *over-coding* (Bruce et al., 2016). *Over-coding* is the process in which many different codes are assigned in order the break down the story into much smaller and more "manageable" chunks (Bruce et al., 2016). In contrast, the aim in narrative analysis and discourse analysis is to keep stories intact to preserve and examine the wealth of storied detail contained in it. The initial analysis procedure begins with a process known as *indwelling*. *Indwelling* involves reading the data (usually interview transcriptions) to familiarize one's self with the data, and making note of initial impressions (Smith, 2016). The next step is to identify the story or stories found in the actual data they've reviewed. To help with this, researchers can scan the text to search for shifts in conversation, or specific language or phrases that depict the beginning or end of a story such as "It all started with . . ." or "that's why I left." The next step is to identify narrative themes and thematic relationships that exist within the context of the stories that are presented. This involves highlighting significant statements or quotes that highlight the explicit content, discourse, and context of each story. In studies of addiction, these themes may include stories related to the onset (e.g., first drug initiation experience, first binge/purge episode), progression (e.g., substance use trajectories), or recovery process (e.g., treatment-seeking behaviors, first discussion of problematic behavior with a friend or family member) of addiction.

The final step is to identify the structure of the narratives. The focus here is to understand "how" a story is put together (Bruce et al., 2016). This involves identifying the core narratives and dominant narrative structure of each interview. Such segments provide an understanding of the *structure* (how narrative accounts are put together) and *function* (purpose they serve) of the phenomenon under study (Creswell, 2013). Recursive reading of the interview transcripts helps researchers identify features of the narratives in relation to temporality such as descriptions of routines, any iterative activities, or perspectives of past and future. After these coding procedures are complete, researchers then regroup to compare themes and perspectives. The final product in discourse and narrative analysis is an in-depth, exhaustive description of the phenomenon.

Narrative and discourse analyses have been used to identify salient features of the lived experience of substance users. For example, Kougiali et al. (2017) examined the directionality of recovery from addiction using the personal narratives of twenty-one active drug users and users in recovery. In this, researchers found personal trajectories from addiction to recovery to be constructed as discontinuous and nonlinear, and contain long-lasting patterns of repeated, interchangeable episodes of relapse (Kougiali et al., 2017). Similarly, Martin and Stenner (2004) used discourse analysis to reveal information about the social constructions of heroin use by reviewing three interview accounts with heroin users. Here, they discovered three primary subject categories that appeared to underpin heroin initiation including peer pressure, response to distress, and risk appraisal. Altogether, narrative and discourse analyses allow addictions researchers to comprehensively understand the "big picture" of experiences or events as participants understand them. The primary advantage of these methods is their ability to preserve the integrity of personal biographies by examining the linguistics and life stories of individuals as a whole.

Grounded Theory Analysis

Grounded theory (GT) analysis refers to the generation of theoretical propositions through the processes of induction and iteration (Rhodes & Coomber, 2010). GT is distinct from other forms of qualitative analysis by its emphasis on theoretical sampling and constant comparison. According to Seale (1999), "theoretical sampling involves choosing cases to study, people to interview, settings to observe, with a view of finding things that might challenge the limitations of existing theory, forcing the researcher to change it in order to incorporate new phenomena." In theoretical sampling, coding is conducted until saturation has been reached. Saturation refers to the point that researchers reach when they no longer need to proceed in further sampling to acquire information about a particular topic or theory (Glaser & Strauss, 1967). Explicit guidelines for determining theoretical saturation are lacking; thus, researchers have to support their claims of saturation by an explanation of how they achieved saturation, including clear evidence. Constant comparison in GT involves the selection of comparison groups to help generate ideas about the specific properties or attributes of a specific theory or construct (Glaser & Strauss, 1967). The rationale for selecting comparison groups is their theoretical relevance for fostering the development of emergent categories or themes in qualitative analysis.

Coding procedures in GT include open coding, axial coding, and selective coding. Open coding is conducted first, and involves breaking down, examining, comparing, conceptualizing and categorizing data (Strauss & Corbin, 1990). The main questions of interest are "What is happening in the data?" and "What construct or idea is this representative of?" (Glaser & Strauss, 1967). Axial coding refers to the process of putting the data back together in new ways after open coding. This is done by utilizing a coding paradigm involving conditions, context, action/interactional strategies, and consequences. Finally, selective coding involves identifying the core category or concept that explains how axial code categories relate. During the GT analysis process, data coding guides the subsequent theoretical sampling process. After collecting additional data, researchers use the insights collected from the initial coding frame to inform the next iteration of data collection until a strong theoretical understanding of an event, object, setting, or phenomenon has emerged.

In addictions research, grounded theory analyses allow researchers to generate theory that closely approximates the reality it represents, rather than testing predefined theories. The inductive nature of the method is advantageous in its flexibility and openness and opportunity for investigators to follow leads gained from the data itself. This approach can also assist analysts in breaking the biases and assumptions often created in the scientific research process (Haralson, 2013).

Thematic Analysis

Thematic analysis in qualitative research can be approached in a variety of ways; however, in addictions research it most typically adopts a "framework analysis" approach (Rhodes & Coomber, 2010). The purpose of thematic analysis is to identify patterns of meaning across a dataset that provide an answer to the research question being identified and addressed. Patterns are identified through a rigorous process of data familiarization, data coding, theme development, and revision. Thematic analysis in addictions research typically follows a five-phase process. This includes: (1) familiarization with the data (through reading and rereading the data, listening to audio recordings, writing field notes, and generating analytical memos); (2) identification of thematic framework; (3) coding (through creating a succinct code book and identifying important features of the data that might be relevant to answering the research questions); (4) charting (organizing the details of codes by theme or case); and (5) interpretation (making sense of the associations found in the dataset).

Coding in thematic analysis uses first-level and second-level coding procedures. First-level coding involves making broad or general descriptive categories that may be used as a coding frame. For example, in a study of online gaming addicts, first-level codes may be as broad as "playing reasons" or "functionality of gaming." Second-level coding involves breaking down the first-level code categories into smaller units of meaning or themes. For example, "social support" or "feelings of control" might serve as second-level codes within the first-level code "playing reasons."

Qualitative Contributions to Substance and Behavioral Addictions Research

Qualitative research has made several significant contributions to the field of substance and behavioral addictions research. Specifically, qualitative approaches have added to the advanced understanding of how wider social, historical, and economic forces shape the everyday realities lived by addicts. Several of these contributions are discussed under the headings of: describing the development of addictions; measuring risk behaviors; reaching and researching hard-to-reach populations; evaluating treatment and intervention programs; investigating barriers to treatment services; understanding motivations for treatment; understanding attitudinal and emotional components of addiction; and formulating diagnostic criteria. Most of the examples provided below pertain to substance abuse, about which most of the qualitative work has been completed.

Describing the Development of Addictions

One goal for scientists engaging in qualitative research is to understand trajectories of addiction including initiation, progression, maintenance, and cessation/recovery. For instance, Mars et al. (2014) documented transitions from prescription opiate pills to injecting heroin by interviewing users and dealers in San Francisco and Philadelphia. Through the use of in-depth, semistructured interviews, researchers discovered a series of racial and demographic differences in transition patterns. Across both cities, younger heroin injectors (twenty to tweny-nine years old) were more likely to report dependence on prescription opioids prior to their heroin initiation, while older initiates (over thirty years old) reported graduating to heroin from other drugs such as cannabis, methamphetamine, and cocaine. Younger pill initiates described their typical pathway toward injection to begin with chewing and snorting pharmaceutical opioids, followed by noninjection heroin use, usually by inhalation (sniffing) or smoking, followed by injection heroin use. Additionally they found that injectors who begin their opiate-using careers with prescription opioids were more likely to be white in comparison to those who transitioned from other drugs.

Similarly, Lankenau et al. (2012) discovered three general trajectories toward injection heroin use amongst a sample of young injection drug users (sixteen to twenty-five years old) : (1) users who injected a prescription opioid before first use or injection heroin episode; (2) users who injected heroin before injecting or using opioids; and (3) users who never injected opioids. Those who injected a prescription opioid prior to injecting heroin described injection to be facilitated by the ease of accessibility to opioids within one's immediate social environment (e.g., family, friends). Additionally they reported withdrawal from opioids as a rationale for injection initiation. In a number of cases, they reported the desire to experiment with a prescription opioid to be fueled by financial incentives and the personal value of being able to trade and sell their personal prescriptions for financial gain. Qualitative studies such as these allow addiction researchers to better understand the contextual and environmental factors that inhibit or accelerate transitions to different drugs. Such information is crucial in the formation of treatment techniques and prevention efforts.

Measuring Risk Behaviors

Qualitative research has contributed to the understanding and development of measures for identifying risk in different substance using populations. For example, an early qualitative study conducted by Needle and colleagues (1998) expanded on the work of epidemiologic data to identify sources of HIV disease transmission among people who inject drugs (PWID). Using systematic field observations of fifty-four different drug injection episodes, researchers examined multiperson use of drug injection equipment, paraphernalia, and transfer of drug solutions to help understand the behavioral transactions that potentiate infectious disease risk. What they found by being in the presence of PWID during their injection episodes was that risk practices associated with the spread of infectious diseases among injection drug users spanned beyond the sharing of needles or syringes. Additionally, the multiperson use of drug paraphernalia (e.g., cookers, cotton, and water) and the transfer of drug solutions contributed to high disease risk. Findings from this study informed the development of questionnaires used to measure disease risk as well as the expansion of services provided at needle exchange sites to include cottons, cookers, and sterile water in addition to sterile syringes/needles.

In a participant observation ethnography looking at health behaviors of heroin users living on the streets of San Francisco, researchers identified differences in risk behaviors between white and African American men (Bourgois et al., 2006). In terms of poly-substance use, white men were more likely to use heroin in conjunction with inexpensive fortified wine, whereas African American men commonly supplemented their heroin with crack. Additionally, white men experienced greater difficulty finding veins to use when injecting, and often injected directly under the skin, resulting in more frequent occurrences of abscesses compared to African American men. Understanding these ethnic differences among street-based heroin injectors has led to the advancement of culturally tailored screening tools for risk assessment. Furthermore, clinical practices and protocols have benefited from qualitative methodologies such as these by providing a theoretical understanding of the social, cultural, institutional, and historical forces that contribute to negative health behaviors.

Reaching and Researching Hard-to-Reach Populations

Without adequate record of the illicit drug industry, local drug markets and people involved in them are largely excluded in social science research. Moreover, the illegality and stigma associated with substance-related activities and populations suggests the existence of difficult-to-reach and hidden populations (Neale et al., 2005). Qualitative research approaches (e.g., ethnographies or interviews) conducted in field settings where substances are consumed and distributed increase researcher's insight into hard-to-reach populations. For example, ethnographic analyses of drug use amongst populations marginalized on the basis of race/ethnicity, gender, and/or social class have evidenced rich information about the social meanings of drug use from the eyes of participants (Bourgois, 1995; Maher, 1997; Sterk, 2008). These accounts featuring participants' experiences in crack-houses, shooting galleries, and homes of drug users, have uncovered valuable information about the broader social-structural forces that play a part in drug-related harms (Bourgois, 2000; Parkin, 2015; Rhodes & Moore, 2001).

Knowledge of females with sex addictions and/or hypersexual disorders has been relatively limited among healthcare professionals and addictions scientists. This is primarily due to rigid societal beliefs surrounding the acceptance of problematic sexual behaviors among women. As a result, women with sexual addictions have become a fairly difficult population to reach. Qualitative researchers have attempted to narrow this gap through the use of case studies, personal stories, and narratives documenting gender-specific contextual and behavioral dynamics of addiction (Dhuffar & Griffiths, 2015; Klausner & Hasselbring, 1990; Schneider, O'Leary & Jenkins, 1995). For example, in a study by Klausner and Hasselbring (1990), women differed in their behavioral manifestation and socialization of exhibitionism: the purposeful and goal-oriented act of intending to attract attention to oneself. In females, exhibitionism was considered a socially acceptable part of seduction, and frequently involved excessive amounts of time dedicated to attracting a sexual partner. Such processes involved spending inordinate amounts of time shopping for seductive outfits, bathing and shaving with special care, and cleaning and ordering their living space. Conversely, male exhibitionists who expressed acts of fantasy and seduction in the initial process of attracting a sexual partner were often perceived by women as perverted. Instead, the expression of preoccupations and fantasies toward one's sexual partner occurred after multiple sexual encounters with someone.

Similarly, Dhuffar and Griffiths (2015) conducted a study aimed at understanding the lived experiences of sex addiction among females. Using an adopted interpretive phenomenological framework, the authors investigated the experiences and conceptualizations of women during the onset, progression, and recovery of sex addiction. Uncovered themes included: focus on the self as a sex addict (intrusive thoughts), uncontrollable desires (loss of control and the "high" and/or "pursuit" or acting out), uncontrollable feelings (sexual acts providing an escape from feeling down or depressed to feelings of enjoyment and content), derision (internal conflict and feelings of shame and guilt), and self-help, treatment, and recovery (factors that facilitated the progression from self-help and treatment seeking to recovery). These studies shed light to the wealth of qualitative methods in allowing for a deep understanding of how gender specific social processes effect the addiction's cycle. Such information has contributed to clinicians' insight into the multiple presentations of sex addiction in females, further highlighting the idea that phases in addiction are embedded within specific social and cultural contexts.

Evaluation of Treatment and Intervention Programs

While quantitative approaches to the evaluation of treatment and intervention services have focused on outcome variables such as tracking efficiency, adherence to medication, and accountability (e.g., number of days spent in the hospital), qualitative research methods have been increasingly used to understand and interpret the meaning behind the numbers (Rhodes & Coomber, 2010). Specifically, the aim of qualitative research is not to show that a treatment or intervention is ineffective, but to stress the importance of exploring and conceptualizing how a person changes, not only whether or not they do so, and factors that influence positive treatment outcomes (Nichter et al., 2004). Such information provides a wider and more nuanced understanding of how programs are implemented, how they are perceived by service users, and how they could be improved (Nichter et al., 2004). For example, Woo et al. (2017) completed a study of stigma experienced by patients receiving methadone maintenance treatment (MMT). By obtaining information regarding common public misconceptions of MMT and stigma-reduction strategies, researchers were able to gain a deeper understanding of the role society and culture played in program implementation. Given the heterogeneity of real-world community contexts, qualitative research designs such as these can provide a more informative and cost-effective way to evaluate and reform treatment and intervention programs (e.g., improve accessibility, retention, and treatment outcomes in MMT).

Investigating Barriers to Treatment Services

Qualitative research has also made important contributions to the emerging literature on barriers to treatment services by exploring users' views and experiences accessing a diverse range of specialist addiction and generic health and social care services (Nichter et al., 2004). For example, in Neale, Shepard and Tompkins' (2007) study on injection drug-users' suggestions for improving engagement in treatment services, participants revealed that providing a larger quantity and wider range of services, providing better operating existing services, and hiring less-judgmental staff would improve engagement into treatment. Additionally, some heroin injectors stated that they disliked methadone treatment because that substitute was highly addictive and had side effects (Neale et al., 2007). These findings illustrate the importance of qualitative research in the context of service improvisations through the observation of client perspectives. Thus, future research such as this is integral to the treatment and comprehensive care of all substance using populations.

Understanding Motivations for Treatment

Qualitative research has also been useful in analyzing motivations for treatment of substance use and behavioral addictions. Cornelius et al., (2017) used qualitative interviews to analyze treatment motivation and pressures to enter treatment among caregivers and adolescents in substance-use disorder treatment. They found that intrinsically motivated treatment (in contrast to coerced treatment) was associated with higher treatment engagement. Additionally, parenting involving competency and autonomy building in adolescents led to the promotion of internal motivations to seek treatment. Latuskie et al. (2019) conducted focus group interviews with pregnant women with substance-use disorders to explore reasons for continued or discontinued use. Based on personal narratives of women's first-hand experiences, results revealed positive relationships with service providers, positive personal relationships, and self-efficacy to play an important role in the decision to stop using substances. Themes that emerged from stories of women who persisted to use substances were distrust of healthcare professionals, external stressors, and low perceived self-efficacy to quit. Qualitative studies such as these have resulted in deeply rooted perceptions of factors that facilitate and hinder positive treatment outcomes in people with addictions.

Understanding Attitudinal and Emotional Components of Addiction

Qualitative research has been utilized to characterize the multifaceted role of regret in people with shopping/compulsive buying disorders. For example, Dittmar (2001) used in-depth interviews and shopping diaries to identify the role of regret in impulse purchases expressed before, during, and after a purchasing event in male and female excessive shoppers. Through in-depth thematic analysis, the authors discovered five central themes that emerged from the data: (1) the actual good/product bought plays a role in the regret process because of its unsatisfactory performance or low quality that is unsuited for the buyer's purpose; (2) consumers express regret regarding the money they've spent for their spending patterns in general, but not for the actual items they've bought; (3) consistent with the dual-self model proposed by Shefrin and Thaler (1988), regret was expressed as an internal conflict between the desire for short-term gratification and the longing for more long-term rational planning; (4) females expressed regret in terms of feelings of guilt when purchasing items for themselves but not for others; and (5) some respondents experienced regret because they viewed the products they bought to be disappointing in terms of expected psychological benefits. Altogether, the authors asserted that these multidimensional aspects of regret should be strongly considered when studying shopping addiction.

Formulating Diagnostic Criterion

Qualitative research has been critical to the formation of diagnostic criteria in the field of behavioral additions. For example, qualitative techniques have been used to emphasize the psychological features of exercise dependence, such as experience of withdrawal symptoms, including anxiety and depression when unable to exercise (Bamber et al., 2000; Cripps, 1995; Sachs & Pargman, 1979; Seheult, 1995). Such approaches have largely informed the development of numerous questionnaires used to measure exercise dependence such as the exercise dependence questionnaire and the obligatory exercise questionnaire (Blumenthal, O'Toole & Chang, 1984; Ogden, Veale & Summers, 1997). Bamber et al. (2000) explored the relationship between exercise dependence, psychological distress, and disordered eating in a sample of female subjects who screened positive for problem eating patterns and exercise dependence. Through semistructured qualitative interviews, researchers discovered that women with exercise dependence behaved differently than women with comorbid exercise and eating disorders. Moreover, exercise-dependent women did not exhibit the sorts of personality profiles, high levels of neuroticism, addictiveness, and impulsivity and the levels of psychological distress that are characteristic of other dependencies. This deviation from the typical behavioral pattern of addiction gave rise to the notion that exercise dependence should be classified as an independent pathology that can be diagnosed on its own, as well as an associated feature of an underlying eating disorder. Such information has strengthened the empirical base of exercise dependence.

Conclusions

Qualitative research has added to the advanced understanding of substance and behavioral addictions by iterating individual perspectives, social meanings, and the specific conditions in which different addictive behaviors occur. It has made major contributions to the field of addictions research regarding research on hard-to-reach and marginalized populations, evaluating treatment and intervention services, investigating barriers to treatment programs, conceptualizing motivational and emotional components of addiction, and aiding in the formulation of diagnostic criterion. Policy makers, researchers, and health practitioners can benefit by learning the research methodologies and practices used in qualitative research. Specifically, these tools help to explore and demonstrate how particular knowledge production, practice, and subjectivity come to be taken as real. Additionally, they can assist in prevention efforts and the expanding interest of qualitative approaches as means of investigating and resolving the complexities of addictions (Rhodes & Moore, 2001).

Although qualitative research methods within the addictions have gained increased acceptance in recent years, research into substance and behavioral addictions is still primarily dominated by quantitative methodologies (Nichter et al., 2004). Nevertheless, this chapter reinforces the importance of qualitative research in theory development, treatment/intervention development, and capturing the richness of human experience in addiction populations. Future research of this nature is needed to promote the development and implementation of efficacious forms of treatment and assist in the comprehensive care of substance-abusing and behavioral addiction populations.

REFERENCES

Adelman, C. (1993). Kurt Lewin and the origins of action research. *Educational Action Research*, **1**(1), 7–24.

Agar, M. (1973). *Ripping and Running: A Formal Ethnography of Urban Heroin Users*. New York: Academic Press.

Agar, M. (1986). *Speaking of Ethnography (Volume 2)*. Beverly Hills, CA: Sage.

Angrosino, M. (2007). *Doing Ethnographic and Observational Research*. Thousand Oaks, CA: Sage.

Bamber, D., Cockerill, I. M., Rodgers, S. & Carroll, D. (2000). "It's exercise or nothing": A qualitative analysis of exercise dependence. *British Journal of Sports Medicine*, **34**(6), 423–430.

Becker, H. S. (1953). Becoming a marihuana user. *American Journal of Sociology*, **59** (3), 235–242.

Bernard, H. R. & Bernard, H. R. (2013). *Social Research Methods: Qualitative and Quantitative Approaches*. Thousand Oaks, CA: Sage.

Bourgois, P. (1995). *In Search of Respect: Selling Crack in El Barrio*. Cambridge: Cambridge University Press.

Bourgois, P. (2000). Disciplining addictions: The bio-politics of methadone and heroin in the United States. *Culture, Medicine and Psychiatry*, **24**(2), 165–195.

Bourgois, P., Martinez, A., Kral, A., et al. (2006). Reinterpreting ethnic patterns among white and African American men who inject heroin: A social science of medicine approach. *PLoS Medicine*, **3**(10), e452.

Binde, P. (2016). Gambling-related embezzlement in the workplace: A qualitative study. *International Gambling Studies*, **16**(3), 391–407.

Blumenthal, J. A., O'Toole, L. C. & Chang, J. L. (1984). Is running an analogue of anorexia nervosa?: An empirical study of obligatory running and anorexia nervosa. *JAMA*, **252**(4), 520–523.

Bruce, A., Beuthin, R., Sheilds, L., Molzahn, A. & Schick-Makaroff, K. (2016). Narrative research evolving: Evolving through narrative research. *International Journal of Qualitative Methods*, **15**(1), 1609406916659292.

Bryman, A. (2017). Quantitative and qualitative research: Further reflections on their integration. In: J. Brannen (Ed.), *Mixing Methods: Qualitative and Quantitative Research*. London: Routledge, pp. 57–78.

Burton, D. (2004). Community-based participatory research on smoking cessation among Chinese Americans in Flushing, Queens, New York City. *Journal of Inter-professional Care*, **18**, 443–445.

Cornelius, T., Earnshaw, V. A., Menino, D., Bogart, L. M. & Levy, S. (2017). Treatment motivation among caregivers and adolescents with substance use disorders. *Journal of Substance Abuse Treatment*, **75**, 10–16.

Creswell, J. W. (2013). *Qualitative Inquiry and Research Design: Choosing among Five Approaches* (3rd edition). Sage Publications.

Cripps, B. (1995). Exercise addiction and chronic fatigue syndrome: Case study of a mountain biker. *Exercise Addiction: Motivation for Participation in Sport and Exercise*. Leicester: The British Psychological Society, pp. 22–33.

Curtis, C. & Davis, C. (2014). A qualitative study of binge eating and obesity from an addiction perspective. *Eating Disorders*, **22**(1), 19–32.

Czarniawska, B. (2004). *Narratives in Social Science Research*. Sage.

De Quincey, T. (2013). *Confessions of an English Opium-Eater and Other Writings*. Oxford University Press.

Denzin, N. K. & Lincoln, Y. S. (Eds.). (2011). *The Sage Handbook of Qualitative Research*. Sage.

Dingle, G. A., Cruwys, T. & Frings, D. (2015). Social identities as pathways into and out of addiction. *Frontiers in Psychology*, **6**, 1795.

Dittmar, H. (2001). Impulse buying in ordinary and "compulsive" consumers. In E. U. Weber, J. Baron & G. Loomes (Eds.), *Cambridge Series on Judgement and Decision Making. Conflict and Tradeoffs in Decision Making*. New York, NY: Cambridge University Press, pp. 110–135.

Dhuffar, M. K. & Griffiths, M. D. (2015). Understanding conceptualisations of female sex addiction and recovery using interpretative phenomenological analysis. *Psychology Research*, **5**(10), 585–603.

Engels, F. (2005). The condition of the working class in England. In: Michael Purdy & David Banks (Eds.) *The Sociology and Politics of Health*. London: Routledge, pp. 22–27.

Flick, U. (2013). *The SAGE Handbook of Qualitative Data Analysis*. Sage.

Garcia, V. & Gonzalez, L. (2011). Participatory research challenges in drug abuse studies among transnational Mexican migrants. *The Open Anthropology Journal*, **4**, 3–11. http://doi.org/10.2174/1874912701104010003

Gardner, S. (2004). Participatory action research helps now. *The Education Digest*, **70** (3), 51.

Glaser, B. G. & Strauss, A. L. (1967). *The Discovery of Grounded Theory: Strategies for Qualitative Research*. New York: Aldine.

Geraghty, J. (2012). Smoking behaviour and interaction: The observation process in research. *British Journal of Nursing*, **21**(5), 286–291. doi:10.12968/bjon.2012.21.5.286

Gergen, K. J. & Gergen, M. M. (1983). The social construction of helping relationships. *New Directions in Helping*, **1**, 143–163.

Gewurtz, R., Moll, S., Poole, J. M. & Gruhl, K. R. (2016). Qualitative research in mental health and mental illness. In: O. Karin, A. Richard & Z. Izabela (Eds.) *Handbook of Qualitative Health Research for Evidence-Based Practice*. New York, NY: Springer, pp. 203–223.

Graham, M. D., Young, R. A., Valach, L. & Alan Wood, R. (2008). Addiction as a complex social process: An action theoretical perspective. *Addiction Research & Theory*, **16**(2), 121–133.

Green, A. R., Larkin, M. & Sullivan, V. (2009). Oh stuff it! The experience and explanation of diet failure: An exploration using interpretative phenomenological analysis. *Journal of Health Psychology*, **14** (7), 997–1008.

Haralson, D. (2013). *Grief reactions to drug loss: A grounded theory approach.* Doctoral dissertation, Colorado State University Libraries.

Howard, M., McMillen, C., Nower, L., et al. (2002). Denial in addiction: Toward an integrated stage and process model – Qualitative findings. *Journal of Psychoactive Drugs*, **34**(4), 371–382.

Jamshed, S. (2014). Qualitative research method – Interviewing and observation. *Journal of Basic and Clinical Pharmacy*, **5**(4), 87–88. http://doi.org/10.4103/0976-0105.141942

Jones, S. (1985). *Depth Interviewing: Applied Qualitative Research*. Aldershot, UK: Gower, pp. 45–55.

Kelly, P. J. (2005). Practical suggestions for community interventions using participatory action research. *Public Health Nursing*, **22**: 65–73. doi: 10.1111/j.0737-1209.2005.22110

Klausner, M. & Hasselbring, B. (1990). *Aching for Love: The Sexual Drama of the Adult Child: Healing Strategies for Women*. San Francisco: Harper.

Koch, T., Selim, P. & Kralik, D. (2002). Enhancing lives through the development of a community-based participatory action research program. *Journal of Clinical Nursing*, **11**, 109–117.

Kougiali, Z. G., Fasulo, A., Needs, A. & Van Laar, D. (2017). Planting the seeds of change: Directionality in the narrative construction of recovery from addiction. *Psychology & Health*, **32**(6), 639–664.

Lankenau, S. E., Teti, M., Silva, K., et al. (2012). Initiation into prescription opioid misuse amongst young injection drug users. *International Journal of Drug Policy*, **23**(1), 37–44.

Latuskie, K. A., Andrews, N. C., Motz, M., et al. (2019). Reasons for substance use continuation and discontinuation during pregnancy: A qualitative study. *Women and Birth*, **32**(1), e57–e64.

Li, W., O'Brien, J. E., Snyder, S. M. & Howard, M. O. (2015). Characteristics of internet addiction/pathological internet use in U.S. university students: A qualitative-method investigation. *PLoS ONE*, **10**(2), e0117372. http://doi.org/10.1371/journal.pone.0117372

Lima-Rodríguez, J. S., Guerra-Martín, M. D., Domínguez-Sánchez, I. & Lima-Serrano, M. (2015). Alcoholic patients' response to their disease: Perspective of patients and family. *Revista Latino-Americana de Enfermagem*, **23**(6), 1165–1172. http://doi.org/10.1590/0104-1169.0516.2662

Lindesmith, A. R. (1947). *Opiate Addiction*. Principia Press.

Maher, L. (1997). *Sexed Work: Gender, Race, and Resistance in a Brooklyn Drug Economy*. Oxford: Clarendon.

Martin, A. & Stenner, P. (2004). Talking about drug use: What are we (and our participants) doing in qualitative research? *International Journal of Drug Policy*, **15**, 395–405.

Mars, S. G., Bourgois, P., Karandinos, G., Montero, F. & Ciccarone, D. (2014). "Every 'never'I ever said came true": Transitions from opioid pills to heroin injecting. *International Journal of Drug Policy*, **25**(2), 257–266.

Mason, J. (1996). *Qualitative Researching*. Sage.

Mathur, M. (2009). Socialisation of street children in India: A socio-economic profile. *Psychology and Developing Societies*, **21**(2), 299–325.

Mendenhall, T., Harper, P., Stephenson, H. & Santo Haas, G. (2011). The SANTA Project (Students against Nicotine and Tobacco

Addiction): Using community-based participatory research to reduce smoking in a high-risk young adult population. *Action Research*, **9**(2), 199-213.

Miles, M. & Huberman, A. (1994). *Qualitative Data Analysis: An Expanded Source Book.* Sage.

Moskalewicz, M. (2016). Lived time disturbances of drug addiction therapy newcomers: A qualitative, field phenomenology case study at Monar-Markot Center in Poland. *International Journal of Mental Health and Addiction*, **14**(6), 1023–1038. doi:10.1007/s11469-016-9680-4

Neale, J., Allen, D. & Coombes, L. (2005). Qualitative research methods within the addictions. *Addiction*, **100**, 1584–1593. doi:10.1111/j.1360-0443.2005.01230

Neale, J., Nettleton, S. & Pickering, L. (2014). Gender sameness and difference in recovery from heroin dependence: A qualitative exploration. *International Journal of Drug Policy*, **25** (1), 3–12.

Neale, J., Shepard, L. & Tompkins, C. N. E. (2007). Factors that help injecting drug users to access and benefit from services: A qualitative study. *Substance Abuse Treatment, Prevention, and Policy*, **2**, 31.

Needle, R. H., Coyle, S., Cesari, H., et al. (1998). HIV risk behaviors associated with the injection process: Multiperson use of drug injection equipment and paraphernalia in injection drug user networks. *Substance Use & Misuse*, **33**(12), 2403–2423.

Nichter, M., Quintero, G., Nichter, M., Mock, J. & Shakib, S. (2004). Qualitative research: contributions to the study of drug use, drug abuse, and drug use (r)-related interventions. *Substance Use & Misuse*, **39**(10–12), 1907–1969.

Nurani, L. (2008). Critical review of ethnographic approach. *Jurnal Sosioteknologi*, **7**(14), 441–447.

Ogden, J., Veale, D. & Summers, Z. (1997). The development and validation of the Exercise Dependence Questionnaire. *Addiction Research*, **5**(4), 343–355.

Orosz, J. (1997). Qualitative Data Analysis: An Expanded Sourcebook (2nd edition). *Public Administration Review*, **57**(6), 543.

Parkin, S. (2015). Colliding intervention in the spatial management of street-based injecting and drug-related litter within settings of public convenience (UK). *Space and Polity*, 1–20.

Preble, E. & Casey, J. J. (1969). Taking care of business – The heroin user's life on the street. *International Journal of the Addictions*, **4**(1), 1–24.

Reinarman, C. (2005). Addiction as accomplishment: The discursive construction of disease. *Addiction Research & Theory*, **13**(4), 307–320.

Rhodes, T. & Coomber, R. (2010). Qualitative methods and theory in addictions research. In: G. Miller, J. Strang & P. Miller (Eds.), *Addiction Research Methods.* Chichester: Wiley-Blackwell, pp. 59–78.

Rhodes, T. & Moore, D. (2001). On the qualitative in drugs research: Part one. *Addiction Research & Theory*, **9**(4), 279–297.

Ronel, N. & Libman, G. (2003). Eating disorders and recovery: Lessons from Overeaters Anonymous. *Clinical Social Work Journal*, **31**, 155–171.

Rossol, J. (2001). The medicalization of deviance as an interactive achievement: The construction of compulsive gambling. *Symbolic Interaction*, **24**(3), 315–341. doi:10.1525/si.2001.24.3.315

Russell-Mayhew, S., von **Ranson, K. M. & Masson, P. C.** (2010). How does Overeaters Anonymous help its members? A qualitative analysis. *European Eating Disorders Review*, **18**, 33–42.

Sachs, M. L. & Pargman, D. (1979). Running addiction: A depth interview examination. *Journal of Sport Behavior*, **2**(3), 143–155.

Saldanha, K., D'Souza, B. & Madangopal, D. (2018). "It's only a game of chance": A portrait of gambling among street children in Mumbai. *Journal of Adolescent Research*, **33** (6), 699–724.

Schensul, J. J., Chandran, D., Singh, S. K., et al. (2010). The use of qualitative comparative analysis for critical event research in alcohol and HIV in Mumbai, India. *AIDS and Behavior*, **14**(Supplement 1), S113–S125. doi:10.1007/s10461-010-9736-6

Schneider, J. A., O'Leary, A. & Jenkins, S. R. (1995). Gender, sexual orientation, and disordered eating. *Psychology and Health*, **10** (2), 113–128.

Seale, C. (1999). Grounding theory. *The Quality of Qualitative Research*, 87–105.

Seheult, C. (1995). Hooked on the "buzz": history of a bodybuilding addict. *Exercise Addiction: Motivation for Participation in Sport and Exercise.* Leicester: The British Psychological Society, pp. 40–44.

Shannon, K., Bright, V., Allinott, S., et al. (2007). Community-based HIV prevention research among substance-using women in survival sex work: The Maka Project Partnership. *Harm Reduction Journal*, **4**(1), 20.

Shefrin, H. M. & Thaler, R. H. (1988). The behavioral life-cycle hypothesis. *Economic Inquiry*, **26**(4), 609–643.

Simmons, J. (2006). The interplay between interpersonal dynamics, treatment barriers, and larger social forces: An exploratory study of drug-using couples in Hartford, CT. *Substance Abuse Treatment and Prevention Policy*, **1**, 12. doi:10.1186/1747-597x-1-12

Simmons, J. & McMahon, J. M. (2012). Barriers to drug treatment for IDU couples: The need for couple-based approaches. *Journal of Addictive Diseases*, **31**(3), 242–257. doi:10.1080/10550887.2012.702985

Simmons, J. & Singer, M. (2006). I love you . . . and heroin: Care and collusion among drug-using couples. *Substance Abuse Treatment and Prevention Policy*, **1**, 7. doi:10.1186/1747-597x-1-7

Simmons, J., Rajn, S. & McMahon, J. M. (2012). Retrospective accounts of injection initiation in intimate partnerships. *International Journal of Drug Policy*, **23**, 303–311.

Smith, B. (2016). Narrative analysis. *Analysing Qualitative Data in Psychology*, **2**, 202–221.

Sterk, C. (2008). *Fast Lives: Women Who Use Crack Cocaine.* Temple University Press.

Strauss, A. & Corbin, J. (1990). *Basics of Qualitative Research.* Sage Publications.

Tsark, J. (2001). A participatory research approach to address data needs in tobacco use among Native Hawaiians. *Asian American/Pacific Islander Journal of Health*, **9**, 40–48.

Wan, C. S. & Chiou, W. B. (2006). Why are adolescents addicted to online gaming? An interview study in Taiwan. *CyberPsychology & Behavior*, **9**(6), 762–776.

Woo, J., Bhalerao, A., Bawor, M., et al. (2017). "Don't Judge a Book Its Cover": A qualitative study of methadone patients' experiences of stigma. *Substance Abuse: Research and Ttreatment*, **11**, 1178221816685087. doi:10.1177/1178221816685087

Part III

Levels of Analysis and Etiology

10 Neurobiology of Substance Addictions

Nina C. Christie, MA, and Antoine Bechara, PhD

Introduction

The triadic neural model of addiction synthesizes decades of competing research ideas in to a single comprehensive model. This model is composed of (a) an amygdala-striatal *impulsive* system, (b) a prefrontal cortical *reflective* system, and (c) an insular-dependent *interoceptive* system. The amygdala-striatal (impulsive) system was the first of the three systems to come under empirical review. The impulsive system is responsible for mediating automatic behavior and directing attention toward salient cues; it influences motivation through mesolimbic dopamine circuits, which play a vital role in the neurobiology of drugs of abuse (Pierce & Kumaresan, 2006). This impulsive mesolimbic dopamine (DA) system is responsible for forming habitual behaviors and transitioning drug use from recreational to compulsive use through Pavlovian and instrumental learning (Everitt & Robbins, 2005). This type of associative learning and habit formation is linked to context-dependent feelings of craving (Volkow et al., 2008). The impulsive system is responsible primarily for "wanting" associated with addictive substances, rather than the subjective "liking" associated with a particular drug (Berridge, Robinson & Aldridge, 2009; Robinson et al., 2005). The second cognitive system implicated in this triadic model is the prefrontal cortex. Historically, addiction has been studied as a subcortical problem resulting from abnormalities in the DA system. More recent research has brought the prefrontal cortex to the forefront of discussion on the neurobiology of addictive substances. The ventromedial prefrontal cortex and the orbitofrontal cortex play an important role in long-term goal setting, decision-making and impulse control (Schoenbaum & Shaham, 2008; Schoenbaum, Roesch & Stalnaker, 2006; Volkow & Fowler, 2000). Deficits in these processes – goal-setting, decision-making, and implicit cognition – have direct implications for addiction and contribute to the continuation of drug use despite negative consequences (Bechara, Noel & Crone, 2006).

One of the latest discoveries implicated a third neural system – the insular system – in the neurobiology of substance addictions (Droutman, Read & Bechara, 2015; Naqvi & Bechara, 2009). Historically, the insula has been known to receive interoceptive signals from the body, and is a necessary component for the experience of emotion and self-awareness (Craig, 2009, 2010). Recently, the insula has been studied in relation to substance addictions with an increasingly nuanced understanding of individual insular subregions (Droutman et al., 2015). The insular cortex can be activated either by homeostatic imbalance (such as withdrawal from alcohol), or by reward cues (such as an environmental context predicting drug use; Naqvi & Bechara, 2009). Neural pathways enable the brain to detect changes going on in the body – and then make that information consciously available to an individual. The same pathways that signal satiety after eating a large dinner signal the conscious feeling of withdrawal from heroin. The insula translates these bottom-up, interoceptive signals into what is subjectively experienced as an urge or craving. These subjective feelings then potentiate the activity of the impulsive system, while weakening or hijacking the goal-driven cognitive resources that are necessary for normal operation of the reflective system. Given the role that these three key neural systems play, it has been proposed that addiction could be a result of abnormal functioning in one or more of these three cognitive systems: amygdala-striatum, prefrontal cortex, and insular cortex (Noël, Brevers & Bechara, 2013). The current chapter addresses the neurocognitive mechanisms associated with each of these three neural systems.

First, we address the neurobiological underpinnings of drugs of abuse in the impulsive system, focusing on the unique psychobiological effects of each substance as well as their common neural pathway. Then, we focus on the reflective system, evaluating how the prefrontal cortex directs cognitive efforts and regulates the impulsive system – and importantly how substances of abuse alter this function. Third, we discuss the insular cortex and its role in communicating information about homeostasis and bodily state changes to the brain, and how this can enhance the role of the impulsive system while attenuating the role of the reflective system. Lastly, we transition from the neurobiological correlates to focus on broader social systems, discussing the role that individual differences and societal perceptions of drugs play in addiction.

Substances of Abuse and Dopamine: The Impulsive System

Substances of abuse can produce a wide array of subjective feelings and behaviors. Generally, different drugs produce differential subjective feelings: even the language used by individuals who use drugs varies depending on the substance. For example, the high from opiates is sometimes called the "heroin hug" with absolute advocacy ("The Heroin Hug | Absolute Advocacy," n.d.; an organization focused on mental health services and addiction) describing the heroin high as follows:

> Imagine being wrapped in the world's biggest, warmest, most welcoming hug. Now, imagine having access to that hug at almost any time.

On the other hand, the Drug Policy Alliance ("What does it feel like to use cocaine? | Drug Policy Alliance," n.d.) describes the cocaine high like this:

> People who use cocaine describe a feeling of alertness, power and energy. They are likely to feel more confident and excited. They may also experience anxiety, paranoia and agitation.

Substances of abuse also produce objectively different physiological changes. Methamphetamine causes an increase in heart rate, dilated pupils, and increased body temperature (Hassan et al., 2016), whereas heroin causes constriction of the pupils and decreases respiration (Baca & Grant, 2007). While these drugs are producing different physiological effects, the neurobiological systems underpinning drug seeking behavior are more uniform. All substances of abuse produce an increase in mesolimbic DA transmission, specifically in the nucleus accumbens, the region at the base of the striatum that receives projections from the ventral tegmental area, or VTA (Oswald et al., 2005).

Dopamine is implicated in a wide array of functions ranging from motor control via the nigrostriatal pathway, to motivation and reward via the mesolimbic pathway. Dopamine plays a common role in each of these seemingly unrelated functions; it aids synaptic plasticity and shapes neural pathways (Molina-Luna et al., 2009). The collection of dopaminergic cells related to motivated behavior are known as the mesolimbic dopamine system: this system is made up of cells originating in the VTA, which sends projections to several different brain regions including the nucleus accumbens (NAcc).

Studies looking at the mechanisms of action of various classes of drugs revealed that the mesolimbic DA pathway is a common denominator for the reward produced by diverse drug classes: stimulants, opiates, ethanol, and cannabinoids. Drugs in each of these classes increase mesolimbic DA transmission, and thus have the potential to be abused.

Stimulants

The stimulant drug category includes several psychoactive substances, such as cocaine, methamphetamine, caffeine, and nicotine. These substances operate on the mesolimbic DA system through different mechanisms while producing the same effects. The reinforcing effects of DA were under study as early as the 1970s (Phillips & Fibiger, 1979). A primary reason that stimulant drugs are so reinforcing is the speed at which these drugs increase DA levels and subsequently leave the brain. While it is generally agreed that mesolimbic dopamine is the neural mechanism underlying drug-seeking behavior (or wanting), studies suggest that dopamine may also be linked to the subjective high or euphoria associated with the ingestion of a drug. For example, as the amount of extracellular DA in the system increases, the subjective "high" increases based on self-report measures (Di Chiara et al., 2004). Additionally, subjective feelings of euphoria, novelty, or exploration closely follow the curve of the extracellular DA concentrations over time. In a PET imaging study on healthy volunteers, as DA spiked, subjective feelings of euphoria increased. After about twenty to thirty minutes, when DA levels decreased (and the cocaine was metabolized), feelings of euphoria also subsided (Volkow et al., 2004). Beyond the direct effects of the drug, environmental cues that a person learns to associate with cocaine use can come to elicit a spike in extracellular DA – even prior to the administration of the drug (Nestler, 2005). This mechanism is thought to be part of the reason for the intense urges and cravings that often result when a drug user views images of people, places, or paraphernalia associated with use.

Cocaine is a stimulant drug that acts on the brain by blocking DA transporters (DATs) that are responsible for clearing extracellular DA from synapses (Nestler, 2005). The net result is an increase DA in the mesolimbic DA system through the disruption of dopamine reuptake processes in the synapse. *Methamphetamine* is another well-known stimulant drug, and it is the most powerful in terms of overall increase in extracellular mesolimbic DA. Methamphetamine interrupts normal functioning of DA transporters (DATs); similar to the effect of cocaine, these transporters are rendered unable to remove extracellular DA from the synapse. In addition to disrupting DATs, methamphetamine *also* causes an increase in the release of dopamine (Nash & Yamamoto, 1992). The net result is excess DA for a prolonged period of time (Fleckenstein et al., 1997). Chronic use of methamphetamine damages DATs – at least temporarily – which raises the risk of neurotoxicity for an individual. After prolonged abstinence from the drug, (typically at least three years in humans) there is evidence that some transporters can become functional once again (Volkow et al., 2001). The combination of DAT disruption and increased DA release yields an increase in synaptic dopamine over ten times the amount seen in a dose of cocaine. Thus, methamphetamine is considered to be the stimulant with the highest addictive potential. Similar to other stimulants, chronic use of methamphetamine leads to context and expectation effects on extracellular DA levels; these effects result in increased dopaminergic output when a person using is in a context where they expect to receive a dose of the drug, regardless of whether or not they actually use (Lin, Pan & Yeh, 2007). This evidence indicates that there are biological changes in the brain that are sensitive not only to the chemical properties of the drug itself, but also to the environmental circumstances that are predictive of the drug.

Besides cocaine and methamphetamine, there are other common substances (e.g., caffeine and nicotine) in the stimulant category that exert an indirect effect, rather than a direct effect, on dopamine neurotransmission. *Caffeine* is considered to be a stimulant drug, but it is not clinically considered to be an addictive substance. Caffeine binds to adenosine receptors, specifically A2A receptors (Huang et al., 2005). When caffeine floods into the brain, adenosine is unable to bind to those receptors; under normal conditions, adenosine inhibits the transmission of dopamine and glutamate in the striatum, making the individual feel tired (Porkka et al., 1997). Glutamate is the primary excitatory neurotransmitter, and along with dopamine, is inhibited when adenosine binds to A2A receptors. Thus, when caffeine – an antagonist – takes the place of adenosine at these receptors, glutamate and dopamine are both disinhibited and the net result is an indirect increase in dopamine (along with a boost of wakefulness). Caffeine indirectly increases dopaminergic signaling in the nucleus accumbens, which is a primary dopaminergic target for drugs of abuse (Solinas et al., 2002). Caffeine users are also susceptible to context and expectation effects: in a context where an individual typically consumes caffeine, she may experience an increase in mesolimbic dopamine regardless of caffeine consumption – similar to how context effects increase dopaminergic signaling in methamphetamine users (Kaasinen et al., 2004). *Nicotine* is also considered a stimulant drug; it increases mesolimbic dopamine through excitation of nicotinic receptors that are found on the surface of mesolimbic dopamine neurons in the ventral tegmental area (VTA) (Brody et al., 2009; Corrigall et al., 1994; Dani, 2003; Pidoplichko et al., 1997). Thus, the mesolimbic dopamine brain regions (particularly dopaminergic signals to the nucleus accumbens) seem to play a key role in the rewarding feelings triggered by (a) cues associated with substances of abuse, (b) the use of these substances, and (c) remedying the subjective feelings of dysregulation that come with acute withdrawal (de la Fuente-Fernández et al., 2002).

Opioids

The term "opiates" is usually used when describing natural molecules, such as endorphins and enkephalins, while the term "opioids" is usually used to apply to synthetic chemicals created to emulate natural opiates. Here, we will use the term opioids to describe both natural and synthetic molecules. Opioids are drugs that act on different types of opioid receptors throughout the brain, namely mu, delta, or kappa receptors. These receptors are the target of endogenous opioids – typically endorphins, dynorphins, and enkephalins. The most well-known class of endogenous opioids is endorphins; they are released during exercise, excitement, orgasm, and pain. They are often referred to as "natural painkillers"

(Koneru, Satyanarayana & Rizwan, 2009). Opioid drugs, such as heroin, morphine, fentanyl, and oxycodone bind to opioid receptors and produce intense feelings of euphoria. While the analgesic properties of opioids are linked to pain pathways in the brain, their addictive properties – including subjective pleasure (see Warlow & colleagues, 2020) – are attributed to their effects that lead to an increase in mesolimbic DA (Herz, 1997; Tanda, Pontieri & Di Chiara, 1997). Opioid receptors are abundantly available on GABA (the primary inhibitory neurotransmitter) neurons in the VTA.

Opioids bind to mu-receptors which inhibit GABAergic neurons that normally suppress dopaminergic cell firing in the VTA. This inhibition of GABA neurons leads to an increase in the firing rate of these now uninhibited dopaminergic cells in the VTA (Wise, 1996). This increased DA neuron firing in the VTA directly increases DA release in the nucleus accumbens (Spanagel, Herz & Shippenberg, 1992). Opioid receptor subtypes other than the mu-opioid receptors do not demonstrate this same effect on mesolimbic DA: there is even evidence indicating kappa-opioid receptors may act in opposition to mu-opioid receptors via down-regulation of DA production in the nucleus accumbens (Spanagel et al., 1992). Mirroring the different effects on dopaminergic output, binding at each receptor type also produces different subjective feelings and experiences. People report feelings of euphoria when opioids bind to delta- and mu-receptors, but report feelings of dysphoria when opioids bind to kappa-receptors; these differences in subjective experience may correspond to the respective upregulation and down-regulation of mesolimbic DA neurotransmission.

Opioids are also subject to expectation effects on experience during use, for both medical and recreational purposes. Opioids are given as pain relief in medical environments: individual expectations alter both subjective and objective measures of efficacy of a mu-opioid agonist. In an experimental setting, individuals were given opioid analgesics under three conditions (Bingel et al., 2011). The first group was told to expect no analgesic results, the second group to expect positive analgesic results, and the third group was told to expect negative analgesic results. Participants in the first condition were expecting no analgesia and they experienced positive pain relief symptoms, demonstrating the physiological impact of the drug alone. However, the second group expected positive analgesic results, they experienced additional positive pain relief symptoms. Lastly, in participants with negative analgesic expectations, pain intensity returned to baseline levels as though they had not received the drug at all (Bingel et al., 2011). Psychological expectations have profound effects on the subjective experience of the drug.

Environmental cues are strongly associated with craving in opioid addiction, just as they are in stimulant use. PET imaging shows that current heroin users have increased blood flow to mesolimbic brain regions associated with dopaminergic signaling when they are shown drug-related cues; this indicates that the brain is pre-emptively expecting to receive heroin, and it could be a major factor contributing to high rates of relapse (Sell et al., 2000). While opioids have their own pharmacological systems and exert unique pharmacological effects, they share with other drugs of abuse a common denominator – the mesolimbic DA system.

Alcohol

Alcohol is generally considered a depressant because of how it affects GABAergic systems, leading to a state of relaxation and drowsiness (Hill & Toffolon, 1990; Marinkovic, Halgren & Maltzman, 2004; Paraskevaides et al., 2010). Alcohol also exerts other effects, particularly on (a) the glutamate system, leading to staggering, slurred speech, and memory blackouts and (b) the opioid system, acting as a painkiller, and giving an a euphoric "high" (Hill & Toffolon, 1990; Marinkovic et al., 2004; Paraskevaides et al., 2010). Alcohol can also act as a stimulant through its actions on both norepinephrinergic and dopaminergic systems. Administration of ethanol, like other drugs of abuse, increases mesolimbic DA levels (Gessa et al., 1985). Thus, the effects of alcohol reach nearly every part of the central nervous system through interactions with dopamine, GABA, glutamate, and norepinephrine: it impairs sensory and motor functions, memory, and language processes all while stimulating the reward system via mesolimbic dopamine disruptions (Hill & Toffolon, 1990; Marinkovic et al., 2004; Paraskevaides et al., 2010). Alcohol increases the release of mesolimbic DA partially through the release of endogenous opioids that upregulate DA production in the VTA (Herz, 1997).

Chronic use of alcohol produces its own unique set of symptoms: people who are in recovery from alcohol use disorders have down-regulated D2 receptor sensitivity, which contributes to an increased salience of and attentiveness toward alcohol and alcohol-related cues. Heightened attention toward these cues is correlated with an increase in subjective craving and desire to use alcohol (Heinz et al., 2004). Specifically, these drug-related cues induce DA release in the mesolimbic DA system via activation of the anterior cingulate and medial prefrontal cortex, which both focus attention toward rewarding cues. This combination increases the risk for relapse in a person who is abstaining from alcohol (Heinz et al, 2004). The dysfunction following chronic alcohol abuse – in the form of down-regulated D2 receptor sensitivity – plays a role in increasing the risk for relapse (Volkow et al., 1996).

Alcohol exerts its reinforcing and euphoric effects via increases in the mesolimbic DA system, like other drugs of abuse. Also similar to other drugs of abuse, DA plays a role in the risk for relapse in people with alcohol use disorders. This is in part due to changes in the brain that rise from increased dopaminergic signaling, which increases synaptic plasticity: the brain is slower to make synaptic changes during a period of sobriety than it is during an initial period of drug use. This leads to a fast cycle of becoming sensitized to the rewarding effects of the drug, and a slower cycle during which the brain recovers from the chronic drug abuse.

Cannabinoids

Cannabis is commonly known as marijuana, weed, or pot. The main psychoactive compound in cannabis is tetrahydrocannabinol (THC). Cannabis is used recreationally for its mental and physical effects, such as a "high" or "stoned" feeling, but it is also used for medicinal and spiritual purposes. THC exerts its most prominent effects via its actions on two types of cannabinoid receptors (a) the CB1 receptor, which is found primarily in the brain as well as in some peripheral tissues and (b) the CB2 receptor, which is found primarily in peripheral tissues, but is also expressed in brain cells. THC appears to alter mood and cognition through its agonist actions on CB1 receptors (Gessa et al., 1998).

While cannabinoids have their own pharmacological pathways, they are also linked to the mesolimbic DA system. Similar to alcohol and opioids, CB1 receptors are found on GABA neurons as well as with mu-opioid receptors in the VTA (Melis et al., 2004; Shen et al., 1996). Activation of CB1 receptors disinhibits the VTA dopamine neurons and increases dopaminergic signaling in a manner similar to the activation of mu-opioid receptors (Tanda et al., 1997). Endogenous cannabinoids induce long-term depression of synaptic plasticity, and exogenous cannabinoids alter this normal functioning by binding to CB1 and CB2 receptors, allowing for an increase in synaptic plasticity that then alters the reward system in the brain (Robbe et al., 2002).

Cannabis is a topic of controversy primarily because of its political status. Marijuana was classified as a Schedule I drug by the United States government; this label indicates that cannabis has a high potential for abuse and no medical benefit – despite scientific evidence for its therapeutic potential (Pertwee, 2010). There is evidence that cannabinoids can reduce pain and inflammation, although more studies are needed on the impact of smoking cannabis, which is the most common form of ingestion (Turcotte et al., 2016). Cannabis has less potential for abuse than opioids, which are commonly prescribed for pain management, thus more research is also needed on the relative merits of cannabinoids to manage chronic pain. However, it is not the case that cannabis has no abuse potential: research on the effects of cannabinoids on the mesolimbic DA system have shown that reward circuitry is activated with cannabis use, which is the common denominator for all substances of abuse (Gardner, 2002).

Summary: Common Innervation of the Impulsive System

While different classes of drugs each have their own unique pharmacological properties, all drugs of abuse ultimately increase mesolimbic DA signaling during use, leading to a deficit in mesolimbic DA release during withdrawal and prolonged abstinence (Rossetti, Hmaiden & Gessa, 1992). The amygdala plays a key role in linking environmental cues to activity of the mesolimbic DA system, thereby eliciting reward reactions not only from the ingestion of a substance, but also from expectations and cues predictive of the delivery of the substance (Ito et al., 2002; Schultz, 1998). Thus the amygdala-striatal impulsive neural system is critical for the incentive motivational effects of a variety of nonnatural rewards (e.g., psychoactive drugs) and natural rewards (e.g., food). This neural system also plays a critical role in learning implicit associations as well as the transference of reward-seeking from a controlled, intentional behavior to an automatic, habitual behavior. In our own research, we have referred to this neural system as the "impulsive" system, and we have shown that it becomes hyperactive and begins to exaggerate the incentive value of rewards in individuals with substance-abuse problems (Bechara, 2005).

Several lines of basic research on drug addiction led to the same conclusion that continued drug use results in the strengthening of motivation-relevant associative memories which promote continued use, determining that this relatively spontaneous process begins to govern behavior. For instance, Everitt and colleagues (2008) argued that dopaminergic activity in the nucleus accumbens reinforces the repetition of behaviors and supports the encoding and processing of proximal stimuli associated with the rewarding experience. Neutral stimuli (such as a particular color of paint) associated with appetitive behaviors (such as drug use), come to represent and cue the appetitive behavior. For example, think about how some people associate a movie theater with buttery popcorn. After many exposures, a person may crave a salty, fatty snack simply upon seeing a movie theater, or even a movie trailer. As cue → behavior → outcome associations are strengthened, patterns of associations signal and drive the behavior without the need for reflective processes to be involved (see Stacy, Pike & Lee, 2020). Cues can then trigger an essentially "automatic" pattern of activation in memory that can be described in various neural network or connectionist models. A similar conclusion was obtained by the incentive sensitization theory (Robinson & Berridge, 1993). This theory suggests that, through repetition of rewarding appetitive experiences, the mesocorticolimbic circuitry is sensitized and mediates motivational processes by attributing incentive salience to reward-related stimuli (e.g., drug-related cues). Cues associated with reward are then able to elicit "wanting" for a specific reward.

Overall, research on the neurobiology of drug addiction shows that increased mesolimbic dopamine activity reinforces the repetition of behaviors, which influences learning, attentional processes, and the strengthening of associations of reinforcing effects (Stacy & Weirs, 2010; Watson et al., 2012). Once a strong habit is formed, cues elicit the habit regardless of anticipated outcomes. Habits become automatic and difficult to change. Another pivotal feature of habit systems is that participants do not necessarily know what triggers their habits, and cues can elicit a behavior entirely outside of conscious awareness (Stacy & Weirs, 2010; Watson et al., 2012).

Addiction and the Prefrontal Cortex: The Reflective System

While over thirty years of research has yielded a remarkable success in understanding the subcortical neural mechanisms that motivate behaviors toward reward, especially drugs, very little attention was paid to the importance of the prefrontal cortex in the decision to take drugs in the first place. Indeed, one fundamental difference between animal paradigms and the human addiction model is that, in the case of humans, the initiation and escalation of drug use is often done with a prior knowledge of the potential negative consequences associated with drug use. In other words, the use of drugs in humans is associated with a conflict: the immediate pleasurable effects of the drug versus the possibility of punishment by the law, parents, schoolteachers, or other authorities.

Indeed, addiction is more than an increase in mesolimbic dopamine that causes a person to pursue drugs at the cost of social status, financial stability, and familial relations. Addiction goes beyond an imbalance of dopaminergic signaling in subcortical regions. The prefrontal cortical system is important for self-regulation and the ability to predict consequences of behavior. In our explanation and research on the addiction process, the prefrontal cortex becomes hypoactive. In comparison to the role of the mesolimbic dopamine signals in the striatum and amygdala, this "reflective" system is slower, requiring conscious thought and deliberation (Noël et al., 2013). When the prefrontal cortex is compromised, it is difficult to control automatic and habitual behaviors that are formed by an overactive impulsive system. The automatic habitual system increases attention to drug cues, because those cues serve as predictors that a spike in mesolimbic DA circuits is imminent: the problem is that it makes abstinence from drugs more difficult. In the case of addiction, it is particularly disadvantageous to rely on habitual behaviors and impulses, and thus the role of the prefrontal cortex becomes even more valuable. When this system is functioning normally, it allows a person to pursue long-term goals flexibly (Goldstein & Volkow, 2011). This is in contrast to the more rigid subcortical reward system in which anything that immediately increases mesolimbic DA is the primary motivation to pursue a goal. This may have worked efficiently when fatty foods and sex were the primary causes of increased dopaminergic signaling, but it does not fare well for the individual who is pursuing methamphetamine or gambling at the cost of other natural rewards like time with family, dinner, or earning a paycheck.

The prefrontal cortex is at the root of self-control in addiction. One metric to estimate self-control in the laboratory is through an individual's capacity to inhibit prepotent motor responses using the stop-signal or go/no-go tasks (Noël et al., 2013). People with a substance use disorder consistently show behavioral impairments in both tasks: in stop-signal tasks they show a larger latency in motor response inhibition, and in go/no-go tasks they show more errors of commission wherein they press a button when the instruction is to withhold a response (Monterosso et al., 2005). Additionally, brain imaging studies show hypoactivation in regions associated with error detection, namely the anterior cingulate cortex, indicating a lack of prefrontal cortical activation when it comes to behavioral inhibition in people with a substance-use disorder (Fu et al., 2008; Hester & Garavan, 2004).

This hypoactivation in prefrontal cortical circuits could exacerbate the problems that arise from hyperactivation of the impulsive system. These are competing systems, and in people with an addiction, the impulsive system becomes much stronger while the reflective system simultaneously becomes weaker: this likely compromises the self-control of individuals who are attempting to remain abstinent in a range of substance addictions including nicotine (Krishnan-Sarin et al., 2007), cocaine (Garavan & Hester, 2007), and alcohol (Bowden-Jones et al., 2005). It is important to note here that it is not simply the case that people with an addiction are left without a reflective prefrontal cortical system: there is a painstaking amount of planning and coordinating required for a person to get their next "score," and people who are daily users are able to maintain this detailed schedule of seeking, finding, purchasing, and then using with a high degree of success despite the barriers set out by law enforcement, family, friends, and jobs. The prefrontal cortical system is "hijacked," and people go from thinking of a wide variety of tasks or natural rewards to thinking relentlessly of drugs and the cycle of seeking, finding, purchasing, and using.

Beyond a purely motor definition of self-control, the important ability to make decisions that are costly in the short-term but that yield long-term benefits (e.g., remaining sober while mourning a death in the family) is impaired in people with an addiction. Delay discounting is the term used for the phenomenon that there is value in immediacy: five dollars now is better than five dollars in one week. There is a tradeoff between smaller-sooner rewards and larger-later rewards in everyday life, and these tradeoffs can become extreme in people with an addiction (see Jarmolowicz & Schneider, 2020). Behavior on delay discounting tasks, in which people are asked to choose between a smaller sum of money today, or a larger sum of money at a later date, is a measure of impulsivity (Ainslie, 1975). Individuals with an addiction systematically devalue delayed rewards at a faster rate than controls: they are more likely to act on impulse (Kirby, Petry & Bickel, 1999). The prefrontal cortex, responsible for rational decision-making, is implicated in delay discounting behavior. People in these situations are asked to decide between different amounts of money at different times. It is not a habit-driven choice; they are tasked with making a deliberate decision based on the nondrug options in front of them. There is a difference in the way that people with an addiction behave in this situation based on activity in the prefrontal cortex. An fMRI study by Monterosso and colleagues demonstrated that methamphetamine users recruited similar levels of neural activation during easy and difficult choices, whereas nonusers recruited little activation during easy choices and selectively utilized neural resources more for the difficult choices (Monterosso et al., 2007). This indicates that rather than a complete inability to use prefrontal brain regions, people using drugs are more likely to have higher levels of neural activation, specifically in the left dorsolateral prefrontal cortex, even for decisions which should be relatively simple to make. Participants with an addiction need more resources to make the same decisions as healthy controls, and this is may be a compensatory mechanism for the lack of efficiency in these neural networks.

The prefrontal cortex is important for working memory (Hinson, Jameson & Whitney, 2003). Deficits in either cortical volume or dopamine transporter operations impairs working memory and may help to explain the findings on delay-discounting behaviors in people with an addiction. A behavioral measure of decision-making in populations with an addiction is the Iowa Gambling Task (IGT). A person must make decisions with uncertainty in the context of punishment and reward: some of the choices yield positive short-term results (high reward) but predict poor long-term results (high punishment), whereas others produce small short-term rewards (low reward) but predict long-term positive results (low punishment). To perform well, participants must forgo short-term benefits for long-term benefits – something that individuals suffering from addiction are characteristically unable to do successfully (Bechara, 2004). Participants with an addiction who complete the IGT demonstrate preferences for short-term high-rewarding stimuli, with the end result being a net loss (Grant, Contoreggi & London, 2000; Noël et al., 2013). Decreased gray matter volume in prefrontal cortical regions, including the orbitofrontal cortex, ventromedial prefrontal cortex (vmPFC), and anterior cingulate is found in chronic drug users. This decrease is found in people who are using methamphetamine (Thompson et al., 2004), heroin (Yuan et al., 2009), alcohol (Mechtcheriakov et al., 2007), and cocaine (Fein, Di Sclafani & Meyerhoff, 2002). The orbitofrontal cortex (OFC) is distinguished by its connectivity to other subcortical structures – notably the amygdala and nucleus accumbens, which both play a role in associative learning (Schoenbaum et al., 2006). Because of these connections, the OFC is implicated in the ability to predict future outcomes based on associations: it can use the value of expected versus actual outcomes to guide executive functions, including decision-making. Drugs alter this system, taking the OFC "offline," which may account for the high delay-discounting rates and maladaptive decision-making patterns found in people with drug addictions (Schoenbaum et al., 2006).

In addition to deficits in the connection between associative learning and executive functioning, somatic states mediated by the prefrontal cortex also play a major role in drug addiction, withdrawal, and relapse. Prefrontal brain regions trigger somatic states from thoughts and memories, which can be in conflict with one another. Euphoric recall of the experience of using would produce a positive signal, whereas the negative consequences of use (e.g., being involved in a car accident or fighting with a loved one) would produce a negative signal. Negative events typically do not occur simultaneously with drug administration: the negative consequences of drug use are almost always delayed relative to the positive experience. The tendency to discount events does not only include rewards, discounting punishments that are delayed in time is still delay discounting. In the brain, the net result is either a positive or a negative signal (Bechara, 2004). Because of delay discounting, this net signal with drug use is more likely to be positive because the euphoric feelings typically precede any negative consequences of use. The vmPFC links both memories and associations to these emotional responses, and if this region and the OFC are impaired, the ability to make decisions based on past associations and future goals becomes even more difficult.

Previously well-adapted individuals display a marked inability to conform to social conventions and make adaptive decisions in their personal lives following damage to the vmPFC (Bechara et al., 1997). Emotion is an integral part of decision-making, and the impairments in the prefrontal cortex in populations with addictions yields problems both in executive functioning and in the synthesis of emotions and memories. Damage to the OFC and vmPFC lead to the increased salience of drugs and drug-related cues (Goldstein & Volkow, 2011). This increase in attention to drug cues is accompanied by a negative prediction error, in which the predicted value of the drug is greater than the experienced value. Each time a person thinks of using – or sees a drug cue – they expect to have a positive experience. In summary, dysfunction in the reflective PFC system could lead to impaired response inhibition and heightened salience attribution toward high short-term rewards in individuals with an addiction.

Goldstein & Volkow proposed a model of addiction, the impaired response inhibition and salience attribution model (iRISA) syndrome to characterize the attention and behavioral deficits found in addicted populations (2011). They outline nine processes that are disrupted in addiction, and discuss which prefrontal regions are implicated in each process. The nine processes are: (1) self-control and behavioral monitoring, (2) emotion regulation, (3) motivation, (4) awareness/interoception, (5) attention and flexibility, (6) working memory, (7) learning and memory, (8) decision-making and valuation, and (9) salience attribution. For self-control and behavioral monitoring, people with addiction display higher than average levels of impulsivity, compulsivity, and risk-taking as well as deficits in error prediction and detection. The prefrontal regions associated with these processes are the anterior cingulate, medial PFC (mPFC), and ventrolateral PFC (vlPFC). Emotion regulation problems, such as enhanced reactivity to stress and inability to suppress emotional intensity, are associated with the OFC, vmPFC and the anterior cingulate cortex. Motivational deficits are characterized by increased motivation to seek drugs at the cost of other goals alongside a decreased motivation to pursue alternate rewards; these effects are mediated by the OFC, vmPFC, anterior cingulate cortex, and the dorsolateral PFC (dlPFC). Problems in awareness and interoception include reduced satiety when presented with the same amount of drug (tolerance), or the denial of an illness or need for treatment with functional deficits in the anterior cingulate, OFC, mPFC, and vlPFC. Attentional deficits include inflexibility in goals, with cognitive resources developing a myopic focus on drug-seeking behaviors and attention increasingly focused on drug-related cues and are related to problems in the dlPFC, anterior cingulate, inferior frontal gyrus, and the vlPFC. Working memory is compromised, with memory formation biased toward stimuli that represent drug use, and away from alternative experiences or tasks. Learning and memory more generally are implicated, such that the associated learning between drugs and drug-cues releases DA; this yields an increase in synaptic plasticity, creating very powerful associations that are difficult to unlearn, while simultaneously making it difficult to learn the associated value of rewards from nondrug reinforcers. This process is mediated by the dlPFC, OFC, and anterior cingulate. Abhorrent decision-making is common among chronic drug users: high rates of delay discounting, inaccurate predictions of future consequences, and the lack of planning and goal formation are all problems related to deficits in the OFC, vmPFC, and dlPFC. Lastly, in salience attribution, drug and drug-related cues are sensitized such that any nondrug rewards are devalued and negative prediction error ensues (i.e., actual experience – expected experience = negative). These prediction errors are overlooked, and the incentive to use again remains high even though the actual experience is repeatedly less satisfying than the individual predicted.

These processes that are disrupted in individuals with an addiction have clear ties to observed behavior in this population, but they are not solely the result of activation in the prefrontal cortex. Error prediction when the expected reward is less than the actual reward, as is the case for people in the beginning stages of drug use, is related to the activity of midbrain dopamine neurons (Bayer & Glimcher, 2005). Successful emotion regulation is accomplished by the interaction between prefrontal and subcortical regions: separate pathways from the vlPFC to the amygdala and nucleus accumbens are found to mediate negative emotion and positive emotion, respectively (Wager et al., 2008). Motivation has complex neuroanatomical substrates; areas including the nucleus accumbens and ventral pallidum are critical components for the motivation to actively work toward a goal, such as procuring drugs (Koob & Volkow, 2010). Conscious awareness of internal cues, or interoception, is mediated by the insular cortex (Naqvi & Bechara, 2009). Attention and cognitive flexibility are controlled primarily by the prefrontal cortex, but when this system is compromised, basal ganglia structures come to the foreground and direct attention toward habitual behaviors (e.g., drug use) that require little input from the PFC (Belin et al., 2009). Working memory is primarily dependent on the integrity of PFC functions, but evidence shows that adrenergic signaling from the amygdala during times of stress plays a role in the ability of the PFC to perform this function (Roozendaal et al., 2004). Learning and memory formation are moderated by a wide range of subcortical structures beyond prefrontal cortical regions, areas including the amygdala, hippocampus, and basal ganglia all seem to play a role in these functions (Robbins et al., 2008). Decision-making and valuation at the level of the prefrontal cortex allows for the synthesis of multiple, contradicting sources of information to be considered prior to choosing one course of action; the subcortical structures, such as the basal ganglia, allow for decision-making and valuation of stimuli and cues on a less sophisticated level (Belin et al., 2009). Lastly, salience attribution is a problem in this population as the salience of drugs and drug-related cues increases and overshadows that of natural rewards; this process is mediated by mesocorticolimbic circuitry (Robinson & Berridge, 2001). Overall, the PFC is implicated across a variety of symptoms seen in individuals with a substance addiction.

Addiction and the Insular Cortex

Based on more recent evidence, a long-forgotten structure, the insular cortex, has emerged as a neural structure that plays a key role in interoceptive representations generated from drug-related cues (e.g., smoking). We have speculated that this function extends to other biological urges as well – such as hunger elicited by food cues. We have argued that activity in the insular cortex elicited by homeostatic imbalance, such as deprivation states or reward cues, serves to sensitize the motivational circuits that propel individuals toward reward (the habit or impulsive system), and to "hijack" the prefrontal cortical system, preventing it from using the cognitive resources necessary to exert self-control to resist reward (Naqvi & Bechara, 2009).

The insula lies deep within the brain underneath the frontal and parietal lobes (Figure 10.1). Research on the insula in recent years has uncovered its role in communicating interoceptive cues to the brain – cues that are critical for the subjective experience of emotional states. Interoception is the neural mapping of changes to homeostasis: changes in pain, temperature, taste, inflammation, and sensual touch are all related to survival. Interoception is the conscious awareness of these

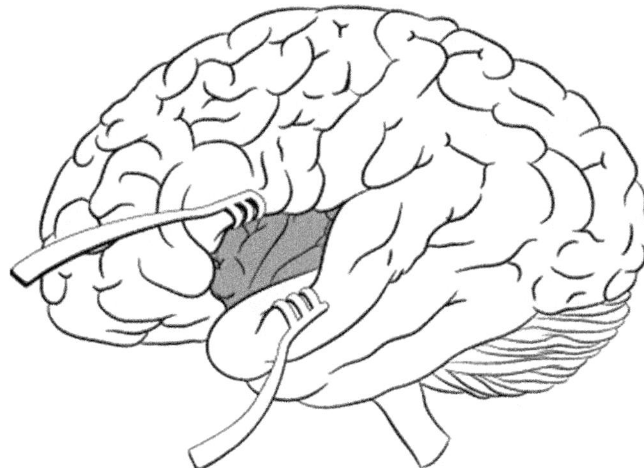

Figure 10.1 A schematic presentation of a human brain showing the insula highlighted in gray

changes (Craig, 2009). In addition to their relevance for survival, interoceptive cues processed through the insula have inherent hedonic value, such that the subjective experience is either positive or negative. Specifically, brain imaging studies have identified the right anterior insula as the area where these interoceptive stimuli come to conscious awareness (Critchley et al., 2004). More recently, the role of the insula in the context of addiction has been given special attention. Interoceptive cues may be the basis for the experience of craving and the urge to use a drug (Gray & Critchley, 2007). Homeostasis is particularly relevant in a population of substance users, as the use of drugs alters a person's physiological processes: craving, relapse, and withdrawal are all characterized by a desire – emotional, behavioral, or physiological – to use a substance. Interviews with people who have an addiction reveal that people often feel that they need to use in order to "feel normal" (Khantzian, 1987). It is likely that this phenomenon is related to interoceptive cues signaling a homeostatic imbalance in the body.

Despite the commonality that drugs of abuse share – namely the increase in mesolimbic DA – each ritual associated with individual drugs has a distinct effect on the body that can contribute to its subjective emotional meaning (Bechara & Naqvi, 2004). Smoking cigarettes produces its own set of interoceptive cues; increased heart rate, autonomic effects from nicotine felt with each drag, sensory effects on the airway, and the taste of tobacco combine to form the unique experience of smoking a cigarette or vaping. Injecting heroin produces a different set of cues; piercing the skin, decreased respiration, and subjective feelings of warmth. Snorting cocaine produces a bitter taste, increased heart rate, and a harsh sensation in the nose and throat. Drinking alcohol has a strong taste and smell, feelings of warmth, and a depression of central nervous system activity. Each drug changes homeostasis and leads to increased activation in the insular cortex, which translates these interoceptive state changes into consciousness (Gasquoine, 2014). Interoceptive cues are not just a small part in the big picture of maintaining addiction: there is evidence that they may be a necessary component. Most of this work has been done in cigarette smokers with an emphasis on the rewarding effects of airway sensory stimulation. Feelings of satiation and a reduction in craving for cigarettes is found in smokers following airway sensory replacement, even without nicotine (Naqvi & Bechara, 2005; Westman, Behm & Rose, 1995). Furthermore, the rewarding effects from airway sensation may be even more powerful than nicotine in reducing craving and subjective reports of urges to smoke (Johnson, Bickel & Kirshenbaum, 2004; Westman, Behm & Rose, 1996).

These interoceptive cues are important for addiction, particularly when they reach conscious awareness. These cues are sent from different areas throughout the body and up to the thalamus, which then relays this information to the insular cortex where conscious awareness begins. The hedonic information that accompanies these cues is not currently thought to be insular-dependent, although the mechanism for how that information is assigned is not yet known. It is likely that the insula sends signals to the amygdala and the OFC to attach corresponding positive and negative valuation to interoceptive signals (Baxter & Murray, 2002; Kringelbach, 2005). The insula is functionally connected to both mesolimbic brain structures and prefrontal cortices; this functional position is critical for its ability to mediate the corresponding impulsive (mesolimbic) and reflective (prefrontal) systems. Activity in the insular cortex is correlated with subjective ratings of the magnitude of urges to use substances including cigarettes, alcohol, heroin, and cocaine (Naqvi & Bechara, 2010; Schmidt et al., 2014), and there is evidence that increased insular activation in response to reward is genetic (Villafuerte et al., 2012). Increased insular activation is correlated with multiple factors in addiction, including (a) attentional bias toward drug-related cues and an increased risk for relapse (Janes et al., 2010), (b) decreased inhibitory functioning in the presence of drug cues (Kaufman et al., 2003), and (c) higher levels of dependence, e.g., on nicotine in smokers (Goudriaan et al., 2010).

The critical role of the insula was assessed in patients with insular lesions: the primary question asks if the insula is a necessary component in maintaining an addiction. A study by Naqvi and colleagues found that, among patients with brain damage and concurrent cigarette addiction, those with damage to the insula were more likely to quit smoking easily, without relapse, and without the persistent urge to smoke (2007). The insula influences these behaviors by responding to interoceptive signals that arise from imbalances in homeostasis coming from changes such as deprivation from drugs, lack of sleep, or increased stress. The insula takes these homeostatic changes and translates them into subjective emotional experiences: in the case of addiction, that emotional experience is an intense craving to use. Beyond that, the insular cortex increases the motivational drive to engage in drug use via two separate mechanisms: (1) upregulating or sensitizing the impulsive striatal/amygdala system and (2) simultaneously diverting attention and decision-making processes from other goals and focusing these cortical resources on the goal of obtaining and using drugs (Wang et al., 2012). The metaphor of drugs "hijacking" the brain fits well: interoceptive signals to the insula are able to "hijack" the reflective prefrontal system of the brain, diverting cognitive resources away from future-oriented goals and toward the immediate goals of the impulsive system – big, fast increases in mesolimbic DA and reward produced by drugs of abuse (Figure 10.2). This seems to be likely given that people with chronic substance use consistently make suboptimal choices (Bechara et al., 2001). A seemingly paradoxical issue arises here: chronic substance users are seemingly successful in repeatedly securing funds to purchase the drug, finding a time and place to use the drug (which if illicit is not an easy feat), and subsequently repeating this process when dealers and suppliers change, funds become seemingly unattainable, or locations are raided. These behaviors demonstrate an ability to plan ahead and make goal-oriented decisions as mentioned previously. However, these decisions to pursue immediate reward often come at the expense of forfeiting future rewards, and people with substance use disorders typically display higher discounting rates than other populations (Amlung et al., 2016; Clewett et al.,

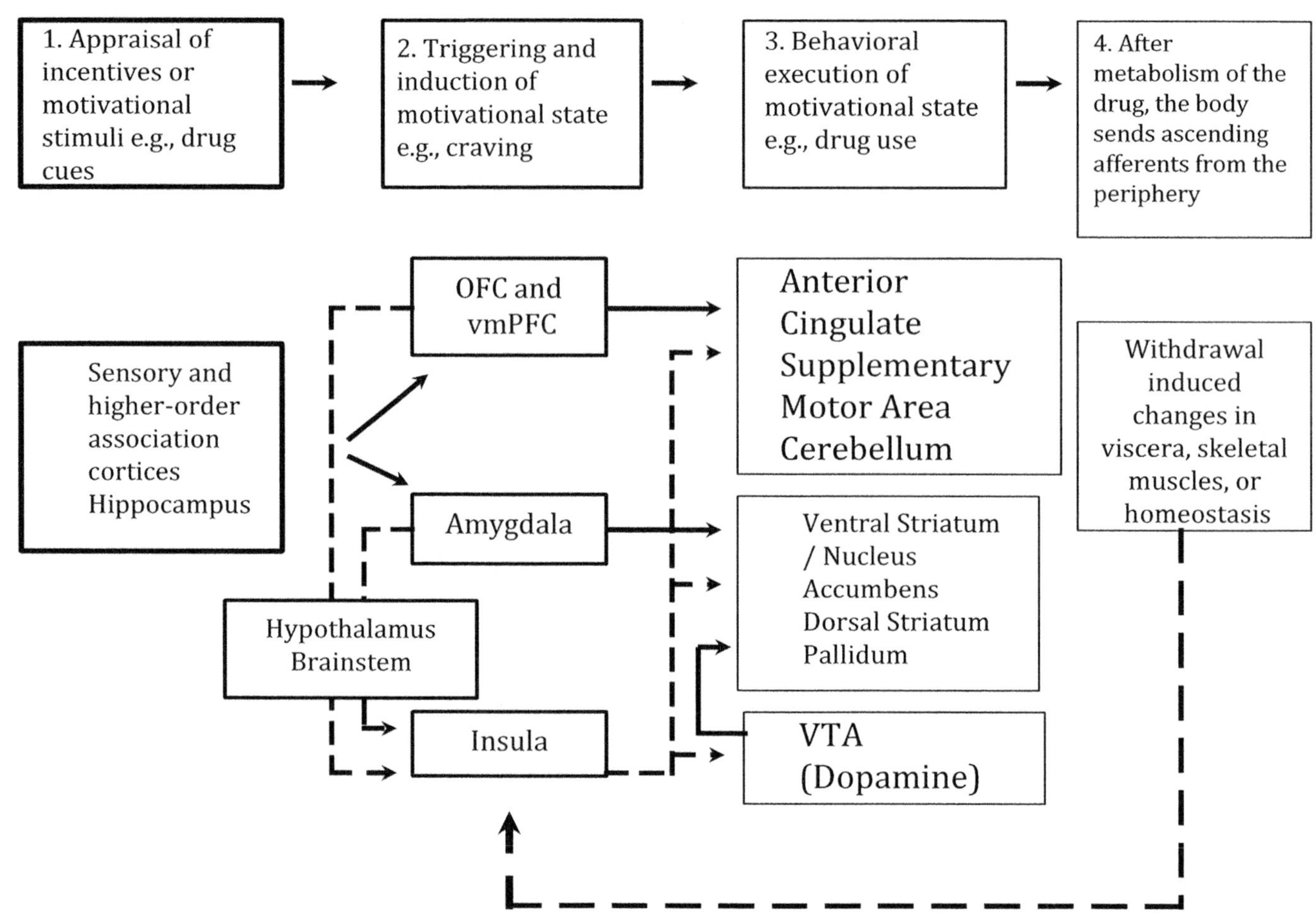

Figure 10.2 A schematic neurological model illustrating a proposed functional role for three key neural systems in addiction. (1) The amygdala-striatal neural system, which we have termed the "impulsive system," excites the traditional reward system involved in the execution of motivational states to seek drugs, such as the ventral striatum/ nucleus accumbens and the mesolimbic dopamine system. (2) The medial orbitofrontal/ ventromedial prefrontal cortex (OFC/VMPC) is a key structure in a neural system we have termed the "reflective system," which forecasts the future consequences of a behavior such as seeking drugs. (3) The proposed functional role of the insula is bolded and dashed

2014). More work needs to be done to discriminate between higher delay discounting rates (preference for immediate rewards at the expense of future larger rewards) and the seemingly paradoxical ability for chronic substance users to make effective decisions regarding personal drug use.

Incentive stimuli (e.g., drug cues) generate motivation in the animal (or human) and instigate approach responses in relation to themselves through the "impulsive system." However, internal factors associated with deprivation states (such as withdrawal) are viewed as a "gate" that determines how effective the incentive input is in exciting the motivational circuits that "pull" and "steer" the animal (or human) toward the appropriate goal object. This process, we propose, is dependent on the insula. Feedback loops arising from the body, reflecting the status of the viscera and homeostasis, and mediated through the insula, will adjust the strengths of the conflicting signals, thereby sensitizing the impulsive system, and potentially overriding the inhibitory control of the reflective system. Recently, rather than overriding the prefrontal inhibitory system, it has been thought that the insula may be subverting the decision-making processes and abilities of the reflective system away from "normal functioning" and into formulating plans for action to seek and procure drugs.

Drug use does not have an objectively positive interoceptive valuation: piercing the skin with a needle causes pain, sensory effects of smoking on airways indicate possible harm to the body, drinking hard liquor burns, and the harsh sensation in the nose and throat from snorting cocaine is not in and of itself pleasurable. However, with repeated exposure to drugs, these cues transform from negative into positive signals. Pleasure derived from these inherently negative interoceptive experiences is a form of emotional learning: a learned association that becomes even more salient through DA-dependent synaptic plasticity (Naqvi & Bechara, 2009). These synaptic changes that alter the valuation of interoceptive cues are found in both the amygdala and the vmPFC, the impulsive and the reflective systems. These neural changes occur after chronic drug use, and the structural changes to the insula and vmPFC remain present in former cocaine users even years into abstinence (Franklin et al., 2002). The insula not only drives motivation toward the pleasurable effects of the drug (whether that is intrinsic pleasure via increased dopaminergic output or associated pleasure via emotional learning and synaptic plasticity), it also plays a role in avoiding punishment. The insula is involved in the emotional experience of pain, which is present in addiction through the negative interoceptive cues associated with drug use (Singer, Critchley & Preuschoff, 2009). The motivation to avoid pain is a contributor to the maintenance of addiction primarily via withdrawal symptoms. Withdrawal is a compilation of negative interoceptive cues associated with the lack of drugs in the body and brain. It is not only painful, but can even be lethal for some drugs if not treated appropriately (Carlson et al., 2012). Functional neuroimaging also provides supporting evidence that the insula is involved in the motivation to avoid unpleasant stimuli (Samanez-Larkin et al., 2008; Seymour et al., 2007).

The discovery of the important role of the insula in smoking addiction does not undermine the seminal work generated to date on the roles of other components in the neural circuitry implicated in addiction (or impulse control disorders more generally), especially the roles of mesolimbic dopamine and the prefrontal cortex. Addressing the role of the insula complements prior work and advances our efforts to find novel therapeutic approaches for treating several impulse control disorders, including breaking the cycle of addiction. Stimulation of future research on the insula has a number of practical implications for clinical studies. The most obvious is that therapeutically modulating the function of the insula may make it easier to overcome addiction and other impulse control problems. This could be accomplished through the design of new pharmacological therapies that target receptors within the insula. Invasive techniques such as deep brain stimulation are also an option. However, non-invasive methods such as repetitive transcranial magnetic stimulation may be promising once the techniques are modified so that they can reach deeper brain structures, such as the insula.

Not All People Are the Same: Individual Differences

While individuals with substance use disorders reveal impairments in their vmPFC functions when we look at them as a large group, looking at individual differences supports a seemingly obvious intuition that not all individuals with an addiction are the same. We compared patients with damage (lesions) to their vmPFC who were not substance abusers to individuals diagnosed with substance dependence (DSM-IV terminology) who do not have brain lesions (Bechara et al., 2001). When comparing the behavioral and physiological profiles of these two groups, we find that only some individuals with substance dependence match the profiles of vmPFC lesion patients, while many others do not. We have suggested that these individuals who more closely match vmPFC patients are characterized by insensitivity to future consequences – they are oblivious to future consequences, positive and negative, and are strongly guided by immediate prospects. The key problem in this subgroup is a dysfunction in their "reflective," prefrontal cortex-dependent, neural system. Another subgroup of substance-dependent individuals matched with vmPFC patients in their behavioral performance (i.e., they seek immediate reward but disregard delayed punishment), yet they demonstrate differences in their physiological profiles (i.e., they show exaggerated physiological responses to reward). This group is suggested to be hypersensitive to reward, so that the prospect of drugs outweighs the prospect of future consequences. The key problem in this subgroup is a dysfunction in their impulsive system. These differences may have implications for prognosis, and they provide testable hypotheses that can be addressed in future research: individuals with substance dependence who closely match vmPFC patients may have a harder time recovering from addiction and remaining abstinent in comparison to those who only partially match the vmPFC patients. One subgroup of individuals with substance dependence appeared normal and did not show behavioral or physiological signs of decision-making deficits. This suggests that not every drug user has impaired decision-making. We have described these individuals as "functional addicts," because a closer inspection of their everyday lives showed that they have suffered minimal social and psychological harm as a consequence of their drug use, (i.e., the ability to keep their job). This subgroup labeled "functional addicts" can be viewed as those who will seek drugs and plan out how and when to use, but this group will tend to seek drugs within what society might deem reasonable means. This subgroup is characterized by a certain threshold for drug use – a point at which procuring or using the drug is no longer worth the cost (economically, socially, or psychologically).

A more intriguing finding is that when we test a large sample of the "normal" population on the IGT, there is a small subgroup that achieves scores that are comparable to those of patients with vmPFC lesions. This raises the question of whether these individuals are predisposed to, or at higher risk of, addiction, than individuals with normal decision-making capabilities. We suggest that the underlying neural basis for this predisposition, or vulnerability, is poor mechanisms of decision-making and impulse control. This suggestion is reasonable in light of the evidence that one risk factor for addiction is hereditary, and genes can act in general fashion (e.g., the serotonin transporter gene) to predispose individuals to multiple, as opposed to specific, drug addictions (Goldman, Oroszi & Ducci, 2005). Perhaps future research using neuroimaging techniques that focus on relationships among (i) genotypes related to specific neurotransmitter systems (e.g., serotonin transporter gene), (ii) level of neural activity in specific neural circuits, and (iii) quality of choice on complex laboratory tasks of decision-making could reveal whether genetic factors lead to suboptimal function in specific neural systems, especially those involving decision-making, that are then expressed in real-life as a variety of behaviors reflecting poor decision-making.

However, not all risk factors are genetic; other factors could be environmental, or the product of gene–environment interactions. The potential for harm in the form of brain development remains relatively high, if an individual had abused drugs during adolescence. Indeed, evidence suggests that the functions of the prefrontal cortex may not develop fully until the age of 25; until that time, the development of neural connections that underlie decision-making and the ability to control powerful temptations is still taking place (Crews, He & Hodge, 2007). Therefore, exposing the prefrontal cortex to drugs before its maturity could be harmful to decision-making, akin to exposing a fetus to drugs during pregnancy. Beyond neurotoxicity to the brain from drug use, an important risk factor for addiction is the incidence of a traumatic brain injury (TBI). People who use substances are at a higher risk of experiencing a TBI, and research indicates that TBI may be a risk factor for the later onset of substance use disorders, although the evidence is still limited at this point (Bjork & Grant, 2009; Graham & Cardon, 2008).

Overall, there are substantial differences within people who develop substance use disorders behaviorally, functionally, physiologically, and genetically. Future research will help us to further individualize diagnoses and prognoses for this population to better treat these individuals.

The Relative Addictive Potential of Different Drugs: Societal Influences

Beyond neurobiology, there are societal trends across time and place indicating that certain drugs are "more addictive" than others. There is evidence to support that the perceived risk of a drug affects its use among the population (Bachman, Johnston & O'Malley, 1990). Currently, in the United States, we are facing an unprecedented number of deaths and reported substance use disorders involving opioids, with the

National Institute on Drug Abuse (NIDA) reporting over 30,000 opioid-related fatal overdoses in 2015 alone. Between 2001 and 2016, the United States opiate-related mortality rate increased by 345 percent (Gomes et al., 2018). Public policy recommendations from Gomes and colleagues include targeted programs to improve addiction care, as well as improving access and availability of harm reduction programs. It may seem that opioids are the most addictive substance in history. However, when we look back at the early 1980s, we see a very different story.

Cocaine was the most widely used illicit substance in the United States, and a 1986 Gallup Poll indicates that people felt that crack cocaine and other forms of cocaine were the most serious problem that society was facing in comparison to alcohol, heroin, and other drugs of abuse (Robinson, 2002). However, this problem was not equally prevalent throughout the population: blue-collar workers, men, and minorities were at a higher risk for mortality related to drug use – indicating that there is a relationship between public policies, social factors, and the severity of problems caused by drug use (Harlow, 1990). Cocaine had traditionally been a drug used mostly by the upper social class, but the introduction of crack cocaine (a cheaper and more potent substrate) resulted in a historical period effect wherein lower social classes began to use the drug at a much higher rate (Miech, Chilcoat & Harder, 2005). During this time, public attitude shifted, and the perceived risk of cocaine began to rise; use began to decline in the late 1980s and early 1990s, and according to NIDA has continued to go down as recently as 2013. This is not necessarily a cause for celebration: in the past decade, the number of people who have tried illicit drugs has increased, risk of infection (commonly Hepatitis C and HIV) from intravenous (IV)-drug use has increased, and risk of fatal overdose has increased (Hasin et al., 2015; Rudd et al., 2016; Spiller et al., 2015).

In contrast to the decline of cocaine use, the use of marijuana has been steadily on the rise since 2007 and is the most likely drug for first time users to try, according to NIDA. New state laws legalizing marijuana are likely to further increase the use of recreational marijuana, even as it remains federally illegal. Of even greater concern to public health, heroin and IV-drug use is also on the rise; the risk for infection and death from opioids is increasingly problematic as more potent synthetic opioids, such as fentanyl, go on the market. In contrast to cocaine use, which shifted from higher to lower socioeconomic circles, heroin has moved from urban areas with minority populations into suburban and rural areas with primarily white populations (Cicero et al., 2014). Fifty years ago, heroin users were primarily minority young adolescent males from low-income urban areas: today, users are more likely to be white, middle-class, either male or female, and in their early twenties (Cicero et al., 2014). Part of this change has been attributed to the marked increase in the abuse of prescription drugs, such as OxyContin (Compton & Volkow, 2006; Grau et al., 2007). The perceived risk of prescription drug use is lower than that of illicit substances. People tend to feel that prescription abuse is low-risk because doctors, the FDA, and the government have deemed prescribed opioids safe for human use (Daniulaityte, Falck & Carlson, 2012). Among people in treatment for drug abuse, 75 percent of heroin users stated that their first regular opioid was a prescription drug, in contrast to fifty years ago where over 75 percent of people in treatment stated that their first regular opioid was heroin (Cicero et al., 2014). Pharmaceutical companies tried to reduce the addictive liability of these drugs by making them more difficult to snort, inject, and breakdown. However, instead of quitting the substance, users turned to heroin, which created an entirely new problem (Cicero et al., 2014).

These two historical case studies on cocaine and heroin demonstrate important concepts to consider for the neurobiology of addiction. Drugs that vary in their subjective effect on the user (e.g., heroin and cocaine) do not have inherently differential liabilities for abuse among specific populations. Rather, it is more useful to look at public opinion, risk perception, drug policies, and public health when trying to determine what certain demographic and historical trends might mean. Looking at the failed "War on Drugs" that began in the 1980s in response to the crack cocaine crisis; the USA is now dealing with the aftermath: increased potential harm via injection, increased potency of commercially available substances, and an increase in the abuse of prescription drugs. The addictive potential for drugs does not rely solely upon their unique properties, but rather upon their shared neurobiological effects: increases in dopaminergic signaling, decreases in prefrontal cortical activity, and changes in the conscious valuation of interoceptive states.

Conclusions

Addiction occurs when there is an imbalance between three interacting neural systems: (1) a hyperactive, striatum-dependent (mesolimbic dopamine) neural system that promotes impulsive, automatic, and habitual behaviors; (2) a hypoactive, prefrontal cortex dependent neural system that reinforces the ability to inhibit impulses and resist stimuli that are rewarding in the short term, but lead to negative consequences in the long term; and (3) a relatively newly discovered system that seems to play a key role in modulating these previously described systems, the insular cortex, which is involved in translating homeostatic and interoceptive signals triggered by deprivation, or by exposure to reward cues, into craving and what may become subjectively experienced as an intense "urge" for a reward. The consequences of overactivation of the insular cortex are the intensification of the impulsive (striatum dependent) system and weakening of the reflective (prefrontal cortex dependent) system. These three interacting systems may also play a role in behavioral addictions as natural rewards – including sex and increased resources (money) – become problematic when they are pursued excessively, producing addictive behaviors such as gambling or sex addiction (see Turel & Bechara, 2016; Vaccarro & Potenza, 2020). These neurobiological studies have strong implications for researching new strategies to disrupt the vicious cycle of addiction.

REFERENCES

Ainslie, G. (1975). Specious reward: a behavioral theory of impulsiveness and impulse control. *Psychological Bulletin*, **82**(4), 463–496. http://doi.org/10.1037/h0076860

Amlung, M., Vedelago, L., Acker, J., Balodis, I. & MacKillop, J. (2017). Steep delay discounting and addictive behavior: a meta-analysis of continuous associations. *Addiction*, 112(1), 51–62. https://doi.org/10.1111/add.13535

Baca, C. T. & Grant, K. J. (2007). What heroin users tell us about overdose. *Journal of Addictive Diseases*, **26**(4), 63–68. http://doi.org/10.1300/J069v26n04_08

Bachman, J. G., Johnston, L. D. & O'Malley, P. M. (1990). Explaining the recent decline in cocaine use among young adults: further evidence that perceived risks and disapproval lead to reduced drug use. *Journal of Health and Social Behavior*, **31**(2), 173. http://doi.org/10.2307/2137171

Baxter, M. G. & Murray, E. A. (2002). The amygdala and reward. *Nature Reviews Neuroscience*. https://doi.org/10.1038/nrn875

Bayer, H. M. & Glimcher, P. W. (2005). Midbrain dopamine neurons encode a quantitative reward prediction error signal. *Neuron*, **47**(1), 129–141. http://doi.org/10.1016/J.NEURON.2005.05.020

Bechara, A. (2004). The role of emotion in decision-making: evidence from neurological patients with orbitofrontal damage. *Brain and Cognition*, **55**(1), 30–40.

Bechara, A. (2005). Decision making, impulse control and loss of willpower to resist drugs: a neurocognitive perspective. *Nature Neuroscience*, **8**(11), 1458–1463. http://doi.org/10.1038/nn1584

Bechara, A. & Naqvi, N. (2004). Listening to your heart: interoceptive awareness as a gateway to feeling. *Nature Neuroscience*, **7**(2), 102–103. http://doi.org/10.1038/nn0204-102

Bechara, A., Damasio, H., Tranel, D. & Damasio, A. R., et al. (1997). Deciding advantageously before knowing the advantageous strategy. *Science*, **275**(5304), 1293–1295. http://doi.org/10.1126/science.275.5304.1293

Bechara, A., Dolan, S., Denburg, N., et al. (2001). Decision-making deficits, linked to a dysfunctional ventromedial prefrontal cortex, revealed in alcohol and stimulant abusers. *Neuropsychologia*, **39**(4), 376–389. http://doi.org/10.1016/S0028-3932(00)00136-6

Belin, D., Jonkman, S., Dickinson, A., Robbins, T. W. & Everitt, B. J. (2009). Parallel and interactive learning processes within the basal ganglia: relevance for the understanding of addiction. *Behavioural Brain Research*, **199** (1), 89–102. http://doi.org/10.1016/J.BBR.2008.09.027

Berridge, K. C., Robinson, T. E. & Aldridge, J. W. (2009). Dissecting components of reward: "liking," "wanting," and learning. *Current Opinion in Pharmacology*, **9**(1), 65–73. http://doi.org/10.1016/J.COPH.2008.12.014

Bingel, U., Wanigasekera, V., Wiech, K., et al. (2011). The effect of treatment expectation on drug efficacy: imaging the analgesic benefit of the opioid remifentanil. *Science Translational Medicine*, **3**(70), 70ra14. http://doi.org/10.1126/scitranslmed.3001244

Bjork, J. M. & Grant, S. J. (2009). Does traumatic brain injury increase risk for substance abuse? *Journal of Neurotrauma*, **26** (7), 1077–1082. http://doi.org/http://dx.doi.org/10.1089/neu.2008.0849

Bowden-Jones, H., McPhillips, M., Rogers, R., Hutton, S. & Joyce, E. (2005). Risk-taking on tests sensitive to ventromedial prefrontal cortex dysfunction predicts early relapse in alcohol dependency: a pilot study. *The Journal of Neuropsychiatry and Clinical Neurosciences*, **17**(3), 417–420. https://doi.org/10.1176/jnp.17.3.417

Brody, A. L., Mandelkern, M. A., Olmstead, R. E., et al. (2009). Ventral striatal dopamine release in response to smoking a regular vs a denicotinized cigarette. *Neuropsychopharmacology*, **34**(2), 282–289. http://doi.org/10.1038/npp.2008.87

Carlson, R. W., Kumar, N. N., Wong-Mckinstry, E., et al. (2012). Alcohol withdrawal syndrome. *Critical Care Clinics*, **28**(4), 549–585. http://doi.org/10.1016/J.CCC.2012.07.004

Cicero, T. J., Ellis, M. S., Surratt, H. L. & Kurtz, S. P. (2014). The changing face of heroin use in the United States. *JAMA Psychiatry*, **71**(7), 821. http://doi.org/10.1001/jamapsychiatry.2014.366

Clewett, D., Luo, S., Hsu, E., et al. (2014). Increased functional coupling between the left fronto-parietal network and anterior insula predicts steeper delay discounting in smokers. *Human Brain Mapping*. https://doi.org/10.1002/hbm.22436

Compton, W. M. & Volkow, N. D. (2006). Abuse of prescription drugs and the risk of addiction. *Drug and Alcohol Dependence*, **83**, S4–S7. http://doi.org/10.1016/j.drugalcdep.2005.10.020

Corrigall, W. A., Coen, K. M. & Adamson, K. L. (1994). Self-administered nicotine activates the mesolimbic dopamine system through the ventral tegmental area. *Brain Research*, **653**(1–2), 278–284. http://doi.org/10.1016/0006-8993(94)90401-4

Craig, A. D. (2009). How do you feel – now? The anterior insula and human awareness. *Nature Reviews Neuroscience*, 10(1), 59–70. http://doi.org/10.1038/nrn2555

Craig, A. D. (2010). The sentient self. *Brain Structure and Function*, **214**(5–6), 563–577. http://doi.org/10.1007/s00429-010-0248-y

Crews, F., He, J. & Hodge, C. (2007). Adolescent cortical development: a critical period of vulnerability for addiction. *Pharmacology Biochemistry and Behavior*, **86**(2), 189–199. http://doi.org/10.1016/J.PBB.2006.12.001

Critchley, H. D., Wiens, S., Rotshtein, P., Öhman, A. & Dolan, R. J. (2004). Neural systems supporting interoceptive awareness. *Nature Neuroscience*, **7**(2), 189–195. http://doi.org/10.1038/nn1176

Dani, J. A. (2003). Roles of dopamine signaling in nicotine addiction. *Molecular Psychiatry*, **8** (3), 255–255. Retrieved from http://go.galegroup.com/ps/anonymous?id=GALE%7CA189963416&sid=googleScholar&v=2.1&it=r&linkaccess=fulltext&issn=13594184&p=AONE&sw=w&authCount=1&isAnonymousEntry=true

Daniulaityte, R., Falck, R. & Carlson, R. G. (2012). "I'm not afraid of those ones just 'cause they've been prescribed": perceptions of risk among illicit users of pharmaceutical opioids. *International Journal of Drug Policy*, **23**(5), 374–384. http://doi.org/10.1016/j.drugpo.2012.01.012

de la Fuente-Fernández, R., Phillips, A. G., Zamburlini, M., et al. (2002). Dopamine release in human ventral striatum and expectation of reward. *Behavioural Brain Research*, **136**(2), 359–363. http://doi.org/10.1016/S0166-4328(02)00130-4

Di Chiara, G., Bassareo, V., Fenu, S., et al. (2004). Dopamine and drug addiction: the nucleus accumbens shell connection. *Neuropharmacology*, **47**, 227–241. http://doi.org/10.1016/J.NEUROPHARM.2004.06.032

Droutman, V., Read, S. J. & Bechara, A. (2015). Revisiting the role of the insula in addiction. *Trends in Cognitive Sciences*, **19**(7), 414–420. http://doi.org/10.1016/J.TICS.2015.05.005

Everitt, B. J. & Robbins, T. W. (2005). Neural systems of reinforcement for drug addiction: from actions to habits to compulsion. *Nature Neuroscience*, **8**(11), 1481–1489. http://doi.org/10.1038/nn1579

Everitt, B. J., Belin, D., Economidou, D., et al. W. (2008). Review: neural mechanisms underlying the vulnerability to develop compulsive drug-seeking habits and addiction. *Philosophical Transactions of the Royal Society of London. Series B, Biological Sciences*, **363**(1507), 3125–3135. http://doi.org/10.1098/rstb.2008.0089

Fein, G., Di Sclafani, V. & Meyerhoff, D. J. (2002). Prefrontal cortical volume reduction associated with frontal cortex function deficit in 6-week abstinent crack-cocaine dependent men. *Drug and Alcohol Dependence*, **68**(1), 87–93. http://doi.org/10.1016/S0376-8716(02)00110-2

Fleckenstein, A. E., Metzger, R. R., Wilkins, D. G., Gibb, J. W. & Hanson, G. R. (1997). Rapid and reversible effects of methamphetamine on dopamine transporters. *Journal of Pharmacology and Experimental Therapeutics*, **282**(2), 834–838. Retrieved from http://jpet.aspetjournals.org/content/282/2/834.abstract

Franklin, T. R., Acton, P. D., Maldjian, J. A., et al. (2002). Decreased gray matter concentration in the insular, orbitofrontal, cingulate, and temporal cortices of cocaine patients. *Biological Psychiatry*, **51**(2), 134–142. http://doi.org/10.1016/S0006-3223(01)01269-0

Fu, L. ping, Bi, G. Hua, Zou, Z. tong, et al. (2008). Impaired response inhibition function in abstinent heroin dependents: an fMRI study. *Neuroscience Letters*, **438**(3), 322–326. https://doi.org/10.1016/j.neulet.2008.04.033

Garavan, H. & Hester, R. (2007). The role of cognitive control in cocaine dependence. *Neuropsychology Review*. https://doi.org/10.1007/s11065-007-9034-x

Gardner, E. L. (2002). Addictive potential of cannabinoids: the underlying neurobiology. *Chemistry and Physics of Lipids*, 121, 267–290. http://doi.org/10.1016/S0009-3084(02)00162-7

Gasquoine, P. G. (2014). Contributions of the insula to cognition and emotion. *Neuropsychology Review*, **24**(2),77–87. http://doi.org/10.1007/s11065-014-9246-9

Gessa, G., Melis, M., Muntoni, A. & Diana, M. (1998). Cannabinoids activate mesolimbic dopamine neurons by an action on cannabinoid CB1 receptors. *European Journal of Pharmacology*, **341**(1), 39–44. http://doi.org/10.1016/S0014-2999(97)01442-8

Gessa, G. L., Muntoni, F., Collu, M., Vargiu, L. & Mereu, G. (1985). Low doses of ethanol activate dopaminergic neurons in the ventral tegmental area. *Brain Research*, **348**(1), 201–203. http://doi.org/10.1016/0006-8993(85)90381-6

Goldman, D., Oroszi, G. & Ducci, F. (2005). The genetics of addictions: uncovering the genes. *Nature Reviews Genetics*, **6**(7), 521–532. http://doi.org/10.1038/nrg1635

Goldstein, R. Z. & Volkow, N. D. (2011). Dysfunction of the prefrontal cortex in addiction: neuroimaging findings and clinical implications. *Nature Reviews Neuroscience*. https://doi.org/10.1038/nrn3119

Gomes, T., Tadrous, M., Mamdani, M. M., Paterson, J. M. & Juurlink. D. N. (2018). The burden of opioid-related mortality in the United States. *JAMA Network Open*, **1**(2), e180217. doi:10.1001/jamanetworkopen.2018.0217

Goudriaan, A. E., De Ruiter, M. B., Van Den Brink, W., Oosterlaan, J. & Veltman, D. J. (2010). Brain activation patterns associated with cue reactivity and craving in abstinent problem gamblers, heavy smokers and healthy controls: an fMRI study. *Addiction Biology*, **15**(4), 491–503. https://doi.org/10.1111/j.1369-1600.2010.00242.x

Graham, D. P. & Cardon, A. L. (2008). An update on substance use and treatment following traumatic brain injury. *Annals of the New York Academy of Sciences*, **1141**, 148–162. http://doi.org/10.1196/annals.1441.029

Grant, S., Contoreggi, C. & London, E. D. (2000). Drug abusers show impaired performance in a laboratory test of decision making. *Neuropsychologia*. https://doi.org/10.1016/S0028-3932(99)00158-X

Grau, L. E., Dasgupta, N., Harvey, A. P., et al. (2007). Illicit use of opioids: is OxyContin® a "gateway drug"? *American Journal on Addictions*, **16**(3), 166–173. http://doi.org/10.1080/10550490701375293

Gray, M. A. & Critchley, H. D. (2007). Interoceptive basis to craving. *Neuron*, 54(2), 183–186. http://doi.org/10.1016/j.neuron.2007.03.024

Harlow, K. C. (1990). Patterns of rates of mortality from narcotics and cocaine overdose in Texas, 1976–87. *Public Health Reports (Washington, D.C. : 1974)*, **105**(5), 455–462. Retrieved from www.ncbi.nlm.nih.gov/pubmed/2120721

Hasin, D. S., Saha, T. D., Kerridge, B. T., et al. (2015). Prevalence of marijuana use disorders in the United States between 2001–2002 and 2012–2013. *JAMA Psychiatry*, **72**(12), 1235. http://doi.org/10.1001/jamapsychiatry.2015.1858

Hassan, S. F., Wearne, T. A., Cornish, J. L. & Goodchild, A. K. (2016). Effects of acute and chronic systemic methamphetamine on respiratory, cardiovascular and metabolic function, and cardiorespiratory reflexes. *The Journal of Physiology*, **594**(3), 763–780. http://doi.org/10.1113/JP271257

Heinz, A., Siessmeier, T., Wrase, J., et al. Correlation between dopamine D2 receptors in the ventral striatum and central processing of alcohol cues and craving. *American Journal of Psychiatry*, **161**(10), 1783–1789. http://doi.org/10.1176/ajp.161.10.1783

Herz, A. (1997). Endogenous opioid systems and alcohol addiction. *Psychopharmacology*, **129**(2), 99–111. http://doi.org/10.1007/s002130050169

Hester, R. & Garavan, H. (2004). Executive dysfunction in cocaine addiction: evidence for discordant frontal, cingulate, and cerebellar activity. *Journal of Neuroscience*, **24**(49), 11017–11022. https://doi.org/10.1523/JNEUROSCI.3321-04.2004

Hill, J. C. & Toffolon, G. (1990). Effect of alcohol on sensory and sensorimotor visual functions. *Journal of Studies on Alcohol*, **51**(2), 108–113. http://doi.org/10.15288/jsa.1990.51.108

Hinson, J. M., Jameson, T. L. & Whitney, P. (2003). Impulsive decision making and working memory. *Journal of Experimental Psychology: Learning, Memory, and Cognition*, **29**(2), 298–306. http://doi.org/10.1037/0278-7393.29.2.298

Huang, Z.-L., Qu, W.-M., Eguchi, N., et al. (2005). Adenosine A2A, but not A1, receptors mediate the arousal effect of caffeine. *Nature Neuroscience*, **8**(7), 858–859. http://doi.org/10.1038/nn1491

Ito, R., Dalley, J. W., Robbins, T. W. & Everitt, B. J. (2002). Dopamine release in the dorsal striatum during cocaine-seeking behavior under the control of a drug-associated cue. *The Journal of Neuroscience*, **22**(14), 6247 LP-6253. Retrieved from www.jneurosci.org/content/22/14/6247.abstract

Janes, A. C., Pizzagalli, D. A., Richardt, S., et al. (2010). Neural substrates of attentional bias for smoking-related Cues: an fMRI study. *Neuropsychopharmacology*. https://doi.org/10.1038/npp.2010.103

Jarmolowicz, D. P. & Schneider, T. D. (2020). Behavioral economics and addictive disorders. In S. Sussman (Ed.) *The Cambridge Handbook of Substance and Behavioral Addictions*. Cambridge, UK: Cambridge University Press, pp. 12–22.

Johnson, M. W., Bickel, W. K. & Kirshenbaum, A. P. (2004). Substitutes for tobacco smoking: A behavioral economic analysis of nicotine gum, denicotinized cigarettes, and nicotine-containing cigarettes. *Drug and Alcohol Dependence*, **74**(3), 253–264. http://doi.org/10.1016/j.drugalcdep.2003.12.012

Kaasinen, V., Aalto, S., Nagren, K. & Rinne, J. O. (2004). Expectation of caffeine induces dopaminergic responses in humans. *European Journal of Neuroscience*, **19**(8), 2352–2356. http://doi.org/10.1111/j.1460-9568.2004.03310.x

Kaufman, J. N., Ross, T. J., Stein, E. A. & Garavan, H. (2003). Cingulate hypoactivity in cocaine users during a GO-NOGO task as revealed by event-related functional magnetic resonance imaging. *Journal of Neuroscience*, **23**(21), 7839–7843. https://doi.org/10.1523/jneurosci.23-21-07839.2003

Khantzian, E. J. (1987). The self-medication hypothesis of addictive disorders: focus on heroin and cocaine dependence. In *The Cocaine Crisis*. Boston, MA: Springer US, pp. 65–74. http://doi.org/10.1007/978-1-4613-1837-8_7

Kirby, K. N., Petry, N. M. & Bickel, W. K. (1999). Heroin addicts have higher discount rates for delayed rewards than non-drug-using controls. *Journal of Experimental Psychology: General*, **128**(1), 78–87. http://doi.org/10.1037/0096-3445.128.1.78

Koneru, A., Satyanarayana, S. & Rizwan, S. (2009). Endogenous opioids: their physiological role and receptors. *Global Journal of Pharmacology*, **3**(3), 149–153. Retrieved from https://pdfs.semanticscholar.org/e83a/851842f363f7e7f561c5ca465df9578d6bbc.pdf

Koob, G. F. & Volkow, N. D. (2010). Neurocircuitry of addiction. *Neuropsychopharmacology*, **35**(1), 217–238. http://doi.org/10.1038/npp.2009.110

Kringelbach, M. L. (2005). The human orbitofrontal cortex: linking reward to hedonic experience. *Nature Reviews Neuroscience*, **6**(9), 691–702. http://doi.org/10.1038/nrn1747

Krishnan-Sarin, S., Reynolds, B., Duhig, A. M., et al. (2007). Behavioral impulsivity predicts treatment outcome in a smoking cessation program for adolescent smokers. *Drug and Alcohol Dependence*, **88**(1), 79–82. https://doi.org/10.1016/j.drugalcdep.2006.09.006

Lin, S.-K., Pan, W. H. T. & Yeh, P.-H. (2007). Prefrontal dopamine efflux during exposure to drug-associated contextual cues in rats with prior repeated methamphetamine. *Brain Research Bulletin*, **71**(4), 365–371. http://doi.org/10.1016/J.BRAINRESBULL.2006.10.001

Marinkovic, K., Halgren, E. & Maltzman, I. (2004). Effects of alcohol on verbal processing: An event-related potential study. *Alcoholism: Clinical & Experimental Research*, **28**(3), 415–423. http://doi.org/10.1097/01.ALC.0000117828.88597.80

Mechtcheriakov, S., Brenneis, C., Egger, K., et al. (2007). A widespread distinct pattern of cerebral atrophy in patients with alcohol addiction revealed by voxel-based morphometry. *Journal of Neurology, Neurosurgery, and Psychiatry*, **78**(6), 610–614. http://doi.org/10.1136/jnnp.2006.095869

Melis, M., Pistis, M., Perra, S., et al. (2004). Endocannabinoids mediate presynaptic inhibition of glutamatergic transmission in rat ventral tegmental area dopamine neurons through activation of CB1 receptors. *The Journal of Neuroscience: The Official Journal of the Society for Neuroscience*, **24**(1), 53–62. http://doi.org/10.1523/JNEUROSCI.4503-03.2004

Miech, R. A., Chilcoat, H. & Harder, V. S. (2005). The increase in the association of education and cocaine use over the 1980s and 1990s: Evidence for a "historical period" effect. *Drug and Alcohol Dependence*, **79**(3), 311–320. http://doi.org/10.1016/J.DRUGALCDEP.2005.01.022

Molina-Luna, K., Pekanovic, A., Röhrich, S., et al. (2009). Dopamine in motor cortex is necessary for skill learning and synaptic plasticity. *PLoS ONE*, **4**(9), e7082. http://doi.org/10.1371/journal.pone.0007082

Monterosso, J. R., Ainslie, G., Xu, J., et al. (2007). Frontoparietal cortical activity of methamphetamine-dependent and comparison subjects performing a delay discounting task. *Human Brain Mapping*, **28**(5), 383–393. http://doi.org/10.1002/hbm.20281

Monterosso, J. R., Aron, A. R., Cordova, X., Xu, J. & London, E. D. (2005). Deficits in response inhibition associated with chronic methamphetamine abuse. *Drug and Alcohol Dependence*. https://doi.org/10.1016/j.drugalcdep.2005.02.002

Naqvi, N. H. & Bechara, A. (2005). The airway sensory impact of nicotine contributes to the conditioned reinforcing effects of individual puffs from cigarettes. *Pharmacology Biochemistry and Behavior*, **81**(4), 821–829. http://doi.org/10.1016/j.pbb.2005.06.005

Naqvi, N. H. & Bechara, A. (2009). The hidden island of addiction: the insula. *Trends in Neurosciences*, **32**(1), 56–67. http://doi.org/10.1016/j.tins.2008.09.009

Naqvi, N. H. & Bechara, A. (2010). The insula and drug addiction: an interoceptive view of pleasure, urges, and decision-making. *Brain Structure and Function*, **214**(5–6), 435–450. http://doi.org/10.1007/s00429-010-0268-7

Naqvi, N. H., Rudrauf, D., Damasio, H. & Bechara, A. (2007). Damage to the insula disrupts addiction to cigarette smoking. *Science (New York, N.Y.)*, **315**(5811), 531–534. http://doi.org/10.1126/science.1135926

Nash, J. F. & Yamamoto, B. K. (1992). Methamphetamine neurotoxicity and striatal glutamate release: comparison to 3, 4-methylenedioxymethamphetamine. *Brain Research*, **581**(2), 237–243. http://doi.org/10.1016/0006-8993(92)90713-J

Nestler, E. J. (2005). The neurobiology of cocaine addiction. *Science & Practice Perspectives*, **3**(1), 4–10. Retrieved from www.ncbi.nlm.nih.gov/pubmed/18552739

Noël, X., Brevers, D. & Bechara, A. (2013). A triadic neurocognitive approach to addiction for clinical interventions. *Frontiers in Psychiatry*, **4**, 179. http://doi.org/10.3389/fpsyt.2013.00179

Oswald, L. M., Wong, D. F., McCaul, M., et al. (2005). Relationships among ventral striatal dopamine release, cortisol secretion and subjective responses to amphetamine. *Neuropsychopharmacology*, **30**(4), 821–832. http://doi.org/10.1038/sj.npp.1300667

Paraskevaides, T., Morgan, C. J. A., Leitz, J. R., et al. (2010). Drinking and future thinking: acute effects of alcohol on prospective memory and future simulation. *Psychopharmacology*, **208**(2), 301–308. http://doi.org/10.1007/s00213-009-1731-0

Pertwee, R. (2010). S.27.01 Pharmacological actions of cannabinoids. *European Neuropsychopharmacology*, **20**, S205. http://doi.org/10.1016/S0924-977X(10)70232-7

Phillips, A. G. & Fibiger, H. C. (1979). Decreased resistance to extinction after haloperidol: implications for the role of dopamine in reinforcement. *Pharmacology Biochemistry and Behavior*, **10**(5), 751–760. http://doi.org/10.1016/0091-3057(79)90328-9

Pidoplichko, V. I., DeBiasi, M., Williams, J. T. & Dani, J. A. (1997). Nicotine activates and desensitizes midbrain dopamine neurons. *Nature*, **390**(6658), 401–404. http://doi.org/10.1038/37120

Pierce, R. C. & Kumaresan, V. (2006). The mesolimbic dopamine system: the final common pathway for the reinforcing effect of drugs of abuse? *Neuroscience & Biobehavioral Reviews*, **30**(2), 215–238. http://doi.org/10.1016/J.NEUBIOREV.2005.04.016

Porkka-Heiskanen, T., Strecker, R., Thakkar, M., Bjorkum, A. & Greene, R. (1997). Adenosine: a mediator of the sleep-inducing effects of prolonged wakefulness. *Science*, **276**(5316), 1265–1268. http://doi.org/10.1126/science.276.5316.1265

Robbe, D., Kopf, M., Remaury, A., Bockaert, J. & Manzoni, O. J. (2002). Endogenous cannabinoids mediate long-term synaptic depression in the nucleus accumbens. *Proceedings of the National Academy of Sciences of the United States of America*, **99**(12), 8384–8. http://doi.org/10.1073/pnas.122149199

Robbins, T. W., Ersche, K. D. & Everitt, B. J. (2008). Drug addiction and the memory systems of the brain. *Annals of the New York Academy of Sciences*, **1141**(1), 1–21. http://doi.org/10.1196/annals.1441.020

Robinson, J. (2002). *Decades of Drug Use: The '80s and '90s*. Retrieved January 10, 2018, from http://news.gallup.com/poll/6352/decades-drug-use-80s-90s.aspx

Robinson, S., Sandstrom, S. M., Denenberg, V. H. & Palmiter, R. D. (2005). Distinguishing whether dopamine regulates liking, wanting, and/or learning about rewards. *Behavioral Neuroscience*, **119**(1), 5–15. http://doi.org/10.1037/0735-7044.119.1.5

Robinson, T. E. & Berridge, K. C. (1993). The neural basis of drug craving: an incentive-sensitization theory of addiction. *Brain Research Reviews*, **18**(3), 247–291. http://doi.org/10.1016/0165-0173(93)90013-P

Robinson, T. E. & Berridge, K. C. (2001). Incentive-sensitization and addiction. *Addiction*, **96**(1), 103–114. http://doi.org/10.1046/j.1360-0443.2001.9611038.x

Roozendaal, B., McReynolds, J. R. & McGaugh, J. L. (2004). The basolateral amygdala interacts with the medial prefrontal cortex in regulating glucocorticoid effects on working memory impairment. *The Journal of Neuroscience*, **24**(6), 1385 LP–1392. Retrieved from www.jneurosci.org/content/24/6/1385.abstract

Rossetti, Z. L., Hmaidan, Y. & Gessa, G. L. (1992). Marked inhibition of mesolimbic dopamine release: a common feature of ethanol, morphine, cocaine and amphetamine abstinence in rats. *European Journal of Pharmacology*, **221**(2–3), 227–234. http://doi.org/10.1016/0014-2999(92)90706-A

Rudd, R. A., Aleshire, N., Zibbell, J. E. & Matthew Gladden, R. (2016). Increases in drug and opioid overdose deaths – United States, 2000–2014. *American Journal of Transplantation*, **16**(4), 1323–1327. http://doi.org/10.1111/ajt.13776

Samanez-Larkin, G. R., Hollon, N. G., Carstensen, L. L. & Knutson, B. (2008). Individual differences in insular sensitivity during loss: anticipation predict avoidance learning: research report. *Psychological Science*, **19**(4), 320–323. http://doi.org/10.1111/j.1467-9280.2008.02087.x

Schmidt, A., Borgwardt, S., Gerber, H., et al. (2014). Acute effects of heroin on negative emotional processing: relation of amygdala activity and stress-related responses. *Biological Psychiatry*, **76**(4), 289–296. http://doi.org/10.1016/j.biopsych.2013.10.019

Schoenbaum, G. & Shaham, Y. (2008). The role of orbitofrontal cortex in drug addiction: a review of preclinical studies. *Biological Psychiatry*, **63**(3), 256–262. http://doi.org/10.1016/J.BIOPSYCH.2007.06.003

Schoenbaum, G., Roesch, M. R. & Stalnaker, T. A. (2006). Orbitofrontal cortex, decision-making and drug addiction. *Trends in Neurosciences*, **29**(2), 116–124. http://doi.org/10.1016/j.tins.2005.12.006

Schultz, W. (1998). Predictive reward signal of dopamine neurons. *Journal of Neurophysiology*, **80**(1), 1–27. http://doi.org/10.1152/jn.1998.80.1.1

Sell, L. A., Morris, J. S., Bearn, J., et al. (2000). Neural responses associated with cue evoked emotional states and heroin in opiate addicts. *Drug and Alcohol Dependence*, **60**(2), 207–216. http://doi.org/10.1016/S0376-8716(99)00158-1

Seymour, B., Daw, N., Dayan, P., Singer, T. & Dolan, R. (2007). Differential encoding of losses and gains in the human striatum. *Journal of Neuroscience*, **27**(18), 4826–4831. http://doi.org/10.1523/JNEUROSCI.0400-07.2007

Shen, M., Piser, T. M., Seybold, V. S., et al. (1996). Cannabinoid receptor agonists inhibit glutamatergic synaptic transmission in rat hippocampal cultures. *The Journal of Neuroscience : The Official Journal of the Society for Neuroscience*, **16**(14), 4322–4334. Retrieved from www.ncbi.nlm.nih.gov/pubmed/8699243

Singer, T., Critchley, H. D. & Preuschoff, K. (2009). A common role of insula in feelings, empathy and uncertainty. *Trends in Cognitive Sciences*, **13**(8), 334–340. http://doi.org/10.1016/j.tics.2009.05.001

Solinas, M., Ferré, S., You, Z.-B., et al. (2002). Caffeine induces dopamine and glutamate release in the shell of the nucleus accumbens. *The Journal of Neuroscience*, **22**(15), 6321 LP-6324. Retrieved from www.jneurosci.org/content/22/15/6321.abstract

Spanagel, R., Herz, A. & Shippenberg, T. S. (1992). Opposing tonically active endogenous opioid systems modulate the mesolimbic dopaminergic pathway (mirodialysis/nucleus accumbens/dopamine release and metabolism/opiate dependence). *Pharmacology*, **89**, 2046–2050. Retrieved from www.pnas.org/content/89/6/2046.full.pdf

Spiller, M. W., Broz, D., Wejnert, C., Nerlander, L., Paz-Bailey, G., Centers for Disease Control and Prevention (CDC), & National HIV Behavioral Surveillance System Study Group. (2015). HIV infection and HIV-associated behaviors among persons who inject drugs – 20 cities, United States, 2012. *Morbidity and Mortality Weekly Report*, **64**(10), 270–275. Retrieved from www.ncbi.nlm.nih.gov/pubmed/25789742

Stacy, A. W. & Wiers, R. W. (2010). Implicit cognition and addiction: a tool for explaining paradoxical behavior. *Annual Review of Clinical Psychology*, **6**(1), 551–575. http://doi.org/10.1146/annurev.clinpsy.121208.131444

Stacy, A. W., Pike, J. & Lee, A. Y. (2020). Multiple memory systems, addiction, and health habits: new routes for translational science. In S. Sussman (Ed.) *The Cambridge Handbook of Substance and Behavioral Addictions*. Cambridge, UK: Cambridge University Press, pp. 152–170.

Tanda, G., Pontieri, F. E. & Di Chiara, G. (1997). Cannabinoid and heroin activation of mesolimbic dopamine transmission by a common mu1 opioid receptor mechanism. *Science (New York, N.Y.)*, **276**(5321), 2048–50. http://doi.org/10.1126/SCIENCE.276.5321.2048

The Heroin Hug | Absolute Advocacy. (n.d.). Retrieved January 10, 2020, from www.absoluteadvocacy.org/the-heroin-hug/

Thompson, P. M., Hayashi, K. M., Simon, S. L., et al. (2004). Structural abnormalities in the brains of human subjects who use methamphetamine. *The Journal of Neuroscience*, **24**(26), 6028 LP-6036. Retrieved from www.jneurosci.org/content/24/26/6028.abstract

Turcotte, C., Blanchet, M.-R., Laviolette, M. & Flamand, N. (2016). Impact of cannabis, cannabinoids, and endocannabinoids in the lungs. *Frontiers in Pharmacology*, **7**, 317. http://doi.org/10.3389/fphar.2016.00317

Turel, O. & Bechara, A. (2016). A triadic reflective-impulsive-interoceptive awareness model of general and impulsive information system use: behavioral tests of neuro-cognitive theory. *Frontiers in Psychology*, **7**, 601. http://doi.org/10.3389/fpsyg.2016.00601

Vaccarro, A. G. & Potenza, M. N. (2020). Neurobiological foundations of behavioral addictions. In S. Sussman (Ed.) *The Cambridge Handbook of Substance and Behavioral Addictions*. Cambridge, UK: Cambridge University Press, pp. 136–151.

Villafuerte, S., Heitzeg, M. M., Foley, S., et al. (2012). Impulsiveness and insula activation during reward anticipation are associated with genetic variants in GABRA2 in a family sample enriched for alcoholism. *Molecular Psychiatry*, **17**(5), 511–519. http://doi.org/10.1038/mp.2011.33

Volkow, N. D. & Fowler, J. S. (2000). Addiction, a disease of compulsion and drive: involvement of the orbitofrontal cortex. *Cerebral Cortex*, **10**(3), 318–325. http://doi.org/10.1093/cercor/10.3.318

Volkow, N. D., Chang, L., Wang, G.-J., et al. (2001). Loss of dopamine transporters in methamphetamine abusers recovers with protracted abstinence. *The Journal of Neuroscience*, **21**(23), 9414–9418. Retrieved from www.jneurosci.org/content/21/23/9414.abstract

Volkow, N. D., Fowler, J. S., Wang, G.-J. & Swanson, J. M. (2004). Dopamine in drug abuse and addiction: results from imaging studies and treatment implications. *Molecular Psychiatry*, **9**(6), 557–569. http://doi.org/10.1038/sj.mp.4001507

Volkow, N. D., Wang, G.-J., Fowler, J. S., et al. (1996). Decreases in dopamine receptors but not in dopamine transporters in alcoholics. *Alcoholism: Clinical and Experimental Research*, **20**(9), 1594–1598. http://doi.org/10.1111/j.1530-0277.1996.tb05936.x

Volkow, N. D., Wang, G.-J., Telang, F., et al. (2008). Dopamine increases in striatum do not elicit craving in cocaine abusers unless they are coupled with cocaine cues. *NeuroImage*, **39**(3), 1266–1273. http://doi.org/10.1016/J.NEUROIMAGE.2007.09.059

Wager, T. D., Davidson, M. L., Hughes, B. L., Lindquist, M. A. & Ochsner, K. N. (2008). Prefrontal-subcortical pathways mediating successful emotion regulation. *Neuron*, **59**(6), 1037–1050. http://doi.org/10.1016/J.NEURON.2008.09.006

Wang, Y., Zhu, L., Zou, Q., et al. (2018). Frequency dependent hub role of the dorsal and ventral right anterior insula. *NeuroImage*, **165**, 112–117. https://doi.org/10.1016/j.neuroimage.2017.10.004

Warlow, S. M., et al. (2020). Sensitization of incentive salience and the transition to addiction. In S. Sussman (Ed.) *The Cambridge Handbook of Substance and Behavioral*

Addictions. Cambridge, UK: Cambridge University Press, pp. 23–37.

Watson, P., de **Wit, S.**, **Hommel, B. & Wiers, R. W.** (2012). Motivational mechanisms and outcome expectancies underlying the approach bias toward addictive substances. *Frontiers in Psychology*, **3**, 440. http://doi.org/10.3389/fpsyg.2012.00440

Westman, E. C., Behm, F. M. & Rose, J. E. (1995). Airway sensory replacement combined with nicotine replacement for smoking cessation: a randomized, placebo-controlled trial using a citric acid inhaler. *Chest*, **107**(5), 1358–1364. http://doi.org/10.1378/CHEST.107.5.1358

Westman, E. C., Behm, F. M. & Rose, J. E. (1996). Dissociating the nicotine and airway sensory effects of smoking. *Pharmacology Biochemistry and Behavior*, **53**(2), 309–315. http://doi.org/10.1016/0091-3057(95)02027-6

What does it feel like to use cocaine? | Drug Policy Alliance. (n.d.). Retrieved January 9, 2020, from www.drugpolicy.org/drug-facts/cocaine/what-cocaine-feels-like

Wise, R. A. (1996). Neurobiology of addiction. *Current Opinion in Neurobiology*, 6(2), 243–251. http://doi.org/10.1016/S0959-4388(96)80079-1

Yuan, Y., Zhu, Z., Shi, J., et al. (2009). Gray matter density negatively correlates with duration of heroin use in young lifetime heroin-dependent individuals. *Brain and Cognition*, **71**(3), 223–228. http://doi.org/10.1016/J.BANDC.2009.08.014

11 Neurobiological Foundations of Behavioral Addictions

Anthony G. Vaccaro, MRes, and Marc N. Potenza, MD, PhD

Introduction: Behavioral Addictions

Several decades ago, the term *addiction* was used at times to refer exclusively to excessive/interfering patterns of substance use behaviors. However, this notion has been challenged more recently, with some nonsubstance use behaviors (e.g., gambling, gaming) being recognized as addictive behavior disorders by the World Health Organization in the eleventh edition of the *International Classification of Diseases* (ICD-11; see https://icd.who.int/browse11/l-m/en#/http://id.who.int/icd/entity/1041487064, accessed January 31, 2019). Although cognitive and epidemiological research showed some initial evidence for classifying some nonsubstance-related behaviors as addictions, neurobiological data have been more recently obtained to further support similarities. In the past two decades, neurobiological studies on behaviors such as gambling, video gaming, and pornography use, among others, have increased, allowing problematic engagement of these behaviors to be compared to substance addictions. Gambling disorder has, since 2013, been categorized together with substance use disorders in the *Diagnostic and Statistical Manual of Mental Disorders* (DSM; currently DSM-5) based on existing evidence, and Internet Gaming Disorder is recognized in DSM-5 as a possible condition warranting additional research. In this chapter, the current state of the neurobiological literature on nonsubstance addictions will be reviewed, with special attention as to how their neurobiological correlates relate to substance addictions.

Gambling Disorder

Gambling involves risking something of value for the hopes of receiving something more valuable. Gambling behaviors appear to predate written record (Schwartz, 2013). While most people gamble, a minority develops problems relating to gambling. It is estimated that up to approximately 5 percent of gamblers may go on to develop gambling problems (Potenza, 2013a), with lifetime prevalence of gambling disorder in the United States estimated at 0.4–0.6 percent and past-year prevalence estimated at 0.2–0.3 percent (Kessler et al., 2008; Petry, Stinson & Grant, 2005).

The recognition of problematic gambling as a psychiatric condition is not new. Pathological gambling was added to DSM-III in 1980 and classified as an "Impulse Control Disorder Not Elsewhere Classified." When gambling was initially added to this category, its classification was largely based on clinical observations. As more empirical research was performed on pathological gambling, findings suggested that the cognitive mechanisms associated with pathological gambling were more complex and involved more than impulsivity. Neurobiological research supported this notion, showing parallels between the neurocognitive correlates of substance use disorders and pathological gambling, including compulsive features and correlates of craving, reward processing, executive control and other constructs (Leeman & Potenza, 2012). In light of accumulating neurobiological evidence, gambling disorder was reclassified in DSM-5 in the category of Substance-Related and Addictive Disorders as the only nonsubstance-related disorder in the category.

The DSM-5 criteria for gambling disorder include: (1) the need to gamble for more money over time; (2) irritability when reducing gambling; (3) unsuccessful attempts to curb gambling behaviors; (4) preoccupation and persistent thoughts about gambling; (5) gambling as a coping mechanism for relieving stress, anxiety or dysphoria; (6) chasing one's losses by gambling in an attempt to win back what was recently lost gambling; (7) lying to conceal gambling behavior; (8) jeopardizing relationships or career or educational opportunities due to gambling; and (9) relying on others for money to relieve desperate financial situations due to gambling (American Psychiatric Association, 2013). An exclusionary criterion exists, stating that gambling is not better explained by manic behavior. An individual is required to meet four or more of the inclusion criteria to receive a diagnosis of gambling disorder. Many of the inclusion criteria are adapted from substance use disorders, and, as can be seen in the rest of this section, the neurobiology of gambling disorder shares similarities with those of substance use disorders.

Neurochemistry of Gambling Disorder

Multiple neurochemical systems have been implicated in gambling disorder. Several relevant neurotransmitter systems are reviewed below.

Dopamine. Dopamine has been relatively extensively researched in addictive behaviors. Dopaminergic mesolimbic circuitries have been proposed as the underlying substrates of reward expectation and motivation toward addictive stimuli (Everitt & Robbins, 2005). The extent to which dopamine contributes prominently to gambling disorder has been debated (Potenza, 2013b, 2018). Between-group differences in D2-like dopamine receptors in the striatum that early studies posited may be central to addictions have not been observed in individuals with gambling disorder (Nutt et al., 2015), with a possible exception being in Parkinson's disease (Steeves et al., 2009), a disorder characterized by loss of dopaminergic neurons. In Parkinson's disease, D2-like dopamine agonists have been associated with pathological gambling (Lee et al., 2010; Weintraub & Claassen, 2017; Weintraub et al., 2010; Voon et al., 2011). However, other factors have also been associated with gambling disorders and other impulse control disorders/behaviors in individuals with Parkinson's disease. These factors include age of Parkinson's disease onset, personal history of an impulse control disorder prior to Parkinson's disease onset, marital status and geographic location (Potenza, 2013b). As such, the etiology of gambling disorder in Parkinson's disease is likely complex and multifactorial. Consistently, potential relationships between mesolimbic dopamine and addictive behaviors are arguably more nuanced than originally conceived. A [^{11}C]raclopride positron emission topography (PET) study found that upon winning slot-machine rewards, individuals with gambling disorder had similar levels of striatal dopamine release as healthy control subjects, but in the group with gambling disorder the level of dopamine released correlated with gambling severity (Joutsa et al., 2012). This evidence is arguably counter to reward deficiency hypotheses that may attribute tolerance to decreased dopamine release. Ventral striatal dopamine release during the Iowa Gambling Task has also been found to positively correlate with excitement level in pathological gamblers (Linnet et al., 2011).

Other studies have focused not on the concentration of mesolimbic released dopamine, but on its binding efficiency, and the availability of receptors for binding. A [^{11}C]-raclopride PET study of D(2)/D(3) receptor availability in the striatum found no differences between individuals with and without pathological gambling, in contrast to previous studies of drug addictions (especially to stimulants), although impulsivity was correlated with receptor availability in the group with pathological gambling (Clark et al., 2012). A separate study using a D3-preferring ligand found that D2-like receptor density positively correlated with the severity of pathological gambling (Boileau et al., 2013). While the D3 dopamine receptor has been proposed to be linked to relapse, and reward-induced and stress-induced motivation toward addictive stimuli in substance use disorders (Heidbreder et al., 2005), the above findings should be viewed very cautiously as they typically involve very small samples, do not observe between-group differences (and when observed have at times not been replicated; Potenza (2018), and when reporting positive findings, typically involve correlations with small within-group samples.

Serotonin. Serotoninergic functioning has been implicated in gambling disorder. Individuals with pathological gambling as compared to those without have been found to have lower cerebrospinal fluid levels of a serotonin metabolite (5-HIAA; Nordin & Eklundh, 1999). Other work has investigated directly how serotonergic drugs may induce neuroendocrine changes. When a 0.5 mg/kg oral dose of meta-chlorophenylpiperazine (m-CPP), a drug predominantly acting as a partial agonist at 5HT2 and 5HT1 receptors, was administered to twenty-six individuals with pathological gambling and twenty-six individuals without the condition in a double-blind, placebo-controlled manner, individuals with pathological gambling exhibited a subjective "high" 180 minutes after administration, unlike healthy control subjects (Pallanti et al., 2006). Furthermore, plasma testing showed that individuals with pathological gambling had significantly higher m-CPP-induced prolactin release, and this release correlated with problem-gambling severity as measured by the Yale–Brown Obsessive Compulsive Scale modified for Pathological Gambling (PG-YBOCS). These data suggest that differences exist in biochemical and subjective responses to serotonergic drugs in individuals with pathological gambling, but do not address specifically where in the neurotransmitter systems such differences may arise. A recent PET study using [^{11}C]-N,N-dimethyl-2-(2-amino-4-methylphenyl thio)benzylamine (a serotonin transporter tracer) failed to find differences in serotonin transporter binding between individuals with and without pathological gambling (Majuri et al., 2017a, 2017b). A PET study using [^{11}C]P943, a selective partial serotonin antagonist tracer, found that the density of 1B serotonin receptors in the ventral striatum and anterior cingulate cortex (ACC) correlated with problem-gambling severity as measured by the South Oaks Gambling Screen, although group differences between individuals with and without pathological gambling behaviors were not observed in this small, preliminary study (Potenza et al., 2013b).

Norepinephrine. Several studies have implicated norepinephrine in gambling disorder, possibly as a means of increased arousal during gambling contexts. Individuals with pathological gambling have been found to have higher cerebrospinal fluid concentrations of 3-methoxy-4-hyroxyphenylglycol, a norepinephrine metabolite (Roy et al., 1988). The level of cerebrospinal fluid MHPG in individuals with pathological gambling has also been found to correlate with levels of extraversion as measured by the Eyesenk Personality Questionnaire (Roy, De Jong & Linnoila, 1989). In a task-based study, both individuals with and without pathological gambling demonstrated increased norepinephrine at the start of gambling activities; however, individuals with pathological gambling maintained higher norepinephrine levels through the entire gambling session (Meyer et al., 2004).

Opioids. Data suggest differences in endogenous opioid activity in gambling disorder. Individuals with pathological gambling may have blunted opioid release and lower receptor availability when compared to individuals without pathological gambling (Majuri et al., 2017; Mick et al., 2016). These preliminary studies suggest possible mechanisms by which opioid receptor antagonists may operate in gambling disorder (see the pharmacological treatment section below).

Pharmacological Treatment of Gambling Disorder

There are currently no medications with an indication from the US Food and Drug Administration (FDA) for gambling disorder. Trials have been conducted investigating various pharmacotherapies for gambling disorder, and initial guidelines based on cooccurring disorders have been proposed (Bullock & Potenza, 2012; Yip & Potenza, 2014).

Dopaminergic. Dopaminergic antagonists have not been found to have clinical utility in treating gambling disorder. Two double-blind trials of olanzapine, a D2-like dopamine receptor antagonist, found no differences in improvement between active and placebo groups (Fong et al., 2008; McElroy et al., 2008). A study investigating the effects of haloperidol, another D2-like dopamine receptor antagonist, found increases in gambling motivations in individuals with pathological gambling, though not in participants without the disorder (Zack & Poulos, 2007). Another medication with dopaminergic properties is bupropion, a drug that is a dopamine-norepineprhine reuptake inhibitor. A twelve-week flexible-dose randomized double-blind trial of bupropion found moderate improvement in both the active and placebo group, and no significant differences between the groups (Black et al., 2007).

Serotoninergic. Selective serotonin reuptake inhibitors (SSRIs) have been found to have mixed results in reducing symptoms of pathological gambling. Early studies involved fluvoxamine. An initial single-blind placebo-controlled trial with a mean dosage of 220 mg/day found a 25 percent decrease in PG-YBOCS scores at eight weeks, and seven out of ten active condition patients achieved abstinence (Hollander et al., 1998). Subsequent double-blind trials provided some additional support, suggesting that patients in the active group may improve more robustly and rapidly than those in the placebo group (Blanco et al., 2002; Hollander et al., 2000). However, in the Blanco et al. trial, differences between groups did not reach significance. Similarly, two double-blind placebo-controlled randomized trials of paroxetine have found mixed results on efficacy, with the eight-week trial showing significant improvement compared to the placebo group at a mean dosage of 51 mg (Kim et al., 2002) while the sixteen-week trial at a comparable mean dosage of 50 mg found no significant differences between the active and placebo groups (Grant et al., 2003). A clinical trial of sertraline, which lasted six months at a mean dosage of 95 mg, failed to find significant differences between the active and placebo groups (Saiz-Ruiz et al., 2005). A trial was conducted of escitalopram among individual with cooccurring anxiety and gambling disorders. A thirteen-subject open-label trial of escitalopram found that within eight weeks on a mean dosage of 25 mg, 61.5 percent of participants had >30 percent improvement on the PG-YBOCS, and individuals demonstrated average decreases of 82.8 percent on the Hamilton Anxiety Scale (Grant & Potenza, 2006). The >30 percent improvement group was then included in an eight-week double-blind placebo-controlled discontinuation phase. The patients assigned to the active escitalopram group maintained gains in problem-gambling and anxiety domains, whereas the individual assigned to placebo reported reoccurrence of symptoms after four weeks. Although these results appear initially promising, the sample size was particularly small. A subsequent trial comparing cognitive-behavioral therapy (CBT) to CBT with escitalopram found that after sixteen weeks, there were no significant differences in improvement in problem-gambling severity or craving between those taking escitalopram during CBT and those who did not take it (Myrseth et al., 2011). These findings suggest that escitalopram may not augment the outcome beyond improvements related to CBT alone, and/or that escitalopram may be most efficacious among individuals with cooccurring anxiety disorders. Additional research is needed to investigate these and other possibilities.

Glutamatergic. The dietary supplement N-acetyl cysteine, which may operate in part via upregulation of glutamate transporters in individuals with addictions (McClure et al., 2014), has been found in preliminary studies to have some efficacy in the treatment of gambling disorder. An initial eight-week open label trial found that sixteen out of twenty-seven patients with pathological gambling experienced a reduction of >30 percent on the PG-YBOCS at a mean dose of approximately 1,500 mg (Grant, Kim & Odlaug, 2007). Thirteen of the sixteen responders were then included in a randomized six-week double-blind placebo-controlled discontinuation phase. After the six weeks, five out of the six participants on N-acetyl cysteine maintained improvements in gambling symptoms, while only two of the seven in the placebo group did. A subsequent twelve-week randomized double-blind placebo-controlled trial investigated N-acetyl cysteine as a means of augmenting imaginal desensitization in comorbid nicotine dependence and gambling disorder (Grant et al., 2014). After six weeks, those in the active group experienced significantly larger improvements than those in the placebo group on the Fagerström Test for Nicotine Dependence, though after the subsequent six weeks the improvements from the imaginal desensitization were equal in both groups. During the three-month follow-up, those who took N-acetyl cysteine demonstrated significantly less problem-gambling severity (as measured by the PG-YBOCS). This finding suggests that N-acetyl cysteine may aid long-term cognitive-behaviorally induced improvements in gambling disorder. Imbalance of synaptic and extra-synaptic glutamate has been proposed as a driving mechanism of long-term drug-seeking behaviors, suggesting that targeting glutamate uptake may be a shared mechanism to target for pharmacological treatment of gambling and substance use disorders (Reissner & Kalivas, 2010). This approach may be particularly useful for treating patients with cooccurring gambling and substance addictions.

Glutamatergic antagonists have shown mixed results in the treatment of gambling disorder. A seventeen-week double-blind placebo-controlled trial of amantadine in patients with Parkinson's disease and pathological gambling found that seven patients reported stopping all gambling behaviors, and an additional five showed 80 percent improvement on the PG-YBOCS after two weeks (Thomas et al., 2010). However, this study initially had seventeen participants, and five dropped out before being included in these results, raising questions as to the robustness or replicability of the findings. A fourteen-week double-blind study for topiramate for individuals with gambling disorder and without Parkinson's disease found no significant differences in improvement between the active and placebo groups on the PG-YBOCS, and a slight trend ($p < 0.1$) of increased improvement on the Barratt Impulsiveness Scale (Berlin et al., 2013).

Opioidergic. Unlike dopaminergic antagonists, opioid receptor antagonists have been shown to in some studies to improve gambling symptomology (Kim, 1998). Naltrexone in particular may be an effective treatment for gambling disorder. The first double-blind randomized placebo-controlled trial of naltrexone in gambling disorder was conducted at an average dosage of 188 mg/day and concluded with an analyzable sample of twenty-five participants in the placebo group and twenty in the active group (Kim et al., 2001). This study showed significant improvements in the active group compared to the placebo group, and this finding was replicated in a subsequent trial where naltrexone was found to specifically reduce gambling urges (Grant et al., 2008a). Significantly, a large four-year follow-up study compared individuals with pathological gambling who had been treated for two years with either naltrexone, topirimate, escitalopram, or bupropion, and their status two years after ceasing treatment (Rosenberg, Dinur & Dannon, 2013). While patients in all groups had significant improvements, the naltrexone group had a significantly lower drop-out rate, as well as significantly larger improvements compared to bupropion on the Hamilton Depression Scale, significantly larger improvements compared to escitalopram and topirimate on the Hamilton Anxiety Scale, and significantly larger improvements on a measure of general well-being compared to bupropion and topirimate. Thus, targeting opioid functioning may be the most effective pharmacotherapy for gambling disorder based on current evidence, and may improve symptomology in multiple domains.

Nalmefene, another opioid antagonist, has also been found in placebo-controlled trials to be associated with better treatment outcomes (Grant et al., 2006, 2010), and opioid antagonists in general have been found to be most effective among individuals with gambling disorder for those with strong cravings and those with family histories of substance use disorders like alcoholism (Grant et al., 2008b). These findings resonate with those in the substance use disorder literature given FDA indications of naltrexone for opioid and alcohol use disorders and the impact of opioid antagonists on reducing cravings; thus there may exist shared biological mechanisms targeted by opioid antagonists across addictive disorders (Yip & Potenza, 2014). A recently published study of dually diagnosed individuals with alcohol dependence also supported that naltrexone may be a preferential treatment with respect to targeting problem-gambling severity, lending further support to this notion (Grant et al., 2017).

EEG Studies of Gambling Disorder

A few studies have examined electrophysiological correlates of pathological gambling. A small early study included eight men with a history of gambling disorder who had since ceased gambling, and eight matched healthy control subjects (Goldstein et al., 1985). The men performed tasks involving sorting nonsense shapes into categories, spelling words with physical letters, describing a procedure, and imagining a scene. In each task, individuals with pathological gambling were found to experience more activity in the opposite hemisphere as compared to the control subjects. More recent work has focused on cue-related and reward-related electrophysiological differences. Individuals with pathological gambling have been found to have higher-amplitude late positive potentials when viewing gambling-related images compared to healthy control subjects (Wölfling et al., 2011). In another study, Hewig and colleagues examined changes in reward-related amplitude during the course of a blackjack game (Hewig et al., 2010). While scalp readings were similar between subjects with and without pathological gambling at the beginning of the game, once the score was 16, individuals with gambling problems were significantly more likely to "hit" rather than "bust." When comparing electrical activity in subjects with and without pathological gambling 300 ms after choosing to "hit" with a score of 16, those with gambling problems had larger amplitudes over a large portion of the scalp. This finding suggests that subjects with and without pathological gambling may most be distinguished not in the processing of a rewarding outcome, but rather in the processing of the expectation of a reward. These findings resonate with fMRI findings suggesting neural differences in subjects with and without pathological gambling during the anticipation phase of reward processing on the monetary incentive delay task (Balodis & Potenza, 2015; Balodis et al., 2012). A prediction-related phenomenon, known as the "near-miss effect," has demonstrated similar electrophysiological patterns as during the blackjack task. The "near-miss effect" is a slot-machine-related phenomenon where a losing display shares features with a winning one, suggesting an illusion of nearly winning. A MEG study comparing oscillatory effects after near misses found that individuals with pathological gambling experienced greater theta band oscillatory activity in the insula and right orbitofrontal cortex (OFC) compared to healthy control subjects (Dymond et al., 2014). The extent of this oscillatory activity also correlated with the severity of gambling problems. The OFC and insula have been implicated in expectation-based reward-seeking, suggesting this oscillatory activity may be reinforcing of reward seeking tendencies (Moorman & Aston-Jones, 2014).

Functional MRI Studies of Gambling Disorder

Functional MRI (fMRI) offers a means of researching neural correlates of gambling behaviors with a more localized focus than EEG. Using fMRI, gambling disorder has been associated with differences in the neural correlates of multiple cognitive processes (Moccia et al., 2017). Here, we review some main domains that have been researched in gambling disorder using fMRI.

Reward Processing in Gambling Disorder. Reward processing in gambling disorder has been studied by investigating neurocognitive correlates of reward-related cues (to invoke anticipatory reward responses) and of receiving the reward itself. With reward-related cues, relevant imagery or audio may be used to induce craving. The earliest cue-based fMRI study of gambling disorder compared neural activity in individuals with pathological gambling and healthy control subjects upon watching videos of simulated interpersonal interactions designed to elicit gambling urges (Potenza et al., 2003a, 2003b). This study found reduced activity in the ventromedial prefrontal cortex (PFC) in individuals with pathological gambling compared to healthy control subjects. Blunted ventromedial PFC and orbital frontal cortex (OFC) in response to gambling cues has been found in multiple studies of cue reactivity, as well as studies of win-/loss-related activities (Balodis et al., 2012; Kober et al., 2016; Reuter et al., 2005; de Ruiter et al., 2009; Worhunsky et al., 2014). These results are consistent with findings of blunted frontostriatal activity during reward anticipation in substance addictions (Beck et al., 2009; Garrison et al., 2017).

However, more dorsal regions of the medial PFC, as well as the dorsolateral PFC, have been reported to be overactive in individuals with pathological gambling in response to gambling-related cues (Crockford et al., 2005). In a study of twenty-eight individuals with pathological gambling, thirty with cocaine dependence, and forty-five healthy control subjects, elevated activity in the anterior cingulate cortex (ACC) and dorsal regions of medial PFC were observed in individuals with pathological gambling when viewing gambling-specific cues, and this activity may be associated with the increased subjective craving rates reported in this group in response to gambling videos (Kober et al., 2016). Interestingly, while cocaine-dependent subjects experienced a similar craving preference for cocaine-related videos, the neural correlates of this increased craving response were in a more ventral region of medial PFC, consistent with prior studies using a similar task (Wexler et al., 2001). This study also reported some of the first neurocognitive gender-related differences in gambling disorder, showing that women with pathological gambling had gambling-cue-related increased activity in the insula and caudate (an area of the dorsal striatum), whereas men with pathological gambling did not. Another recent study on cue reactivity and craving in gambling disorder supplemented BOLD (blood oxygenation level dependent) measures of regional reactivity with functional connectivity measures. Nineteen individuals in treatment for gambling disorder and nineteen healthy control subjects viewed gambling cues, food cues, and neutral-relaxing cues, and rated their levels of craving (Limbrick-Oldfield et al., 2017). Individuals with pathological gambling had gambling-cue-specific increased activity in the left insula and ACC, and the subjective level of craving correlated with the degree of activity in the insula and ventral striatum. Notably, the level of craving also negatively correlated with functional connectivity between the ventral striatum and medial PFC, and this finding may reflect less prefrontal control over craving (Goldstein & Volkow, 2011).

Decision-Making and Executive Function in Gambling Disorder. The Iowa Gambling Task (IGT) is used to evaluate how risk/reward decision-making may be learned over time, involving the weighing of risks and rewards for optimal choices (Bechara et al., 1994; Brevers et al., 2013). Along with poorer task performance that may be due to increased risk-taking, increased impulsivity, and less loss-induced behavioral changes, individuals with pathological gambling have been found to exhibit during IGT performance relatively decreased activity in regions including the ventromedial PFC, OFC, and dorsolateral PFC (Tanabe et al., 2007; Brevers et al., 2016), and relatively increased activity in the ventral striatum (Brevers et al., 2016). The ventral striatum has also been found to show increased functional connectivity with the posterior cingulate cortex, occipital gyrus, and temporal gyrus during IGT performance in individuals with pathological gambling compared to control subjects (Brevers et al., 2016). Interestingly, hypoactivation of the OFC does not hold for all aspects of the IGT. Specifically, during high-risk decisions on the IGT, individuals with pathological gambling, compared to matched healthy control subjects, have been found to exhibit hyperactivation of the OFC, caudate, and amygdala (Power, Goodyear & Crockford, 2012). It is possible that this may reflect a mechanism for tolerance in gambling disorder, where smaller-risk decisions for smaller rewards become less salient over time, increasing the salience and reward expectation for higher-risk choices. It should be noted that some studies have found that individuals with gambling disorder do not differ from those without on IGT performance, with neural correlates of reward processing on the prospect phase of the monetary incentive delay task in regions including the ventral striatum associating with IGT performance in a sample with and without gambling disorder (Balodis et al., 2018).

Another line of research has investigated delay discounting in pathological gambling. Delay discounting refers to weighing between smaller, sooner rewards and the prospect of larger, later rewards (i.e., "one marshmallow now, or five marshmallows later"), and has been found to be a relevant to substance addictions and gambling disorder (Andrade & Petry, 2012). In one study of delay discounting, sixteen individuals with pathological gambling and sixteen control subjects made choices between smaller immediate rewards, larger rewards after a delay, or larger rewards with a risk element to them (Miedl, Peters & Buchel, 2012). Problem-gambling severity was measured by the *Kurzfragebogen zum Glücksspielverhalten*, a German gambling questionnaire. When weighing between immediate or delayed rewards, problem-gambling severity negatively correlated with activity in the OFC, ventral striatum, and rostral ACC, suggesting a weaker representation of the reward value brought by waiting. These correlations were not found for probabilistic discounting (weighing between small reward or risking for a larger one), possibly suggesting that gambling disorder involves larger deficits in temporal elements of reward valuation than probability-based ones. This finding aligns with previous work, which has found that the preference for impulsive choices over delayed rewards correlates with the magnitude of activity in the ventral striatum during such choices (Hariri et al., 2006).

Delay discounting in gambling disorder may relate to impaired reinforcement learning. During delay discounting, ventral striatal activity has been found to scale not only with the preference for immediate versus delayed rewards, but also with differential feedback response for positive versus negative results (Hariri et al., 2006). Individuals with pathological gambling may perseverate after losses, and this perseveration has been correlated with decreased activity in the ventromedial PFC (de Ruiter et al., 2009). These results suggest that individuals with pathological gambling may have deficits in learning from negative reinforcement, similar to individuals with substance use disorders (Tanabe et al., 2007). This finding may relate to experiences of individuals with Parkinson's disease undergoing levodopa treatment (Gescheidt et al., 2013), who may develop gambling problems (van Eimeren et al., 2010; Voon et al., 2017). The relatively blunted activation in the ventromedial PFC may be consistent across gambling and substance use disorders (Tanabe et al., 2007).

Individuals with pathological gambling may also have deficits in cognitive control. Individuals with pathological gambling show differences related to impulse control on behavioral tasks (Lawrence et al., 2009). Individuals with pathological gambling have demonstrated greater deactivation of the ventromedial PFC during the Stroop color-word interference task (Potenza et al., 2003a), and Stroop-related brain activity in the ventromedial PFC and ventral striatum has been linked to treatment outcomes in preliminary studies (Potenza et al., 2013a).

Structural and Diffusion MRI in Gambling Disorder

Aside from functional differences, neurostructural correlates of pathological gambling have also been investigated. An early whole-brain study using voxel-brain morphometry compared individuals with pathological gambling, alcohol use disorder, and neither disorder, found volumetric differences for those with alcohol use disorder compared to the other two groups in various regions, but no significant differences between individuals with and without pathological gambling (van Holst et al., 2012). These findings resonate with that investigating individuals with pathological gambling, cocaine dependence, and neither disorder that similarly found between-group differences related to the PFC and specifically in the cocaine-dependent group (Yip et al., 2018). In the same study, impulsivity measures were related to smaller volumes of largely subcortical structures including the amygdala and hippocampus, suggesting that transdiagnostic measures and diagnostic measures relate differently to brain structures. A study involving thirty-two individuals with, and forty-seven without, pathological gambling that focused on the amygdala and hippocampus found that individuals with pathological gambling had smaller gray-matter volumes in the left hippocampus and right amygdala, and this related to higher scores on the Behavioral Inhibition Scale and Behavioral Activation Scale (Rahman, Xu & Potenza, 2014).

Studies using diffusion-based MRI techniques have implicated white-matter tracts in gambling disorder. Several studies have found decreased fractional anisotropy in the corpus callosum of individuals with pathological gambling as compared to those without (Joutsa et al., 2011; Yip et al., 2013), and in one study this was related to scores on the Behavioral Activation System Fun-Seeking subscale (Yip et al., 2013). The internal capsule and both anterior and posterior radiations from the thalamus have been implicated in studies of pathological gambling, albeit in different manners with primary tracts implicated in some but not other studies (Joutsa et al., 2011; Yip et al., 2017). In the 2017 study by Yip and colleagues, the pathological gambling and cocaine use disorder groups were found to differ from control subjects in secondary (crossing) fibers, with findings suggesting reduced white matter integrity in the left internal capsule, posterior thalamic radiation, and corona radiata. This finding suggests that white-matter integrity in these regions may transcend substance and behavioral addictions, and not a specific neurotoxic effect of drug exposure.

Heritability of, and Genetics in, Gambling Disorder

Twin studies provide an opportunity for estimating genetic and environmental contributions to gambling disorder and cooccurring conditions. Data from 3,359 male twin pairs from the Vietnam Era Twin Registry estimated that genetic factors accounted for approximately 34 percent to 54 percent of the variance for experiencing a DSM-III-R diagnosis of pathological gambling (Eisen et al., 1998). The same data have been used to investigate the cooccurrence of gambling and substance use disorders (Xian et al., 2014), with findings suggesting that all of the overlaps between gambling and stimulant use disorders were related to shared genetic factors, while overlaps with arguably more socially accepted drugs (cannabis, tobacco) included both genetic and environmental contributions. Similarly, twin studies also suggest shared genetic and environmental contributions to the cooccurrence between gambling and alcohol use disorder (Slutske et al., 2000), with findings extending to women (Slutske et al., 2013). Shared genetic contributions have also been identified between gambling and affective disorders such as major depression and generalized anxiety disorder, with environmental contribution also implicated in the co-occurrence between gambling and panic disorders (Giddens et al., 2011; Potenza et al., 2005).

Some studies have investigated the molecular genetics of gambling disorder. Candidate gene approaches have investigated specific genes with mixed findings in small samples (Lim et al., 2012; Lobo et al., 2007, 2010). Several genome-wide association studies have been conducted in gambling disorder with the two studies to date not having identified regions reaching genome-wide significance (Lang et al., 2016; Lind et al., 2013). However, in one study, a polygenic risk score for alcohol use disorder was linked to gambling disorder (Lang et al., 2016). Additionally, allelic variants with functional enzymatic correlates have been investigated in gambling disorder, with findings suggesting that allelic variants of the gene (*COMT*) coding for catechol-O-methyl transferase may operate through fronto-parietal mechanisms and link to treatment outcome with a catechol-O-methyl transferase inhibitor tolcapone (Grant et al., 2013). Additionally, an allelic variant of the gene (*DBH*) coding for dopamine beta-hydroxylase, an enzyme that converts dopamine to norepinephrine, has been linked across individuals with and without gambling disorder to subjective and neural correlates of emotional processing, suggesting a transdiagnostic mechanism for emotional dysregulation relevant to gambling disorder and other addictions (Yang et al., 2016).

Internet Gaming Disorder (IGD)

In the internet addiction literature, there has been debate as to whether the internet should be the focus of an addiction, whether activities conducted on the internet are addictive, or the term "addiction" should apply to such behaviors at all (Griffiths, King & Demetrovics, 2014). Some consider internet behaviors such as gaming and cybersex as subtypes of internet addiction (Young, 2009). Below we will describe neurobiological research into internet use behaviors; Internet Gaming Disorder (IGD), in particular.

Internet Gaming Disorder (IGD): "Condition for Further Study"

In 2012, one billion people played online games, making internet gaming a highly prevalent activity (Kuss, 2013). While gaming is not inherently problematic for most, some studies estimate that between 4 percent and 20 percent of the adult and adolescent population may develop problems related to gaming (Yau et al., 2012). Research into IGD has been in part prompted by gaming-related harms experienced around the world that have in part led to the development of rehabilitation centers (Hayoun, 2014). IGD was introduced in Section III of DSM-5 as a "condition for further study," and has been approved by the secretariat of the World Health Organization for inclusion in ICD-11. This announced inclusion has sparked debate in the field as to the existence of IGD, and whether the benefits of classifying it and providing care for those experiencing impairments may outweigh the fear of stigmatizing nonproblematic gaming (Aarseth et al., 2017; Dullur & Starcevic, 2017; King et al., 2018). The criteria used for IGD in ICD-11 are: (1) "impaired control over gaming"; (2) "increasing priority given to gaming to the extent that gaming takes precedence over other life interests and daily activities"; and (3) "continuation or escalation of gaming despite the occurrence of negative consequences" (ICD-11). These criteria mirror those for gambling disorder in the ICD-11. The criteria used in the DSM-5 for IGD are similar but are more closely linked to the DSM-5 criteria for gambling disorder, with criteria focused on using gaming to escape from dysphoric states, preoccupation, withdrawal, tolerance, repeated unsuccessful attempts to cut back or quit, and lying to conceal gaming behavior (APA, 2013). While the criteria in ICD-11 may be considered broad, the DSM-5 criteria have been criticized by some as having domains that may be more questionable in their relevance to IGD, such as tolerance which may not be based on increasing time spent gaming (King & Delfabbro, 2016; King, Herd & Delfabbro, 2017).

Part of the reason IGD was not included in the main text of DSM-5 was related to the limited data available during the DSM-5 workgroup discussions. Multiple instruments have been used to evaluate IGD, which may contribute to wide prevalence estimates and other debated aspects (King et al., 2013; Petry & O'Brien, 2013). While the generation of IGD criteria is helpful for promoting consistency across studies and geographic jurisdictions, more research is needed into the reliability, validity, and clinical utility of the specific criteria and overall construct. The DSM-5 calls for further neurobiological research into IGD as a means of evaluating the similarities between its underlying neurofunctional correlates and those of other addictions. The next section reviews neurobiological research of IGD.

Neurochemistry and Pharmacology of IGD

Dopamine has been investigated in IGD. Individuals with IGD may have lower dopamine receptor availability in the caudate and right putamen and less expression of dopamine transporters than healthy control subjects (Kim et al., 2011). Using a candidate gene approach, the TaqIA1 allele of the *DRD2* gene has been associated with IGD and greater reward dependence (Han et al., 2007). While lower receptor availability may be a risk-factor, it is also possibly a developmental progression within the disorder, as the availability of dopamine receptors in the striatum has been correlated with the years of excessive gaming (Tian et al., 2014).

Pharmacological Treatment of IGC

Few investigations of pharmacological treatments for IGD have been conducted. In a study of bupropion and escitalopram (Song et al., 2016), 119 individuals with IGD were treated either with bupropion, escitalopram, or a placebo, and multiple measures were assessed at the beginning of treatment and six weeks later. Individuals were evaluated with psychometric assessments including the Clinical Global Impression-Severity Scale, Young's Internet Addiction Scale, Beck Depression Inventory, ADHD (attention deficit hyperactivity disorder) Rating Scale, and Behavioral Inhibition System and Behavioral Activation System Scale. While both medications were found to lead to improvements on all scales, bupropion was correlated with greater improvements on all scales except the Beck Depression Inventory.

Treatment of Comorbid Conditions. Several pharmacological studies have examined the treatment of cooccurring disorders and IGD. Bupropion was found to be helpful in the treatment of cooccurring major depressive disorder and IGD during an eight-week active treatment period (Han & Renshaw, 2012). However, four weeks after treatment ended, while IGD features such as amount of time spent gaming continued to decrease, symptoms of major depressive disorder, such as decreased mood, often recurred.

ADHD may frequently cooccur with IGD. A study of methylphenidate treatment in children with ADHD and IGD found improvement of both ADHD and IGD symptoms, and improvement correlated across domains

(Han et al., 2009). A study of atomoxetine and methylphenidate in the treatment of adolescents with comorbid IGD and ADHD found that both medications were related to improvement of impulsivity and measures of gaming behaviors, and neither was more effective than the other (Park et al., 2016). However, only methylphenidate was found to improve ADHD symptoms. These data appear to suggest that while the symptoms of ADHD are correlated with problematic gaming, they are not equivalent phenomena.

EEG studies of IGD

Brain-based electrophysiological studies have been conducted on IGD. One resting-state study found decreased absolute power for beta bands and increased power for gamma bands for individuals with IGD as compared to those without IGD (Choi et al., 2013). These differences were associated with both impulsivity and IGD severity. A study comparing resting-state coherence in individuals with IGD, alcohol use disorder and neither disorder found that intrahemispheric gamma coherence was related to IGD regardless of level of impulsivity (Park, et al., 2017a, 2017b). More specifically, right fronto-central gamma coherence correlated with IGD severity as measured by the Internet Addiction Test. Other EEG studies have found further differences between individuals with IGD and alcohol use disorder, such as lower absolute beta power during resting-state in IGD subjects (Son et al., 2015). These data suggest neurobiological distinctions between alcohol use disorder and IGD, and specifically that the beta band may be a correlate of IGD. The beta band has also been found to have greater absolute power in temporal regions in individuals with ADHD and IGD (Park et al., 2017a, 2017b). Furthermore, the beta band has higher intrahemispheric coherence in fronto-temporo-parieto-occipital areas in individuals with major depressive disorder and IGD (Youh et al., 2017), relative to individuals with only ADHD and major depressive disorder, respectively.

Resting-state EEG has also been used in conjunction with treatment responses in IGD. Twenty individuals with IGD were assessed before and after six months of treatment with an SSRI (Kim et al., 2017). Higher theta activity at baseline was prospectively related to symptom improvement (based on Internet Addiction Test scores), and that improvement correlated with decreased delta activity after six months of treatment. While the change in delta activity may be attributed to the improvement of general depression and anxiety symptoms, adjusting for improvements in these areas (as measured by the Beck Depression Inventory and Beck Anxiety Inventory) did not change the theta band finding.

How event-related potentials may be modified by the presence of rewarding gaming stimuli has been investigated in IGD, for example, during navigation of a reward-based virtual maze in an attempt to find as many rewards as possible in twenty minutes (Duven et al., 2015). Individuals with IGD exhibited a larger N100 with longer latency, and smaller P200 and P300, in the left hemisphere and midline, upon finding rewards in the maze. These results were interpreted to represent possible tolerance to gaming rewards, or perhaps rewards in general. A subsequent study found further evidence for the P300's relevance to reward processing in IGD, finding lower amplitudes for gaming cues during No/Go trials of a Go No/Go task (Balconi, Venturella & Finocchiaro, 2017).

Functional MRI studies of IGD

Multiple neurocognitive domains, including reward processing, decision-making, executive function, and social cognition, have been investigated in IGD (Yao et al., 2017). In this section, we review the IGD fMRI literature in these domains.

Reward Processing in IGD. In a study of cue-induced craving, thirty-nine males with IGD and twenty-three without IGD viewed images related to internet gaming, those related to general internet use, and degraded mosaic images and subsequently rated how strongly the image induced a subjective craving (Liu et al., 2017a, 2017b). The severity of problematic internet use in the IGD group was measured by the Chinese Internet Addiction Scale (Chen et al, 2003), and all subjects were evaluated for exclusionary psychiatric histories by interview. When contrasting activations to gaming-related cues and general internet cues, individuals with IGD exhibited more activity in the ventral and dorsal striatum, while healthy control subjects exhibited more activity in the insula. Self-reported intensity of craving in IGD patients correlated positively with the dorsal striatum and negatively with left ventral striatal activity. These results resonate with some found in studies of substance use disorders, where the progression of the disorder has been proposed to involve cue processing shifting from the ventral to dorsal striatum (Everitt & Robbins, 2013).

Frontostriatal circuitry has been implicated in multiple cue-reactivity studies of IGD (Ko et al., 2009, 2013a, 2013b; Sun et al., 2012) and may track with levels of subjective craving (Han et al., 2010; Zhang et al., 2016). However, increased activity of the insula and decreased connectivity of the insula with the precuneus was found to be associated with behavioral-intervention-related reductions in subjective craving, suggesting that the frontostriatal regions may be more related to cue reactivity than to the experience of craving (Zhang et al., 2016). This supports previous findings suggesting that subjective craving and cue-reactivity for behavioral addictions and for substance use disorders are related but separate phenomena (Goudriaan et al., 2010; Sun et al., 2012).

Decision-Making and Executive Function in IGD. In risk-based valuation-decision tasks, individuals with IGD may make riskier choices compared to healthy control subjects. During risky decisions, individuals with IGD have been reported to exhibit less activity in regions such as the dorsolateral PFC, inferior frontal gyrus, and precentral gyrus, and more activity in the inferior frontal cortex, ACC, and insula (Dong & Potenza, 2016; Lin et al., 2015; Qi et al., 2015; Wang et al., 2017). These findings suggest that specific regions or circuits may not be as strongly engaged during the processing of risk during decision-valuation processes in individuals with IGD. Upon experiencing losses in these types of tasks, IGD participants have shown more activity in the left dorsolateral PFC and inferior frontal gyrus (Dong et al., 2013) and OFC (Dong, Huang & Du, 2011; Liu et al., 2017a) and less activity in the ACC and posterior cingulate cortex (Dong et al., 2011, 2013). These findings suggest that reward-seeking circuitries may be less affected by losses in individuals with IGD, raising the possibility that error-monitoring may be impaired in IGD. Upon experiencing wins, IGD participants show decreased activity in the caudate and posterior cingulate cortex and increased activity in the OFC (Dong et al., 2011, 2013). These findings suggest differences in activations in reward-related regions as have been implicated in studies of other addictive disorders (Blum et al., 2015).

Two executive-function tasks include the Stroop and Go/No-Go tasks. During Stroop performance, individuals with IGD show relatively increased activation of regions including the dorsolateral PFC, ACC, precuneus, and superior and medial areas of the temporal gyrus (Dong, et al., 2012a, 2012b, 2014); however, weaker functional connectivity has been reported between these regions in association with IGD (Yuan et al., 2016). These results are accompanied with worse task performance and suggest an attempt to compensate for reduced connectivity. The results from Go/No-Go tasks mirror those of Stroop studies, in regards to worse performance and more neural activity compared to healthy controls (Dong et al., 2015). During No-Go trials of Go/No-Go tasks, individuals with IGD have been found to show relatively increased activity in the dorsolateral PFC, ACC, and various areas of the parietal lobe during No-Go trials (Ding et al., 2014; Liu et al., 2014). Another study found less activity in the pre-supplementary motor area (pre-SMA) region during Go/No-Go tasks in IGD subjects compared to healthy control subjects (Chen et al., 2015). After No-Go trials in a task using gaming cues as a distractor, IGD subjects showed neural activity that has been linked in other studies to heightened reward-seeking and decreased error monitoring, such as greater OFC and dorsolateral PFC activity and decreased insula activity (Ko et al., 2014; Liu et al., 2014).

Social Cognition in IGD. Several studies have investigated self-perception, identification, and immersion, factors proposed to link to gaming in Massively Multiplayer Online Role-Playing Games (MMORPGs) versus other genres (Eichenbaum et al., 2015; Na et al., 2017). In MMORPGs, players may immerse themselves in a virtual world through an avatar and play in real-time with many other players. Some qualities of this genre have been linked to problematic gaming, with some individuals using MMORPGs as proxies for social interaction (Cole & Griffiths, 2007) and as a means of escape (Schimmenti et al., 2012).

One study related to immersion used a task where participants clicked the mouse while watching an animation of a ball being thrown among virtual avatars (Kim et al., 2012). In some blocks, participants were instructed to click as the ball was caught and thrown by a specific avatar, as if they were the agent controlling the avatar, while in a control condition they were instructed to click as the ball was in midair between two players. During these trials, the animation would shift back and forth between a first-person view and third-person view of the avatar, requiring the participant to reassign where in space they were labeling themselves as the agent. By isolating activity related to the shift in agency, individuals with IGD were observed to activate the insula and left temporo-parietal junction more so than healthy control subjects. This finding was interpreted as individuals with IGD showing stronger immersion and disembodiment from themselves while playing avatar-based games. Other studies have found similar results, suggesting that individuals with IGD may self-identify more strongly with their avatars than individuals without IGD, showing greater activity in self-related neural regions such as the medial temporal gyrus, precuneus, and angular gyrus (Dieter et al., 2015; Leménager et al., 2014). Individuals with IGD may demonstrate brain activities suggestive of identifying less so with their physical real self than do comparison subjects, as reflected by less angular gyrus activity on self-perception tasks (Leménager et al., 2014).

Structural and Diffusion MRI Studies of IGD

A coordinate-based meta-analysis of voxel-based morphometry studies of individuals with IGD found on average lower gray-matter volume in the left dorsolateral PFC, right putamen, OFC, ACC, and SMA, compared to healthy control subjects (Yao et al., 2017). Cortical thickness in many of these regions has also been found to be thinner in individuals with IGD as compared to healthy control subjects, and this decreased cortical thickness has been correlated with lower cognitive control on Stroop tasks (Yuan et al., 2013). Cortical thickness has also been found to be relatively increased in the left precentral cortex, precuneus, and medial temporal cortex in individuals with IGD (Yuan et al., 2013). These regions are similar to those functionally implicated in altered immersive experience while gaming (Dieter et al., 2015; Leménager et al., 2014). Data suggest white-matter connectivity and integrity differences in IGD. Increased fractional anisotropy within the posterior limb of the internal capsule has been found to correlate with the duration of IGD (Yuan et al., 2011), and greater fractional anisotropy in the thalamus has been found to correlate with the severity of IGD (Dong et al., 2012b). Decreased fractional anisotropy in individuals with IGD as compared to those without has been found in the OFC, corpus callosum, cingulum, inferior fronto-occipital fasciculus, and external capsule, although left external capsule fractional anisotropy correlated negatively with scores on Young's Internet Addiction Scale (Lin et al., 2012). Broadly, IGD may be associated with increased local white-matter integrity, in particular in subcortical and brainstem structures, and decreased intercortical and intraregional white-matter integrity. However, it is unclear if these changes are vulnerability factors for IGD or a result of IGD.

Pornography and Cybersexual Disorders

Although gaming has been a significant focus of internet addiction research in recent years, other behaviors warrant consideration, including pornography use. It is estimated that as much as 30 percent of bandwidth on the internet is related to pornography viewing (The Huffington Post, 2013). Like IGD, problematic pornography use is not an official disorder in the DSM-5; unlike IGD, it was not proposed as a condition for further study, and has no consistent proposed diagnostic criteria. Criteria for hypersexual disorder were proposed for DSM-5, but were not included in the main text or section of the DSM-5 (Kafka, 2010). A field trial for hypersexuality disorder was conducted (Reid et al., 2012), with the proposed criteria for hypersexuality disorder including specifications for cybersex (use of the internet to meet sexual partners and/or engage in "virtual sex") and pornography. The criteria for hypersexual disorder shared similarities with those for other addictive behaviors, including repetitive engagement and urges for the relevant sexual stimuli, significant functional or self-perceived impairments due to these urges, and difficulties limiting or ceasing the behavior. As with gaming, the internet may serve as a medium that increases usage, via such mechanisms as accessibility, availability and affordability (Kor et al., 2013). Compulsive sexual behavior disorder has been included in ICD-11 as an impulse-control disorder (Kraus et al., 2018), although some findings suggest that some forms of compulsive sexual behavior disorder, like problematic pornography use, may not track closely with measures of impulsivity (Bőthe et al., 2019). The ICD-11 criteria for compulsive sexual behavior disorder include: (1) "persistent pattern of failure to control intense, repetitive sexual impulses or urges resulting in sexual behavior"; (2) this repetitive failure manifesting over a period of six months or more and leading to "marked distress or significant impairment in personal, family, social, educational, occupational, or other important areas of functioning"; (3) distress that is not "entirely related to moral judgements and disapproval about sexual impulses, urges, or behaviors"; and (4) no diagnosis of paraphilic disorder. The ICD-11 does not specifically mention cybersex and problematic pornography use subtypes, though compulsive sexual behavior disorder may be heterogeneous with respect to specific problematic sexual urges/behaviors and other features (Derbyshire & Grant, 2015).

While neurobiological research on problematic pornography use is relatively limited, studies using visually presented sexual stimuli suggest that pathways relevant to reward and salience processing may relate importantly to compulsive sexual behavior disorder. A systematic review of forty neuroscience studies on visually presented sexual stimuli found consistencies between their biological correlates and those for other positive hedonic stimuli, including ventral striatal activation (Gola et al., 2016). It is not clear the extent to which these findings may reflect the viewing of pornographic material as a reward being sought or if it reflects a cue for the reward of sexual activity, or some other possibility (Georgiadis & Kringelbach, 2012). Gola and colleagues note that whether visually presented sexual stimuli are considered cues or rewards may differ depending on context, especially in laboratory settings where the stimuli does not lead to sexual activity, and in these contexts may be more likely to be considered the reward itself (2016).

Pharmacological Treatment of Cybersexual Behaviors

There are limited data on neurochemical factors linked to problematic pornography use. If compulsive sexual behavior disorder is similar to other addictive behaviors, differences may be hypothesized in specific neurotransmitter systems (e.g., opioidergic). Current data on potential neurochemical mechanisms is largely derived from case reports of pharmacological treatments.

Preliminary data suggest that naltrexone, an opioid receptor antagonist, may have promise in treating problematic pornography use. One case report describes a patient ceasing excessive pornography viewing and cybersexual activity while being treated with oral naltrexone (Bostwick & Bucci, 2008). The patient had reported severe urges to engage in sexual behavior on the internet from the age of ten years through his mid-to-late twenties, leading to marital difficulties and multiple job losses. While previously treated with therapy and SSRIs, the patient reported that these treatments helped with depressive symptoms and only temporarily helped with impulse control or cravings. After starting with naltrexone, the patient reported decreased urges and pleasure from viewing cybersexual material, better impulse control as the dose was increased, and eventual sustained remission at a dose of 50 mg/day. Another case report involved a patient with problematic pornography use who entered into treatment and received cognitive behavioral therapy which led to reductions in pornography consumption (Kraus et al., 2015). In the setting of decreased pornography viewing, the patient reported increased craving. Naltrexone was introduced, leading to decreased craving in the setting of persistent reductions in use. A third case report for a patient with comorbid tobacco and pornography addiction also suggests benefits of naltrexone (Capurso, 2017). The patient reported urges throughout the day for both cigarettes and pornography, failures to reduce the use of both, and time spent watching pornography as increasing. At a dose of 50 mg/day of naltrexone, the patient reduced both tobacco and pornography use to less than 30 percent of usage prior to treatment. Owing to reported anhedonia, the patient eventually stopped taking naltrexone, and both tobacco and pornography use returned to their original levels. Based on naltrexone's mechanism of action with respect to indirect modulation of mesolimbic reward systems through GABAergic interneurons, problematic pornography use may involve multiple neurotransmitter systems, and future studies should examine further potential contributions from opioidergic, GABAergic, dopaminergic and other neurotransmitter systems.

Changes in sexual urges and behavior and anxiety have been suggested in a case series of the SSRI paroxetine in the treatment of problematic pornography use (Gola & Potenza, 2016). While treatment with paroxetine were associated with reductions in anxiety and pornography consumption, after several months on 20 mg/day of paroxetine, all three patients reported engagement in new compulsive sexual behaviors separate from pornography use. The patients began partaking in such behaviors as marital affairs and prostitution. These findings suggest that while modulating serotonergic pathways with SSRIs may reduce anxiety, they may also increase sexual risk-taking, possibly through amygdalar mechanisms (Gola, Miyakoshi & Secousse, 2015), and this possibility warrants direct examination.

EEG Studies of Cybersexual Behaviors

During EEG, individuals with problematic pornography use demonstrated smaller late positive potential amplitudes upon viewing sexually desirable images compared to those who did not report problematic use (Prause et al., 2015). The authors interpret this effect to "disprove" problematic pornography use from being considered as an addictive behavior, as late positive potential amplitude in response to relevant cues is generally higher in both substance and behavioral addictions (Dunning et al., 2011; Moeller et al., 2012; Thalemann, Wölfling & Grüssier, 2007; Wölfling et al., 2011). However, Gola in his commentary on this study, notes a possible misinterpretation of the sexually desirable images as cues, instead as the reward itself (2016). If the late positive potential in this study is interpreted as the reward value of viewing the pornographic images, this would be consistent with models of other addictions, where the reward value decreases, leading to tolerance (Berridge, 2012; Robinson et al., 2016). It is also worth noting that individual classification of problematic pornography use in this study was based on self-perception, which may make this group not equivalent to a clinical population with compulsive sexual behavior disorder and raises questions regarding the precise characteristics of the group. For example, diagnosing problematic pornography use based on self-perception may not screen out individuals who report distress related to moral disapproval of their urges and behaviors, which is an exclusionary factor for compulsive sexual behavior disorder in ICD-11 (Kraus et al., 2018).

Structural and Functional MRI Studies on Cybersexual Behaviors

Structural and functional differences in the brain have been associated with problematic pornography use. Smaller gray-matter volume in the right caudate has been associated with increased pornography use in young males without diagnosed psychiatric disorders (Kühn & Gallinat, 2014). In this same group, resting-state functional activity between the right caudate and left dorsolateral PFC was negatively correlated with the amount of time spent watching pornography weekly. Along with these task-independent changes, the amount of time spent watching pornography negatively correlated with blood oxygenation level dependent (BOLD) reactivity in the putamen upon viewing visually presented sexual stimuli. Individuals with problematic pornography use, compared to those without, have also been found to have greater BOLD reactivity in the left caudate, right dorsolateral PFC, right dorsal ACC, right supramarginal gyrus, and bilateral thalamus upon viewing pornographic stimuli (Seok & Sohn, 2015). The dorsal ACC has been implicated in problematic pornography use in association with cue reactivity to sexual images (Voon et al., 2014). The dorsal ACC's role in cue reactivity in problematic pornography use may relate to conditioning and novelty preference. Dorsal ACC activity has been found to correlate with preference for novel sexual images in individuals with compulsive sexual behavior, and this in turn has been correlated with increased habituation of the dorsal ACC to sexual vs. monetary images (Banca, et al., 2016).

The ventral striatum appears to contribute importantly to problematic pornography use. The magnitude of BOLD activity ventral striatum in response to pornographic cues was larger in individuals with compulsive sexual behaviors or problematic pornography use, compared to healthy control subjects, in multiple studies (Brand et al., 2016; Gola et al., 2017; Voon et al., 2014). One study used a modified monetary incentive delay task involving sexual and monetary cues and rewards. In doing so, the sexual cues induced stronger ventral striatum activity in men with problematic pornography use, and the pornographic image as a sexual reward, did not differ from responses from healthy control males. However, sexual as compared to monetary rewards elicited greater ventral striatal activation in both men with and without problematic pornography use. Voon and colleagues found that functional connectivity between the dorsal ACC, ventral striatum, and amygdala was more strongly correlated with sexual desire ("how much did this video increase your desire?") in the compulsive sexual behavior group than in the control group, but that this was not true for reward value ("how much did you like this video?"). These findings overall support problematic pornography use as sharing similarities with substance addictions and other behavioral addictions within craving and reward models of addiction (Berridge, 2012; Robinson et al., 2016).

Conclusions

Nonsubstance behaviors are now beginning to be considered in the context of an addiction framework. Neurobiological research has found similarities between substance use disorders and behavioral addictions involving gambling, gaming and compulsive sexual behaviors. Existing data demonstrate some similarities in neurochemical, neurofunctional, and neuropathological features, and thus expand the range of addictive behaviors. Larger-scale studies are needed.

REFERENCES

Aarseth, E., Bean, A. M., Boonen, H., et al. (2017). Scholars' open debate paper on the World Health Organization ICD-11 Gaming Disorder proposal. *Journal of Behavioral Addictions*, **6**(3), 267–270.

Andrade, L. F. & Petry, N. M. (2012). Delay and probability discounting in pathological gamblers with and without a history of substance use problems. *Psychopharmacology*, **219**(2), 491–499.

American Psychiatric Association. (2013). *Diagnostic and Statistical Manual of Mental Disorders* (5th edition). Arlington, VA: American Psychiatric Publishing.

Balconi, M., Venturella, I. & Finocchiaro, R. (2017). Evidences from rewarding system, FRN and P300 effect in internet-addiction in young people. *Brain Sciences*, **7**(7). doi: 10.3390/brainsci7070081

Balodis, I. M., Kober, H., Worhunsky, P. D., et al. (2012). Diminished frontostriatal activity during processing of monetary rewards and losses in pathological gambling. *Biological Psychiatry*, **71**(8), 749–757.

Balodis, I. M., Linnet, J., Arshad, F., et al. (2018). A preliminary study relating neural processing of reward and loss prospect to risky decision-making in individuals with and without gambling disorder. *International Gambling Studies*, **18**(2), 269–285.

Balodis, I. M. & Potenza, M. N. (2015). Anticipatory reward processing in addicted populations: a focus on the monetary incentive delay task. *Biological Psychiatry*, **77**, 434–444.

Banca, P., Morris, L. S., Mitchell, S., et al. (2016). Novelty, conditioning and attentional bias to sexual rewards. *Journal of Psychiatric Research*, **72**, 91–101.

Bechara, A., Damasio, A. R., Damasio, H. & Anderson, S. W. (1994). Insensitivity to future consequences following damage to human prefrontal cortex. *Cognition*, **50**(1–3), 7–15.

Beck, A., Schlagenhauf, F., Wustenberg, T., et al. (2009). Ventral striatal activation during reward anticipation correlates with impulsivity in alcoholics. *Biological Psychiatry*, **66**(8), 734–742.

Berlin, H. A., Braun, A., Simeon, D., et al. (2013). A double-blind, placebo-controlled trial of topiramate for pathological gambling. *The World Journal of Biological Psychiatry: The Official Journal of the World Federation of Societies of Biological Psychiatry*, **14**(2), 121–128.

Berridge, K. C. (2012). From prediction error to incentive salience: mesolimbic computation of reward motivation. *European Journal of Neuroscience*, **35**(7), 1124–1143.

Black, D. W., Arndt, S., Coryell, W. H., et al. (2007). Bupropion in the treatment of pathological gambling: a randomized, double-blind, placebo-controlled, flexible-dose study. *Journal of Clinical Psychopharmacology*, **27** (2), 143–150. https://doi.org/10.1097/01.jcp.0000264985.25109.25

Blanco, C., Petkova, E., Ibanez, A. & Saiz-Ruiz, J. (2002). A pilot placebo-controlled study of fluvoxamine for pathological gambling. *Annals of Clinical Psychiatry: Official Journal of the American Academy of Clinical Psychiatrists*, **14**(1), 9–15.

Blum, K., Thanos, P. K., Oscar-Berman, M., et al. (2015). Dopamine in the brain: hypothesizing surfeit or deficit links to reward and addiction. *Journal of Reward Deficiency Syndrome*, **1**(3), 95–104.

Boileau, I., Payer, D., Chugani, B., et al. (2013). The D2/3 dopamine receptor in pathological gambling: a positron emission tomography study with [11C]-(+)-propyl-hexahydro-naphtho-oxazin and [11C]raclopride. *Addiction*, **108**(5), 953–963.

Bőthe, B., Tóth-Király, I., Orosz, G., et al. (2019). Revisiting the role of impulsivity and compulsivity in problematic sexual behaviors. *Journal of Sex Research*, 56(2), 166–179.

Bostwick, J. M. & Bucci, J. A. (2008). Internet sex addiction treated with naltrexone. *Mayo Clinic Proceedings*, **83**(2), 226–230.

Brand, M., Snagowski, J., Laier, C. & Maderwald, S. (2016). Ventral striatum activity when watching preferred pornographic pictures is correlated with symptoms of Internet pornography addiction. *NeuroImage*, **129**, 224–232.

Brevers, D., Bechara, A., Cleeremans, A. & Noel, X. (2013). Iowa Gambling Task (IGT): twenty years after – gambling disorder and IGT. *Frontiers in Psychology*, **4**, 665.

Brevers, D., Noel, X., He, Q., Melrose, J. A. & Bechara, A. (2016). Increased ventral-striatal activity during monetary decision making is a marker of problem poker gambling severity. *Addiction Biology*, **21**(3), 688–699.

Bullock, S. A. & Potenza, M. N. (2012). Pathological gambling: neuropsychopharmacology and treatment. *Current Psychopharmacology*, **1**(1). doi: 10.2174/2211556011201010067

Capurso, N. A. (2017). Naltrexone for the treatment of comorbid tobacco and pornography addiction. *The American Journal on Addictions*, **26**(2), 115–117.

Chen, C.-Y., Huang, M.-F., Yen, J.-Y., et al. (2015). Brain correlates of response inhibition in Internet gaming disorder. *Psychiatry and Clinical Neurosciences*, **69**(4), 201–209.

Chen, S. H., Weng, L. J., Su, Y. J., Wu, H. M. & Yang, P. F. (2003). Development of a Chinese Internet addiction scale and its psychometric study. *Chinese Journal of Psychology*, **45**, 279–294.

Choi, J.-S., Park, S. M., Lee, J., et al. (2013). Resting-state beta and gamma activity in Internet addiction. *International Journal of Psychophysiology: Official Journal of the International Organization of Psychophysiology*, **89**(3), 328–333.

Clark, L., Stokes, P. R., Wu, K., et al. (2012). Striatal dopamine D(2)/D(3) receptor binding in pathological gambling is correlated with mood-related impulsivity. *NeuroImage*, **63**(1), 40–46.

Cole, H. & Griffiths, M. D. (2007). Social interactions in massively multiplayer online role-playing gamers. *Cyberpsychology & Behavior: The Impact of the Internet, Multimedia and Virtual Reality on Behavior and Society*, **10**(4), 575–583.

Crockford, D. N., Goodyear, B., Edwards, J., Quickfall, J. & el-Guebaly, N. (2005). Cue-induced brain activity in pathological gamblers. *Biological Psychiatry*, **58**(10), 787–795.

de Ruiter, M. B., Veltman, D. J., Goudriaan, A. E., et al. (2009). Response perseveration and ventral prefrontal sensitivity to reward and punishment in male problem gamblers and smokers. *Neuropsychopharmacology: Official Publication of the American College of Neuropsychopharmacology*, **34**(4), 1027–1038.

Derbyshire, K. L. & Grant, J. E. (2015). Compulsive sexual behavior: a review of the literature. *Journal of Behavioral Addictions*, **4** (2), 37–43.

Dieter, J., Hill, H., Sell, M., et al. (2015). Avatar's neurobiological traces in the self-concept of massively multiplayer online role-playing game (MMORPG) addicts. *Behavioral Neuroscience*, **129**(1), 8–17.

Ding, W., Sun, J., Sun, Y.-W., et al. (2014). Trait impulsivity and impaired prefrontal impulse inhibition function in adolescents with internet gaming addiction revealed by a Go/No-Go fMRI study. *Behavioral and Brain Functions*, **10**, 20.

Dong, G., Devito, E. E., Du, X. & Cui, Z. (2012a). Impaired inhibitory control in "internet addiction disorder": a functional magnetic resonance imaging study. *Psychiatry Research*, **203**(2–3), 153–158.

Dong, G., DeVito, E., Huang, J. & Du, X. (2012b). Diffusion tensor imaging reveals thalamus and posterior cingulate cortex abnormalities in internet gaming addicts. *Journal of Psychiatric Research*, **46**(9), 1212–1216.

Dong, G., Hu, Y., Lin, X. & Lu, Q. (2013). What makes Internet addicts continue playing online even when faced by severe negative consequences? Possible explanations from an fMRI study. *Biological Psychology*, **94**(2), 282–289.

Dong, G., Huang, J. & Du, X. (2011). Enhanced reward sensitivity and decreased losssensitivity in Internet addicts: an fMRI study during a guessing task. *Journal of Psychiatric Research*, **45**(11), 1525–1529.

Dong, G., Lin, X. & Potenza, M. N. (2015). Decreased functional connectivity in an executive control network is related to impaired executive function in Internet gaming disorder. *Progress Neuro-Psychopharmacol Biol Psychiatry*, **57**, 76–85.

Dong, G., Lin, X., Zhou, H. & Lu, Q. (2014). Cognitive flexibility in internet addicts: fMRI evidence from difficult-to-easy and easy-to-difficult switching situations. *Addictive Behaviors*, **39**(3), 677–683.

Dong, G. & Potenza, M. N. (2016). Risk-taking and risky decision-making in Internet gaming disorder: implications regarding online gaming in the setting of negative consequences. *Journal of Psychiatric Research*, **73**, 1–8.

Dullur, P. & Starcevic, V. (2017). Internet gaming disorder does not qualify as a mental disorder. *Australian & New Zealand Journal of Psychiatry*, **52**(2), 110–111.

Dunning, J. P., Parvaz, M. A., Hajcak, G., et al. (2011). Motivated attention to cocaine and emotional cues in abstinent and current cocaine users – an ERP study. *European Journal of Neuroscience*, **33**(9), 1716–1723.

Duven, E. C. P., Muller, K. W., Beutel, M. E. & Wolfling, K. (2015). Altered reward processing in pathological computer gamers – ERP-results from a semi-natural gaming-design. *Brain and Behavior*, **5**(1), 13–23.

Dymond, S., Lawrence, N. S., Dunkley, B. T., et al. (2014). Almost winning: induced MEG theta power in insula and orbitofrontal cortex increases during gambling near-misses and is associated with BOLD signal and gambling severity. *NeuroImage*, **91**, 210–219.

Eichenbaum, A., Kattner, F., Bradford, D., Gentile, D. A. & Green, C. S. (2015). role-playing and real-time strategy games associated with greater probability of Internet Gaming Disorder. *Cyberpsychology, Behavior and Social Networking*, **18**(8), 480–485.

Eisen, S. A., Lin, N., Lyons, M. J., et al. (1998). Familial influences on gambling behavior: an analysis of 3359 twin pairs. *Addiction*, **93**(9), 1375–1384.

Everitt, B. J. & Robbins, T. W. (2005). Neural systems of reinforcement for drug addiction: from actions to habits to compulsion. *Nature Neuroscience*, **8**(11), 1481–1489.

Everitt, B. J. & Robbins, T. W. (2013). From the ventral to the dorsal striatum: devolving views of their roles in drug addiction. *Neuroscience and Biobehavioral Reviews*, **37**(9 Pt A), 1946–1954.

Fong, T., Kalechstein, A., Bernhard, B., Rosenthal, R. & Rugle, L. (2008). A double-blind, placebo-controlled trial of olanzapine for the treatment of video poker pathological gamblers. *Pharmacology, Biochemistry, and Behavior*, **89**(3), 298–303.

Garrison, K. A., Yip, S. W., Balodis, I. M., et al. (2017). Reward-related frontostriatal activity and smoking behavior among adolescents in treatment for smoking cessation. *Drug and Alcohol Dependence*, **177**, 268–276.

Georgiadis, J. R. & Kringelbach, M. L. (2012). The human sexual response cycle: brain imaging evidence linking sex to other pleasures. *Progress in Neurobiology*, **98**(1), 49–81.

Gescheidt, T., Marecek, R., Mikl, M., et al. (2013). Functional anatomy of outcome evaluation during Iowa Gambling Task performance in patients with Parkinson's disease: an fMRI study. *Neurological Sciences: Official Journal of the Italian Neurological Society and of the Italian Society of Clinical Neurophysiology*, **34**(12), 2159–2166.

Giddens, J. L., Xian, H., Scherrer, J. F., Eisen, S. A. & Potenza, M. N. (2011). Shared genetic contributions to anxiety disorders and pathological gambling in a male population. *Journal of Affective Disorders*, **132**, 406–412.

Gola, M. (2016). Decreased LPP for sexual images in problematic pornography users may be consistent with addiction models. Everything depends on the model. (Commentary on Prause, Steele, Staley, Sabatinelli, & Hajcak, 2015). *Biological Psychology*, **120**, 156–158.

Gola, M., Miyakoshi, M. & Sescousse, G. (2015). Sex, impulsivity, and anxiety: interplay between ventral striatum and amygdala reactivity in sexual behaviors. *Journal of Neuroscience*, **35**(46), 15227–15229.

Gola, M. & Potenza, M. N. (2016). Paroxetine treatment of problematic pornography use: a case series. *Journal of Behavioral Addictions*, **5**(3), 529–532.

Gola, M., Wordecha, M., Marchewka, A. & Sescousse, G. (2016). Visual sexual stimuli – cue or reward? A perspective for interpreting brain imaging findings on human sexual behaviors. *Frontiers in Human Neuroscience*, **10**, 402.

Gola, M., Wordecha, M., Sescousse, G., et al. (2017). Can pornography be addictive? An fMRI study of men seeking treatment for problematic pornography use. *Neuropsychopharmacology: Official Publication of the American College of Neuropsychopharmacology*, **42**(10), 2021–2031.

Goldstein, L., Manowitz, P., Nora, R., Swartzburg, M. & Carlton, P. L. (1985). Differential EEG activation and pathological gambling. *Biological Psychiatry*, **20**(11), 1232–1234.

Goldstein, R. Z. & Volkow, N. D. (2011). Dysfunction of the prefrontal cortex in addiction: neuroimaging findings and clinical implications. *Nature Reviews. Neuroscience*, **12**(11), 652–669.

Goudriaan, A. E., De Ruiter, M. B., Van Den Brink, W., Oosterlaan, J. & Veltman, D. J. (2010). Brain activation patterns associated with cue reactivity and craving in abstinent problem gamblers, heavy smokers and healthy controls: an fMRI study. *Addiction Biology*, **15**, 491–503.

Grant, J. E., Kim, S. W. & Hartman, B. K. (2008b). A double-blind, placebo-controlled study of the opiate antagonist naltrexone in the treatment of pathological gambling urges. *The Journal of Clinical Psychiatry*, **69**(5), 783–789.

Grant, J. E., Kim, S. W., Hollander, E. & Potenza, M. N. (2008a). Predicting response to opiate antagonists and placebo in the treatment of pathological gambling. *Psychopharmacology*, **200**, 521–527.

Grant, J. E., Kim, S. W. & Odlaug, B. L. (2007). N-acetyl cysteine, a glutamate-modulating agent, in the treatment of pathological gambling: a pilot study. *Biological Psychiatry*, **62**(6), 652–657.

Grant, J. E., Kim, S. W., Potenza, M. N., et al. (2003). Paroxetine treatment of pathological gambling: a multi-centre randomized controlled trial. *International Clinical Psychopharmacology*, **18**(4), 243–249.

Grant, J. E., Odlaug, B. L., Chamberlain, S. R., et al. (2013). A proof of concept study of tolcapone for pathological gambling: relationships with COMT genotype and brain activation. *European Neuropsychopharmacology*, **23**(11), 1587–1596.

Grant, J. E., Odlaug, B. L., Chamberlain, S. R., et al. (2014). A randomized, placebo-controlled trial of N-acetylcysteine plus imaginal desensitization for nicotine-dependent pathological gamblers. *The Journal of Clinical Psychiatry*, **75**(1), 39–45.

Grant, J. E., Odlaug, B. L., Potenza, M. N., Hollander, E. & Kim, S. W. (2010). A multi-center, double-blind, placebo-controlled study of the opioid antagonist nalmefene in the treatment of pathological gambling. *British Journal of Psychiatry*, **197**, 330–331.

Grant, J. E. & Potenza, M. N. (2006). Escitalopram treatment of pathological gambling with co-occurring anxiety: an open-label pilot study with double-blind discontinuation. *International Clinical Psychopharmacology*, **21**(4), 203–209.

Grant, J. E., Potenza, M. N., Hollander, E., et al. (2006). A multicenter investigation of the opioid antagonist nalmefene in the treatment of pathological gambling. *American Journal of Psychiatry*, **163**, 303–312.

Grant, J. E., Potenza, M. N., Kraus, S. W. & Petrakis, I. L. (2017). Naltrexone and disulfiram treatment response in veterans with alcohol dependence and co-occurring gambling problems. *Journal of Clinical Psychiatry*, **78**(9), e1299–e1306.

Griffiths, M. D., King, D. L. & Demetrovics, Z. (2014). DSM-5 internet gaming disorder needs a unified approach to assessment. *Neuropsychiatry*, **4**(1), 1–4.

Han, D. H., Kim, Y. S., Lee, Y. S., Min, K. J. & Renshaw, P. F. (2010). Changes in cue-induced, prefrontal cortex activity with video-game play. *Cyberpsychology, Behavior and Social Networking*, **13**(6), 655–661.

Han, D. H., Lee, Y. S., Na, C., et al. (2009). The effect of methylphenidate on Internet video game play in children with attention-deficit/hyperactivity disorder. *Comprehensive Psychiatry*, **50**(3), 251–256.

Han, D. H., Lee, Y. S., Yang, K. C., et al. (2007). Dopamine genes and reward dependence in adolescents with excessive internet video game play. *Journal of Addiction Medicine.*, **1**, 133–138.

Han, D. H. & Renshaw, P. F. (2012). Bupropion in the treatment of problematic online game play in patients with major depressive disorder. *Journal of Psychopharmacology*, **26** (5), 689–696.

Hariri, A. R., Brown, S. M., Williamson, D. E., et al. (2006). Preference for immediate over delayed rewards is associated with magnitude of ventral striatal activity. *The Journal of Neuroscience: The Official Journal of the Society for Neuroscience*, **26**(51), 13213–13217.

Hayoun, M. (2014). *China: Inside an Internet gaming disorder rehab center*. Aljazeera America.

Heidbreder, C. A., Gardner, E. L., Xi, Z.-X., et al. (2005). The role of central dopamine D3 receptors in drug addiction: a review of pharmacological evidence. *Brain Research. Brain Research Reviews*, **49**(1), 77–105.

Hewig, J., Kretschmer, N., Trippe, R. H., et al. (2010). Hypersensitivity to reward in problem gamblers. *Biological Psychiatry*, **67**(8), 781–783.

Hollander, E., DeCaria, C. M., Finkell, J. N., et al. (2000). A randomized double-blind fluvoxamine/placebo crossover trial in pathologic gambling. *Biological Psychiatry*, **47** (9), 813–817.

Hollander, E., DeCaria, C. M., Mari, E., et al. (1998). Short-term single-blind fluvoxamine treatment of pathological gambling. *The American Journal of Psychiatry*, **155**(12), 1781–1783.

Huffington Post (2013). Porn sites get more visitors each month than Netflix, Amazon and Twitter combined.

Joutsa, J., Johansson, J., Niemela, S., et al. (2012). Mesolimbic dopamine release is linked to symptom severity in pathological gambling. *NeuroImage*, **60**(4), 1992–1999.

Joutsa, J., Saunavaara, J., Parkkola, R., Niemela, S. & Kaasinen, V. (2011). Extensive abnormality of brain white matter integrity in pathological gambling. *Psychiatry Research*, **194**(3), 340–346.

Kessler, R. C., Hwang, I., LaBrie, R., et al. (2008). DSM-IV pathological gambling in the National Comorbidity Survey Replication. *Psychological Medicine*, **38**(9), 1351–1360.

Kafka, M. P. (2010). Hypersexual disorder: a proposed diagnosis for DSM-V. *Archives of Sexual Behavior*, **39**(2), 377–400.

Kim, S. H., Baik, S. H., Park, C. S., et al. (2011). Reduced striatal dopamine D2 receptors in people with Internet addiction. *Neuroreport*, **22**(8), 407–411.

Kim, S. W. (1998). Opioid antagonists in the treatment of impulse-control disorders. *The Journal of Clinical Psychiatry*, **59**(4), 159–164.

Kim, S. W., Grant, J. E., Adson, D. E. & Shin, Y. C. (2001). Double-blind naltrexone and placebo comparison study in the treatment of pathological gambling. *Biological Psychiatry*, **49**(11), 914–921.

Kim, S. W., Grant, J. E., Adson, D. E., Shin, Y. C. & Zaninelli, R. (2002). A double-blind placebo-controlled study of the efficacy and safety of paroxetine in the treatment of pathological gambling. *The Journal of Clinical Psychiatry*, **63**(6), 501–507.

Kim, Y. J., Lee, J.-Y., Oh, S., et al. (2017). Associations between prospective symptom changes and slow-wave activity in patients with Internet gaming disorder: a resting-state EEG study. *Medicine*, **96**(8), e6178.

Kim, Y.-R., Son, J.-W., Lee, S.-I., et al. (2012). Abnormal brain activation of adolescent internet addict in a ball-throwing animation task: possible neural correlates of disembodiment revealed by fMRI. *Progress in Neuro-Psychopharmacology & Biological Psychiatry*, **39**(1), 88–95.

King, D. L. & Delfabbro, P. H. (2016). Defining tolerance in Internet Gaming disorder: Isn't it time?. *Addiction*, **111**(11), 2064–2065.

King, D. L., Delfabbro, P. H., Potenza, M. N., et al. (2018). Internet gaming disorder should qualify as a mental disorder. *Australian & New Zealand Journal of Psychiatry*, **52**(7), 615–617.

King, D. L., Haagsma, M. C., Delfabbro, P. H., Gradisar, M. & Griffiths, M. D. (2013). Toward a consensus definition of pathological video-gaming: a systematic review of psychometric assessment tools. *Clinical Psychology Review*, **33**(3), 331–342.

King, D. L., Herd, M. C. & Delfabbro, P. H. (2017). Tolerance in Internet gaming disorder: a need for increasing gaming time or something else? *Journal of Behavioral Addictions*, **6**(4), 525–533.

Ko, C.-H., Hsieh, T.-J., Chen, C.-Y., et al. (2014). Altered brain activation during response inhibition and error processing in subjects with Internet gaming disorder: a functional magnetic imaging study. *European Archives of Psychiatry and Clinical Neuroscience*, **264**(8), 661–672.

Ko, C.-H., Liu, G.-C., Hsiao, S., et al. (2009). Brain activities associated with gaming urge of online gaming addiction. *Journal of Psychiatric Research*, **43**(7), 739–747.

Ko, C.-H., Liu, G.-C., Yen, J.-Y., et al. (2013a). Brain correlates of craving for online gaming under cue exposure in subjects with Internet gaming addiction and in remitted subjects. *Addiction Biology*, **18**(3), 559–569.

Ko, C.-H., Liu, G.-C., Yen, J.-Y., et al. (2013b). The brain activations for both cue-induced gaming urge and smoking craving among subjects comorbid with Internet gaming addiction and nicotine dependence. *Journal of Psychiatric Research*, **47**(4), 486–493.

Kober, H., Lacadie, C. M., Wexler, B. E., et al. (2016). Brain activity during cocaine craving and gambling urges: an fMRI study. *Neuropsychopharmacology: Official Publication of the American College of Neuropsychopharmacology*, **41**(2), 628–637.

Kor, A., Fogel, Y., Reid, R. & Potenza, M. N. (2013). Should hypersexual disorder be classified as an addiction? *Sexual Addiction Compulsivity*, **20**, 27–47.

Kraus, S. W., Krueger, R. B., Briken, P., et al. (2018). Compulsive sexual behaviour disorder in the ICD-11. *World Psychiatry*, **17**, 109-110.

Kraus, S. W., Meshberg-Cohen, S., Martino, S., Quinones, L. J. & Potenza, M. N. (2015). Treatment of compulsive pornography use with naltrexone: a case report. *American Journal of Psychiatry*, **172**(12), 1260–1261.

Kühn, S. & Gallinat, J. (2014). Brain structure and functional connectivity associated with pornography consumption: the brain on porn. *JAMA Psychiatry*, **71**(7), 827–834.

Kuss, D. J. (2013). Internet gaming addiction: current perspectives. *Psychology Research and Behavior Management*, **6**, 125–137.

Lang, M., Leménager, T., Streit, F., et al. (2016). Genome-wide association study of pathological gambling. *European Psychiatry*, **36**, 38–46.

Lawrence, A. J., Luty, J., Bogdan, N. A., Sahakian, B. J. & Clark, L. (2009). Problem gamblers share deficits in impulsive decision-making with alcohol-dependent individuals. *Addiction*, **104**(6), 1006–1015.

Lee, J.-Y., Kim, J.-M., Kim, J. W., et al. (2010). Association between the dose of dopaminergic medication and the behavioral disturbances in Parkinson disease. *Parkinsonism & Related Disorders*, **16**(3), 202–207.

Leeman, R. F. & Potenza, M. N. (2012). Similarities and differences between pathological gambling and substance use disorders: a focus on impulsivity and compulsivity. *Psychopharmacology*, **219**(2), 469–490.

Leménager, T., Dieter, J., Hill, H., et al. (2014). Neurobiological correlates of physical self-concept and self-identification with avatars in addicted players of Massively Multiplayer Online Role-Playing Games (MMORPGs). *Addictive Behaviors*, **39**(12), 1789–1797.

Lim, S., Ha, J., Choi, S.-W., Kang, S.-G. & Shin, Y.-C. (2012). Association study on pathological gambling and polymorphisms of dopamine D1, D2, D3, and D4 receptor genes in a Korean population. *Journal of Gambling Studies*, **28**(3), 481–491.

Limbrick-Oldfield, E. H., Mick, I., Cocks, R. E., et al. (2017). Neural substrates of cue reactivity and craving in gambling disorder. *Translational Psychiatry*, **7**(1), e992.

Lin, F., Zhou, Y., Du, Y., et al. (2012). Abnormal white matter integrity in adolescents with internet addiction disorder: a tract-based spatial statistics study. *PLoS ONE*, **7**(1), e30253.

Lin, X., Zhou, H., Dong, G. & Du, X. (2015). Impaired risk evaluation in people with Internet gaming disorder: fMRI evidence from a probability discounting task. *Progress in Neuro-Psychopharmacology & Biological Psychiatry*, **56**, 142–148.

Lind, P. A., Zhu, G., Montgomery, G. W., et al. (2013). Genome-wide association study of a quantitative disordered gambling trait. *Addiction Biology*, **18**(3), 511–522.

Linnet, J., Moller, A., Peterson, E., Gjedde, A. & Doudet, D. (2011). Dopamine release in ventral striatum during Iowa Gambling Task performance is associated with increased excitement levels in pathological gambling. *Addiction*, **106**(2), 383–390.

Liu, G.-C., Yen, J.-Y., Chen, C.-Y., et al. (2014). Brain activation for response inhibition under gaming cue distraction in internet gaming disorder. *The Kaohsiung Journal of Medical Sciences*, **30**(1), 43–51.

Liu, L., Xue, G., Potenza, M. N., et al. (2017a). Dissociable neural processes during risky decision-making in individuals with Internet-gaming disorder. *NeuroImage. Clinical*, **14**, 741–749.

Liu, L., Yip, S. W., Zhang, J.-T., et al. (2017b). Activation of the ventral and dorsal striatum during cue reactivity in Internet gaming disorder. *Addiction Biology*, **22**(3), 791–801.

Lobo, D. S. S., Souza, R. P., Tong, R. P., et al. (2010). Association of functional variants in the dopamine D2-like receptors with risk for gambling behaviour in healthy Caucasian subjects. *Biological Psychology*, **85**(1), 33–37.

Lobo, D. S. S, Vallada, H. P., Knight, J., et al. (2007). Dopamine genes and pathological gambling in discordant sib-pairs. *Journal of Gambling Studies*, **23**(4), 421–433.

Majuri, J., Joutsa, J., Johansson, J., et al. (2017a). Dopamine and opioid neurotransmission in behavioral addictions: A comparative PET study in pathological gambling and binge eating. *Neuropsychopharmacology: Official Publication of the American College of Neuropsychopharmacology*, **42**(5), 1169–1177.

Majuri, J., Joutsa, J., Johansson, J., et al. (2017b). Serotonin transporter density in binge eating disorder and pathological gambling: a PET study with [(11)C]MADAM. *European Neuropsychopharmacology: The Journal of the European College of Neuropsychopharmacology*, **27**(12), 1281–1288.

McClure, E. A., Gipson, C. D., Malcolm, R. J., Kalivas, P. W. & Gray, K. M. (2014). Potential role of N-acetylcysteine in the management of substance use disorders. *CNS Drugs*, **28**(2), 95–106.

McElroy, S. L., Nelson, E. B., Welge, J. A., Kaehler, L. & Keck, P. E. J. (2008). Olanzapine in the treatment of pathological gambling: a negative randomized placebo-controlled trial. *The Journal of Clinical Psychiatry*, **69**(3), 433–440.

Meyer, G., Schwertfeger, J., Exton, M. S., et al. (2004). Neuroendocrine response to casino gambling in problem gamblers. *Psychoneuroendocrinology*, **29**(10), 1272–1280.

Mick, I., Myers, J., Ramos, A. C., et al. (2016). Blunted endogenous opioid release following an oral amphetamine challenge in pathological gamblers. *Neuropsychopharmacology: Official Publication of the American College of Neuropsychopharmacology*, **41**(7), 1742–1750.

Miedl, S. F., Peters, J. & Buchel, C. (2012). Altered neural reward representations in pathological gamblers revealed by delay and probability discounting. *Archives of General Psychiatry*, **69**(2), 177–186.

Moccia, L., Pettorruso, M., De Crescenzo, F., et al. (2017). Neural correlates of cognitive control in gambling disorder: a systematic review of fMRI studies. *Neuroscience and Biobehavioral Reviews*, **78**, 104–116.

Moeller, S. J., Hajcak, G., Parvaz, M. A., et al. (2012). Psychophysiological prediction of choice: relevance to insight and drug addiction. *Brain* **135**(11), 3481–3494. doi:10.1093/brain/aws252

Moorman, D. E. & Aston-Jones, G. (2014). Orbitofrontal cortical neurons encode expectation-driven initiation of reward-seeking. *The Journal of Neuroscience: The Official Journal of the Society for Neuroscience*, **34**(31), 10234–10246.

Myrseth, H., Molde, H., Støylen, I., et al. (2011). A pilot study of CBT versus escitalopram combined with CBT in the treatment of pathological gamblers. *International Gambling Studies* **11**(1), 121–141.

Na, E., Choi, I., Lee, T.-H., et al. (2017). The influence of game genre on Internet gaming disorder. *Journal of Behavioral Addictions*, 1–8.

Nordin, C. & Eklundh, T. (1999). Altered CSF 5-HIAA disposition in pathologic male gamblers. *CNS Spectrums*, **4**(12), 25–33.

Nutt, D. J., Lingford-Hughes, A., Erritzoe, D. & Stokes, P. R. (2015). The dopamine theory of addiction: 40 years of highs and lows. *Nature Reviews Neuroscience*, **16**(5), 305.

Pallanti, S., Bernardi, S., Quercioli, L., DeCaria, C. & Hollander, E. (2006). Serotonin dysfunction in pathological gamblers: increased prolactin response to oral m-CPP versus placebo. *CNS Spectrums*, **11**(12), 956–964.

Park, J. H., Hong, J. S., Han, D. H., et al. (2017a). Comparison of QEEG findings between adolescents with attention deficit hyperactivity disorder (ADHD) without comorbidity and ADHD comorbid with Internet Gaming Disorder. *Journal of Korean Medical Science*, **32**(3), 514–521.

Park, S. M., Lee, J. Y., Kim, Y. J., et al. (2017b). Neural connectivity in Internet gaming disorder and alcohol use disorder: a resting-state EEG coherence study. *Scientific Reports*, **7**(1), 1333.

Park, J. H., Lee, Y. S., Sohn, J. H. & Han, D. H. (2016). Effectiveness of atomoxetine and methylphenidate for problematic online gaming in adolescents with attention deficit hyperactivity disorder. *Human Psychopharmacology: Clinical and Experimental*, **31**(6), 427–432.

Petry, N. M. & O'Brien, C. P. (2013). Internet gaming disorder and the DSM-5. *Addiction*, **108**(7), 1186–1187.

Petry, N. M., Stinson, F. S. & Grant, B. F. (2005). Comorbidity of DSM-IV pathological gambling and other psychiatric disorders: results from the National Epidemiologic Survey on Alcohol and Related Conditions. *The Journal of Clinical Psychiatry*, **66**(5), 564–574.

Potenza, M. N. (2013a). Neurobiology of gambling behaviors. *Current Opinion in Neurobiology*, **23**(4), 660–667.

Potenza, M. N. (2013b) How central is dopamine to pathological gambling or gambling disorder? *Frontiers in Behavioral Neuroscience* **7**,206. (PMC3870289)

Potenza, M. N. (2018) Searching for replicable dopamine-related findings in gambling disorder. *Biological Psychiatry*, **83**, 984–986.

Potenza, M. N., Balodis, I. M., Franco, C. A., et al. (2013a). Neurobiological considerations in understanding behavioral treatments for pathological gambling. *Psychology of Addictive Behaviors: Journal of the Society of Psychologists in Addictive Behaviors*, **27**(2), 380–392.

Potenza, M. N., Leung, H.-C., Blumberg, H. P., et al. (2003a). An fMRI Stroop task study of ventromedial prefrontal cortical function in pathological gamblers. *The American Journal of Psychiatry*, **160**(11), 1990–1994.

Potenza, M. N., Steinberg, M. A., Skudlarski, P., et al. (2003b). Gambling urges in pathological gambling: a functional magnetic resonance imaging study. *Archives of General Psychiatry*, **60**(8), 828–836.

Potenza, M. N., Walderhaug, E., Henry, S., et al. (2013b). Serotonin 1B receptor imaging in pathological gambling. *The World Journal of Biological Psychiatry: The Official Journal of the World Federation of Societies of Biological Psychiatry*, **14**(2), 139–145.

Potenza, M. N., Xian, H., Shah, K. R., Scherrer, J. F. & Eisen, S. A. (2005). Shared genetic contributions to pathological gambling and major depression in men. *Archives of General Psychiatry*, **62**, 1015–1021.

Power, Y., Goodyear, B. & Crockford, D. (2012). Neural correlates of pathological gamblers preference for immediate rewards during the Iowa Gambling Task: an fMRI study. *Journal of Gambling Studies*, **28**(4), 623–636.

Prause, N., Steele, V. R., Staley, C., Sabatinelli, D. & Hajcak, G. (2015). Modulation of late positive potentials by sexual images in problem users and controls inconsistent with "porn addiction." *Biological Psychology*, **109**, 192–199.

Qi, X., Du, X., Yang, Y., et al. (2015). Decreased modulation by the risk level on the brain activation during decision making in adolescents with internet gaming disorder. *Frontiers in Behavioral Neuroscience*, **9**, 296.

Rahman, A. S., Xu, J. & Potenza, M. N. (2014). Hippocampal and amygdalar volumetric differences in pathological gambling: a preliminary study of the associations with the behavioral inhibition system. *Neuropsychopharmacology: Official Publication of the American College of Neuropsychopharmacology*, **39**(3), 738–745.

Reid, R. C., Carpenter, B. N., Hook, J. N., et al. (2012). Report of findings in a DSM-5 field trial for hypersexual disorder. *The Journal of Sexual Medicine*, **9**(11), 2868–2877.

Reissner, K. J. & Kalivas, P. W. (2010). Using glutamate homeostasis as a target for treating addictive disorders. *Behavioural Pharmacology*, **21**(5-6), 514–522.

Reuter, J., Raedler, T., Rose, M., et al. (2005). Pathological gambling is linked to reduced activation of the mesolimbic reward system. *Nature Neuroscience*, **8**(2), 147–148.

Robinson, M. J., Fischer, A. M., Ahuja, A., Lesser, E. N. & Maniates, H. (2016). Roles of "wanting" and "liking" in motivating behavior: Gambling, food, and drug addictions. *Current Topics in Behavioral Neuroscience*, **27**, 105–136.

Rosenberg, O., Dinur, L. K. & Dannon, P. N. (2013). Four-year follow-up study of pharmacological treatment in pathological gamblers. *Clinical Neuropharmacology*, **36**(2), 42–45.

Roy, A., Adinoff, B., Roehrich, L., et al. (1988). Pathological gambling: a psychobiological study. *Archives of General Psychiatry*, **45**(4), 369–373.

Roy, A., De Jong, J. & Linnoila, M. (1989). Extraversion in pathological gamblers: correlates with indexes of noradrenergic function. *Archives of General Psychiatry*, **46**(8), 679–681.

Saiz-Ruiz, J., Blanco, C., Ibanez, A., et al. (2005). Sertraline treatment of pathological gambling: a pilot study. *The Journal of Clinical Psychiatry*, **66**(1), 28–33.

Schimmenti, A., Guglielmucci, F., Barbasio, C. & Granieri, A. (2012). Attachment disorganization and dissociation in virtual worlds: a study on problematic Internet use among players of online role playing games. *Clinical Neuropsychiatry*, **9**(5), 187–195.

Schwartz, D. G. (2013). *Roll the Bones: The History of Gambling.* Las Vegas, NV: Winchester Books.

Seok, J. W. & Sohn, J. H. (2015). Neural substrates of sexual desire in individuals with problematic hypersexual behavior. *Frontiers in Behavioral Neuroscience*, **9**, 321.

Slutske, W. S., Eisen, S., True, W. R., et al. (2000). Common genetic vulnerability for pathological gambling and alcohol dependence in men. *Archives of General Psychiatry*, **57**(7), 666–673.

Slutske, W. S., Ellingson, J. M., Richmond-Rakerd, L. S., Zhu, G. & Martin, N. G. (2013). Shared genetic vulnerability for disordered gambling and alcohol use disorder in men and women: evidence from a national community-based Australian Twin Study. *Twin Research and Human Genetics: The Official Journal of the International Society for Twin Studies*, **16**(2), 525–534.

Son, K.-L., Choi, J.-S., Lee, J., et al. (2015). Neurophysiological features of Internet gaming disorder and alcohol use disorder: a resting-state EEG study. *Translational Psychiatry*, **5**, e628.

Song, J., Park, J. H., Han, D. H., et al. (2016). Comparative study of the effects of bupropion and escitalopram on Internet gaming disorder. *Psychiatry and Clinical Neurosciences*, **70**(11), 527–535.

Steeves, T. D. L., Miyasaki, J., Zurowski, M., et al. (2009). Increased striatal dopamine release in Parkinsonian patients with pathological gambling: a [11C] raclopride PET study. *Brain*, **132**(5), 1376–1385.

Sun, Y., Ying, H., Seetohul, R. M., et al. (2012). Brain fMRI study of crave induced by cue pictures in online game addicts (male adolescents). *Behavioural Brain Research*, **233** (2), 563–576.

Tanabe, J., Thompson, L., Claus, E., et al. (2007). Prefrontal cortex activity is reduced in gambling and nongambling substance users during decision-making. *Human Brain Mapping*, **28**(12), 1276–1286.

Thalemann, R., Wölfling, K. & Grüsser, S. M. (2007). Specific cue reactivity on computer game-related cues in excessive gamers. *Behavioral Neuroscience*, **121**(3), 614.

Thomas, A., Bonanni, L., Gambi, F., Di Iorio, A. & Onofrj, M. (2010). Pathological gambling in Parkinson disease is reduced by amantadine. *Annals of Neurology*, **68**(3), 400–404.

Tian, M., Chen, Q., Zhang, Y., et al. (2014). PET imaging reveals brain functional changes in internet gaming disorder. *European Journal of Nuclear Medicine and Molecular Imaging*, **41** (7), 1388–1397.

van Eimeren, T., Pellecchia, G., Cilia, R., et al. (2010). Drug-induced deactivation of inhibitory networks predicts pathological gambling in PD. *Neurology*, **75**(19), 1711–1716.

van Holst, R. J., de Ruiter, M. B., van den Brink, W., Veltman, D. J. & Goudriaan, A. E. (2012). A voxel-based morphometry study comparing problem gamblers, alcohol abusers, and healthy controls. *Drug and Alcohol Dependence*, **124**(1–2), 142–148.

Voon, V., Mole, T. B., Banca, P., et al. (2014). Neural correlates of sexual cue reactivity in individuals with and without compulsive sexual behaviours. *PLoS ONE*, **9**(7), e102419.

Voon, V., Napier, T. C., Frank, M. J., et al. (2017). Impulse control disorders and levodopa-induced dyskinesias in Parkinson's disease: an update. *The Lancet. Neurology*, **16**(3), 238–250.

Voon, V., Sohr, M., Lang, A. E., et al. (2011). Impulse control disorders in Parkinson disease: a multicenter case-control study. *Annals of Neurology*, **69**(6), 986–996.

Wang, Y., Wu, L., Wang, L., et al. (2017). Impaired decision-making and impulse control in Internet gaming addicts: evidence from the comparison with recreational Internet game users. *Addiction Biology*, **22**(6), 1610–1621.

Weintraub, D. & Claassen, D. O. (2017). Impulse control and related disorders in Parkinson's disease. *International Review of Neurobiology*, **133**, 679–717.

Weintraub, D., Koester, J., Potenza, M. N., et al. **for the DOMINION Study Group** (2010). Impulse control disorders in Parkinson's disease: a cross-sectional study of 3,090 patients. *Archives of Neurology*, **67**, 589–595.

Wexler, B. E., Gottschalk, C. H., Fulbright, R. K., et al. (2001). Functional magnetic resonance imaging of cocaine craving. *American Journal of Psychiatry*, **158**(1), 86–95.

Wölfling, K., Morsen, C. P., Duven, E., et al. (2011). To gamble or not to gamble: at risk for craving and relapse–learned motivated attention in pathological gambling. *Biological Psychology*, **87**(2), 275–281.

Worhunsky, P. D., Malison, R. T., Rogers, R. D. & Potenza, M. N. (2014). Altered neural correlates of reward and loss processing during simulated slot-machine fMRI in pathological gambling and cocaine dependence. *Drug and Alcohol Dependence*, **145**, 77–86.

Xian, H., Giddens, J. L., Scherrer, J. F., Eisen, S. A. & Potenza, M. N. (2014). Environmental factors selectively impact co-occurrence of problem/pathological gambling with specific drug-use disorders in male twins. *Addiction*, **109**(4), 635–644.

Yang, B.-Z., Balodis, I. M., Lacadie, C. M., Xu, J. & Potenza, M. N. (2016). A preliminary study of DBH (encoding dopamine beta-hydroxylase) genetic variation and neural correlates of emotional and motivational processing in individuals with and without pathological gambling. *Journal of Behavioral Addictions*, **5**(2), 282–292.

Yao, Y.-W., Liu, L., Ma, S.-S., et al. (2017). Functional and structural neural alterations in Internet gaming disorder: a systematic review and meta-analysis. *Neuroscience and Biobehavioral Reviews*, **83**, 313–324.

Yau, Y. H. C., Crowley, M. J., Mayes, L. C. & Potenza, M. N. (2012). Are Internet use and video-game-playing addictive behaviors? Biological, clinical and public health implications for youths and adults. *Minerva Psychiatrica*, **53**(3), 153–170.

Yip, S. W., Lacadie, C., Xu, J., et al. (2013). Reduced genual corpus callosal white matter integrity in pathological gambling and its relationship to alcohol abuse or dependence. *The World Journal of Biological Psychiatry: The Official Journal of the World Federation of Societies of Biological Psychiatry*, **14**(2), 129–138.

Yip, S. W., Morie, K. P., Xu, J., et al. (2017). Shared microstructural features of behavioral and substance addictions revealed in areas of crossing fibers. *Biological Psychiatry. Cognitive Neuroscience and Neuroimaging*, **2** (2), 188–195.

Yip, S. W. & Potenza, M. N. (2014). Treatment of gambling disorders. *Current Treatment Options in Psychiatry*, **1**(2), 189–203.

Yip, S. W., Worhsunky, P. D., Xu, J., et al. (2018). Gray-matter relationships to diagnostic and transdiagnostic features of drug and behavioral addictions. *Addiction Biology*, **23**(1), 394–402.

Youh, J., Hong, J. S., Han, D. H., et al. (2017). Comparison of electroencephalography (EEG) coherence between major depressive disorder (MDD) without comorbidity and MDD comorbid with Internet Gaming Disorder. *Journal of Korean Medical Science*, **32**(7), 1160–1165.

Young, K. (2009). Internet addiction: diagnosis and treatment considerations. *Journal of Contemporary Psychotherapy*, **39**(4), 241–246.

Yuan, K., Cheng, P., Dong, T., et al. (2013). Cortical thickness abnormalities in late adolescence with online gaming addiction. *PLoS ONE*, **8**(1), e53055.

Yuan, K., Qin, W., Wang, G., Zeng, F., Zhao, L., Yang, X., . . . **Tian, J.** (2011). Microstructure abnormalities in adolescents with internet addiction disorder. *PLoS ONE*, *6*(6), e20708.

Yuan, K., Qin, W., Yu, D., et al. (2016). Core brain networks interactions and cognitive control in internet gaming disorder individuals in late adolescence/early adulthood. *Brain Structure & Function*, **221** (3), 1427–1442.

Zack, M. & Poulos, C. X. (2007). A D2 antagonist enhances the rewarding and priming effects of a gambling episode in pathological gamblers. *Neuropsychopharmacology: Official Publication of the American College of Neuropsychopharmacology*, **32**(8), 1678–1686.

Zhang, J.-T., Yao, Y.-W., Potenza, M. N., et al. (2016). Effects of craving behavioral intervention on neural substrates of cue-induced craving in Internet gaming disorder. *NeuroImage. Clinical*, **12**, 591–599.

12 Multiple Memory Systems, Addiction, and Health Habits: New Routes for Translational Science

Alan W. Stacy, PhD, James Russell Pike, MBA, and Anna Yu Lee, BS

Introduction

Memory system approaches rely heavily on converging findings from neuroscience and allied multidisciplinary areas. These approaches are relevant to all behaviors and habits, with the addictions as a special case. Memory processes govern the encoding, retention, retrieval, or accessibility of experiences, and the conversion of experiences into a variety of tendencies, actions, cognitions, and affective states that reflect these experiences. These processes affect how experiences are converted into future actions. Previous experiences cannot affect later behavior unless they are registered and retained in the brain in some form, and the memory literature and work at the neural level provides a thorough, rigorous, multilevel and biologically plausible framework to enhance understanding of health habits of all kinds. Because of the rich array of basic research findings on memory, an effective application of research on multiple memory systems to addiction may require more than attention to the addiction literature alone. Thus, this chapter addresses a wide range of findings on application of memory systems to addiction and suggests new routes for the study and application of some of the more poorly understood processes. This work falls into the realm of Type 1 translational research (Fishbein et al., 2016), in which basic research is harnessed in hopes of developing new innovations in understanding, prediction, and intervention. To accomplish these goals, this chapter provides a primer on existing memory system theories, highlights findings from relevant prospective research on habit and addictive behaviors, clarifies some of the primary differences across disciplines, and provides examples of new routes for translational science.

Contemporary memory system approaches were motivated initially by early clinical findings from human patients with brain damage and from a series of studies on nonhuman animals. The most frequently cited early clinical case involved patient HM, who presented with a particular form of amnesia in which new information could not be consciously or deliberately recalled (Scoville & Milner, 1957). Other than impairment in conscious or deliberate recall of new events, HM appeared to show normal or mostly normal levels of other forms of memory involving common facts, retention of learned habits, and other forms of memory for knowledge learned prior to neurosurgery for a serious medical issue. Because of uncontrollable seizures, major sections of the hippocampal region within the medial temporal lobe had been surgically resected. In addition to research with HM and similar patients studied at that time (Scoville & Milner, 1957), subsequent studies have confirmed that patients with impaired conscious recollection and lesions within this particular region of the brain retain normal performance on a variety of memory-related tasks that do not require recollection of a previous event (Levy, Stark & Squire, 2004; Schacter, 1985; Shimamura & Squire, 1984; Vaidya et al., 1995). Many of these studies have attempted to determine experimentally through manipulation of memory materials, instructions, and other experimental procedures what forms of memory were impaired or retained in these patients. The most common conclusion across several decades is that lesions or other abnormalities within the medial temporal lobe, including the hippocampus and related structures, are most likely to have led to impairment in this form of memory. Studies using a range of experimental designs have addressed other memory disorders as well, implicating different forms of memory and different neural circuits. For example, patients with Parkinson's disease typically have been found to develop impairments in the learning of new habits, with normal performance on tests of conscious recollection often termed explicit memory (Knowlton, Mangels & Squire, 1996; Packard & Knowlton, 2002). Alzheimer's patients, however, have not shown impairments in this form of habit memory (Eldridge, Masterman & Knowlton, 2002), despite decline in several other forms of memory over time. Additional dissociations in memory processes are found in patients with semantic dementia and Huntington's disease (Gabrieli et al., 1997; Vallet et al., 2017).

Animal research in rodents (White & McDonald, 2002; White, Packard & McDonald, 2013) and nonhuman primates (Rolls, 2000) also has studied the neural basis of different forms of learning and memory. This research experimentally manipulates different processes through varying the conditions of learning, as well as more invasive techniques such as infusion, lesion, or electrical stimulation. There are consistent commonalities across humans and other species at least regarding several of the regions and circuits involved in different forms of memory (White et al., 2013). Some research in this area has paid particular attention to memory systems involved in drug use and addiction, a topic that will be addressed in more detail below. Implications for a range of addictions and health habits will be suggested.

Acknowledgements The authors thank Kyla Mcilwee and Daniel Woytowich for helpful comments on this manuscript. Research reported in this publication was supported in part by the National Institute of Child Health and Human Development (NICHD) in conjunction with the US Food and Drug Administration (FDA) Center for Tobacco Products (R01HD077560) and the National Institute on Drug Abuse (R01DA033871). The content is solely the responsibility of the authors and does not necessarily represent the official views of the National Institutes of Health or the Food and Drug Administration.

Memory System Theories: A Primer Based on Research in Humans and Other Mammals

Declarative and Nondeclarative Memory Systems: Introduction and Terminology

The most frequently cited memory system approach was proposed by Squire and his colleagues (Squire, 2009; Squire & Knowlton, 1995; Squire, Knowlton & Musen, 1993). Squire used some of the findings briefly outlined above as well as many other findings to argue for two general categories and a number of more specific forms of memory. One category is declarative memory, which covers memory processes that involve conscious recollection of a specific event (episodic memory) as well as recall of commonly known facts and other semantic knowledge (semantic memory). Episodic memory is essentially compatible with typical colloquial discussions of memory: conscious memory for previous events or occurrences. The other category is nondeclarative (or procedural) memory, which involves other forms of memory that individuals have no conscious or introspective access to. These nondeclarative forms of memory reflect habits, classical conditioning, evaluative preferences, priming, and the development of many forms of skills.

An important distinction related to Squire's framework is the distinction between implicit and explicit memory. Implicit memory is a term first made popular by Graf and Schacter (Graf & Schacter, 1985), and was the first widely influential definition of any form of implicit cognition after about 1980. They suggested that "implicit memory is revealed when performance on a task is facilitated in the absence of conscious recollection" (p. 501). Explicit memory is essentially the same as episodic memory in Squire's terminology. Implicit memory has been further divided into different types, sometimes classified as conceptually driven (based on meaning or relations) or data driven (based on superficial or perceptual features). For the goals of the present chapter, perhaps the most important source of confusion across these terms has to do with how semantic or conceptual processes are construed and categorized. In Squire's nomenclature, semantic memory *content* that is accessible to consciousness falls under the umbrella of declarative memory. However, this does not imply that semantic memory *processes* are similarly accessible. Squire recognizes that priming, an ostensibly inaccessible process in his category of nondeclarative memory, can involve not only perceptual features but also semantic or conceptual ones. Indeed, many studies on implicit memory since the 1980s have engaged conceptual, semantic, or associative processes to study effects on indirect tests of memory; that is, tests that do not typically engage declarative memory since they do not require deliberate recollection of a previous event or conscious consideration of facts. For example, studies in amnesic patients (participants with impaired explicit memory) have found that presentation of a word list primes (facilitates) scores on a later test of implicit conceptual memory that requests free top-of-mind responses to cue words. The cue words are not the same words presented in the initial list but are *associatively related* to the words in that list (Levy et al., 2004; Schacter, 1985; Shimamura & Squire, 1984; Vaidya et al., 1995). The probabilities of "target" responses (words from the original word list) on this test are substantially higher than baseline associative response probabilities (free response probabilities without presentation of an earlier word list). These results have revealed an implicit form of memory for the list. In some studies, comparisons are made with nonamnesic participants, who show equivalent levels of priming but no deficits in explicit memory. Studies conducted with amnesic patients, and with adequate control of materials and participant selection, make it difficult to argue for effects of deliberate or conscious recollection.

On the surface, effects of priming using indirect tests that rely on conceptually driven processes may not be easy to completely reconcile with Squire's procedural (nondeclarative) system, since this form of priming often involves processing of meaning and/or associations that are, at least in some sense, accessible and can be "declared." However, this form of priming also spontaneously (i.e., without deliberation, explicit attempt at recall, or substantial effort) facilitates responses in the absence of ability to remember a recent event. In other words, the event or the process leading to the response does not need to be accessed or understood. In a different but related paradigm in cognitive science, often termed *semantic priming*, the presentation of a word or letter string on a computer screen (e.g., doctor) very rapidly facilitates the processing of a strongly related concept presented next (e.g., nurse). The two words are presented nearly simultaneously, with a very short interstimulus interval (e.g., 250 ms). The most frequently studied task asks for a *lexical decision*, in which the participant merely indicates with a keyboard press whether the second letter string is a word or not (yes or no). The typical finding is that a strongly related word will speed up processing beyond a baseline or comparison condition, as measured with response latency (Hutchison et al., 2008). The effects occur very rapidly and are often inferred as being automatic. People may not be able to declare the nature of this process and are not known to recall all or even any of the events that may have led to the strong relationship responsible for the findings. Yet, people realize relationships between many strongly associated concepts, even though they may not be aware of the automatic or implicit priming memory mechanisms that such relationships foster. As the word *doctor* primes *nurse*, *dog* primes *cat*, *chair* primes *table*, and in some people a word or phrase such as *Friday night* or *party* may, without any deliberation, rapidly prime thoughts of drinking alcohol, using party drugs, risky sexual behavior, or binge eating. Indeed, a variety of cues or "triggers" are known to be important in drug use and other risky behaviors, involving, for example: situational and social cues, affect, and drug paraphernalia (Back et al., 2014; Frankland, Bradley & Mogg, 2016; Oliver, Jentink, Drobes & Evans, 2016; Shono, Ames & Stacy, 2016; Shono et al., 2018; Sussman et al., 2001). In the present framework, cues should not be conceptualized as only conditioned or discriminative stimuli leading to a conditioned or instrumental response. The cues are likely to be relevant at a broader (or more distributed) level, and even at early stages of habit formation before commonly measured physiological symptoms of reactivity to cues (Garland et al., 2012) emerge. Priming effects that occur in everyday life are likely to color how one cognition flows to another (one's train of thought), how one behavior is engaged in but not another, what outcomes are considered, and so on. Indeed, research in social psychology has shown how various manipulations of events and stimuli prime subsequent behavior in remarkable ways (Bargh, Chen & Burrows, 1996).

Although Squire and some others classify all forms of priming as a nondeclarative process, some researchers may infer that priming does not ever manifest any conscious access to relevant content. Yet, many of the priming studies just cited require content to come to mind as part of the test of priming effects, even some studies authored by Squire that focused on nondeclarative processes. Thus, while the process of priming is nondeclarative or implicit, access to content *can be* part of the manifestation or measurement of this process. In some experimental paradigms, related content may not come to mind, whereas in other priming paradigms content does come to mind. Further, the power of strong relationships or associations in memory has been demonstrated in priming effects, but people can be generally aware of differences in such relationships. This is not inconsistent with the view that these associations can also operate (essentially) reflexively and are not necessarily brought to mind or consciously considered at behavior decision points. Similarly, conceptual or semantic processes are involved in priming, but the contents of semantic memory can obviously be involved in conscious thought. The contention that processes that are unconscious at some level can have a wide variety of manifestations, including conscious access to some related content, is generally consistent with the idea that such processes have many "flavors" (Bargh & Morsella, 2008) or variations (Moors, Spruyt & De Houwer, 2010).

Thought Experiments: Priming as a Nondeclarative Process in a Motivational Theory of Addiction

Thought experiments also illustrate how priming may operate rapidly in a *process* that is not accessible to awareness, while related content may or may not come to mind. Imagine someone with strong associations in memory between seeing a glass of wine (or seeing a sweet food) and reaching for it. In the present perspective the strength of the association between a glass of wine and reaching for it not only influences motivational processes postulated in contemporary models of addiction (e.g., Berridge & Robinson, 2016), but also influences the strength of a conceptual or semantic priming process and the rapid accessibility of conscious thoughts related to the wine. It is possible that if the individual is right next to the wine bar with full glasses immediately available, with only a short reach required, the reach might happen so fast that content (a reflection about wine) does not come to mind before the reach. This would be consistent with an automatic motivational process that Berridge and Robinson (Berridge & Robinson, 2016) term incentive-sensitization, in which drug cues trigger unconscious "wanting" that is supported by the mesolimbic motivational system (MMS). This system is involved in drug use, as well as other appetitive and potentially addictive behaviors such as sugar consumption and sex (Mahler & Berridge, 2012). The MMS has even been linked to gambling (Robinson et al., 2014). Yet, although not addressed by Berridge and Robinson, it is quite possible that MMS effects that foster behavior (e.g., approaching wine or a sweet food) are accompanied by one or both of the cognitive processes just outlined. Again, the priming literature suggests these include: (a) a rapid, nondeclarative, initially unconscious form of conceptual/semantic priming and (b) subsequent access to conscious thoughts activated by priming. Such priming may further propel people to engage in the behavior, especially in particular situations.

A second example provides the reasoning. In a twist to the first example, the wine bar (or dessert tray) is across the room but visible. The individual may automatically orient toward the bar (or tray) because of the incentive properties of the appetitive cue in accord with MMS effects and likely a parallel process of priming and related attentional processes. But since an immediate automatic motor response is likely too simple for complex navigation across a room full of people, associated primed thoughts (e.g., "there's a path to the wine") likely would spontaneously pop to mind assisting a circuitous route through friends to the object of attraction. Yet, Berridge and Robinson's model implies that cognitive priming must not be very relevant to addictions, which they clearly contend are governed by unconscious wanting *independent from cognitive processes*. However, on the basis of the large literature on priming, there is little reason to believe that people would not also experience rapid cognitive priming effects that act in parallel with motivational systems.

Rapid priming effects may even help engage motivational systems. Indeed, involvement of a form of conceptual/semantic priming is likely relevant to the rapid registration and interpretation of a drug (or other) situation through neocortical sensory and multisensory regions that associate cues to a drug context so that the MMS system is triggered by the situation. After all, to be a powerful trigger for drug use (or any other behavior), such a situation must be recognized with a relevant (e.g., drug or food related) meaning – spontaneous meaning analysis is well supported by interconnected neocortical regions (Binder & Desai, 2011). These neocortical priming effects, as well as stimulus-response (S-R) habit associations addressed below, seem likely to be involved in all habitual behaviors in humans, leading to rapid activation of a particular behavioral option when cues trigger the right meaning. Priming effects, whether classified as unconscious activation or more conscious but quite rapid accessibility of specific content, do not require involvement of the MMS or pharmacological effects. However, in the framework advanced here, MMS effects characterizing addiction would be expected to further triangulate neural systems on a particular behavior once the meaning of the cue is registered and to substantially influence motivational direction and urgency.

These contentions have implications for translational science. There needs to be a bridge between work on conceptual/semantic priming, on the one hand, and research on the MMS and related motivation systems. The current state of the literature is missing this linkage. The implications span theory, methods, and intervention. For example, if conceptual priming is indeed involved, then new routes for intervention could harness the power of associative learning involved in priming effects. Hypothesis tests would likely use imaging methods focused on new regions of interest (ROIs), experimental manipulations of priming, and/or validated measures of nondeclarative cognitive processes.

Habit: A Procedural System Distinct from Declarative Memory

In a classic study of different forms of memory in amnesic and Parkinson's patients, Knowlton and colleagues (Knowlton et al., 1996) found evidence of a double dissociation in which amnesic patients, with damage in the medial temporal lobe, showed severely impaired explicit memory for a training trial, but normal learning on a classification test that requires gradual learning of associations. On the other hand, Parkinson's patients, with damage to the neostriatum (part of the basal ganglia), failed to learn on the classification test but had intact explicit memory for the training episode. The classification test is analogous to habit learning experiments in nonhuman animals, in which the striatum has been strongly implicated in habit learning. Knowlton and colleagues concluded that the two memory systems are separate and parallel and that the neostriatal system is important for not only motor learning but also nonmotor habits that require the learning of new associations. A number of additional studies lend credence to the view that the habit system is distinct from other memory systems across multiple species of mammals in addition to humans (Packard & Goodman, 2013; Packard & Knowlton, 2002; Yin & Knowlton, 2006b). For example, Packard and Knowlton (2002) reviewed lesion and drug studies in monkeys and rats, neuropsychological studies in humans with basal ganglia dysfunction, and neuroimaging studies in humans without dysfunctions. Resolving some contradictions in this literature, they concluded that the basal ganglia and medial temporal lobe are normally activated simultaneously during learning but that the memory systems supported by these regions can act either cooperatively or competitively depending on the learning situation. For instance, Foerde, Knowlton and Poldrack (2006) found that in a nonpatient sample the probabilistic classification task appeared to be learned through the declarative system unless the task was accompanied by engagement in a second simultaneous, distracting task. In that case, the results suggested it was learned through the habit system as in Knowlton et al. (1996). The general implication is that the operation of different memory systems depends on the particular learning situation as well as the neuropsychological well-being of the individual.

More recently, White, Packard and McDonald (2013) reviewed much of the rodent research on multiple memory systems and documented fundamental distinctions among the habit memory system (that supports S-R associations represented in the dorsal striatum), hippocampus (supporting stimulus–stimulus associations), and amygdala (supporting conditioned cue preference). In their comprehensive review, they also found that the engagement of different memory systems was highly dependent on the experimental task, as well as related factors such as learning history in other tasks, cue and context manipulations, and even individual differences. Generally consistent with White, Packard and colleagues, Yin and Knowlton (2006a) highlighted evidence that, in addictive behaviors, control of behavior evolves with repeated experiences from a form of memory that is essentially declarative in nature (and involves relationships between actions and outcomes or A-O associations) to one that is controlled by a circuit involving the dorsolateral striatum that represents S-R associations that control habit. In nonhuman animals, the research groups studying this issue find that outcomes of behavior can be "devalued," in which they no longer are contingent on a behavior, and the habit system still propels the behavior once enough learning trials have established the S-R association. This parallels the observation in humans that addicts continue to take drugs even when tolerance to reinforcing drug effects has developed and many negative outcomes have occurred through drug use. Some perspectives suggest that at some point in addiction drug users no longer even like the drug (Berridge & Robinson, 2016). However, it is not clear if this is because of the typical cues of questioning addicts when they are outside of the drug situation (e.g., in treatment or when abstinent, when negative outcomes are quite salient), or the result of questioning in the absence of drug cues that trigger liking; people can strongly like *and* dislike something (cf. Cacioppo & Gardner, 1999) and have different feelings or cognitions manifested in different situations.

Everitt and Robbins (2016) recently provided a major review of their work and other accumulating evidence that generally concurs with Yin and Knowlton and others working on the neural basis of habit for the past several decades. On the basis of human and nonhuman animal research, Everitt and Robbins argue for an additional step beyond habit in drug addiction in some individuals, in which top-down executive control is impaired by continued drug use. Executive control may be degraded through damage to the ventromedial prefrontal cortex, involved in affective decision-making and reward-processing (Bechara, 2005; Noël, Brevers & Bechara, 2013), as well as regions associated with inhibitory control (Ames et al., 2014a) or working memory (Yan et al., 2014). Under any of these conditions of impaired executive function, people may find it particularly difficult to resist impulses originating from the habit system, providing one explanation of why some people appear so compulsive in their drug use and relapse after even an extended period of abstinence. However, some evidence suggests that deficits in affective decision making may precede and facilitate formation of addictive behaviors, while "colder" (less emotional) forms of executive processing (working memory) may be a result of harmful drug effects (Yan et al., 2014). An example of a dual-process model addressed later in this chapter proposes that executive functions and automatic associative processes underlying habit interact in their effects on many behaviors. Though drug use may degrade some functions, individual differences may have important effects on a wide range of appetitive behaviors even in the absence of impairment from drug use or other sources. Nevertheless, at some point in trajectories of heavy use of many drugs, neuroadaptation in a variety of circuits occurs (Koob & Le Moal, 2008; Koob & Volkow, 2016; Volkow, Koob & McLellan, 2016), leading to, for example, aversive states during drug withdrawal and even after long periods of abstinence. Such states and similar ones, such as stress, may act as powerful cues for relapse.

The most comprehensive approach to intervention in habit processes has been championed by Wood and her colleagues (Neal, Wood & Drolet, 2013; Ouellette & Wood, 1998; Wood & Neal, 2007). Although these strategies may be most relevant to addictive behaviors before extensive neuroadaptation and compulsion has occurred, the work is highly relevant if one considers that new healthy habits for alternative behaviors likely need to be developed among those with any degree of habit, compulsion, or even initial trials involving an unhealthy, habit forming behavior. Thus, habit approaches can be readily translated to prevention as well as treatment. Perhaps the most important translational message from the basic research reviewed in this chapter is that as a new behavior continues unimpeded, neural mechanisms foster habit development that can become independent of the outcomes and may be completely independent from any other variables of focus in prevention science and traditional prediction or survey research. Preventive strategies, whether primary or secondary, must compete with the powerful habit engine and likely consider the variables that propel habit, such as the cues or situations associated with drug use or other health behaviors in memory and the learning experiences that encode these associations. In the habit perspective in this chapter, preventive actions taught in a program must also somehow engage habit instigation processes if preventive steps are to compete with the instigation of harmful habits. Wood and colleagues are among the very small minority of researchers taking habit processes translated from basic research seriously in interventions and offer many routes for novel intervention.

A Revision of Memory Systems: An Emphasis on Memory Consolidation or Transfer

Henke (2010) suggested a revision of Squire's original framework, in which multiple memory systems are still prominent but are categorized quite differently. Instead of distinguishing memory systems based primarily on conscious access, she argues for a distinction based on processing operations typical of the system. In her framework and review, the hippocampus is responsible for the "rapid encoding of flexible associations even without consciousness" (p. 526). The neocortex, basal ganglia, and cerebellum support slower encoding of associations that are much more rigid. Memory for events with spatial, temporal, and featural properties of any type are encoded through the hippocampus, with likely feedback loops involving neocortex bringing meaning to the events. Memory supporting categories, habits, classical conditioning, new semantic learning, and skill or other procedural learning operates through the slower, gradual processes. Although consciousness may be more relevant in the hippocampal system than the others, Henke reviewed evidence that the hippocampus can be involved in particular forms of unconscious memory. The take-home message is that there is not a one-to-one or perfect correspondence between consciousness and the hippocampus or medial temporal lobe. According to Henke, these cognitive operations have to do more with modes of processing than with consciousness. In health research, modes of processing are not trivial, since interventions may need to compete with modes of processing that normally control habit as well as spontaneous cognitions that might precede or propel habit engagement and even initial trial of a substance.

One of the most important implications of Henke's framework in terms of health behavior is her focus on interactions between two systems: the hippocampus complex and neocortex. She argues that cycles of retrieval of information and processing help information first learned through the hippocampal system become "semanticized," that is, regularized and generalized in a form supported by the neocortex. Episodic memories, acquired from exposure to similar events, can then accumulate as a more general form of memory within the semantic system. Based in part on this view, an intervention promoting cycles of retrieval and semanticization has recently shown promise for HIV and hepatitis screening behavior (Stacy, Nydegger & Shono, 2019); encoding was verified through comprehensive and objective manipulation checks. A form of semantic learning may also occur independently from the hippocampus, through many trials and a very gradual learning process.

To be clear about effects on semantic memory, it is important to underscore that semantic forms of memory can generalize across different modalities or attributes (e.g., visual, tactile, auditory, affective, motoric, olfactory, and linguistic features). The concept of "dog" must be learned, and different experiences are eventually semanticized through experiences with the sight, sound, and feel of a dog in early childhood, or through hearing or reading about these perceptual attributes. The different experiences form connections across different regions of the neocortex, each specializing in different modalities. Yet, a unitary concept that transcends any particular dog emerges. This concept is supported, at least in part, by a distributed neural connective architecture within the neocortex, though it may also be supported by a convergence zone or amodal hub within the anterior temporal lobes that processes inputs from different modalities through a common set of neurons (Patterson, Nestor & Rogers, 2007). The representation of a concept usually has some similarity across individuals within a shared culture, but also marked individual differences in strength of connections across modalities, salient features, and other attributes that represent the concept. There is no reason that concepts about alcohol, tobacco, other drugs, or other addictive behaviors are not similarly semanticized through repeated episodic learning, which can occur through all sorts of vicarious sources well before a drug or behavior is ever tried. After an addictive behavior is engaged in repeatedly, there is also no reason to expect that the representation of a behavior-related concept (such as a situation to eat a sweet food or use a drug) does not also change, supported by underlying changes in connection weights within neocortex and possibly other regions. As suggested in the earlier discussion, the identification of a relevant or associated situation must be important to cue-dependent motivation in addiction.

Memory Systems Involving Rewards and Punishers

Roll's (2000) view of memory systems, based mostly on research in nonhuman primates, adheres to Squire's framework but provides a detailed summary of the representation of reinforcement and stimulus-reinforcement association learning, which is quite relevant to addiction. He argues for the pivotal importance of a system involving the orbitofrontal cortex and amygdala, as have investigators conducting human research (e.g., Noël et al., 2013). In common with many other investigators, he argues that learning relevant to behavior and its correlates involves the modification of connection weights among neurons. The amygdala and orbitofrontal cortex receive input from sensory regions (e.g., taste, olfactory, and visual cortices) that initially process a stimulus in the environment; then these two "evaluative" regions process whether a stimulus is associated with rewards or punishers. Connections engaging the basal ganglia provide goals for motor responses.

Rather than reiterate all the details and other neural processes covered in Roll's framework, we focus instead on several different aspects of evaluative processes that should be considered for the purpose of this chapter. The evaluative system involving the amygdala and orbitofrontal cortex receives input from diverse sensory areas. Recall that there is some evidence in humans that unimodal sensory and motor areas in the neocortex converge in some fashion in humans to manifest "concepts," or amodal representations that transcend any particular example (or exemplar). As suggested earlier, this may occur either through connections among the unimodal regions and/or through a region specializing in amodal convergence that represents concepts (Patterson et al., 2007). Further, individual differences in connection weights within neocortical regions can readily lead to individual differences in the characteristics or qualities of represented concepts. Regarding rewarding properties of drug use or other behaviors, many concepts likely are associated with (or characterized by) evaluative features even if an individual has never actually engaged in a behavior related to the concept (e.g., as learned vicariously). Evaluation probably occurs at the concept level; indirect or vicarious learning experiences could readily associate the concept with positive or negative characteristics that may not be felt directly but can be thought about or imagined. Without engaging in the behavior, these characteristics may be represented only at a "cold" (nonemotional) cognitive level, or in some instances vicarious learning might engage the evaluative system outlined by Rolls, Bechara and colleagues, and others. However, even at a cold conceptual level, which can still spontaneously influence one's train of thought through priming, activation of a set of relationships in memory may affect the decision to try a drug or initiate another addictive behavior for the first time or at least "prepare" an individual to more readily accept (or reject) a drug or to participate in another addictive behavior in certain situations (e.g., a party with friends). These likely processes have not apparently been studied by neuroscientists conducting research on the development of habits and addiction; that research has focused mostly on later stages of addiction and studies in nonhuman animals. Moreover, when research on health behavior or addiction epidemiology has focused on evaluative constructs, it has typically focused on self-reported survey-based evaluative constructs (e.g., attitudes, beliefs, values, etc.), rather than multiple memory system research of focus in this chapter. Though it is reasonable to hypothesize that relationships in conceptual or semantic memory affect initial trials of most behaviors, with respect to drug use subsequent trials provide direct experience that can engage a variety of pharmacologic and related neuroadaptive effects outlined by Rolls and many others (Berridge & Robinson, 2016; Everitt & Robbins, 2016; Kandel & Kandel, 2014; Koob & Volkow, 2016; Rolls, 2000; Volkow et al., 2016). As outlined earlier, strong effects on the MMS also occur with experience with appetitive behaviors such as food and sex (Mahler & Berridge, 2012). The thought or sight of a drug or other appetitive cue can then attain a "special" motivational, incentive, or affective status, while the habit processes outlined earlier are also engaged. The arguments about conceptual priming processes are advanced here because there is likely a relationship between conceptual or associative learning before trial of a new behavior, and in subsequent trials of the new behavior, involving the underlying circuits connecting conceptual and reward learning, as well as the processes leading to continued use and addiction. There is a growing number of ways to study these processes in humans within memory system frameworks that have neural plausibility. This is a virtually untapped route for advancing understanding of the development of appetitive habits of all kinds and may provide new routes for intervention.

Prospective Findings Relevant to Habit

Variables that might reveal the operation of the habit system researched extensively in neuroscientific studies are not frequently the focal point of prospective or epidemiologic research on drug use or other health behaviors. However, meta-analyses of these studies have demonstrated the power of possible proxy measures for habit. Although there is no claim of isomorphism between neural systems of habit and these proxy measures, the following findings coupled with the compelling body of neural research suggest that the detailed study of habit should be much more common across disciplines in health and addiction research, extending to epidemiologic inquiry.

Predictive Effects of Past Behavior on Future Behavior

On the surface, prospective or longitudinal research on addictions may not seem relevant to neural models of memory systems. However, prior behavior (including drug use) is often the strongest predictor of future behavior in such studies (Derzon & Lipsey, 1999; Hagger et al., 2016; McEachan et al., 2011), and past behavior has sometimes been used as a direct measure of habit (Landis, Triandis & Adamopoulos, 1978). Past behavior is usually quite predictive independent of whether the behavior is desirable, such as condom use (Albarracin et al., 2001; Stacy, Stein & Longshore, 1999) and physical activity (McEachan et al., 2011), or undesirable, such as binge-eating or various forms of drug use (Derzon & Lipsey, 1999; Stacy, Bentler & Flay, 1994). Such strong autoregressive relationships may hinder the success of interventions ranging from the treatment of opiate addiction (Brewer et al., 1998) to eliminating doping in athletic competitions (Ntoumanis et al., 2014).

At least on the surface, the argument that the autoregressive path between past and future behavior reflects effects of habit processes seems to be one of the plausible explanations. Especially for drugs with stronger addictive properties, past behavior may be a potent proxy measure for habit and predictor of future behavior, even when there is a strong rationale for change such as pregnancy (Moore et al., 1996). In many instances, it is difficult to consistently find other constructs that predict behavior beyond the autoregressive effect of past behavior. If other variables are predictive once past behavior is included in the analysis, the other variables often pale in comparative effect size. This effect is compatible with the notion that past behavior is at least partially a reflection of habit processes, which are perpetuated through the neural processes studied by investigators such as Knowlton, Yin, White, Packard, and others. At some point in a trajectory of drug or other addiction, S-R learning supported by the habit system allows behavior-related cues to automatically foster the behavior. At this point, when the drug or other object of desire is not readily available, conceptually based associations supported by the neocortex are likely to be engaged, probably spontaneously, so the drug or other object (e.g., sweet food) can be sought out. For example, a friend's apartment or a convenience store might immediately pop to mind; this location would have been initially represented through the hippocampus but could become essentially automatized in cognition. It also may be involved in conditioned cue preference, since the friend's house could become a conditioned stimulus associated with reward. If a location for the object does not automatically come to mind, then deliberate recollective attempts likely occur, mediated through the hippocampus, to remember where the object has been occasionally obtained in the past. Incentive salience is also likely to become a powerful force at some point after continued drug use or engagement in other appetitive behaviors. However, gradual S-R learning through the basal ganglia might be more in line with the frequently continuous, though skewed, distribution of previous drug use in its prediction of future drug use observed in many prospective studies. Although strong psychoactive properties of some drugs, some routes of administration, and certain individual differences could greatly speed up this process, and even one-trial learning may be possible (Rolls, 2000), habit perspectives do not require psychoactive effects for gradual habit learning. Such perspectives help explain strong autoregressive effects, cue effects, behavioral persistence, and resistance to change even for behaviors that have no pharmacological implications, such as physical activity and the use of seat belts or dental floss. As suggested earlier, however, drug use at the extreme end of the spectrum can engender a compulsive form of behavior likely affected by neural processes beyond habit. Nevertheless, habit processes are fundamental and have a broad base of multimethod and even multispecies support, with strong neural plausibility and relative simplicity. It is difficult to find this range of multimethod and multispecies support for other constructs popular in theories applied to the epidemiology of addictive behaviors.

Another reasonable set of interpretations of the common autoregressive effect of previous behavior is that the effect appears only because the underlying processes, or other variables, are not measured in the study (see Figure 12.1). The autoregressive effect could be explained by these unmeasured variables or a range of other effects, such as the following relationships that could be added to Figure 12.1 in a series of more complex models:

(1) A correlation between a detailed measurement of habit processes (or other processes, such as genetic predisposition) and past behavior could explain away the predictive effect of past behavior. If so, then estimating correlations among the predictors on the left side of Figure 12.1 would make the path denoted with the solid line nonsignificant. At least one of the paths depicted with a dashed or dotted line would become significant.

(2) Habit processes or other processes could affect both previous behavior and future behavior, in which past behavior is found to be either a mediator (intervening predictor), or an epiphenomenal correlate that has no effect once these predictive effects are considered in the analysis.

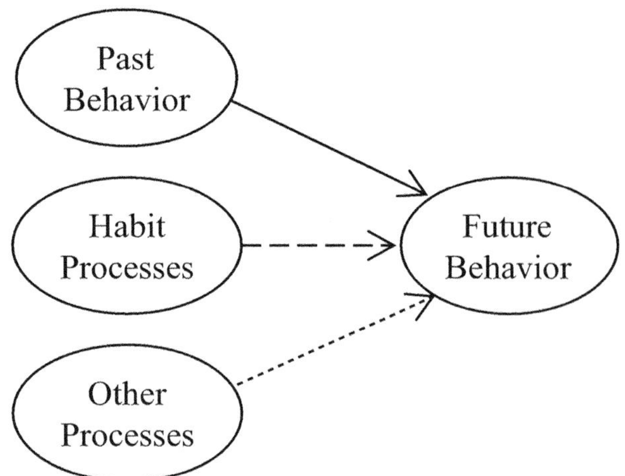

Note. Solid line depicts typically strong predictive effect of past behavior on future behavior. Dashed line depicts hypothetical effect of habit processes in the brain that have not been measured in epidemiologic studies. Dotted line depicts possible effects of other processes (see text).

Figure 12.1 Path diagram of effects of past behavior and unmeasured correlates

(3) An assumption that past behavior closely parallels the effect of the neural process of habit outlined in this chapter would assume that the two are very strongly correlated and either one would predict future behavior. In that case, past behavior would be a good proxy measure for, or indicator of, the habit processes supported by neural circuits: they could then be considered indicators of the same latent construct.

(4) Past behavior and underlying habit processes may be seen as distinct constructs but may have reciprocal effects over time, in which engagement in the behavior affects neural processes, those processes propel future behavior, engagement in the behavior again affects neural processes, and so on. Specific processes underlying a reciprocal process could be explained by several of the neural approaches outlined in this chapter.

Although there is presently no way to differentiate between these alternatives in previous epidemiological inquiry, the autoregressive effect is more robust and common than perhaps any other effect in prospective studies of health behavior. Yet, this effect is usually ignored or sometimes not measured at all, and many of the most commonly used health behavior theories do not address it. When past behavior or habit is addressed, it is usually not considered in a theoretical manner or in any detail. Multiple system approaches to memory, and assessment techniques that provide ways to measure underlying associations in memory, provide an avenue to take these consistent longitudinal effects more seriously and offer clear routes for translational science for those willing to study the basic literature.

Predictive Effects of Declarative Measures of Habit

Another way to potentially address habit in prospective research is to use self-reported introspective (or declarative) reports of habit phenomena and gauge subsequent predictive effects. Verplanken and Orbell (2003) developed such a scale referred to as the Self-Report Habit Index (SRHI). This index assesses agreement with three domains of behavior patterns involving repetition, perceived automaticity (e.g., doing without thinking), and identity. Although, like simple measures of past behavior, declarative or self-report measures of habit are not indirect measures that are known to measure implicit or unconscious influences, it seems likely that people have some accessible knowledge of some aspects of their previous behaviors. A more recent meta-analysis (Gardner, de Bruijn & Lally, 2011) demonstrated that the SRHI was a significant and sizable predictor of dietary behavior and physical activity. However, many of the studies in the meta-analysis were cross-sectional, in which the habit index was used to predict a measure of past behavior. Although used less frequently in addiction research, initial prospective studies suggest that the SRHI is equally predictive of future smoking (Orbell & Verplanken, 2010) and binge drinking (Gardner, de Bruijn & Lally, 2012; Norman, 2011). Implicit in some of the SRHI content is the apparent assumption that habit should be defined at the extreme end of habit development when little interferes temporally with S-R reactions, such as when one brushes his or her teeth when a toothbrush is in one's hand, or when one puts on a seat belt after hearing a car's auditory signal. However, habit can be defined on a continuum from no S-R associations, to weak associations, moderate associations, and so on. Also, thoughts may frequently intervene even in strong habits. An automatic thought may pop to mind about putting on a seat belt in the car before one automatically reaches for the seat belt. A thought about having a drink must intervene before driving to a store to purchase alcohol, unless one assumes that this process is fully unconscious. Thus, it is not clear whether a measure of past behavior or the SRHI scale is a better proxy reflection of the likely continuous nature of habit and habit development, from weak to strong habits and weak to strong S-R associations. It is possible since the SRHI yields a continuous or at least ordinal measure despite some of its content, and it may be a quite good proxy measure. Again, it has been found to be a good predictor of behavior.

In the approach that brings neocortical sources of priming into the picture, people would be expected to develop some associations between regularly experienced characteristics they exhibit and their behavior. Through the processes outlined by Henke, repeated experiences like these would eventually lead to semanticization of those experiences. Semanticization and resultant spontaneously or automatically accessible associations in memory can readily affect answers on a self-reported survey (e.g., through the availability heuristic; Tversky & Kahneman, 1973), though many other cognitive processes that cannot be identified in a traditional survey study can also lead to these self-reports. Indeed, traditional survey measures (including virtually all measures of attitudes, beliefs, all types of expectations/expectancies, intentions, personality scales that list behaviors, and even perceived norms) that mention the target behavior or something similar to it may correlate with behavior through a number of unrecognized processes: semantic or episodic memory activity, priming, intensive deliberation and search processes engaging multiple prefrontal circuits (such as those involved in language, working, memory, and decision processing), framing and self-presentation processes, and so on, despite common assumptions about such measures as reflections of their target construct. Because of mention of behavior, most or possibly all such measures (dating back to the 1950s and earlier; Rotter, 1954) likely will be better predictors of behavior than many other measures that do not directly ask for self-reflections about the behavior. Different nuances in referring to behavior could readily lead to apparently independent prediction. Nonetheless, the prospective effects reported above are of relevance and future research might investigate further what underlying processes govern self-reports about past behavior and habit. At this point, the face validity and predictive effects of either type of measure (declarative or nondeclarative) should not be taken as sufficient evidence to determine underlying processes, and it requires more than psychometrics to fully validate measures and their interpretation.

Study of Nondeclarative Processes in Prospective Research on Addictive Behaviors

Examples of Measures and Findings

Another set of epidemiologic findings relevant to memory system views of addiction is the predictive effects of variables designed to tap into implicit memory or nondeclarative systems that do not depend on conscious recollection or deliberation, such as those already introduced. Within this class of measure, several different types of assessments have been used to assess associations in memory relevant to drug use. One example is the Implicit Association Test (IAT) (Greenwald, McGhee & Schwartz, 1998; Greenwald, Nosek & Banaji, 2003; Nosek, Greenwald & Banaji, 2005, 2007). Most versions of the IAT assess through a series of reaction time (RT) trials whether people more strongly associate a target behavior with positive or negative attributes; this yields an indirect measure of attitude toward the target behavior. Other IATs assess associations of a behavior with other attributes, like arousal or excitement (Wiers et al., 2005). Although a complete review is beyond the scope of this chapter, it is notable that several longitudinal studies have shown the IAT predicts future use of tobacco (Chassin et al., 2010; Sherman et al., 2009; Spruyt et al., 2015) and alcohol (Lindgren et al., 2016; Thush & Wiers, 2007; Thush et al., 2008; Wiers et al., 2005). A recent novel and promising version of the IAT indirectly addresses self-identity, measuring the association of the target drug with "me" compared to "not me" (Lindgren et al., 2016, 2017). In a rigorous eight-wave prospective study of college students, the drinking-identity IAT significantly predicted alcohol consumption and drinking problems, even after adjusting for previous alcohol use, other versions of the IAT, and explicit cognition variables (Lindgren et al., 2016). Although an excitement IAT (Wiers et al., 2005) was also predictive, only the identity IAT was predictive after twenty-one months. Another of several other examples of an IAT is the approach IAT (Palfai & Ostafin, 2003), but it was not as predictive as other IAT tests in the Lindgren study. Overall, addiction or drug related IATs have shown enough consistency in prediction to warrant their continued refinement and use. Neural correlates of drug IATs are beginning to be investigated (Ames et al., 2013, 2014b).

Another example of an indirect assessment of association in memory is word association tests that do not mention the target behavior and do not depend on recollection or causal judgements. These tests have been modeled after tests used in cognitive neuroscience to study memory systems, memory impairments such as amnesia, and implicit memory. The assessment uses simple top-of-mind instructions, typically asking participants to write the first word or behavior that comes to mind in response to a given cue. The cue can be either a single word, short phrase, or picture, which in addiction research can usefully denote a temporal (e.g., Friday night), spatial (at a restaurant), social (with friends or a group), or affect-related (fun) feature. This measure has been found to be predictive of future use of alcohol (Ames et al., 2017; Kelly, Masterman & Marlatt, 2005; Krank et al., 2005; Salemink & Wiers, 2014; Thush et al., 2007; Van Der Vorst et al., 2013) and marijuana (Ames et al., 2017; Shono et al., 2018). When asking for a top-of-mind action or behavior, this form of word association is termed *verb generation* (VG) in cognitive neuroscience. In neuropsychological studies of VG, the most compelling evidence of memory in the absence of conscious recollection of the task comes from amnesic participants. Seger and colleagues (Seger et al., 1997) found that amnesic participants and participants without memory impairment (controls) revealed equivalent levels of priming in a VG task, even though the amnesic participants scored significantly worse than controls on a test of conscious recollection (recognition). Complementary findings in neural imaging suggest that, as noted by Seger and colleagues (Seger et al., 1997), brain regions typically activated in VG (Crescentini, Shallice & Macaluso, 2010; Raichle et al., 1994) are distinct from those activated during explicit memory retrieval (Cabeza & Nyberg, 2000). Indeed, VG assessments and other indirect measures of associations in memory have been long implicated in the operation of implicit conceptual memory (Seger, Rabin, Desmond & Gabrieli, 1999). However, the nature of the processing in response to VG depends on the strength of association of the cue and a response or previous experience with cue-response combinations. Neural imaging work on VG is consistent with this interpretation, with attenuation of activation within the left inferior frontal gyrus when highly associated action words are generated (Burton & Martin, 2006) and decreased activation in left inferior prefrontal cortex, anterior cingulate gyrus, and right cerebellum in response to repetition of cues (Raichle et al., 1994). Repetition also facilitates response time (Seger et al., 2000). A typical finding is that extensive activation in left prefrontal regions (Buckner et al., 2000; Seger et al., 2000; Thompson-Schill, D'Esposito & Kan, 1999) decreases with stronger association strength, spontaneity, or repetition, suggesting more efficiency and less processing in these regions. The pattern of results is consistent with other streams of research suggesting changes from predominantly effortful or control-related processes to more automatic (or implicit) processes as experience increases (Chein & Schneider, 2005; Schneider & Chein, 2003). Recent neuropsychological findings studying free word association without manipulating a previous priming trial are also compatible (Sheldon, Romero & Moscovitch, 2013). Despite the predictive effects of VG and other word production tasks on addictive behaviors, and independent studies on neural correlates of VG, no neural imaging methods have been applied to addiction-related VG or similar word production association tasks. The integration of these two streams of research could be quite informative and provide important routes for understanding and applying nondeclarative cognitive processes in theory and intervention.

One of the most recent innovations in this measurement area has been use of the affect misattribution procedure (AMP) in addiction research (Payne et al., 2016). The AMP can be considered a type of priming assessment, since the computerized procedure first presents an image of an alcoholic or soft drink almost immediately followed by a Chinese pictograph. Participants press one of two keys indicating whether they think the pictograph is less or more pleasant than the average pictograph presented. Importantly, participants are warned to avoid being influenced by the prime. Because the pairing of pictographs with different beverage images is arbitrary, priming effects on the pleasantness judgments are thought to represent an automatic carryover effect of affect generated from the prime. In a unique analysis of potentially different prospective effects of implicit processes in initial nondrinkers versus drinkers, Payne and his colleagues (Payne et al., 2016) found that scores on the AMP predicted alcohol consumption one year later in over 800 adolescents from the southeastern United States. In another study that examined initial nondrinkers, Van Der Vorst colleagues (Van Der Vorst et al., 2013) found that associations in memory assessed indirectly with word association predicted the onset of drinking in over 1,000 Canadian adolescents. Both studies demonstrated that direct drinking experience was not necessary to reveal predictive effects of associations

Table 12.1 Some indirect tests of association and example citation on substance use

Reaction time tests	
Implicit Association Test (IAT)	(Lindgren et al., 2016)
Extrinsic Affective Simon Test (EAST)	(de Jong et al., 2007)
Affective Priming	(Glock, Klapproth & Müller, 2015)
Semantic Priming - Lexical Decision	(Zack, Poulos & Woodford, 2006)
Dissociation in Semantic Priming and Explicit Memory	(Ray et al., 2004)
Semantic Priming - Word Naming	(Weingardt, Stacy & Leigh, 1996)
Word production	
Verb Generation - Controlled Association	(Shono et al., 2018)
Free Word Association	(Van Der Vorst et al., 2013)
Continuous Word Association	(Szalay, Strohl & Doherty, 1999)
Episodic memory tests	
Illusory Memory in Recognition	(Reich, Goldman & Noll, 2004)
Process Dissociation	(Fillmore, Vogel-Sprott & Gavrilescu, 1999)
Other examples	
Affect Misattribution Procedure (AMP)	(Payne et al., 2016)
Approach-Avoidance Task	(Wiers et al., 2009)

Note. Examples are restricted to indirect measures of association, mostly with support from basic research.

in memory, thought to reflect processes that operate implicitly or at least relatively spontaneously.

Table 12.1 lists measurement strategies already discussed as well as additional examples that have been applied to addictive behaviors. The list is not exhaustive, with only a small sample of the many important contributions. Although it is beyond the scope of this chapter to review more of the promising findings, nearly all of the listed strategies have been translated from basic research on memory, cognitive neuroscience, or from studies in social psychology that have strongly implicated the assessments with implicit or non-declarative processes. By providing falsifiable measurement tools, these assessments allow research to go well beyond mere speculations about the possibility of automatic or implicit cognitive processes, automatic action schemata, or similar reasonable ideas in the literature (Yalachkov, Kaiser & Naumer, 2015). The survey, epidemiologic, and intervention literatures rarely address this class of measure, but the strategies receive a wide range of experimental support from basic research and do not rely on psychometrics alone. Interestingly, some of the strategies rely on experimental manipulation of materials on explicit or direct tests of memory, such as recognition or cued recall. In these instances, inferences of implicit or automatic processes are derived on the basis of effects of variation in the structure of materials (e.g., pattern of associations in presented words), other manipulations, or sometimes calculation of separate implicit and explicit components of memory. Such effects are consistent with multiple memory system views that focus on cross-system interactions (Henke, 2010). In any case, many of these measurement strategies, and the theories underlying them, should receive greater attention in research on health habits and addiction because they provide new routes for innovation. Only a few have been studied in terms of neural systems of memory, a potentially fundamental direction for future research.

Revisiting Definitions Within a Historical Context

There are several notable differences in some of the research just summarized, regarding conceptual focus, measurement procedures, and even definitions. Research on implicit or automatic processes in memory research and cognitive neuroscience has remained an essentially distinct area from study of these processes in social psychology, though there have been some cross-disciplinary influences. Research on addictive and health-related behaviors has translated both of these areas, though implicit attitude approaches in social psychology (Greenwald & Banaji, 1995) probably have received the most attention in health research. In basic cognitive and neuroscientific research, Graf and Schacter's definition of implicit memory (Graf & Schacter, 1985) has been widely influential, as was the earlier study and definition of automatic and controlled processes (Schneider & Shiffrin, 1977; Shiffrin & Schneider, 1977). However, vigorous research on implicit processes in cognition was produced earlier during the 1950s and 1960s, exemplified especially by the powerful concept of implicit associative response (IAR). IAR was a major influence in research on verbal learning (Underwood, 1965) and originates in the foundational work of Bousfield and colleagues (Bousfield, Whitmarsh & Danick, 1958). This early work using IAR concepts relied heavily on indirect measurement techniques to estimate association strength and to then predict the operation of the implicit response, which helped spawn subsequent work across several decades of cognitive research (Cabeza & Lennartson, 2005; Deese, 1962; Robinson & Roediger, 1997; Underwood, Reichardt & Malmi, 1975) and some of the health-related research shown in Table 12.1. Wide use of scientific indexes of association strength began in early foundational research on IAR and related topics such as memory intrusions (now classified as illusory memory) (Deese, 1959; Underwood, 1965), semantic generalization (Cramer, 1970b), and mediated priming (Cramer, 1970a). More contemporary research has found that association strength significantly predicts semantic priming at the item level (Hutchison et al., 2008), effects that are usually inferred as automatic. In extra-list cued recall, in which recall cues are provided that are related in various ways to previously presented materials, the pattern of responses is well predicted from various association parameters and effects of the parameters are inferred as reflections of implicit association processes (Nelson et al., 1998). In contemporary illusory memory paradigms derived from the original work of Deese (1959), the associative connection of study lists has been found to be the best predictor of variability in false recall (r = 0.73) in multiple regression analyses (Roediger et al., 2001). Health research using indexes of association strength championed initially by IAR research, and now commonly used in cognitive neuroscience, is a reasonable direction buttressed by a rich and powerful but virtually unrecognized potential in this domain.

Social psychological definitions of implicit processes also provide a promising continued direction, though this area has a somewhat divergent history (Payne & Gawronski, 2010). Greenwald is often cited in this literature for the original definition of implicit cognition (Greenwald & Banaji, 1995), in which, similar to Graf and Schacter, traces of past experience that are unavailable to introspection or self-report influence performance. However, Greenwald goes further and equates a psychological construct (such as attitude) with past experience, suggesting that in implicit cognition the construct and its content are not identified or are inaccurately identified. Interestingly, this assertion does not obviously cover many of the effects demonstrated across independent studies on implicit memory or on automatic processes involved in semantic memory. In many such studies, the target content comes to mind, but the source of the content does not. For example, amnesic patients identified to have impaired explicit memory usually show normal levels of implicit memory on indirect tests, which do not request the participant to think back to a previous event. The same participants, when properly selected for the particular types of amnesia, show severely impaired explicit memory. They cannot remember the event, yet exposure to the event brought content to mind, or affected that content, during a subsequent indirect test that (to them) is unrelated to the previous exposure. As revealed earlier, these patients are known to have intact systems of other forms of memory such as semantic and habit memory and have no known lesions in the neocortex or the basal ganglia. In nonpatient populations, many other experimental investigations of implicit memory also require that content comes to mind, even though recollection about a previous event is not requested. In these paradigms the participants are aware of the *content* during their response on the memory test, but not the *source* of the content or how the content is accessed. This is completely in line with Graf and Schacter's definition of implicit memory and with the use of IAR concepts. Just because content may pop to mind to influence a response does not mean that the activation or accessibility of that content was not influenced by an implicit or automatic process, using definitions from cognitive science. Indeed, to the present authors it is quite possible that many of the most powerful implicit processes do spontaneously trigger content that comes to mind while influencing behavior, but in a reflexive manner that is not dependent on deliberation, extensive thought, or explicit recall. This does not discount the importance of implicit content that is not even brought to mind (not introspectively identified) or that may be quite different from conscious content, influencing behavior without any type of awareness of that content (Young et al., 2014). It also does not discount the importance of some of the ingenious paradigms that are difficult for participants to control during test administration, such as several versions of the IAT used in addiction research. Characteristics such as speed or spontaneity, effort or deliberation, controllability, awareness of the source of memory or thought, and awareness of the process constitute different flavors of implicit and automatic processes, and it is not scientifically known which flavor or combination is most relevant to behavior. As mentioned above, even paradigms that use tests of explicit memory, but experimentally vary association parameters in the materials, have found important effects of processes that can be readily defined as implicit or automatic. Yet, research using quite different procedures from social psychology, such as the IAT and AMP, may reveal different aspects of implicit cognition that are important for a complete understanding of the full range of important processes. The historical context, as well as the widely distributed nature of relevant neural processes, reveals that a far greater range of validated concepts and tests from basic research should be studied in research on addictions and health behavior, rather than emphasis on only a small range from one or two most recently popular subdisciplines.

A Note About Working Memory and Dual Processes

Working memory (WM) is generally defined as one of the critical executive functioning processes (Fuster, 2001) and more specifically defined as a process for temporary maintenance and manipulation of information (Baddeley, 2001). Neural research has made progress on delineating relevant circuits and regions (Eriksson et al., 2015; Kharitonova, Winter & Sheridan, 2015). While WM is not usually addressed in terms of the previously outlined multiple memory systems, its conceptual and empirical relevance to health behaviors has received increasing research attention. People vary in levels of WM capacity; this implies individual differences in capacities to maintain and manipulate information, especially during short periods of time. Higher levels of WM capacity may therefore help people think more effectively or adaptively about behaviors before acting.

In prospective research, lower levels of WM have been associated with: higher levels of follow-up alcohol use among a community sample of adolescents (Khurana et al., 2012), higher levels of alcohol problems among adolescents from special education schools (Peeters et al., 2014), escalation in cannabis use among heavy cannabis users (Cousijn et al., 2014), increases in sexual risk-taking among a community sample of adolescents (Khurana et al., 2015), and increased risk for substance use disorder among a community sample of adolescents (Khurana et al., 2017). For the most part, these studies indicated small effect sizes ($r < -0.14$). The exception to this trend was a study on heavy cannabis users (Cousijn et al., 2014), which indicated a large effect size ($r = -0.54$).

Some dual-process models of addictive behaviors propose an interaction between executive functions and the effects of implicit associations on addictive behaviors. In these models, executive functions such as WM are part of a system of controlled, or "reflective," processes which moderate the automatic, or "impulsive" pathways between implicit approach action tendencies and substance use (Wiers & Stacy, 2006). As depicted in Figure 12.2, these functions may enhance one's ability to direct attentional resources toward the suppression of impulses to

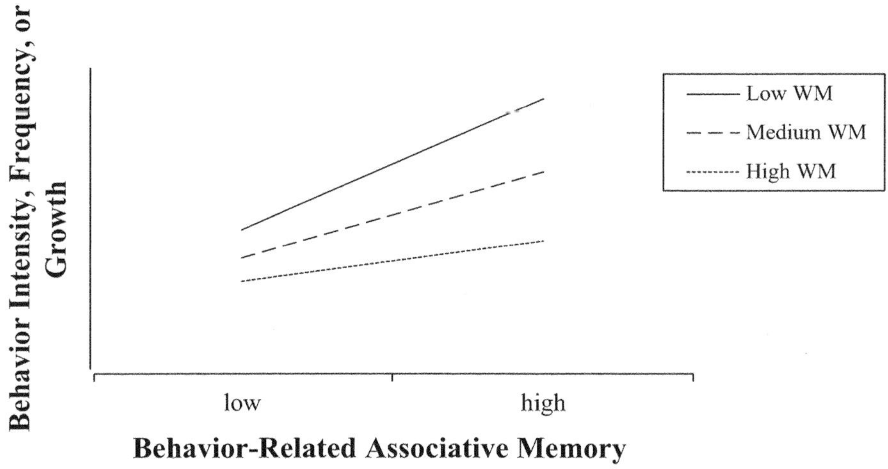

Figure 12.2 Working memory (WM) moderates effects of associative memory on addictive behavior

engage in unhealthy behaviors such that those higher in WM show less of an effect of associations in memory (Stacy, Ames & Knowlton, 2004). In research on addictive behaviors, this interaction model was initially supported in studies on WM in at-risk youth (Grenard et al., 2008; Thush et al., 2008). However, in a recent meta-analysis of this interaction effect, the results were mixed, with four out of eleven studies supporting the hypothesized interaction (Ames et al., 2020). Thus, the findings to date suggest that a dual-process model focusing on WM adds complexity that may not be necessary, since a simpler model focusing on associations in memory as a direct-effect predictor is usually more well supported within the realm of memory system approaches.

A New Translation: Episodic Memory, Semantic/ Conceptual Systems, and Health Behavior

Beyond Language but Before Habit and Addiction

As addressed earlier, Henke's (Henke, 2010) review supports the idea that learned information of all types initially encoded through episodic or explicit memory can become "semanticized" (generalized and semi-permanent) under appropriate conditions, likely involving cycles of retrieval of previously learned information and repeated, somewhat regular experiences. In her terms, the manifestations of information encoded as episodic memory, supported by the hippocampus and related systems, can emerge ("transfer" or "consolidate") in a more general, cross-modal semantic form of memory supported by neocortical circuits. However, in some of the literature, semantic memory is restricted to memories triggered by language alone (Binder, Desai, Graves & Conant, 2009). Yet, there are many phenomena supported in part through the neocortex, and partially accessible through language in humans, that are not solely engaged via the language route, such as nonverbal visual or tactile perception and affective or motivational states. In the nonhuman primate literature, it is common to talk of "conceptual" processes, which is also a frequent term in research on human memory. When language is not a focus, either because of the species or the research design, a form of generalized memory across modalities supported by diverse regions of neocortex has been documented, such as perceptual–motor associations (Hoshi & Tanji, 2007; Ishida et al., 2016). Because these are multisensory memory phenomena that are generalized in some sense (i.e., revealed through probing of diverse sensory modalities) and much more permanent than episodic memories, it makes sense to classify this form of knowledge as conceptual or semantic. The word "dog" does not have to be heard, read, or spoken to bring forth a motor tendency to either approach or avoid the animal – it could be a bark, the sight, or accidental touch of a dog, and it could be any type of dog, not just one based on previous experience. In response to any sort of perceptual cue, the word "dog" is no doubt rapidly accessed in memory along with other learned associations, including those connected to motor or premotor regions. It is doubtful that the word "dog" by itself would always strongly activate perceptual and motoric associations, unless it is in the right context of meaning, such as suddenly hearing "here comes a dog." Individual differences in learning can be prominent, affecting whether motoric and emotion-related modalities are strongly associated with the concept or its subcategories. Similarly, behavior-related concepts such as "beer," "hit," "doughnut," and "chocolate" are also represented and connected across modalities, with large individual differences. They too can share characteristics across linguistic, perceptual, and sometimes motoric and emotion features. As suggested in a comprehensive meta-analysis of the neural underpinnings of language-based semantic knowledge (Binder et al., 2009), presentation of words may not be sufficient to detect subtle activation of motor or perceptual regions or circuits. Advances in imaging methods and better coverage of words or phrases most likely to be associated with perceptual–motor responses may eventually yield a more complete understanding. Nevertheless, to restrict conceptual knowledge supported by neocortex to only those phenomena that can be activated solely through language misses perhaps some of the most important neocortical influences on behavior and the initial learning of new habits. In our reading of the literature, the semantic, or if you prefer a different terminology, conceptual system represents associations in memory that are typically more regularized, generalized, and permanent than those supported by the hippocampus. This neocortical system supports language associations as well, in parallel with diverse sensory and motor associations, and language is just one of the many modes supported.

Despite her compelling review, Henke (Henke, 2010) did not address habit or the linkages between neocortical processes and behavior. This is the missing link most relevant to the current chapter. One might ask: why would regularized relationships, associations, and meanings (either emotionally "hot" or "cold") that have become spontaneously accessible/generated through neocortical circuits not be relevant to behavior? Do people not usually think, at least a little, about a behavior before first trying it, and if so, where do the thoughts come from? Why might a teenager try a drink of alcohol, but probably not try a drink of dirty water, if offered by a friend? Is this likely effect entirely unconscious and not able to be "declared" or is it spontaneous, quite influential, but with accessed content that becomes declarable after automatic activation? Although constructs from traditional surveys have been routinely used in attempts to explain behavior choices like this and many others, some might argue that memory system approaches supported with multiple, independent methods across species, studied at levels from neural to cognitive and behavioral, should be at least as prominent in both epidemiologic and experimental or intervention research. Why have memory system approaches been rarely applied to addictive behaviors and relevant behavior choices outside of neuroscience? One may speculate that the neuroscientists in the area have not typically worked on behavioral interventions or applied their work to areas such as behavioral epidemiology or prevention science, and the intervention and prevention experts have focused on prevailing approaches and paradigms in their field rather than translation of consistent findings from basic research on memory systems. There need to be bridges between these research areas.

Neural Circuits Linking the Basal Ganglia to Premotor Cortex: An Example

There are a variety of ways in which memories that can be defined as semantic or conceptually driven, supported by the neocortex, have a strong potential to affect behavior and instigate habit development. Although there is continued fruitful study of circuits that may be defined as "hot," or emotional, such as those involving the ventromedial prefrontal cortex and amygdala (Bechara, 2005), there is far less attention in addiction research to a range of other circuits and processes that are likely highly relevant, especially to the first trial of a drug and the very beginning of habit formation. Here is highlighted just one example of this class of process, focusing on the premotor cortex and basal ganglia (BG). Research on circuits connecting the BG to the premotor and motor cortex may provide impetus for investigation of a problem not typically addressed in habit research: How do learned associations and conceptual meanings get translated to initial trials of a behavior? Neural and behavioral research on habit, as well as research on the neuronal effects of psychoactive drugs, helps one to understand how a behavior, once tried, may either slowly or rapidly become a habit or addiction. However, the link between cognition and that first action is usually discussed theoretically in the context of traditional survey-based constructs (e.g., measured as attitudes, expectancies, norms, beliefs, or personality traits) or more rarely in terms of problems in functioning of executive or decision systems either due to individual differences or lack of full cortical maturation in adolescence or young adulthood (Bechara, 2005). Memory systems supporting learned relations or associations, meanings, habit, and linkages across neural systems are not addressed in either survey research or in most research on executive functions, trial of a new behavior, or survey literature on habit formation.

There are biologically plausible ways in which learned associations and meanings registered only through indirect experiences, supported by multisensory and motor circuits in the neocortex, can impact motor responses, i.e., behavior and habit. First, a number of studies using fMRI in humans (Oguri et al., 2013) and diverse neural methods in nonhuman primates (Ishida et al., 2016; Wang et al., 2017) reveal substantial connectivity between BG and cortical motor areas such as the premotor cortex. Further, in humans the premotor cortex is part of a widespread, distributed cortical network thought to underlie semantic or conceptual memory and processing, linking multiple sensory regions, motor regions, and language areas together. In nonhuman primates, the premotor cortex has been associated with decision making prior to action and preparatory motor responses (Coallier, Michelet & Kalaska, 2015; Mirabella, Pani & Ferraina, 2011). In a recent review article, Hélie and colleagues (Hélie, Ell & Ashby, 2015) argued that the findings support BG as serving a "training" function, in which BG modulates the learning of associations across diverse cortical areas. Through experience coupled with input from the BG, the associations are strengthened and can become automatic in their effects via Hebbian learning (a type of associative learning). The premotor cortex is an important part of this BG-cortico circuitry, specializing in associations involving behavior. A recent review of relevant cue reactivity studies supports its potential importance in drug use (Yalachkov et al., 2015).

The premotor cortex, as well as the visual cortex, also has been studied in imagery tasks related to behavior and in intervention research, revealing effects of imagery on neural activation patterns. This is relevant to addiction and other health behavior in part because individually imagined cues (e.g., going to a bar looking for a drug) may overlap well with actual visual cues perceived in the environment. Indeed, visual imagery activates a number of neural regions in common with visual perception, "standing-in" for visual perception (Kosslyn, Ganis & Thompson, 2001), and a number of studies also support neural commonalities across motor imagery and movement (Miller et al., 2010; Wei & Luo, 2009). Related studies show that motor imagery engages not only the premotor cortex but also connected regions (Pilgramm et al., 2016; Wriessnegger et al., 2016; Zabicki et al., 2017) and that neurofeedback during motor imagery modulates neural activity in this region (Marins et al., 2015; Pilgramm et al., 2016). Behavioral effects have been uncovered in studies of skill acquisition in sports (Robin et al., 2007) and rehabilitation (Hovington & Brouwer, 2010), revealing benefits of motor imagery for improving motor preparation and behavior performance. There is no reason to believe that when imagery is used spontaneously by an individual outside of the lab or treatment situation, such as when someone is contemplating a future action and engaging in concrete (i.e., imageable) thoughts, that the premotor cortex would not be similarly engaged. Though the imagery "trial" originates in individual thought, the trial is essentially an episodic event encoded through hippocampal and related circuits like other episodic events: the trial features are encoded as a form of memory usually classified as explicit memory. If the individual repeats a similar trial with some regularity, the episodic memory can eventually become semanticized. It is not difficult to imagine an adolescent or young adult considering a future behavior, going through an imagined scenario on mind involving the cue (e.g., party situation) and behavior (e.g., drug use), repeating the scenario in imagery a number of times, and developing a spontaneous tendency (supported by neural processes involving semanticization) toward the behavior that is more reflexive than presumed in traditional health behavior theory popular in public health. Resulting associative memories could become spontaneous enough to make the behavior a highly accessible and likely behavioral option in the future, under the right conditions or set of cues. If the behavior is engaged in, then habit memory, supported by additional neural regions, can begin to strengthen like a snowball rolling down the hill. The growing, vigorous interest in the neural processes underlying motor imagery and behavioral implications is just one example of a wide range of recent work in embodied cognition (Glenberg, Witt & Metcalfe, 2013).

The premotor cortex is just one example from a set of related circuits involved in widely distributed semantic or conceptual processing, and as such constitutes only one of a number of plausible regions of interest for new discoveries linking episodic, semantic, and habit memory (cf. Yalachkov et al., 2015). Many other regions and circuits supporting this sort of processing are relevant to the transition across initial learning, first few trials of a behavior, and the early stages of habit formation. These processes are even relevant among compulsive drug users, especially when other processes must intervene when a desired drug is not immediately available to manifest immediate S-R habit system effects. The processes are also relevant to formation of heathy habits that may interfere with, or replace, substance use or another unhealthy appetitive behavior as the most salient (or at least competitive) alternative behavior. Hypotheses for specific patterns of changes in neural activity, concomitant changes in associations in memory regarding cues and motor responses, and behavioral effects can be derived from previous work on the premotor cortex, other regions likely involved in semantic and image processing, and embodied cognition. One issue for future research is that the widely distributed (multisensory) semantic system is probably engaged almost continually, except during certain stages of sleep. Gross approximations of neural activity such as fMRI may frequently have difficulty detecting differences in activity engaged by an appetitive cue if most any cue leads to semantic processing. Yet, the pattern of activation at more subtle levels that define different meanings could be quite different across these cues. Pattern differences, in turn, would lead to whether motor and subcortical processes are engaged. Recently, some neural research has reported effects of drug cues on multisensory and distributed motor processing, suggesting that the approach should receive greater attention (Hanlon et al., 2014; Yalachkov et al., 2015).

Relation to Other Approaches

There are of course many approaches to addiction and health behavior not addressed in this chapter. Many of them could be seen as in some way relevant to multiple memory system approaches, but only a few are listed here. First, the topic of *behavioral economics* is highly related because this area suggests a wide range of processes that appear to be automatic or at least spontaneous and operate without a requirement for deliberation or rational agency. Further, rather than a list of unrelated biases, Kahneman (2003, 2011) argues convincingly that most judgement and decision biases uncovered in behavioral economics are manifestations of an underlying automatic associative system, or System I in his terminology; in the neural perspectives discussed in this chapter, System I actually comprises a set of nondeclarative memory systems.

Regarding so-called *explicit cognitions*, in the present approach self-reports of cognitions on traditional attitude, expectancy, or belief surveys likely reflect a complex array of difficult-to-pinpoint activity across neural systems coupled with manifestations of the availability heuristic (Tversky & Kahneman, 1973), self-perceptions, and "online" judgments that depend strongly on priming effects from the structure of the survey and order of survey items. Similar to this reasoning, Kahneman (2011) argues that such reflections engage a set of heterogeneous processes (he refers to as System II) that require effort and cognitive resources yet are heavily influenced by automatic biases that color content and judgments through System I. Although the source of responses to measures of explicit cognition and even the actual meaning or construct validity of these measures is usually quite unclear from a neural or multimethod perspective, some recent progress has been made in linking explicit cognitions to neural processes (Cristofori & Grafman, 2017; Luttrell et al., 2016; Wing et al., 2018). In comments that support traditional surveys of explicit cognition, Blanton and colleagues (Blanton, Burrows & Jaccard, 2016) recently suggested that indirect measures, many of which have received support across independent methods in basic research, and explicit or direct survey measures, many of which mention the target behavior and thus may be *inevitably* predictive of the behavior, should be routinely compared to adequately judge indirect measures and implicit processes. However, to insist on such comparisons in most research would take critical focus away from improving how indirect assessments can best tap into the different associations that are represented in different neural systems. No traditional survey measure is a validated assessment of associations in memory or other concepts from the basic research outlined in this chapter. To harness the potential of a multiple memory system approach as a unique research domain in this area, it is necessary to: conduct research on validated indirect assessments of associations in memory, translate additional measures from basic research in cognitive neuroscience, and study underlying processes taking into account findings from multiple methods and even different species. One caveat is that a multiple memory system approach is concerned with all types of associations in memory, not just evaluative or attitudinal associations receiving the most focus in research on implicit social cognition. In the present approach, all associations in memory guide the flow of cognition, color one's train of thought, and influence behavior, not just those restricted to attitudinal or goal-related content. Interestingly, the traditional conception of attitude is not obligatory in such an approach, and a *bipolar* view of affect would be incompatible though Cacioppo and colleague's neurobiologically plausible view of affect or emotion as *bivalent* is compatible (Cacioppo & Berntson, 1999; Cacioppo & Gardner, 1999): bivalent affect implies that positive and negative affect operate independently.

Beyond the consideration of traditional constructs and measures, some indirect tests of cognition not addressed in this chapter, like the addiction Stroop, are usually assumed to assess *attentional processes*, rather than memory. However, even among these tests some theories suggest the possibility of a basis in associative memory or related conditioning processes (for major review, see Cox, Fadardi & Pothos, 2006). Indeed, a fast-acting memory process is likely required to guide selective attention (Cowan, 1988). In the present approach, the important evidence-based effects of certain types of attentional bias retraining procedures (Bazzaz, Fadardi & Parkinson, 2017; Ziaee et al., 2016) may be mediated by the development of S-R habit associations that help direct attention away from a problematic stimulus; during training, these associations may strengthen, consolidate, or transfer across memory systems through mechanisms outlined by Henke (2010) and Knowlton and colleagues (1996).

Finally, there have been valiant attempts to develop *single system models of memory and cognition* on the basis of basic research (Hintzman, 1986; Hommel & Wiers, 2017; Reder, Park & Kieffaber, 2009). Although the neurobiological plausibility of such models appears to be limited, some single system models could be readily reconceptualized as a way to model multiple memory systems at a higher level of analysis. In Hintzman's powerful model, associations in memory are represented by episodic memory traces that share common features. Having many memory traces that have, for example, encoded *party* with marijuana use, *Friday night* with drinking alcohol, or *feeling good* with opiates, creates a strong association between the members of the encoded pair of features, and the sum of such memory traces with common features is activated by cues to emerge as an *echo* in working memory; the echo is essentially a holistic representation of the constituent memories, and can be classified as a concept, schema, or other generalized representation. Though not addressed by Hintzman, different types of features are likely supported through different memory systems. As an example, source memory including the spatial-temporal context of an event could be encoded primarily through the hippocampal system, allowing for explicit recall of a previous event. If the system is impaired, then the relevant feature would not be encoded in the memory trace, though unimpaired systems would allow for other types of encoding of the event. The feature supported by the impaired hippocampal system would essentially get a weight of zero in a computational model of the process. In such a simple adjustment of Hintzman's model, many findings on amnesic and other neuropsychological populations could be explained within a single computational system that adjusts weights given to different neural subsystems or circuits depending on their functional integrity and activity. Engagement in appetitive behaviors such as drug use, sex, or eating sweet foods alters neural activity in subsystems that might also affect these weights. Although the validity of the adjusted model has not been tested, this example illustrates how multiple memory systems might be incorporated into a single more general model that is nonetheless subserved by multiple memory systems.

Conclusions

Multiple memory system approaches are useful for understanding addictions and for the development of new hypotheses and research that can substantially advance theory and help promote the discovery of new intervention routes. This chapter provides just one view of an important sample of the relevant literature, providing examples of not only what already has been learned, but also what has not. In particular, while plausibly of major importance, some memory systems have not been applied to addiction in any explicit way. The importance of associations in memory, found to be predictive of many different cognitive responses in basic research across five decades, as well as predictive of addictive behaviors in prospective work, is compatible with multiple-memory system views of health behavior and suggest that implicit associations are key elements in the establishment and maintenance of addictions and habits. The focus on associations is consistent with neural models of memory systems and more generally on the connective nature of brain circuitry, neural plasticity, and effects of learning on the weight of connections across neural circuits. Associations in memory influence spontaneous thoughts, how different situations trigger different thoughts and differential access to competing content and tendencies, what behaviors are in one's consideration set and are most salient in a given moment, and what cognitions, even if previously learned to some degree, are not even brought to mind or thought about in many everyday situations. These processes normally operate without awareness of their effects, though they govern content that pops to mind, influencing the flow of cognition including thoughts about imminent actions. One might ask, can people even think of a behavior or alternative that is not accessed in memory in some form? Do reflexive thoughts, likely based on associations, not usually precede the decision of an addict to seek a drug of choice or a binge eater to choose a certain food? Even if so, this does not rule out more "robotic" forms of association governed by strong habits. As an example, an alcoholic may reflexively reach out for a drink in sight, possibly without conscious thought. Even then, it is likely on the basis of memory system views that a distributed set of associations that bring actions and related thoughts to mind is also activated, likely in parallel (cf. Ray et al., 2004). If an object (e.g., drug or food) of choice is not immediately available, then a simple, and possibly unconscious, habit reflex (e.g., a conditioned response) to reach for the object is unlikely to work alone. The multiple memory system approach is just one example of translation of readily available basic research on memory and cognition that is quite different from any prevailing theory popular in public health areas. Such approaches derived from basic experimental research suggest an entirely different set of constructs, variables, and methods as compared to the prevailing Zeitgeist in health behavior research on cognitive processes and provide neurally plausible routes for developing new explanatory hypotheses and new routes for intervention.

REFERENCES

Albarracín, D., Johnson, B. T., Fishbein, M. & Muellerleile, P. A. (2001). Theories of reasoned action and planned behavior as models of condom use: A meta-analysis. *Psychological Bulletin*, **127**(1), 142–161.

Ames, S. L., Grenard, J. L., He, Q., et al. (2014b). Functional imaging of an alcohol-Implicit Association Test (IAT). *Addiction Biology*, **19** (3), 467–481. doi:10.1111/adb.12071

Ames, S. L., Grenard, J. L., Stacy, A. W., et al. (2013). Functional imaging of implicit marijuana associations during performance on an Implicit Association Test (IAT). *Behavioural Brain Research*, **256**, 494–502. doi:10.1016/j.bbr.2013.09.013

Ames, S. L., Wong, S. W., Bechara, A., et al. (2014a). Neural correlates of a Go/No Go task with alcohol stimuli in light and heavy young drinkers. *Behavioural Brain Research*, **274**, 382–389

Ames, S. L., Xie, B., Aragon, J. & Stacy, A. W. (2020). Moderating effects of control functions on implicit cognitive processes in health behavior: A meta-analysis. *Submitted for publication.*

Ames, S. L., Xie, B., Shono, Y. & Stacy, A. W. (2017). Adolescents at risk for drug abuse: A 3-year dual-process analysis. *Addiction*, **112**(5), 852–863. doi:10.1111/add.13742

Baddeley, A. D. (2001). Is working memory still working? *American Psychologist*, **11**, 851–864. doi:10.1037/0003-066X.56.11.851

Back, S. E., Gros, D. F., McCauley, J. L., et al. (2014). Laboratory-induced cue reactivity among individuals with prescription opioid dependence. *Addictive Behaviors*, **39**(8), 1217–1223. doi:10.1016/j.addbeh.2014.04.007

Bargh, J. A., Chen, M. & Burrows, L. (1996). Automaticity of social behavior: Direct effects of trait construct and stereotype activation on action. *Journal of Personality and Social Psychology*, **71**(2), 230–244.

Bargh, J. A. & Morsella, E. (2008). The unconscious mind. *Perspectives on Psychological Science*, **3**(1), 73–79.

Bazzaz, M. M., Fadardi, J. S. & Parkinson, J. (2017). Efficacy of the attention control training program on reducing attentional bias in obese and overweight dieters. *Appetite*, **108**, 1–11. doi:10.1016/j.appet.2016.08.114

Bechara, A. (2005). Decision making, impulse control and loss of willpower to resist drugs: A neurocognitive perspective. *Nature Neuroscience*, **8**(11), 1458–1463. doi:10.1038/nn1584

Berridge, K. C. & Robinson, T. E. (2016). Liking, wanting, and the incentive-sensitization theory of addiction. *American Psychologist*, **71** (8), 670–679. doi:10.1037/amp0000059

Binder, J. R. & Desai, R. H. (2011). The neurobiology of semantic memory. *Trends in Cognitive Sciences*, **15**(11), 527–536. doi:10.1016/j.tics.2011.10.001

Binder, J. R., Desai, R. H., Graves, W. W. & Conant, L. L. (2009). Where is the semantic system? A critical review and meta-analysis of 120 functional neuroimaging studies. *Cerebral Cortex*, **19**(12), 2767–2796. doi:10.1093/cercor/bhp055

Blanton, H., Burrows, C. N. & Jaccard, J. (2016). To accurately estimate implicit influences on health behavior, accurately estimate explicit influences. *Health Psychology*, **35**(8), 856–860. doi:10.1037/hea0000348; 10.1037/hea0000348.supp (Supplemental).

Bousfield, W. A., Whitmarsh, G. A. & Danick, J. J. (1958). Partial response identities in verbal generalization. *Psychological Reports*, **4**(3), 703–713.

Brewer, D. D., Catalano, R. F., Haggerty, K., Gainey, R. R. & Fleming, C. B. (1998). A meta-analysis of predictors of continued drug use during and after treatment for opiate addiction. *Addiction*, **93**(1), 73–92. doi:10.1046/j.1360-0443.1998.931738.x

Buckner, R. L., Koutstaal, W., Schacter, D. L. & Rosen, B. R. (2000). Functional MRI evidence for a role of frontal and inferior temporal cortex in amodal components of priming. *Brain: A Journal of Neurology*, **123**(3), 620–640.

Burton, P. C. & Martin, R. C. (2006). Semantic retrieval versus selection in verb generation: An fMRI investigation. Paper presented at the *47th Annual Meeting of the Psychonomic Society*, Houston, Texas.

Cabeza, R. & Lennartson, E. R. (2005). False memory across languages: Implicit associative response vs fuzzy trace views. *Memory*, **13**(1), 1–5.

Cabeza, R. & Nyberg, L. (2000). Imaging cognition II: An empirical review of 275 PET and fMRI studies. *Journal of Cognitive Neuroscience*, **12**(1), 1–47.

Cacioppo, J. T. & Berntson, G. G. (1999). The affect system: Architecture and operating characteristics. *Current Directions in Psychological Science*, **8**, 133–137.

Cacioppo, J. T. & Gardner, W. L. (1999). Emotion. *Annual Review of Psychology*, **50**, 191–214.

Chassin, L., Presson, C. C., Sherman, S. J., Seo, D.-C. & Macy, J. T. (2010). Implicit and explicit attitudes predict smoking cessation: Moderating effects of experienced failure to control smoking and plans to quit. *Psychology of Addictive Behaviors*, **24**(4), 670–679. doi:10.1037/a0021722

Chein, J. M. & Schneider, W. (2005). Neuroimaging studies of practice-related change: fMRI and meta-analytic evidence of a domain-general control network for learning. *Cognitive Brain Research*, **25**(3), 607–623.

Coallier, É, Michelet, T. & Kalaska, J. F. (2015). Dorsal premotor cortex: Neural correlates of reach target decisions based on a color-location matching rule and conflicting sensory evidence. *Journal of Neurophysiology*, **113**(10), 3543–3573. doi:10.1152/jn.00166.2014

Cousijn, J., Wiers, R. W., Ridderinkhof, K. R., et al. (2014). Effect of baseline cannabis use and working-memory network function on changes in cannabis use in heavy cannabis users: A prospective fMRI study. *Human Brain Mapping*, **35**(5), 2470–2482. doi:10.1002/hbm.22342

Cowan, N. (1988). Evolving conceptions of memory storage, selective attention, and their mutual constraints within the human information-processing system. *Psychological Bulletin*, **104**(2), 163–191. doi:10.1037/0033-2909.104.2.163

Cox, W. M., Fadardi, J. S. & Pothos, E. M. (2006). The addiction-Stroop test: Theoretical considerations and procedural recommendations. *Psychological Bulletin*, **132** (3), 443–476. doi:10.1037/0033-2909.132.3.443

Cramer, P. (1970a). Associative strength as a determinant of mediated priming. *Journal of Verbal Learning and Verbal Behavior*, **9**(6), 658–664. doi:http://dx.doi.org/10.1016/S0022-5371(70)80029-9

Cramer, P. (1970b). Semantic generalization: Demonstration of an associative gradient. *Journal of Experimental Psychology*, **84**(1), 164–172. doi:10.1037/h0028935

Crescentini, C., Shallice, T. & Macaluso, E. (2010). Item retrieval and competition in noun and verb generation: An fMRI study. *Journal of Cognitive Neuroscience*, **22**(6), 1140–1157. doi:10.1162/jocn.2009.21255.

Cristofori, I. & Grafman, J. (2017). Neural underpinnings of the human belief system. In H. Angel, L. Oviedo, R. F. Paloutzian, et al. (Eds.), *Processes of Believing: The Acquisition, Maintenance, and Change in Creditions*. Cham, Switzerland: Springer International Publishing, pp. 111–123. doi:10.1007/978-3-319-50924-2_8

de Jong, P. J., Wiers, R. W., van de Braak, M. & Huijding, J. (2007). Using the Extrinsic Affective Simon Test as a measure of implicit attitudes towards alcohol: Relationship with drinking behavior and alcohol problems. *Addictive Behaviors*, **32**(4), 881–887. doi:10.1016/j.addbeh.2006.06.017

Deese, J. (1959). On the prediction of occurrence of particular verbal intrusions in immediate recall. *Journal of Experimental Psychology*, **58**(1), 17–22.

Deese, J. (1962). On the structure of associative meaning. *Psychological Review*, **69**(3), 161–175. doi:10.1037/h0045842

Derzon, J. H. & Lipsey, M. W. (1999). Predicting tobacco use to age 18: A synthesis of longitudinal research. *Addiction*, **94**(7), 995–1006. doi:10.1046/j.1360-0443.1999.9479955.x

Eldridge, L. L., Masterman, D. & Knowlton, B. J. (2002). Intact implicit habit learning in Alzheimer's disease. *Behavioral Neuroscience*, **116**(4), 722–726.

Eriksson, J., Vogel, E.K., Lansner, A., Bergström, F. & Nyberg, L. (2015). Neurocognitive architecture of working memory. *Neuron*, **88**(1), 33–46. doi:10.1016/j.neuron.2015.09.020

Everitt, B. J. & Robbins, T. W. (2016). Drug addiction: Updating actions to habits to compulsions ten years on. *Annual Review of Psychology*, **67**, 23–50. doi:10.1146/annurev-psych-122414-033457

Fillmore, M. T., Vogel-Sprott, M. & Gavrilescu, D. (1999). Alcohol effects on intentional behavior: Dissociating controlled and automatic influences. *Experimental and Clinical Psychopharmacology*, **7**(4), 372–378.

Fishbein, D. H., Ridenour, T. A., Stahl, M. & Sussman, S. (2016). The full translational spectrum of prevention science: Facilitating the transfer of knowledge to practices and policies that prevent behavioral health problems. *Translational Behavioral Medicine*, **6**(1), 5–16. doi:10.1007/s13142-015-0376-2

Foerde, K., Knowlton, B. J. & Poldrack, R. A. (2006). Modulation of competing memory systems by distraction. *PNAS Proceedings of the National Academy of Sciences of the United States of America*, **103**(31), 11778–11783. doi:10.1073/pnas.0602659103

Frankland, L., Bradley, B. P. & Mogg, K. (2016). Time course of attentional bias to drug cues in opioid dependence. *Psychology of Addictive Behaviors*, **30**(5), 601–606. doi:10.1037/adb0000169; 10.1037/adb0000169.supp (Supplemental)

Fuster, J. M. (2001). The prefrontal cortex – An update: Time is of the essence. *Neuron*, **30**, 319–333.

Gabrieli, J. D. E., Stebbins, G. T., Singh, J., Willingham, D. B. & Goetz, C.G. (1997). Intact mirror-tracing and impaired rotary-pursuit skill learning in patients with Huntington's disease: Evidence for dissociable memory systems in skill learning. *Neuropsychology*, **11**(2), 272–281. doi:10.1037/0894-4105.11.2.272

Gardner, B., de Bruijn, G. & Lally, P. (2011). A systematic review and meta-analysis of applications of the Self-Report Habit Index to nutrition and physical activity behaviours. *Annals of Behavioral Medicine*, **42**(2), 174–187. doi:10.1007/s12160-011-9282-0

Gardner, B., de Bruijn, G. & Lally, P. (2012). Habit, identity, and repetitive action: A prospective study of binge-drinking in UK students. *British Journal of Health Psychology*, **17**(3), 565–581. doi:10.1111/j.2044-8287.2011.02056.x

Garland, E. L., Franken, I. H., Sheetz, J. J. & Howard, M. O. (2012). Alcohol attentional bias is associated with autonomic indices of stress-primed alcohol cue-reactivity in alcohol-dependent patients. *Experimental and Clinical Psychopharmacology*, **20**(3), 225–235. doi:10.1037/a0027199

Glenberg, A. M., Witt, J. K. & Metcalfe, J. (2013). From the revolution to embodiment: 25 years of cognitive psychology. *Perspectives on Psychological Science*, **8**(5), 573–585. doi:10.1177/1745691613498098

Glock, S., Klapproth, F. & Müller, B. C. N. (2015). Promoting responsible drinking? A mass media campaign affects implicit but not explicit alcohol-related cognitions and attitudes. *British Journal of Health Psychology*, **20**(3), 482–497. doi:10.1111/bjhp.12130

Graf, P. & Schacter, D. L. (1985). Implicit and explicit memory for new associations in normal and amnesic subjects. *Journal of Experimental Psychology: Learning, Memory, and Cognition*, **11**(3), 501–518.

Greenwald, A. G. & Banaji, M. R. (1995). Implicit social cognition: Attitudes, self-esteem, and stereotypes. *Psychological Review*, **102**(1), 4–27.

Greenwald, A. G., McGhee, D. E. & Schwartz, J. L. K. (1998). Measuring individual differences in implicit cognition: The Implicit Association Test. *Journal of Personality and Social Psychology*, **74**(6), 1464–1480.

Greenwald, A. G., Nosek, B. A. & Banaji, M. R. (2003). Understanding and using the Implicit Association Test: I. An improved scoring algorithm. *Journal of Personality and Social Psychology*, **85**(2), 197–216.

Grenard, J. L., Ames, S. L., Wiers, R. W., et al. (2008). Working memory capacity moderates the predictive effects of drug-related associations on substance use. *Psychology of Addictive Behaviors*, **22**(3), 426–432. doi:10.1037/0893-164X.22.3.426

Hagger, M. S., Chan, D. K. C., Protogerou, C. & Chatzisarantis, N. L. D. (2016). Using meta-analytic path analysis to test theoretical predictions in health behavior: An illustration based on meta-analyses of the theory of planned behavior. *Preventive Medicine*, **89**, 154–161. doi:10.1016/j.ypmed.2016.05.020

Hanlon, C. A., Dowdle, L. T., Naselaris, T., Canterberry, M. & Cortese, B. M. (2014). Visual cortex activation to drug cues: A meta-analysis of functional neuroimaging papers in addiction and substance abuse literature. *Drug and Alcohol Dependence*, **143**, 206–212. doi:10.1016/j.drugalcdep.2014.07.028

Hélie, S., Ell, S. W. & Ashby, F. G. (2015). Learning robust cortico-cortical associations with the basal ganglia: An integrative review. *Cortex: A Journal Devoted to the Study of the Nervous System and Behavior*, **64**, 123–135. doi:10.1016/j.cortex.2014.10.011

Henke, K. (2010). A model for memory systems based on processing modes rather than consciousness. *Nature Reviews Neuroscience*, **11**(7), 523–532. doi:10.1038/nrn2850

Hintzman, D. L. (1986). "Schema abstraction" in a multiple-trace memory model. *Psychological Review*, **93**(4), 411–428.

Hommel, B. & Wiers, R. W. (2017). Towards a unitary approach to human action control. *Trends in Cognitive Sciences*, **21**(12), 940–949. doi:10.1016/j.tics.2017.09.009

Hoshi, E. & Tanji, J. (2007). Distinctions between dorsal and ventral premotor areas: Anatomical connectivity and functional properties. *Current Opinion in Neurobiology*, **17**(2), 234–242. doi:10.1016/j.conb.2007.02.003

Hovington, C. L. & Brouwer, B. (2010). Guided motor imagery in healthy adults and stroke: Does strategy matter? *Neurorehabilitation and Neural Repair*, **24**(9), 851–857. doi:10.1177/1545968310374190

Hutchison, K. A., Balota, D. A., Cortese, M. J. & Watson, J. M. (2008). Predicting semantic priming at the item level. *The Quarterly Journal of Experimental Psychology*, **61**(7), 1036–1066. doi:10.1080/17470210701438111

Ishida, H., Inoue, K., Takada, M. & Hoshi, E. (2016). Origins of multisynaptic projections from the basal ganglia to the forelimb region of the ventral premotor cortex in macaque monkeys. *European Journal of Neuroscience*, **43**(2), 258–269. doi:10.1111/ejn.13127

Kahneman, D. (2003). A perspective on judgment and choice: Mapping bounded rationality. *American Psychologist*, **58**(9), 697–720.

Kahneman, D. (2011). *Thinking, Fast and Slow* (1st edition). New York, NY: Farrar, Straus and Giroux.

Kandel, E. R. & Kandel, D. B. (2014). A molecular basis for nicotine as a gateway drug. *The New England Journal of Medicine*, **371**(10), 932–943. doi:10.1056/NEJMsa1405092

Kelly, A. B., Masterman, P. W. & Marlatt, G. A. (2005). Alcohol-related associative strength and drinking behaviours: Concurrent and prospective relationships. *Drug and Alcohol Review*, **24**(6), 489–498.

Kharitonova, M., Winter, W. & Sheridan, M. A. (2015). As working memory grows: A developmental account of neural bases of working memory capacity in 5- to 8-year old children and adults. *Journal of Cognitive Neuroscience*, **27**(9), 1775–1788. doi:10.1162/jocn_a_00824

Khurana, A., Romer, D., Betancourt, L. M., et al. (2012). Working memory ability predicts trajectories of early alcohol use in adolescents: The mediational role of impulsivity. *Addiction*, **108**, 506–515.

Khurana, A., Romer, D., Betancourt, L. M., et al. (2015). Stronger working memory reduces sexual risk taking in adolescents, even after controlling for parental influences. *Child Development*, **86**(4), 1125–1141. doi:10.1111/cdev.12383

Khurana, A., Romer, D., Betancourt, L. M. & Hurt, H. (2017). Working memory ability and early drug use progression as predictors of adolescent substance use disorders. *Addiction*, **112**(7), 1220–1228. doi:10.1111/add.13792

Knowlton, B. J., Mangels, J. A. & Squire, L. R. (1996). A neostriatal habit learning system in humans. *Science*, **273**(5280), 1399–402.

Koob, G. F. & Le Moal, M. (2008). Addiction and the brain antireward system. *Annual Review of Psychology*, **59**, 29–53. doi:10.1146/annurev.psych.59.103006.093548

Koob, G. F. & Volkow, N. D. (2016). Neurobiology of addiction: A neurocircuitry analysis. *The Lancet Psychiatry*, **3**(8), 760–773. doi:10.1016/S2215-0366(16)00104-8

Kosslyn, S. M., Ganis, G. & Thompson, W. L. (2001). Neural foundations of imagery. *Nature Reviews Neuroscience*, **2**(9), 635–642. doi:10.1038/35090055

Krank, M., Wall, A.-M., Stewart, S. H., Wiers, R. W. & Goldman, M. S. (2005). Context effects on alcohol cognitions. *Alcoholism: Clinical & Experimental Research*, **29**(2), 196–206. doi:10.1097/01.ALC.0000153545.36787.C8

Landis, D., Triandis, H. C. & Adamopoulos, J. (1978). Habit and behavioral intentions as predictors of social behavior. *The Journal of Social Psychology*, **106**(2), 227–237. doi:10.1080/00224545.1978.9924174

Levy, D. A., Stark, C. E. L. & Squire, L. R. (2004). Intact conceptual priming in the absence of declarative memory. *Psychological Science*, **15**(10), 680–686. doi:10.1111/j.0956-7976.2004.00740.x

Lindgren, K. P., Neighbors, C., Gasser, M. L., Ramirez, J. J. & Cvencek, D. (2017). A review of implicit and explicit substance self-concept as a predictor of alcohol and tobacco use and misuse. *The American Journal of Drug and Alcohol Abuse*, **43**(3), 237–246. doi:10.1080/00952990.2016.1229324

Lindgren, K. P., Neighbors, C., Teachman, B. A., et al. (2016). Implicit alcohol associations, especially drinking identity, predict drinking over time. *Health Psychology*, **35**(8), 908–918. doi:10.1037/hea0000396; 10.1037/hea0000396.supp (Supplemental).

Luttrell, A., Stillman, P. E., Hasinski, A. E. & Cunningham, W. A. (2016). Neural dissociations in attitude strength: Distinct regions of cingulate cortex track ambivalence and certainty. *Journal of Experimental Psychology: General*, **145**(4), 419–433. doi:10.1037/xge0000141; 10.1037/xge0000141.supp (Supplemental).

Mahler, S. V. & Berridge, K. C. (2012). What and when to "want"? Amygdala-based focusing of incentive salience upon sugar and sex. *Psychopharmacology*, **221**(3), 407–426. doi:10.1007/s00213-011-2588-6

Marins, T. F., Rodrigues, E. C., Engel, A., et al. (2015). Enhancing motor network activity using real-time functional MRI neurofeedback of left premotor cortex. *Frontiers in Behavioral Neuroscience*, **9**. doi:10.3389/fnbeh.2015.00341

McEachan, R. R. C., Conner, M., Taylor, N. J. & Lawton, R. J. (2011). Prospective prediction of health-related behaviours with the Theory of Planned Behaviour: A meta-analysis. *Health Psychology Review*, **5**(2), 97–144. doi:10.1080/17437199.2010.521684

Miller, K. J., Schalk, G., Fetz, E. E., et al. (2010). Cortical activity during motor execution, motor imagery, and imagery-based online feedback. *Proceedings of the National Academy of Sciences of the United States of America*, **107**(9), 4430–4435. doi:10.1073/pnas.0913697107

Mirabella, G., Pani, P. & Ferraina, S. (2011). Neural correlates of cognitive control of reaching movements in the dorsal premotor cortex of rhesus monkeys. *Journal of Neurophysiology*, **106**(3), 1454–1466. doi:10.1152/jn.00995.2010

Moore, P. J., Turner, R., Park, C. L. & Adler, N. E. (1996). The impact of behavior and addiction on psychological models of cigarette and alcohol use during pregnancy. *Addictive Behaviors*, **21**(5), 645–658. doi:10.1016/0306-4603(95)00100-X

Moors, A., Spruyt, A. & De Houwer, J. (2010). In search of a measure that qualifies as implicit: Recommendations based on a decompositional view of automaticity. In B. Gawronski & B. K. Payne (Eds.), *Handbook of Implicit Social Cognition: Measurement, Theory, and Applications*. New York, NY: The Guilford Press, pp. 19–37.

Neal, D. T., Wood, W. & Drolet, A. (2013). How do people adhere to goals when willpower is low? The profits (and pitfalls) of strong habits. *Journal of Personality and Social Psychology*, **104**(6), 959–975. doi:10.1037/a0032626

Nelson, D. L., McKinney, V. M., Gee, N. R. & Janczura, G. A. (1998). Interpreting the influence of implicitly activated memories on recall and recognition. *Psychological Review*, **105**(2), 299–324. doi:10.1037/0033-295X.105.2.299

Noël, X., Brevers, D. & Bechara, A. (2013). A neurocognitive approach to understanding the neurobiology of addiction. *Current Opinion in Neurobiology*, **23**(4), 632–638. doi:10.1016/j.conb.2013.01.018

Norman, P. (2011). The theory of planned behavior and binge drinking among undergraduate students: Assessing the impact of habit strength. *Addictive Behaviors*, **36**(5), 502–507. doi:10.1016/j.addbeh.2011.01.025

Nosek, B. A., Greenwald, A. G. & Banaji, M. R. (2005). Understanding and using the Implicit Association Test: II. Method variables and construct validity. *Personality and Social Psychology Bulletin*, **31**(2), 166–180.

Nosek, B. A., Greenwald, A. G. & Banaji, M. R. (2007). The Implicit Association Test at age 7: A methodological and conceptual review. In J. A. Bargh (Ed.), *Automatic Processes in Social Thinking and Behavior*. New York, NY: Psychology Press Ltd, pp. 265–292.

Ntoumanis, N. D., Ng, J. Y. Y., Barkoukis, V. & Backhouse, S. (2014). Personal and psychosocial predictors of doping use in physical activity settings: A meta-analysis. *Sports Medicine*, **44**(11), 1603–1624. doi:10.1007/s40279-014-0240-4

Oguri, T., Sawamoto, N., Tabu, H., et al. (2013). Overlapping connections within the motor cortico-basal ganglia circuit: fMRI-tractography analysis. *Neuroimage*, **78**, 353–362. doi:10.1016/j.neuroimage.2013.04.026

Oliver, J. A., Jentink, K. G., Drobes, D. J. & Evans, D. E. (2016). Smokers exhibit biased neural processing of smoking and affective images. *Health Psychology*, **35**(8), 866–869. doi:10.1037/hea0000350; 10.1037/hea0000350.supp (Supplemental).

Orbell, S. & Verplanken, B. (2010). The automatic component of habit in health behavior: Habit as cue-contingent automaticity. *Health Psychology*, **29**(4), 374–383. doi:10.1037/a0019596

Ouellette, J. & Wood, W. (1998). Habit and intention in everyday life: The multiple processes by which past behavior predicts future behavior. *Psychological Bulletin*, **124**(1), 54–74. doi:10.1037//0033-2909.124.1.54

Packard, M. G. & Goodman, J. (2013). Factors that influence the relative use of multiple memory systems. *Hippocampus*, **23**(11), 1044–1052. doi:10.1002/hipo.22178

Packard, M. G. & Knowlton, B. J. (2002). Learning and memory functions of the basal ganglia. *Annual Review of Neuroscience*, **25**(1), 563–593. doi:10.1146/annurev.neuro.25.112701.142937

Palfai, T. P. & Ostafin, B. D. (2003). Alcohol-related motivational tendencies in hazardous drinkers: Assessing implicit response tendencies using the modified-IAT. *Behaviour Research and Therapy*, **41**(10), 1149–1162.

Patterson, K., Nestor, P. J. & Rogers, T. T. (2007). Where do you know what you know? The representation of semantic knowledge in the human brain. *Nature Reviews Neuroscience*, **8**(12), 976–987. doi:10.1038/nrn2277

Payne, B. K. & Gawronski, B. (2010). A history of implicit social cognition: Where is it coming from? Where is it now? Where is it going? In B. Gawronski & B. K. Payne (Eds.), *Handbook of Implicit Social Cognition: Measurement, Theory, and Applications* . New York, NY: The Guilford Press, pp. 1–15.

Payne, B. K., Lee, K. M., Giletta, M. & Prinstein, M. J. (2016). Implicit attitudes predict drinking onset in adolescents: Shaping by social norms. *Health Psychology*, **35**(8), 829–836. doi:10.1037/hea0000353; 10.1037/hea0000353.supp (Supplemental).

Peeters, M., Monshouwer, K., Janssen, T., Wiers, R. W. & Vollebergh, W. A. M. (2014). Working memory and alcohol use in at-risk adolescents: A 2-year follow-up. *Alcoholism: Clinical & Experimental Research*, **38**(4), 1176–1183. doi:10.1111/acer.12339

Pilgramm, S., de **Haas, B., Helm, F.**, et al. (2016). Motor imagery of hand actions: Decoding the content of motor imagery from brain activity in frontal and parietal motor areas. *Human Brain Mapping*, **37**(1), 81–93. doi:10.1002/hbm.23015

Raichle, M. E., Fiez, J. A., Videen, T. O., et al. (1994). Practice-related changes in human brain functional anatomy during nonmotor learning. *Cerebral Cortex*, **4**(1), 8–26. doi:10.1093/cercor/4.1.8

Ray, S., Bates, M. E. & Ely, B. M. (2004). Alcohol's dissociation of implicit and explicit memory processes: Implications of a parallel distributed processing model of semantic priming. *Experimental and Clinical Psychopharmacology*, **12**(2), 118–125.

Reder, L. M., Park, H. & Kieffaber, P. D. (2009). Memory systems do not divide on consciousness: Reinterpreting memory in terms of activation and binding. *Psychological Bulletin*, **135**(1), 23–49. doi:10.1037/a0013974

Reich, R. R., Goldman, M. S. & Noll, J. A. (2004). Using the false memory paradigm to test two key elements of alcohol expectancy theory. *Experimental and Clinical Psychopharmacology*, **12**(2), 102–110.

Robin, N., Dominique, L., Toussaint, L., et al. (2007). Effect of motor imagery training on service return accuracy in tennis: The role of imagery ability. *International Journal of Sport and Exercise Psychology*, **5**(2), 175–186.

Robinson, M. J. F., Anselme, P., Fischer, A. M. & Berridge, K. C. (2014). Initial uncertainty in Pavlovian reward prediction persistently elevates incentive salience and extends sign-tracking to normally unattractive cues. *Behavioural Brain Research*, **266**, 119–130. doi:10.1016/j.bbr.2014.03.004

Robinson, K. J. & Roediger, H. L. (1997). Associative processes in false recall and false recognition. *Psychological Science*, **8**(3), 231–237.

Roediger, H. L., Watson, J. M., McDermott, K. B. & Gallo, D. A. (2001). Factors that determine false recall: A multiple regression analysis. *Psychonomic Bulletin & Review*, **8**(3), 385–407.

Rolls, E. T. (2000). Memory systems in the brain. *Annual Review of Psychology*, **51**, 599–630. doi:10.1146/annurev.psych.51.1.599

Rotter, J. B. (1954). *Social Learning and Clinical Psychology*. Englewood Cliffs, NJ: Prentice-Hall, Inc. doi:10.1037/10788-000

Salemink, E. & Wiers, R. W. (2014). Alcohol-related memory associations in positive and negative affect situations: Drinking motives, working memory capacity, and prospective drinking. *Psychology of Addictive Behaviors*, **28** (1), 105–113. doi:10.1037/a0032806

Schacter, D. L. (1985). Priming of old and new knowledge in amnesic patients and normal subjects. *Annals of the New York Academy of Sciences*, **444**, 41–53.

Schneider, W. & Chein, J. M. (2003). Controlled & automatic processing: Behavior, theory, and biological mechanisms. *Cognitive Science*, **27** (3), 525–559. doi:10.1016/S0364-0213(03)00011-9

Schneider, W. & Shiffrin, R. M. (1977). Controlled and automatic human information processing: I. Detection, search, and attention.

Psychological Review, **84**(1), 1–66. doi:10.1037/0033-295X.84.1.1

Scoville, W. B. & Milner, B. (1957). Loss of recent memory after bilateral hippocampal lesions. *Journal of Neurology, Neurosurgery & Psychiatry*, **20**(1), 11–21. doi:10.1136/jnnp.20.1.11

Seger, C. A., Desmond, J. E., Glover, G. H. & Gabrieli, J. D. (2000). Functional magnetic resonance imaging evidence for right-hemisphere involvement in processing unusual semantic relationships. *Neuropsychology*, **14**(3), 361–369.

Seger, C. A., Rabin, L. A., Desmond, J. E. & Gabrieli, J. D. (1999). Verb generation priming involves conceptual implicit memory. *Brain and Cognition*, **41**(2), 150–177. doi:10.1006/brcg.1999.1116

Seger, C. A., Rabin, L. A., Zarella, M. M. & Gabrieli, J. D. E. (1997). Preserved verb generation priming in global amnesia. *Neuropsychologia*, **35**(8), 1069–1074. doi:10.1097/OLQ.0b013e318214bb70

Sheldon, S., Romero, K. & Moscovitch, M. (2013). Medial temporal lobe amnesia impairs performance on a free association task. *Hippocampus*, **23**(5), 405–412. doi:10.1002/hipo.22099

Sherman, S. J., Chassin, L., Presson, C., Seo, D.-C. & Macy, J. T. (2009). The intergenerational transmission of implicit and explicit attitudes toward smoking: Predicting adolescent smoking initiation. *Journal of Experimental Social Psychology*, **45**(2), 313–319. doi:10.1016/j.jesp.2008.09.012

Shiffrin, R. M. & Schneider, W. (1977). Controlled and automatic human information processing: II. Perceptual learning, automatic attending and a general theory. *Psychological Review*, **84**(2), 127–190. doi:10.1037/0033-295X.84.2.127

Shimamura, A. P. & Squire, L. R. (1984). Paired-associate learning and priming effects in amnesia: A neuropsychological study. *Journal of Experimental Psychology: General*, **113**(4), 556–570. doi:10.1037/0096-3445.113.4.556

Shono, Y., Ames, S. L. & Stacy, A. W. (2016). Evaluation of internal validity using modern test theory: Application to word association. *Psychological Assessment*, **28**(2), 194–204. doi:10.1037/pas0000175

Shono, Y., Edwards, M. C., Ames, S. L. & Stacy, A. W. (2018). Trajectories of cannabis-related associative memory among vulnerable adolescents: Psychometric and longitudinal evaluations. *Developmental Psychology*, **54**(6), 1148–1158. doi:10.1037/dev0000510

Spruyt, A., Lemaigre, V., Salhi, B., et al. (2015). Implicit attitudes towards smoking predict long-term relapse in abstinent smokers. *Psychopharmacology*, **232**(14), 2551–2561. doi:10.1007/s00213-015-3893-2

Squire, L. R. (2009). Memory and brain systems: 1969–2009. *The Journal of Neuroscience*, **29** (41), 12711–12716. doi:10.1523/JNEUROSCI.3575-09.2009

Squire, L. R. & Knowlton, B. J. (1995). Memory, hippocampus, & brain systems. In M. Gazzaniga (Ed.), *The Cognitive Neurosciences*. Cambridge, MA: MIT Press, pp. 825–837.

Squire, L. R., Knowlton, B. & Musen, G. (1993). The structure and organization of memory. *Annual Review of Psychology*, **44**, 453–495.

Stacy, A. W., Ames, S. L. & Knowlton, B. J. (2004). Neurologically plausible distinctions in cognition relevant to drug use etiology and prevention. *Substance Use & Misuse*, **39**(10–12), 1571–1623.

Stacy, A. W., Bentler, P. M. & Flay, B. R. (1994). Attitudes and health behavior in diverse populations: Drunk driving, alcohol use, binge eating, marijuana use, and cigarette use. *Health Psychology*, **13**(1), 73–85. doi:10.1037/0278-6133.13.1.73

Stacy, A. W., Nydegger, L. A. & Shono, Y. (2019). Translation of basic research in cognitive science to HIV risk: A randomized controlled trial. *Journal of Behavioral Medicine*, **42**, 440–451.

Stacy, A. W., Stein, J. A. & Longshore, D. (1999). Habit, intention, and drug use as interactive predictors of condom use among drug abusers. *AIDS and Behavior*, **3**(3), 231–241.

Sussman, S., Ames, S. L., Dent, C. W. & Stacy, A. W. (2001). Self-reported high-risk locations of drug use among drug offenders. *American Journal of Drug and Alcohol Abuse*, **27**(2), 281–299.

Szalay, L. B., Strohl, J. B. & Doherty, K. T. (1999). *Psychoenvironmental Forces in Substance Abuse Prevention*. Dordrecht, the Netherlands: Kluwer Academic Publishers.

Thompson-Schill, S. L., D'Esposito, M. & Kan, I. P. (1999). Effects of repetition and competition on activity of left prefrontal cortex during word generation. *Neuron*, **23**(3), 513–522.

Thush, C. & Wiers, R. W. (2007). Explicit and implicit alcohol-related cognitions and the prediction of future drinking in adolescents. *Addictive Behaviors*, **32**(7), 1367–1383. doi: S0306-4603(06)00299-1 [pii] 10.1016/j.addbeh.2006.09.011

Thush, C., Wiers, R. W., Ames, S. L., et al. (2007). Apples and oranges? Comparing indirect measures of alcohol-related cognition predicting alcohol use in at-risk adolescents. *Psychology of Addictive Behaviors*, **21**(4), 587–591.

Thush, C., Wiers, R. W., Ames, S. L., et al. (2008). Interactions between implicit and explicit cognition and working memory capacity in the prediction of alcohol use in at-risk adolescents. *Drug and Alcohol Dependence*, **94**(1–3), 116–124. doi:S0376-8716(07)00432-2 [pii] 10.1016/j.drugalcdep.2007.10.019

Tversky, A. & Kahneman, D. (1973). Availability: A heuristic for judging frequency and probability. *Cognitive Psychology*, **5**(2), 207–232. doi:10.1016/0010-0285(73)90033-9

Underwood, B. J. (1965). False recognition produced by implicit verbal responses. *Journal of Experimental Psychology*, **70**(1), 122–129.

Underwood, B. J., Reichardt, C. S. & Malmi, R. A. (1975). Sources of facilitation in learning conceptually structured paired-associate lists. *Journal of Experimental Psychology: Human Learning and Memory*, **1**(2), 160–166. doi:10.1037/0278-7393.1.2.160

Vaidya, C. J., Gabrieli, J. D.E., Keane, M. M. & Monti, L. A. (1995). Perceptual and conceptual memory processes in global amnesia. *Neuropsychology*, **9**(4), 580–591.

Vallet, G. T., Hudon, C., Bier, N., et al. (2017). A semantic and episodic memory test (SEMEP) developed within the embodied cognition framework: Application to normal aging, Alzheimer's disease and semantic dementia. *Frontiers in Psychology*, **8**. doi:10.3389/fpsyg.2017.01493

Van Der Vorst, H., Krank, M. D., Engels, R. C. M. E., et al. (2013). The mediating role of alcohol-related memory associations on the relation between perceived parental drinking and the onset of adolescents' alcohol use. *Addiction*, **108**(3), 526–533. doi:10.1111/add.12042

Verplanken, B. & Orbell, S. (2003). Reflections on past behavior: A self-report index of habit strength. *Journal of Applied Social Psychology*, **33**(6), 1313–1330. doi:10.1007/s12160-011-9305-x

Volkow, N. D., Koob, G. F. & McLellan, A. T. (2016). Neurobiologic advances from the brain disease model of addiction. *The New England Journal of Medicine*, **374**(4), 363–371. doi:10.1056/NEJMra1511480

Wang, J., Johnson, L. A., Jensen, A. L., et al. (2017). Network-wide oscillations in the parkinsonian state: Alterations in neuronal activities occur in the premotor cortex in parkinsonian nonhuman primates. *Journal of Neurophysiology*, **117**(6), 2242–2249. doi:10.1152/jn.00011.2017

Wei, G. & Luo, J. (2010). Sport expert's motor imagery: Functional imaging of professional motor skills and simple motor skills. *Brain Research*, **1341**, 52–62. doi:10.1016/j.brainres.2009.08.014

Weingardt, K. R., Stacy, A. W. & Leigh, B. C. (1996). Automatic activation of alcohol concepts in response to positive outcomes of alcohol use. *Alcoholism: Clinical and Experimental Research*, **20**(1), 25–30.

White, N. M. & McDonald, R. J. (2002). Multiple parallel memory systems in the brain of the rat. *Neurobiology of Learning and Memory*, **77** (2), 125–184. doi:10.1006/nlme.2001.4008

White, N. M., Packard, M. G. & McDonald, R. J. (2013). Dissociation of memory systems: The story unfolds. *Behavioral Neuroscience*, **127** (6), 813–834. doi:10.1037/a0034859

Wiers, R. W., Rinck, M., Dictus, M. & van den Wildenberg, E. (2009). Relatively strong automatic appetitive action-tendencies in male carriers of the OPRM1 G-allele. *Genes, Brain & Behavior*, **8**(1), 101–106. doi:10.1111/ j.1601-183X.2008.00454.x

Wiers, R. W. & Stacy, A. W. (2006). Implicit cognition and addiction. *Current Directions in Psychological Science*, **15**(6), 292–296.

Wiers, R. W., van de Luitgaarden, J., van den Wildenberg, E. & Smulders, F. T. Y. (2005). Challenging implicit and explicit alcohol-related cognitions in young heavy drinkers. *Addiction*, **100**(6), 806–819. doi:10.1111/ j.1360-0443.2005.01064.x

Wing, E. A., Iyengar, V., Hess, T. M., et al. (2018). Neural mechanisms underlying subsequent memory for personal beliefs: An fMRI study. *Cognitive, Affective & Behavioral Neuroscience*, **18**(2), 216–231. doi:10.3758/ s13415-018-0563-y

Wood, W. & Neal, D. T. (2007). A new look at habits and the habit-goal interface. *Psychological Review*, **114**(4), 843–863. doi:2007-13558-001 [pii] 10.1037/0033-295X.114.4.843

Wriessnegger, S. C., Steyrl, D., Koschutnig, K. & Müller-Putz, G. R. (2016). Cooperation in mind: Motor imagery of joint and single actions is represented in different brain areas. *Brain and Cognition*, **109**, 19–25. doi:10.1016/ j.bandc.2016.08.008

Yalachkov, Y., Kaiser, J. & Naumer, M.J. (2015). The role of sensory and motor brain regions in drug-cue reactivity. In S. J. Wilson (Ed.), *The Wiley Handbook on the Cognitive Neuroscience of Addiction*. Wiley-Blackwell, pp. 175–194.

Yan, W., Li, Y., Xiao, L., et al. (2014). Working memory and affective decision- making in addiction: A neurocognitive comparison between heroin addicts, pathological gamblers and healthy controls. *Drug and Alcohol Dependence*, **134**, 194–200. doi:10.1016/j. drugalcdep.2013.09.027

Yin, H. H. & Knowlton, B. J. (2006a). Addiction and learning in the brain. In R. W. Wiers & A. W. Stacy (Eds.), *Handbook of Implicit Cognition and Addiction*. Thousand Oaks, CA: SAGE Publications, pp. 167–184.

Yin, H. H. & Knowlton, B. J. (2006b). The role of the basal ganglia in habit formation. *Nature Reviews Neuroscience*, **7**(6), 464–476. doi:10.1038/nrn1919

Young, K. A., Franklin, T. R., Roberts, D. C. S., et al. (2014). Nipping cue reactivity in the bud: Baclofen prevents limbic activation elicited by subliminal drug cues. *The Journal of Neuroscience*, **34**(14), 5038–5043. doi:10.1523/ JNEUROSCI.4977-13.2014

Zabicki, A., de **Haas, B.**, **Zentgraf, K.**, et al. (2017). Imagined and executed actions in the human motor system: Testing neural similarity between execution and imagery of actions with a multivariate approach. *Cerebral Cortex*, **27**(9), 4523–4536. doi:10.1093/cercor/ bhw257

Zack, M., Poulos, C. X. & Woodford, T. M. (2006). Diazepam dose-dependently increases or decreases implicit priming of alcohol associations in problem drinkers. *Alcohol and Alcoholism*, **41**(6), 604–610. doi:10.1093/ alcalc/agl076

Ziaee, S. S., Fadardi, J. S., Cox, W. M. & Yazdi, S. A. A. (2016). Effects of attention control training on drug abusers' attentional bias and treatment outcome. *Journal of Consulting and Clinical Psychology*, **84**(10), 861–873. doi:10.1037/a0040290

13 The Role of Culture in Addiction

Beth R. Hoffman, PhD, and Jennifer B. Unger, PhD

Introduction

The relationship between culture and addiction is complicated. First, culture itself is complex; it encompasses the languages, customs, beliefs, values, knowledge, memories, and ways of understanding the world transmitted among members of a group. Addiction is no less complicated a concept, one we can identify by common features but that remains a mystery in terms of the mechanisms driving behavior (Sussman & Sussman, 2011).

Second, it is difficult to study one's own culture as the belief systems and thought patterns of the culture are internally ingrained. Assessments often tend to be of objects or services of one's cultural grouping (e.g., books read, stories told, humor, community organizations, languages spoken), and may or may not tap unique qualities of one's culture. Third, culture impacts one via a set of personal experiences and interactions that is also affected by individual characteristics (Eckersley, 2005). As a result, the impacts of culture on behaviors vary across individuals (Eckersley, 2005).

Finally, the culture in which one lives affects what one considers an addiction, who is more at risk for addiction, and how addiction is treated. Many risk factors are addiction-specific, though some risk factors are universal. For example, addictive behaviors are more common for people with a history of childhood abuse or neglect, and parents with addictions are more likely to abuse and/or neglect children (McCrory & Mayes, 2015). This pattern of abuse/neglect and addiction may be considered as cultural at the micro level, as the behaviors are learned within the culture of the family.

The most current version of the *Diagnostic and Statistical Manual of the American Psychiatric Association* (DSM-5, 2013) has, for the first time, defined addiction without referring to substance use. Rather, conditions with evidence that the behavior leads to activation of neurological "reward systems" of addiction are included as "substance-related and addictive disorders." This decision has resulted in the tentative exclusion of certain conditions (compulsive buying and compulsive sexual behavior, among others) as addictions due to a lack of evidence that these conditions activate the required neurological processes (Piquet-Pessôa et al., 2014). The DSM undergoes periodic revision based on the evolution of scientific knowledge and popular opinions about normative versus aberrant behaviors, which is also part of culture. This entails the inclusion and exclusion of diagnoses over time. One could argue that the collection of information is culturally based, affects what phenomena are salient, what researchers choose to study, which unexamined biases underlie research assumptions, and which research is funded. A notable example is the exclusion of homosexuality from the DSM-II in 1973, after appearing as a disorder in the DSM-I. This was based in part upon research indicating that homosexuality does not negatively impact quality of life, as was previously assumed (Drescher, 2015), and in part on the efforts of gay members of the American Psychological Association and other gay activists who advocated for the diagnosis to be dropped (Spiegel, 2002).

Popular culture (e.g., current film, television, web content, music, and other multimedia) also affects what is considered an addiction. Treatment of addiction is a lucrative industry, despite low success rates for treatment programs. Self-help books, treatment centers, and pharmaceutical companies (who develop and sell drugs to treat addiction) all benefit from the addiction industry. Culture also influences beliefs about what types of addictive behaviors and experiences are normative versus nonnormative: for example, nicotine addiction used to be commonplace enough that hospital waiting rooms were filled with smoke and ashtrays. Now a smoker must smoke only in designated outdoor areas in most US states and in many countries worldwide. Meanwhile, Western society encourages and even celebrates addictions to caffeine, work, overeating, and exercise (Wilkerson, 2015).

Since culture is difficult to define, it makes sense to examine it through more concrete aspects of identity that are affected by culture. Culturally based personal identity factors such as ethnicity, gender, nationality and sexual identity may impact an individual's exposure to or likelihood of developing an addiction, and these factors may also interact. In addition, the historical context of an addictive behavior plays a role in whether society considers the behavior worth studying, the legality of the behavior, whether engaging in the behavior is accepted within society, and who is allowed to engage in the behavior.

This chapter will examine how culture impacts specific addictions, separately, within the cultural contexts of ethnicity, gender, nationality, sexuality and history of the addiction. Studies were collected systematically from CINAHL and PsycINFO using the following keywords: culture, history, race, ethnicity, gender, nationality, lesbian, gay, bisexual, transgender, compulsive buying, workaholism, work addiction, gambling disorder, internet addiction, drug addiction, alcohol addiction, nicotine addiction, opiate addiction, marijuana addiction, methamphetamine addiction, compulsive exercise, food addiction, love addiction, and sex addiction. These searches yielded 143 articles, which were screened to determine whether they fit the scope of this review. Additional articles were collected based on references in other collected articles. In total, ninety articles were retained for the purpose of this review. The information available for each varies based on trends in research and how recently an addiction has been identified, as well as the factors outlined above. Table 13.1 provides a summary of each of nine addictions discussed and key cultural differences by ethnic, national, gender, or sexual orientation; as well as a synopsis on the role of history in the addiction.

Shopping

Historical Context

The definition of compulsive buying first appeared in 1987 as "inappropriate, typically excessive, and clearly disruptive to the lives of individuals who appear impulsively driven to consume" (Faber, O'Guinn &

Table 13.1 Summary of key cultural findings by addiction

	History of the disorder	Ethnic comparisons	National comparisons	Gender comparisons	Sexual identity comparisons
Shopping	-	-	No differences in shopping addiction rates across countries (Kwak et al., 2004; Maraz et al., 2016).	Higher rates of shopping addiction in women (Black, 2007; Maraz et al., 2016).	-
Work	Working hours peaked in the 1800s, decreased due to mechanization and labor organizing. Increasing among certain industries (white collar, transportation) since the 1970s (Golden, 2009; Whaples, 2001).	No differences in work addiction rates between US blacks and whites (Aziz et al., 2010)	Confusianism ideals contribute to higher rates of overwork in East Asian cultures (Kang et al., 2017; Stankov, 2010). No differences in antecedents to workaholism in Turkish professors and studies done on Western populations (Burke et al., 2008).	Similar prevalence of work addiction by gender but different expression of traits by males and females (Burke, 1999; Romeo et al., 2014)	-
Gambling	Long history of gambling in Persian (Parhami et al., 2012) and Chinese (Raylu & Oei, 2004) cultures.	Gambling forbidden by Muslim religion (Parhami et al., 2012). Whites have lower gambling rates than marginalized and aboriginal groups in the USA, New Zealand & Australia (Barnes et al., 2017; Ministry of Health, 2009). Blacks and NA/AI populations have twice the rate of disordered gambling of other US groups (Luczak et al., 2017).	Legality affects gambling rates (Kwak et al., 2004). Brazilian gamblers differ from US gamblers in age and marital status (Medeiros et al., 2015b).	Men in Brazil and USA prefer table games, women preferred EGM (Medeiros et al., 2016).	-
Internet	Addiction first identified in 1996 (Griffiths, 1996; Young, 1996, 2017).	-	Poor self-concept leads to internet addiction in the US but not in the UAE (Quinones & Kakabadse, 2015).	Males more likely to exhibit internet addiction in Turkey; no gender differences in Poland and the Ukraine (Blachnio et al., 2016).	-
Substances	Use by soldiers during wartime linked with subsequent increase in use in general community in USA (American Cancer Society, 2017; Russon et al., 2011; Shrem & Halkitis, 2008).	In USA, highest substance use by multiracial groups, and American Indians (Jamal et al., 2016; Luczak et al., 2017). Differences in substance use by ethnic groups within racial categories (Caetano et al., 1998; Luczak et al., 2017).	-	Asian women use tobacco at lower rates than males in the USA (Maxwell et al., 2012).	High rates of meth use among MSM (Halkitis et al., 2001).
Exercise	Development of the "thin ideal" of the 1960s, leading to a more toned ideal after 2000 (Thompson et al., 2004).	In the USA, Asians have higher rate of body dissatisfaction, but no difference in compulsive exercising compared to others (Kelly et al., 2015).	Differences in compulsive exercise scale based on country of residence for Turkish males and females living in Europe (Yildiz et al., 2017).	Males have higher rates of compulsive exercise than females (Guidi et al., 2009).	-

Table 13.1 (*cont.*)

	History of the disorder	Ethnic comparisons	National comparisons	Gender comparisons	Sexual identity comparisons
Food	See above.	No difference in binge eating by race/ethnicity in US male college students (Kelly et al., 2015). Whites higher rates of binge eating than Blacks among US women 45–64 (Flint et al., 2014).	–	No difference in food addiction rates by gender (Sanlier et al., 2017).	More food addiction and symptoms in LGB individuals, unless controlling for age and BMI (Rainey et al., 2018).
Sex	Reaction to the free love movement of the 1960s and 1970s, arose with increase in labeling of addictions in the 1980s (Irvine, 1995).	–	–	–	–
Love	–	–	–	–	–

Krych, 1987). Two years later, Faber and O'Guinn (1989) had modified their definition to just two criteria: repetitive purchasing behavior that an individual is powerless to stop and that the individual considers problematic. The condition was listed in the DSM-IV as a "culture-bound disorder" (Babbar, 2007; Black, 2007) but removed from the DSM-5 due to a lack of evidence that compulsive buying fits the characteristics of addiction (Piquet-Pessôa et al., 2014).

No articles were found examining the history of shopping addiction (as separate from the history of the diagnosis). This may be related to a lack of study in this area, as the field of shopping addiction is still nascent. It may also be due to a lack of concern that shopping is a maladaptive behavior given its prevalence in society.

Ethnic Comparisons

To date, there exist no studies examining ethnic differences among those with shopping addiction. One may speculate that this sort of addiction exists across ethnic groups, given that there exist disposable income and available objects to purchase.

Cross-National Comparisons

Compulsive buying is impossible without certain culturally based elements. These include a market driven economy, a range of goods available for purchase, sufficient disposable income, and leisure time (Black, 2007). In other words, compulsive buying is most prevalent among individuals in wealthier countries or among wealthier individuals in developing countries.

There have been few cross-national studies of compulsive buying. One study found no difference in predictors of compulsive buying and the comorbidity of compulsive buying and other compulsive behaviors between samples in South Korea and the United States (Kwak, Zinkhan & Roushanzamir, 2004). A meta-analysis of factors predicting compulsive buying across studies from sixteen countries found no differences in rates of compulsive buying across cultures (Maraz et al., 2016).

Gender Comparisons

Several studies have suggested that women are more likely to be compulsive shoppers than are men. Gendered differences in compulsive shopping may depend on the measures used, as some studies have found evidence for similar rates of compulsive shopping among males and females (Koran et al., 2006) while others have found overwhelmingly more women reporting compulsive shopping (Dittmar, 2004). If it exists, the relationship may be due to it being more socially acceptable for women to shop, while men are more likely to "collect" (Black, 2007). In a study examining the interaction of age and gender, younger females were more at risk of compulsive buying than other groups (Maraz et al., 2016). Differences in age may be developmental or may be generational, and thus due to culture. Youth and beauty are valued in many cultures, which may lead young women to buy compulsively to enhance people's perception of their value in society.

Sexual Identity Comparisons

To date, no studies have examined whether shopping addiction differs by sexual identity. One may speculate that differences, should they exist, are complex and difficult to understand, as with other cultural variables pertaining to shopping addiction.

Work Addiction

Historical Context

Work addiction, or workaholism, has been a concept in culture since its first use in 1971 (Oates, 1971). The term is a portmanteau of work and alcoholism, pointing to the parallels between work addiction and alcohol addiction. Though definitions vary, the two defining characteristics of work addiction are: (1) a compulsion to work and (2) willingness to prolong work at the expense of other commitments and enjoyment of work (Aziz et al., 2010; Baruch, 2011). As the culture of the United States values work and technology increasingly allows work to encroach into nonwork hours, an identity as a workaholic may not be much of a stigma and may be seen by some as a positive characteristic, or at least more equivalent to chocoholism than alcoholism (Baruch, 2011).

Though the concept of workaholism is fairly recent, working long hours at a job is not a new phenomenon. In the USA, weekly working hours peaked in 1830 around seventy hours per week (US Department of the Interior, 1883; Whaples, 2001); a combination of mechanization and labor rights movements stimulated a decline in work hours through the remainder of the ninteenth and into the twentieth century (Brody, 1989; Golden, 2009; Whaples, 2001). The Great Depression brought fewer work days and shorter shifts (Hunnicutt, 1988), leading to the passing of the Fair Labor Standards Act in 1938, which established the standard forty-hour workweek with overtime at a rate of "time-and-a-half" for overtime hours. The workweek length remained relatively stable until the 1970s. Since then, workers in white collar jobs, sales, and transportation workers have been working longer hours, on average (e.g., Golden, 2009). US workers spend more hours at work than do workers in many Western European countries (Altonji & Oldham, 2003; Alesina et al., 2005; Ueberfeldt, 2006).

Ethnic Comparisons

While there are some differences across groups, cross-cultural studies indicate that the primary components of workaholism are present across racial and ethnic groups. There is no difference in work addiction between black and white workers in the southeast USA, though there are differences based on job type; i.e., middle managers had higher work addiction scores than did nonmanagers (Aziz et al., 2010).

Cross-National Comparisons

A study of Turkish professors found that antecedents of workaholic behavior were similar to those found in similar studies in Western countries. However, work enjoyment was the greatest predictor of psychological well-being for the Turkish sample, differing from other studies which found drive to work predicting psychological well-being in Western samples (Burke, Koyoncu & Fiksenbaum, 2008).

In East Asian cultures like those of China, Japan, and Korea, working excessive hours and other workaholic tendencies are the norm, to the extent that there is a term in Japanese, "karoshi," for death from overwork. Kang, Matusik and Barclay (2017) suggest that these intense work environments arise from modern interpretations of Confucian cultural ideas, as Confucianism is a dominant background culture in these countries (just as Judeo-Christian cultural ideas have permeated culture in the United States and Western Europe). For example, Confucianism emphasizes personal effort and responsibility, along with forgiveness for failure. In modern society, competition for resources in Confucian cultures has led to an increasing emphasis on personal effort, leading to workaholic tendencies (Stankov, 2010). Further, Confucian culture values harmony and coherence in one's personal settings, such as family and work environments. Therefore, workers entrenched in Confucian thought may accept overtime work as a way to benefit their coworkers (Kang et al., 2017).

Gender Comparisons

Several studies have examined the role of gender in workaholism. Burke (1999) did not find a difference of the prevalence of workaholics by gender, despite males being older, more educated, making more money, and being in their jobs longer. However, Burke (1999) did find a difference in the expression of workaholism by gender, where females are more likely than men to experience perfectionism and work stress. A study of Brazilian managers found that males were more than females likely to put energy into work over relationships (Romeo et al., 2014), providing support to the idea that there is a difference in gender expression of work addiction but not in prevalence.

Sexual Identity Comparisons

No studies to date have indicated a difference in work addiction based on sexual identity. We speculate that there is no plausible reason for such variation to exist.

Gambling

Historical Context

The practice and methods of gambling are historically tied to certain cultures (Parhami et al, 2012; Raylu & Oei 2004) and forbidden in others (for example, Muslim societies; Parhami et al., 2012). For example, Persia is the birthplace of backgammon and poker, which are still popular among present-day Persians, as are other die and board games (Parhami et al., 2012). This is despite waxing and waning legality, depending on the regime's adherence to Islamic values (Parhami et al., 2012). Parhami and colleagues (2012) recorded a prevalence of problem gambling (PG) among Persian-Americans at 7 percent, considerably higher than the 1.2 percent PG rate of the general population.

Ethnic Comparisons

In the USA, problem gambling rates are higher among black, Asian American, and Native American groups than they are among whites (Barnes, Welte & Tidwell, 2017; Luczak et al., 2017). In general, studies of New Zealand and Australia (Ministry of Health, 2009) mirror these results: whites have lower rates of gambling than other ethnic groups, and aboriginal groups have twice the PG rates of whites in each country. Several factors may account for this disparity, such as lower socioeconomic status (Raylu & Oei, 2004), leading to gambling out of desperation to make money or out of a lack of understanding of the statistical odds stacked against them, coping with discrimination and other stressors, and genetics. Aside from noncultural factors, magical thinking (belief in luck or fate) is more common in American Indian cultures and may contribute to the higher problem gambling (PG) rates (Raylu & Oei, 2004). In this case, one would expect that other cultures that engage in magical thinking would also demonstrate increased rates of gambling.

National Comparisons

Culture affects gambling rates via several factors. A culturally imposed family structure may also perpetuate gambling, as children are likely to emulate a gambling patriarch, especially if the society is highly patrilineal, such as in China, where gambling has historically been prevalent (Raylu & Oei, 2004). The legality of gambling within a country also affects gambling rates (Kwak et al., 2004). Cameroon and Senegal legalized lotteries in the 1990s as a way of increasing revenue, despite majority Muslim populations (Brenner, Lipeb & Servet, 1996; Raylu & Oei, 2004).

A team of researchers has studied cross-cultural differences between problem gamblers in the USA and Brazil (Medeiros et al., 2015a, 2015b, 2016). Brazilian gamblers with PG are more likely to be married, start gambling and develop symptoms of PG at an older age, and express less of an urge to gamble than do US problem gamblers (Medeiros et al., 2015b). The older age of onset and progression to PG may be due to the more enduring legality (and therefore access) to gambling in the USA; most onset for the Brazilian sample occurred between 1993 and 2004, when bingo venues were legal in Brazil (Medeiros et al., 2015b).

Gender Comparisons

The study discussed above also examined gender difference in gambling disorder expression. Type of game preferred differed by gender, but not by country; men preferred table games (such as poker and craps) while women preferred electronic gaming machines, which are potentially a more addictive means of gambling (Medeiros et al., 2016). Aside from cultural norms of casino gambling as a man's providence, one possible explanation for this is that electronic gaming machines and other solitary gambling activities like bingo is a less immersive experience, allowing women to chat with others nearby. On the other hand, men may be more attracted to casino games with direct competition (like poker) due to the effects of higher testosterone levels, which affect tendencies for both competition and riskier financial decisions (Stenstrom & Saad, 2011).

Sexual Identity Comparisons

To date, no studies have examined the role of sexual identity on gambling addiction. It is possible that prevalence of gambling addiction, along with alcohol, tobacco and other substance abuse (ATOD), is relatively high among LGBT populations (e.g., REFS), as there is some cooccurrence of gambling with ATOD. However, there is a need for research on this topic.

Internet Addiction

Historical Context

Accounts of excessive internet use first appeared in the 1990s, almost as early as the advent of the internet itself. However, it was not until 1996 that the phenomenon was first mentioned in scholarly literature (Griffiths, 1996; Young, 1996, 2017). Definitions of internet addiction vary. Initially, Young (1996) divided internet addiction into five types: cybersexual addiction, cyberrelational addiction, net compulsion, information overload and computer addiction. Tao and colleagues (2010) proposed a "2+1" criteria for internet addiction disorder (IAD): subjects must show symptoms of preoccupation and withdrawal along with one of five other possible symptoms, along with criteria involving duration of the disorder and interruption of daily life. The DSM-5 lists internet gaming as a "Condition for Further Study," but not internet use in general (APA, 2013; Block, 2008). This condition does not include internet gambling, which is considered a part of the criteria for Gambling Disorder.

Controversies remain regarding the nature and classification of IAD. While definitions of IAD allow us to identify those suffering from the condition, it is unclear what aspect of internet use is proving addictive. Critics state that the internet is merely a means of communication, and those who are "addicted" to the internet are actually addicted to their internet activities of gambling, watching pornography, shopping, or other potentially "problem" behaviors (Chakraborty, Basu & Kumar, 2010). In terms of classification, IAD is comorbid with anxiety and depression (Ha et al., 2006), leading some to propose it is not an addiction after all (Chakraborty et al., 2010). Bax (2016) maintains that IAD may have many of the same effects as other addictions but its etiology is different, stemming from a need for acceptance and self-expression that often occurs after a childhood with rejection, high levels of stress, or physical and/or mental trauma. Naydanova and Beal (2016) categorized excessive internet use as either a harmonious (beneficial) or obsessive (addictive) internet passion; they found that harmonious passion (i.e., intrinsic enjoyment of internet use) was associated with higher self-worth, while obsessive passion (i.e., using the internet to gain approval of others via postings) was negatively associated with self-worth.

Ethnic Comparisons

No studies to date have examined ethnic differences of internet addiction within a country. There are differences in ethnicity by country, which are presented below.

Cross-National Comparisons

Culture plays a role in a society's perception of the utility of the internet as well as in proclivity to excessive internet use. Studies comparing British and Chinese students indicate that the British students see the internet as an educational tool while the Chinese students use the internet to express individuality (Li & Kirkup, 2007). A subsequent study of Facebook addiction in these three countries revealed that emotional stability and conscientiousness were negatively associated with Facebook addiction in all three countries, though the relationship of other personality characteristics (such as extraversion, openness, and agreeableness) to IAD varied by country (Blachnio et al., 2017). A comparative study of residents in the USA and the United Arab Emirates (UAE) revealed that a poor concept of self-concept combined with low social support leads to compulsive internet use in the USA but not in the UAE (Quinones & Kakabadse, 2015). A study of high-school students in the USA and Russia yielded similar relationships between excessive internet use and self-worth for participants from the two countries (Naydanova & Beal, 2016). This may be related to the high individualistic nature of the USA compared to the greater collectivist nature of the UAE and Russia (Hofstede Insights, n.d.). The collectivist culture may provide a buffer against the negative impacts of negative feelings about oneself, protecting against excessive internet use.

Internet addiction disorder (IAD) and related disorders are a growing concern among certain countries due to ease of internet access and the young age of onset (King et al., 2017). Approaches for counteracting excessive internet use vary by culture, with East Asian cultures favoring school-based prevention and technological tools for reducing internet use (e.g., software that blocks certain websites or limits time spent online), while researchers in Western countries such as the United States, Spain, and Germany suggest milder approaches such as workshops and online education (King et al., 2017). For example, South Korea, Japan, and China have taken a top-down approach to combating excessive internet use via policy change; charging multiple government ministries with addressing the problem (King et al., 2017) and providing a direct pathway for incorporating prevention efforts in public schools via policy. This is despite evidence that the prevalence of IAD may be lower than thought, with a rate of 2.7 percent among South Korean students (Seok & DaCosta, 2012). Meanwhile, the USA, UK, and Australia do not recognize IAD or Gaming Disorder officially, addressing these as hazards to health due to the sedentary behaviors of many with excessive internet use (King et al., 2017). Perhaps the collectivist nature of Eastern countries leads them to view excessive internet use as a removal from general society and thus a threat, while more individualistic Western societies do not have this concern about their citizens.

Gender Comparisons

In Turkey males are more likely to indicate IAD, while there is no gender difference present in Poland and the Ukraine (Blachnio et al., 2016). No other studies have yielded gender comparisons in IAD.

Sexual Identity Comparisons

No known studies have examined sexual identity as a factor in IAD. We believe there is no reason to assume differences.

Substance Addiction

Historical Context

The history of substance addiction goes as far back as there have been psychotropic substances to ingest. The first recorded instance of problematic substance use is in the *Odyssey*, where Odysseus recounts when his crew meets the lotus-eaters, who offered the lotus fruit to his men. Upon eating the fruit, the men forgot about home and did not wish to leave, but only wanted to eat more of the fruit (Homer, 1919).

Among licit substances (such as alcohol and tobacco), marketing and use are linked to culture in the form of advertisements, depiction in popular media, and related health messages. Use during wartime, whether sanctioned by the military or not, is also a factor affecting a substance's acceptance by the culture. Tobacco has been integral to US culture, as a commodity in the colonies (Virginia, in particular) in exchange for European luxury goods, and in the Revolutionary War, when its sale funded the war effort. The US War Department, who bought all Bull Durham tobacco to ship to soldiers overseas, facilitated tobacco use by soldiers in World War I. As a result, almost all World War I veterans were addicted to cigarettes (nicotine). By World War II, cigarettes were included in soldiers' rations (Russo et al., 2011). This adoption of tobacco use by several generations of veterans, along with pervasive cigarette advertising on TV, radio, film and in print, led to widespread tobacco use, nicotine addiction, and an unprecedented increase in lung cancer in the second half of the twentieth century (American Cancer Society, 2017). The military gave methamphetamine to soldiers during several conflicts, including World War II, the Korean War, and the Vietnam War to increase wakefulness and efficiency. The first illicit production of the drug began in the 1950s by motorcycle gangs, many of whom were veterans (Shrem & Halkitis, 2008). There have been three periods of increased amphetamine use in US culture, each of which can be tied to a US foreign conflict: post World War II, late 1960s to early 1970s (Vietnam war), and mid 1990s (Gulf War; Shrem & Halkitis, 2008).

Ethnic Comparisons

Surveillance studies of substance use have demonstrated differences in use by race/ethnicity. In general, rates for multiracial groups, American Indians, and whites are high (depending on the substance) and Asians are lowest in substance use across the board (Jamal et al., 2016; Luczak et al., 2017; Center for Behavioral Health Statistics and Quality, 2017). Cultural differences also exist by race/ethnicity within the greater US culture, as black smokers are less likely to smoke with friends than are white smokers (Finkenauer et al., 2009), which may lead to greater tobacco use and addiction among white smokers. The tobacco industry also has targeted specific racial/ethnic groups in an attempt to increase their tobacco use. For example, the tobacco industry has a long history of marketing menthol cigarettes to black Americans; to the point where menthol cigarettes have actually become associated with black culture (Gardiner, 2004).

However, substance use literature reminds us that the monolithic labels we use to describe race/ethnicity groups (black, Asian, Hispanic/Latino, etc.) often mask more specific cultural differences (Luczak et al., 2017). For example, Cuban Americans have lower rates of alcohol consumption than other Hispanic/Latino ethnic groups; Chinese and Japanese adults in are Los Angeles more likely to drink than are Filipino or Korean adults (Alegria et al., 2007; Caetano, Clark & Tam, 1998). Acculturation affects substance use rates as well; as people immigrate and adapt to a new dominant culture their substance abuse risk trends toward that of the new culture (Martinez et al., 2016). For example, foreign-born Latinos show lower rates of substance use disorders than to those born in the United States (Alegria et al., 2007).

Cross-National Comparisons

The extent to which a culture is individualist or collectivist will affect whether substance use occurs alone or with others (Lv et al., 2016). Eckersley (2005) proposes that the materialism and individualism of Western culture leads to high rates of substance use: materialism is fueled by a dissatisfaction with oneself, which can be resolved by consuming more products, including drugs; individualism leads to a feeling of isolation from others, leading to consumption of substances that lower defenses and promote feelings of unity. There are also cultural differences in neurological responses to substance cues among addicts (Lv et al., 2016).

Gender Comparisons

While few studies examine differences in addiction, evidence does indicate greater illicit drug use among males than among females in the USA (Center for Behavioral Health Statistics and Quality, 2017). There are gender differences in tobacco use among several Asian cultures, with higher smoking prevalence among Korean, Vietnamese, and Filipino men, lower prevalence among Chinese men, and very low prevalence among women of most Asian subgroups (Maxwell et al., 2012).

Sexual Identity Comparisons

There still remains a lack of understanding about whether substance addiction varies as a result of sexual identity, though there does appear to be a relatively high prevalence of ATOD misuse among LGBT populations. Methamphetamine use has been high in prevalence among men who have sex with men (MSM) since at least the mid 1990s (Halkitis et al., 2001). These men state that they use methampetamines for a variety of reasons, including increasing sexual desire as well as a means of coping with the stress of a positive HIV status or of social pressure, and as a means of avoiding conflict (Shrem & Halkitis, 2008). The use of methamphetamines among MSM goes hand-in-hand with high-risk sexual behavior, leading to increased rates of HIV and other sexually transmitted infections, as well as the problems associated with chronic methamphetamine use and dependence (Shrem & Halkitis, 2008).

Compulsive Exercising

Historical Context

Compulsive exercising is a persistent urge to exercise that interferes with daily life even when an injury or other condition indicates against it (Meyer et al., 2011). This behavior is seen often among bulimia patients, who engage in compulsive exercising as a compensatory (calorie-burning) behavior. Compulsive exercising among bulimia patients can lead to increased comorbidity of depression and increase the severity of the bulimia condition (Homan, 2010).

Since the 1960s the "thin ideal" has been a fixture in Western culture, leading to excessive dieting and exercise by those wishing to attain this ideal. Since 2000, the "thin ideal" has shifted from the heroin chic of the 1900s to a more toned and athletic appearance (as opposed to simply slender; Thompson et al., 2004). This "athletic ideal" has led to increased rates of compulsive exercising for those who endorse it, over those endorsing merely a thin ideal (Homan, 2010). Though research has yet to link excessive exercising to the "thin ideal," pressure from family, friends and media to attain this ideal has been linked to eating disorders (Goodwin, Heycroft & Meyer, 2011; Stice & Agras, 1998) and compulsive exercise leads to eating disorders (Meyer et al., 2011).

Ethnic Comparisons

There may be cultural differences in acceptance of the "thin ideal," as African-American men tend to prefer a larger body size than do whites; though data with other racial/ethnic groups is, as of yet, inconsistent (Ricciardelli et al., 2007). Future research will clarify whether differences in compulsive exercise and factors predicting compulsive exercise vary by race/ethnicity and nationality. A study of racial/ethnic differences among American male college students indicated that Asian males have more body image concerns than do white or black males; however, there was no difference in compulsive exercise rates between racial/ethnic groups (Kelly et al., 2015).

National Comparisons

Yildiz and colleagues (2017) studied Turkish nationals living in Turkey and in several countries throughout Europe (Germany, the Netherlands, Belgium, and Norway). Results indicated that there was a difference in compulsive exercise based on country of residence (Yildiz et al., 2017).

Gender Comparisons

Though females are considered "typical" eating disorder patients, there is also rising societal pressure for males to attain the toned, muscular ideal. In fact, college-age males exhibited higher rates of compulsive exercise than did females in at least one study (Guidi et al., 2009). A study of adolescents in the UK found that males are more likely to be influenced by significant others to become more muscular and both males and females were influenced by media messages of the "thin ideal" (Goodwin et al., 2011).

Sexual Identity Comparisons

There are no studies on exercise addiction and sexual minority status. We fail to conjecture why any such differences would exist.

Food Addiction

Historical Context

The field of food addiction is nascent, with many researchers still assessing whether food addiction is a valid construct (Ziauddeen & Fletcher, 2013). Food is necessary to sustain life, and it is difficult to draw clear boundaries between appropriate eating, excessive eating, and addictive eating. Studies examining culture and food addiction have focused on how an endorsement of food addiction affects other people's perceptions of the individual. For example, Latner and colleagues (2014) found that bias toward a fictional overweight woman was lower if the woman was described as having a food addiction. Other food addiction research hints at the role of identifying addictions in policy creation, as a study of US adults revealed that belief in food addiction as a valid construct resulted in increased support of obesity-related policies, regardless of political party affiliation (Schulte, Tuttle & Gearhardt, 2016).

Ethnic Comparisons

Most studies indicate no racial/ethnic differences in binge eating (Kelly et al., 2015), though Flint and colleagues (2014) did find that whites have higher rates of binge-eating disorder than blacks in a sample of forty-five- to sixty-four-year-old women. There is a relationship between compulsive exercise and binge eating (Kelly et al., 2015), suggesting that there might be one underlying condition (such as body image disorder) driving both behaviors, or that the two conditions are comorbid.

Cross-National Comparisons

No studies to date have examined differences in food addiction by country.

Gender Comparisons

Thus far, most studies have not found gender differences in food addiction (Sanlier et al., 2017).

Sexual Identity Comparisons

Rainey et al. (2018) found that lesbian, gay and bisexual (LGB) individuals reported more food addiction and a greater number of symptoms in univariate analyses. However, food addiction was no longer associated with LGB status when controlling for BMI and age.

Sexual Addiction

Historical Context

Much like with food addiction, sexual addiction research has been the subject of a debate about the validity of the construct. The definition of sexual addiction is also complicated by shifting ideas about appropriate sexual behavior and frequency, which vary across cultures and subcultural groups (e.g., LGBT communities) and shifting ideas of morality (Reay, Attwood & Gooder, 2013). Sexuality is inherently cultural in that naming of a sexually related concept alters that which is named by adding a moral context (Cryle 2009a, 2009b; Laquer, 2009) and also determines how society approaches it in terms of policy and treatment (Goodman, 2001). For example, in the instance of a legal infraction for sexual behavior, defining sexual compulsion as an impulse control problem provokes a more penalty-driven reaction than does defining it as an addiction (Goodman, 2001), which elicits more sympathy and calls for treatment.

The term sexual addiction first came into use in the 1970s and 1980s. Irvine (1995) asserts that this occurred as a reaction to the "free" sexuality of the 1960s and 1970s. The 1980s also saw a trend in labeling of compulsions as addictions in the 1980s, a combination of a need for a medical diagnosis to validate the need for treatment (and third party financial support for treatment), narratives of individuals' experiences with addiction, among other cultural influences, such as a fear of sexual behavior stemming from the HIV epidemic (Irvine, 1995).

The classification of sexual addiction has been contentious. Goodman (2001) has discussed the categorization of sexual compulsion as an addiction rather than an impulse disorder. He defines addiction as a failure to control a behavior and continuing the behavior despite negative consequences, which differs from impulse disorder in that addiction is motivated by a desire to relieve the anxiety or dysphoria of cravings while impulse disorder is related to a desire to experience certain arousing sensations (Goodman, 2001). He then proceeds to list similarities of sexual addiction to substance addiction, including the course and progression of the condition, personal descriptions for both of cravings and loss of control, and presence of tolerance, withdrawal, and relapse with both conditions (Goodman, 2001). Despite this intellectually thorough categorization, self-diagnosed patients did not show signs of addictive tendencies, obsessiveness or compulsion: hallmarks of those with compulsive behavioral disorders (Reay et al., 2013; Reid & Carpenter, 2009).

It would seem that sexual compulsive disorder, as proposed by Coleman (2003), might be a better term. Coleman (2003) defined compulsive sexual disorder as the presence of recurrent, intense sexual fantasies, urges, and behaviors that cause distress and affect daily functioning. However, the DSM specifies that compulsive behavior cannot be gratifying or pleasurable on its own merit, which would exclude intrusive sexual behavior from classification as a compulsion (Goodman, 2001). Further, sexual compulsions do not respond to antidepressants in a similar manner to OCD symptoms, providing neurological support (Goodman, 2001) for the argument that sex addiction is not a compulsion.

If not a clear addiction or compulsion, perhaps one should consider "out of control sexual behavior" (Bancroft & Vudakinovic, 2004) to explain the phenomenon under study. This term is very dependent on culture, as standards within the culture will determine what is considered out of control: is it behavior at the extreme edge of normal, or does it differ from normal behavior in some substantial, qualitative manner (Bancroft & Vudakinovic, 2004)? For example, there are different standards for what constitutes an appropriate frequency of sexual activity depending on whether relationships are homosexual or heterosexual (Wall, Stephenson & Sullivan, 2013). There are gender differences in what constitutes problematic sexual behavior as well; women indicating sexual behavior as "out of control" were more likely than other women to have ten or more sexual partners, concurrent relationships, less satisfaction with their current relationship, and to have sex with a partner met on the internet. Men with "out of control" behavior were more likely than other men to pay for sex (Skegg et al., 2010). Finally, many more people may experience what they consider to be "out of control" behavior than may consider it problematic. The majority of people in a cohort from Dunedin, New Zealand, indicated an incident of problematic sexual behavior did not negatively affect their lives (Skegg et al., 2010).

Given this lack of clarity in the scientific community regarding the nature of sexual addiction, it is unsurprising that the lay public is just as confused. Since most people labeled as sex addicts self-diagnosed (Reay et al., 2013), this is particularly problematic. A study of thirty-one self-identified sex addicts who attended Sex Addicts Anonymous (SAA) meetings or were sex addiction patients at a clinic yielded a variety of sexual behaviors, including exhibitionism, pedophilia and voyeurism. Some patients reported obsessive-compulsive disorder with a compulsive masturbation component. Two SAA participants did not report behavior that they couldn't control, but rather behaviors they'd like to do but society prohibited (Bancroft & Vudakinovic, 2004). In other words, their self-diagnosed behavior did not fit the criteria for the condition.

Ethnic, Cross-National, Gender, and Sexual Identity Comparisons

No studies to date have examined comparisons of sexual addiction by ethnicity, nationality, gender, or sexual identity. Such work is needed.

Love Addiction

Passionate love is a universal concept found in all cultures and throughout history. Modern culture is replete with love songs, romantic comedies, and romance novels depicting idealized (and often dysfunctional) stories of love. This intense, all-consuming love parallels an addiction to substances in terms of an intoxicating early period of infatuation with the loved one and feelings of irritability, sadness, and emptiness, similar to withdrawal, when the loved one is gone (Reynaud et al., 2010). Despite this, the field of love addiction is relatively new, and few studies have codified whether love addiction is actually addiction, let alone any cultural elements of love addiction. As for sex addiction, many love addicts are self-identified and attendees of one of the thousands of Sex and Love Addiction Anonymous meetings worldwide (Reynaud et al., 2010).

Ethnic, Cross-National, Gender, and Sexual Identity Comparisons

Given the early stage of this field of study, no studies to date have examined comparisons of love addiction by ethnicity, nationality, gender, or sexual identity. Research is needed.

Conclusions

Identifying and validating addictions is still underway for certain addictions, including food, love and sex addiction. Coleman (2003) distinguishes addictions as separate from behaviors that are developmentally appropriate (including both human and relationship development), not pathological, and not at conflict with one's values. These criteria, while useful for defining addiction as a concept, do not provide clarity about how to distinguish addiction. Values, particularly, vary from person to person. Who should determine if one's behaviors are against a set of values – the person engaging in the behavior, the person making the diagnosis, or the prevailing society? What happens as values shift?

It seems that there is a spectrum from biology to culture as a contributor to addiction: as more biological mechanisms are established, culture is less considered to be associated with that addiction (e.g., see Luczak et al., 2017). Labeling someone as an addict may generate more sympathy for that person than does labeling them a criminal, so the shifting field of addiction has the potential to impact how we address crime, punishment, and rehabilitation. The label of addiction can also be a way of avoiding responsibility, or may be perceived as such by the public, as in the case of Harvey Weinstein entering a facility for sex addiction rehabilitation after decades of sexual misconduct (Welch, 2017). However, identifying addiction can also increase public support of people with those addictions and of policies to combat these addictions, as described above in the case of food addiction.

Ultimately, addiction and culture are inexorably intertwined. The research for many addictions is in the early stages, and much remains to be learned about cultural predictors of addictions as well as cultural comparisons of addictions. Understanding the extent of their interaction and the degree to which culture affects addiction will be essential to the future of addiction studies, as well as to policy, public health, and criminology studies.

REFERENCES

Alegria, M., Mulvaney-Day, N., Torres, M., et al. (2007). Prevalence of psychiatric disorders across Latino subgroups in the United States. *American Journal of Public Health*, **97**, 68–75.

Alesina, A., Glaeser, E. & Sacerdote, B. (2005). Work and leisure in the US and Europe: Why so different? *NBER Maroeconomic Annual*, 20, 1-64.

Altonji, J. & Oldham, J. (2003). Vacation laws annual work hours. *Economic Perspectives: Federal Reserve Bank of Chicago*, Fall, 19–29.

American Cancer Society (2017). *Cancer Facts & Figures 2017.*

American Psychiatric Association (2013). *Diagnostic and Statistical Manual of Mental Disorders* (5th edition). Arlington, VA: American Psychiatric Publishing.

Aziz, S., Adkins, C. T., Walker, A. G. & Wuensch, K. L. (2010). Wokaholism and work-life imbalance: Does cultural origin influence the relationship? *International Journal of Psychology*, 45(1), 72–79.

Babbar, I. (2007). Correspondence: Compulsive buying – A culture-bound disorder? *International Journal of Social Psychiatry*, **53** (2), 189–190.

Bancroft, J. & Vukadinovic, Z. (2004). Sexual addiction, sexual compulsivity, sexual impulsivity, or what? Toward a theoretical model. *The Journal of Sex Research*, **41**(3), 225–234.

Barnes, G. M., Welte, J. W. & Tidwell, M. O. (2017). Gambling involvement among Native Americans, Blacks, and whites in the United States. *The American Journal on Addictions*, **26**, 713–721.

Baruch, Y. (2011). The positive wellbeing aspects of workaholism in cross cultural perspective: The chocoholism metaphor. *Career Development International*, 16(6), 572–591.

Bax, T. (2016). "Internet gaming disorder" in China: Biomedical sickness or sociological badness? *Games and Culture*, **11** (3), 233–255.

Blachnio, A., Przepiórka, A., Senol-Durak, E., Durak, M. & Sherstyuk, L. (2016). The role of self-esteem in Internet addiction: A comparison between Turkish, Polish and Ukrainian samples. *European Journal of Psychiatry*, **30**(2), 149–155.

Blachnio, A., Przepiórka, A., Senol-Durak, E., Durak, M. & Sherstyuk, L. (2017). The role of personality traits in Facebook and Internet addictions: A study on Polish, Turkish and Ukrainian samples. *Computers in Human Behavior*, **68**, 269–275.

Black, D. W. (2007). A review of compulsive buying disorder. *World Psychiatry*, **6**, 14–18.

Block, J. J. (2008). Issues for DSM-V: Internet addiction. *American Journal of Psychiatry*, **165** (3), 306–307.

Brenner, G. A., Lipeb, M. & Servet, J. (1996). Gambling in Cameroon and Senegal: A response to crisis? In J. McMillen (Ed.), *Gambling Cultures: Studies in History and Interpretation*. New York: Routledge, Taylor & Francis Group.

Brody, D. (1989). Time and work during early American industrialism. *Labor History*, **30**(1), 5–46.

Burke, R. J. (1999). Workaholism in organizations: Gender differences. *Sex Roles*, **41**(5/6), 335–345.

Burke, R. J., Koyuncu, M. & Fiksenbaum, L. (2008). Workaholism, work and extra-work satisfactions and psychological well-being among professors in Turkey. *Cross-cultural Management: An International Journal*, **15**(4), 353–366.

Caetano, R., Clark, C. L. & Tam, T. (1998). Alcohol consumption among racial/ethnic minorities: Theory and research. *Alcohol Health and Research World*, **22**(4), 233–241.

Center for Behavioral Health Statistics and Quality (2017). *Results from the 2016 National Survey on Drug Use and Health: Detailed Tables*. Rockville, MD: Substance Abuse and Mental Health Services Administration.

Chakraborty, K., Basu, D. & Kumar, V. (2010). Internet addiction: Consensus, controversies and the way ahead. *East Asian Archives of Psychiatry*, **20**, 123–132.

Coleman, E. (2003). Compulsive sexual behavior: What to call it, how to treat it? *SIECUS Report*, **31**(5), 12–16.

Cryle, P. (2009a). Interrogating the work of Thomas W. Laqueur. *Sexualities*, **12**(4), 411–417.

Cryle, P. (2009b). *Les Choses et les Mots*: Missing words and blurry things in the history of sexuality. *Sexualities*, **12**(4), 437–450.

Dittmar, H. (2004). Understanding and diagnosing compulsive buying. In R. H. Coombs (Ed.), *Handbook of Addictive Disorders*. Wiley, pp. 411–450.

Drescher, J. (2015). Queer diagnoses revisited: The past and future of homosexuality and gender diagnoses in DSM and ICD. *International Review of Psychiatry*, **27**(5), 386–395.

Eckersley, R. M. (2005). "Cultural fraud": The role of culture in drug abuse. *Drug and Alcohol Review*, **24**, 157–163.

Faber, R. J. & O'Guinn, T. C. (1989). Classifying compulsive consumers: Advances in the development of a diagnostic tool. *Advances in Consumer Research*, **16**, 738–744.

Faber, R .J., O'Guinn, T. C. & Krych, R. (1987). Compulsive consumption. *Advances in Consumer Research*, **14**, 132–135.

Finkenauer, R., Pomerleau, C. S., Snedecor, S. M. & Pomerleau, O. F. (2009). Race differences in factors relating to smoking initiation. *Addictive Behaviors*, **34**, 1056–1059.

Flint, A.J., Gearhardt, A. N., Corbin, W. R., et al. (2014). Food-addiction scale measurement in 2 cohorts of middle-aged and older women. *American Journal of Clinical Nutrition*, **99**, 578–586.

Gardiner, P. S. (2004). The African Americanization of menthol cigarette use in the United States. *Nicotine and Tobacco Research*, **6**(S1), S55–65.

Golden, L. (2009). A brief history of long work time and the contemporary sources of overwork. *Journal of Business Ethics*, **84**, 217–227.

Goodman, A. (2001). What's in a name? Terminology for designating a syndrome of driven sexual behavior. *Sexual Addiction & Compulsivity*, **8**, 191–213.

Goodwin, H., Haycraft, E. & Meyer, C. (2011). Sociocultural correlates of compulsive exercise: Is the environment important in fostering a compulsivity towards exercise among adolescents? *Body Image*, **8**, 390–395.

Griffiths, M. (1996). Gambling on the Internet: A brief note. *Journal of Gambling Studies*, **12** (4), 471–473.

Guidi, J., Pender, M., Hollon, S. D., et al. (2009). The prevalence of compulsive eating and exercise among college students: An exploratory study. *Psychiatry Research*, **165**, 154–162.

Ha, J. H., Yoo, H. J., Cho, I. H., et al. (2006). Psychiatric comorbidity assessed in Korean children and adolescents who screen positive for Internet addiction. *Journal of Clinical Psychiatry*, 67, 821–826.

Halkitis, P. N., Parsons, J. T. & Stirratt, M. J. (2001). A double epidemic: Crystal methamphetamine drug use in relation to HIV transmission among gay men. *Journal of Homosexuality*, **41**(2), 17–35.

Hofstede Insights (n.d.). *Country Comparison*. Retrieved from www.hofstede-insights.com/country-comparison/russia,the-united-arab-emirates,the-usa/.

Homer (1919). *The Odyssey with an English Translation* by A. T. Murray, in two volumes. Cambridge, MA:, Harvard University Press; London: William Heinemann, Ltd.

Homan, K. (2010). Athletic-ideal and thin-ideal internalization as prospective predictors of body dissatisfaction, dieting, and compulsive exercise. *Body Image*, **7**, 240–245.

Hunnicutt, B. (1988). *Work Without End: Abandoning Shorter Hours for the Right to Work*. Philadelphia: Temple University Press.

Irvine, J. M. (1995). Reinventing perversion: Sex addiction and cultural anxieties. *Journal of the History of Sexuality*, **5**(3), 429–450.

Jamal, A., King, B. A., Neff, L. J., et al. (2016). Current cigarette smoking among adults – United States, 2005–2015. *Morbidity and Mortality Weekly Report*, **65**(44), 1205–1211.

Kang, J. H., Matusik, J. G. & Barclay, L. A. (2017). Affective and normative motives to work overtime in Asian organizations: Four cultural orientations from Confucian ethics. *Journal of Business Ethics*, 140, 115–130.

Kelly, N. R., Cotter, E. W., Tanofsky-Kraff, M. & Mazzeo, S. E. (2015). Racial variations in binge eating, body image concerns, and compulsive exercise among men. *Psychology of Men & Masculinity*, **16**(3), 326–336.

King, D. L., Delfabbro, P. H., Doh, Y. Y., et al. (2017). Policy and prevention approaches for disordered and hazardous gaming and Internet use: An international perspective. *Prevention Science*, **19**(2), 233–249.

Koran, L. M., Faber, R. J., Aboujaoude, E., Large, M. D. & Serpe, R. T. (2006). Estimated prevalence of compulsive buying behavior in the United States. *American Journal of Psychiatry*, 163, 1806–1812.

Kwak, H., Zinkhan, G. M. & Roushanzamir, E. P. (2004). Compulsive comorbidity and its psychological antecedents: A cross-cultural comparison between the US and South Korea. *The Journal of Consumer Marketing*, **21**(6), 418–434.

Laqueur, T. W. (2009). Sexuality and the transformation of culture: The *Longue Durée*. *Sexualities*, **12**(4), 418–436.

Latner, J. D., Puhl, R. M., Murakami, J. M. & O'Brien, K. S. (2014). Food addiction as a causal model of obesity. Effects on stigma, blame, and perceived psychopathology. *Appetite*, **77C**, 77–82.

Li, N. & Kirkup, G. (2007). Gender and cultural differences in Internet use: A study of China and the UK. *Computers & Education*, **48**, 301–317.

Lv, W., Wu, Q., Liu, X., et al. (2016). Cue reactivity in nicotine and alcohol addiction: A cross-cultural view. *Frontiers in Psychology*, **7**, e1–e7.

Luczak, S. E., Khoddam, R., Yu, S., et al. (2017). Prevalence and co-occurrence of addictions in U.S. ethnic/racial groups. Implications for genetic research. *The American Journal on Addictions*, **26**, 424–436.

Maraz, A., Griffiths, M. D. & Demetrovics, Z. (2016). The prevalence of compulsive buying: A meta-analysis. *Addiction*, **111**, 408–419.

Martinez, M. J., Huang, S., Estrada, Y., Sutton, M. Y. & Prado, G. (2016). The relationship between acculturation, ecodevelopment, and substance use among Hispanic adolescents. *Journal of Early Adolescence*, **37**(7), 948–974.

Maxwell, A. E., Crespi, C. M., Alano, R. E., Sudan, M. & Bastani, R. (2012). Health risk behaviors among five Asian American subgroups in California: Identifying intervention priorities. *Journal of Immigrant and Minority Health*, **14**, 890–894.

McCrory, E. J. & Mayes, L. (2015). Understanding addiction as a developmental disorder: An argument for a developmentally informed multilevel approach. *Current Addiction Reports*, **2**, 326–330.

Medeiros, G. C., Leppink, E. W., Redden, S. A., et al. (2016). A cross-cultural study of gambling disorder: A comparison between women from Brazil and the United States. *Revista Brasileira de Psiquiatria*, **38**, 53–57.

Medeiros, G. C., Leppink, E. W., Yaemi, A., et al. (2015a). Electronic gaming machines and gambling disorder: A cross-cultural comparison between treatment-seeking subjects from Brazil and the United States. *Psychiatry Research*, **230**(2), 430–435.

Medeiros, G. C., Leppink, E., Yaemi, A., et al. (2015b). Gambling disorder in older adults: A cross-cultural perspective. *Comprehensive Psychiatry*, **58**, 116–121.

Meyer, C., Taranis, L., Goodwin, H. & Haycraft, E. (2011). *European Eating Disorders Review*, **19**, 174–189.

Ministry of Health (2009). *A Focus on Problem Gambling: Results of the 2006/07 New Zealand Health Survey*. Wellington: Ministry of Health.

Naydanova, E. & Beal, B. D. (2016). Harmonious and obsessive Internet passion, competence, and self-worth: A study of high school students in the United States and Russia. *Computers in Human Behavior*, **64**, 88–93.

Oates, W. (1971). *Confessions of a Workaholic: The Facts about Work Addiction*. New York: World.

Parhami, I., Siani, A., Campos, M.D., et al. & **UCLA Gambling Studies Program** (2012). Gambling in the Iranian-American community and an assessment of motives: A case study. *International Journal of Mental Health and Addiction*, **10**, 710–721.

Piquet-Pessôa, M., Ferreira, G. M., Melca, I. A. & Fontenelle, L. F. (2014). DSM-5 and the decision not to include sex, shopping or stealing as addictions. *Current Addiction Reports*, **1**, 172–176.

Quinones, C. & Kakabadse, N. K. (2015). Self-concept clarity, social support, and compulsive Internet use: A study of the US and the UAE. *Computers in Human Behavior*, **44**, 347–356.

Rainey, J. C., Furman, C. R. & Gearhardt, A. N. (2018). Food addiction among sexual minorities. *Appetite*, **120**, 16–22.

Raylu, N. & Oei, T. P. (2004). Role of culture in gambling and problem gambling. *Clinical Psychology Review*, **23**, 1087–1114.

Reay, B., Attwood, N. & Gooder, C. (2013). Inventing sex: The short history of sex addiction. *Sexuality and Culture*, **17**, 1–19.

Reid, R. C. & Carpenter, B. N. (2009). Exploring relationships of psychopathology in hypersexual patients using the MMPI-2. *Journal of Sex & Marital Therapy*, **35**, 294–310.

Reynaud, M., Karila, L., Blecha, L. & Benyamina, A. (2010). Is love passion an addictive disorder? *The American Journal of Drug and Alcohol Abuse*, 36, 261–267.

Ricciardelli, L. A., McCabe, M. P., Williams, R. J. & Thompson, J. K. (2007). The role of ethnicity and culture in body image and disordered eating among males. *Clinical Psychology Review*, **27**, 582–606.

Romeo, M., Yepes-Baldó, M., Berger, R. & Da Costa, F. F. (2014). Workaholism in Brazil: Measurement and individual differences. *Addiccionese*, **26**(4), 312–320.

Russo, P., Nastrucci, C., Alzetta, G. & Szalai, C. (2011). Tobacco habit: Historical, cultural, neurobiological, and genetic features of people's relationship with an addictive drug. *Perspectives in Biology and Medicine*, **54**(4), 557–577.

Sanlier, N., Varli, S. N., Macit, M. S., Mortas, H. & Tatar, T. (2017). Evaluation of disordered eating tendencies in young adults. *Eating and Weight Disorders*, **22**, 623–631.

Schulte, E. M., Tuttle, H. M. & Gearhardt, A. N. (2016). Belief in food addiction and obesity-related policy support. *PLoS ONE*, **11** (1), e0147557.

Seok, S. & DaCosta, B. (2012). The world's most intense online gaming culture: Addiction and high-engagement prevalence rates among South Korean adolescents and young adults. *Computers in Human Behavior*, **22**(6), 2143–3151.

Shrem, M. T. & Halkitis, P. N. (2008). Methamphetaine abuse in the United States: Contextual, psychological and sociological considerations. *Journal of Health Psychology*, **13**(5), 669–679.

Skegg, K., Nada-Raja, S., Dickson, N. & Paul, C. (2010). Perceived "out of control" sexual behavior in a cohort of young adults from the Dunedin Multidisciplinary Health and Development Study. *Archives of Sex Behavior*, **39**, 968–978.

Spiegel, A. (2002, January 18). 81 words. *This American Life*. Radio episode retrieved from www.thisamericanlife.org/204/81-words

Stankov, L. (2010). Unforgiving Confucian culture: A breeding ground for high academic achievement, test anxiety and self-doubt? *Learning and Individual Differences*, 20, 555–563.

Stenstrom, E. & Saad, G. (2011). Testosterone, financial risk-taking, and pathological gambling. *Journal of Neuroscience, Psychology, and Economics*, **4**(4), 254–266.

Stice, E. & Agras, W. S. (1998). Predicting onset and cessation of bulimic behaviors during adolescence: A longitudinal grouping analysis. *Behavior Analysis*, **29**, 257–276.

Sussman, S. & Sussman, A. N. (2011). Considering the definition of addiction. *International Journal of Environmental Research and Public Health*, **8**, 4025–4038.

Tao, R., Huang, X., Wang, J., et al. (2010). Proposed diagnostic criteria for internet addiction. *Addiction*, **105**, 556–564.

Thompson, J. K., van den Berg, P., Roehrig, M., Guarda, A. S. & Heinberg, L. J. (2004). The sociocultural attitudes towards appearance scale-3 (SATAQ-3): Development and validation. *International Journal of Eating Disorders*, **35**, 293–304.

Ueberfeldt, A. (2006). *Working time over the 20th century*. Bank of Canada Working Paper, 2006–2018.

United States, Department of Interior, Census Office (1883). *Report on the Statistics of Wages in Manufacturing Industries*, by Joseph Weeks, 1880 Census, Vol. 20. Washington: GPO.

US Mortality Volumes 1930 to 1959 and US Mortality Data 1960 to 2014, National Center for Health Statistics, Centers for Disease Control and Prevention. (OR Cancer Facts and Figures 2017, American Cancer Society)

Wall, K. M., Stephenson, R. & Sullivan, T. S. (2013). Frequency of sexual activity of most recent male partner among young, Internet-using men who have sex with men in the United States. *Journal of Homosexuality*, **60** (10), 1520–1538.

Welch, A. (2017). The problem with Harvey Weinstein's sex addiction claim. CBS News, November 6, 2017. Retrieved January 17, 2018 from www.cbsnews.com/news/sex-addiction-claims-harvey-weinstein-kevin-spacey/.

Whaples, R. (2001). Hours of work in US history. EH.Net Encyclopedia, April 14, 2001. Retrieved June 6, 2018 from http://eh.net/encyclopedia/hours-of-work-in-u-s-history/.

Wilkerson, M. (2015). America's five most socially acceptable addictions. Substance.com, January 14, 2015. Retrieved February 1, 2018 from www.substance.com/americas-five-most-socially-acceptable-addictions/18305/.

Yildiz, M., Bingöl, E., Şahan, H., Bayköse, N. & Şenel, E. (2017). A cross-cultural approach to sport psychology: Is exercise addiction a determinant of life quality? *Sport Journal*, **1**, 1–10.

Young, K. S. (1996). Internet addiction: The emergence of a new clinical disorder. *CyberPsychology & Behavior*, **1**(3), 237–244.

Young, K. S. (2017). The evolution of Internet addiction. *Addictive Behaviors*, **64**, 229–230.

Ziauddeen, H. & Fletcher, P. C. (2013). Is food addiction a valid and useful concept? *Obesity Reviews*, **14**, 19–28.

14 The Physical and Social Environments as Determinants of Health: Implications for Substance and Behavioral Addictions

Robert W. Strack, PhD, MBA, Muhsin Michael Orsini, EdD,
D. Rose Ewald, MPH, and Lawrence M. Scheier, PhD

Introduction

Organization of the spaces in which people live, work, and play affects the way they function and thrive. This can be as trivial as having a neatly arranged bedroom or living room, or it can extend to include the office workspace, mass transit used to access work, and the local parks where one may enjoy recreation and health maintenance. All of these "structural" factors impinge on one's daily routine and can influence health. Operationally speaking, urban planners and public health advocates label these physical and spatial features as the *built environment* (BE). One only has to consider neighborhoods characterized by vacant dilapidated buildings, unkempt parks, dense residential spaces cluttered with litter, and poorly maintained bicycle paths or running trails to appreciate how this must influence the residents' health and well-being. Add to the equation transportation deficiencies for commuting to work and a limited mix of employment options, and the impact of environmental constraints is even more pronounced (Braveman & Egerter, 2013; Federal Reserve System & Brookings Institution, 2008; Sharkey, 2013).

Contextual factors that influence human behaviors encompass the *physical environment* (e.g., natural and built environments), the *social environment* (e.g., social support, norms, beliefs and attitudes), as well as the potential nuances of objective (actual) versus subjective (perceived) environments (Glanz & Kegler, 2008; Sallis, Owen & Fisher, 2008). Put quite simply, behavior is not solely the product of a rational motivated actor, operating independently from his or her environment; rather, it is also a function of edifices, neighborhoods, and public spaces, as well as the inhabitants, community norms, and the social capital they generate. As discussed by Hoffman and Unger in Chapter 13 on the role of culture in addiction, this perspective suggests that the environment is persuasive, and can control, manage, and shape behavior and well-being in its own right.

Society's inclination for "health individualism" results in an overemphasis on solutions that expect individuals to moderate their own behaviors (Goldberg, 2012; Higgs et al., 2009; Hughes, 2007; Ulijaszek & McLennan, 2016). This approach fails fully to appreciate the profound influence that shifts in the social and ecological environments have had on collective health, inclusive of a broad array of addictions. Complex problem behaviors that lead to addiction and dependence often defy amelioration or prevention and have no single solution. As discussed in this chapter, addictive behaviors have as much to do with the environmental contexts surrounding individuals as with their unique biological factors, specific brain mechanisms, and psychogenic causes. Any attempt to address addiction at either individual or population levels would benefit from careful consideration of the social and contextual influences surrounding addictions. Interventions informed by this understanding are more likely to be efficacious than those solely targeted toward individual biology, motivations, or attitudes. As the Institute of Medicine (IOM) (2000) affirmed:

> To prevent disease, we increasingly ask people to do things that they have not done previously, to stop doing things they have been doing for years, and to do more of some things and less of other things. . . . It is unreasonable to expect that people will change their behavior easily when so many forces in the social, cultural, and physical environment conspire against such change (p. 4).

Ecologically informed strategies that acknowledge and address growing awareness of connections between socioeconomic, cultural, political, environmental, organizational, psychological, and biological determinants of health and illness will hold a greater promise for success than those limited in scope to the laboratory of the individual.

In this chapter, we discuss the relationship between physical and social environments (PSE), health, and the behavior of humans. We begin by presenting a theoretical framework supporting a multidimensional conceptualization of the environment. We broaden this conceptual perspective to include social determinants of health, incorporating into this framework the people relied upon for one's daily social commerce, the domestic groups that form one's local friendship network, and the day-to-day transactions in one's residential neighborhood. We then focus on the influential role of the PSE on the consumption of alcohol, tobacco, and other substances; food, eating behaviors, and addictions contributing to the current obesity epidemic; and a selection of other behavioral addictions. The chapter closes by discussing methodological considerations and implications for professional practice.

Theory and Conceptualization of the Physical and Social Environments (PSE)

Operationally defining the PSE and conceptualizing how it operates to influence behavior requires a theoretical framework (Perdue, Gostin & Stone, 2003; Renalds, Smith & Hale, 2010). Unlike a building perched on an unmoving foundation, the effect of the environment is not static by any means. Rather, the PSE is dynamic, moving, intertwined with many different factors, and constantly exerting an influence. Conceptual frameworks for understanding the PSE rely mainly on dynamical systems approaches to explain how they influence behavior. Dynamical systems approaches (von Bertalanffy, 1968), whether drawing from ecological (Bronfenbrenner, 1977; McLeroy et al., 1988), transactional (Sameroff, 2010), or reciprocal interactional (Lerner & Kauffman, 1985; Scarr & McCartney, 1983) perspectives, posit that human behavior reflects a myriad of contextual influences. Stated differently, the "parts cannot be separated from wholes" (Sameroff, 2010, p. 7), thus requiring that one not focus on distinguishing the noise from the signal, but rather seek to understand the signal in the context of the noise.[1]

Whether unintentional or by design, built and social environments influence the human experience. A core premise of dynamical systems views, and threaded throughout this chapter, is the notion of a "reciprocal" relation between individuals and groups (the *agent*) and their external PSE (the *exposure*). In other words, individuals thrive within a certain socio-physical milieu through which they transact to produce behavior (Stokols & Shumaker, 1981). This milieu, described as the *agent–exposure interface*, becomes central to understanding the causal linkages between humans and their environs and the effect this has on behavior. This approach is meant to challenge the rational decision-making paradigm and broaden the lens of diagnosis, prevention, and treatment of the addictions.

One way of conceptualizing the PSE is to recognize that it represents a shift from emphasizing "downstream" factors mainly concerned with the individual as a responsible party for his/her own behavior to focus on "upstream" factors including the physical and spatial layout of a community and normative social influences (Braveman, Egerter & Williams, 2011). While the downstream has been associated with methodologic individualism, the upstream includes physical features of the environment (e.g., roads, buildings, food sources, and parks), economic factors (income, wealth, and education), and social transactions that transpire on a daily basis (i.e., people milling about). Upstream factors also characterize neighborhoods based on residential stability, whether residents perceive it as "safe," brimming with economic and social resources (employment, housing, and safety), and the quality of social interactions that promote neighborhood cohesion. The latter PSE feature emphasizes "bonding" and forming trustworthy networks that provide a form of social capital (Ferlander, 2016; Song, 2011). This change in perspective can be summarized as "rather than regarding lifestyle as the prime cause of health problems, we need to analyze the determinants of lifestyle" (Freudenberg, 2007).

Empirical Studies of the PSE

Studies of the PSE and health in numerous fields have examined such topics as whether mass transportation (Winters et al., 2010) or bicycling paths (Moudon et al., 2006) influence commutation behavior, pedestrian walkability studies (Giles-Corti & Donovan, 2003; Leyden, 2003), physical layout and activity (Handy et al., 2002), and whether additional street lighting makes neighborhood residents feel safe enough to walk or exercise outdoors at night (Wood et al., 2008). Research on the PSE also extends to include the degree to which access to healthy food options impact dietary patterns and obesity (Larson, Story & Nelson, 2009).

In each of these examples, the complexion of a neighborhood, its physical spaces and spatial layout, provides a window from which to view a person's choices regarding their health and well-being. This has been the focus of *smart growth* strategies (Dalbey, 2008; Hutch et al., 2011) that consider the effects of housing access, transportation, land use, housing density, open space, sidewalk utilization, food outlets, proximity to shopping, local community investment strategies, and recreation as they influence decisions to exercise, eat well, and form enduring bonds with neighbors. Encouraging stronger bonds reflects a growing need to overcome social isolation, particularly among residents of disadvantaged neighborhoods, or the disabled or elderly, and can promote social cohesion and garner a sense of community (Kawachi, 1999; Putnam, 2000; Victor et al., 2000).

Numerous studies have now linked neighborhood social and physical disorganization with both adverse mental (Latkin & Curry, 2003; Leventhal & Brooks-Gunn, 2003) and medical health outcomes (Latkin & Curry, 2003; Renalds et al., 2010). Two examples of the latter include associations between where one lives and risk of cardiovascular disease (Cubbin, Hadden & Winkleby, 2001; Diez-Roux, 2004; Hankey, Marshall & Brauer, 2012) and Type 2 diabetes (Chaix et al., 2011). Added to this body of work, there is evidence obtained from space, place, and crime studies (Perkins et al., 1993; Wilcox, Quisenberry & Jones, 2016) and, more recently, studies conducted both in the USA (Satcher, Okafor & Dill, 2012) and abroad (Burns & Snow, 2012) emphasizing the role of the BE in sexual health.

A handful of studies have examined the role of the PSE in fostering drug use and have demonstrated an increase in drug overdoses in the context of physical qualities of the neighborhood (Cerdá et al., 2013; Hembree et al., 2005), the association of negative BE characteristics on alcohol consumption (Bernstein et al., 2007), and the importance of social environments for understanding differences in youth cannabis use (Hyshka, 2013). The study by Hembree et al. (2005) showed a positive association between drug overdose death and physical features of the neighborhood environment (i.e., external factors including building decay and proper upkeep as well as internal maintenance factors affecting heat, water, toilets, and cleanliness). Bernstein et al. (2007) surveyed 1570 residents of the fifty-nine community districts that constitute New York City and found that various physical features of the BE (rundown nature of buildings, maintenance, heating, and water problems) were associated with increased odds of heavy drinking (five or more drinks in one sitting). These models adjusted for depression and many of the demographic factors (age, income, race, education, and marital status) that are likely to contribute to where a person lives and also influence their alcohol consumption.

More than Bricks and Mortar: A Social Determinant Perspective on Health

The combined emphasis of the PSE on both physical and social determinants necessitates a more elaborate model. This is reflected in the work of Northridge and colleagues, who blend urban planning, sociology, and a public health perspective into a Social Determinants of Health and Environmental Health Promotion conceptual model (Northridge, Sclar & Biswas, 2003; Schulz & Northridge, 2016). According to this framework, the built environment is construed as buildings, spaces, and products modified by people inclusive of land use, transportation, services, pubic resources, zoning regulations, and edifices, all designed to incorporate multiple levels of influence.[2] However, separate from the BE is the social context, including community investment, policies, ordinance enforcement, community capacity, civic participation, and quality of education, the latter of which represents a capital investment in the future. Both the physical and social environmental contexts are hypothesized to influence more proximal

[1] This is perhaps best stated by Sameroff (2010), when discussing the perennial nature–nurture question and how to address rectifying problems with children, who wrote, "it is both child and parent, but it also neurons and neighborhoods, synapse and schools, proteins and peers, and genes and governments" (p. 7).

[2] Environmental factors like toxins and biological pollutants are considered part of the "natural" environment.

factors including stressors that occur in the environment, neighborhood and workplace, violent crime and safety, police response, financial insecurity, environmental toxins, and health and resource disparities that may exist because of race, gender, or nationality (Braveman et al., 2011; Freudenberg et al., 2015; Gostin & Martinez, 2004).

The social determinants of health (SDoH) are thus a framework that views the PSE as nonmedical factors that interact to affect health outcomes and behavioral choices. When the environment is unhealthy, there is also a direct effect on the physiological stress response, resulting in production of excess cortisol that has further detrimental health effects. The interactions between environmental effects and behavioral choices and health outcomes are depicted in Figure 14.1, and form the basis of the evidence provided in this chapter linking PSEs as key determinants of our health (Ewald, Strack & Orsini, 2019).

Within this framework, it becomes clear that the SDoH affect all people, but not equally. Disadvantaged neighborhoods often lack the assets that are necessary to support good health, resulting in significant inequities that can lead to profound social, economic, and health consequences for the residents (American Public Health Association [APHA], 2016). The association of adverse health outcomes with neighborhood-level poverty and deprivation persists after adjustment for individual-level factors (Adler et al., 1993; Diez-Roux, 1998), suggesting that the influence of neighborhood conditions on personal health behaviors and addictions related to alcohol and drug use, smoking, physical activity, and dietary habits is independent of individual SES (APHA, 2016).

A study of over 57,000 youth found that poorer child health was strongly associated with accumulated social disadvantage, reflected by poverty, low parental education, living in a single-parent family, and minority race/ethnic status. This study evaluated the effect of these factors on child health status and found that low income accounted for most of the morbidity and mortality disparities associated with race and ethnic status. The remaining three factors were found to be independent and cumulative, in that they additively and exponentially increased risk of poor child health status. Thus, they did not act as separate proxies for a single underlying disadvantage. Of note, these disadvantages were not ameliorated or eliminated when the child had health insurance or access to healthcare. The authors concluded that the physical, developmental, and psychological disadvantages experienced by poor children could be explained by cumulative environmental and psychosocial exposures, and these effects carry over throughout childhood and into adulthood (Bauman, Silver & Stein, 2006). Studies such as these influence our understanding of the protective as well as risk-engendering influences that place and social order have on human behaviors, addictions, and health.

Operational Definitions of Social Determinants

There are a number of different perspectives regarding how to construct and operationally define SDoH . The World Health Organization (WHO) defines SDoH as the conditions of daily life and the environmental and structural factors that produce health-damaging or enhancing

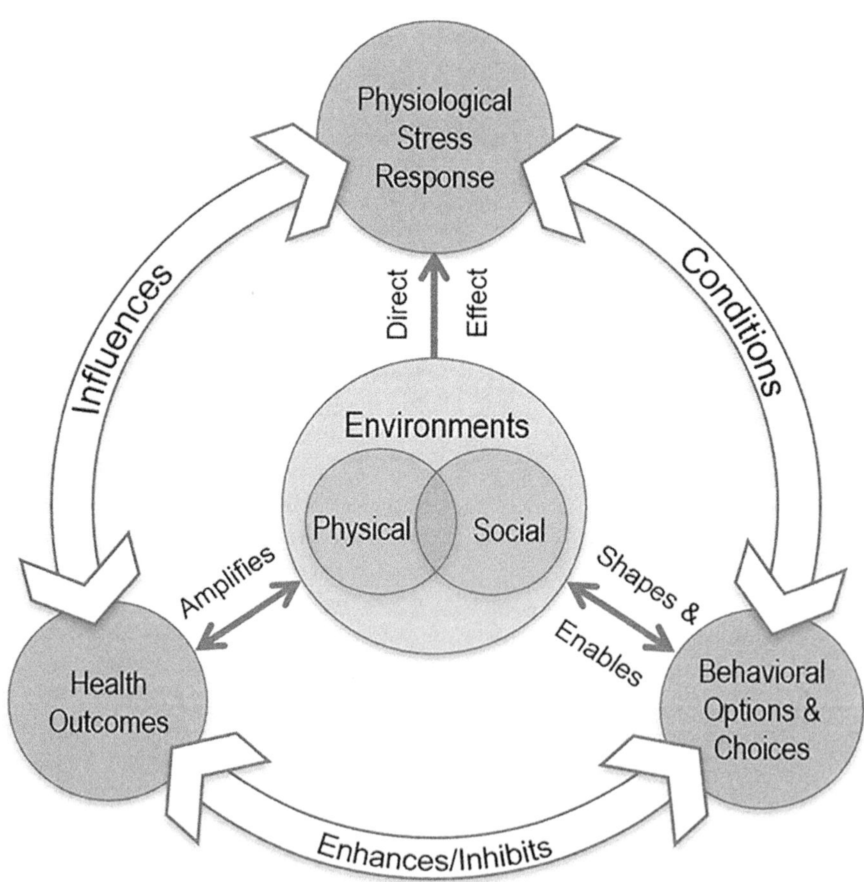

Figure 14.1 How the physical and social environment affects human behaviors and health.

experiences (Commission on Social Determinants of Health, 2008). Social determinants encompass five key areas that influence health in different ways: health and healthcare, education, economic stability, social and community context, and neighborhood and built environment (Healthy People 2020, 2017). The Public Health Institute ([PHI], 2015) review of twenty-two SDoH frameworks found that even while variations in terminology and definitions were present, SDoH were consistently recognized as the broad set of influences that shape individual and population health. In general, the common threads involved influences that "reach far beyond the healthcare system, and include structural drivers (e.g., the inequitable distribution of power, money, opportunity, and resources) and conditions of daily life (e.g., the environments in which people are born, live, work, play, worship, and age)" (Davis, Rivera & Parks, 2015, p. 3). The PHI (2015) report also differentiates social determinants into discrete categories involving: (a) physical conditions and built environment, (b) resource and services environment, and (c) social environment. Each of these is briefly described below.

Physical conditions include water, soil, and air quality, and hazardous substances from the natural environment (PHI, 2015), and the *built environment* describes the physical structures and design elements of a neighborhood, including land use, housing, sidewalks, street quality, connectivity, green spaces, and retail mix (Suglia et al., 2016). The *resource and services environment* refers to those aspects of the natural and built environment that provide services and access to resources to the public, such as parks and public recreation areas; light rail, bus, and other public transportation systems; child-care centers and schools; grocery, convenience, and liquor stores; fast food restaurants, exercise facilities, and other retail businesses (PHI, 2015). *Social environment* includes the *socioeconomic* conditions of the community, which refers to the level of education and financial condition of the residents themselves, both individually and collectively, as well as the *normative characteristics* of a neighborhood, which can be defined as the social relationships and social processes between the people and groups who live and work there (Carroll-Scott et al., 2013).

All of these social determinant influences are construed as "bidirectional" with the health of the community influencing both proximal (e.g., ongoing crime) and distal (e.g., natural environment) causes. One can illustrate the two-way effects[3] using examples from the literature. For example, studies have linked hazards and poor safety features in domestic residential buildings with the prevalence of accidents and crime. Likewise, radon, mold, and damp living conditions have been associated with high rates of respiratory disease, and communicable diseases have been found to occur in overcrowded housing. In these cases, social conditions and health are impacted by the physical environment. These "interfaces" are the targets of interventions, usually in the form of policy and legal initiatives which provide better housing facilities to the poor, who are disproportionately affected by PSE conditions (Curtis, Cave & Coutts, 2002).

Health and well-being are also influenced through public policies regarding housing and education, the social hierarchy relative to income distribution and workplace control, the effect of discrimination and social networks on social relationships, and the role of cultural norms (Galea & Vlahov, 2002), as well as neighborhood crime and safety, segregation, and social norms developed over time (Suglia et al., 2016). Specific to addictive behaviors, public policies can greatly influence the PSE and either enhance or suppress the exposure to influences that lead to the adoption or continuation of addictions. Recognizing the combined influences of these factors on health risks, the *risk environment framework* defines the risk environment as "the space – whether social or physical – in which a variety of factors interact to increase the chances of drug-related harm" (Rhodes, 2002, p. 88).

The bidirectional influence of the PSE is perhaps seen most clearly in neighborhoods with high rates of substance use and visible sex-trade activity. Moreover, the close ties between the economic, political, and moral interests of a community are reflected in zoning regulations that congregate strip clubs, bars, motels, and rooming houses in designated geographic zones, often near commercial areas or economically depressed neighborhoods. Policing practices often restrict these immoral or illegal behaviors and lead to geographic concentrations of marginalized populations, already stratified by economic, racial, ethnic, and gender barriers (Deering et al., 2014; Draus, Roddy & Asabigi, 2015). Draus et al. (2015) report that it is the combined effects of local zoning and policing practices, client/customer behaviors, cultural norms, and economic imperatives that produce an environment conducive to sex-trade work. While these factors produce the physical and structural aspects of sex-trade work, the social environmental aspects are primarily produced by gender and power inequities, with women historically having fewer financial options than men and frequently needing to support children. It is perhaps no surprise that women turned to sex work as the best available strategy for meeting daily survival needs.

Spatial isolation in the physical, structural, and social environments increases health risks among drug users and sex workers, including increased risk of contracting HIV. Health risks are increased when sex workers barter sex for drugs or engage in sex while high, because they are less likely to follow safe-sex practices. Where sex work and drug use overlap, sex workers are at a disadvantage when negotiating terms, are less able to assess drug quality, and may share drug use equipment (Deering et al., 2014). The risk environment thus encompasses the bidirectional nature of the PSE, reflecting not only the risk behaviors of the individual and their vulnerability to drug-related harm, but the myriad social, physical, and structural determinants of harm that contribute to and reinforce risk behaviors, drug use, and health inequalities (Deering et al., 2014; Rhodes, 2002). These bidirectional influences of PSE on human behavior and health are illustrated in Figure 14.1, with PSE shaping and enabling our behavioral options and choices as well as positively or negatively amplifying health outcomes directly.

Social Determinant Influence on Social Capital and Collective Efficacy

In addition to the physical environment, the social environment provides a basis for social capital and collective efficacy; these assets combine to provide benefits to individual residents and the community as a whole (Cohen, Inagami & Finch, 2008). Social hierarchies that evolve in response to characteristics such as SES may influence social support and can increase psychological vulnerabilities. The psychosocial stressors associated with income disparity can lead to increased tension and violence between individuals. Such factors increase the potential for substance use and abuse and erode social trust. Neighborhoods with lower social capital and less collective efficacy experience higher rates of

[3] This relationship can be portrayed in the same way as "reciprocal determinism" is used in Bandura's (1986) model of social learning theory to capture cycles of mutual influence characterizing interdependencies.

violence and homicide, and greater potential for drug use and abuse, whereas neighborhoods with greater collective efficacy can discourage undesirable behaviors before they escalate and thus reduce or prevent these outcomes. The degree of collective efficacy in a neighborhood is directly related to the ability of the residents to respond to visible signs of social disorder (Galea, Rudenstine & Vlahov, 2005; Vaeth, Wang-Schweig & Caetano, 2017). Here again, the bidirectional nature of the PSE and its influences on addictions reinforces the importance of SDoH.

Social Capital

Studies of the PSE are rooted in the concept of *social capital* as a contributor to health and well-being (Song, 2011). For instance, there is evidence that socioeconomic status in the form of poverty or social disadvantage is related to health outcomes (Evans & Kantrowitz, 2002; Kawachi, 1999), including obesity (Beech et al., 2011) and children's health (Bauman et al., 2006), as well as psychological functioning (Kessler & Cleary, 1980; Mulatu & Schooler, 2002). *Social capital* refers to the resources available that help individuals prosper and can include community organizational features like libraries as places to learn, community involvement (i.e., civic participation, also called *bonding* social capital) to improve political stature, and social networks that can be mobilized in support of the individual (Coleman, 2000; Ferlander, 2016).[4] According to Coleman (2000), social capital must be productive and achieve the aims of its social actors to achieve certain goals, economic or otherwise. Putnam (2000) augments this by suggesting that "norms of trustworthiness" are part of social capital as these expectations of reciprocity motivate people to create enduring social ties within the realms of community activities (e.g., faith-based organizations) and commerce (e.g., trusting bankers to underwrite new local community business growth), and provide access to a network of supportive friendships (i.e., tangible support).

A body of work has examined social capital in relation to mental health, distress, and other health outcomes. Several studies have shown that socially isolated, lower income individuals in race-stratified neighborhoods that lack access to interpersonal supports have higher rates of psychological distress (Irwin et al., 2008; Mitchell & LaGory, 2002).[5] Both US and international studies reinforce that the lack of social capital in terms of human resources (friendships) and connection to the community (civic participation) is related to distress or poor health, even when controlling for the usual contextual and individual-level risk factors (Kim, Subramanian & Kawachi, 2006; Yip et al., 2007; Ziersch, Baum & Putland, 2005). Social capital plays a prominent role by boosting self-esteem and reinforcing coping resources, which enable individuals to deal with stress and provocation from the environment.

Collective Efficacy

While exposure to features in the PSE can influence both the experience and perception of social interactions, the blending of these factors leads to the development of collective efficacy (Cohen et al., 2008). *Collective efficacy* has been defined as social cohesion among neighbors within a community combined with a willingness to intervene to promote the common good (Sampson, Raudenbush & Earls, 1997) and represents a group's capacity to achieve collective goals that are not imposed by regulations or outside forces (Galea et al., 2005). Collective efficacy or social trust does not refer to specific networks or individual ties to them; rather it is an aggregate of individual perceptions of the social environment in a neighborhood. Neighborhoods characterized by high collective efficacy feel safe, and foster resident familiarity through increased social interaction. Residents of such neighborhoods are capable of effectively maintaining social controls exercised through development plans, effective police regulation, pedestrian-friendly neighborhoods and civic pride. Neighborhoods characterized by loose social ties and lacking efficacy are more likely to be unsafe and dangerous and have high numbers of alcohol outlets and desolate or rundown parks. Each of these consequences of poor PSEs greatly influences the select architectural layout of the community and detrimentally alters behavioral choices (Hansen, Skov & Skov, 2016).

To illustrate the influence of PSE and social determinants on human behaviors and health, one can examine evidence from the literature that demonstrates the relationship between PSE and substance use and addiction. We extend this discussion to include the environment's influence on eating addictions, including eating behaviors that affect obesity, as well as other behavioral addictions.

PSE Studies, Substance Use, and Addiction

PSE studies that focus on unique neighborhood features have generally emphasized various facets of social cohesion, social disorganization, and other social determinants that render one neighborhood more or less vulnerable to drug use outcomes (Bernstein et al., 2007; Tucker et al., 2013; Wilson et al., 2016). One way to capture these relations is to examine spatial relationships between alcohol retail outlet density and consumption practices.[6] Density studies acknowledge that individuals drink alcohol partly because of internal motivations (i.e., personality factors like self-esteem or depression) but also consider the role of distinct neighborhood features that reflect BE pressures and availability.

Consumption of Alcohol

The literature on geospatial relationships infers that, independent of internal motivations, there are *place characteristics* that influence

[4] Song (2011), among others, takes the view that social capital is a network resource phenomenon distinct from social cohesion, social integration, and social support. The socioeconomic assets and means that social networks provide through close associates (monetary wealth, occupation, and education) enhance ones' social capital.

[5] This should include mention of the classic study by Brown and Harris (1978) of poor women residing in the Outer Hebrides, a remote collection of islands located on the northwest edge of Scotland, that established both protective and damaging effects from social networks on psychiatric outcomes like depression and anxiety.

[6] We have purposely avoided focusing on studies that examine community-based environmental prevention strategies (i.e., responsible beverage service, shoulder tap and commercial regulatory policies, compliance and roadside sobriety checks, and social host ordinances). This decision was based on the fact these efforts target "features" of the environment but in most cases not the physical BE itself. A more thorough understanding of these environmental prevention approaches can be found in Treno et al. (2015).

whether neighborhood residents will engage in high-risk behaviors, including alcohol misuse and excessive or binge drinking. Place characteristics are direct proxies for the BE because they include both physical features of the environment (e.g., the density of retail outlets selling alcohol and their physical proximity to residences) as well as social determinants, which can include social mingling that occurs outside of nightclubs, adherence to zoning regulations, decision-making by planning commissions when they confer licensing on establishments that serve alcohol, and police activity related to loitering and public nuisance complaints for intoxicated patrons (Nowell et al., 2006; Treno et al., 2007).

In the case of alcohol outlet density studies, the high prevalence of retail outlets located in a particular neighborhood creates a normative climate that condones use of alcohol, making it relatively easy to obtain (e.g., purchasing liquor while walking home from work or school) and socially acceptable (e.g., drinking in local pubs and bars). The results of these studies are consistent with *availability theory* positing that in the absence of normative constraints, drinking increases with the proliferation of sales outlets, resulting in an increase in the number of heavy drinkers, and also increases in drinking-related consequences (Stockwell & Gruenewald, 2004).[7]

Alcohol Outlet Density

Several factors may contribute to inconsistent findings from studies of alcohol density and consumption (Livingston, Chikritzhs & Room, 2007). The variation of study designs may contribute to different findings; most studies have relied on cross-sectional designs hindering their ability to render causal assertions. Outlet types have also varied considerably, with some studies focusing on pubs, bars, and nightclubs, while others emphasize off-premise alcohol sales, which can include supermarkets and convenience stores in some US locales. Furthermore, studies vary in the composition of outcomes, including self-reported consumption, consumption calculated based on per capita sales, and alcohol-related harms, the latter exemplified by motor vehicle accidents (Treno et al., 2007) and pedestrian injury collisions (LaScala, Johnson & Gruenewald, 2001). Notwithstanding these differences, it is known that alcohol retail density is greater in poor, racial minority, and disadvantaged communities (Bernstein et al., 2007; Pollack et al., 2005), and is independently associated with greater alcohol consumption among both adults and adolescents (Gruenewald, Ponicki & Holder, 1993; Milam et al., 2014; Scribner, Cohen & Fisher, 2000).

In one study, Scribner et al. (2000) showed that the effect of alcohol outlet density (liquor and convenience stores) on consumption (number of drinks in the past week) can be explained entirely through neighborhood factors (all persons within a particular census tract reside in a high outlet density zone) rather than individual-level processes (individual's proximity to retail outlet), controlling for demographics and individual level norms and consumption. At the aggregate census tract level, drinking norms were more supportive of consumption in areas with low mean distances to alcohol outlets and the same held for rates of consumption, with low mean distance to the closest alcohol outlet leading to higher consumption. Schonlau and colleagues (2008) used aggregated mean distance to alcohol retail outlets by census tract in their study conducted in Los Angeles County and southern Louisiana. For Louisiana residents only, the models revealed that the number of retail outlets was associated with twelve-month and ninety-day ethanol consumption (computed based on the average ethanol content of a drink, for drinks per day in the past year and previous ninety days).

There is also the possibility that proscriptive norms differ based on land use, with higher tolerance for drinking in some locales than others. For example, some neighborhoods willingly support local pubs as long as there are restrictions on hours of operation and public loitering. This stands in contrast to residential areas that border closely to restaurants that serve alcohol. A few small neighborhood pubs are quite different from ten pubs, bars, or restaurants in close proximity that may transform an area into an entertainment district. Retail establishments choosing to locate near each other, called *commercial bunching* as discussed by Livingston et al. (2007), may produce an increase in alcohol-related harms among specific subgroups; most notably individuals at high risk for excessive drinking (and this effect may be masked by larger null population effects that fail to address subgroups based on consumption practices). Taverns and sports bars that provide food and alcohol incentives in the form of happy hours, ladies drink for free, and cheap well drinks on football nights are likely to attract younger male patrons who engage in heavy drinking, which leads to disinhibition (i.e., promoting aggression and violent acts). This is an example that epitomizes the spatial relations between alcohol outlet density and high-risk drinking, where people and place come together in a perfect storm to create opportunities for excessive drinking (Livingston et al., 2007).

The notion of high-risk subgroups raises another important concern. Do researchers find that alcohol retail density contributes to consumption in populations that are more prone to drink (i.e., problem drinkers, people attending sporting events, or among high-risk groups)? One way to address this concern is to examine whether alcohol retail outlets and liquor sales influence college student drinking. It is not uncommon to find college youth drinking at football tailgating parties and fraternity or sorority events (Sher, Bartholow & Nanda, 2001). Moreover, national surveillance data indicate that young adulthood corresponds with peak alcohol consumption including alcohol misuse and binge drinking (Schulenberg et al., 2017). As a result, establishing linkages between college drinking and alcohol density has been a focal topic both in the USA (Wechsler et al., 2002; Weitzman et al., 2003), a country with a zero tolerance policy for underage drinking, and other countries that favor harm reduction approaches (Kypri et al., 2008). Several environmental considerations have been examined, including deterrence strategies, restrictions in sales of alcohol, limited licensing, and changes to the physical environment through restriction of off-premise retail outlets (Chaloupka & Wechsler, 1996; Toomey, Lenk & Wagenaar, 2007).

Consumption of Tobacco and Other Substances

Alcohol outlets are frequently also tobacco outlets and provide opportunities for purchase and sale of illicit drugs (Milam et al., 2016). Greater frequency of youth smoking is significantly associated with increased density of tobacco outlets within one mile of children's homes, and

[7] This does not factor into the equation the price, utility, opportunity cost and other "economic" factors that behavioral economists have cited as crucial to understanding consumption practices (e.g., Stockwell & Gruenewald, 2004). It also does not address the potential for reciprocal causation where availability stimulates consumption, but consumption also fosters increased sales with the potential for increasing the number of institutions selling spirits at reduced cost to meet commodity demand.

schools in neighborhoods that have the highest tobacco outlet density (five or more outlets within half a mile of the school) also have a higher prevalence of current smokers (Lipperman-Kreda et al., 2014). Alcohol and tobacco advertising, as a specific component of the PSE, is frequently targeted to racially segregated neighborhoods, as well as schools with more racial/ethnic minority students (e.g., Hispanic), which spurs use of tobacco products (Milam et al., 2014; Vaeth et al., 2017). Children are three times more likely to pass an alcohol or tobacco billboard when walking or commuting to school in mostly racial/ethnic minority neighborhoods than in mostly Caucasian neighborhoods (Milam et al., 2014). Exposure to the promotion of unhealthy products is directly related to behavioral uptake. The relationship of a tobacco prompting PSE on tobacco use behaviors is additionally complicated with the added reciprocal influence of a smoker's social network also contributing to the uptake and continuation of tobacco use. Each of these PSE influences are critical for our understanding of the etiology of individual tobacco use and supports the use of environmental strategies for addressing tobacco addiction. Higher smoking rates are associated with neighborhoods segregated by SES (Galea et al., 2005). As a marker for deprivation, SES is such a strong predictor of tobacco use that smoking prevalence can be used to identify disadvantaged populations. SES is believed to explain the difference in smoking cessation rates between 1973 and 1996, which were virtually unchanged for the poor but doubled for the most affluent during the same time period (Cummings, Fong & Borland, 2009).

Examining the public health efforts surrounding the USA's reduction in tobacco use provides a rich illumination of a powerful multilevel approach that specifically targeted an array of physical and social environments associated with tobacco use, resulting in tobacco use rates dropping from 42 percent in 1965 to only 15 percent in 2015 (Centers for Disease Control and Prevention [CDC], 2007). While the addictive properties of nicotine are well-established scientifically, it is likely that most individuals have now come to appreciate the influences of manipulating environmental triggers that promote health and/or discourage the uptake of tobacco products. Physical and social environmental changes, such as smoke-free zones, taxation policies, restaurant smoking bans and restrictions, and social norming campaigns, have all interacted to yield a remarkable public health success. These findings strongly support the importance of PSE studies in both the understanding of tobacco use etiology, and prevention and treatment modalities.

The Role of Population Density

In addition to the density of alcohol and tobacco retail outlets, the influence of the PSE is also affected by population density. The local neighborhood environment directly influences youth risk behaviors, including drug and alcohol use and abuse; however, there are notable differences between urban and rural behavior patterns, which change over time (Galea et al., 2005). Recent surveillance data in the USA indicates that rural adolescents may use substances at the same or higher rates than their urban counterparts and that, in addition to alcohol, the use of methamphetamine, smokeless tobacco, and inhalants is higher among rural youth (Warner, 2016). A large national survey of adolescents conducted in 2000 suggested that heroin use was comparable between urban and rural areas and that other forms of illicit drug use were more likely in urban environments (Galea et al., 2005). The same survey was conducted again in 2012 and found that perceived ease of access to illicit drugs, including marijuana, LSD, ecstasy, and cocaine, was greater among urban students in more densely populated areas, which may reflect greater availability, greater prevalence of use, or both. Perceived ease of access to alcohol was found to be about the same for both rural and urban adolescents, increasing from about 25 percent of middle school students to about 60 percent of high-school students. There was a correlation between perceived ease of access and actual use of alcohol by rural adolescents, and compared to urban youth, actual alcohol and tobacco use by rural adolescents was higher (Warren, Smalley & Barefoot, 2015).

In contrast to other illicit drug use, rates of use and misuse of prescription opioids for nonmedical purposes is somewhat higher in rural areas, which have a higher proportion of older residents, possibly as a result of more young people leaving for school or work opportunities (Brooks et al., 2017). Here again, the same mechanisms of the PSE influencing behavioral choices leading to addictions are also present when one examines opioid use. With the greater number of close kinship ties in rural communities, it is easier for rural adolescents to obtain these drugs with or without a prescription (Brooks et al., 2017; Keyes et al. 2014). One study found that 62 percent of rural adolescents obtained prescription opioids through diversion from friends and family members and 23 percent obtained them from physicians (Monnat & Rigg, 2016). Curiously, although rural adolescents perceive prescription opioids as more harmful than other prescription medications, such as amphetamines, they also perceive the use of prescription opioids as less harmful than other drugs, except alcohol and marijuana. This may be because prescription opioids can be taken orally, without the need for needles, smoking, or snorting, and therefore have less stigma associated with them, or because adolescents using prescription opioids have observed others taking these drugs and are familiar with their effects (Keyes et al., 2014).

PSE Studies, Eating Behaviors, and Obesity

Unlike consumption of other substances, it is not possible to entirely abstain from food consumption. The downside of the need to eat is that the foods we consume are increasingly more highly processed and studies continue to highlight the impact of industry-orchestrated changes of our food environment on our collective health (Popkin, 2006; WHO & Food and Agriculture Organization of the United Nations, 2003). The manipulation of fats, sugars, flavor enhancers, and caffeine have greatly increased the consumption of foods containing highly saturated fats and refined sugar, increased the profits of food companies, and coincided with a dramatic rise in obesity rates (Gearhardt et al., 2011; Monteiro et al., 2011). The result of these industry changes is the increased consumption of readily available, energy-dense but nutrient-poor foods at the expense of healthier options (Gearhardt et al., 2012; Gearhardt, Corbin & Brownell, 2009).

Considerable evidence shows that blended food products containing highly palatable stimuli contribute to addictive-type eating behaviors in humans. The evidence suggests that, while these food formulations may not result in a physiological addiction to the substances in food, there is frequently a neurobiological response in the brain reward centers that is similar to that seen with substance addictions (Burrows et al., 2017; Davis, 2013; Olsen, 2011; Schreiber, Odlaug & Grant, 2013). For this reason, eating behaviors such as binge eating, compulsive overeating, and food cravings are frequently described as food addictions. Food addiction is a topic of intense debate and research which is further discussed by Schulte, Schiestl and Gearhardt in Chapter 28, but there is no debate that these highly processed foods are now known to be a significant contributor to the unhealthy eating behaviors of humans and can contribute to obesity. While eating behaviors have a significant influence on the choices that lead to the consumption of various foods, the situation is further complicated by the fact that food choices change as a result of stress (Zellner et al., 2006), and psychosocial stressors have been linked with childhood obesity (Gundersen et al., 2011). Food choices can contribute to obesity in other ways as well.

A promising area of behavioral research involves the application of behavioral economics to understand how environmental availability and other factors influence the food choices we make daily (as illustrated in Figure 14.1). Consumers' food choices are influenced by ready availability, convenience, low price, large portion sizes, and food preferences based on habits, which can become automatic (beneath the radar of consciousness) or "default" choices. Making different, healthier food choices requires conscious effort and deliberate actions, and the ability to delay immediate gratification in favor of long-term health (Roberto & Kawachi, 2014). Healthy eating involves food choices frequently made in an environment that promotes unhealthy choices. Research has shown that small changes to promote healthier foods, such as price discounts or product positioning for ease of access, increased visibility, or greater convenience, can nudge consumers to make healthier choices (Jilcott Pitts et al., 2016; Just & Gabrielyan, 2016).

An obesogenic environment occurs when neighborhood environmental conditions encourage lifestyles and habits that promote the development of obesity; such an environment includes cultural and social pressure for eating energy-dense foods, ready availability and access to such foods, and limited opportunities or encouragement to engage in physically active behavior during work or leisure time, or while commuting (Corrêa, Schmitz & Vasconcelos, 2015). Obesity is also influenced by a variety of other factors in the residential environment that influence behaviors, including neighborhood crime rate; integrated parks, green spaces, lighting, bike paths, and sidewalks; convenient, robust public transportation; the availability of recreational facilities, primary care practices, and obesity counseling centers; and the density of food outlets, including quality grocery stores, farmer's markets, and fast food restaurants (Beech et al., 2011; Rahman, Cushing & Jackson, 2011).

Retail Food and Fast Food Outlet Density

Residents of neighborhoods that have short supplies of healthy foods, or what are called "food deserts" have very limited access to nutritious foods at reasonable prices, consume fewer fruits and vegetables and more dietary fats, have a poorer diet quality, and are more likely to be overweight or obese (Corrêa et al., 2015; Galvez, Pearl & Yen, 2010). The USDA defines a *food desert* as a census tract in which the poverty rate is at least 20 percent and, for at least 33 percent of the residents, the nearest large grocery store or supermarket is more than one mile away, if metropolitan, or more than ten miles away, if nonmetropolitan (Casazza et al., 2015). Fast food density's influence on behavior is similar to those referenced earlier for alcohol outlet density. Fast food restaurants are more highly concentrated in low-income neighborhoods around schools, and sodas and fast food are more available than fruits and vegetables. Perhaps not surprisingly, students had healthier diets and lower BMI scores if they attended schools that were further away from fast food restaurants and convenience stores (Corrêa et al., 2015).

It is clear that the environment actively shapes one's eating behaviors and habits. One has only to recognize government-sponsored referendums, such as Healthy People 2020 (2017), and efforts by the CDC (2009), the National Prevention Strategy (National Prevention Council, 2012), and the National Institutes of Health (NIH) Strategic Plan (Obesity Research Task Force, 2011) to appreciate the concerted national responses to the unhealthy environments contributing to the obesity crisis (and potentially facilitating binge eating or even food addiction disorder). Collectively, these institutions recognize that a range of individual, social, economic, and environmental factors contribute to obesity. There is sufficient evidence to associate the detrimental effects of unhealthy and unsupportive PSE in a neighborhood with residents' sometimes-addictive behaviors, excessive consumption of unhealthy foods, extreme amounts of screen time, and lack of activity. It is essential to continue to expand the public's understanding of the PSE surrounding the food they eat and the degree to which they build physical activity into their daily lives, as each is critical for addressing obesity as a nation.

PSE Studies and Other Behavioral Addictions

As with substance use, eating behaviors, food choices, obesity, and physical activity, PSE also plays a role in other activities and can lead to problem behaviors and behavioral addictions. Addictions to substances and to behaviors like eating, sex, and gambling predate the invention of the telephone, television, computers, or the internet. Behavioral addictions to television, smartphones, and the internet (and their content) have only become possible since these technologies became widely available. These technologies have enabled unlimited access to and virtual participation in activities that formerly required in-person participation (e.g., gambling, sports, game playing, dating, and other social activities) and either in-person or mail-order purchases (e.g., pornography, shopping). These technologies have also created the potential for new addictive behaviors, such as texting, use of social media for chatting, and live streaming videos. Part of the challenge of researching behavioral addictions that involve the use of the internet or other "mobile" technologies is distinguishing between harmless behavior and problem or pathological behavior.

The field of behavioral addictions is rapidly evolving, and this is reflected in recent changes in the fifth edition of the *Diagnostic and Statistical Manual of Mental Disorders* (DSM-5), which now includes a new category *Substance-Related and Addictive Disorders* with two subcategories: *Substance-Related Disorders* and *Non-Substance-Related Disorders*. Gambling behaviors are listed in the *Non-Substance-Related Disorders* subcategory, based on the strength of evidence indicating activation of the same central pathways in the brain and behavioral symptoms similar to those of substance addictions (American Psychiatric Association [APA], 2013). At the time of the DSM-5 publication, the evidence was not strong enough to include internet gaming, eating behaviors/obesity, sex addiction, or shopping addiction in the *Non-Substance-Related Disorders* subcategory (Hebebrand et al., 2014); however, Internet Gaming Disorder (IGD) was listed as a condition for further study (Sussman et al., 2018).

Impulse Control and our Understanding of Addictions

Research into behavioral addictions is complicated by the fact that excessive behaviors are associated with impaired impulse control (Fattore, 2014) as well as psychiatric conditions such as obsessive-compulsive disorder, ADHD, anxiety, and depression (Andreassen et al., 2016). Individuals may experience more than one problem behavior at the same time, which can reinforce each other, alternate with each other, or mask one another (Konkolÿ Thege, Hodgins & Wild, 2016). Similar regions of the brain are activated by pathological or problem behaviors and substance addictions (Fattore, 2014); when they co-occur, it is more difficult to provide effective treatment (Konkolÿ Thege et al., 2016). There is also strong evidence that these same regions of the brain undergo physiological remodeling (including new neural pathways) when exposed to chronic stressors in the PSE during childhood and adolescence, a time when the brain is still developing (Everitt & Robbins, 2016; Ewald et al., 2019). As illustrated in Figure 14.1, the direct effects of PSE on individual physiological stress responses and associated brain remodeling, are important elements for the diagnosis and treatment of addictions. These brain changes are associated with impaired impulse control and may predispose individuals to addictive behaviors or substance addiction (Everitt & Robbins, 2016; Ewald et al., 2019). There is much to be resolved before there is clear understanding of the causes of behavioral addictions.

Debate continues among researchers about potential behavioral addictions, including online gaming addiction (considered legitimate), pornography, sex, and television addictions (considered controversial), and shoplifting, tanning, and love addictions (considered highly speculative) (Konkolÿ Thege et al., 2016). The term *addiction* is often used to describe excessive work and exercise behaviors, but these behaviors may also arise in conjunction with psychiatric or eating disorders (Andreassen et al., 2016; Cook, Hausenblas & Freimuth, 2014). Until screening instruments are fully validated and consensus reached on diagnostic criteria, there will continue to be debate about the nature of behavioral addictions. There is a paucity of research regarding the effect of the BE and the PSE on the individual engaging in most of these behaviors. Nevertheless, it is instructive to explore what is known.

Gambling

Gambling behavior can range from occasional or social participation, to frequent participation (at least twice a week), problem gambling, and pathological gambling, as defined in the DSM (Welte et al., 2016a). Gambling participation and gambling frequency do not necessarily equate with problem or pathological gambling. *Problem gambling* is associated with severe adverse consequences but does not meet any of the DSM criteria (Nowak & Aloe, 2014). *Pathological gambling* generally begins during adolescence or childhood, but there are gender differences in the timing and its progression. Males start gambling at a significantly younger age than females, but once females do start gambling, they progress to pathological gambling at a much faster rate than males. About 10 percent of women who are pathological gamblers finance their addiction through prostitution (Fattore, 2014).

Research findings are inconsistent regarding problem or pathological gambling behaviors. Although frequency of gambling participation is greater in areas where casinos are located, many cross-sectional studies have found that risk of problem or pathological gambling increased with closer proximity to a casino during the first year after a casino opened (Tong & Chim, 2013; Welte et al., 2016a); however, other studies have found an inverse relationship, and some found no relationship between proximity and problem or pathological gambling (Sévigny et al., 2008; Tong & Chim, 2013). Studies that examined the prevalence of problem or pathological gambling before and after casinos opened consistently found that proximity to a casino did not result in higher prevalence rates for local residents (Sévigny et al., 2008; Welte et al., 2016b), leading some to suggest that the novelty of the initial exposure is followed by adaptations in behavior or loss of interest (Sévigny et al., 2008; Tong & Chim, 2013; Welte et al., 2016b). In states with more types of legalized gambling, there is no significant association between the prevalence of problem gambling and the number of types of gambling, but the number of years of exposure to various forms of gambling is associated with increased rates of problem gambling (Welte et al., 2016b).

Problem and pathological gambling behaviors can occur with any type of gambling activity, even in the absence of gambling venues like casinos or race tracks. In addition to casino gambling, noncasino gambling can include games of chance (e.g., cards, dice, bingo, charitable gambling, raffles, office pools), games of skill (e.g., golf, billiards), sports betting, horse or dog racing (on- or off-track), lotteries, video lottery terminals or gambling machines, and internet gambling (Welte et al., 2016b). Sports gambling, such as fantasy football leagues and basketball playoff brackets, has become increasingly popular in recent years. Legalized gambling activity has been normalized and incorporated into daily life in the form of popular televised poker competitions (Lee, Lemanski & Jun, 2008), as well as internet gambling, state lotteries, and scratch-off tickets (Nowak & Aloe, 2014), which are readily available at most convenience stores and gas stations. These changes in the number of venues for legal gambling create opportunities that make gambling easier, while at the same time making it more difficult to determine the extent of problem and pathological gambling in the general population.

College students are highly susceptible to gambling for a variety of reasons. They are "a population group specifically targeted by the media, a vast number of whom have the resources, proximity, and free time to become involved" and who are not averse to engaging in risky behaviors (Nowak & Aloe, 2014, p. 822). Several studies have reported that the majority (72 percent to 80 percent) of college students have a significantly increased risk of problem gambling when compared to the general population (6 percent to 8 percent versus 2 percent to 4 percent, respectively; Sherba & Gersper, 2017). A meta-analysis retrieving data from eighteen studies and an aggregate of over 13,000 college students estimated that 10.23 percent were probable pathological gamblers (Nowak & Aloe, 2014). This prevalence reflects the fact that gambling, once dependent on physical access or interactions in the BE, has been enabled and exacerbated by the development of the internet, cell phones, and other digital technology, which are used extensively by college students.

Internet and Other Technology

Summarizing the literature on internet and video game addiction (IVGA) Sussman and colleagues (2018) wrote that "a wide variety of online activities are engaging enough to be potentially addictive, including video games, social media, smartphone use, texting, streaming videos, and online pornography" (p. 308). Research into IVGA and its subtypes is ongoing, and the subtype of video game addictions known as IGD "concerns only addiction to online video gaming and excludes that of other potentially addictive screen habits included in IVGA" (p. 309). The most popular types of online video games are role-playing games, such as massive multiplayer online games or MMOs, multiplayer online battle arena games, "shooters," and real-time strategy games (Sussman et al., 2018).

Because the use of internet and online technology is not dependent on specific locations in the BE (unless internet or Wi-Fi service is only available in certain locations), other PSE factors appear to make a greater contribution to the risk for development of IVGA. Sussman et al. (2018) reported that IVGA appears to be associated with alcohol use, ADHD, depression, and anxiety. Psychosocial factors associated with development of IVGA in adolescents include "poor family support, poor family relationships, high family conflict, and poor psychosocial support" (p. 313). Severity of IVGA is mitigated by greater social support and parental involvement and exacerbated by poor parental mental health. The risk of developing IVGA is higher for males in relation to computer gaming and higher for females in relation to social networking or smart phone use (Sussman et al., 2018).

Media Exposure and Physical Activity

The reach of media exposure on behaviors goes beyond gaming practice and is increasingly impacting the behavioral choices made for leisure time activities, which have become a significant environmental influence among youth. Children spend an average of nearly four hours a day being sedentary while playing video games and utilizing electronic media, all of which decreases free time available for physical activity. The increasing screen time exposes them to advertising that is specifically tailored to children, and much of what they see promotes unhealthy foods. In the USA, 75 percent of food manufacturer's advertising budgets, and 95 percent of the fast food industry's advertising budgets, are spent on television advertising, and many food manufacturers target additional advertising to children through direct product placement in children's movies, by partnering with toy companies, and by creating kids' clubs and featuring video games on their websites. Compared to their white counterparts, low-income racial/ethnic minority children watch more movies and television, and there are more food commercials on television shows that target African American audiences; these programs are also more likely to promote fast foods, candy, and soda than programs for more general audiences (Hillier, 2008).

Methodological Considerations

Research and measurement challenges will continue to be an issue in exploring the connection between the PSE and human behaviors. For instance, alcohol outlet density studies should continue to expand development of PSE theories to guide discovery in the field. Many investigators used, as a weak metric, administrative data to obtain the number of outlets in a designated geospatial area, and coupled this with information about distances between business entities and per capita consumption based on aggregate alcohol sales. This generates demand curves and economic models as plausible explanations for why increasing outlet density is associated with increased consumption and alcohol-related harms. This same lack of specificity affects any transactional or "ecological" models of behavior that rely on multiple levels of influence. Quite frankly, outside of a few mentions of criminological, availability, or social disorganization theories, there is heavy reliance on pure conjecture to establish why specific features of the PSE like alcohol outlet density are related to consumption and alcohol-related harms. At the individual level, there is little in the way of testable hypotheses showing connections between different levels of influence and how they shape behavior. The precise mechanisms that motivate behaviors leading to consumption are rarely, if ever, modeled. Studies are needed to identify the actual underlying mechanisms driving consumption in order to move away from correlational studies to the production of more "causal" evidence.

Within studies of alcohol density, many study designs utilized multi-level hierarchical linear modeling to tease apart the relative contributions of individual versus aggregate neighborhood effects on consumption. From an analysis point of view, the study design controls for spatial autocorrelation, which arises from underlying similarity that occurs within members from the same geographical space (i.e., neighborhood), and that can occur between adjacent or neighboring blocks. The lack of independence between members within neighborhoods can occur because they share physical parameters that define neighborhoods (i.e., distributive traffic patterns or physical street layout, proximity to industry or mass transportation) or social determinants (i.e., low-income projects or elderly housing) (Chaix et al., 2011; Getis, 2010).[8]

No matter how they are structured, studies examining whether the BE and likewise neighborhood factors affect health behaviors and addictions are not without their drawbacks. Two important methodological issues raised include the lack of control for both selective participation and selection bias (Diez-Roux, 2004; Leventhal & Brooks-Gunn, 2003) leading to distortion of effects and also the complex multi-level and reciprocal nature of these effects that make it hard to determine causation.[9] The latter is often called a "reflection" or endogeneity problem because many researchers construe neighborhood contextual effects as the sum of all the individual-level effects (i.e., SES is often used as a proxy to measure the aggregate neighborhood attribute of wealth). This has also been discussed as the *ecological fallacy* (Diez-Roux, 1998) because inferences are being made from one level (individual) to another (aggregate neighborhood) and may not hold in situ outside of statistical models.

[8] The problem of clustering among adjoining neighborhoods is termed spatial autocorrelated measurement error (Moran coefficient) and corresponds statistically with the intraclass correlation coefficient. In either case, in a hierarchically clustered design some portion of variance in the outcome is accounted for by the larger aggregate collection (i.e., neighborhoods distinguished by block or census tract) and some portion is accounted for by members that are found residing within the aggregate (block or census tract). Failure to address these different variance components could lead to biased estimates of effects (i.e., inflated standard errors).

[9] A good deal of social epidemiology relies on the assumption that an individual can be transported from one neighborhood to another with little effect of this relocation on the outcome under study (units can be exchanged, assuming control for individual-level differences). However, individual-level characteristics in the form of predisposing factors (spatial proximity to hospital for sicker people) may confound (or mediate) neighborhood "selection," thus introducing a modicum of bias into the equation. Greenland and Robins (1986) discuss this epidemiological confounding in greater detail (and also see Diez-Roux, 1998, for a similar discussion).

Conclusions

The environmental contexts that surround humans, whether defined as physical, built, social, or perceived have an enormous influence on the cognitions, opportunities, motivations, and behaviors of humans. The challenges professionals face in assessing and intervening to address the consequences of human behaviors, inclusive of addictions, is limited by their ability to understand the complex interactions of said environments on socially constructed lives. This chapter has attempted to call attention to the all-too-common narrow lens focused on the moral character or biological shortcomings of individuals who are ultimately nested within larger social structures. The theoretical perspectives and examples of physical and social environmental influences on human behavior are provided to illuminate and encourage a broadening of perspective to consider these systemic and powerful influences.

The growing awareness of the influence that environmental contexts have on human behavior will continue to evolve as governments, organizations, and professions increasingly prioritize investigation and targeted efforts for shaping healthier physical and social environments. Governmental and philanthropic funding geared toward systemic and structural environmental changes would hasten the ability to build the etiologic knowledge and practice base required for these more efficacious social and physical environment strategies.

Within professional practice, addressing addictive behaviors will not reach the level of effectiveness desired without intervention efforts that include consideration of built and social environmental influences. This is particularly important in light of the neurobiological evidence associating environmental stressors with physiological changes in brain structures that precede addictive behaviors. Here, it is important that addiction experts augment and strengthen efforts to identify upstream factors that influence behavior. This effort can then be integrated with what is known about social determinants that influence health. This emphasis requires professions to revisit professional values and statements of purpose. Revised professional statements may encourage the rethinking of professional preparation programs, and subsequent professional practices and obligations to incorporate social and physical influences in the current addictions etiology, prevention, and treatment models and practices.

A minimum outcome of considering built and social environmental influences would be a burgeoning cadre of health and addictions professionals with sensitized appreciation of some of the PSEs that influence health-related behaviors and health status itself. With expanded understanding, clinicians and healthcare settings may be able to strengthen routine care by developing health-promotion strategies that embrace new partnerships for ameliorating or mitigating the social determinants that are shown to be most important and changeable (Gottlieb, Sandel & Adler, 2013). Because addressing social determinants and altering physical and social environments are beyond health care setting's typical practice, these professionals can advocate for expanded research to continue exploration of causal mechanisms and effective strategies. With increased awareness of the PSE influence on addictions, professionals can use their informed and expert voice to educate and advocate for policy makers to address the detrimental social influences causing ill health in society (Gruen, Pearson & Brennan, 2004).

Not only does this broader lens of health behavior and addictions causality remove the often-unjust onus on individuals, it also points to a growing literature that continues to demonstrate the key factors that influence all human behavior on a daily basis. Addressing social ills from both a personal responsibility (individual agency) as well as a social responsibility (collective agency) perspective provides the best hope for shaping the PSE, behaviors, and health (Blacksher & Lovasi, 2012). It also provides a plethora of new opportunities for understanding human suffering on a larger scale, rather than individual by individual, which should be seen as a welcomed addition to one's professional tool kit. As long as problems of human behavior are defined at an individual level, practitioners will be burdened with simply pulling people from the river rather than looking upstream to more clearly see what is responsible for pushing people into harm's way.

REFERENCES

Adler, N. E., Boyce, W. T., Chesney, M. A., Folkman, S. & Syme, S. L. (1993). Socioeconomic inequalities in health: No easy solution. *Journal of the American Medical Association*, **269**(24), 3140–3145. https://doi.org/10.1001/jama.193.03500240084031

American Psychiatric Association (2013). *Diagnostic and Statistical Manual of Mental Disorders* (5th edition). Washington, DC: American Psychiatric Association.

American Public Health Association [APHA] (2016). *Opportunities for health collaboration: Leveraging community development investments to improve health in low-income neighborhoods.* Retrieved October 17, 2017, from www.apha.org/policies-and-advocacy/public-health-policy-statements/policy-database/2017/01/17/opportunities-for-health-collaboration

Andreassen, C. S., Griffiths, M. D., Sinha, R., Hetland, J. & Pallesen, S. (2016). The relationships between workaholism and symptoms of psychiatric disorders: A large-scale cross-sectional study. *PLoS ONE*, **11**(5), e0152978. https://doi.org/10.1371/journal.pone.0152978

Bandura, A. (1986). *Social Foundations of Thought and Action: A Social Cognitive Theory.* Englewood Cliffs, NJ: Prentice-Hall.

Bauman, L. J., Silver, E. J. & Stein, R. E. K. (2006). Cumulative social disadvantage and child health. *Pediatrics*, **117**(4), 1321–1328. https://doi.org/10.1542/ped.2005-1647

Beech, B. M., Fitzgibbon, M. L., Resnicow, K. & Whitt-Glover, M. C. (2011). The impact of socioeconomic factors and the built environment on childhood and adolescent obesity. *Childhood Obesity*, **7**(1), 19–24. https://doi.org/10.1089/chi.2011.0106

Bernstein, K. T., Galea, S., Ahern, J., Tracy, M. & Vlahov, D. (2007). The built environment and alcohol consumption in urban neighborhoods. *Drug and Alcohol Dependence*, **91**(2–3), 244–252. https://doi.org/10.1016/j.drugalcdep.2007.06.006

Blacksher, E. & Lovasi, G. S. (2012). Place-focused physical activity research, human agency, and social justice in public health: Taking agency seriously in studies of the built environment. *Health & Place*, **18**(2), 172–179. https://doi.org/10.1016/j.healthplace.2011.08.019

Braveman, P. A. & Egerter, S. (2013). *Overcoming obstacles to health in 2013 and beyond.* Robert Wood Johnson Foundation Commission to Build a Healthier America. Retrieved from https://www.rwjf.org/en/library/research/2013/06/overcoming-obstacles-to-health-in-2013-and-beyond.html

Braveman, P. A., Egerter, S. & Williams, D. R. (2011). The social determinants of health: Coming of age. *Annual Review of Public Health*, **32**(1), 381–398. https://doi.org/10.1146/annurev-publhealth-031210-101218

Bronfenbrenner, U. (1977). Toward an experimental ecology of human development. *American Psychologist*, **32**(7), 513–531. https://doi.org/10.1037/0003-066X.32.7.513

Brooks, B., McBee, M., Pack, R. & Alamian, A. (2017). The effects of rurality on substance use disorder diagnosis: A multiple-groups latent class analysis. *Addictive Behaviors*, **68**, 24–29. https://doi.org/10.1016/j.addbeh.2017.01.019

Brown, G. W. & Harris, T. O. (1978). *Social Origins of Depression: A Study of Psychiatric Disorder in Women.* New York: Free Press.

Burns, P. A. & Snow, R. C. (2012). The built environment & the impact of neighborhood characteristics on youth sexual risk behavior in Cape Town, South Africa. *Health & Place*, **18**(5), 1088–1100. https://doi.org/10.1016/j.healthplace.2012.04.013

Burrows, T., Skinner, J., McKenna, R. & Rollo, M. (2017). Food addiction, binge eating disorder, and obesity: Is there a relationship? *Behavioral Sciences*, **7**(3), bs7030054. https://doi.org/10.3390/bs7030054

Carroll-Scott, A., Gilstad-Hayden, K., Rosenthal, L., et al. (2013). Disentangling neighborhood contextual associations with child body mass index, diet, and physical activity: The role of built, socioeconomic, and social environments. *Social Science & Medicine*, **95**, 106–114. https://doi.org/10.1016/j.socscimed.2013.04.003

Casazza, K., Brown, A., Astrup, A., et al. (2015). Weighing the evidence of common beliefs in obesity research. *Critical Reviews in Food Science and Nutrition*, **55**(14), 2014–2053. https://doi.org/10.1080/10408398.2014.922044

Centers for Disease Control and Prevention [CDC] (2007). Cigarette smoking among adults – United States, 2006. *Morbidity and Mortality Weekly Report*, **56**(44), 1157–1161. Retrieved from http://www.jstor.org/stable/23318296

Centers for Disease Control and Prevention [CDC] (2009). *Recommended Community Strategies and Measurements to Prevent Obesity in the United States: Implementation and Measurement Guide* (Vol. MMWR 2009). Atlanta, GA: US Dept of Health & Human Services.

Cerdá, M., Ransome, Y., Keyes, K. M., et al. (2013). Revisiting the role of the urban environment in substance use: The case of analgesic overdose fatalities. *American Journal of Public Health*, **103**(12), 2252–2260. https://doi.org/10.2105/AJPH.2012.301347

Chaix, B., Billaudeau, N., Thomas, F., et al. (2011). Neighborhood effects on health: Correcting bias from neighborhood effects on participation. *Epidemiology*, **22**(1), 18–26. https://doi.org/10.1097/EDE.0b013e3181fd2961

Chaloupka, F. J. & Wechsler, H. (1996). Binge drinking in college: The impact of price, availability, and alcohol control policies. *Contemporary Economic Policy*, **14**(4), 112–124. https://doi.org/10.1111/j.1465-7287.1996.tb00638.x

Cohen, D. A., Inagami, S. & Finch, B. (2008). The built environment and collective efficacy. *Health & Place*, **14**(2), 198–208. https://doi.org/10.1016/j.healthplace.2007.06.001

Coleman, J. S. (2000). Social capital in the creation of human capital. In E. L. Lesser (Ed.), *Knowledge and Social Capital: Foundations and Applications.* Boston: Butterworth-Heinemann, pp. 17–41.

Commission on Social Determinants of Health (2008). *Closing the Gap in a Generation: Health Equity Through Action on the Social Determinants of Health. Final Report of the Commission on Social Determinants of Health.* Retrieved from World Health Organization: www.who.int/social_determinants/thecommission/finalreport/en/

Cook, B., Hausenblas, H. & Freimuth, M. (2014). Exercise addiction and compulsive exercising: Relationship to eating disorders, substance use disorders, and addictive disorders. In T. Brewerton & D. A. Baker (Eds.), *Eating Disorders, Addictions and Substance Use Disorders.* Berlin, Heidelberg: Springer. https://doi.org/10.1007/978-3-642-45378-6_7

Corrêa, E. N., Schmitz, B. de A. S. & Vasconcelos, F. de A. G. de. (2015). Aspects of the built environment associated with obesity in children and adolescents: A narrative review. *Revista de Nutrição*, **28**(3), 327–340. https://doi.org/10.1590/1415-52732015000300009

Cubbin, C., Hadden, W. C. & Winkleby, M. A. (2001). Neighborhood context and cardiovascular disease risk factors: The contribution of material deprivation. *Ethnicity & Disease*, **11**(4), 687–700.

Cummings, K. M., Fong, G. T. & Borland, R. (2009). Environmental influences on tobacco use: Evidence from societal and community influences on tobacco use and dependence. *Annual Review of Clinical Psychology*, **5**, 433–458. https://doi.org/10.1146/annurev.clinpsy.032408.153607

Curtis, S., Cave, B. & Coutts, A. (2002). Is urban regeneration good for health? Perceptions and theories of the health impacts of urban change. *Environment & Planning C: Government & Policy*, **20**(4), 517–534. https://doi.org/10.1068/c02r

Dalbey, M. (2008). Implementing smart growth strategies in rural America: Development patterns that support public health goals. *Journal of Public Health Management and Practice*, **14**(3), 238–243. https://doi.org/10.1097/01.PHH.0000316482.65135.e8

Davis, C. (2013). Compulsive overeating as an addictive behavior: Overlap between food addiction and binge eating disorder. *Current Obesity Reports*, **2**(2), 171–178. https://doi.org/10.1007/s13679-013-0049-8

Davis, R., Rivera, D. & Parks, L. F. (2015). *Moving from Understanding to Action on Health Equity: Social Determinants of Health Frameworks and THRIVE.* Retrieved from www.preventioninstitute.org/publications/moving-understanding-action-health-equity-social-determinants-health-frameworks-and

Deering, K. N., Rusch, M., Amram, O., et al. (2014). Piloting a "spatial isolation" index: The built environment and sexual and drug use risks to sex workers. *International Journal of Drug Policy*, **25**(3), 533–542. https://doi.org/10.1016/j.drugpo.2013.12.002

Diez-Roux, A. V. (1998). Bringing context back into epidemiology: Variables and fallacies in multilevel analysis. *American Journal of Public Health*, **88**(2), 216–222. https://doi.org/10.2105/AJPH.88.2.216

Diez-Roux, A. V. (2004). Estimating neighborhood health effects: The challenges of causal inference in a complex world. *Social Science & Medicine*, **58**(10), 1953–1960. https://doi.org/10.1016/S0277-9536(03)00414-3

Draus, P., Roddy, J. & Asabigi, K. (2015). Streets, strolls and spots: Sex work, drug use and social space in Detroit. *International Journal of Drug Policy*, **26**(5), 453–460. https://doi.org/10.1016/j.drugpo.2015.01.004

Evans, G. W. & Kantrowitz, E. (2002). Socioeconomic status and health: The potential role of environmental risk exposure. *Annual Review of Public Health*, **23**(1), 303–331. https://doi.org/10.1146/annurev.publhealth.23.112001.112349

Everitt, B. J. & Robbins, T. W. (2016). Drug addiction: Updating actions to habits to compulsions ten years on. *Annual Review of Psychology*, **67**, 23–50. https://doi.org/10.1146/annurev-psych-122414-033457

Ewald, D. R., Strack, R. W. & Orsini, M. M. (2019). Rethinking addiction. *Global Pediatric Health*, **6**, 1–16. https://doi.org/10.1177/2333794X18821943

Fattore, L. (2014). Sex differences in addictive disorders. *Frontiers in Neuroendocrinology*, **35**(3), 272–284. https://doi.org/10.1016/j.yfrne.2014.04.003

Federal Reserve System & Brookings Institution (2008). *The Enduring Challenge of Concentrated Poverty in America: Case Studies from Communities Across the U.S.*,

In D. Erickson, C. Reid, L. Nelson, A. O'Shaughnessy & A. Berube (Eds.). Washington, DC: Federal Reserve System. Retrieved from www.federalreserve.gov/publications.htm

Ferlander, S. (2016). The importance of different rorms of social capital for health. *Acta Sociologica*, **50**(2), 115–128. https://doi.org/10.1177/0001699307077654

Freudenberg, N. (2007). From lifestyle to social determinants: New directions for community health promotion research and practice. *Preventing Chronic Disease*, **4**(3). Retrieved from www.cdc.gov/pcd/issues/2007/jul/06_0194.htm

Freudenberg, N., Franzosa, E., Chisholm, J. & Libman, K. (2015). New approaches for moving upstream: How state and local health departments can transform practice to reduce health inequalities. *Health Education & Behavior*, **42**(1), 46S–56S. https://doi.org/10.1177/1090198114568304

Galea, S. & Vlahov, D. (2002). Social determinants and the health of drug users: Socioeconomic status, homelessness, and incarceration. *Public Health Reports*, **117** (Supplement 1), S135–S145.

Galea, S., Rudenstine, S. & Vlahov, D. (2005). Drug use, misuse, and the urban environment. *Drug and Alcohol Review*, **24**(2), 127–136. https://doi.org/10.1080/09595230500102509

Galvez, M. P., Pearl, M. & Yen, I. H. (2010). Childhood obesity and the built environment. *Current Opinion in Pediatrics*, **22**(2), 202–207. https://doi.org/10.1097/MOP.0b013e328336eb6f

Gearhardt, A. N., Bragg, M. A., Pearl, R. L., et al. (2012). Obesity and public policy. *Annual Review of Clinical Psychology*, **8**(1), 405–430. https://doi.org/10.1146/annurev-clinpsy-032511-143129

Gearhardt, A. N., Corbin, W. R. & Brownell, K. D. (2009). Food addiction: An examination of the diagnostic criteria for dependence. *Journal of Addiction Medicine*, **3**(1), 1–7. https://doi.org/10.1097/ADM.0b013e318193c993

Gearhardt, A. N., Grilo, C. M., DiLeone, R. J., Brownell, K. D. & Potenza, M. N. (2011). Can food be addictive? Public health and policy implications. *Addiction*, **106**(7), 1208–1212. https://doi.org/10.1111/j.1360-0443.2010.03301.x

Getis, A. (2010). Spatial autocorrelation. In M. M. Fischer & A. Getis (Eds.), *Handbook of Applied Spatial Analysis*. Berlin, Heidelberg: Springer Berlin Heidelberg, pp. 255–278. https://doi.org/10.1007/978-3-642-03647-7_14

Giles-Corti, B. & Donovan, R. J. (2003). Relative influences of individual, social environmental, and physical environmental correlates of walking. *American Journal of Public Health*, **93** (9), 1583–1589. https://doi.org/10.2105/AJPH.93.9.1583

Glanz, K. & Kegler, M. C. (2008). *Environments: Theory, Research and Measures of the Built Environment*. Division of Cancer Control and Population Sciences, National Cancer Institute. Retrieved from https://cancercontrol.cancer.gov/brp/research/constructs/environments.html

Goldberg, D. S. (2012). Social justice, health inequalities and methodological individualism in US health promotion. *Public Health Ethics*, **5**(2), 104–115. https://doi.org/10.1093/phe/phs013

Gostin, L. O. & Martinez, R. M. (2004). The future of the public's health: Vision, values, and strategies. *Health Affairs*, **23**(4), 96–107. https://doi.org/10.1377/hlthaff.23.4.96

Gottlieb, L., Sandel, M. & Adler, N. E. (2013). Collecting and applying data on social determinants of health in health care settings. *JAMA Internal Medicine*, **173**(11), 1017–1020. https://doi.org/10.1001/jamainternmed.2013.560

Greenland, S. & Robins, J. M. (1986). Identifiability, exchangeability, and epidemiological confounding. *International Journal of Epidemiology*, **15**(3), 413–419.

Gruen, R. L., Pearson, S. D. & Brennan, T. A. (2004). Physician-citizens - Public roles and professional obligations. *Journal of the American Medical Association*, **291**(1), 94–98. https://doi.org/10.1001/jama.291.1.94

Gruenewald, P. J., Ponicki, W. R. & Holder, H. D. (1993). The relationship of outlet densities to alcohol consumption: A time series cross-sectional analysis. *Alcoholism: Clinical and Experimental Research*, **17**(1), 38–47. https://doi.org/10.1111/j.1530-0277.1993.tb00723.x

Gundersen, C., Mahatmya, D., Garasky, S. & Lohman, B. (2011). Linking psychosocial stressors and childhood obesity. *Obesity Reviews*, **12**(5), e54–e63. https://doi.org/10.1111/j.1467-789X.2010.00813.x

Handy, S. L., Boarnet, M. G., Ewing, R. & Killingsworth, R. E. (2002). How the built environment affects physical activity: Views from urban planning. *American Journal of Preventive Medicine*, **23**(2), 64–73. https://doi.org/10.1016/S0749-3797(02)00475-0

Hankey, S., Marshall, J. D. & Brauer, M. (2012). Health impacts of the built environment: Within-urban variability in physical inactivity, air pollution, and ischemic heart disease mortality. *Environmental Health Perspectives*, **120**(2), 247–253. https://doi.org/10.1289/ehp.1103806

Hansen, P. G., Skov, L. R. & Skov, K. L. (2016). Making healthy choices easier: Regulation versus nudging. *Annual Review of Public Health*, **37**(1), 237–251. https://doi.org/10.1146/annurev-publhealth-032315-021537

Healthy People 2020 (2017). *Social determinants of health*. Retrieved October 23, 2017, from www.healthypeople.gov/2020/topics-objectives/topic/social-determinants-of-health

Hebebrand, J., Albayrak, Ö., Aden, R., et al. (2014). "Eating addiction," rather than "food addiction," better captures addictive-like eating behavior. *Neuroscience and Biobehavioral Reviews*, **47**, 295–306. https://doi.org/10.1016/j.neubiorev.2014.08.016

Hembree, C., Galea, S., Ahern, J., et al. (2005). The urban built environment and overdose mortality in New York City neighborhoods. *Health & Place*, **11**(2), 147–156. https://doi.org/10.1016/j.healthplace.2004.02.005

Higgs, P., Leontowitsch, M., Stevenson, F. & Rees Jones, I. (2009). Not just old and sick - the "will to health" in later life. *Ageing and Society*, **29**(5), 687–707. https://doi.org/10.1017/S0144686X08008271

Hillier, A. (2008). Childhood overweight and the built environment: Making technology part of the solution rather than part of the problem. *Annals of the American Academy of Political and Social Science*, **615**(1), 56–82. https://doi.org/10.1177/0002716207308399

Hughes, K. (2007). Migrating identities: The relational constitution of drug use and addiction. *Sociology of Health & Illness*, **29**(5), 673–691. https://doi.org/10.1111/j.1467-9566.2007.01018.x

Hutch, D. J., Bouye, K. E., Skillen, E., et al. (2011). Potential strategies to eliminate built environment disparities for disadvantaged and vulnerable communities. *American Journal of Public Health*, **101**(4), 587–595. https://doi.org/10.2105/AJPH.2009.173872

Hyshka, E. (2013). Applying a social determinants of health perspective to early adolescent cannabis use - An overview. *Drugs: Education, Prevention and Policy*, **20**(2), 110–119. https://doi.org/10.3109/09687637.2012.752434

Institute of Medicine. (2000). *Promoting Health: Intervention Strategies from Social and Behavioral Research*. Washington, DC: National Academies Press. https://doi.org/10.17226/9939

Irwin, J., LaGory, M., Ritchey, F. & Fitzpatrick, K. (2008). Social assets and mental distress among the homeless: Exploring the roles of social support and other forms of social capital on depression. *Social Science & Medicine*, **67**(12), 1935–1943. https://doi.org/10.1016/j.socscimed.2008.09.008

Jilcott Pitts, S. B., Wu, Q., Sharpe, P. A., et al. (2016). Preferred healthy food nudges, food store environments, and customer dietary practices in 2 low-income southern communities. *Journal of Nutrition Education and Behavior*, **48**(10), 735–742. https://doi.org/10.1016/j.jneb.2016.08.001

Just, D. R. & Gabrielyan, G. (2016). Why behavioral economics matters to global food policy. *Global Food Security*, **11**, 26–33. https://doi.org/10.1016/j.gfs.2016.05.006

Kawachi, I. (1999). Social capital and community effects on population and individual health. *Annals of the New York Academy of Sciences*, **896**(1), 120–130. https://doi.org/10.1111/j.1749-6632.1999.tb08110.x

Kessler, R. C. & Cleary, P. D. (1980). Social class and psychological distress. *American Sociological Review*, **45**(3), 463–478. https://doi.org/10.2307/2095178

Keyes, K. M., Cerdá, M., Brady, J. E., Havens, J. R. & Galea, S. (2014). Understanding the rural-urban differences in nonmedical prescription opioid use and abuse in the United States. *American Journal of Public Health*, **104**(2), 52–59. https://doi.org/10.2105/AJPH.2013.301709

Kim, D., Subramanian, S. V & Kawachi, I. (2006). Bonding versus bridging social capital and their associations with self rated health: A multilevel analysis of 40 US communities. *Journal of Epidemiology and Community Health*, **60**(2), 116–122. https://doi.org/10.1136/jech.2005.038281

Konkolÿ Thege, B., Hodgins, D. C. & Wild, T. C. (2016). Co-occurring substance-related and behavioral addiction problems: A person-centered, lay epidemiology approach. *Journal of Behavioral Addictions*, **5**(4), 614–622. https://doi.org/10.1556/2006.5.2016.079

Kypri, K., Bell, M. L., Hay, G. C. & Baxter, J. (2008). Alcohol outlet density and university student drinking: A national study. *Addiction*, **103**(7), 1131–1138. https://doi.org/10.1111/j.1360-0443.2008.02239.x

Larson, N. I., Story, M. T. & Nelson, M. C. (2009). Neighborhood environments: Disparities in access to healthy foods in the U.S. *American Journal of Preventive Medicine*, **36**(1), 74–81. https://doi.org/10.1016/j.amepre.2008.09.025

LaScala, E. A., Johnson, F. W. & Gruenewald, P. J. (2001). Neighborhood characteristics of alcohol-related pedestrian injury collisions: A geostatistical analysis. *Prevention Science*, **2**(2), 123–134. https://doi.org/10.1023/A:1011547831475

Latkin, C. A. & Curry, A. D. (2003). Stressful neighborhoods and depression: A prospective study of the impact of neighborhood disorder. *Journal of Health and Social Behavior*, **44**(1), 34–44. https://doi.org/10.2307/1519814

Lee, H.-S., Lemanski, J. L. & Jun, J. W. (2008). Role of gambling media exposure in influencing trajectories among college students. *Journal of Gambling Studies*, **24**(1), 25–37. https://doi.org/10.1007/s10899-007-9078-0

Lerner, R. M. & Kauffman, M. B. (1985). The concept of development in contextualism. *Developmental Review*, **5**(4), 309–333. https://doi.org/10.1016/0273-2297(85)90016-4

Leventhal, T. & Brooks-Gunn, J. (2003). Moving to opportunity: An experimental study of neighborhood effects on mental health. *American Journal of Public Health*, **93**(9), 1576–1582. https://doi.org/10.2105/AJPH.93.9.1576

Leyden, K. M. (2003). Social capital and the built environment: The importance of walkable neighborhoods. *American Journal of Public Health*, **93**(9), 1546–1551. https://doi.org/10.2105/AJPH.93.9.1546

Lipperman-Kreda, S., Mair, C., Grube, J. W., et al. (2014). Density and proximity of tobacco outlets to homes and schools: Relations with youth cigarette smoking. *Prevention Science*, **15**(5), 738–744. https://doi.org/10.1007/s11121-013-0442-2

Livingston, M., Chikritzhs, T. & Room, R. (2007). Changing the density of alcohol outlets to reduce alcohol-related problems. *Drug and Alcohol Review*, **26**(5), 557–566. https://doi.org/10.1080/09595230701499191

McLeroy, K. R., Bibeau, D., Steckler, A. & Glanz, K. (1988). An ecological perspective on health promotion programs. *Health Education & Behavior*, **15**(4), 351–377. https://doi.org/10.1177/109019818801500401

Milam, A. J., Furr-Holden, C. D. M., Cooley-Strickland, M. C., Bradshaw, C. P. & Leaf, P. J. (2014). Risk for exposure to alcohol, tobacco, and other drugs on the route to and from school: The role of alcohol outlets. *Prevention Science*, **15**(1), 12–21. https://doi.org/10.1007/s11121-012-0350-x

Milam, A. J., Johnson, S. L., Furr-Holden, C. D. M. & Bradshaw, C. P. (2016). Alcohol outlets and substance abuse amongh high schoolers. *Journal of Community Psychology*, **44**(7), 819. https://doi.org/10.1002/jcop.21802

Mitchell, C. U. & LaGory, M. (2002). Social capital and mental distress in an impoverished community. *City & Community*, **1**(2), 199–222. https://doi.org/10.1111/1540-6040.00017

Monnat, S. M. & Rigg, K. K. (2016). Examining rural/urban differences in prescription opioid misuse among US adolescents. *Journal of Rural Health*, **32**(2), 204–218. https://doi.org/10.1111/jrh.12141

Monteiro, C. A., Levy, R. B., Claro, R. M., de Castro, I. R. R. & Cannon, G. (2011). Increasing consumption of ultra-processed foods and likely impact on human health: Evidence from Brazil. *Public Health Nutrition*, **14**(1), 5–13. https://doi.org/10.1017/S1368980010003241

Moudon, A. V., Lee, C., Cheadle, A. D., et al. (2006). Operational definitions of walkable neighborhood: Theoretical and empirical insights. *Journal of Physical Activity and Health*, **3**(Supplement 1), S99–S117. https://doi.org/10.1123/jpah.3.s1.s99

Mulatu, M. S. & Schooler, C. (2002). Causal connections between socio-economic status and health: Reciprocal effects and mediating mechanisms. *Journal of Health and Social Behavior*, **43**(1), 22–41. https://doi.org/10.2307/3090243

National Prevention Council. (2012). *National Prevention Council Action Plan: Implementing the National Prevention Strategy*. Washington, DC: National Prevention Council. Retrieved from http://purl.fdlp.gov/GPO/gpo50605

Northridge, M. E., Sclar, E. D. & Biswas, P. (2003). Sorting out the connections between the built environment and health: A conceptual framework for navigating pathways and planning healthy cities. *Journal of Urban Health*, **80**(4), 556–568. https://doi.org/10.1093/jurban/jtg064

Nowak, D. E. & Aloe, A. M. (2014). The prevalence of pathological gambling among college students: a meta-analytic synthesis, 2005–2013. *Journal of Gambling Studies*, **30**(4), 819–843. https://doi.org/10.1007/s10899-013-9399-0

Nowell, B. L., Berkowitz, S. L., Deacon, Z. & Foster-Fishman, P. (2006). Revealing the cues within community places: Stories of identity, history, and possibility. *American Journal of Community Psychology*, **37**(1–2), 29–46. https://doi.org/10.1007/s10464-005-9006-3

Obesity Research Task Force (2011). *Strategic Plan for NIH Obesity Research*. Rockville, MD: National Institutes of Health (NIH Publication No. 11-5493). Retrieved from https://obesityresearch.nih.gov/about/StrategicPlanforNIH Obesity Research Full-Report_2011.pdf

Olsen, C. M. (2011). Natural rewards, neuroplasticity, and non-drug addictions. *Neuropharmacology*, **61**(7), 1109–1122. https://doi.org/10.1016/j.neuropharm.2011.03.010

Perdue, W. C., Gostin, L. O. & Stone, L. A. (2003). Public health and the built enviromnent: Historical, empirical, and theoretical foundations for an expanded role. *Journal of Law, Medicine & Ethics*, **31**(4), 557–566. https://doi.org/10.1111/j.1748-720X.2003.tb00123.x

Perkins, D. D., Wandersman, A., Rich, R. C. & Taylor, R. B. (1993). The physical environment of street crime: Defensible space, territoriality and incivilities. *Journal of Environmental Psychology*, **13**(1), 29–49. https://doi.org/10.1016/S0272-4944(05)80213-0

Pollack, C. E., Cubbin, C., Ahn, D. & Winkleby, M. (2005). Neighbourhood deprivation and alcohol consumption: Does the availability of alcohol play a role? *International Journal of Epidemiology*, **34**(4), 772–780. https://doi.org/10.1093/ije/dyi026

Popkin, B. M. (2006). Global nutrition dynamics: The world is shifting rapidly toward a diet linked with noncommunicable diseases. *American Journal of Clinical Nutrition*, **84**(2), 289–298. https://doi.org/10.1093/ajcn/84.1.289

Public Health Institute [PHI] (2015). *Making the case for linking community development and health: A resource for those working to improve low-income communities and the lives of the people living in them.* Public Health Institute. Retrieved from www.phi.org/resources/?resource=making-the-case-for-linking-community-development-and-health

Putnam, R. D. (2000). *Bowling Alone: The Collapse and Revival of American Community.* New York: Simon & Schuster.

Rahman, T., Cushing, R. A. & Jackson, R. J. (2011). Contributions of built environment to childhood obesity. *Mount Sinai Journal of Medicine*, **78**(1), 49–57. https://doi.org/10.1002/msj.20235

Renalds, A., Smith, T. H. & Hale, P. J. (2010). A systematic review of built environment and health. *Family and Community Health*, **33**(1), 68–78. https://doi.org/10.1097/FCH.0b013e3181c4e2e5

Rhodes, T. (2002). The risk environment: A framework for understanding and reducing drug-related harm. *International Journal of Drug Policy*, **13**(2), 85–94. https://doi.org/10.1016/S0955-3959(02)00007-5

Roberto, C. A. & Kawachi, I. (2014). Use of psychology and behavioral economics to promote healthy eating. *American Journal of Preventive Medicine*, 47(6), 832–837. https://doi.org/10.1016/j.amepre.2014.08.002

Sallis, J. F., Owen, N. & Fisher, E. B. (2008). Ecological models of health behavior. In K. Glanz, B. K. Rimer & K. Viswanath (Eds.), *Health Behavior and Health Education: Theory, Research, and Practice* (4th edition). San Francisco, CA: Jossey-Bass, pp. 465–485.

Sameroff, A. (2010). A unified theory of development: A dialectic integration of nature and nurture. *Child Development*, **81**(1), 6–22. https://doi.org/10.1111/j.1467-8624.2009.01378.x

Sampson, R. J., Raudenbush, S. W. & Earls, F. (1997). Neighborhoods and violent crime: A multilevel study of collective efficacy. *Science*, **277**(5328), 918–924. Retrieved from www.jstor.org/stable/2892902

Satcher, D., Okafor, M. & Dill, L. J. (2012). Impact of the built environment on mental and sexual health: Policy implications and recommendations. *ISRN Public Health*, **2012** (9), 1–7. https://doi.org/10.5402/2012/806792

Scarr, S. & McCartney, K. (1983). How people make their own environments: A theory of genotype → environment effects. *Child Development*, **54**(2), 424–435. https://doi.org/10.2307/1129703

Schonlau, M., Scribner, R., Farley, T. A., et al. (2008). Alcohol outlet density and alcohol consumption in Los Angeles county and southern Louisiana. *Geospatial Health*, **3**(1), 91–101. https://doi.org/10.4081/gh.2008.235

Schreiber, L. R. N., Odlaug, B. L. & Grant, J. E. (2013). The overlap between binge eating disorder and substance use disorders: Diagnosis and neurobiology. *Journal of Behavioral Addictions*, **2**(4), 191–198. https://doi.org/10.1556/JBA.2.2013.015

Schulenberg, J. E., Johnston, L. D., O'Malley, P. M., et al. (2017). *Monitoring the Future National Survey Results on Drug Use, 1975–2016: Volume II, College Students and Adults Ages 19–55.* Ann Arbor: Institute for Social Research, The University of Michigan. Retrieved from http://monitoringthefuture.org/pubs.html#monographs

Schulz, A. & Northridge, M. E. (2016). Social determinants of health: Implications for environmental health promotion. *Health Education & Behavior*, **31**(4), 455–471. https://doi.org/10.1177/1090198104265598

Scribner, R. A., Cohen, D. A. & Fisher, W. (2000). Evidence of a structural effect for alcohol outlet density: A multilevel analysis. *Alcoholism: Clinical and Experimental Research*, **24**(2), 188–195. https://doi.org/10.1111/j.1530-0277.2000.tb04590.x

Sévigny, S., Ladouceur, R., Jacques, C. & Cantinotti, M. (2008). Links between casino proximity and gambling participation, expenditure, and pathology. *Psychology of Addictive Behaviors*, **22**(2), 295–301. https://doi.org/10.1037/0893-164X.22.2.295

Sharkey, P. (2013). *Stuck in Place: Urban Neighborhoods and the End of Progress Toward Racial Equality.* Chicago: The University of Chicago Press.

Sher, K. J., Bartholow, B. D. & Nanda, S. (2001). Short- and long-term effects of fraternity and sorority membership on heavy drinking: A social norms perspective. *Psychology of Addictive Behaviors*, **15**(1), 42–51. https://doi.org/10.1037/0893-164X.15.1.42

Sherba, R. T. & Gersper, B. E. (2017). Community college and university student gambling beliefs, motives, and behaviors. *Community College Journal of Research and Practice*, **41**(12), 823–841. https://doi.org/10.1080/10668926.2016.1233142

Song, L. (2011). Social capital and psychological distress. *Journal of Health and Social Behavior*, **52**(4), 478–492. https://doi.org/10.1177/0022146511411921

Stockwell, T. & Gruenewald, P. J. (2004). Controls on the physical availability of alcohol. In N. Heather & T. Stockwell (Eds.), *The Essential Handbook of Treatment and Prevention of Alcohol Problems.* Hoboken, NJ: Wiley, pp. 213–233.

Stokols, D. & Shumaker, S. A. (1981). People in places: A transactional view of settings. In J. H. Harvey (Ed.), *Cognition, Social Behaviour and the Environment.* Hillsdale, NJ: Lawrence Erlbaum Assoc., pp. 441–488.

Suglia, S. F., Shelton, R. C., Hsiao, A., et al. (2016). Why the neighborhood social environment is critical in obesity prevention. *Journal of Urban Health*, **93**(1), 206–212. https://doi.org/10.1007/s11524-015-0017-6

Sussman, C. J., Harper, J. M., Harper, J. M., Stahl, J. L. & Weigle, P. (2018). Internet and video game addictions: Diagnosis, epidemiology, and neurobiology. *Child and Adolescent Psychiatric Clinics of North America*, **27**(2), 307–326. https://doi.org/10.1016/j.chc.2017.11.015

Tong, H. H. & Chim, D. (2013). The relationship between casino proximity and problem gambling. *Asian Journal of Gambling Issues and Public Health*, **3**(1), 1–17. https://doi.org/10.1186/2195-3007-3-2

Toomey, T. L., Lenk, K. M. & Wagenaar, A. C. (2007). Environmental policies to reduce college drinking: An update of research findings. *Journal of Studies on Alcohol and Drugs*, **68**(2), 208–219. https://doi.org/10.15288/jsad.2007.68.208

Treno, A. J., Gruenewald, P. J., Grube, J. W., Saltz, R. F. & Paschal, M. J. (2015). Environmental approaches to prevention: A community-based perspective. In R. K. Ries, D. A. Fiellin, S. C. Miller & R. Saitz (Eds.), *The ASAM Principles of Addiction Medicine* (5th edition). Philadelphia, PA: Wolters Kluwer Health.

Treno, A. J., Johnson, F. W., Remer, L. G. & Gruenewald, P. J. (2007). The impact of outlet densities on alcohol-related crashes: A spatial panel approach. *Accident Analysis and Prevention*, **39**(5), 894–901. https://doi.org/10.1016/j.aap.2006.12.011

Tucker, J. S., Pollard, M. S., de la **Haye, K., Kennedy, D. P. & Green, H. D.** (2013). Neighborhood characteristics and the initiation of marijuana use and binge drinking. *Drug and Alcohol Dependence*, **128** (1–2), 83–89. https://doi.org/10.1016/j.drugalcdep.2012.08.006

Ulijaszek, S. J. & McLennan, A. K. (2016). Framing obesity in UK policy from the Blair years, 1997–2015: The persistence of individualistic approaches despite overwhelming evidence of societal and economic factors, and the need for collective responsibility. *Obesity Reviews*, **17**(5), 397–411. https://doi.org/10.1111/obr.12386

Vaeth, P. A. C., Wang-Schweig, M. & Caetano, R. (2017). Drinking, alcohol use disorder, and treatment access and utilization among U.S. racial/ethnic groups. *Alcoholism: Clinical and Experimental Research*, **41**(1), 6–19. https://doi.org/10.1111/acer.13285

Victor, C., Scambler, S., Bond, J. & Bowling, A. (2000). Being alone in later life: Loneliness, social isolation and living alone. *Reviews in Clinical Gerontology*, **10**(4), 407–417. https://doi.org/10.1017/S0959259800104101

von Bertalanffy, L. (1968). *General System Theory: Foundations, Development, Applications*. New York: George Braziller.

Warner, T. D. (2016). Up in smoke: Neighborhood contexts of marijuana use from adolescence through young adulthood. *Journal of Youth Adolescence*, **45**(1), 35–53. https://doi.org/10.1007/s10964-015-0370-5

Warren, J. C., Smalley, K. B. & Barefoot, K. N. (2015). Perceived ease of access to alcohol, tobacco and other substances in rural and urban US students. *Rural and Remote Health*, **15**(4), 1–10. Retrieved from www.rrh.org.au/journal/article/3397

Wechsler, H., Lee, J. E., Nelson, T. F. & Kuo, M. (2002). Underage college students' drinking behavior, access to alcohol, and the influence of deterrence policies. Findings from the Harvard School of Public Health College Alcohol Study. *Journal of American College Health*, **50**(5), 223–236. https://doi.org/10.1080/07448480209595714

Weitzman, E. R., Folkman, A., Folkman, K. L. & Wechsler, H. (2003). The relationship of alcohol outlet density to heavy and frequent drinking and drinking-related problems among college students at eight universities. *Health & Place*, **9**(1), 1–6. https://doi.org/10.1016/S1353-8292(02)00014-X

Welte, J. W., Barnes, G. M., Tidwell, M.-C. O., Hoffman, J. H. & Wieczorek, W. F. (2016a). The relationship between distance from gambling venues and gambling participation and problem gambling among U.S. adults. *Journal of Gambling Studies*, **32**(4), 1055–1063. https://doi.org/10.1007/s10899-015-9583-5

Welte, J. W., Tidwell, M.-C. O., Barnes, G. M., Hoffman, J. H. & Wieczorek, W. F. (2016b). The relationship between the number of types of legal gambling and the rates of gambling behaviors and problems across U.S. states. *Journal of Gambling Studies*, **32**(2), 379–390. https://doi.org/10.1007/s10899-015-9551-0

Wilcox, P., Quisenberry, N. & Jones, S. (2016). The built environment and community crime risk interpretation. *Journal of Research in Crime and Delinquency*, **40**(3), 322–345. https://doi.org/10.1177/0022427803253801

Wilson, N., Syme, S. L., Boyce, W. T., Battistich, V. A. & Selvin, S. (2016). Adolescent alcohol, tobacco, and marijuana use: The influence of neighborhood disorder and hope. *American Journal of Health Promotion*, **20**(1), 11–19. https://doi.org/10.4278/0890-1171-20.1.11

Winters, M., Brauer, M., Setton, E. M. & Teschke, K. (2010). Built environment influences on healthy transportation choices: Bicycling versus driving. *Journal of Urban Health*, **87**(6), 969–993. https://doi.org/10.1007/s11524-010-9509-6

Wood, L., Shannon, T., Bulsara, M., et al. (2008). The anatomy of the safe and social suburb: An exploratory study of the built environment, social capital and residents perceptions of safety. *Health & Place*, **14**(1), 15–31. https://doi.org/10.1016/j.healthplace.2007.04.004

World Health Organization & Food and Agriculture Organization of the United Nations (2003). *Diet, nutrition and the prevention of chronic diseases. Report of a joint WHO/FAO expert consultation*. Geneva, Switzerland: World Health Organization (Technical Report Series 916). Retrieved from www.who.int/nutrition/publications/obesity/WHO_TRS_916/en/

Yip, W., Subramanian, S. V., Mitchell, A. D. & Lee, D. T. S. (2007). Does social capital enhance health and well-being? Evidence from rural China. *Social Science & Medicine*, **64**(1), 35–49. https://doi.org/10.1016/j.socscimed.2006.08.027

Zellner, D. A., Loaiza, S., Gonzalez, Z., et al. (2006). Food selection changes under stress. *Physiology & Behavior*, **87**(4), 789–793. https://doi.org/10.1016/j.physbeh.2006.01.014

Ziersch, A. M., Baum, F. E. & Putland, C. (2005). Neighbourhood life and social capital: The implications for health. *Social Science & Medicine*, **60**(1), 71–86. https://doi.org/10.1016/j.socscimed.2004.04.027

Part IV

Prevention and Treatment

15 Adolescent Drug Misuse Prevention: Challenges in School-Based Programming

Lawrence M. Scheier, PhD

Introduction

School-based drug prevention is now approaching its fifth decade of existence, and now faces a critical juncture. This crossroads of sorts arises because we have amassed a considerable literature detailing what works, for whom, and under what conditions. Nevertheless, we still find the American public somewhat reticent to implement drug prevention programs utilizing the school as a venue (Ringwalt et al., 2011). Added to this is an undercurrent suggesting that programs developed in rigorous research trials and supported by ample funding, may not be implemented with fidelity in "real-world" conditions (e.g., Gottfredson & Gottfredson, 2002). This is somewhat alarming given that pertinent information regarding evidence-based programs is readily available to school districts through various government sponsored websites.[1] Moreover, most purveyors of drug prevention programs provide ample support for implementation including heavy doses of teacher training (Kealey et al., 2000), including coaching (Reinke et al., 2014) and technical assistance all aimed at preserving implementation fidelity. More importantly, under various federal guidelines, schools are mandated to implement evidence-based programs. Congressional acts including the Drug-Free Schools and Communities Act (DFSCA, 1987) and subsequent refinements in the No Child Left Behind Act (NCLB, 2001) and it successor legislation the Every Student Succeeds Act (ESSA, 2015) stipulate that schools receiving federal support must implement evidence-based drug-use prevention programs.

In order to better understand what makes school-based drug prevention work, this chapter explores several different themes related to program construction, delivery, evaluation, and implementation. I begin with an overview of drug epidemiology obtained from one of the annual nationally representative surveys. These numbers provide a framework for understanding the extent of drug use as a health problem, and provide support for why drug prevention focuses primarily on "gateway" drugs including alcohol, cigarettes, and marijuana. I also cover major theories of human motivation that guides current drug prevention frameworks. One important topic that has received a great deal of attention revolves around "cultural adaptation" and what makes programs culturally sound. I use an example of a culturally grounded program to flesh out this discussion and attend to some of the key issues that need to be addressed when designing programs for racial or ethnic minority groups. I also attend to durability of program effects, consider mediation of effects, and the need for longitudinal follow-up to establish if programs can sustain their impact over an extended period of time, garnering support for their economic vitality. I also examine, albeit briefly, factors that influence program implementation including teachers who are the primary focus of delivery, and capacity building, which has been shown to influence program outcomes.

[1] Three relevant examples of Federally sponsored websites for obtaining information on school-based EBPs include: (1) National Registry of Evidence-based Prevention Programs (http://nrepp.samhsa.gov/), (2) California Evidence-Based Clearinghouse for Child Welfare (CEBC; www.cebc4cw.org/), and (3) Blueprints for Healthy Youth Development (www.blueprintsprograms.com). Budget cutbacks in the Trump administration have eliminated NREPP as a function of SAMHSA; however, the website reviewing evidence-based programs remains intact.

Ignoring the Evidence does not Make Sense

Perhaps some of the reasons for shying away from implementing school-based drug prevention is rooted in scholarly findings that reinforce that highly popular programs like DARE do not achieve their desired outcomes (Clayton, Cattarello & Johnstone, 1996; Lynam et al., 1999; Rosenbaum, Gordon & Hanson, 1998) or at best have quite modest effects (Ennett et al., 1994). Despite the moribund evidence, DARE still remains incredibly visible nationwide (Birkeland, Murphy-Graham & Weiss, 2005; Caputi & McLellan, 2017). As I explore in this chapter, and have mentioned elsewhere (Scheier, 2015), there is consistent evidence supporting a handful of well-designed, well-implemented, multicomponent programs with long-term findings supporting favorable prevention outcomes. This is countered, however, by evaluation findings, like those reported for DARE during the program's early stages, which do not support long-term favorable findings. Even alternative programs delivered through the DARE police officer networks have not fared well (Sloboda et al., 2009). To be fair, the program has undergone considerable revision to update the core curriculum (Hecht et al., 2003, Kulis et al., 2007) with preliminary positive short-term effects reported on putative mediators for the elementary school version (Day et al., 2017). However, additional evaluation findings reported by independent investigators remain mixed even with the refinements (Vincus et al., 2010) further bringing into question its suitability for large-scale dissemination (Caputi & McLellan, 2017).

Drug Epidemiology: Prevalence Rates of Drug Use

Understanding the complex relations between schools and drug prevention requires that we first assess the magnitude of the drug problem. The federal government monitors drug trends among youth using several different surveillance strategies. There are household surveys that produce a nationally representative sample including ages twelve to eighteen (Center for Behavioral Health Statistics and Quality, 2016), as well as nationally representative school-based surveys like the Monitoring the Future Study (MTF; Miech et al., 2017) targeting secondary school students, and the Youth Risk Behavior Surveillance Survey targeting sixth- to twelfth-grade students (Kann et al., 2015), the latter also including questions probing exposure to, and commission of, violent activities. There are also nationally representative surveys focusing exclusively on tobacco products (Office on Smoking and Health, 2015) and furthermore, the Bureau of Labor Statistics survey of labor force activity among youth that includes questions about alcohol and drug use (Jackson & Schulenberg, 2013). The different approaches utilize slightly different survey methodologies and canvass different aspects of the population. They also differ because youth truant or absent from school may be delinquent and failure to include high-risk youth may downwardly bias prevalence estimates (e.g., Kogan et al., 2005; Townsend, Flisher & King, 2007).

The MTF survey is one of the more featured national surveys, and has been used over a considerable time span to guide our nation's response to the youth drug problem. The survey reports drug prevalence estimates based on eighth-, tenth-, and twelfth-grade students and has been expanded to include a longitudinal study of college youth. Routine implementation of the MTF survey to surveil youth drug involvement commenced in the mid 1970s (Johnston, Bachman & O'Malley, 1977). A careful examination of historical trends shows that prevalence rates for high-school seniors were relatively high in the late 1970s, hovering around 92.5 percent, 24.3 percent, and 56.4 percent, for lifetime use of alcohol, cigarettes, and marijuana, respectively, and the same numbers were 71.2 percent, 38.4 percent, and 35.4 percent for past thirty-day use.[2] Fast forward thirty years, and the same numbers based on the most recent surveillance data (Johnston et al., 2018) indicates that lifetime rates are 61.5 percent, 26.6 percent, and 45 percent for the same three drugs, and 33.2 percent, 9.7 percent, and 22.9 percent for past thirty-day use, respectively.[3] These numbers are based on a total of 43,700 youth attending secondary school, 13,500 of whom are in the twelfth grade. Importantly, showcasing the twelfth-grade prevalence rates does not negate there are major historical shifts in consumption for the other age groups, with a lowering of the age of first use, and higher prevalence rates for some drugs than observed historically.

Indeed, in the ensuing forty years between these two time frames we have witnessed downturns in rates for some drugs, minor sampling fluctuation in others, and even notable upticks in some drug types.[4] Any period, age, or class "cohort" effects exemplifying downturns in consumption are often met quickly thereafter with increasing rates in subsequent years or the introduction of new drug types (e.g., "roofies" or date rape drugs, MDMA or ecstasy) that have demanded our nation's attention. In some cases, small fluctuations in rates of drug use reflect secular trends for a particular age group (seniors versus eighth and tenth graders) that soon dissipates. Overall, 1970 or 2017, still a sizable percentage of US youth have tried alcohol, with more than 25 percent having smoked cigarettes, and slightly under 50 percent reporting having tried marijuana before they leave high school. This is the type of information that fuels the USA's public health agenda and that has seen a dramatic increase in the funding portfolio of the nation's premiere institute that tackles the drug abuse problem.

Budgetary Considerations

The National Institute of Drug Abuse (NIDA), which funds a considerable portion of the US drug prevention activities, came about in the mid 1970s as part of congressional legislation. Public Law 93-282, or what is called the "Comprehensive Alcohol Abuse and Alcoholism Prevention, Treatment, and Rehabilitation Act Amendments," established the Alcohol, Drug Abuse, and Mental Health Administration (ADAMHA), a governing body that supervised and coordinated the functions of the National Institute of Mental Health, NIDA, and the National Institute of Alcoholism and Alcohol Abuse. Coinciding with this legislative act, the various programs and responsibilities of the Division of Narcotic Addiction and Drug Abuse (DNADA) and the Special Action Office for Drug Abuse Prevention (SAODAP) were moved to NIDA. Section 204 of this law, enacted on May 14, 1974, gave NIDA a permanent statutory basis, and established it as a freestanding Institute operating within the National Institutes of Health. In this time span, from the late 1970s to the current date, the budget of NIDA has soared from roughly 39 million dollars to over 1,077,550 billion dollars in the fiscal year (FY) 2017.[5] Prevention receives a lion's share of this budget, although it is hard to tease apart expenditures specific for prevention activities as they permeate the entire NIDA portfolio.[6] What can be gathered from these statistics is that the problem of youth drug abuse is both trenchant and costly whether one examines direct prevention expenditures or societal costs (e.g., Caulkins et al., 2004).

Theoretical Foundations of Drug Prevention

Most current prevention programs are guided in some part by a knowledge of risk and protective factors related to drug use (Hawkins, Catalano & Miller, 1992). This effort is supplemented by theoretical guidance primarily taken from social learning theory (Bandura, 1977) and self-efficacy theory (Bandura, 1997). The basic premise behind social learning theory is that learning occurs in one of two ways; either from direct role modeling or vicariously. Direct role modeling involves an actor that

[2] I used the 1977 data to correspond to a thirty-year gap to the current year. The first MTF assessment of high-school seniors was conducted in 1975, data were collected on eighth and tenth graders beginning in 1991.

[3] There are some slight methodological differences in the manner which surveys were handled in 1977 versus 2017. These include the methodology for handling weighting of survey responses and adjustments for the design effects, as well as the formatting of questions and the drug types covered. This is typical for a survey spanning such a long time frame, but a careful examination of prevalence before and after any item wording changes show there is little disruption in the pattern of findings for lifetime and thirty-day point estimates.

[4] This does not negate various drug crises and epidemics that emerged among young adults and adolescents including cocaine and crack in the 1980s, opiates more recently, and various other drugs that emerged in the 1990s (e.g., Rohypnol, GHB, and ecstasy). However, as we explore later in this chapter, the focus of primary prevention still rests primarily with deterring use of the three "gateway" drugs (Kandel, 2002).

[5] www.drugabuse.gov/about-nida/legislative-activities/budget-information/fiscal-year-2017-budget-information-congressional-justification-national-institute-drug-abuse. The 2018 budget saw a slight downturn to 865,000,000 under the current Trump administration.

[6] Public Law 96-181, passed in 1979 and called the "Drug Abuse Prevention, Rehabilitation, and Treatment Act," mandated that at least 7 percent in FY 1980 and 10 percent in FY 1981 of NIDA's Community Programs budget be spent on prevention.

is regarded favorably (i.e., older brother) and this exemplar models a behavior that is immediately demonstrated and followed by positive reinforcement. In the case of smoking, drinking, or using illicit substances, the role model, usually a person with high social status or value (older person, or a music icon glorified in the media) will engage in the behavior and this is coupled with immediate reinforcement. A media depiction of a valued social actor smoking cigarettes or drinking alcohol is highly persuasive to a young and impressionable child. The persuasive message reverberates around "looking cool" and being older, more adult-like, providing reinforcement for the behavior. Psychological inoculation theory (Evans et al., 1978; Flay, 1985) and even persuasive communication theory (McGuire, 1966) both build off the premise that one can slowly and incrementally build resistance to peer pressures to smoke and drink and teach youth to recognize false messages in media, entertainment, and television that promote drug use (i.e., actors that drink alcohol to relieve stress sends a message about coping).

Vicarious learning does not require the individual engage in the behavior first-hand; rather they can "watch" and learn. Based on extensive research (e.g., Bandura, 1965; Bandura, Ross & Ross, 1961; Bandura & Walters, 1963), a series of experiments showed that young children can view aggression being modeled by either adults or their same-age peers and then become more aggressive themselves when put into the same situation (i.e., these imitative responses were examined in experimental conditions using film-mediated aggression as children watched either adults or their peers act aggressively toward a "bobo" doll and then saw the "actors" rewarded and given candy for being aggressive). The coupling of reinforcement with behavior was "viewed" from a distance but was still quite persuasive. This is the same explanation given for youth watching their peers smoke or drink and then associating these behaviors with the subsequent rewards (e.g., looking older, making friends, being social). The fact that youth don't directly engage in the behavior does not stop them from learning the benefits of such behaviors. Associations like this are the foundation of "expectancies," laid down in memory, and the resulting reinforcement contingencies become hard to break.

Self-Efficacy Theory

Self-efficacy theory (Bandura, 1986, 1997) takes a somewhat different point of view and, while it incorporates some of the basic tenets of social learning theory, suggests additional reasons why youth may use drugs. According to self-efficacy theory, youth are susceptible to drug offers because they lack certain requisite skills to effectively deter negative peer pressure. Their vulnerability arises because they lack "confidence" in their ability to refuse drug offers and thus succumb to peer pressure. Botvin (2000) has outlined a case where youth low in self-esteem and lacking social skills, and who ruminate over their social status (i.e., neglected by their peers), are more likely to accept drug offers when given the opportunity in the presence of their socially valued peers (i.e., this boosts their self-esteem and positive regard among peers).

Drug-use prevention programs that incorporate self-efficacy theory blend social skills training with generic competence enhancement strategies to strengthen youths' confidence or sense of mastery (Griffin & Botvin, 2004). The increased sense of mastery that comes from practice fuels an expectancy; the latter is reflected by a series of mental contingencies ("if I do this then that"). These contingencies arise from past effort, the contexts surrounding this effort, and the product or "outcome" that is produced. Knowing they possess the right skill to resolve a problem, an individual will "believe" they can execute a particular task. In a self-efficacy formulation, the individual develops a cognitive schema or mental picture that they can mobilize the required skills and mastery to effectively meet the situational demands or engage the task at hand. This cognitive assessment fuels an "efficacy expectation" that determines whether or not the individual will engage in the behavior. Separate from an efficacy expectancy, an outcome expectancy then involves a determination of what will happen if the efficacy expectation comes to fruition and the person engages (the perception that reasonable goals can be obtained through mastery and effort). Skill acquisition is always based on knowledge and obtained through strategy development (i.e., repeated practice resulting in valid performance evaluations). The individual that practices accumulates sufficient experience (mastery) and then "knows" they can resolve the task, essentially motivating them to engage in it. The efficacy formulation then becomes a judgment of the individual's ability to produce certain outcomes (i.e., "if I say no to a drug offer, what will happen and how will I feel?"). In current prevention programs, the use of behavioral rehearsal, positive reinforcement, role playing, and group activities are all intended to draw from the theoretical adage that practice leads to confidence. More-confident youth will likely refuse drug offers and turn down peer offers to use drugs or engage in deviant behaviors. Confidence begets a course of action (i.e., motivation) and increases the likelihood the individual will be persistent even in the face of impediments (i.e., peer pressure), because the person believes they can obtain favorable outcomes based on past performance.

Many early versions of generic "life skills" prevention programs utilized self-efficacy theory as a framework to guide intervention strategies targeting competence and social skills (e.g., Botvin & Dusenbury, 1987; Pentz, 1983). The basic tenets of these programs suggest that social skills in the form of assertiveness training and techniques to reduce social anxiety will foster social efficacy and improve a youth's chances to refuse drug offers, without feeling their peers will reject them. In the case of multimodal programs, life skills including decision-making, goal-adaptation, problem-solving, self-management, and anxiety-reducing techniques (i.e., progressive relaxation) are posited to help youth combat the vicissitudes of adolescent development (i.e., storm and stress). These strategies are often coupled with techniques to promote school bonding, normative education (correcting misperceptions regarding how many peers or adults really smoke cigarettes), and lifestyle incongruence (i.e., who I want to be); with the goal of developing prosocial and conventional behaviors (e.g., Hansen, 2015). In theory, youth exposed to these programs will be better situated to deal with stressful situations beginning with drug offers, or given their own curiosity to use, and eventually including other situations that crop up and that may require garnering confidence to use condoms or avoid high-risk situations including unprotected sex (e.g., Griffin, Botvin & Nichols, 2006) and excessive drinking, even when the latter is legal for them (e.g., Griffin, Botvin & Nichols, 2004).

Cultural Adaptation: Are Culture and Development Independent?

In recent years, several authors have addressed the issue of "cultural adaptation," or finding a fit between a program and the host audience where it is slated for delivery. Weighing heavily on this debate is the issue of "surface" versus "deep" structure changes that may be necessitated in any adaptation (Greenfield, 2000; Resnicow et al., 2000). In order to fully grasp the flavor of this debate, one must first establish that a program has core components or "active ingredients," which reflect the underlying logic model. These components are direct reflections of theoretical underpinnings that represent the proposed mechanisms of behavior change (discussed above in terms of social learning and self-efficacy theory). Axioms, syntax, and postulates are the "glue" that connect the fabric of theory and intervention modalities with specific "teachable" strategies that target reduced vulnerability. For instance, using the examples elaborated in the theoretical section above, a program based on self-efficacy theory would include core components that build confidence, social efficacy (i.e., refusal skills), generic life, and coping skills. The actual intervention modalities might include behavioral rehearsal, and role-playing skits, all coupled with feedback and positive reinforcement after demonstrating newly acquired social skills (i.e., assertiveness). Eventually, with increasing mastery, and spurred on by their own confidence, youth will learn to "just say no" when offered drugs, or refuse to believe false media impressions that smoking cigarettes is "cool." In the simplest context, their increased confidence will cement indelible linkages between skills, beliefs, and behavior that reduces risk and promotes protection against drug use.

The essential question at the heart of the deep versus surface structure debate, is whether these theoretically driven core components need to be modified to suit a unique cultural or host setting. Any type of adaptation, cultural or otherwise, is going to modify or fine tune some aspect of the program. The crux of the debate revolves around whether these adjustments are meant to create novel program delivery and implementation schemes, or are meant to restructure core components. Resnicow et al. (2000) depicts *surface structure* changes as finding ways to match program content (delivery and types of activities) to cultural mores, including "people, places, language, music, foods, brand names, locations, and clothing" (p. 273) that are consistent with the beliefs and cultural mores of the target audience. Product brands (i.e., cigarettes or alcohol beverage types) can vary considerably between cultures as can media outlets, resulting in changes to program content to accentuate familiar cultural outlets.[7] At face value, surface structure entails adaptations to make a program more receptive, enhance the content's comprehension, and increase acceptance through relevance (reducing incongruity).

A *deep structure* change, on the other hand, involves revamping the program content and maybe even the program logic model in ways that can address differences in cultural views. The focus of deep structure change is on "*construal* " or how a particular culture, based on its history and perceptions, views health behaviors (e.g., certain cultures believe that disease is a burden placed on the individual by God). In the USA these views can include perceptions of racism, oppression, and economic opportunity for African-Americans, and acculturative influences (cultural stress) and ethnic identity in the case of Latino populations (e.g., Meca, Reinke & Scheier, 2017; Romero & Roberts, 2003). Furthermore, the messages tailored for Latino populations can capitalize on existing traditions including *familismo*, *respeto*, *dignidad*, and *simpatía*, all of which can be incorporated into prevention materials using telenovas (short stories) that appeal to the target population.

Gemeinschaft and Gesellschaft

To better appreciate what is meant by "*cultural views* " one can turn to theories of social change in human development (e.g., Greenfield, 2009). This perspective frames cultural differences by the concepts of *Gemeinschaft* and *Gesellschaft*, both of which are used to describe sociocultural ecologies. Gemeinschaft refers to "community" and is often used to characterize tribal customs in relatively poor, closely knit "back and hip" cultures (i.e., Africa). This includes "swaddling" a child in some type of portable carrier and working in an agrarian setting with the child nearby. The child is kept in close physical proximity during the day and this can extend to sleeping arrangements in the home where multiple individuals from an extended family share a common room. Gesellschaft, on the other hand, refers to dominant societal views regarding child rearing and that are often captured in more technologically oriented, urban societies, with clear division of labor and a less communal sense of child rearing and life. This would entail the Eurocentric view where parents' ethnotheories hold that children must learn to achieve autonomy, self-reliance, and independence as heralded virtues that are products of parental socialization. Children have their own bedrooms, are told to occupy themselves or play with siblings, and adult privacy is highly valued. In Gesellschaft social groups, the concept of child rearing involves parents who engage fee-for-service childcare including dropping off the child at a facility for the duration of the day (where all meals and naps are managed) and returning late in the day to retrieve the child.

Taken together, both social ecologies are a prelude to understanding the roots of "socialization" and the cognitive blueprint people use to articulate personal meaning. As Greenfield suggests, the former ecology is "folk" (collectivist) that prioritizes an interdependent family whereas the latter is "urban" (individualistic) that prioritizes self-hood and achievement. In order to garner success, cultural adaptations of drug prevention need to reconcile these two different "ecologies" that underlie socialization (i.e., values and learning styles), and address the different cultural pathways they produce in development (Greenfield et al., 2003). What may come of this is a better understanding of factors that contribute to racial or ethnic differences and more importantly what we often mistake as "demographic differences" that are the result of social class stratification, the digital divide, social complexity, family rearing, and values clarification.

Case Example

An example can help to highlight the intrinsic value of the deep versus surface structure debate. Suppose a parent–child drug prevention program includes two modules: one emphasizing social assertiveness (i.e., refusal skills) as a prelude to building social efficacy, and a second component emphasizing parental monitoring. Both components have sizable literatures supporting their inclusion in drug prevention. The program is being readied for implementation on a Native American Indian reservation and the program developer meets with local tribal stakeholders in advance of the scheduled training. In the weeks preceding implementation, the tribal representative reviewed the program

[7] In striving to clarify what cultural sensitivity means, Resnicow and colleagues define cultural competence as the capacity for the practitioner to deliver a culturally sensitive program, where the latter encompasses the norms, values, and beliefs, experiences, behaviors, social, and historical forces that affect the design, delivery, and evaluation of a program.

content and now comments to the developer that the program "won't work in this tribe." The developer is shocked to hear this retort as the program is "evidence-based" and has been tested for its effectiveness with racial and ethnic minority youth in New York City as well as other contexts. The tribal representative then explains to the developer that children are not permitted to speak back to their authorities and the "social assertiveness" component will foment trouble within the tribe. Even if the program component is meant to teach refusal skills, the close overlap between the contexts of peer-to-peer and child-to-parent relations will be problematic, particularly if children become more (inappropriately) assertive in front of their elders. This is an example of conflicting values that can be problematic for psychoeducational interventions.

After further discussion, the tribal representative suggests that the component addressing parental monitoring won't work either. Again, the developer is amazed by this feedback, as this strategy is incredibly effective in most drug prevention programs, not only his own. At this point, the tribal representative suggests that parental monitoring in their tribe is shared by many individuals, supporting the "pluralistic" approach they take to accommodate their reliance on subsistence agrarian farming and ranching. Many parents are gone for long periods of time while they take the farm animals to graze at higher mountainous elevations on their tribal lands. Their absence shifts parenting to the elders, who won't stand for some of the more "democratic" parenting principles taught in the program.[8]

As this example provides, there may be a lack of "fit" between a particular program (and its core components) and the host setting. This fit is what Resnicow and colleagues meant by "*cultural sensitivity*" and the need to modify program components. Changing surface features of the program, particularly how it is delivered, may not sufficiently address the reality that deep structures need to be changed. In essence, the program may require revamping to address the underlying socialization processes particular to a social group. Unfortunately, the prevention community focuses mostly on surface changes that strive to modify existing programs and achieve "fit" in primarily lower-income racial and ethnic minority communities. This is a big part of the fidelity versus fit debate (Castro, Barrera & Martinez, 2004), which may miss the mark if cultural adaptation requires "*deep*" changes in structural factors that affect socialization (i.e., Greenfield's view of cultural pathways driven partly by sociodemographics, values, learning templates, and development). A program that is kept primarily intact without pressing accommodation to its basic core components, is seeking to define cultural sensitivity based on surface structure changes (e.g., Kumpfer et al., 2002). This strategy may fall short for dissemination of programs outside of the USA in societies that are more collectivist (i.e., emphasize the importance of the group over the individual) or even within the USA to communities that reflect rich traditional "mores" carried over from participants' original countries (e.g., Muslims originating from Africa or the Middle East, or Latinos migrating from Mexico; or some American Indian lifestyles).

[8] Greenfield (2009) provides an excellent example of how shifting from a Gemeinschaft to a Gesellschaft environment for Mexicans immigrating from rural poor communities to Los Angeles in the 1990s created strife between local teachers and parents, because of their different learning and cultural styles. The result was to place child-rearing practices in the crosshairs with children forced to negotiate conflicting values because of this ecological transition and the intergenerational pressures caused by different belief and value systems.

To achieve a better appreciation of cultural adaptation, programs need to tackle the thorny issue of "deep structures" with greater scientific scrutiny and intensity. This means recognizing the deeply intertwined nature of culture, mind, and behavior (Bateson, 1972; Berry, 1976). According to these views, culture is a generative *process* rather than merely a collection of independent variables. In many respects researchers have failed to assess this process in a fundamentally sound way. Culture must be seen as "symbolic"; in other words, as a lens through which one can understand personal subjective meaning. A major point of departure for many cultures is the respective emphasis on individualism versus collectivism (i.e., relationship between self and group) and how these unique approaches to personal meaning color value systems and world views (i.e., *weltanshauung*). Reconciling the powerful influence of socialization as "organized cultural experiences" will go a long way to resolving whether a program can maintain its strong ties to psychological theories of human behavior while at the same time maintaining the integrity of the program in different cultural settings.

Examples of Cultural Adaptations

As many first-generation drug prevention programs moved from efficacy to effectiveness, developers initiated empirical studies to assess the relevance of program materials earmarked for racial and ethnic minority groups. Two, in particular, the *Life Skills Training* program (*LST*) and the *keepin' it REAL* program (*kiR*) bridged the cultural gap by reformulating their programs, albeit using different strategies. In the case of *LST*, the program developer mapped ways to make surface structure changes that involved program implementation (i.e., delivery) without changes to the core components and then tested the culturally focused program in a relatively large school-based sample of inner-city, ethnic and racial minority youth (Botvin et al., 1994, 1995). Program content was evaluated by Hispanic cultural experts, reading specialists, health educators, and urban minority students. Empirical findings confirm that the surface structure modifications were done reasonably well (using myths, language and idiomatic expressions relevant to African-American or Hispanic youth). Follow-up studies of these predominantly minority samples reveal lower rates of cigarette smoking initiation and escalation among treated compared to control girls over a two-year period (Botvin et al., 1999). Likewise, using the same data, Botvin and colleagues (2001a, 2001b) showed that binge drinking rates were lower in treated students compared to controls at both one-year and two-year follow-up.

A different approach to cultural adaptation is exemplified by the *keepin' it REAL* (*kiR*) school-based drug prevention program, which has been culturally adapted for implementation with different minority groups, including African-American and Mexican-American youth (Harthun et al., 2009; Hecht et al., 2003). The adaptation involves "*cultural grounding*" (Hecht & Krieger, 2006), an approach that combines community-based participatory research methods with various elements of communication competence theory (Spitzberg & Cupach, 1984). The strength of this approach is that it recognized that antidrug and prosocial behavior messages need to be relevant, flexible, context specific, and consistent with the language and values of the intended target population. To do this, the prevention messages must emanate from within the culture; based on the core values and communication styles of the intended audience. This "emic" or grounded type of approach uses focus groups, narrative and community stakeholder interviews to produce something "*from kids through kids to kids*" (Hecht & Krieger, 2006, p. 307). At a fundamental level, the program examines the contexts in which youth are offered drugs, the language they use during these encounters (i.e., methods of refusing offers, or communicating about the drugs), and the different communication styles that ethnic, gender, and racial groups utilize to effectively navigate day-to-day social interactions and normative peer pressure. This was the basis for the acronym "REAL" capturing *"refuse, explain, avoid, and leave"* as viable social resistance strategies employed by youth and that resonate with their cultural values rather than reflecting ideas formulated by adult curriculum developers.

The active ingredients of *kiR* emphasize *knowledge* (i.e., information regarding drug effects but taught using narratives as "stories"), *motivation* (i.e., emphasizing descriptive, injunctive, and personal norms), *skills* (refusal, stress management, decision-making, and effective social interactions), and *outcomes* (consequences of drug use for self and others). The instructional modalities include ten lessons that are taught by classroom teachers backed by five videos that depicts resistance skills in real-life situations (written by and filmed with high-school youth from Phoenix, Arizona, role playing as the actors). There are also community PSAs and school-based booster activities (twelve additional school activities offered in the eighth grade) that resonate the antidrug themes.[9]

Space limitations preclude a complete review of all the empirical findings related to *keepin' it REAL*. There is evidence from several randomized trials with extended follow-up showing positive program effects with intervention youth having a slower rate of growth in alcohol and marijuana use (Hecht, Graham & Elek, 2006).[10] Kulis et al. (2007) showed that *kiR* significantly decreased the likelihood of alcohol use and separately discontinued alcohol use (user transitioning to nonuser) in treated versus control youth. Recently, *kiR* has been tested in a randomized effectiveness trial with Mexican youth (Kulis et al., 2005) and also in rural settings (Colby et al., 2013). Findings from both of these studies continue to reinforce the efficacy of the program. An enhanced acculturation version of the basic program has also shown favorable effects (e.g., Elek, Wagstaff & Hecht, 2010). A small-scale pilot study examining the effectiveness of a translated version (Mexican Spanish) provided evidence of declines in alcohol and marijuana, but not for cigarettes in treated versus control students.

The core strategies of *kiR* have recently been incorporated into the basic fabric of the national DARE elementary (*EkiR*)[11] school drug prevention program. Analyses based on a quasi-experimental matching design indicates favorable immediate short-term effects on target social and emotional learning skills (i.e., proximal mediators). However, changes in mediators did not translate to reduced behavioral outcomes; most likely given the young age of the sample, very low base rates, and lack of variability in the outcomes (Day et al., 2017).

Strategies for Program Evaluation

An important element to any program evaluation is to show that the program worked in the manner hypothesized. This is termed a manipulation check and has also been called treatment construct validity (McCaul & Glasgow, 1985). Manipulation checks involve determining whether the intervention activities influenced the target risk mechanisms (hypothesized mediators), and then subsequently whether effects on mediators translate into behavior change (e.g., Judd & Kenny, 1981). Although the intervention targets drug use as its principal outcome,[12] the generative mechanisms that underlie these behavior changes are posited to occur through intervening mechanisms, which reflect processes within the individual that place them at risk and are the real "targets" of the intervention. Generally, mediators involve some form of social skills, competencies (i.e., self-management), norms (i.e., beliefs in the prevalence of drug use), lifestyle values, or cognitions related to drug use (i.e., expectancies regarding the perceived effects of drug use). Although somewhat oversimplified, following exposure to an intervention, mediators like drug refusal assertiveness skills are posited to change, resulting in less vulnerability to use drugs.

In the traditional language of mediation, the "$\alpha\beta$" effect captures the program's effect on the outcome "generated" through the mediator. According to this formulation, "α" is the path from intervention to mediator assessing action theory and "β" designates the path from mediator to outcome assessing conceptual theory (Chen, 1990). Further decomposition of the total effects produces the direct effect (τ'), adjusted for the "$\alpha\beta$" indirect effect. A significant indirect effect should reduce the overall direct effect as this variance gets partitioned.[13] Tests of mediation have been an indispensable tool to establish the magnitude of program effects (e.g., MacKinnon & Dwyer, 1993; MacKinnon & Lockwood, 2003).[14]

[9] The program is somewhat more complex than can be explained here and for purposes of brevity, I provided only topical highlights. A more detailed elaboration of program content can be found in Gosin, Marsilgia and Hecht (2003).

[10] The way the authors modeled growth, they included Time 1 as a covariate in one model and averaged the three subsequent time points as the intercept (reflecting average recent use). They also modeled Time 1 as part of the growth trajectory and then used the intercept to predict the slope term. In either case, prevention effects were favorable on average recent use and likewise on growth in recent use, the latter modeled based on all four data collections including the preintervention point.

[11] The elementary school version utilizes prevention strategies culled from social emotional learning theory (Durlak et al., 2015), an evidence-based approach that fosters positive adaptation, prosocial behavior, and academic achievement among younger children.

[12] In the absence of mediation, a significant direct effect could represent *"social diffusion"* where the precise mechanisms for active ingredients are not elaborated. Two things come to mind here. First, certain mechanisms of change have not been elaborated in the proposed logic model, but the effects are "real" just not disclosed (or modeled). In other words, crucial and relevant variables have been omitted (this is consistent with the Law of Indirect Effect). Second, some would lodge a complaint against the position that mediation is not essential to support program outcomes. This view is entirely "atheoretical" and given the heavy reliance on theory for drug prevention, such an outcome would not pass muster in light of the published Standards of Evidence (Flay et al., 2005).

[13] MacKinnon (2000) demonstrates that a significant direct effect is not required to establish mediation. Also, the direct effect can diminish in magnitude or be reduced to zero. Significance of the mediated effect is based on the square root of the variance term for $\alpha\beta$, which produces confidence intervals around the standard error of the mediated effect and can be based on the first-order Taylor series or the multivariate delta method.

[14] For the sake of brevity, the chapter does not attend to moderation, which is also a formidable part of program evaluation. Stacy et al. (1992), for instance, have shown that self-efficacy moderates the effect of social influences on cigarette smoking such that students low in susceptibility to peer social influence may not need to learn refusal assertion.

Importantly, Hansen and McNeal (1996) remind us that there is a "limiting" effect in mediation analyses. This arises because the maximum expected program effect on the behavioral outcome is tied mathematically to the relationship between the intervention and the targeted mediator(s). In other words, axiomatically speaking, the intervention is intended to change a youth's skills, beliefs, attitudes, and norms, and not directly influence their behavior (i.e., a social diffusion effect). The action theory portion of the indirect effect (α) will be quite telling in how large the overall program effect will be, because a strong intervention will change the mediator to a large degree but have little influence on the second stage in the sequence (β) corresponding to the effect of the mediator on the outcome. Hansen and McNeal couch this relationship in terms of the *Law of Maximum Expected Potential Effect*, which traces the "flow" of multiplying the indirect path from intervention to mediator by the path from the mediator to the outcome. A well-crafted intervention affects the "α" path but not the "β" path, the latter is relatively immutable to prevention effects.[15] Thus, effects sizes are more sensitive to changes that occur with the program's effect on the mediator rather than the mediator's effect on the behavioral outcome.

Although at face value specification of mediating effects would seem quite simple, it has been quite troublesome for the field of drug prevention for several reasons. First, many program evaluations omit testing the "causal chain" that involves positing the full intervention–mediation–outcome relations (e.g., Furr-Holden et al., 2004). There are a myriad of reasons for this omission. In some cases, base rates for drug use are incredibly low, which is quite symptomatic with elementary school interventions. Statistically speaking, with restricted variances it is hard to demonstrate effects of the mediator on the behavioral outcomes. When this occurs, investigators will resort to testing intervention effects on proxy measures including "intentions" to use drugs. As the cohort matures, effects on behavioral outcomes can be modeled in subsequent years, and with sufficient follow-up, prevention models can be extended to include additional high-risk behaviors (illicit drug use, unprotected sex, multiple sex partners and HIV risk, drunk driving, binge drinking, to name a few), a point to which we will return in the section addressing durable program effects. Notwithstanding, failing to model mediators, or modeling them without sufficient temporal lags, will unduly influence model parameters.

Other reasons include failing to specify mediation entirely and only examining direct effects, the latter emphasizing whether the intervention reduces drug prevalence rates. This is usually a first pass with many programs, to justify continued implementation for funding agencies and to maintain participation among the schools themselves. Subsequent publications then dissect intervention effects through mediation analyses. In some cases, an investigator will posit contemporaneous relations between mediator and outcome. This strategy obfuscates causal relations (e.g., Longshore et al., 2007). The study of Project ALERT with middle-school youth examined mediation from seventh grade to ninth grade; however, the outcome and mediator were temporally related, negating the possibility to examine true "intervening mechanisms" and disentangle contemporaneous relations (for additional mediation analyses experiencing the same temporality problem see also, Orlando et al., 2005). In effect, the designs used in these studies place the mediator too close in time to the outcome, not allowing sufficient time for development and consolidation of the target behaviors (i.e., skills). Only with repeated practice, reinforcement, and continued refinement can youth gain the required mastery to assert themselves socially and refuse drug offers or obtain better decision-making skills. The desired intervention effects may not occur when the mediator is assessed in the same time frame as the outcome.

In some cases, intervention effects take time to mature and youth require sufficient time to practice their newly acquired skills. Across several studies, many youth reported that they "get" the program, but didn't find opportunities to exercise their newfound skills. With time, their development catches up with program content (i.e., prevention may exert a "sleeper effect") and they find greater utility for the skills taught, greater opportunity to implement them, and greater understanding of the ramifications of drug use and negative peer influence.

There is also the issue that a single nomothetic mediation framework may not adequately apply to all students. In other words, youth may differ in the quality of their "vulnerability." For instance, one youth may lack social skills and find it hard to refuse drug offers, while another youth possesses adequate social skills, can refuse drug offers, but faces more active drug use norms among their immediate peer group (i.e., normative expectations are driven through peer socialization). In this case, intervention effects may vary between individuals and would apparently be tied inextricably to mediator status (e.g., low versus high social skills). This more complicated picture requires an alternative person-centered framework to adequately express program effects (Collins, Graham & Flaherty, 1998). Lanza and Rhoades (2013) suggest using latent class analysis to model intervention effects (with mediation) and avoid pitfalls of low power and a high Type I error rate normally encountered with subgroup analyses. Such analyses can guide the search for prevention effects according to possible unobserved qualities of the mediator (qualitatively different patterns in social skills) and on the basis of multiple dimensions (youth varying in their endorsement of peer norms) that may have gone undetected by the naked eye or using traditional linear regression approaches.

Prevention Examples of Mediation

The literature now contains several examples of investigators assessing mediation for both tobacco interventions (e.g., MacKinnon, Taborga & Morgan-Lopez, 2002) as well as gateway drugs (DeGarmo et al., 2009; Harrington et al., 2001; Liu, Flay & Aban Aya Investigators, 2009; MacKinnon, Weber & Pentz, 1989; MacKinnon et al., 1991; McNeal et al., 2004; Scheier, Botvin & Griffin, 2001). In addition to standard regression approaches, analytic frameworks for testing mediation have included growth modeling (e.g., Simons-Morton et al., 2005), and latent-variable structural equation modeling (e.g., Orlando et al., 2005; Scheier et al., 2001). Although these represent only a handful of the studies examining mediation in prevention, they showcase major features of mediation using a wide range of analytic techniques and with different programs.

In general, findings from mediation studies are quite encouraging with evidence accumulating that program effects follow the stated logic models. Indeed, programs based in social learning theory have demonstrated that intervention effects on drug use outcomes were, in most

Furthermore, there is now sufficient evidence showing that a more complete understanding of moderators of program effects is essential to understand how many drug prevention programs "work" (e.g., Donaldson, 2001; Hansen et al., 1991; Mason et al., 2009; Sussman et al., 2012).

15 Mason and Spoth (2012) suggest this may not always be the case.

cases, entirely mediated by peer influence variables (norms). Resistance self-efficacy was also a potent mediator in most cases for cigarettes and in some cases for alcohol. Orlando et al. (2005) showed that positive alcohol beliefs (expectancies or perceived benefits) significantly mediated intervention effects on intentions to drink and both past month alcohol use and misuse. All intervention effects were in the hypothesized direction. Using data from the *Life Skills Training* intervention discussed earlier, Scheier et al. (2001) showed that a latent variable reflecting "social competence" (i.e., social skills and refusal efficacy) mediated intervention effects on multiple drug use (alcohol, cigarettes, and marijuana). The analyses were temporally sequenced using seventh-grade baseline measures, mediators assessed in the eighth grade, and follow-up conducted in the ninth and tenth grades. Social competence (defense of rights, social efficacy, and refusal efficacy) also mediated intervention effects when the models were restricted to only alcohol users or likewise only cigarette users in an effort to test whether the intervention could disrupt developmental progression. Again, all effects were favorable, showing that increased level of social competence was associated with less multiple drug use among all types of users (controlling for baseline levels), less drug use among those students who reported only using alcohol at baseline, and less alcohol use in the ninth grade and less multiple drug use in the tenth grade among students who were only using cigarettes at baseline. The lagged design used in this study reinforces the program having durable effects on putative mediators that cast their effect forward in time to later behavior. However, it is worth noting that the authors did not test "cohort" effects and whether these effects were age-graded or only for the cohort followed longitudinally.

Testing Multicomponent Programs

West and Aiken (1997) provide several examples of how manipulation checks in the context of mediation can be used to detect optimal program components. Their approach relies on componential or dismantling designs to detect individual effects of active ingredients with multicomponent programs. This is an important experimental feature that can also serve as a reminder that program effects can be dormant for a certain time period and then surface later in developmentally appropriate periods (Sussman, 2017). This is to be expected, as youth may require time to practice and consolidate new behavioral skills. Drug refusal skills may only be operative if youth are offered drugs, which is highly unlikely to occur in the elementary school years, but more likely to occur when these youth reach middle or junior high school. Furthermore, one component can be highly active at one point but wane in its influence over time. This, too, might be expected in drug prevention programs targeting elementary school youth that emphasize peer norms, which may not be active for that age period as many youth don't actually smoke cigarettes or drink alcohol at this young age. However, by the time these same youth enter middle or junior high school more of their peers are actually using drugs and norm setting may be a more useful ingredient in drug prevention. The notion of what garners program effects is also germane to multimodality programs that may combine different arms, for example, using PSAs and media outlets, community efforts to raise awareness, and a school-based component. These complex designs make it almost impossible to detect what specific modality had the biggest effect, but the ability to tease apart component effects has been demonstrated with tobacco use prevention systems (Sussman et al., 2013).

Decomposition of effects with multiple components can be useful to signify dormant or null effects of a particular component. Dismantling designs also provide a concrete means of detecting iatrogenic or counter-intuitive effects that inadvertently increase drug use. Using program components that don't vitiate the intended prevention effects is costly because of resource and time constraints. Realistically, most developers of multicomponent programs are reluctant to shave off pieces of the intervention under the assumption there are "synergistic" effects between components. In this case, special designs like stepped-wedge regression, Latin square, or fractional factorial designs are needed to tease apart functional active ingredients from ineffectual components.

Establishing Durable Program Effects

A pressing concern in drug prevention is the durability of program effects. Although most programs can demonstrate some short-term changes in behaviors or likewise changes in the target risk factors, creating wide utilization and dissemination of programs require that these effects must be sustained over an extended period. This is especially true if we think about the context of drug prevention. Most school-based programs are delivered in middle or junior high school, with program content focusing on social and personal skills, values, and beliefs, peer norms, and resistance to media influences. The anticipated effect of the program many not take hold until years to come when drug use becomes more prevalent and youth find themselves in situations that require knowing, for instance, how to refuse drug offers. In their review of twenty-five tobacco and other drug prevention programs, Skara and Sussman (2003) showed that many programs do achieve immediate effects that convey to future years supporting long-term (more than two years) and consistent program effects. This finding is consistent with the premise of psychological inoculation that was part of many early smoking prevention trials (Evans et al., 1978).

The framework for understanding the literature examining durable program effects can be divided into two essential groups: (1) programs that have tested effects within the first year or two after implementation, which may be called "short-term" longitudinal effects, and (2) programs that have extended longitudinal follow-up to three or more years post-implementation. A few comments about the unique challenges facing longitudinal follow-ups are in order. First and foremost there is the expense of conducting longitudinal studies, which requires tremendous resources to locate youth both during the school semester (many youth change schools) and in some cases even after they have left the school system. Generally speaking, when conducting longitudinal prevention trials, funding agencies like NIDA or NIAAA usually provide money for five years of study. This is based on the premise of a start-up year for recruitment of schools, three years of intervention (seventh to ninth grade), and then a one-year follow-up. However, extending funding beyond this term requires additional rationally sound arguments embedded in grant applications for why the cohort should be followed coupled with good review scores that hold up to scrutiny in Advisory Council meetings.

There is also the concern over attrition (participation bias) that can occur as a result of inefficient tracking efforts and how this can affect both internal and external validity. Although social security numbers provide a formidable means of tracking individuals through various commercial, financial, and government databases, privacy concerns often prevent this personally identifiable information from being provided in drug prevention trials. This adds to the burden of tracking youth based only on school location and early contact information. The tracking process can now be augmented with the advent of social media (i.e., Facebook, Snapchat or Instagram), which makes it easier to find highly mobile participants. There is also concern with inflation of Type I error rates consistent with designating multiple outcomes (what has been called "statistical fishing" requiring the need to control familywise error rates), and selection bias (who can be found after many years of noncontact?), to name a few (Hill et al., 2016). The inflated Type I error rates often occur as researchers extend the search for program effects to correlated behaviors. For instance, developers of a middle-school alcohol or drug prevention program might want to consider whether the intervention also reduces risky behaviors like unprotected sex (Griffin et al., 2006) or drunk driving (Griffin et al., 2004; Shope et al., 2001) in young adulthood. This brings to mind that the original logic model to account for behaviors at a much earlier age may no longer hold, with potentially new mediators and outcomes needed to address the underlying causal mechanisms. This may require reformulation and developmental extension of the underlying prevention model.[16] This type of thinking has yielded developmental cascade models for both etiology (e.g., Eiden et al., 2016) and prevention (Patterson, Forgatch & DeGarmo, 2010) that reflect the need for extending logic models.

Findings from Longitudinal Follow-up Studies

A few longitudinal studies can be illustrative both for cigarette smoking, and separately for alcohol and other drug use. Turning first to smoking prevention trials, two longitudinal studies in particular deserve to be mentioned as they represent the vanguard for how longitudinal follow-up studies "*should*" be conducted. The first is a smoking prevention study conducted in Finland, called the North Karelia Youth Project (Vartiainen et al., 1998), a school- and community-based smoking intervention that tracked youth for fifteen years posttest. Interestingly, the actual intervention was of relatively short duration relative to other programs. Only ten sessions were involved, spread out from seventh to ninth grade. Also, the sample size was relatively small, encompassing 903 youth spread out over three experimental conditions including a minimal contact control group. Still, the concerted tracking efforts resulted in an overall retention rate of 71 percent, highest (77 percent) in the control condition. The fifteen-year follow-up included a survey sent home and a nurse conducting a cardiovascular risk factor assessment that took place in a local health center. These types of programs work well if the population relies on health centers or community health workers for provision of services.

Using students as the unit of analysis, the intervention had favorable effects at two-year (age fifteen), three-year (age sixteen), four-year (age seventeen), and eight-year (age twenty-one) posttests with reduced levels of smoking (use vs. nonuse, low levels, and daily) in the health education and teacher-led conditions, up to the four-year follow-up, compared to controls (Vartiainen et al., 1986). At the eight-year follow-up, the teacher-led condition showed favorable reductions in smoking compared to controls (Vartiainen et al., 1990). However, no significant differences by condition existed at the fifteen-year follow-up when the sample members were roughly twenty-eight years of age (although the pattern of findings remained intact with higher levels and rates of smoking among controls). Nonsmokers, however, were less likely to become smokers in the two experimental conditions compared to controls ($p < 0.05$). With school as the unit of analysis, to control for clustering effects and inflated Type I error rates, the intervention schools had significantly lower lifetime and monthly mean smoking prevalence rates compared to control schools ($p < 0.05$).

The Hutchinson Smoking Prevention Project (HSPP) provides a second example of a longitudinal smoking prevention trial (Peterson et al., 2000a). This fifteen-year study commenced in the third grade and involved a rigorous group-randomized matched-pair experimental design (Mann et al., 2000; Peterson et al., 2000b). The intervention was based on social-learning theory, and was characterized by high adherence, dosage, and participation (retention rates surpassed 90 percent) with no evidence of contamination across schools. Curricular features of the program included norm setting, refusal skills training to boost self-efficacy, identifying negative social influences in the media, values clarification, rewarding nonsmoking motivations, and securing positive family influences. More extensive information on the in-service teacher training, curriculum content, process evaluation, use of bogus pipeline procedures for biochemical validation of saliva cotinine, and analysis schemes can be found in Kealey et al. (2000) and Peterson et al. (2000b). Despite extensive attention paid to numerous important features of study execution and implementation in the real world, analyses provided no evidence of program efficacy at the fifteen-year follow-up. This included daily smoking prevalence, current smoking, cumulative smoking, and grade of initiation to smoking. There was, however, a slight significant difference favoring the intervention for number of cigarettes smoked per day among daily smokers. The nonsignificant longitudinal effects remained consistent two years post high school.

Sussman et al. (2001) suggested that the results of HSPP need to be interpreted within the context of a compendium of hundreds of other studies, which collectively provided compelling evidence that some school-based prevention approaches are effective. Moreover, they offered a rationale for the inconsistent findings in the field. For example, HSPP was conducted at small schools in primarily rural settings with primarily white youth. Moreover, the study did not include several relevant components that undergird the social influence approach and that are critical to obtaining prevention effects. Examples include listening and communication skills, decision-making, and making a commitment to a drug-free lifestyle.

In contrast to the smoking prevention trials based solely on social learning theory, longitudinal follow-up of multimodal drug and alcohol prevention programs have yielded more promising findings. For instance, Hawkins et al. (2001, 2008) reported on long-term follow-up from the Seattle Social Development Project (SSDP). Based on theories of delinquency, the SSDP reinforces the importance of bonding to school as a protective factor (i.e., youth identify with and adopt conventional behaviors through attachment to important and prosocial role models) and was launched in elementary school with youth followed initially up to age eighteen (Hawkins et al., 1999). Initial findings reported favorable treatment effects in several problem behavior domains (delinquency,

[16] Reformulation of the underlying logic model may also require a new "theory" driving the prevention model. For instance, a social learning formulation may work for middle-school youth with a focus on peer influence, norm setting, and refusal skills. However, as these same youth enter young adulthood the reasons for continued drug use may tap further into personality (risk taking or emotional distress) and require a secondary formulation that includes emotion focused coping, self-medication, or interactional continuity to account for continued life's problems.

drinking, sexual behavior, pregnancy, and school misbehavior). Subsequently, Hawkins et al. (2001) examined intervention effects on school bonding using growth modeling with an elementary-school cohort followed until age eighteen. In these analyses, a full intervention condition was treated in Grades 1–6, a delayed or late-intervention condition was treated in Grades 5 and 6, and the control condition received no exposure. The full intervention condition had the highest mean level of school bonding at age eighteen. In addition, while levels of school bonding declined for the delayed condition and controls, the same rate of growth significantly differed for the full intervention group, accelerating in a cuplike fashion at age sixteen. The experimental differences in school bonding emerged around age thirteen, a year after the intervention had concluded (i.e., providing some evidence of dormant effects).

Subsequent follow-up of the same cohorts at ages twenty-four and twenty-seven (>90 percent retention) provided evidence of sustained intervention effects on several important domains of interest (Hawkins et al., 2008). Multivariate analyses showed that full intervention group participants had higher SES scores (education and income at age twenty-seven), fewer mental health disorder symptoms at ages twenty-four and twenty-seven, and lower prevalence of being diagnosed with an STD at ages twenty-four and twenty-seven, compared to controls. No effects were observed for the substance abuse measures and the findings for criminal activity were counter to hypotheses, with higher rates in the full intervention group.

Conclusions

In this chapter, I have tried to present a fair appraisal of school-based drug prevention. This included reviewing the state-of-the-art in drug prevention with a careful eye cast to the theoretical principles that drive these programs, mediating mechanisms, cultural adaptations, and evaluation criteria. While this only presents a topical view of the field (it is a very complex thing to prevent drug use), addressing these major concerns should give the reader some inkling of what is required to develop, implement, evaluate, and disseminate drug prevention to the point where it has a certain heuristic value to address the larger issue of youth health promotion. One of the first things one considers when wanting to prevent something is "what causes it?" and this has been a difficult question to resolve for drug prevention field (Scheier, 2010). Like any epidemiological question regarding the proliferation of a disease, one attempts to address immediate causes of drug use and then focus on precipitating events. In the long run, this has led the field to the current point where most state-of-the-art programs are multicomponent, focusing on a compilation of social or generic life skills, decision-making, normative education, values clarification, cognitive misperceptions and providing some information about the consequences of drug use. The fact that most current drug prevention programs focus on a multitude of skills, beliefs, values, and attitudes does not by any means indicate that program developers do not have a sense of the causes of drug use; only that they recognize the complexity of the problem.

A persistent theme in the drug abuse literature is that many programs that get implemented have little if any evidence that they actually work. This issue has been raised particularly with DARE, given its prominence and wide uptake in the school systems. In truth, the field has benefited somewhat from the lack of concrete evidence supporting some programs. This has urged prevention scientists to move beyond what Kuhn (1970) termed "normal science" and find ways to push the event horizon and secure both conceptual and methodological advances. The current zeitgeist was fueled initially by the clarion call for credible scientific evidence, relying more on rigorous evaluation criteria (Flay et al., 2005), and establishing new benchmarks addressing "what works and for whom." Program developers have become, in essence, more scientific and this has been quite promising and most helpful (Hansen, 2015).

Along the way, there has been a branching of sorts, with the field taking on new issues relevant to implementation and dissemination. We now have a better sense of why certain school-based programs may not work and what impediments need to be addressed. This has come partly as a result of several seminal studies that examined more carefully what actually happens when a program is introduced and delivered in a school setting. For instance, what do the teachers think of the program and what actually happens in the classroom? Teachers are vital contributors to the school climate and play an integral role in the diffusion of any innovation, regardless of purpose (e.g., Beets et al., 2008; LaRusso, Romer & Selman, 2008). In particular, research has shown that their perception of organizational factors (support from the administration) and school climate factors (e.g., Payne, Gottfredson & Gottfredson, 2006) influences fidelity of implementation (Pas, Waasdorp & Bradshaw, 2015; Rohrbach, Graham & Hansen, 1993).

This type of evidence has encouraged program developers to think about not only the putative causes of drug use, but to extend their prevention models and also consider the framework of implementation, acknowledging that teachers modify content (adaptation) to suit the needs of their classroom and fit the program to the population they are tasked with teaching. As Ringwalt et al. (2004) have suggested, these slight modifications can be desirable given that in many cases teachers tweak the program to incorporate their students' unique cultural or sociodemographic contexts and in some cases adapt programs to the students' learning styles. More importantly, these types of contextual considerations have placed the discussion of fidelity versus fit (e.g., Castro et al., 2004) on the front burner, as more and more program developers see their programs undergoing modest changes when they transition from efficacy to effectiveness trials.

When it comes to teachers, programs are implemented with considerable advance thought given to their work situation, competing demands on their time, and importantly their resolve to teach the designated program in light of other curricular obligations. Added to this, research now shows the importance of securing stakeholder "buy-in" at the organizational (principals and district superintendents) level, which can lend precious support to the teachers in light of their time commitment. There is also recognition that diffusion of innovations involving school-based drug prevention requires a modicum of behavior change on the part of teachers (e.g., Kealey et al., 2000). Conceivably, many teachers may find the interactive delivery methods for drug-use prevention quite different from curricular instructional methods used for teaching routine coursework. As a result, there are lapses where teachers may resort to tried and true or familiar methods that deviate somewhat from the methods proposed in the teacher intervention workbooks. Regardless, recent studies of program integrity lends support to several teacher-related factors improving program outcomes including adherence, dosage, and whether the teacher is enthusiastic, involves their students, and effectively uses interactive teaching methods (e.g., Giles, Harrington & Fearnow-Kenney, 2001; Hansen et al., 1991; Ringwalt et al., 2003; Rohrbach et al., 1993). Even more importantly, when it comes to the question of "who should deliver drug prevention?" additional research shows that teachers fare quite well in achieving desired program outcomes when compared to trained health specialists (Rohrbach et al., 2007).

Even with these studies in hand, there remain additional questions. For one thing, what constitutes sufficient training for those tasked with implementing drug prevention in the schools? Research initiatives that have examined implementation fidelity consistently note deviations in the amount of program that gets delivered. This occurs despite extensive documentation of the program training methods, extensive technical assistance (Katz & Wandersman, 2016), and intensive training (with behavioral rehearsal, feedback, and simulations of what will transpire in the actual classroom), the latter taking place over the course of several days prior to program implementation. During these training sessions, participants receive exposure to curriculum objectives, program theory, drug use trends, and receive instruction in interactive teaching methods. Less examined, however, is how much training is both necessary and sufficient to boost adherence (e.g., Durlak & Dupree, 2008). Relatively little is known about which specific features of the context influence teacher adherence the most, administrative support, features of the school (i.e., organizational climate, racial composition, average class size), mutable characteristics of the students (i.e., engagement or conversely their delinquent behaviors), or individual differences in the teachers (e.g., experience, race, gender, grade taught, education, program-related beliefs, perceived organizational supports, and untapped motivational factors).

From an intervention point of view, one should consider if there are definitive steps to improve the overall quality of program delivery. This would require experimental manipulations with interventions at more than one level, including staging a drug prevention program for students and separately a teacher training initiative focusing on skills required to enhance program delivery. A simple design would pit routine teacher training against "enhanced" teacher training (and perhaps a third "booster" condition; see, for example, Pas et al., 2015) and then evaluate the effect of this treatment on program outcomes. Added to these concerns, one needs to consider capacity building at the district or community level to ensure adequate resources are provided to the teachers. Teachers are often strained in their capacity to teach and the addition of extra drug prevention sessions may be rebuffed if there is no administrative support. In the long run, ensuring teacher investment in program overtures and providing equivalent dosage to all recipients is crucial to ensuring the full program content is delivered and in a consistent manner. This goes a long way to rule out confounding by exposure and also to eliminate competing explanations for program failure. To achieve these goals, systematic studies that break down "implementation" into active kernels are needed and this has to be part of the science of prevention in order to better understand real-world drug prevention program effects (e.g., Berkel et al., 2011).

REFERENCES

Bandura, A. (1965). Influence of models' reinforcement contingencies on the acquisition of imitative responses. *Journal of Personality and Social Psychology*, **1**, 589–595.

Bandura, A. (1977). *Social Learning Theory*. Englewood Cliffs. NJ: Prentice-Hall.

Bandura, A. (1986). *Social Foundations of Thought and Action: A Social Cognitive Theory*. Englewood Cliffs, NJ: Prentice-Hall.

Bandura, A. (1997). *Self-Efficacy: The Exercise of Control*. New York, NY: W. W. Freeman & Co.

Bandura, A., Ross, D. & Ross, S. A. (1961). Transmission of aggression through imitation of aggressive models. *Journal of Abnormal and Social Psychology*, **63**, 575–582.

Bandura, A. & Walters, R. H. (1963). *Social Learning and Personality Development*. New York, NY: Holt, Rinehart & Winston.

Bateson, G. (1972). *Steps to an Ecology of Mind*. Chicago, IL: University of Chicago Press.

Beets, M. W., Flay, B. R., Vuchinich, S., et al. (2008). School climate and teachers' beliefs and attitudes associated with implementation of the Positive Action Program: A diffusion of innovations model. *Prevention Science*, **9**, 264–275.

Berkel, C., Mauricio, A. M., Schoenfelder, E. & Sandler, I. N. (2011). Putting the pieces together: An integrated model of program implementation. *Prevention Science*, **12**, 23–33.

Berry, J. W. (1976). *Human Ecology and Cognitive Style: Comparative Studies in Cultural and Psychological Adaptation*. New York, NY: Sage/Hasted.

Birkeland, S., Murphy-Graham, E. & Weiss, C. (2005). Good reasons for ignoring good evaluation: The case of the drug abuse resistance education (D.A.R.E.) program. *Evaluation and Program Planning*, **28**, 247–256.

Botvin, G. J. (2000). Preventing drug abuse in schools: Social and competence enhancement approaches targeting individual-level etiological factors. *Addictive Behaviors*, **25**, 887–897.

Botvin, G. J. & Dusenbury, L. (1987). Life Skills Training: A psychoeducational approach to substance abuse prevention. In C. A. Maher & J. E. Zins (Eds.), *Psychoeducational Interventions in Schools: Methods and Procedures for Enhancing Student Competence*. Elmford, NY: Pergamon Press Inc., pp. 46–65.

Botvin, G. J., Griffin, K. W., Diaz, T. & Ifill-Williams, M. (2001a). Drug abuse prevention among minority adolescents: Posttest and one-year follow-up of a school-based preventive intervention. *Prevention Science*, **2**, 1–13.

Botvin, G. J., Griffin, K. W., Diaz, T. & Ifill-Williams, M. (2001b). Preventing binge drinking during early adolescence: One- and two-year follow-up of a school-based preventive intervention. *Psychology of Addictive Behaviors*, **15**, 360–365.

Botvin, G. J., Griffin, K. W., Diaz, T., Miller, N. & Ifill-Williams, M. (1999). Smoking initiation and escalation in early adolescent girls: One-year follow-up of a school-based prevention intervention for minority youth. *Journal of the American Medical Women's Association*, **54**, 139–143.

Botvin, G. J., Schinke, S. P., Epstein, J. A. & Diaz, T. (1994). Effectiveness of culturally focused and generic skills training approaches to alcohol and drug abuse prevention among minority youth. *Psychology of Addictive Behaviors*, **8**, 116–127.

Botvin, G. J., Schinke, S. P., Epstein, J. A., Diaz, T. & Botvin, E. M. (1995). Effectiveness of culturally focused and generic skills training approaches to alcohol and drug abuse prevention among minority adolescents: Two-year follow-up results. *Psychology of Addictive Behaviors*, **9**, 183–194.

Caputi, T. L. & McLellan, T. (2017). Truth and D.A.R.E.: Is D.A.R.E's new Keepin' it REAL curriculum suitable for American nationwide implementation? *Drugs, Education, Prevention and Policy*, **24**, 49–57.

Castro, F. G., Barrera, M. & Martinez, C. R. (2004). The cultural adaptation of prevention interventions: Resolving tensions between fidelity and fit. *Prevention Science*, **5**, 41–45.

Caulkins, J. P., Pacula, R. L., Paddock, S. & Chiesa, J. (2004). What we can—and cannot—expect from school-based drug prevention. *Drug and Alcohol Review*, **23**, 79–87.

Center for Behavioral Health Statistics and Quality (2016). *Key substance use and mental health indicators in the United States: Results from the 2015 National Survey on Drug Use and Health* (HHS Publication No. SMA 16-4984, NSDUH Series H-51). Retrieved from www.samhsa.gov/data/

Chen, H. T. (1990). *Theory Driven Evaluation.* Newbury Park, CA: Sage.

Clayton, R. R., Cattarello, A. M. & Johnstone, B. M. (1996). The effectiveness of Drug Abuse Resistance Education (Project DARE): 5-year follow-up results. *Preventive Medicine,* **25,** 307–318.

Colby, M., Hecht, M. L., Miller-Day, M., et al. (2013). Adapting school-based substance use prevention curriculum through cultural grounding: A review and exemplar of adaptation processes for rural schools. *American Journal of Community Psychology,* **51,** 190–205.

Collins, L. M., Graham, J. W. & Flaherty, B. P. (1998). An alternative framework for defining mediation. *Multivariate Behavioral Research,* **33,** 295–312.

Day, L. E., Miller-Day, M., Hecht, M. L. & Fehmie, D. (2017). Coming to the new D.A.R.E.: A preliminary test of the officer-taught elementary keepin' it REAL curriculum. *Addictive Behaviors,* **74,** 67–73.

DeGarmo, D. S., Eddy, J. M., Reid, J. B. & Fetrow, R. A. (2009). Evaluating mediators of the impact of the Linking the Interests of Families and Teachers (LIFT) multimodal preventive intervention on substance use initiation and growth across adolescence. *Prevention Science,* **10,** 208–220.

DFSCA (1987). Drug-Free Schools and Community Act, 1987, Pub. Law. No. 101-226 § 103 stat.

Donaldson, S. I. (2001). Mediator and moderator analysis in program development. In S. Sussman (Ed.), *Handbook of Program Development for Health Behavior Research and Practice.* Thousand Oak, CA: Sage Publications, pp. 470–500.

Durlak, J. A., Domitrovich, C. E., Weisberg, R. P. & Gullotta, T. P. (Eds.) (2015). *Handbook of Social and Emotional Learning.* New York, NY: Guilford Press.

Durlak, J. A. & DuPre, E. P. (2008). Implementation matters: A review of research on the influence of implementation on program outcomes and the factors affecting implementation. *American Journal of Community Psychology,* **41,** 327–350.

Eiden, R. D., Lessard, J., Colder, C. R., et al. (2016). Developmental cascade model for adolescent substance use from infancy to late adolescence. *Developmental Psychology,* **52,** 1619–1633.

Elek, E., Wagstaff, D. A. & Hecht, M. L. (2010). Effects of the 5th and 7th grade enhanced version of the keepin' it REAL substance use prevention curriculum. *Journal of Drug Education,* **40,** 61–79.

Ennett, S. T., Tobler, N. S., Ringwalt, C. L. & Flewelling, R. L. (1994). How effective is drug abuse resistance education? A meta-analysis of Project DARE outcome evaluations. *American Journal of Public Health,* **84,** 1394–1401.

ESSA (2015). Every Student Succeeds Act of 2015, Pub. Law. No. 114-95 § 114 stat.

Evans, R.I., Rozelle, R.M., Mittelmark, M.B., et al. (1978). Deterring the onset of smoking in children: Knowledge of immediate physiological effects and coping with peer pressure, media pressure, and parent modeling. *Journal of Applied Social Psychology,* **8,** 126–135.

Flay, B. R. (1985). Psychosocial approaches to smoking prevention: A review of findings. *Health Psychology,* **4,** 449–488.

Flay, B. R., Biglan, A., Boruch, R. F., et al. (2005). Standards of evidence: Criteria for efficacy, effectiveness and dissemination. *Prevention Science,* **6,** 151–175.

Furr-Holden, C. D. M., Ialongo. N. S., Anthony, J. C., Petras, H. & Kellam, S. G. (2004). Developmentally inspired drug prevention: Middle school outcomes in a school-based randomized prevention trial. *Drug and Alcohol Dependence,* **73,** 149–158.

Giles, S. M., Harrington, N. G. & Fearnow-Kenney, M. (2001). Evaluation of the All Stars program: Student and teacher factors that influence mediators of substance use. *Journal of Drug Education,* **31,** 385–397.

Gosin, M., Marsiglia, F. F. & Hecht, M. L. (2003). *keepin' it R.E.A.L.*: A drug resistance curriculum tailored to the strengths and needs of pre-adolescents of the southwest. *Journal of Drug Education,* **33,** 119–142.

Gottfredson, D. C. & Gottfredson, G. D. (2002). Quality of school-based prevention programs: Results from a national survey. *Journal of Research in Crime and Delinquency,* **39,** 3–35.

Greenfield, P. M. (2009). Linking social change and developmental change: Shifting pathways of human development. *Developmental Psychology,* **45,** 401–418.

Greenfield, P. M. (2000). Three approaches to the psychology of culture: Where do they come from? Where can they go? *Asian Journal of Social Psychology,* **3,** 223–240.

Greenfield, P. M., Keller, H., Fuligni, A. & Maynard, A. (2003). Cultural pathways through universal development. *Annual Review of Psychology,* **54,** 461–490.

Griffin, K. W. & Botvin, G. J. (2004). The prevention and treatment of adolescent drug abuse. In P. Allen-Meares & M. W. Fraser (Eds.), *Intervention with Children and Adolescents: An Interdisciplinary Perspective.* Boston, MA: Allyn & Bacon, pp. 335–355.

Griffin, K. W., Botvin, G. J. & Nichols, T. R. (2004). Long-term follow-up effects of a school-based drug abuse prevention program on adolescent risky drinking. *Prevention Science,* **5,** 207–212.

Griffin, K. W., Botvin, G. J. & Nichols, T. R. (2006). Effects of a school-based drug abuse prevention program for adolescents on HIV risk behavior in young adulthood. *Prevention Science,* **7,** 103–112.

Hansen, W. B. (2015). All Stars: A conceptual history. In L. M. Scheier (Ed.), *Handbook of Drug Abuse Prevention Research, Intervention Strategies, and Practice.* Washington, DC: American Psychological Association, pp. 197–216.

Hansen, W. B. & McNeal, R. B. (1996). The law of maximum expected potential effect: Constraints placed on program effectiveness by mediator relationships. *Health Education Research: Theory & Practice,* **11,** 501–507.

Hansen, W. B., Graham, J. W., Wolkenstein, B. H. & Rohrbach, L. A. (1991). Program integrity as a moderator of prevention program effectiveness: Results for fifth-grade students in the adolescent alcohol prevention trial. *Journal of Studies on Alcohol and Drugs,* **52,** 568–579.

Harrington, N. G., Giles, S. M., Hoyle, R. H., Feeney, G. J. & Yungbluth, S. C. (2001). Evaluation of the All Stars character education and problem behavior prevention program: Effects on mediator and outcome variables for middle school students. *Health Education & Behavior,* **28,** 533–546.

Harthun, M. L., Dustman, P. A., Reeves, L. J., Marsiglia, F. F. & Hecht, M. L. (2009). Using community-based participatory research to adapt *keepin' it REAL*: Creating a socially, developmentally, and academically appropriate prevention curriculum for 5th graders. *Journal of Alcohol and Drug Education,* **53,** 12–38.

Hawkins, J. D., Catalano, R. F., Kosterman, R., Abbott, R. D. & Hill, K. G. (1999). Preventing adolescent health-risk behavior by strengthening protection during childhood. *Archives of Pediatrics & Adolescent Medicine,* **153,** 226–234.

Hawkins, J. D., Catalano, R. F. & Miller, J. Y. (1992). Risk and protective factors for alcohol and other drug problems in adolescence and early adulthood: Implications for substance abuse prevention. *Psychological Bulletin,* **112,** 64–105.

Hawkins, J. D., Guo, J., Hill, K. G., Battin-Pearson, S. & Abbott, R. D. (2001). Long-term effects of the Seattle Social Development Intervention on school bonding trajectories. *Applied Developmental Science*, **5**, 225–236.

Hawkins, J. D., Kosterman, R., Catalano, R. F., Hill, K. G. & Abbott, R. D. (2008). Effects of social development intervention in childhood 15 years later. *Archives of Pediatric and Adolescent Medicine*, **16**, 1133–1141.

Hecht, M. L. & Krieger, J. L. R. (2006). The principle of cultural grounding in school-based substance abuse prevention. *Journal of Language and Social Psychology*, **25**, 301–319.

Hecht, M. L., Graham, J. W. & Elek, E. (2006). The drug resistance strategies intervention: Program effects on substance use. *Health Communication*, **20**, 267–276.

Hecht, M. L., Marsiglia, F. F., Elek, E., et al. (2003). Culturally grounded substance use prevention: An evaluation of the *keepin' it R.E.A.L.* curriculum. *Prevention Science*, **4**, 233–248.

Hill, K. G., Woodward, D., Woelfel, T., Hawkins, J. D. & Green, S. (2016). Planning for long-term follow-up: Strategies learned from longitudinal studies. *Prevention Science*, **17**, 806–818.

Jackson, K. M. & Schulenberg, J. E. (2013). Alcohol use during the transition from middle school to high school: National panel data on prevalence and moderators. *Developmental Psychology*, **49**, 2147–2158.

Johnston, L. D., Bachman, J. G. & O'Malley, P. M. (1977). *Drug Use Among American High School Students, 1975–1977* (DHEW Publication No. [ADM] 78-619). Rockville, MD: National Institute on Drug Abuse, 256 pages.

Johnston, L. D., Miech, R. A., O'Malley, P. M., et al. (2018). *Monitoring the Future National Survey Results on Drug Use: 1975–2017: Overview, Key Findings on Adolescent Drug Use*. Ann Arbor, MI: Institute for Social Research, University of Michigan.

Judd, C. M. & Kenny, D. A. (1981). Process analysis: Estimating mediation in treatment evaluations. *Evaluation Review*, **5**, 602–619.

Kandel, D. B. (Ed.) (2002). *Stages and Pathways of Drug Involvement: Examining the Gateway Hypothesis*. New York, NY: Cambridge University Press.

Kann, L., McManus, T., Harris, W. A., et al. (2015). Center for Disease Control and Prevention, Youth Risk Behavior Surveillance - United States, 2015. *Morbidity and Mortality Weekly Report, Surveillance Summaries*, **65**(6), 1–173.

Katz, J. & Wandersman, A. (2016). Technical assistance to enhance prevention capacity: A research synthesis of the evidence base. *Prevention Science*, **17**, 417–428.

Kealey, K. A., Peterson, A. V., Gaul, M. A. & Dinh, K. (2000). Teacher training as a behavior change process: Principles and results from a longitudinal study. *Health Education and Behavior*, **27**, 64–81.

Kogan, S. M., Luo, Z., Brody, G. H. & Murry, V. M. (2005). The influence of high school dropout on substance use among African American youth. *Journal of Ethnicity in Substance Abuse*, **4**, 35–51.

Kuhn, T. S. (1970). *The Structure of Scientific Revolutions* (2nd edition). Chicago, IL: University of Chicago Press.

Kulis, S., Marsiglia, F. F., Elek, E., Dustman, P., Wagstaff, D. A. & Hecht, M. L. (2005). Mexican/Mexican American adolescents and keepin' it REAL: An evidence-based substance use prevention program. *Children & Schools*, **27**, 133–145.

Kulis, S., Nieri, T., Yabiku, S., Stromwall, L. K. & Marsiglia, F. F. (2007). Promoting reduced and discontinued substance use among adolescent substance users: Effectiveness of a universal prevention program. *Prevention Science*, **8**, 35–49.

Kumpfer, K. L., Alvarado, R., Smith, P. & Bellamy, N (2002). Cultural sensitivity and adaptation in family-based prevention interventions. *Prevention Science*, **3**, 241–246.

Lanza, S. T. & Rhoades, B. L. (2013). Latent class analysis: An alternative perspective on subgroup analysis in prevention and treatment. *Prevention Science*, **14**, 157–168.

LaRusso, M. D., Romer, D. & Selman, R. L. (2008). Teachers as builders of respectful school climates: Implications for adolescent drug use norms and depressive symptoms in high school. *Journal of Youth and Adolescence*, **37**, 386–398.

Liu, L. C., Flay, B. R. & Aban Aya Investigators (2009). Evaluating mediation in longitudinal multivariate data: Mediation effects for the Aban Aya Youth Project drug prevention program. *Prevention Science*, **10**, 197–207.

Longshore, D., Ellickson, P. L., McCaffrey, D. F. & St. Clair, P. A. (2007). School-based drug prevention among at-risk adolescents: Effects of ALERT Plus. *Health Education & Behavior*, **34**, 651–668.

Lynam, D. R., Milich, R., Zimmerman, R., et al. (1999). Project DARE: No effects at 10-year follow-up. *Journal of Consulting and Clinical Psychology*, **67**, 590–593.

MacKinnon, D. P. (2000). Contrasts in multiple mediator models. In J. Rose, L. Chassin, C. C. Presson & S. J. Sherman (Eds.) *Multivariate Applications in Substance Use Research: New Methods for New Questions*. Mahwah, NJ: Lawrence Erlbaum, pp. 141–160.

MacKinnon, D. P. & Dwyer, J. H. (1993). Estimation of mediated effects in prevention studies. *Evaluation Review*, **17**, 144–158.

MacKinnon, D. P., Johnson, C. A., Pentz, M. A., et al. (1991). Mediating mechanisms in a school-based drug prevention program: First year effects of the Midwestern Prevention Project. *Health Psychology*, **10**, 164–172.

MacKinnon, D. P. & Lockwood, C. M. (2003). Advances in statistical methods for substance abuse prevention research. *Prevention Science*, **4**, 155–171.

MacKinnon, D. P., Taborga, M. P. & Morgan-Lopez, A. A. (2002). Mediation designs for tobacco prevention research. *Drug and Alcohol Dependence*, **68**, S69–S83.

MacKinnon, D. P., Weber, M. D. & Pentz, M. A. (1989). How do school-based drug prevention programs work and for whom? *Drugs and Society*, **3**, 125–143.

Mann, S. L., Peterson, A. V., Marek, P. M. & Kealey, K. A. (2000). The Hutchinson Smoking Prevention Project Trial: Design and baseline characteristics. *Preventive Medicine*, **30**, 485–495.

Mason, W. A. & Spoth, R. L. (2012). Sequence of alcohol involvement from early onset to young adult alcohol abuse: Differential predictors and moderation by family-focused preventive intervention. *Addiction*, **107**, 2137–2148.

Mason, W. A., Kosterman, R., Haggerty, K. P., et al. (2009). Gender moderation and social developmental mediation of the effect of a family-focused substance use prevention intervention on young adult alcohol abuse. *Addictive Behaviors*, **34**, 599–605.

McCaul, K. D. & Glasgow, R. E. (1985). Preventing adolescent smoking: What have we learned about treatment construct validity? *Health Psychology*, **4**, 361–387.

McGuire, W. J. (1966). Attitudes and opinions. *Annual Review of Psychology*, **17**, 475–514.

McNeal, R. B., Hansen, W. B., Harrington, N. G. & Giles, S. M. (2004). How All Stars works: An examination of program effects on mediating variables. *Health Education Quarterly*, **31**, 165–178.

Meca, A., Reinke, L. G. & Scheier, L. M. (2017). Acculturation and tobacco/illicit drug use in Hispanic youth. In S. J. Schwartz, and J. B. Unger (Eds.), *The Oxford Handbook of Acculturation and Health*. New York, NY: Oxford University Press, pp. 281–299.

Miech, R. A., Johnston, L. D., O'Malley, P. M., et al. (2017). *Monitoring the Future National Survey Results on Drug Use, 1975–2016: Volume I, Secondary School Students*. Ann Arbor, MI: Institute for Social Research, The University of Michigan. Available at http://monitoringthefuture.org/pubs.html#monographs

NCLB (2001). No Child Left Behind Act of 2001, Pub. Law. No. 107-110, 20 U.S.C. § 6319 stat.

Office on Smoking and Health (2015). *National Youth Tobacco Survey*. Centers for Disease Control and Prevention, National Center for

Chronic Disease Prevention and Health Promotion. Atlanta, GA: US Department of Health and Human Services.

Orlando, M., Ellickson, P. L., McCaffrey, D. F. & Longshore, D. L. (2005). Mediation analysis of a school-based drug prevention program: Effects of Project ALERT. *Prevention Science*, **6**, 35–46.

Pas, E. T., Waasdorp, T. E. & Bradshaw, C. P. (2015). Examining contextual influences on classroom-based implementation of positive behavior support strategies: Findings from a randomized controlled effectiveness trial. *Prevention Science*, **16**, 1096–1106.

Patterson, G. R., Forgatch, M. S. & DeGarmo, D. S. (2010). Cascading effects following intervention. *Development and Psychopathology*, **22**, 949–970.

Payne, A. A., Gottfredson, D. C. & Gottfredson, G. D. (2006). School predictors of the intensity of implementation of school-based prevention programs: Results from a national study. *Prevention Science*, **7**, 225–237.

Pentz, M. A. (1983). Prevention of adolescent substance abuse through social skill development. In T. J. Glynn, C. G. Leukefeld & J. B. Ludford (Eds.), *Preventing Adolescent Drug Abuse: Intervention Strategies*. Washington, DC: NIDA Research Monograph, pp. 195–232.

Peterson, A. V., Kealey, K. A., Mann, S. L., Marek, P. M. & Sarason, I. G. (2000a). Hutchinson Smoking Prevention Project: Long-term randomized trial in school-based tobacco use prevention—Results on smoking. *Journal of the National Cancer Institute*, **92**, 1979–1991.

Peterson, A. V., Mann, S. L., Kealey, K. A. & Marek, P. M. (2000b). Experimental design and methods for school-based randomized trials: Experience from the Hutchinson Smoking Prevention Project (HSPP). *Controlled Clinical Trials*, **21**, 144–165.

Reinke, W. M., Stormont, M., Herman, K. C. & Newcomer, L. (2014). Using coaching to support teacher implementation of classroom-based interventions. *Journal of Behavioral Education*, **23**, 150–167.

Resnicow, K., Soler, R. E., Braithwaite, R. L., Ahluwalia, J. S. & Butler, J. (2000). Cultural sensitivity in substance use prevention. *Journal of Community Psychology*, **28**, 271–290.

Ringwalt, C. L., Ennett, S., Johnson, R., et al. (2003). Factors associated with fidelity to substance use prevention curriculum guides in the nation's middle schools. *Health Education & Behavior*, **30**, 375–391.

Ringwalt, C. L., Vincus, A., Ennett, S., Johnson, R. & Rohrbach, L. A. (2004). Reasons for teachers' adaptation of substance use prevention curricula in schools with non-white student populations. *Prevention Science*, **5**, 61–67.

Ringwalt, C. L., Vincus, A., Hanley, S., et al. (2011). The prevalence of evidence-based drug use prevention curricula in U.S. middle schools in 2008. *Prevention Science*, **12**, 63–69.

Rohrbach, L. A., Dent, C. W., Skara, S., Sun, P. & Sussman, S. (2007). Fidelity of implementation in Project Towards No Drug Abuse (TND): A comparison of classroom teacher and program specialists. *Prevention Science*, **8**, 125–132.

Rohrbach, L. A., Graham, J. G. & Hansen, W. B. (1993). Diffusion of a school-based substance abuse program: Predictors of program implementation. *Preventive Medicine*, **22**, 237–260.

Romero, A. J. & Roberts, R. E. (2003). Stress within a bicultural context for adolescents of Mexican decent. *Cultural Diversity and Ethnic Minority Psychology*, **9**, 171–184.

Rosenbaum, D. P., Gordon, S. & Hanson, S. (1998). Assessing the effects of school-based drug education: A six-year multilevel analysis of project D.A.R.E. *Journal of Research in Crime and Delinquency*, **35**, 381–412.

Scheier, L. M. (2015). Theoretical models of drug use etiology: Foundations of prevention. In L. M. Scheier (Ed.), *Handbook of Adolescent Drug Use Prevention: Research, Intervention Strategies, and Practice*. Washington, DC: American Psychological Association, pp. 67–83.

Scheier, L. M. (Ed.) (2010). *Handbook of Adolescent Drug Use Prevention: Research, Intervention Strategies, and Practice*. Washington, DC: American Psychological Association.

Scheier, L. M., Botvin, G. J. & Griffin, K. W. (2001). Preventive intervention effects on developmental progression in drug use: Structural equation modeling analyses using longitudinal data. *Prevention Science*, **2**, 91–112.

Shope, J. T., Elliott, M. R., Raghunathan, T. E. & Waller, P. F. (2001). Long-term follow-up of a high school alcohol prevention programs' effect on students subsequent driving. *Alcoholism: Clinical and Experimental Research*, **25**, 403–410.

Simons-Morton, B., Haynie, D., Saylor, K., Crump, A. D.,& Chen, R. (2005). Impact analysis and mediation of outcomes: The Going Places Program. *Health Education & Behavior*, **32**, 227–241.

Skara, S. & Sussman, S. (2003). A review of 25 long-term adolescent tobacco and other drug use prevention program evaluations. *Preventive Medicine*, **37**, 451–474.

Sloboda, Z., Stephens, R. C., Stephens, P. C., et al. (2009). The Adolescent Substance Abuse Prevention Study: A randomized field trial of a universal substance abuse prevention program. *Drug and Alcohol Dependence*, **102**, 1–10.

Spitzberg, B. H. & Cupach, W. R. (1984). *Interpersonal Communication Competence*. Beverly Hills, CA: Sage Publications.

Stacy, A. W., Sussman, S., Dent, C. W., Burton, D. & Flay, B. R. (1992). Moderators of peer social influence in adolescent smoking. *Journal of Personality and Social Psychology*, **18**, 163–172.

Sussman, S. (2017). *Substance and Behavioral Addictions: Concepts, Causes, and Cures*. New York, NY: Cambridge University Press.

Sussman, S., Hansen, W. B., Flay, B. R. & Botvin, G. J. (2001). Hutchinson Smoking Prevention Project: Long-term randomized trial in school-based tobacco use prevention-results on smoking. *Journal of the National Cancer Institute*, **93**, 1267.

Sussman, S., Levy, D., Lich, K. H., et al. (2013). Comparing effects of tobacco use prevention modalities: Need for complex systems models. *Tobacco Induced Diseases*, **11**, 1–14.

Sussman, S., Sun, P., Rohrbach, L. A. & Spruijt-Metz, D. (2012). One-year outcomes of a drug abuse prevention program for older teens and emerging adults: Evaluating a motivational interviewing booster component. *Health Psychology*, **31**, 476–485.

Townsend, L., Flisher, A. J. & King, G. (2007). A systematic review of the relationship between high school dropout and substance use. *Clinical Child and Family Psychology*, **10**, 295–317.

Vartiainen, E., Paavola, M., McAlister, A. & Puska, P. (1998). Fifteen-year follow-up of smoking prevention effects in the North Karelia Youth Project. *American Journal of Public Health*, **88**, 81–85.

Vartiainen, E., Pallonen, U., McAlister, A., Koskela, K. & Puska, P. (1986). Four-year follow-up results of the smoking prevention program in the North Karelia Youth Project. *Preventive Medicine*, **15**, 692–698.

Vartiainen, E., Pallonen, U., McAlister, A. & Puska, P. (1990). Eight-year follow-up results of an adolescent smoking prevention program: The North Karelia Youth Project. *American Journal of Public Health*, **80**, 78–79.

Vincus, A. A., Ringwalt, C., Harris, M. S. & Shamblen, S. R. (2010). A short-term, quasi-experimental evaluation of D.A.R.E.'s revised elementary school curriculum. *Journal of Drug Education*, **40**, 37–49.

West, S. G. & Aiken, L. S. (1997). Toward understanding individual effects in multicomponent prevention programs: Design and analysis strategies. In K. J. Bryant, M. Windle & S. G. West (Eds.), *The Science of Prevention: Methodological Advances from Alcohol and Substance Abuse Research*. Washington, DC: American Psychological Association, pp. 167–209.

16 Treatment of Alcohol, Tobacco, and Other Drug (ATOD) Misuse

Steve Sussman, PhD, FAAHB, FAPA, FSPR, and Maria Bolshakova, BS*, *authorship shared equally

Introduction

Addictions typically develop over a several year time-span, and what may have seemed like reasonably acceptable behavior at first may morph into cumulating negative consequences that are inadequately addressed. It is the costs of addiction that lead to cessation attempts. However, recognizing and stopping an alcohol, tobacco, or other drug (ATOD) addiction may require multiple attempts by treatment agents or support persons, much effort on the part of the individual sufferer, and counteraction of the large social climate that helps facilitate and maintain the addiction.

In general, acknowledging that one is suffering from an addiction and in need of some sort of treatment is the first step. Some persons suffering from addiction recover naturally; they may simply "grow out of it" or recognize the need to change and seek out informal channels of assistance. They may quit cold-turkey, read self-help books, follow manuals, or seek out informal support, to do it on their own. In fact, a summary of available literature suggests that one-third of problem ATOD misusers recover on their own without formalized treatment (Heyman, 2013; Sussman, 2017; Toneatto et al., 1999). The number seems to be a bit higher for alcohol abuse, with Cunningham (1999) reporting 54 percent to 88 percent of problem drinkers quitting naturally. Another study found that a third of cocaine and heroin addicts exhibited spontaneous (natural) recovery (Bischof, Rumpf & Ulrich, 2012; Toneatto et al., 1999).

However, many other addicts may not fully process their addiction and related consequences ("denial") or may try to hide from significant others the severity of consequences that their ATOD addiction elicits. Eventually, negatively consequential events may lead one to be more likely to desire to quit or control ATOD use and seek out formalized pathways of assistance. For example, at some point in the addiction "career," health may be affected, and a routine doctor's visit may enlighten the addict as to the severity of the situation (e.g., the initial stages of Alcoholic Liver Disease). As another example, the individual may experience withdrawal symptoms (e.g., finger trembling or extreme sweating after abrupt termination of alcohol use), and reluctantly keep engaging with the drug to avoid withdrawal. The addict may desire to terminate the symptomatology and need the supervision of medical personnel while "getting clean" (e.g., to avoid cholinergic shock effects of alcohol withdrawal). Either of these examples may result in inpatient or outpatient care, depending on severity of the consequences experienced. In more tragic circumstances, an event may occur that dramatically necessitates the person to seek out formalized treatment. For example, experiencing a driving while under the influence (DUI) or a reckless behavior legal charge may result in the person being mandated to some sort of treatment (of course, this can happen even if they are a casual user who made a "mistake").

Oftentimes, an addict's use of the drug and the behaviors associated with use have become more or less automatic for them. They may not recognize or desire to avoid the stimuli that trigger engagement with the addiction and may be susceptible to the immediate gratification of using the drug rather than considering alternative behaviors. Sometimes it takes confrontational input, or even a formal intervention, from family, friends or the workplace to lead a person to realize that their behavior has gotten out of control and developed into a negatively consequential addiction (which is hurting themselves or others).

The *Diagnostic and Statistical Manual of Mental Disorders* (fifth edition) (DSM-5) is a widely recognized tool for diagnosing a variety of mental disorders. In this manual, substance use disorder is defined as a maladaptive pattern of substance use leading to clinically significant impairment or distress and identifies eleven criteria that indicate how these impairments and distress may be manifested (APA, 2013).

(1) Tolerance – the individual needs increased amounts of the substance to achieve the desired effect or will experience the desired effect less when continuing the same dosage.
(2) Withdrawal – physical symptoms that the body experiences in the case of some drugs after abruptly stopping drug use, or using a closely related substance to relieve the symptoms (e.g., taking pain killers as a substitute for heroin).
(3) The individual takes larger amounts of the substance or over a longer period of time than intended.
(4) The individual desires to control their substance use and has not been successful, often with failed attempts in the past (loss of control).
(5) A great deal of time is spent in activities pertaining to the substance, such as obtaining the drugs, using them, and recovering from their effects.
(6) Important activities are neglected or reduced due to the substance use – this could include time spent with family and friends, recreational activities, or missing work.
(7) The individual continues to use the substance although aware that it has a negative and persistent impact on well-being (e.g., continuing to use amphetamines even after having been previously hospitalized for an acute psychotic reaction related to that drug use).
(8) The individual experiences craving related to the drug, contexts of its use, and stimuli associated with use (e.g., upon seeing or imagining a meth pipe).
(9) The individual experiences consequences related to role functioning (e.g., misses school, work, or is unable to do job as a parent).
(10) The individual experiences consequences in social functioning (e.g., friends complain about the drinking or using).
(11) The individual uses in physically hazardous situations (e.g., while driving or operating heavy machinery).

The DSM-5 specifies that the individual must present with at least two or more of these criteria, in a one-year period as a function of recurrent use, to qualify for substance use disorder. As with most mental disorders, substance abuse can act on a large spectrum of daily behavior and lead to impairment in multiple life spheres.

Regardless of how the problem is first recognized and diagnosed, ATOD addiction is extremely difficult to resolve (e.g., relapse rates to near-baseline levels are approximately 66 percent over a one-year period after a first quit attempt, regarding cigarettes, alcohol, marijuana, or heroin; Sussman, 2017). When an addiction involves so many events in someone's life, it can be hard to make the changes necessary for recovery. For instance, certain friends and groups of people may be associated with the ATOD use, which might mean ceasing to see those people anymore, or living with potential temptations that must be dealt with when socializing with these others. There also may be certain places such as bars, casinos, hookah lounges, just to name a few, that an addict would not be able to visit comfortably anymore. For some individuals, their entire daily routine and activities may have to change as they work toward reshaping their addictive patterns. They may be ill-equipped to handle the emotional realities that they must face without the use of substances; including coping with previous traumatic experiences. Up to one-third of ATOD misusers seek out formalized treatment. Some of the remaining persons may experience natural recovery; others may not and continue to accumulate negative consequences throughout their lives; eventually they tend to slow down in their use, develop chronic illnesses, or die (Heyman, 2013).

More on Natural Recovery

There exists evidence to suggest that many young people "grow out" of the addiction as they reach adulthood (Wakefield & Schmitz, 2014). These individuals tend to be less likely to exhibit notable harm to self or others and appear to not to be reliant on ATODs to function comfortably. Various studies also have been conducted to evaluate what factors lead to natural recovery among adults (approximately one-third of those suffering from an ATOD disorder). There is evidence that when problem drug users experience both negative consequences of ATOD use, but also positive alternatives if they stay sober, they may be especially successful in achieving sobriety. Negative consequences include job demotion or loss, getting into trouble with the law, relationships failing, and feeling depressed. Positive alternatives include the desire and possibility to maintain relationships, prospects for a new job, increased stability, or having a child, among other life hurdles (Waldorf, 1983; Waldorf et al., 1992). There is also evidence to suggest that natural recovery may be more realistic for those that experience less severity of problems associated with the drug abuse, whereas those who fall on the upper end of the continuum of problem severity may benefit more from formal treatment (Bischof et al., 2003; Stea, Yakovenko & Hodgins, 2015). One study found three separate groups of spontaneous recoveries using cluster analyses. The first group was characterized as having high severity of dependence, low/few alcohol-related problems, and little social support. The second group had high severity of dependence as well as high/many alcohol-related problems and medium social support, and the third group identified from the analysis had high social support, and low severity of dependence and alcohol-related problems. Those who had low severity or few alcohol-related problems were able to recover with minimal social support, but those with high severity of dependence along with many alcohol-related problems were in need of social support to aid their recovery (Bischof et al., 2003).

Much of the natural recovery literature touches on the idea of social capital. High social capital might be defined as indicating a high degree of social support and few social problems; the individual receives benefits that accrue as the result of personal contacts and social networks (Granfield & Cloud, 2001). Indeed, Granfield and Cloud (2001) found in their qualitative analysis of forty-six naturally recovering addicts that having friends and family members who provided support to them in their crisis rather than condoning their problem drug behavior history was "critical to their natural recovery." Social capital is also important to understand when setting policies concerning drug use, because drug abusers still tend to be sent off to jail for engaging with their addiction, further isolating them from their support network which may do more harm than good (Granfield & Cloud, 2001; Reinarman & Levine, 1997).

To further explore the stages of natural recovery, Mohatt et al. (2008) studied Alaskan Natives who identified as having been problem drinkers but were now abstinent for five or more years. They found a sequence of the recovery process that the participants identified as their general experience with trying to quit naturally. The first step of the process included a reflective stage in which the individual thinks about the consequence of their alcohol use. In the second stage, the individual experiments with sobriety, and typically cycles through phases of attempting to become sober and falling back into problem behavior. The third stage is marked by a final decision to become sober, possibly after many failed attempts.

Stages 4 and 5 are the sobriety stages. Stage 4 includes active coping and dealing with cravings to drink (for some participants). Stage 5 sobriety is characterized by moving beyond simply coping into "living life as it was meant to be lived." These stages obviously do not apply to every addict attempting to recover on one's own, but it provides a heuristic framework to reference when conceptualizing what individuals go through in natural recovery.

Treatment Participation, Attrition, and General Types of Treatment Settings

An estimated 23.5 million people in the USA who are aged twelve years or older need treatment for a substance abuse problem, but only around 2.6 million (11.2 percent) receive treatment at any sort of specialized facility (SAMHSA National Survey on Drug Use and Health, 2017). The prevalence of admissions by type of drug has been shifting recently, considering the recent opioid epidemic and legalization of marijuana. Out of those that seek help for their drug use problem, alcohol abuse, and opioid abuse (including prescription opioids and heroin) both account for 34 percent of treatment admissions. Admission for alcohol abuse has decreased from a high of 41 percent, while opioid abuse has increased from 20 percent in 2008. Marijuana accounts for 14 percent of admissions, stimulants at 9 percent, and cocaine at 5 percent (SAMHSA, Treatment Episode Data Set, TEDS, 2015).

Termination and attrition rates are high – one study reported a 45 percent termination rate within the first month of a hospital-based sample of alcoholics (Gordis et al., 1981), while another study of alcoholism treatment found that 35 percent of clients failed to return after the initial visit in an alcoholism treatment clinic (Rees, 1986). A 30 percent to 40 percent drop-out rate has been consistent for the past forty years (Sussman, 2017). Early attrition from substance abuse treatment is a major issue, as drop-out predicts poor outcomes in treatment (Iguchi & Stilzer, 1991; Stark, 1992). One psychological predictor of early low retention in a residential substance treatment program was the level of psychological distress and distress tolerance, with those who had lower distress tolerance and higher psychological distress being more likely to drop out of treatment early (Daughters et al., 2005). Among methadone maintenance patients admitted to an outpatient clinic for the treatment of opioid abuse disorder, predictors of retention in the program included social stability, previous treatment experience, expectations for reducing drug use, higher methadone dose level, and higher motivation (Simpson & Joe, 1993).

There are specific actions that have been shown to be effective for increasing retention rate. Small, decentralized clinics that employ higher clinic staff: patient ratios tend to have relatively lower drop-out rates. Patient contact that is individualized, fast, warm, and friendly can also go a long way to getting a patient to stay in treatment. Creating friendly and comfortable environments for patients to live and interact with others and having a general presence of social support may help boost patient retention as well (Stark, 1992). Chafetz, Blanc and Hill (1970) also found a few ways to increase patient's show rates to an alcohol clinic following admission to an emergency service at a hospital. The data from a series of experiments indicated that welcoming patients and treating them with respect, decreasing wait times, increasing direct patient contact, dealing with concrete concerns (financial, housing), and coming to the patient's homes all resulted in an increase in initial and long-term attendance at the alcohol clinics. In other words, having staff able to provide genuine and humane treatment, which ensures patients are having their needs met, will lead to lower dropout rates.

Types of Treatment Involvement

Generally, there are *three broad types of formal treatment modalities (settings)* offered for substance abuse: outpatient treatment, inpatient treatment, and partial hospitalization program (i.e., PHP, nonresidential treatment, hospital-based, which provides diagnostic and treatment services on a level of intensity similar to an inpatient program, but on less than a twenty-four-hour basis). For the most severe cases, especially individuals who need to adhere to a detoxification protocol, an inpatient stay, even for a brief time (e.g., a seventy-two-hour hold for alcohol use), may be the most beneficial to address the physical symptoms of the withdrawal. There has not been much evidence found that indicates whether inpatient treatment, outpatient treatment, or partial hospitalization is better in general for quitting a substance, although overall, inpatient programs have demonstrated higher completion rates than outpatient programs (75 percent versus 18 percent; Wickizer et al., 1994).

There have also been individual differences found (Fink et al., 1985). Individuals who are more severely deteriorated and have achieved less social support and stability have been found to benefit more from intensive treatment (Miller & Hester, 1986). However, a majority of addicts may not benefit from a more intensive stay, contingent on the content of the intervention and the treatments offered. There is also the consideration of costs, as substance abuse treatment can run a patient through thousands of dollars rather quickly. Researchers studying the cost-effectiveness of partial hospitalization versus inpatient treatment for the rehabilitation of alcohol abusers found that costs favored partial hospitalization, with outcomes at twenty-four-month follow-up remaining generally the same between inpatient and partial hospitalization groups (Fink et al., 1985). Barnett and Swindle (1997) proposed placing a twenty-one-day limit on length of stay in an inpatient program, as the effectiveness of staying beyond twenty-one days was generally not worth the cost. Certainly, though, programs that follow-up participants at least ninety days show better outcomes (Fletcher, Tims & Brown, 1997).

Health Disparities in Treatment

Recently, special populations (disadvantaged groups) have received more consideration. That is, a tailoring of treatment may be needed for subgroups of addicts. *Women*, for example, are more likely to report a history of sexual abuse and indicate more emotional distress than men (Wallen, 1992), which could be important to address in treatment. Women also have different predictors of treatment retention than men. One study found that women with histories of higher incomes, those who are currently unemployed, are married, or belong to any ethnic category other than African-American, are more likely to remain in treatment (Mertens & Weisner, 2000). Women, in general, demonstrate more efficacious help-seeking behaviors and personal independence than men and may do better (less dropout) in treatment (Florentine et al., 1997), though they may be less likely to reach treatment due to gender-specific concerns (e.g., worry about children being placed in foster care; Sussman & Ames, 2008).

Studies have indicated *racial disparities* in access to treatment. One study found that among those in need of treatment, whites were more likely than African-American or Hispanic participants to be receiving alcohol or drug abuse treatment, and African-Americans were more likely to have no access to drug or alcohol treatment programs. Hispanics also suffered; with an increased likelihood to have delayed care or receiving less care than needed (Wells et al., 2001). Barriers to care include disproportionate lack of alcohol and drug abuse treatment centers in the South and Southwest of the USA, which have large minority populations (McAuliffe & Dunn, 2004). Other barriers to treatment entry include lack of knowledge about services and how to obtain them, concern about costs of treatment, and being unable to find child care while in rehabilitation in the African-American population. Treatment entry concerns among non-black respondents generally have been more psychological (fear of stigmatization, belief that treatment won't work), rather than material (Grant, 1977).

African-Americans and Hispanics are more likely to enter outpatient care than inpatient care, compared to white clients, even after adjusting for addiction characteristics, employment, and other patient-level factors. It is possible that these treatment completion differences can be reduced by actively increasing enrollment of African-American and Hispanic substance abusers into inpatient/residential treatment programs (Bluthenthal, Jacobson & Robinson, 2007). Furthermore, experiences of discrimination while attempting to obtain mental health or substance abuse treatment was reported by African-Americans and Latinos, which was associated with relatively lower perceived helpfulness of treatment ratings for Latinos ($AOR = 0.09$, $p < 0.05$) and early treatment termination for blacks ($AOR = 13.38$, $p < 0.05$); Mays et al., 2017). Indeed, sociocultural and economic factors affect the availability of resources, compliance with medication, and access to social welfare systems, all which may have a profound effect on entering treatment and treatment outcome (Galea & Vlahov, 2002).

Studies have often found racial disparities in treatment outcomes, although specific results have been mixed (McCaul, Svikis & Moore, 2001; Walton et al., 2003; Weisner et al., 2002). African-Americans have been found to have lower treatment completion rates than whites, although some of the variation can be explained by economic differences such as employment, homelessness, and availability of state provided medical insurance. It is interesting to note that these economic differences explain the variation in completion rate more in outpatient care than residential care – 40 percent versus 7 percent (Jacobson, Robinson & Bluthenthal, 2007). Curiously, in one somewhat older study, intensive inpatient *alcohol* treatment completion rates were higher for whites than African-Americans, Hispanics, and Native Americans, whereas intensive inpatient *drug* treatment program completion rates were highest among Hispanic clients, followed by African-American, and Native American clients, with lowest completion among whites (Wickizer et al., 1994). It is not clear how to interpret these results.

There is evidence that different racial groups may respond more positively to certain treatment modalities (Le Fauve et al., 2003; Villanueva et al., 2002), and culturally sensitive programs can help to engage clients and increase retention rates (Petry, 2003; Rouse, Carter & Rodriguez-Andrew, 1995). For example, programs that help enhance ethnic identification and pride may demonstrate better treatment outcomes for ethnic-specific populations (Sussman, 2017). More research is needed to address racial disparities in alcohol and drug abuse treatment, but in the meantime, it may be wise to consider culturally specific features of treatments for minorities.

Shifting Views on Addiction

Alcoholism (and ATOD use in general) is often seen as a sin, or a product of weak will, and thus alcohol abuse treatment can be stigmatizing. Some aspects of treatment including spirituality may appear to provide a redemption-from-sin orientation as well (Sussman et al., 2013). This does not bode well for patients, as those who perceive that there was a greater stigma toward alcohol disorders have been found to be less likely to seek treatment (Keyes et al., 2010). The high rate of relapse, and need for repeated attempts to quit, may reinforce a perception of alcoholics as being evil or weak-willed.

There has relatively recently been a call for substance abuse to be treated more as a chronic condition rather than as a moral failing (McLellan et al., 2000). Notable similarities exist between substance abuse and chronic conditions such as hypertension, diabetes or asthma. In all of these examples, a change in lifestyle is usually needed in order to achieve results. For traditional chronic diseases, these changes include taking prescribed medication, engaging in healthier eating, and exercising; for substance abuse, it means living a life that does not involve drugs or alcohol and learning how to cope and enjoy life without the substance. ATOD treatment nowadays may also include instruction on healthier eating and exercise. It is interesting to note that patients suffering from chronic disease do not do much better in complying with taking their medication and lifestyle changes than individuals with substance use disorders do in maintaining sobriety. McLellan (2002) argues for a continued care approach in substance abuse rehabilitation. Just as with (other) chronic diseases, rather than treating these disorders as ones that can be fixed in one single treatment program, he argues for monitoring of patients. Continuously checking in to see how they are doing with their ongoing and lifetime fight against relapse, and utilizing different sources such as physicians, case workers, and counselors, are ways the continuing care approach may be able to ensure the best chance at one maintaining sobriety.

Assessment

There are many different tools available to clinicians to assess ATOD misuse. *Screening* is a preliminary evaluation to ascertain whether an individual may exhibit classic signs of substance abuse, and may be followed by a *comprehensive assessment*, which is a full and thorough evaluation of the substance abuse problem. The assessment helps to develop a diagnosis and treatment plan for the patient.

Screening helps to identify someone as a potential problem drug user, and oftentimes it is the first step to receiving treatment. Screening can be done by physicians, counselors, family, friends, and even the individual who suspects that he/she may have a problem. While a trained mental health professional is generally the most reliable source for screening, there are many tools available online and free of charge that can be helpful in the initial phase of determining if there is a problem that needs to be addressed. The NIH has multiple tools to help evaluate potential alcohol and drug use available on their website (e.g., see: www.drugabuse.gov/nidamed-medical-health-professionals/tool-resources-your-practice/screening-assessment-drug-testing-resources/chart-evidence-based-screening-tools-adults; accessed March 15, 2018). Some of the most popular self-report instruments are the CAGE or the CRAFFT, the MAST, the NIDA Modified ASSIST Drug Use Screening Tool, and the Substance Abuse Subtle Screening Inventory (SASSI), just to name a few (e.g., see Grigsby et al., 2017). For example the CRAFFT involves six items: the patient reports whether he or she rides in a car (the "C") where the driver is under the influence, uses to relax (the "R"), uses alone (the "A"), forgets a period of time while under the influence (blackouts; the "F"), has received complaints from family or friends regarding drug use (the second "F"), and has gotten into trouble due to drug use (the "T"). The CRAFFT has demonstrated good convergent validity and nearly acceptable internal consistency ($\alpha = 0.68$; see Grigsby et al., 2017).

After a potential substance use problem has been identified, it is best for a trained clinician to administer a full assessment to evaluate the substance use problem and needs for treatment. Assessment tools are either structured or semistructured; structured assessments have a set list of questions to ask the patient and can be useful for someone who is not as well-trained on substance-abuse disorders. Semistructured interviews include open-ended questions, and allow the clinician to get a better understanding of the scope of the problem and details that may be important in the determination of a treatment plan. Questions may detail using history, family conflict and use, employment and social problems due to use, and medical and legal problems due to use (e.g., DUIs, attendance at twelve-step meetings, or hospitalizations related to drug use).

It is also important to include questions about cooccurring conditions; for example, an individual may be addicted to multiple drugs, or they may have comorbid psychiatric issues such as depression, anxiety, or PTSD, as examples. In the USA, generally, an official diagnosis involves use of the *Structured Clinical Interview for the Diagnostic Statistical Manual-V* (SCID-V; APA, 2013), which adheres to the eleven DSM-5 criteria presented at the beginning of this chapter. Patients with cooccurring mental health conditions need to have those issues addressed in treatment as well; dual diagnosis may play a large role in the addiction. Finally, in recent years there has been some research regarding neurocognitive assessment in substance abuse treatment. Neurocognitive tests may be able to present a more objective assessment of impairment than self-report, and there has been some indication in the literature that those in treatment for substance abuse do have impaired neurocognitive performance. It is also interesting to note that treatment may help to repair some of these neurocognitive deficits, a finding that may help to encourage patients to engage in and continue with treatment (Meek, Clark & Solana, 1989).

Recovery Models

If one considers a stepped-care approach to treatment, one might view the addict as transitioning from most informal and least intrusive (e.g., self-help, twelve-step meetings, therapy), to most formal and structured (outpatient, inpatient treatment), until ending up with the treatment that finally arrests the negatively consequential behavior. Of course, there is great variability in application of such an approach. Some addicts may be successful in an informal or outpatient approach, and some may go directly into an inpatient facility if their addiction is severe enough or given the financial opportunity. A stepped-care approach may or may not improve outcomes, though it may save on treatment costs (e.g., see Jaehne et al., 2012).

There are several different recovery models that have been proposed in the literature, but as of now they are generally heuristic in value, without much empirical support. They are useful in assisting clinicians to assess and develop treatment plans for their patients. The general idea behind all of these stages-of-recovery models is that the addict ceases their behavior to arrest the cumulating consequences of their addiction, and then gradually learns how to live their life without the substances (Sussman, 2017). These models also propose that there is a developmental process that fluctuates between individuals and progresses in stages, always with the possibility of relapse (recycling do-loops).

The model of Mueller and Ketcham (1987) proposes three general phases that addicts go through to heal and make changes in their behavior. These phases include stabilization, early recovery, and middle-to-late recovery. Stabilization is the initial phase, which may involve detoxification and the management of withdrawal symptoms for the patient. It also includes assessing any comorbid problems, medical care, and nutritional status assessment. After the stabilization phase, the patient progresses into early recovery, which includes treatment planning and various modes of treatment such as cognitive-behavioral therapy, Motivational Interviewing, skills training, and other types of counseling that will be discussed later in this chapter. Early recovery is the bulk of the treatment setting, which includes the therapy necessary to move forward with sobriety. Middle-to-late recovery in this model deals with the aftercare and relapse prevention; setting up plans and resources that will ensure the best chance for success at maintaining sobriety. This could include outpatient programs or group therapy, living in a sober home, or planning for lifestyle changes that will need to occur after leaving treatment, such as removing oneself from situations that may encourage relapse. An emphasis is then put on learning to live life sober (i.e., in a balanced way) and finding alternate ways to enjoy life and remain healthy.

The Johnson Model (Johnson, 1980) places emphasis on psychological changes that occur in the process of recovery that help to facilitate treatment. This model has four stages of recovery – admission, compliance, acceptance, and surrender. Admission is a distinct phase in this model; the individual accepts that they have a problem with substance abuse and allows themselves to enter into treatment. Compliance indicates a change in the patient's attitude from resisting treatment to complying with the prescribed changes in their lifestyle. Acceptance occurs when the patient takes responsibility for their recovery and gains insight into the severity of their problems. There may be a distinct increase in self-awareness in this stage, as well as self-acceptance. The final phase, surrender, occurs when an individual understands that they may need to be cautious in the future, and take the steps necessary to prevent relapsing such as engaging in outpatient programs, and utilizing the support of others to help them cope with future difficulties.

The Gorski and Miller (1984, 1986) Model follows the same path as the Mueller and Ketcham Model, with a few notable differences. This model includes more molecular developmental periods in the process of recovery that affect physiological changes and produce various goals during each period. These periods include transition, stabilization, early recovery, middle recovery, and late recovery. The transition period is much like the admission and compliance phase in the Johnson Model, as it involves individuals transitioning from using substances to recognizing the need for treatment and setting the goal to pursue an abstinent lifestyle. Stabilization in this model is akin to stabilization mentioned in the Mueller and Ketcham Model, where detoxification, managing withdrawal symptoms, and crisis management are the top priority. Then, there are three periods of recovery, with the early recovery phase focusing on healthy coping by replacing addictive thoughts and behaviors with sobriety-based actions. Middle recovery involves the beginning of living a balanced life without the use of substances and repairing the damage that may have occurred over the lifespan of the addiction. Late recovery may involve personality changes and a deeper understanding of the nature of the addiction, and resolution of family of origin issues. Finally, maintenance is an ongoing process of growth and development that recognizes that there is always the possibility for relapse but ensures that the individual is taking an active part in making sure they do not slip back into their old habits.

Motivation

Motivation plays a key role in the treatment process. Motivation can be viewed in a multitude of ways, and there have been several models of motivation proposed. It may be described as the goal objective (in this case, sobriety) and the amount of work, or energy, that one is willing to put in to obtain the desired goal (Bindra & Stewart, 1966). It could also be seen as an intrapersonal state of readiness to change (DiClemente et al., 1991). There is a common saying of having to "hit rock bottom" to finally be motivated enough to seek help. One study found that hitting rock bottom for participants was more related to the severity of symptoms of anxiety, depression, and other forms of emotional distress rather than traditional drinking severity measures (Ryan, Plant & O'Malley, 1995). Despite the negative consequences that an individual may experience due to the addiction, there is also something to be said about motivation acting separately as a positive driving force toward changing behavior (e.g., hope as a driving force).

The *Transtheoretical Model* of motivation provides a framework as a model of stages of recovery and involves stages of change that progress through establishing a commitment to a goal and providing the energy to complete the goal (e.g., Prochaska & DiClemente, 1982). The patient's state of readiness to change is seen as their motivation to change their behavior. During precontemplation the individual does not plan to change. Contemplation to change and quit ATOD use occurs when costs reliably rise above benefits, and self-revelation processes lead one in a positive direction. Preparation involves planning to quit, and action and maintenance involves techniques of quitting and relapse prevention.

According to one type of *Direction-Energy Model*, motivation occurs when there is a desire for a self-image change, curiosity, and mood enhancement, which all drive the goal of sobriety. The energy required to complete the goal is fulfilled if the individual perceives a match between one's behavioral repertoire with the demands of attaining the goal, social and intrapersonal pressures to change, and how embedded the individual is in the lifestyle which permits a comfortable end goal (Bindra & Stewart, 1966; Sussman, 1996; Sutton & Eiser, 1984).

External and internal motivation is yet another motivation construct discussed in the literature. The *Intrinsic-Extrinsic Motivation Model* asserts that intrinsic motivation (the individual identifying with the desirability of the goal on a person level) leads to more goal achievement than extrinsic, or outside rewards (Curry, Wanger & Grothaus, 1990). However, both sources of motivation should be considered in treatment. Intrinsic motivation may be enhanced by utilizing therapies such as Motivational Interviewing and proximal goal setting (Manderlink & Harackiewicz, 1984). Extrinsic motivation may be utilized by focusing on socioenvironmental elements that combine personal and social goals, and is response-contingent (Fishbein & Ajzen, 1975; Rotter, 1954; Sussman, 2017).

Some research does suggest that patients who have low internal motivation, regardless of whether external motivation was high, have been found to have poorer outcomes (Ryan et al., 1995). Consistent with this theory (of intrinsic versus extrinsic motivation), one may consider the finding in a few studies that individuals referred to treatment through the legal system have been rated as less likely to complete treatment, and show less improvement in psychiatric symptoms and use of alcohol by their clinicians than those coming to treatment of their own accord (Ryan et al., 1995; Wickizer et al., 1994). This may be because of the fact that being court-mandated to therapy is an external pressure (though it is a "teachable moment"), and the individual has no choice other than to attend, even if they may personally not believe it is necessary or desirable.

Treatments

For a patient seeking ATOD treatment, there are many alternative strategies that might be utilized. Some of the different types of treatments available, and the empirical evidence behind using these techniques, will be discussed here. Detoxification and pharmacological approaches, cognitive-behavioral therapy, contingency management, Motivational Interviewing, cue exposure, twelve-step programs, group and family therapy, and some additional approaches (e.g., yoga, complementary medicine) are presented.

Detoxification and Pharmacotherapy

The first line of treatment oftentimes may include detoxification, and/or some sort of pharmacological approach. Detoxification is the process of managing a person's symptoms, including physical and emotional pain, while the body reacts to the withdrawal from the drug. Many people detox off the drug alone, without the help of medical treatment, but that also heavily depends on the drug of abuse. For example, alcohol, opioid, and benzodiazepine withdrawal can be extremely intense and even life threatening. Symptoms may include nausea, vomiting, tremors, anxiety, hallucinations, and seizures.

Alcohol detoxification often involves medical supervision, an IV for fluids to replenish the body, as well as drugs such as Librium or other benzodiazepines (to ease potential cholinergic shock), carbamazepine, naltrexone, SSRIs and buspirone (Julien, 2005). This is not an exhaustive list and there are multiple other drugs that may be combined to offset certain symptoms of the withdrawal. Detoxification usually involves an institutionalized process with a three-to-five-day inpatient stay, and intensive medical management and supervision. Pharmacological approaches are used not only for detox; they can be used in combination with talk-therapy and may even be used as a long-term option to help reduce craving or assist with remaining abstinent.

For *opioid detoxification*, methadone is often used, along with naltrexone, clonidine, buprenorphine, and Darvon. These are examples of drug agonists, which provide similar effects of the drug of choice but produce fewer disabling effects. There has been evidence suggesting that medication-assisted treatment (MAT), particularly methadone and buprenorphine for opioid-use disorder, is beneficial in reducing relapse (for around 50 percent of those who use these aids; Sussman, 2017; Vigezzi et al., 2006). Unfortunately, not all providers have the resources or permission to supply their patients with such drug agonists. On the other hand, drug antagonists block the effects of the drug, so that when the person uses the drug, they do not experience the usual pleasant effects of it (e.g., naloxone and naltrexone); the drugs often are used to prevent relapse after detoxification. Yet, some other pharmacotherapies (e.g., antibuse for alcohol) even produce negative and uncomfortable effects if the drug is taken (see Sussman & Ames, 2008). Sometimes the patient may even be put under sedation, essentially sleeping off the withdrawal, using a procedure deemed "ultra rapid detoxification" (Salimi et al., 2014).

While *nicotine detoxification* may not need medical supervision, individuals seeking to stop smoking will still suffer from unpleasant effects, especially during the first two weeks or so after quitting. Some medications that may ease these symptoms are bupropion SR, varenicline, and various nicotine-containing products (which provide the nicotine effect without intake of tar-related carcinogens) such as nicotine gum, patch, inhaler, nasal sprays, and lozenges (Fiori et al., 2008).

Cognitive-Behavioral Therapy (CBT)

Cognitive-behavioral therapy (CBT) is an intervention that includes changing cognitions that lead to unwanted behavior, as well as impacting the behaviors directly. It can be a powerful tool for treatment of substance abuse and is regarded as an evidence-based approach for ATOD treatment (Carroll et al., 1998; Fiori et al., 2008; Magill & Ray, 2009; Sussman & Ames, 2008). Changing behavior patterns in patients is done through a number of stimulus-organism-response-reinforcement techniques (*SORR*). These techniques involve altering: the presence or salience of the stimuli confronting the person (stimulus control), how the person interprets the stimuli (organism control), the responses of the person to the stimuli (response control), and/or changing the contingencies of reinforcement related to those responses (reinforcement control; Goldfried & Davidson, 1994). CBT typically includes *problem solving*. This approach involves generating a number of alternative options rather than merely engaging in the unwanted behavior, in this case drug/alcohol abuse. Further, problem solving involves examining the pros and cons of each behavioral option and trying to make the best decision based on the available options (Sussman & Ames, 2008).

CBT may also include a component called *cognitive restructuring*, which involves modifying one's inner speech by recognizing and examining negative and self-defeating thought patterns and replacing them with more self-fulfilling and rational cognitions that lead to more positive thoughts and behavior. Some "cognitive errors," or maladaptive ways of thinking that may need to be changed, are all-or-nothing thinking, catastrophizing, overgeneralization, and global judgements, just to name a few (Meichenbaum, 1977).

Self-instructional training is also a part of CBT, and can help those that are very impulsive, with lack of an "inner voice" to guide behavioral regulation. This approach involves recognizing missing cognitions and adding in cognitions through practice (Meichenbaum, 1977). *Social and self-control skills training* is also often implemented in CBT (Grenard et al., 2006), and involves training patients to increase their self-control skills (e.g., stalling, assertiveness training, prosocial coping skills training), conversational and listening skills, anger management, and may involve role-playing social situations (Sussman & Ames, 2008). CBT has been found to be most effective when combined with pharmacological approaches (e.g., regarding tobacco cessation; Fiori et al., 2008).

Residential CBT programs are community-based programs with twenty-four-hour supervised treatment, all the while receiving support from other members of the program. Residential CBT programs generally involve the same principles as regular CBT treatment (the SORR model) such as modifying environmental stimuli, and identification of problems that may threaten sobriety, coping skills training, as well as establishing social connections and support (Sussman & Ames, 2008). As with other programs that utilize CBT, residential CBT programs may provide relapse prevention programming, and may assist in vocational, educational, and nutritional needs through skills development and enhancing access to recovery community resources.

Contingency Management

Contingency management (CM) may assist with enhancing retention in treatment. In this type of program, an operant condition – reinforcement (e.g., money, necessity items) – is provided to patients contingent on performance (e.g., showing up at meetings, not using ATODs). For example, researchers have experimented with an incentive voucher program for cocaine-dependent patients, offering counseling, or counseling combined with incentive vouchers. Half of the participants were offered various amounts of points that translated into retail credit for cocaine-free urinalysis results. Those in the incentive group were significantly more likely to remain abstinent during treatment and at one-year follow-up, compared to those that only received the counseling (70 percent versus 17 percent). In another condition, incentives were offered to one group contingent on drug-free urinalysis while the other group still received the voucher regardless of urinalysis results. Those in the contingency-based incentive group were again more likely to be abstinent from cocaine use (Higgins et al., 1994, 2000). CM shows promise, though it works because contingencies are in place. Once removed, unless behavior becomes contingent on natural reinforcers, behavior may go back to baseline (relapse).

Motivational Interviewing

Motivational Interviewing (MI) combines the principles of cognitive therapy, Carl Roger's client-centered approach, and the Transtheoretical Motivation Model (Miller & Rollnick, 2013). It has been shown to be effective for ATOD treatment in a meta-analysis with treatment and comparison groups, albeit with small effect sizes (0.3 for six to twelve months postprogramming and 0.2 for more than twelve months, and even lower for tobacco cessation). However, when MI was used in conjunction with other programming, such as being used as an initial screening technique or a means of follow-up, effect sizes reached 0.6 (Hettema, Steele & Miller, 2005). Motivational Interviewing may be particularly useful in the initial screening and beginning of the treatment phase, in which therapists help the patient to clarify goals and follow through with their efforts to change behavior (Miller & Rodnick, 2013). It focuses on client-directed changes, and techniques of motivational interviewing are recommended to be highly personalized to the individual (Ray et al., 2014). For patients that are ambivalent about changing their behavior, MI is particularly useful. The client and patient relationship and interactions are of utmost importance in this therapy (Barnett et al., 2014). There are eight central strategies that MI uses to facilitate behavior change.

(1) The therapist giving advice to the patient to start or reinforce new goals.
(2) Removing barriers to change.
(3) Providing positive choice options to the patient.
(4) Decreasing the desirability to continue using the drug.
(5) Showing empathy.
(6) Providing accurate feedback on behavior (e.g., positive reflections by the therapist are more likely to lead to positive change than negative or neutral reflections).
(7) Helping the client clarify their goals by confronting potential discrepancies between their future goals and their current situation.
(8) Supporting the development of the patient's self-efficacy through active helping (Barnett et al., 2014).

Motivational Interviewing is often combined with CBT, and recently there has been a new wave of group MI (Sussman, 2015). With group MI, the therapist must pay attention to the group structure and roles, as well as individual experiences that occur through the group process to ensure adequate facilitation of the group therapy (Engle et al., 2010; Sussman, 2015).

Cue Exposure

Another treatment for ATOD abuse is the cue-exposure and reactivity approach, which is based on classical conditioning/learning models (Yin & Knowlton, 2006). The cue-exposure theory postulates that repeated exposure to drug-related cues automatically results in craving for that drug, or arousal that is uncomfortable, and which may prompt the addict to seek out the drug. Craving is seen as a conditioned response to stimuli, in this case, the drug of choice (Drummond, 2000; Monti, Rohsenow & Hutchison, 2000; Niaura et al., 1988; Rohsenow et al., 1994). There is evidence that shows that when an addict is exposed to drug-related stimuli (versus drug-neutral stimuli), there is a significant increase in self-reports of craving (Carter & Tiffany, 1999). The cue-exposure treatment protocol is used to extinguish the conditioned responses (craving) through unreinforced exposure to conditioned stimuli (drugs/alcohol) which, in turn, should minimize usage of the substance. For instance, an alcohol abuser could be exposed to sights and sounds of alcohol, or may visit a bar with their therapist (in-vivo exposure), or may use imaginal exposure (in-vitro) to visualize drinking-related cues without acting on these cues to extinguish conditioned responding, all the while practising skills to engage in alternative behavior (e.g., relaxation and meditation; Monti et al., 1989). This could prove to be additionally beneficial when the patient leaves treatment and has to face the real world and all of the drug-related stimuli that they may inevitably encounter. There are various problems associated with this treatment such as spontaneous recovery (e.g., later in-vivo exposure to the drug in the same or a new setting, which leads to a return of craving) and generalizability (e.g., extinction of craving in the lab may not generalize to the real world) (Conklin & Tiffany, 2001), but there is evidence for some success of this treatment in problem gambling (Grant & Odlaug, 2014). This approach is also similar to that of exposure-therapy for obsessive-compulsive disorder, phobias, and anxiety, which is considered the gold-standard treatment for those disorders (POTS, 2004); however, more research is needed to better apply the cue exposure paradigm to substance use disorders.

Attentional Retraining

Another approach to changing cue responses is a relatively new technique that is still being investigated, which involves redirecting cognition and attentional cues away from the cue approach behavior (drug-seeking), and on to more neutral stimuli (Cox et al., 2014; Franken, 2003). Attentional retraining involves a visual probe task (dot probe paradigm) that uses target drug-related pictures and drug-neutral images to get patients to implicitly redirect attention away from the drug-related cues and focus on neutral cues instead (e.g., shifting from images of alcohol to soda). This technique has shown some promise (Field & Eastwood, 2005; McGeary et al., 2014), though, overall, results are equivocal at present (Sussman, 2017).

Twelve-Step Programs

Twelve-step programs are often commonly thought of when treatment for substance use is mentioned, which makes sense considering their philosophies are used by over two-thirds of inpatient and outpatient treatment programs in the USA (Sussman, 2010). Alcoholics Anonymous (AA) and Narcotics Anonymous (NA) are the two main ATOD twelve-step programs that exist. They make use of group mutual support meetings and a pathfinder (sponsor) as main source of social support, with regular anonymous meetings where individuals can share their stories of addiction, recovery, relapse, and coping with difficult life events. Twelve-step programs are abstinence-oriented, multidimensional, nonprofit, humanistic, voluntary, involving mutual social support (Galaif & Sussman, 1995; Sussman, 2010; Sussman & Ames, 2008). The programs are independent and self-supporting, do not accept outside donations and do not contribute their opinions to outside issues. The only requirement to join a program is the desire to stop an addiction. Twelve-step programs operate on the classic disease model of addiction. There exist beliefs such as that addicts do not "feel comfortable in their own skin," can fall victim to their inner addict voice, and that generally the addictive behavior is a result of implicit processes that lead to uncontrolled behavior due to an individual's baseline restlessness, irritability, or discontent (RID; Alcoholics Anonymous, 1976; Narcotics Anonymous, 1988). Processes of change include coming to believe in an outside higher power to assist with recovery, becoming aware of wrongs done and making amends, and maintaining a daily spiritual regimen (e.g., meditation and prayer).

Some of the criticisms of twelve-step programs are that they are somewhat "cult-like," with members being dependent on the program itself, and disregarding anyone who may want to take another approach to sobriety (Trimpey, 1989, 1996). There have also been complaints that those who do not embrace all of the twelve steps may feel unwelcome at meetings (Bufe, 1991), and particularly members who do not subscribe to the tenant of believing in a "higher power." Nonreligious and non-spiritual participants may find themselves not progressing in the program as well as others.

Even so, with all of the criticisms that twelve-step programs encounter, there is a plethora of anecdotal support for the programs, and some empirical evidence as well (Ferri, Amato & Davoli, 2006; Kelly et al., 2012). Though there has been little controlled research regarding programs, the available evidence is that abstinence rates among participants is about as high as cognitive-behavioral treatment and Motivational Interviewing (Project MATCH; Connors, 1998).

Anonymity and social support are two very important components of twelve-step programs, which allow members to develop a sense of trust and intimacy with each other. Members work the twelve steps together and encourage each other toward sobriety. *Sober-living homes* are also a part of this notion of peer support, and while they are not an official part of twelve-step programs, many AA and NA programs have members who live together in a house and support each other's sobriety. All of the residents pay their own rent and food costs, but there is usually some communal aspect of living together and making sure all of the residents abstain from drug use. There has been support for the suggestion that these homes are effective for former addicts to maintain sobriety and live in a structured environment (Heslin et al., 2012; Mueller & Jason, 2014). Along with the member meetings and a social network of peers who are there to support individuals and reinforce that they are not alone in their struggle, twelve-step programs encourage self-selecting a sponsor who is an individual who helps the person through recovery and may give them advice and provide additional social support. About 10 percent of people will remain active in AA for several years, and of those who remain active, 50 percent maintain sobriety, especially if they are helping others in recovery or are otherwise active participants (Galaif & Sussman, 1995; Pagano et al., 2004).

Group and Family Therapy

Much like twelve-step programs, *group therapy* is helpful for individuals that benefit from social support and peer feedback, although unlike twelve-step programs group therapy is led by a trained therapist. It can be a less expensive option than individual therapy and allows the therapist to coach and monitor the patients at first, and then move on to discuss more in-depth addiction-related issues. This process also encourages others in the group to voice their thoughts and experiences, allowing intimacy between group participants to form, and members also learn skills in expressing themselves and listening to others (Sussman & Ames, 2008). There is empirical support for group therapy that indicates it is about as effective as individual approaches, and better than self-help groups or less-intensive programming (Stead & Lancaster, 2005; Weiss et al., 2004).

Family therapy also involves social ties but, rather than peer support, family therapy attempts to utilize family members in a systems-type approach to treatment. While there are several types of family therapy models, one major theory behind family therapy is that the addiction does not exist in only the individual sufferer, but rather is part of a system of problematic behavior, some of which stems from the family members and dynamics that are present (Horigian et al., 2015). A well-trained therapist is needed to conduct family therapy sessions to explore problems in family relationships such as inappropriate roles, conflict, and boundary issues (enmeshed, disengaged), with the goal being to utilize the resources and support of the family to help the addict and the family system as a whole to integrate and heal. Oftentimes, there is a barrier of actually enrolling the whole family in treatment, but if the family is willing to participate, there have been successful therapeutic results (Horigian et al., 2015; Rowe, 2012). Family therapy may be particularly helpful for adolescent ATOD abuse (Liddle et al., 2001).

Families may also be helpful in utilizing *behavioral contracting*, which is a type of binding agreement between the addict and another person or persons that includes specific details about behavioral constraints on observable behaviors. It may involve rewards and penalties for conforming to the contract or violating the contract. For example, an individual may set up a contract with the family that stipulates no purchasing of any alcohol, consuming alcohol, going to parties, or going to liquor stores. If anyone in their family notices any type of this behavior, the contract is violated and a predetermined penalty is enacted. Likewise, the contract may include rewards for complying with the contract, such as monetary payouts for not going to risky locations, or for a preagreed on number of months of staying sober. There has been some evidence of this behavioral contracting approach being effective for couples in which one member is alcoholic (O'Farrell & Fals-Stewart, 2000), as well as in chemically dependent patients (Talbot & Crosby, 2001). There are of course drawbacks to this method, as the behavior cannot always be monitored 100 percent, incentives may lose their appeal, such a contract may inadvertently attempt to alter naturally occurring family roles, and the contract most likely will not be able to last forever (Sussman & Ames, 2008).

Additional Therapies

There are numerous other approaches to treatment of addiction that have not yet been studied well enough to provide conclusive evidence of their success. One treatment that has been utilized is *acupuncture*, although the literature shows that it is not considered an effective treatment for substance use (Margolin et al., 2002; Ter Riet, Kleijnen & Knipschild, 1990); yet, some people hope that this treatment may be helpful (which it may be for some people, if nothing more than through a placebo effect). Other approaches warrant further investigation, as some pilot studies have shown them to be effective. For instance, a residential pilot group treatment program was conducted to test the effectiveness of *yoga and meditation mind-body techniques* for substance-use recovery in India. Participants showed improvement on a number of psychological self-report questionnaires (Khalsa et al., 2008). Hatha yoga in methadone maintenance patients was also shown to be as effective as psychodynamic group therapy (Shaffer, LaSalvia & Stein, 1997). A review of yoga and mindfulness practices for treatment in addiction supported these interventions as complementary therapies for treating and preventing addictive behaviors (see Kechter & Black, 2020; Khanna & Greeson, 2013). In a mindfulness training pilot study comparing mindfulness to CBT, results suggested that psychological and physiological indices of stress were reduced for the mindfulness training group, compared to CBT. There were also no differences in treatment satisfaction or drug use between groups (Brewer et al., 2009), indicating mindfulness may serve as another type of therapy to help treat and prevent relapse among alcoholics (Zgierska et al., 2008). A *biofeedback* protocol implemented in inpatient therapy for addiction is also a seldomly explored avenue, which may be considered another complementary medicine type of approach. In one small RCT study of 120 volunteers receiving residential treatment for substance abuse, treatment subjects received forty to fifty sessions of EEG biofeedback (e.g., alpha-theta wave training) and were contrasted with an attention control group (Scott et al., 2005). The treatment subjects remained in treatment longer and achieved higher abstinent rates (77 percent versus 44 percent) at twelve months posttreatment.

Recently, *mHealth (mobile health)* has been considered as a source of treatment or supplemental treatment for mental health and substance-use disorders. This approach generally includes internet-based, text-messaging, or mobile-phone application delivery of services. One recent review found that participants using mHealth as a tool for substance abuse treatment noted the ease and convenience of the interventions, and the majority of studies provided efficacy for the support of these tools (Kazemi et al., 2017). Indeed, considering the cost of traditional rehabilitation and mental health services, a cheaper, more-convenient avenue of intervention delivery may be a solution, especially for those who are not insured. Some other therapies include *art, music, and wilderness training* therapy, which all have some anecdotal evidence of success but are severely lacking in research studies to back up their claim of effectiveness.

Multiple Addictions and Harm Reduction

Oftentimes patients enter treatment with multiple addictions that must all be addressed. Recently, there has been some headway in treatment centers offering programming that manages multiple substance and behavioral addictions (e.g., gambling, gaming). Sometimes one addiction is more severe than the other and may take precedence, and at other times clinicians have pondered whether another addiction might be "left alone." The biggest example of this is cigarette smoking – there are many cases in which a person undergoes inpatient treatment for a drug abuse problem but is still allowed to smoke (Sussman & Ames, 2008). While smoking is also an addiction that is extremely harmful to health, some clinicians believe that it may be more important to deal with the primary addiction and allow the individual to maintain that other habit for the time-being, so as to not completely overwhelm them with a complete overhaul of their lifestyle. This is sometimes referred to as "withdrawal mediation," wherein one addiction takes the place of another one. In this example, someone who is in recovery for alcohol abuse may smoke to cope with or relieve withdrawal from the primary drug of abuse. (Some research, though, suggests that quitting smoking along with alcohol use, for example, leads to no higher relapse than focusing only on alcohol; Sussman & Ames, 2008.)

Table 16.1 Summary of empirical treatment modalities

Treatment method	Description	Focus of treatment	Especially beneficial for
Natural recovery	"Growing out" of addiction without formalized means of treatment.	Quitting cold-turkey, reading self-help books, seeking out informal support.	Individuals who appear to need ATODs less than the typical addict to function comfortably. Individuals experiencing less severity of problems.
Detoxification and pharmacotherapy	Detoxification – managing a person's symptoms, including physical and emotional pain, while the body reacts to the withdrawal of the drug. Pharmacotherapy – supplementing treatment with prescribed drugs.	Usually involves an institutionalized process with a three-to-five-day inpatient stay, and intensive medical management and supervision. Use of medication-assisted therapy such as methadone or buprenorphine for opioid addicts.	Typically used for drugs that produce very strong withdrawal symptoms such as alcohol, benzodiazapenes, and opioids.
Cognitive-behavioral therapy (CBT)	Cognitive-behavioral therapy (CBT) is an intervention that includes changing cognitions that lead to unwanted behavior, as well as the impacting the behaviors directly.	Changing behavior patterns in patients is done through a number of stimulus-organism-response-reinforcement techniques (SORR). CBT also teaches problem-solving techniques, cognitive restructuring, social skills, implementation intentions, and self-instructional training.	Evidence-based approach for all ATOD treatment.
Motivational Interviewing	Combines the principles of cognitive therapy, Carl Roger's client-centered approach, and the Transtheoretical Motivation Model.	Focuses on client-directed changes, and techniques of motivational interviewing are recommended to be highly personalized to the individual.	May be particularly useful in the initial screening and beginning of treatment phase, in which therapists help the patient to clarify goals and follow through with their efforts to change behavior.
Cue-exposure and attentional retraining	Redirecting cognition and attentional cues away from the cue approach behavior (drug-seeking), and on to more neutral stimuli.	The cue exposure treatment protocol is used to extinguish the conditioned responses (craving) through unreinforced exposure to conditioned stimuli (drugs/alcohol) which, in turn, should minimize usage of the substance.	This could prove to be additionally beneficial when the patient leaves treatment and has to face the real world and all of the drug-related stimuli that they will inevitably encounter.
Twelve-step programs	Programs in which anonymous individuals gather and share their stories of addiction, recovery, relapse, and all of the difficulties surrounding their substance use problems.	Twelve-step programs are abstinence-oriented, multidimensional, nonprofit, humanistic, voluntary, and socially supportive. Anonymity and social support are two very important components of twelve-step programs, which allow members to develop a sense of trust and intimacy with each other.	Their philosophies are used by over two-thirds of inpatient and outpatient treatment programs. There is not much empirical evidence for twelve-step programs, but there is a lot of anecdotal support.
Group and family therapy	Group therapy allows for individuals to express their thoughts in a group setting, obtaining feedback from peers. Family therapy attempts to utilize family members in a systems-type approach to treatment.	This process encourages others in the group to voice their thoughts and experiences, allowing intimacy between group participants to form, and members also learn skills in expressing themselves and listening to others.	There is empirical support for group therapy that indicates it is about as effective as individual approaches, and better than self-help groups or less intensive programming.

Notes. We use "addiction" to refer to someone who uses a substance (ATOD) to achieve an appetitive effect, becomes preoccupied with using, loses control over using, and experiences negative consequences (see Sussman & Pakdaman, 2020). An "addict" refers to anyone addicted to an ATOD product.

Marijuana and methadone have also been studied as maintenance drugs for individuals quitting more harmful substances (Marlatt et al., 2012; Pentz et al., 1997; Swartz, 2010). These approaches are examples of harm reduction. *Harm reduction* means accepting that an individual may not be able to quit their addiction all at once, and finding short-term goals for the patient that are acceptable and achievable. It involves slowly changing the dangerous behavior to a less-dangerous one – such as using methadone as a safer substitute for heroin patients, which will hopefully lead to minimal harm or cessation all together (of methadone as well at some point; Duncan et al., 1994; Marlatt, Somers & Tapert, 1993; Pentz et al., 1997). There is also the possibility for some individuals to become controlled users rather than becoming completely abstinent, but it is only a small portion of former addicts that can achieve this with success (approximately 5 percent of alcoholics; Sussman & Ames, 2001).

Relapse Prevention

As mentioned in the beginning of this chapter, relapse rates in addiction recovery are unfortunately very high – a single attempt of quitting a substance results in a 50 percent to 75 percent chance of relapse within a year of the attempt (Heyman, 2013; Sussman & Ames, 2008). Relapse is when an individual who has remained abstinent for some time engages with their addiction once more – it can be a single event (a "lapse"), a binge, or a complete return to the drug-using behavior (a full relapse; Marlatt, 1985). There are often warning signs that a relapse may be likely to happen; for example, changes in thinking, feeling and behavior, avoidance, defensiveness, or loss of control (Gorski & Miller, 1984). Relapse is linked to a failure to avoid settings and situations where substance use might occur, failure to maintain effective coping mechanisms, interpersonal problems, negative affective states, and cravings or intrusive thoughts about the addiction (Hendershot et al., 2011; Marlatt, 1985). Relapse after discharge from treatment is associated with having greater resource needs, involvement in substance-using leisure activities, minority status, and being single (Walton et al., 2003). Some forms of relapse prevention have already been discussed in this chapter, such as sober living homes and support groups, CBT self-management techniques, decision-making, and meditation. When it comes to maintenance of recovery, evidence has shown that participating in some type of outpatient or twelve- step program may benefit individuals (Moos et al., 1999; Ouimette, Moos & Finney, 1998). It may be helpful to have a recovery community to rely on for social support, for guidance, for "safe" fun, and also to act as monitors and "check in" on the progress of the individual.

One can set their own plans to prevent the use of an ATOD by specifying a plan of action, otherwise known as setting an *implementation intention.* The aim is to create an "If X occurs (e.g., the person passes by a bar), then I will perform behavior Y (walk past the bar)" strategy. The goal of implementation intentions is for the cue–response behavior to become automatically initiated over time, with little or no conscious effort given to proceed with the healthier behavior (Gollwitzer, 1999). This may help individuals regulate or control their use of ATODs, especially given that drugs can negatively affect control processes (Prestwich, Conner & Lawton, 2006). Some evidence has shown effects across a variety of health behaviors, including binge and heavy drinking (Haggar et al., 2012; Prestwich et al., 2006). One recent study of treatment-seeking individuals with alcohol use disorder found a significant decrease of 1.09 drinks per day for those in an implementation intervention group versus a 0.29 decrease of daily drinks decrease for the control group (Moody et al., 2018).

With all of the new technologies and apps that exist nowadays, there is also research to be done on the efficacy of technological innovations that may assist relapse prevention, such as *Geographical Information Systems (GIS)-type apps* that have one check-in everyday, set goals, or even monitor locations traversed during the day to ensure the individual is not going near something such as a liquor store or bar (a "slippery slope"). As another example, *internet-based adolescent substance abuse relapse prevention modules* show promise as a supplement to treatment (Trudeau et al., 2017). Inclusion of modules that provide instruction on relapse triggers (e.g., irrational or fearful thinking, negative effect, social pressures), coping with cravings, and planning, can favorably impact drug-use outcomes beyond other treatment provided. Another technology example, *telemedicine,* or two-way, real-time interactive communication between a patient and healthcare provider, represents a rapidly expanding, but still relatively untapped resource to engage children, adolescents, and their family members in treatment-based interventions (Sussman et al., 2018).

One of the key aspects to staying sober is to be able to adequately cope with high-risk situations, which involves maintaining a high level of self-efficacy to stay sober, even under very trying circumstances (Larimer, Palmer & Marlatt, 1999; Marlatt, 1985). It is also important to remind patients that, even if a lapse occurs, it does not mean that all is lost and that the addict will automatically spiral out of control (the abstinence violation effect [AVE]). The goal is for the addict to regain balance as soon as possible. Cognitive restructuring techniques can help to prevent this spiral from happening.

There is still research to be done on effective relapse prevention programming, as the number of people who eventually relapse is still staggeringly high. It may be useful to encourage recovering addicts to lead a healthy holistic lifestyle, to incorporate a healthy diet, exercise, meditate, and make other positive well-being lifestyle changes that may encourage them to remain sober and live their life without using drugs (Hendershot et al., 2011).

Conclusions

Addiction is a lifelong battle, sometimes very easy and sometimes very difficult, that extends beyond completion of treatment. Although much of the research on addiction has helped practitioners gain new perspectives on the disorder and ways to help, the relapse and attrition rates for substance use disorders are regrettably still high. Further research needs to examine barriers to treatment entry, paying particular attention to disparities among genders and races, as well as stigma that pervades perceptions of the disorder. A disease label may or may not decrease stigma; there is always the possibility that the sufferer could be viewed as both "evil" and "sick." Drop-out rates can be lowered by having friendly, supportive staff who are knowledgeable in the field of addiction medicine. More research should be conducted to test the effectiveness of modern therapies. Even though various types of therapy may help in the short term, many individuals still fall back in their old ways and relapse or move on to becoming addicted to a new substance or behavior. Harm-reduction strategies should be further investigated, and a special emphasis should be placed on relapse prevention methods.

REFERENCES

Alcoholics Anonymous (1976). *Alcoholics Anonymous.* New York: Alcoholics Anonymous World Services.

American Psychiatric Association (2013). *Diagnostic and Statistical Manual of Mental Disorders: DSM-V- TR* (5th edition). Arlington, VA: American Psychiatric Publishing.

Barnett, P. G. & Swindle, R. W. (1997). Cost-effectiveness of inpatient substance abuse treatment. *Health Services Research,* **32**(5), 615.

Barnett, E., Spruijt-Metz, D., Moyers, T. B., et al. (2014). Bidirectional relationships between client and counselor speech: The importance of reframing. *Psychology of Addictive Behaviors,* **28**(4), 1212.

Bischof, G., Rumpf, H. J., Hapke, U., Meyer, C. & John, U. (2003). Types of natural recovery from alcohol dependence: A cluster analytic approach. *Addiction,* **98**(12), 1737–1746.

Bischof, G., Rumpf, H. J. & John, U. (2012). Natural recovery from addiction. In H. Shaffer, D. A. LaPlante & S. E. Nelson (Eds.), *APA Handbooks in Psychology®. APA Addiction Syndrome Handbook, Volume 2. Recovery, Prevention, and Other Issues.* Washington, DC: American Psychological Association, pp. 133–155.

Bindra, D. & Stewart, J. (Eds.) (1966). *Introduction to Motivation*. Harmondsworth: Penguin Books.

Bluthenthal, R. N., Jacobson, J. O. & Robinson, P. L. (2007). Are racial disparities in alcohol treatment completion associated with racial differences in treatment modality entry? Comparison of outpatient treatment and residential treatment in Los Angeles County, 1998 to 2000. *Alcoholism: Clinical and Experimental Research*, **31**(11), 1920–1926.

Brewer, J. A., Sinha, R., Chen, J. A., et al. (2009). Mindfulness training and stress reactivity in substance abuse: results from a randomized, controlled stage I pilot study. *Substance Abuse*, **30**(4), 306–317.

Bufe, C. (1991). *Alcoholics Anonymous: Cult or Cure?* San Francisco, CA: Sharp Press.

Carroll, K. M., Connors, G. J., Cooney, N. L., et al. (1998). Internal validity of Project MATCH treatments: Discriminability and integrity. *Journal of Consulting and Clinical Psychology*, **66**(2), 290.

Carter, B. L. & Tiffany, S. T. (1999). Meta-analysis of cue-reactivity in addiction research. *Addiction*, **94**(3), 327–340.

Chafetz, M. E., Blanc, H. T. & Hill, M. J. (1970). *Frontiers of Alcoholism*. New York: Science House.

Conklin, C. A. & Tiffany, S. T. (2001). The impact of imagining personalized versus standardized urge scenarios on cigarette craving and autonomic reactivity. *Experimental and Clinical Psychopharmacology*, **9**(4), 399.

Connors, G. J. (1998). Overview of Project MATCH. *The Addictions Newsletter*, **5**, 4–5.

Cox, W. M., Fadardi, J. S., Intriligator, J. M. & Klinger, E. (2014). Attentional bias modification for addictive behaviors: Clinical implications. *CNS Spectrums*, **19**(3), 215–224.

Cunningham, J. A. (1999). Resolving alcohol-related problems with and without treatment: The effects of different problem criteria. *Journal of Studies on Alcohol*, **60**(4), 463–466.

Curry, S., Wagner, E. H. & Grothaus, L. C. (1990). Intrinsic and extrinsic motivation for smoking cessation. *Journal of Consulting and Clinical Psychology*, **58**(3), 310.

Daughters, S. B., Lejuez, C. W., Bornovalova, M. A., et al. (2005). Distress tolerance as a predictor of early treatment dropout in a residential substance abuse treatment facility. *Journal of Abnormal Psychology*, **114** (4), 729.

DiClemente, C. C., Prochaska, J. O., Fairhurst, S. K., et al. (1991). The process of smoking cessation: an analysis of precontemplation, contemplation, and preparation stages of change. *Journal of Consulting and Clinical Psychology*, **59**(2), 295.

Drummond, D. C. (2000). What does cue-reactivity have to offer clinical research? *Addiction*, **95**(8s2), 129–144.

Duncan, D. F., Nicholson, T., Clifford, P., Hawkins, W. & Petosa, R. (1994). Harm reduction: An emerging new paradigm for drug education. *Journal of Drug Education*, **24** (4), 281–290.

Engle, B., Macgowan, M. J., Wagner, E. F. & Amrhein, P. C. (2010). Markers of marijuana use outcomes within adolescent substance abuse group treatment. *Research on Social Work Practice*, **20**(3), 271–282.

Ferri, M., Amato, L. & Davoli, M. (2006). Alcoholics Anonymous and other 12-step programmes for alcohol dependence. *Cochrane Database of Systematic Reviews*, **3**. Article CD005032.

Field, M. & Eastwood, B. (2005). Experimental manipulation of attentional bias increases the motivation to drink alcohol. *Psychopharmacology*, **183**(3), 350–357.

Fink, E. B., Longabaugh, R., McCrady, B. M., et al. (1985). Effectiveness of alcoholism treatment in partial versus inpatient settings: Twenty-four month outcomes. *Addictive Behaviors*, **10**(3), 235–248.

Fletcher, B. W., Tims, F. M. & Brown, B. S. (1997). Drug Abuse Treatment Outcome Study (DATOS): Treatment evaluation research in the United States. *Psychology of Addictive Behaviors*, **11**(4), 216.

Fiore, M. C., Jaen, C. R., Baker, T., et al. (2008). *Treating Tobacco Use and Dependence: 2008 Update*. Rockville, MD: US Department of Health and Human Services.

Fishbein, M. & Ajzen, I. (1975). *Belief, Attitude, Intention and Behavior: An Introduction to Theory and Research*. Reading, MA: Addison-Wesley.

Florentine, R., Anglin, M. D., Gil-Rivas, V. & Taylor, E. (1997). Drug treatment: Explaining the gender paradox. *Substance Use & Misuse*, **32**(6), 653–678.

Franken, I. H. (2003). Drug craving and addiction: integrating psychological and neuropsychopharmacological approaches. *Progress in Neuro-Psychopharmacology and Biological Psychiatry*, **27**(4), 563–579.

Galaif, E. R. & Sussman, S. (1995). For whom does Alcoholics Anonymous work? *International Journal of the Addictions*, **30**(2), 161–184.

Galea, S. & Vlahov, D. (2002). Social determinants and the health of drug users: Socioeconomic status, homelessness, and incarceration. *Public Health Reports*, **117** (Supplement 1), S135.

Goldfried, M. R. & Davison, G. C. (1994). *Clinical Behavior Therapy (Expanded edition)*. New York: John Wiley & Sons.

Gollwitzer, P. M. (1999). Implementation intentions: Strong effects of simple plans. *American Psychologist*, **54**, 493–503.

Gordis, E., Dorph, D., Sepe, V. & Smith, H. (1981). Outcome of alcoholism treatment among 5578 patients in an urban comprehensive hospital-based program: Application of a computerized data system. *Alcoholism: Clinical and Experimental Research*, **5**(4), 509–522.

Gorski, T. T. & Miller, M. (1984). *The Phases and Warning Signs of Relapse*. Independence, MO: Independence Press.

Gorski, T. T. & Miller, M. (1986). *Staying Sober: A Guide for Relapse Prevention*. Independence, MO: Independence Press.

Granfield, R. & Cloud, W. (2001). Social context and "natural recovery": The role of social capital in the resolution of drug-associated problems. *Substance Use & Misuse*, **36**(11), 1543–1570.

Grant, B. F. (1997). Barriers to alcoholism treatment: Reasons for not seeking treatment in a general population sample. *Journal of Studies on Alcohol*, **58**, 365–371.

Grant, J. E. & Odlaug, B. L. (2014). Diagnosis and treatment of gambling disorder. In *Behavioral Addictions: Criteria, Evidence, and Treatment*. London: Academic Press/ Elsevier, pp. 35–60.

Grenard, J. L., Ames, S. L., Pentz, M. A. & Sussman, S. (2006). Motivational interviewing with adolescents and young adults for drug-related problems. *International Journal of Adolescent Medicine and Health*, **18**(1), 53–68.

Grigsby, T. J., Sussman, S., Chou, C. P. & Ames, S. L. (2017). Assessment of substance misuse. In *Research Methods in the Study of Substance Abuse*. Cham, Switzerland: Springer, pp. 197–233.

Haggar, M. S., Lonsdale, A., Koka, A., et al. (2012). An intervention to reduce alcoholic consumption in undergraduate students using implementation intentions and mental simulations: A cross-national study. *International Journal of Behavioral Medicine*, **19**, 82–96.

Hendershot, C. S., Witkiewitz, K., George, W. H. & Marlatt, G. A. (2011). Relapse prevention for addictive behaviors. *Substance Abuse Treatment, Prevention, and Policy*, **6**, 17.

Heslin, K. C., Singzon, T., Aimiuwu, O., Sheridan, D. & Hamilton, A. (2012). From personal tragedy to personal challenge: responses to stigma among sober living home residents and operators. *Sociology of Health & Illness*, **34**(3), 379–395.

Heyman, G. M. (2013). Quitting drugs: quantitative and qualitative features. *Annual Review of Clinical Psychology*, **9**, 29–59.

Hettema, J., Steele, J. & Miller, W. R. (2005). Motivational interviewing. *Annual Review of Clinical Psychology*, **1**, 91–111.

Higgins, S. T., Budney, A. J., Bickel, W. K., et al. (1994). Incentives improve outcome in outpatient behavioral treatment of cocaine dependence. *Archives of General Psychiatry*, **51**(7), 568–576.

Higgins, S. T., Wong, C. J., Badger, G. J., Ogden, D. E. H. & Dantona, R. L. (2000). Contingent reinforcement increases cocaine abstinence during outpatient treatment and 1 year of follow-up. *Journal of Consulting and Clinical Psychology*, **68**(1), 64–72.

Horigian, V. E., Feaster, D. J., Brincks, A., et al. (2015). The effects of Brief Strategic Family Therapy (BSFT) on parent substance use and the association between parent and adolescent substance use. *Addictive Behaviors*, **42**, 44–50.

Iguchi, M. Y. & Stitzer, M. L. (1991). Predictors of opiate drug abuse during a 90-day methadone detoxification. *The American Journal of Drug and Alcohol Abuse*, **17**(3), 279–294.

Jacobson, J. O., Robinson, P. L. & Bluthenthal, R. N. (2007). Racial disparities in completion rates from publicly funded alcohol treatment: economic resources explain more than demographics and addiction severity. *Health Services Research*, **42**(2), 773–794.

Jaehne, A., Loessl, B., Frick, K., et al. (2012). The efficacy of stepped care models involving psychosocial treatment of alcohol use disorders and nicotine dependence: A systematic review of the literature. *Current Drug Abuse Reviews*, **5**, 41–51.

Johnson, V. E. (1980). *I'll Quit Tomorrow: A Practical Guide to Alcoholism Treatment.* San Francisco, CA: Harper & Row.

Julien, R. M. (2005). *A Primer of Drug Action* (9th edition). New York: W. H. Freeman.

Kazemi, D. M., Borsari, B., Levine, M. J., et al. (2017). A systematic review of the mHealth interventions to prevent alcohol and substance abuse. *Journal of Health Communication*, **22**(5), 413–432.

Kechter, A. & Black, D. S. (2020). Mindfulness-based interventions applied to addiction treatments. In S. Sussman (Ed.), *The Cambridge Handbook of Substance and Behavioral Addictions*, Cambridge, UK: Cambridge University Press, pp. 409–418

Kelly, J. F., Hoeppner, B., Stout, R. L. & Pagano, M. (2012). Determining the relative importance of the mechanisms of behavior change within Alcoholics Anonymous: A multiple mediator analysis. *Addiction*, **107** (2), 289–299.

Khalsa, S. B. S., Khalsa, G. S., Khalsa, H. K. & Khalsa, M. K. (2008). Evaluation of a residential JaKundalini yoga lifestyle pilot program for addiction in India. *Journal of Ethnicity in Substance Abuse*, 7(1), 67–79.

Khanna, S. & Greeson, J. M. (2013). A narrative review of yoga and mindfulness as complementary therapies for addiction. *Complementary Therapies in Medicine*, **21**(3), 244–252.

Larimer, M. E., Palmer, R. S. & Marlatt, G. A. (1999). Relapse prevention: An overview of Marlatt's cognitive-behavioral model. *Alcohol Research and Health*, **23**(2), 151–160.

Le Fauve, C. E., Lowman, C., Litten, R. Z., III & Mattson, M. E. (2003). Introduction: National Institute on Alcohol Abuse and Alcoholism workshop on treatment research priorities and health disparities. *Alcoholism: Clinical and Experimental Research*, **27**, 1318–1320.

Liddle, H. A., Dakof, G. A., Parker, K., et al. (2001). Multidimensional family therapy for adolescent drug abuse: Results of a randomized clinical trial. *The American Journal of Drug and Alcohol Abuse*, **27**(4), 651–688.

Magill, M. & Ray, L. A. (2009). Cognitive-behavioral treatment with adult alcohol and illicit drug users: A meta-analysis of randomized controlled trials. *Journal of Studies on Alcohol and Drugs*, **70**(4), 516–527.

Manderlink, G. & Harackiewicz, J. M. (1984). Proximal versus distal goal setting and intrinsic motivation. *Journal of Personality and Social Psychology*, **47**(4), 918.

Margolin, A., Kleber, H. D., Avants, S. K., et al. (2002). Acupuncture for the treatment of cocaine addiction: A randomized controlled trial. *JAMA*, **287**(1), 55–63.

Marlatt, G. A. (1985). Relapse prevention: Theoretical rationale and overview of the model. In G. A. Marlatt & J. R. Gordon (Eds.), *Relapse Prevention.* New York: Guilford Press, pp. 3–70.

Marlatt, G. A., Larimer, M. E. & Witkiewitz, K. (Eds.) (2012). *Harm Reduction: Pragmatic Strategies for Managing High-Risk Behaviors* (2nd edition). New York: Guilford Press.

Marlatt, G. A., Somers, J. M. & Tapert, S. F. (1993). Harm reduction: Application to alcohol abuse problems. *NIDA Research Monograph*, **137**, 147–166.

Mays, V. M., Jones, A., Delany-Brumsey, A., Coles, C. & Cochran, S. D. (2017). Perceived discrimination in healthcare and mental health/substance abuse treatment among blacks, latinos, and whites. *Medical Care*, **55** (2), 173.

McAuliffe, W. E. & Dunn, R. (2004). Substance abuse treatment needs and access in the USA: Interstate variations. *Addiction*, **99**, 999–1014.

McCaul, M. E., Svikis, D. S. & Moore, R. D. (2001). Predictors of outpatient treatment retention: Patient versus substance use characteristics. *Drug and Alcohol Dependence*, **62**(1), 9–17.

McGeary, J. E., Meadows, S. P., Amir, N. & Gibb, B. E. (2014). Computer-delivered, home-based, attentional retraining reduces drinking behavior in heavy drinkers. *Psychology of Addictive Behaviors*, **28**(2), 559.

McLellan, A. T., O'Brien, C. P., Lewis, D. & Kleber, H. D. (2000). Drug addiction as a chronic medical illness: Implications for treatment, insurance and evaluation. *Journal of the American Medical Association*, **284**, 1689–1695.

McLellan, A. T. (2002). Have we evaluated addiction treatment correctly? Implications from a chronic care perspective. *Addiction*, **97** (3), 249–252.

Meek, P. S., Clark, H. W. & Solana, V. L. (1989). Neurocognitive impairment: The unrecognized component of dual diagnosis in substance abuse treatment. *Journal of Psychoactive Drugs*, **21**(2), 153–160.

Meichenbaum, D. (1977). *Cognitive Behavior Modification: An Integrative Approach.* New York: Plenum.

Mertens, J. R. & Weisner, C. M. (2000). Predictors of substance abuse treatment retention among women and men in an HMO. *Alcoholism: Clinical and Experimental Research*, **24**(10), 1525–1533.

Miller, W. R. & Hester, R. K. (1986). Inpatient alcoholism treatment: Who benefits? *American Psychologist*, **41**(7), 794.

Miller, W. R. & Rollnick, S. (2013). *Motivational Interviewing: Helping People Change* (3rd edition). New York: Guilford Press.

Mohatt, G. V., Rasmus, S. M., Thomas, L., et al. (2008). Risk, resilience, and natural recovery: A model of recovery from alcohol abuse for Alaska Natives. *Addiction*, **103**(2), 205–215.

Monti, P. M., Abrams, D. B., Kadden, R. M. & Cooney, N. L. (1989). *Treating Alcohol Dependence.* New York: Guilford Press.

Monti, P. M., Rohsenow, D. J. & Hutchison, K. E. (2000). Toward bridging the gap between biological, psychobiological and psychosocial models of alcohol craving. *Addiction*, **95**(8s2), 229–236.

Moody, L. N., Tegge, A. N., Poe, L. M., Koffarnus, M. N. & Bickel, W. K. (2018). To drink or to drink less? Distinguishing between effects of implementation intentions on decisions to drink and how much to drink in treatment-seeking individuals with alcohol use disorder. *Addictive Behaviors*, **83**, 64–71.

Moos, R. H., Finney, J. W., Ouimette, P. C. & Suchinsky, R. T. (1999). A comparative evaluation of substance abuse treatment: I. Treatment orientation, amount of care, and 1-year outcomes. *Alcoholism: Clinical and Experimental Research*, **23**(3), 529–536.

Mueller, D. G. & Jason, L. A. (2014). Sober-living houses and changes in the personal networks of individuals in recovery. *Health Psychology Research*, **2**(1), 5–10.

Mueller, L. A. & Ketcham, K. (1987). *Recovering: How to Get and Stay Sober*. New York: Bantam.

Narcotics Anonymous (1988). *Narcotics Anonymous* (5th edition). Van Nuys, CS: Narcotics Anonymous World Services.

Niaura, R. S., Rohsenow, D. J., Binkoff, J. A., et al. (1988). Relevance of cue reactivity to understanding alcohol and smoking relapse. *Journal of Abnormal Psychology*, **97**(2), 133.

O'Farrell, T. J. & Fals-Stewart, W. (2000). Behavioral couples therapy for alcoholism and drug abuse. *Journal of Substance Abuse Treatment*, **18**(1), 51–54.

Ouimette, P. C., Moos, R. H. & Finney, J. W. (1998). Influence of outpatient treatment and 12-step group involvement on one-year substance abuse treatment outcomes. *Journal of Studies on Alcohol*, **59**(5), 513–522.

Pagano, M. E., Friend, K. B., Tonigan, J. S. & Stout, R. L. (2004). Helping other alcoholics in alcoholics anonymous and drinking outcomes: Findings from project MATCH. *Journal of Studies on Alcohol*, **65**(6), 766–773.

Pediatric OCD Treatment Study (POTS) Team. (2004). Cognitive-behavior therapy, sertraline, and their combination for children and adolescents with obsessive-compulsive disorder. *Journal of the American Medical Association*, **292**, 1969–1976.

Pentz, M. A., Sussman, S. & Newman, T. (1997). The conflict between least harm and no-use tobacco policy for youth: Ethical and policy implications. *Addiction*, **92**(9), 1165–1174.

Petry, N. M. (2003). A comparison of African American and non-Hispanic Caucasian cocaine-abusing outpatients. *Drug and Alcohol Dependence*, **69**, 43–49.

Prestwich, A., Conner, M. & Lawton, R. (2006). Implementation intentions: Can they be used to prevent and treat addiction? In R. W. Wiers & A. W Stacy (Eds.), *Handbook on Implicit Cognition and Addiction*. Thousand Oaks, CA: Sage, pp. 455–469.

Prochaska, J. O. & DiClemente, C. C. (1982). Transtheoretical therapy: Toward a more integrative model of change. *Psychotherapy: Theory, Research & Practice*, **19**(3), 276.

Ray, A. E., Kim, S. Y., White, H. R., et al. (2014). When less is more and more is less in brief motivational interventions: Characteristics of intervention content and their associations with drinking outcomes. *Psychology of Addictive Behaviors*, **28**(4), 1026.

Rees, D. W. (1986). Changing patients' health beliefs to improve compliance with alcoholism treatment: A controlled trial. *Journal of Studies on Alcohol*, **47**(5), 436–439.

Reinarman, C. & Levine, H. G. (Eds.) (1997). Real opposition, real alternatives. *Crack in America: Demon Drugs and Social Justice*. University of California Press, p.345.

Rohsenow, D. J., Monti, P. M., Rubonis, A. V., et al. (1994). Cue reactivity as a predictor of drinking among male alcoholics. *Journal of Consulting and Clinical Psychology*, **62**(3), 620.

Rouse, B. A., Carter, J. H. & Rodriguez-Andrew, S. (1995). Race/ethnicity and other sociocultural influences on alcoholism treatment for women. In M. Galanter (Ed.) *Recent Developments in Alcoholism, Volume 12: Alcoholism and Women*. New York: Plenum Press, pp. 343–367.

Rotter, J. B. (1954). *Social Learning and Clinical Psychology*. Englewood Cliffs, NJ: Prentice Hall.

Rowe, C. L. (2012). Family therapy for drug abuse: Review and updates 2003–2010. *Journal of Marital and Family Therapy*, **38**(1), 59–81.

Ryan, R. M., Plant, R. W. & O'Malley, S. (1995). Initial motivations for alcohol treatment: Relations with patient characteristics, treatment involvement, and dropout. *Addictive Behaviors*, **20**(3), 279–297.

Salimi, A., Safari, F., Mohajerani, S. A., et al. (2014). Long-term relapse of ultra-rapid opioid detoxification. *Journal of Addictive Diseases*, **33**(1), 33–40.

Scott, W. C., Kaiser, D., Othmer, S. & Sideroff, S. I. (2005). Effects of an EEG biofeedback protocol on a mixed substance abusing population. *The American Journal of Drug and Alcohol Abuse*, **31**(3), 455–469.

Shaffer, H. J., LaSalvia, T. A. & Stein, J. (1997). Comparing Hatha yoga with dynamic group psychotherapy for enhancing methadone maintenance treatment: A randomized clinical trial. *Alternative Therapies in Health and Medicine*, **3**, 57–67.

Simpson, D. D. & Joe, G. W. (1993). Motivation as a predictor of early dropout from drug abuse treatment. *Psychotherapy: Theory, Research, Practice, Training*, **30**(2), 357–368.

Stark, M. J. (1992). Dropping out of substance abuse treatment: A clinically oriented review. *Clinical Psychology Review*, **12**(1), 93–116.

Stea, J. N., Yakovenko, I. & Hodgins, D. C. (2015). Recovery from cannabis use disorders: Abstinence versus moderation and treatment-assisted recovery versus natural recovery. *Psychology of Addictive Behaviors*, **29** (3), 522–531.

Stead, L. F. & Lancaster, T. (2005). Group behavior therapy programmes for smoking cessation. *Cochrane Database of Systematic Reviews*, **2**. Article CD001007.

Substance Abuse and Mental Health Services Administration, Center for Behavioral Health Statistics and Quality. (2017). *Treatment Episode Data Set (TEDS): 2005–2015*. National Admissions to Substance Abuse Treatment Services. BHSIS Series S-91, HHS Publication No. (SMA) 17-5037. Rockville, MD: Substance Abuse and Mental Health Services Administration (www.samhsa.gov/data/nsduh/reports-detailed-tables-2017-NSDUH; accessed October 23, 2018).

Sussman, S. (1996). Development of a school-based drug abuse prevention curriculum for high-risk youths. *Journal of Psychoactive Drugs*, **28**(2), 169–182.

Sussman, S. (2010). A review of Alcoholics Anonymous/Narcotics Anonymous programs for teens. *Evaluation & the Health Professions*, **33**(1), 26–55.

Sussman, S. (2015). Evaluating the efficacy of Project TND: Evidence from seven research trials. *Handbook of Adolescent Drug Use Prevention: Research, Intervention Strategies, and Practice*. Washington, DC: American Psychological Association.

Sussman, S. (2017). *Substance and Behavioral Addictions: Concepts, Causes, and Cures*. Cambridge: Cambridge University Press.

Sussman, S. Y. & Ames, S. L. (2001). *The Social Psychology of Drug Abuse*. Buckingham: Open University Press.

Sussman, S. & Ames, S. L. (2008). *Drug Abuse: Concepts, Prevention, and Cessation*. Cambridge: Cambridge University Press.

Sussman, S. & Pakdaman, S. (2020). Appetitive needs and addiction. In S Sussman (Ed.), *The Cambridge Handbook of Substance and Behavioral Addictions*. Cambridge, UK: Cambridge University Press, pp. 3–12.

Sussman, S., Cowgill, B., Galstyan, E. & Richardson, J. (2018). Substance abuse. In: S. G. Forman & J. D. Shahidullah (Eds.), *Handbook of Pediatric Behavioral Healthcare: An Interdisciplinary Collaborative Approach*. New York: Springer Publishing Company, pp. 213–227.

Sussman, S., Milam, J., Arpawong, T. E., et al. (2013). Spirituality in addictions treatment: Wisdom to know. . . what it is. *Substance Use & Misuse*, **48**(12), 1203–1217.

Sutton, S. R. & Eiser, J. R. (1984). The effect of fear-arousing communications on cigarette smoking: An expectancy-value approach. *Journal of Behavioral Medicine*, **7**(1), 13–33.

Swartz, R. (2010). Medical marijuana users in substance abuse treatment. *Harm Reduction Journal*, **7**(1), 3.

Talbott, G. D. & Crosby, L. R. (2001). Recovery contracts: Seven key elements. *Addiction*

Recovery Tools: A Practical Handbook. Thousand Oaks, CA: Sage, pp. 127–146.

Ter Riet, G., Kleijnen, J. & Knipschild, P. (1990). A meta-analysis of studies into the effect of acupuncture on addiction. *British Journal of General Practice*, **40**(338), 379–382.

Toneatto, T., Sobell, L. C., Sobell, M. B. & Rubel, E. (1999). Natural recovery from cocaine dependence. *Psychology of Addictive Behaviors*, **13**(4), 259.

Trimpey, J. (1989). *The Small Book: A Revolutionary Alternative for Overcoming Alcohol and Drug Dependence.* New York: Delacorte Press.

Trimpey, J. (1996). *Rational Recovery: The New Cure for Substance Addiction*. New York: Pocket Books.

Trudeau, K. J., Black, R. A., Kamon, J. L. & Sussman, S. (2017). A randomized controlled trial of an online relapse prevention program for adolescents in substance abuse treatment. *Child & Youth Care Forum*, **46**(3),437–454.

Vigezzi, P., Guglielmino, L., Marzorati, P., et al. (2006). Multimodal drug addiction treatment: A field comparison of methadone and buprenorphine among heroin- and cocaine-dependent patients. *Journal of Substance Abuse Treatment*, **31**, 3–7.

Villanueva, M., Tonigan, J. S. & Miller, W. R. (2002). A retrospective study of client-treatment matching: Differential treatment response of Native American alcoholics in Project MATCH [Abstract]. *Alcoholism: Clinical and Experimental Research*, **26** (Supplement 5), 83A.

Wakefield, J. C. & Schmitz, M. F. (2014). How many people have alcohol use disorders? Using the harmful dysfunction analysis to reconcile prevalence estimates in two community surveys. *Frontiers in Psychiatry*, **5**, 10.

Waldorf, D. (1983). Natural recovery from opiate addiction: Some social-psychological process of untreated recovery. *Journal of Drug Issues*, **13**(Spring), 237–280. [Google Scholar]

Waldorf, D., Reinarman, C. & Murphy, S. (1992). *Cocaine Changes: The Experience of Using and Quitting (Volume 49).* Philadelphia: Temple University Press.

Wallen, J. (1992). A comparison of male and female clients in substance abusetreatment. *Journal of Substance Abuse Treatment*, **9**(3), 243–248.

Walton, M. A., Blow, F. C., Bingham, C. R. & Chermack, S. T. (2003). Individual and social/environmental predictors of alcohol and drug use 2 years following substance abuse treatment. *Addictive Behaviors*, **28**(4), 627–642.

Weisner, C., Matzger, H., Tam, T. & Schmidt, L. (2002). Who goes to alcohol and drug treatment? Understanding utilization within the context of insurance. *Journal of Studies on Alcohol*, **63**(6), 673–682.

Weiss, R. D., Jaffee, W. B., Menil de, V. P. & Cogley, C. B. (2004). Group therapy for substance use disorders: What do we know? *Harvard Review of Psychiatry*, **12**(6), 339–350.

Wells, K., Klap, R., Koike, A. & Sherbourne, C. (2001). Ethnic disparities in unmet need for alcoholism, drug abuse, and mental health care. *American Journal of Psychiatry*, **158**(12), 2027–2032.

Wickizer, T., Maynard, C., Atherly, A., et al. (1994). Completion rates of clients discharged from drug and alcohol treatment programs in Washington State. *American Journal of Public Health*, **84**(2), 215–221.

Yin, H. H. & Knowlton, B. J. (2006). Addiction and learning in the brain. In R. W. Wiers & A. W. Stacy (Eds.), *Handbook of Implicit Cognition and Addiction*. Thousand Oaks, CA: Sage Publications, pp. 167–183.

Zgierska, A., Rabago, D., Zuelsdorff, M., et al. (2008). Mindfulness meditation for alcohol relapse prevention: A feasibility pilot study. *Journal of Addiction Medicine*, **2**(3), 165.

17 Prevention and Treatment of "Food Addiction"

Caroline Davis, PhD, and Ashley E. Mason, PhD

Introduction

Any successful effort to mitigate use or engagement in an addiction disorder – initially through *prevention* and/or *early intervention* strategies, and ultimately when *treatment* is the most appropriate option – depends, inevitably, on the manner which one conceptualizes the problematic behavior. Historically, perspectives on addiction have emphasized the immorality of compulsive use of harmful substances – a perspective largely predicated on the assumption of individual psychopathology and one that incorporates various sanctions and frequently diabolical forms of punishments (Robinson & Adinoff, 2016). Another view, which also eschews the "medical" model of addiction, argues that addiction is a voluntary choice – and hence a "bad habit" that derives from a "myopic" view of available, albeit largely delayed, alternative choices that have more adaptive outcomes (Heyman, 2009; Kurti & Dallery, 2012). It is also important to emphasize the sociological tradition, which provides a context to the medical science. Consider drug misuse. Drug use and its consequences are social processes that cannot be separated from the sociopolitical contexts in which they occur (Maher & Dertadian, 2017). In other words, society has important reactions to drug taking that contribute to the user's psychological deterioration that cannot simply be attributed to pharmacological impact of the substance on the body. Likewise, sociopolitical contexts impact the function of persons who participate in other addictions (e.g., sex, gambling), beyond the intrinsic reward involved. Currently, however – and while moral, legal, and sociocultural conceptions of addiction continue to exist – the medicalization of addiction disorders has prevailed for at least the last half century, with claims that addiction is essentially an acquired "brain disease" (e.g., Leshner, 2001; Volkow, Koob & McLellan, 2016; Wise, 2000) with various behavioral markers such as strong cravings, increasing compulsivity, and frequent and chronic relapses after attempts to terminate the behavior. In turn, these symptoms reflect a developing neuropathology where excessive consumption or administration of the substance or behavior fosters escalating conditioned associations with predicting cues, a downregulation of dopaminergic response to the addictive stimulus, and a concomitant downregulation of the cortically driven capacity for self-regulation (Volkow, Wise & Baler, 2017).

Environmental Influences and Psychobiological Risk for Addiction

All forms of mammalian life appear to share the emotional, motivational, and biochemical properties of the mesocorticolimbic dopamine brain reward pathway – evolutionarily ancient neural circuitry that regulates a broad spectrum of natural activities such sexual activity, novelty-seeking, and consumption of energy resources, that are essential for the preservation of the species (Panksepp, Knutson & Burgdorf, 2002; Sussman & Pakdaman, 2020). All drugs of abuse are dopamine agonists – many potent like amphetamine and obtained by direct route of administration –which typically flood the reward pathways. Repetitive and excessive substance abuse tends to cause neurophysiological and neuroplastic adaptations in the common reward pathways, which in turn foster the addictive processes characterized by increasing compulsivity and cravings; see Ouzir and Errami (2016) for a review.

Given the role of psychology, biology, and social influences on substance use, some have proposed compelling evolutionary views on addictive processes. It has been argued that vulnerability to become addicted could have resulted from natural selection for other traits (Hill, 2013). According to the *mismatch hypothesis*, for example, susceptibility to addiction may result from the incongruity between one's current environment and the ancestral one in which the brain's reward pathways developed (Hill, 2013). Such evolutionary arguments are especially apposite for understanding addictive tendencies to certain highly rewarding foods.

Although ultra-processed foods do not produce the intoxication caused by alcohol or the euphoria some experience from stimulant drugs like cocaine, they nevertheless have pronounced parallels with conventional addictive drugs. For instance, both foster cravings, and are associated with compulsivity, and the inability to cut down, even in the face of adverse consequences (Davis & Carter, 2014). Similarly to the downwardly spiraling process of drug addiction, over-stimulation of the mesocorticolimbic pathways in the brain by highly palatable and calorically dense foods contributes, over time to a compulsive pattern of consumption. In turn, the effects of tolerance, deficits in adaptive decision making, and increased impulsive responding may prompt even more frequent and greater intake, both of drugs and of highly rewarding foods (Davis, 2014; Ouzir & Errami, 2016).

Robert Lustig poignantly claimed that "sugar is a gateway drug" (see O'Callaghan, 2017). While adolescence is the most common period of initial drug use, other concomitant factors are known to exacerbate the risk at that period of development including, prominently, traits of impulsivity which manifest behaviorally as insufficient inhibition in risky choices, and poor ability to delay gratification (e.g., Weafer, Mitchell & de Wit, 2014). A recent study – in support of Lustig's contention – found that those who self-reported being "addicted" to a variety of (nondrug) addictive behaviors such as gambling, shopping, sex, eating, and internet activities showed a significantly increased likelihood of future drug use, and the outcome was even stronger when trait impulsivity was added to the model (Chuang et al., 2017). A wealth of previous evidence has demonstrated that a broad range of addictive substances cross-sensitize to each other (Smith et al., 2009). This study extends the findings to behaviors rather than substances, and reinforces the notion that strategies and interventions that target highly impulsive youth – those found frequently in externalizing conditions like ADHD and Cluster B personality disorders – are likely to maximize impact on food addiction.

A Brief History of the Food-Addiction Construct

Notions that certain foods have strong reinforcing properties and can, in some individuals, foster dependence, has a relatively long history –

dating back at least to the eighteenth century, as we have reviewed elsewhere (e.g., Davis, 2014; Davis & Carter, 2014). "Evolutionary Mismatch" viewpoints contend that certain behaviors were enhanced during the hunter-gatherer lifestyle – from which human genetic endowment had its origins – because they bestowed both survival and reproductive advantages to the species (Sussman & Pakdaman, 2020). However, in the context of advanced technology and other rapid environmental changes, these same behaviors have tended to become maladaptive and overexpressed (Davis, 2014).

From Passive Overeating to Addictive Responses to Food

A considerable body of research has endorsed the idea that food addiction is an identifiable clinical entity with many psychobehavioral similarities to convention substance use disorders. For example, those who met the diagnostic criteria of the *Yale Food Addiction Scale* (YFAS) had a significantly greater prevalence of severe depression, more pronounced symptoms of ADHD, more intense food cravings, and greater emotional overeating compared to their obese counterparts (e.g., Davis et al., 2011). They also reported more impulsivity and other addictive personality traits than did their weight-matched controls. Other studies have replicated the links between food addiction and cooccurring mood disorders, in addition to demonstrating associations with psychological and sexual abuse (Nunes-Neto et al., 2018). A recent study, directly comparing women with food addiction to those with substance use disorders, identified similar psychopathological characteristics including posttraumatic stress disorder, depression, and emotional dysregulation (Hardy et al., 2018). And finally, in a nonclinical sample of adults recruited from the community, it was demonstrated that compulsive grazing (i.e., the consumption of relatively small amounts of food over an extended period of time, and the inability to resist such repetitive snacking despite having intentions to stop) was a stronger statistical predictor of food-addiction symptoms than binge-eating behaviors – a finding which has particular relevance for bariatric patients and post-surgical outcomes (Bonder et al., 2018).

Importantly, there is also good evidence that about 50 percent of obese adults diagnosed by the YFAS also meet the DSM-IV criteria for binge-eating disorder (Davis at el., 2011; Gearhardt et al., 2012). An earlier study also found that 92 percent of their female sample met the DSM-IV-TR criteria for substance dependence when the word "food" was substituted for "drug" in a telephone interview (Cassin & von Ranson, 2007). Such investigations, and related work, raise the question of whether food addiction simply reflects a more severe subtype of BED. This issue is especially apropos in light of the clear overlap in the diagnostic criteria of each condition. Not only do they share substantial symptom overlap (Davis et al., 2011; Gearhardt et al., 2012), but there is some preliminary evidence of shared biological underpinnings (Carter et al., 2016; Davis et al., 2014).

In an earlier publication, we proposed a "continuum hypothesis" of overeating whereby a downwardly escalating dimension of excess consumption and behavior is reflected by their increased severity and compulsiveness (Davis, 2013). In other words, occasional overeating can foster more frequent episodes and in some individuals, bouts of binge eating or compulsive grazing behaviors. In clinically significant and severe cases of BED it is argued that the condition resembles an addictive process. Preliminary support for this perspective was obtained in a study a study of overweight men and women who met DSM-IV-TR criteria for BED (Davis, 2013). In the first set of analyses, the researchers compared one group with cooccurring YFAS-diagnosed food addiction and the other without – groups that were equivalent in age and BMI – and found that those with food addiction reported greater emotional and cue-driven overeating, had more severe binge eating and food cravings, and were more sensitive or reactive to the rewarding properties of food. They also had more addictive and impulsive personality traits, and had more elevated symptoms of depression compared to their nonfood addicted BED counterparts.

In the second analysis – and examining the same dependent variables as in the first analysis – the researchers compared the BED group with food addiction to weight- and age-matched adults without BED and without food. Interestingly, these two groups were very similar and only differed significantly on a few variables including that the former group had higher binge-eating scores, elevated food cravings, and higher reports of hedonic eating than the control group. A later study, employing sophisticated psychometric analyses of several popular eating-behaviors questionnaires, concluded that they all share a common construct, which they called "uncontrolled eating" (Vainik et al., 2015). The authors also found that certain questionnaires focus on different levels of severity of the construct, supporting the continuum model of compulsive consumption and its severity. In addition, the uncontrolled eating appeared to be for certain types of foods such as refined sugar, as opposed to merely overeating (see Schulte, Schiestl & Gearhardt, 2020).

Prevention and Early Intervention of Overeating and Obesity

Using sophisticated statistical modeling procedures, it has been estimated that interventions designed to reduce the intake of added sugar intake in the human diet would have substantial health and economic benefits. For instance, a 20 percent reduction in sugar over a twenty-year period is predicted to reduce Type II diabetes and coronary artery disease by 20 percent and 9 percent, respectively (Vreman et al., 2017). Other metabolic complications of obesity have also emerged, at alarmingly rates, in childhood and adolescence over the past generation. Given estimates that children consume more than a third of their daily energy resources in schools, programs and policies aimed at preventing/reducing childhood obesity have begun to target the food environment in educational institutions (Rosettie et al., 2018).

School-Based Programs for the Promotion of Healthy Eating

Over the past half century or so, the largest shift in beverage consumption amongst children and adolescents in the USA has been an increase in sugar-sweetened drinks – such as sodas, sport drinks, and energy drinks – from approximately 87 kcal to 154 kcal per day (Popkin, 2010). By contrast, milk consumption dropped by almost 100 kcal per day during the same time period. Such changes are highly relevant because of the well-established and strong associations among obesity, Type II diabetes, and the intake of sugar-sweetened drinks (Malik, Willett & Hu, 2009), as well as the sound evidence that consumption of sugar-sweetened drinks in childhood and adolescence is positively associated with weight gain during adulthood (Viner & Cole, 2006).

One school-based intervention approach has been to use the taxation of sugar-sweetened drinks as a form of direct economic incentive, because educational institutions are responsible for regulating about a third of children's daily food intake outside of holiday periods. A recent experimental market-place study, using different front-of-package labeling and sugar taxation across conditions, found that increasing price was associated a significant decrease in sugary drink purchase (Acton & Hammond, 2018). The effects of a "high sugar" label were in the positive direction, although the findings did not reach statistical significance. The authors of a current review have also concluded that the taxation approach promises some success in addition to its usefulness in generating extra revenue for educational programs (Yoshida & Simoes, 2018). However, the authors noted that because the taxation strategy faces strong opposition from the food industry, even higher tax rates might be necessary to have a meaningful impact on BMI.

Other policies to improve the diet of children have included providing fresh fruit and vegetables in the schools, and restricting access to sugar-sweetened drinks. However, the efficacy of such interventions is mostly unknown. In a recent study, Rosettie and her colleagues (2018) used comparative risk assessment frameworks to model the impact of these policies. If a food and provision policy were implemented nationally in the USA, daily fruit intake would increase by approximately 25 percent, and sugar-sweetened drink consumption would decrease by about the same amount. There would, however, be little impact on vegetable intake. These results mesh with a meta-analytic study of the effectiveness of various food-environment policies in schools aimed at improving children's dietary behaviors (Micha et al., 2018). Importantly, however, this study did not identify any significant and consistent decrease in children's adiposity as a consequence of newly implemented policy changes.

Regarding the promotion of healthy eating in the schools, it may also be possible to speculate on useful prevention/intervention approaches by extrapolating from educational efforts to prevent other problematic behaviors that are rife in the school system, such as tobacco addiction. For example, evidence suggests that educational programs that emphasize the development of social competence in their curricula produced a significant increase in quit rates compared to those that did not (Hartmann-Boyce et al., 2014). Social and emotional learning programs could help prevent motivational-driven maladaptive behaviors by promoting responsible decision-making and self-control.

Population-Based Strategies for the Prevention of Overeating and Obesity

Enhancing the palatability of foods is at the heart of the food industries' strategies to increase profits at the retail level (see Davis [2014] for a review). For example, the annual intake of sugar has tripled globally in the last half century, because of its broad (over)use in so many processed foods (Lustig, Schmidt & Brindis, 2012). Over the past three to four decades, the proportion of household consumption of *ultra-processed* foods – ones that are made and marketed to be hyperpalatable, visually attractive, and able to be consumed at any time and place – has steadily increased (Monteiro et al., 2017). There is also good evidence that the population prevalence of sugar consumption has been among the most significant predictors of global obesity prevalence, which in turn has been reliably associated with Type 2 diabetes, coronary heart disease, and other aspects of the metabolic syndrome (Siervo et al., 2013).

Of all these added ingredients, many believe that sugar is the primary component contributing to the addictive potential of some foods. For instance, in an examination of the components of a typical "fast food" meal, it was concluded that while added fat and salt tend to increase the salience of the food, it is the sugar and caffeine that foster its compulsive intake and the development of an addictive process regarding its further use (Garber & Lustig, 2011).

It seems that the most problematic sugar physiologically is fructose, which has increased worldwide, at least three-fold in the past century or so (Vos et al., 2008). In addition – and in the quantities it is typically consumed – there are several negative consequences on human metabolic functioning, such as the compromising of normal satiety signals (Lustig, 2013). It has also been claimed that fructose is simply "alcohol without the buzz," because the latter is produced by the fermentation of fructose (Lustig, 2013). Although comparative data are scarce, it is interesting to note that estimates of the population prevalence of YFAS-measured food addiction (Pedram et al., 2013) and alcoholism appear to be similar: between 5 percent and 10 percent of the population (Grant et al., 2004). It has also been found that individual differences in the response to sweet taste are positively correlated with an inclination to drink alcohol to excess, and with the genetic vulnerability for alcoholism (Kampov-Polevoy et al., 2004).

The global risk of noncommunicable diseases has been associated largely with the human consumption of unhealthy commodities such as tobacco, alcohol, and ultra-processed food and beverages. Not surprisingly, debates have ensued about the role that industry monopolies – and multinational corporations that produce and distribute these products – have in the prevention and control of the diseases that they directly or indirectly perpetuate (Moodie et al., 2013). If certain foods can be addictive, this holds implications for public health policies and regulatory agencies (Gearhardt et al., 2011b). Increasing prices and decreasing ease of access to addictive substances has tended to reduce their use (e.g., Martineau et al., 2013), suggesting that taxation is one viable method to target reductions in the use of substances, even at the very highest levels of use (Wagenaar, Salois & Komro, 2009).

Applied to addictive foods, this may indicate that implementing taxes on foods such as sugary candy and soda may reduce consumption (Schulte, Avena & Gearhardt, 2015). However, these measures are often socially unpopular. Moreover, some have claimed that taxation on addictive substances like nicotine has only reduced smoking in higher socioeconomic (SES) groups, and therefore has exacerbated SES inequalities (Riediger & Bombak, 2018). Others point out the fallacy of this assertion, however, and note that although smoking remains higher among lower SES individuals, similar reductions have been achieved across all groups in the past generation, and that lower SES groups often are more responsive to price increases than their counterparts (Hammond, Reid & Jones, 2018). As a consequence of their strong response to price changes, large health benefits often accrue to lower SES consumers. In addition, the potentially greater financial burden on low SES consumers due to high taxation could be offset by pro-poor use of tax revenues (Sassi et al., 2018).

The modern food environment is replete with cues to eat from a myriad of sources: television commercials, billboards observable along the highway, or online advertisements. Experiments altering visibility, proximity, and the arrangement of food in public spaces (e.g., Arno & Thomas, 2016) have demonstrated that individuals are less likely to select calorically rich or "junk" foods compared to those viewed as "healthy options" (Schulte et al., 2015). Given the positive association between impulsivity and addictive behaviors (Davis et al., 2011; Murphy, Stojek & MacKillop, 2014), reducing opportunities to act on impulse in the retail environment, and hence to eat less impulsively, may also assist individuals struggling with addictive-like to better manage their eating behavior.

Reducing daily exposures to cues to eat foods that trigger reward-driven eating may also benefit individuals who do not struggle with addictive tendencies toward food – namely, those who would benefit substantially from weight loss or avoiding future weight gain (Hales et al., 2017). Furthermore, reducing exposure to daily temptations may reduce "self-control depletion," and enhance our abilities to make healthier food choices (Hofmann, Rauch & Gawronski, 2007).

Treatment Directions

Introduction

Equipped with a working model of food addiction, we can consider possible treatments that may be helpful once an individual identifies as having addictive responses to food (Meadows, Nolan & Higgs, 2017). The current state of treatment strategies matches the nascence of the food-addiction construct. Indeed, it is arguable that there are currently no approaches that merit a "gold standard treatment" label. In this section, we provide a broad review of putative treatments in various stages of development, ranging from those that have been tested in human trials to experiments targeting mechanisms for future treatment development, as well as environmental and sociopolitical changes that may not merit a treatment label at all. Although the prevalence of food addiction (as defined by the YFAS) in US women has been estimated at 5.8 percent – with the highest prevalence being among women aged forty-five to sixty-one years (range: 7.4 percent to 9.4 percent; Flint et al., 2014) – food addiction is not currently a diagnosis listed in the DSM-5. We therefore review treatment modalities that target key components of addictive-like eating behaviors, most commonly craving and binge eating (Rogers & Smit, 2000). These therapies have largely been examined among individuals with BED.

Behavioral Treatment Modalities

Treatment strategies targeting core characteristics of addictive-like eating (especially craving, bingeing, and impulsivity) have shown some effectiveness. In particular, researchers have assessed the effects of cognitive behavioral therapy (CBT), as well as acceptance and mindfulness based practices on such symptoms. Abstinence-focused, twelve-step interventions, such as *Overeaters Anonymous* may also hold promise, given studies demonstrating their effectiveness in other addictive disorders (Zemore et al., 2018). However, researchers have yet to rigorously evaluate their effects on addictive-like eating. What follows is a review of treatments that target components of addictive-like eating behavior.

Cognitive-behavioral therapy (CBT) (Grilo et al., 2011) is a therapeutic modality targeting cognitions and behaviors that are believed to maintain compulsive eating patterns. CBT focuses on altering stimuli or cognitively correcting problematic thoughts or feelings that precipitate maladaptive behaviors. In practice, this often includes keeping records or diaries of thoughts, feelings, and situations that occur before, during, and/or after loss-of-control episodes of overeating. This allows individuals to reflect on current ways of responding to these thoughts, feelings, and situations, and to consider alternatives. Although BED and food addiction are distinct constructs (Davis, 2017; Gearhardt et al., 2012), though perhaps with a 50 percent overlap, that have been conceptualized in terms of severity of loss of control overeating (Davis, 2013; Vainik et al., 2015) to date, CBT has not been explicitly investigated among individuals that have been designated as having FA by a particular metric (e.g., YFAS, DSM-5 criteria for substance dependence). Notably, however, enhanced CBT for eating disorders (CBT-E) has been found to reduce binge-eating episodes in the context of BED and bulimia nervosa (Fairburn et al., 2009).

Mindfulness-based techniques such as eating awareness training (MB-EAT; Kristeller & Wolever, 2010) and acceptance-based interventions (e.g., Katterman et al., 2014) focus on the treatment of intractable food cravings and binge eating, mostly in the context of BED (Godfrey, Gallo & Afari, 2015). These models incorporate the following directives: (1) paying attention, on purpose, in the present moment, and nonjudgmentally; (2) adopting an accepting and openness to what is observed; and (3) focusing on the reduction of maladaptive behavioral responses to aversive psychological and/or physiological states (Bishop et al., 2006; Kabat-Zinn & Hanh, 2009). To date, trials employing these techniques have reported clinically significant reductions in binge eating (Godfrey et al., 2015). However, researchers have mostly examined the effects of mindfulness-based methods on food cravings in brief experimental settings with non-clinical samples (e.g., Alberts, Thewissen & Raes, 2012; Lacaille et al., 2014).

Abstinence-focused twelve-step programs, such as *Overeaters Anonymous* and *Food Addicts Anonymous*, are self-help support groups that were initially implemented for individuals with alcohol-use disorders, but later adapted for a broad range of addictive behaviors including overeating (Malenbaum et al., 1988; Yeary, 1987). In this context, these programs are often predicated on the notion that processed foods with high glycemic loads, such as those with added sugar and fat, have addictive-like properties that foster compulsive overeating (Gearhardt et al., 2011a; Schulte et al., 2015). As such, these programs typically promote abstinence from trigger foods (Ronel & Libman, 2003). Although little systematic outcome research has been carried out on these programs, one recent study found that relative to a pretreatment baseline, YFAS scores were significantly lower after one year and marginally lower after five years of group support (Weinstein et al., 2015).

Pharmaceutical Modalities

Pharmaceuticals have long been used to treat binge eating and span several classification types, ranging from selective serotonin reuptake inhibitors (SSRIs) and serotonin and norepinephrine reuptake inhibitors (SNRIs) to anti-epileptics and appetite-suppressing drugs (Reas & Grilo, 2015). Regrettably, this research has yet to identify clear-cut treatment directions, as very few drugs have been studied in multiple confirmatory trials. Moreover, most trials have reported relatively high rates of placebo responders (Brownley et al., 2015).

Recently, there has been a shift toward the investigation of pharmaceuticals that impact areas of the brain implicated in addiction and the regulation of reward (Avena, Murray & Gold, 2013; Rebello & Greenway, 2016). For example, a combination of bupropion, which agonizes the dopamine system, and naltrexone, which antagonizes the opioid system (ContraveTM; Orexigen), has been found to reduce loss of control over eating and to diminish food cravings (Apovian et al., 2013; Greenway et al., 2010). Similarly, lorcaserin (BelviqTM), a serotonergic agonist used in the treatment of obesity (Chan et al., 2013), is associated with reduced food cravings, although these reductions are larger when it is combined with an appetite suppressant (Rebello et al., 2018). Topiramate (TopamaxTM), an anticonvulsant used in the treatment of alcohol and other substance misuse disorders (Shinn & Greenfield, 2010), as well as obesity (Kramer et al., 2011), has also been shown to reduce binge-eating frequency (McElroy et al., 2003). In addition, baclofen, which is commonly used in the treatment of alcohol use disorders (Pierce et al., 2018; Rose & Jones, 2018), has been found to reduce binge eating (Corwin et al., 2012), although confirmatory evidence has mostly come from small samples (e.g., Broft et al., 2007).

The most recently approved medication for BED is Lisdexamfetamine dimesyate (VyvanseTM), a central nervous system stimulant that inhibits dopamine and norepinephrine reuptake and that is commonly used to treat attention-deficit/hyperactivity disorder (ADHD). This medication was FDA approved for BED in the USA in 2015, and in 2017 in Canada. Phase 2 and 3 trials with Vyvanse have shown clear evidence that the drug is effective in reducing binge-eating days in those with moderate to severe BED (Citrome, 2015; McElroy et al., 2015, 2016). It has also been associated with weight loss in those with BED who are overweight or with obesity. Although pharmaceuticals may hold promise in addressing targets in food addiction, evidence to date suggests that combining behavioral interventions, specifically CBT with pharmacotherapy, may yield better results than pharmacotherapy alone (Reas & Grilo, 2015).

Surgical Modalities

Bariatric surgery patients are more likely to present with compulsive overeating and other patterns of problematic eating, and studies are beginning to understand more clearly the impact of surgery on these behaviors (Conceição, Utzinger & Pisetsky, 2015; Ivezaj, Wiedemann & Grilo, 2017). Bariatric surgery has been associated with a reduction in the hedonic drive to eat, and with diminished food cravings (Leahey et al., 2012; Schultes et al., 2010) – especially for "fast foods" and sweets (Pepino et al., 2014a). Another study found that among patients presenting for bariatric surgery, 58 percent met the YFAS criteria for food addiction preoperatively, and at six and twelve months postsurgery this rate was reduced to 7 percent and 14 percent, respectively (Sevinçer et al., 2016). Importantly, however, the amount of missing data at follow-up (63 percent at six months, 76 percent at twelve months) warrants caution in interpreting these findings, although baseline YFAS scores did not differ between dropouts and completers at either time period. Similarly, another study found that 32 percent (n = 14) of individuals who presented for bariatric surgery met the YFAS criteria for food addiction, and that their postoperative weight loss was significantly associated with remission from food addiction (Pepino et al., 2014b).

Data have yet to clarify the mechanisms through which bariatric surgery exerts these effects – factors which may go beyond physiologic changes to the digestive system and may implicate hormone profiles and biological processes that underpin eating behavior (Primeaux et al., 2016). For example, one study found that assessments of microbial environments were able to discriminate between pre- and postsurgery status (Sanmiguel et al., 2017).

In summary, although studies have assessed a variety of behaviors and symptoms from pre- to postbariatric surgery, it will behoove future researchers to increase sample sizes to enhance the reliability of the findings to date. Inclusion of food-addiction symptoms and status in these assessments would also facilitate the implementation of meta-analytic procedures to enhance our understanding of the impact of bariatric surgery on addictive-like eating behaviors.

Cognitive Mechanisms in the Development of Future Treatments

The identification of intervention targets is an essential precursor to the development of successful intervention strategies (Czajkowski et al., 2015). To identify these targets in the context of hedonic overeating, researchers have focused on identifying areas in the brain that are engaged before and during eating. Several studies have demonstrated that visual exposure to highly palatable food and the anticipation of eating such food can activate reward-related regions in the brain, including the striatum, midbrain, amygdala, and orbitofrontal cortex. Such exposure and anticipation can also deactivate regions responsible for inhibitory control. The strength of this pattern of activation/deactivation is positively associated with hedonic overeating and future weight gain (Stice & Yokum, 2016). Individuals with greater food addiction (FA) (as indexed by the YFAS) show similar patterns of neural activation upon food cue exposure as do individuals with substance dependence diagnoses when exposed to substance-related cues (Gearhardt et al., 2011c). More broadly, meta-analytic data have documented similar patterns of neural activation in reward-related regions for cigarette and food cues (Tang et al., 2012).

Cognitive intervention strategies targeting changes in various types of hedonic overeating (e.g., snacking in the absence of hunger, binge eating, uncontrolled eating) have thus paralleled those developed for the treatment of substance dependence. To date, however, these interventions have yielded mixed results, and generally focus on eating behavior in the laboratory or change in weight, rather than changes in measures of FA (Allom, Mullan & Hagger, 2016; Forcano et al., 2018; Jones et al., 2017). Below, we review experimental paradigms focused on putative targets in the treatment of various types of eating beyond caloric needs. We review interventions targeting (1) reflective "top-down" processes characterized by conscious effortful control, and (2) automatic "bottom-up" processes characterized by impulsivity and associative learning (Wiers et al., 2013). We caution that these interventions have not been overtly tested in populations meeting YFAS criteria for food addiction or DSM-5 criteria for substance dependence; however, we discuss them in relation to hedonic overeating where possible.

Reflective processes are explicit, consciously experienced, and top-down processes that allow us to control our behavior in a goal-directed fashion. Laboratory studies show that in general, binge eating is associated with dysregulated reflective processes, such as lower inhibitory control (Balodis et al., 2013) and reduced executive function, including working memory capacity (Duchesne et al., 2010). It follows that researchers have examined cognitive retraining methods such as inhibitory control training (ICT), working memory training (WMT), and episodic future thinking (EFT) as potential interventions.

Automatic processes are implicit, impulsive, and bottom-up processes that result from learned associations: in the context of hedonic overeating, these learned associations are largely between cues for tasty foods and the rewarding effects of eating such foods. Laboratory studies have shown that binge eating is associated with dysregulated automatic processes including altered attentional bias for food cues (Stojek et al., 2018) and greater general and food-related impulsivity (Giel et al., 2017). These associations have led to the development of cognitive interventions focused on retraining attentional focus away from food cues and reducing impulsive eating behavior. Such interventions include cue-specific-ICT (cue-ICT), attentional bias modification (ABM), and approach avoidance training (AAT).

General Inhibitory Control Training (general-ICT)

Reduced generalized inhibitory control, as indexed by tasks such as the Stop Signal Task (Logan, Schachar & Tannock, 1997) has been associated with obesity (Lavagnino et al., 2016), but its associations with binge eating have been mixed. For example, though poorer inhibitory control has been associated with also having a BED diagnosis (Svaldi et al., 2014), it has failed to differentiate between individuals with and without BED (Wu et al., 2013). Inhibitory control training (ICT) targets deficits in inhibitory control by strengthening inhibitory responses to arbitrary cues. Researchers have examined two types of ICT in the context of hedonic overeating and obesity: "general-ICT," which employs nonfood stimuli in the assessment of abilities to inhibit behavioral responding, and "cue-specific-ICT," which differs in that it employs specific cue types (e.g., food- or drug-related cues; see below) and is focused on increasing inhibitory control only in the context of specific cue types. To date, general-ICT has not been consistently associated with reductions in laboratory or real-world hedonic overeating, whereas cue-specific-ICT has shown more promise (Jones et al., 2017). Researchers have thus speculated that general indices of inhibitory control may identify individuals at risk for weight gain over time, but that intervening on inhibitory control in the service of changing eating behavior may require further specificity (i.e., intervention using food-specific inhibitory control training; e.g., Oomen et al., 2018, see below).

Working Memory Training (WMT)

Data have demonstrated associations between reduced working memory capacity, as indexed by tasks such as backward digit span and the N-Back (Pelchat et al., 2004), and hedonic overeating. For example, reduced working memory capacity is associated with binge eating (Duchesne et al., 2010) and loss of control over eating (Manasse et al., 2014). Working memory training (WMT) focuses on improving abilities to retain and report information through memory-related tasks. These abilities are critical in the maintenance of self-regulation and goal-directed behavior, such as refraining from overeating in the pursuit of weight-loss goals. Few studies have investigated WMT in the context of hedonic overeating. However, one study randomized individuals of overweight or obese BMI status to complete up to twenty-five web-based sessions of WMT or a control (sham) training task (maximum one session per day). The WMT group completed tasks that increased in difficulty each day, whereas the control group completed similar tasks that remained easy throughout the intervention, and both groups finished their sessions in an average of thirty-four days. Although both groups evidenced improvements in working memory from pre- to postintervention, these improvements were larger within the WMT group. The WMT group also reported reductions in ruminative thoughts about food and emotional eating (Houben, Dassen & Jansen, 2016). Though many researchers have highlighted the potential importance of WMT in the reduction of overeating (Higgs, Robinson & Lee, 2012; Juarascio et al., 2015), data have yet to show whether WMT can change hedonic overeating outside of the laboratory (Jones et al., 2017).

Episodic Future Training (EFT)

Individuals with obesity evidence greater inabilities to delay gratification as measured by tasks such as delayed discounting (Bickel & Marsch, 2001). Episodic future training (EFT) (Daniel, Stanton & Epstein, 2013) addresses these deficits by engaging the episodic memory network. The EFT paradigm asks the individual to vividly imagine the future during decision making so as to reduce tendencies toward immediate gratification. Although EFT has not been specifically tested in BED or FA, it has been tested among individuals of overweight or obese BMI status. Data have begun to link uncontrolled eating and deficits in episodic memory (Martin, Davidson & McCrory, 2018). Interestingly, cueing episodic memory (historical events) and episodic future thinking (possible future events) yield similar impacts on food intake in the laboratory (Vartanian et al., 2016). In the laboratory, EFT interventions have been found to reduce posttask eating of tasty foods among individuals of overweight or obese BMI status (Daniel et al., 2013). In the field, smartphone-based EFT has been shown to reduce caloric intake during dinner at a public restaurant among women of overweight or obese BMI status (O'Neill, Daniel & Epstein, 2016).

Cue-Specific Inhibitory Control Training

Cue-specific-ICT is a variation of general-ICT that aims to strengthen inhibitory control upon exposure to specific cues (in the present context: food). Cue-specific-ICT thus focuses on both inhibitory processes as well as learned associations between food cues and behavioral responses. Cue-specific-ICT has been found to be more effective than general-ICT in reducing eating in the laboratory (Oomen et al., 2018). Meta-analytic data including studies that used specific cues for food have shown that, relative to a variety of active control groups, cue-specific-ICT groups had significantly larger reductions in short-term eating-related behavior in the laboratory (95 percent CIs [0.19, 0.47]; $Z = 4.57$, $p < 0.001$; $I^2 = 76$ percent; Jones et al., 2016). Although data suggest that cue-ICT can elicit short-term behavior changes in the laboratory, future studies should ascertain how to achieve lasting changes outside of the laboratory.

Attentional Bias Modification (ABM)

Evidence for attentional bias as a mechanism underpinning eating behavior is mixed: some data show that greater attentional bias for food cues is positively associated with greater subsequent eating (Werthmann, Jansen & Roefs, 2015) and some do not (Field et al., 2016). Observed positive associations have fostered the development of attentional bias modification (ABM) interventions. ABM interventions manipulate attentional bias for food cues by training individuals to avoid or attend to certain cues, before assessing motivational states and consummatory behavior. In the context of eating behavior, ABM retrains attention away from appetitive food cues and toward neutral or control alternatives, and study designs often include bogus post-ABM taste tests. Meta-analytic data suggest that ABM paradigms can reduce unhealthy food intake (Turton et al., 2016). Studies contrasting "attend" and "avoid" conditions on subsequent food intake have shown that participants who receive "avoid" training subsequently eat less of the trained food than participants who receive "attend" training; however, most studies lack standard control conditions that do not manipulate attention (Forcano et al., 2018; Jones et al., 2017). Inclusion of standard control conditions will allow for clearer testing of the hypothesis that reducing associations between attentional bias and food can lead to reductions in consumption.

Several ABM studies have included cross-sectional laboratory experiments as well as longitudinal designs, such as multiple training sessions (inside and outside of the laboratory) and assessment sessions after an initial laboratory experiment. For example, one study provided participants with ABM retraining *toward* chocolate cues or retraining *away* from these cues, for either one session or five sessions. At a baseline laboratory visit, those retrained away from chocolate cues evidenced larger reductions in attentional bias for chocolate cues and ate less chocolate, but these effects were no longer evident at assessment one week later. In contrast, participants who went on to receive five total weekly training sessions showed reductions in attentional bias for chocolate cues one week after their final training session (Kemps, Tiggemann & Elford, 2015). Similarly, in a small study of individuals of overweight or obese BMI status, participants received retraining away from food cues in multiple sessions over the course of eight weeks. Although participants evidenced reductions in binge eating, food cravings, and weight, reassessment of attentional bias revealed that results varied by measure: pre–post attention to food cues increased when measured using the Dot Probe task, but did not show this pattern when measured using the Food Stroop task (Boutelle et al., 2016). These results should be interpreted with caution due to study attrition and sample size; however, they suggest that ABM may be a promising intervention for binge eating. Future research should clarify the mechanisms through which ABM exerts effects.

Approach Avoidance Training (AAT)

Individuals with obesity or who report greater trait food craving relative to lean individuals or those with lower trait food craving, respectively, have shown greater approach responses toward food cues (Brockmeyer et al., 2015; Kemps & Tiggemann, 2015). Approach avoidance training (AAT) was developed to retrain automatic approach responses toward appetitive cues into avoid responses. Few data speak to the effects of AAT in the context of hedonic overeating and, in general, data linking AAT to changes in eating behavior are mixed (Becker et al., 2015; Dickson, Kavanagh & MacLeod, 2016; Schumacher, Kemps & Tiggemann, 2016). One study reported that among individuals with obesity, smartphone-delivered AAT reduced approach responses toward unhealthy foods, increased approach responses toward healthy foods, and was associated with weight-loss at an assessment six weeks after a one-week intervention period (Kakoschke et al., 2018). The mixed findings surrounding AAT may be due to strong moderators of AAT intervention effects: for example, individuals with greater impulsivity, relative to those with lower impulsivity, tend to eat more healthy foods after receiving retraining to approach healthy foods (Kakoschke, Kemps & Tiggemann, 2017). AAT interventions may hold promise in reducing maladaptive responding within the modern obesogenic environment; however, they require further testing inside and outside of the laboratory in tandem with careful measurements of potential moderating effects.

Conclusions

The principal conclusion following this review of prevention and treatment strategies for reducing the prevalence of compulsive and excessive overeating – what is commonly known as "food addiction" – is that virtually no direct information is available to inform evidence-based recommendations. Therefore, the review utilized studies based almost entirely on clinical conditions such as obesity and BED.

Regarding treatment, although the field still requires more-focused investigation, perhaps the most promising evidence-based modality occurs in the field of cognitive interventions targeting hedonic overeating. These strategies are theory-driven and align with an experimental-medicine approach toward intervention development (Czajkowski et al., 2015). In addition, future research should carefully assess potential moderators of intervention effects, including impulsivity, dietary restraint, emotional eating, and other factors that differentiate among individuals along the continuum of overeating (Forcano et al., 2018; Vainik et al., 2015). Moving forward, research should also include standardized control groups to allow researchers to test the theoretical bases on which the interventions have been developed. Cognitive interventions for hedonic overeating hold promise in that they may be highly disseminable treatments that are readily accessible via smartphones and other mobile technologies (e.g., O'Neill et al., 2016; Oomen et al., 2018).

Indeed, the use of technology-based treatments is gaining increased popularity among the general population as seen, for example, by the results of a national survey in Germany, where a quarter of the population had a positive opinion about seeking help online in the case of a mental-health problem or emotional distress – with higher rates among those who are frequent users of the internet (Eichenberg, Wolters & Brahler, 2013). Current corroborating research indicates that online self-help programs show encouraging success as subsidiary approaches to in-person interventions, although the challenge is to find improved strategies for increasing motivation to use them (Ludtke et al., 2018). In this regard, a recently published systematic review of current online support availability for food addiction produced some provocative results. Of particular interest are their findings that (i) self-help groups such as twelve-step programs are the main source of available support; (ii) there is very little evidence regarding the success of these putative treatments; and (iii) specialized input from accredited healthcare professionals is very rare in any of these programs (McKenna, Skinner & Burrows, 2018).

Another important target area for future research is the examination of sex/gender differences since disordered eating behaviors and YFAS-diagnosed food addiction occur with greater frequency in females than in males (e.g., Yu et al., 2018). However, although animal studies have clearly shown strong links between drug-seeking and palatable food-seeking behaviors, and that females demonstrate more drug seeking and preference-for-sweets than males, there is limited evidence available to establish whether links between hedonic overeating and drug addiction extend to the human condition (Carroll & Smethells, 2016). Consequently, an important direction for future research includes studies investigating whether sex moderates the efficacy of various preventions, interventions, and treatment strategies for these conditions.

REFERENCES

Acton, R. B. & Hammond, D. (2018). The impact of price and nutrition labelling on sugary drink purchases: results from an experimental marketplace study. *Appetite*, **121**, 129–137.

Alberts, H. J. E. M., Thewissen, R. & Raes, L. (2012). Dealing with problematic eating behaviour. The effects of a mindfulness-based intervention on eating behaviour, food cravings, dichotomous thinking and body image concern. *Appetite*, **58**(3), 847–851.

Allom, V., Mullan, B. & Hagger, M. (2016). Does inhibitory control training improve health behaviour?

A meta-analysis. *Health Psychology Review*, **10** (2), 168–186.

Arno, A. & Thomas, S. (2016). The efficacy of nudge theory strategies in influencing adult dietary behaviour: A systematic review and meta-analysis. *BMC Public Health*, **16**, 676.

Apovian, C. M., Aronne, L., Rubino, D., et al. (2013). A randomized, phase 3 trial of naltrexone SR/bupropion SR on weight and obesity-related risk factors (COR-II). *Obesity*, **21**(5), 935–943.

Avena, N. M., Murray, S. & Gold, M. S. (2013). The next generation of obesity treatments: Beyond suppressing appetite. *Frontiers in Psychology*, **4**, 721.

Balodis, I. M., Molina, N. D., Kober, H., et al. (2013). Divergent neural substrates of inhibitory control in binge eating disorder relative to other manifestations of obesity. *Obesity*, **21**(2), 367–377.

Becker, D., Jostmann, N. B., Wiers, R. W. & Holland, R. W. (2015). Approach avoidance training in the eating domain: Testing the effectiveness across three single session studies. *Appetite*, **85**, 58–65.

Bickel, W. K. & Marsch, L. A. (2001). Toward a behavioral economic understanding of drug dependence: Delay discounting processes. *Addiction*, **96**(1), 73–86.

Bishop, S. R., Lau, M., Shapiro, S., et al. (2006). Mindfulness: A proposed operational definition. *Clinical Psychology: Science and Practice*, **11**(3), 230–241.

Bonder, R., Davis, C., Kuk, J. L. & Loxton, N. J. (2018). Compulsive "grazing" and addictive tendencies towards food. *European Eating Disorders Review*, **26**(6), 569–573.

Boutelle, K. N., Monreal, T., Strong, D. R. & Amir, N. (2016). An open trial evaluating an attention bias modification program for overweight adults who binge eat. *Journal of Behavior Therapy and Experimental Psychiatry*, **52**, 138–146.

Brockmeyer, T., Hahn, C., Reetz, C., Schmidt, U. & Friederich, H.-C. (2015). Approach bias and cue reactivity towards food in people with high versus low levels of food craving. *Appetite*, **95**, 197–202.

Broft, A. I., Spanos, A., Corwin, R. L., et al. (2007). Baclofen for binge eating: An open-label trial. *International Journal of Eating Disorders*, **40**(8), 687–691.

Brownley, K. A., Peat, C. M., Via, M. L. & Bulik, C. M. (2015). Pharmacological approaches to the management of binge eating disorder. *Drugs*, **75**(1), 9–32.

Carroll, M. E. & Smethells, J. R. (2016) Sex differences in behavioral dyscontrol: Role in drug addiction and novel treatments. *Frontiers in Psychiatry*, **6**, article 175.

Carter, A., Hendrikse, J., Lee, N., et al. (2016). The neurobiology of "food addiction" and its implications for obesity treatment and policy. *Annual Review of Nutrition*, **36**, 105–128.

Cassin, S. E. & von Ranson, K. M. (2007). Is binge eating experienced as an addiction? *Appetite*, **49**, 687–690.

Chan, E. W., He, Y., Chui, C. S. L., et al. (2013). Efficacy and safety of lorcaserin in obese adults: A meta-analysis of 1-year randomized controlled trials (RCTs) and narrative review on short-term RCTs. *Obesity Reviews*, **14**(5), 383–392.

Chuang, C.-W. I., Sussman, S., Stone, M. D., et al. (2017). Impulsivity and history of behavioral addictions are associated with drug use in adolescents. *Addictive Behaviors*, **74**, 41–47.

Citrome, L. (2015). Lisdexamfetamine for binge eating disorder in adults: A systematic review of the efficacy and safety profile for this newly approved indication – What is the number needed to treat, number needed to harm and likelihood to be helped or harmed? *International Journal of Clinical Practice*, **69** (4), 410–421.

Conceição, E. M., Utzinger, L. M. & Pisetsky, E. M. (2015). Eating disorders and problematic eating behaviours before and after bariatric surgery: Characterization, assessment and association with treatment outcomes. *European Eating Disorders Review*, **23**(6), 417–425.

Corwin, R. L., Boan, J., Peters, K. F. & Ulbrecht, J. S. (2012). Baclofen reduces binge eating in a double-blind, placebo-controlled, crossover study. *Behavioural Pharmacology*, **23**(5–6), 616–625.

Czajkowski, S. M., Powell, L. H., Adler, N., et al. (2015). From ideas to efficacy: The ORBIT model for developing behavioral treatments for chronic diseases. *Health Psychology: Official Journal of the Division of Health Psychology, American Psychological Association*, **34**(10), 971–982.

Daniel, T. O., Stanton, C. M. & Epstein, L. H. (2013). The future is now: Reducing impulsivity and energy Intake using episodic future thinking. *Psychological Science*, **24**(11), 2339–2342.

Davis, C. (2017). A commentary on the associations among 'food addiction', binge eating disorder, and obesity: Overlapping conditions with idiosyncratic clinical features. *Appetite*, **115**, 3–8.

Davis, C. (2013). Compulsive overeating as an addictive behavior: Overlap between food addiction and binge eating disorder. *Current Obesity Reports*, **2**, 171–178.

Davis, C. (2014). Evolutionary and psychophysiological perspectives on addictive behaviors and addictive substances: Relevance to the 'food addiction' construct. *Substance Abuse and Rehabilitation*, **5**, 129.

Davis, C. & Carter, J. C. (2014). If certain foods are addictive, how might this change the treatment of compulsive overeating and obesity? *Current Addiction Reports*, **1**, 89–95.

Davis, C., Curtis, C., Levitan, R. D., et al. (2011). Evidence that food addiction is a valid phenotype of obesity. *Appetite*, **57**(3), 711–717.

Dickson, H., Kavanagh, D. J. & MacLeod, C. (2016). The pulling power of chocolate: Effects of approach-avoidance training on approach bias and consumption. *Appetite*, **99**, 46–51.

Duchesne, M., Mattos, P., Appolinário, J. C., et al. (2010). Assessment of executive functions in obese individuals with binge eating disorder. *Revista Brasileira de Psiquiatria*, **32**(4), 381–388.

Eichenberg, C., Wolters, C. & Brahler, E. (2013). The internet as a mental health advisor in Germany – Results of a national survey. *PLoS ONE*, **11**,e79206.

Fairburn, C. G., Cooper, Z., Doll, H. A., et al. (2009). Transdiagnostic cognitive-behavioral therapy for patients with eating disorders: A two-site trial with 60-week follow-up. *American Journal of Psychiatry*, **166**(3), 311–319.

Field, M., Werthmann, J., Franken, I., et al. (2016). The role of attentional bias in obesity and addiction. *Health Psychology: Official Journal of the Division of Health Psychology, American Psychological Association*, **35**(8), 767–780.

Flint, A. J., Gearhardt, A. N., Corbin, W. R., et al. (2014). Food-addiction scale measurement in 2 cohorts of middle-aged and older women. *The American Journal of Clinical Nutrition*, **99**(3), 578–586.

Forcano, L., Mata, F., de la Torre, R. & Verdejo-Garcia, A. (2018). Cognitive and neuromodulation strategies for unhealthy eating and obesity: Systematic review and discussion of neurocognitive mechanisms. *Neuroscience & Biobehavioral Reviews*, **87**, 161–191.

Garber, A. K. & Lustig, R. H. (2011). Is fast food addictive? *Current Drug Abuse Reviews*, **4**, 146–162.

Gearhardt, A., Davis, C., Kuschner, R. & Brownell, K. (2011a). The addiction potential of hyperpalatable foods. *Current Drug Abuse Reviews*, **4**(3), 140–145.

Gearhardt, A., Grilo, C. M., DiLeone, R. J., Brownell, K. D. & Potenza, M. N. (2011b). Can food be addictive? Public health and policy implications. *Addiction*, **106**(7), 1208–1212.

Gearhardt, A. N., White, M. A., Masheb, R. M., et al. (2012). An examination of the food addiction construct in obese patients with binge eating disorder. *International Journal of Eating Disorders*, **45**, 657–663.

Gearhardt, A., Yokum, S., Orr, P. T., et al. (2011c). Neural correlates of food addiction. *Archives of General Psychiatry*, **68** (8), 808–816.

Giel, K. E., Teufel, M., Junne, F., Zipfel, S. & Schag, K. (2017). Food-related impulsivity in obesity and binge eating disorder: A systematic update of the evidence. *Nutrients*, **9**(11), 1170.

Godfrey, K. M., Gallo, L. C. & Afari, N. (2015). Mindfulness-based interventions for binge eating: A systematic review and meta-analysis. *Journal of Behavioral Medicine*, **38**(2), 348–362.

Grant, B. F., Dawson, D. A., Stinson, F. S., Chou, S. P. & Dufour, M. C. (2004). The 12-month prevalence and trends in DSM-IV alcohol abuse and dependence: United States 1991-1992 and 2001-2002. *Drug and Alcohol Dependence*, **74**, 223–234.

Greenway, F. L., Fujioka, K., Plodkowski, R. A., et al. (2010). Effect of naltrexone plus bupropion on weight loss in overweight and obese adults (COR-I): A multicentre, randomised, double-blind, placebo-controlled, phase 3 trial. *The Lancet*, **376** (9741), 595–605.

Grilo, C. M., Masheb, R. M., Wilson, G. T., Gueorguieva, R. & White, M. A. (2011). Cognitive-behavioral therapy, behavioral weight loss, and sequential treatment for obese patients with binge-eating disorder: a randomized controlled trial. *Journal of Consulting and Clinical Psychology*, **79**(5), 675–685.

Hales, C. M., Carroll, M. D., Fryar, C. D. & Ogden, C. L. (2017). Prevalence of obesity among adults and youth: United States, 2015-2016. *NCHS Data Brief*, no. 288; DHHS publication; no. (PHS) 2018-1209.

Hammond, D., Reid, J. L. & Jones, A. C. (2018). Setting the record straight on taxation and disparities in smoking. *Canadian Medical Association Journal*, **190**, E964.

Hardy R., Fani, N., Jovanovic, T. & Michopoloulos, V. (2018). Food addiction and substance addiction in women: Common clinical characteristics. *Appetite*, **120**, 367–373.

Hartmann-Boyce, J., Stead, L. F., Cahill, K. & Lancaster, T. (2014). Efficacy of interventions to combat tobacco addiction: Cochrane update of 2013 reviews. *Addiction*, **109**, 1414–1425.

Heyman, G. M. (2009). *Addiction: A Disorder of Choice.* Cambridge, MA: Harvard University Press.

Higgs, S., Robinson, E. & Lee, M. (2012). Learning and memory processes and their role in eating: Implications for limiting food intake in overeaters. *Current Obesity Reports*, **1**(2), 91–98.

Hill, E. M. (2013). Chapter 4—An evolutionary perspective on addiction. *Principles of Addiction Volume 1*. Cambridge, MA: Academic Press, pp. 41–50.

Hofmann, W., Rauch, W. & Gawronski, B. (2007). And deplete us not into temptation: Automatic attitudes, dietary restraint, and self-regulatory resources as determinants of eating behavior. *Journal of Experimental Social Psychology*, **43**(3), 497–504.

Houben, K., Dassen, F. C. M. & Jansen, A. (2016). Taking control: Working memory training in overweight individuals increases self-regulation of food intake. *Appetite*, **105**, 567–574.

Ivezaj, V., Wiedemann, A. A. & Grilo, C. M. (2017). Food addiction and bariatric surgery: a systematic review of the literature. *Obesity Reviews*, **18**(12), 1386–1397.

Jones, A., Di Lemma, L. C. G., Robinson, E., et al. (2016). Inhibitory control training for appetitive behaviour change: A meta-analytic investigation of mechanisms of action and moderators of effectiveness. *Appetite*, **97**, 16–28.

Jones, A., Hardman, C. A., Lawrence, N. & Field, M. (2017). Cognitive training as a potential treatment for overweight and obesity: A critical review of the evidence. *Appetite*, **24**(1), 50–67.

Juarascio, A. S., Manasse, S. M., Espel, H. M., Kerrigan, S. G. & Forman, E. M. (2015). Could training executive function improve treatment outcomes for eating disorders? *Appetite*, **90**, 187–193.

Kabat-Zinn, J. & Hanh, T. N. (2009). *Full Catastrophe Living: Using the Wisdom of Your Body and Mind to Face Stress, Pain, and Illness.* New York: Random House LLC.

Kakoschke, N., Hawker, C., Castine, B., Courten, B. de & Verdejo-Garcia, A. (2018). Smartphone-based cognitive bias modification training improves healthy food choice in obesity: A pilot study. *European Eating Disorders Review*, **26**(5), 526–532.

Kakoschke, N., Kemps, E. & Tiggemann, M. (2017). Impulsivity moderates the effect of approach bias modification on healthy food consumption. *Appetite*, **117**(1), 117–125.

Kampov-Polevoy, A., Lange, L., Bobashev, G., et al. (2004). Sweet-liking is associated with transformation of heavy drinking into alcohol-related problems in young adults with high novelty seeking. *Alcoholism: Clinical and Experimental Research*, **38**, 2119–2126.

Katterman, S. N., Goldstein, S. P., Butryn, M. L., Forman, E. M. & Lowe, M. R. (2014). Efficacy of an acceptance-based behavioral intervention for weight gain prevention in young adult women. *Journal of Contextual Behavioral Science*, **3**(1), 45–50.

Kemps, E. & Tiggemann, M. (2015). Approach bias for food cues in obese individuals. *Psychology & Health*, **30**(3), 370–380.

Kemps, E., Tiggemann, M. & Elford, J. (2015). Sustained effects of attentional re-training on chocolate consumption. *Journal of Behavior Therapy and Experimental Psychiatry*, **49**, 94–100.

Kramer, C. K., Leitao, C. B., Pinto, L. C., et al. (2011). Efficacy and safety of topiramate on weight loss: A meta-analysis of randomized controlled trials. *Obesity Reviews*, **12**(5), e338–e347.

Kristeller, J. L. & Wolever, R. Q. (2010). Mindfulness-based eating awareness training for treating binge eating disorder: The conceptual foundation. *Eating Disorders*, **19** (1), 49–61.

Kurti, A. N. & Dallery, J. (2012). Review of Heyman's addiction: A disorder of choice. *Journal of Applied Behavior Analysis*, **45**, 229–240.

Lacaille, J., Ly, J., Zacchia, N., et al. (2014). The effects of three mindfulness skills on chocolate cravings. *Appetite*, **76**, 101–112.

Lavagnino, L., Arnone, D., Cao, B., Soares, J. C. & Selvaraj, S. (2016). Inhibitory control in obesity and binge eating disorder: A systematic review and meta-analysis of neurocognitive and neuroimaging studies. *Neuroscience & Biobehavioral Reviews*, **68**, 714–726.

Leahey, T. M., Bond, D. S., Raynor, H., et al. (2012). Effects of bariatric surgery on food cravings: do food cravings and the consumption of craved foods "normalize" after surgery? *Surgery for Obesity and Related Diseases: Official Journal of the American Society for Bariatric Surgery*, **8**(1), 84–91.

Leshner, A. I. (2001). Addiction is a brain disease. *Issues in Science and Technology*, **17**, 75–80.

Logan, G. D., Schachar, R. J. & Tannock, R. (1997). Impulsivity and inhibitory control. *Psychological Science*, **8**(1), 60–64.

Ludtke, T., Pult, L. K., Schroder, J., Moritz, S. & Bucke, L. (2018). A randomized controlled trial on a smartphone self-help application (Be Good to Yourself) to reduce depressive symptoms. *Psychiatry Research*, **269**, 753–762.

Lustig, R. H. (2013). Frusctose: It's "alcohol without the buzz". *Advances in Nutrition*, **4**, 226–235.

Lustig, R. H., Schmidt, L. A. & Brindis, C. D. (2012). Public health: The toxic truth about sugar. *Nature*, **482**, 27–29.

Maher, L. & Dertadian, G. (2017). Qualitative research. *Addiction*, **113**, 167–172.

Malenbaum, R., Herzog, D., Eisenthal, S. & Wyshak, G. (1988). Overeaters anonymous: Impact on bulimia. *International Journal of Eating Disorders*, **7**(1), 139–143.

Malik, V. S., Willett, W. C. & Hu, F. B. (2009). Sugar-sweetened beverages and BMI in children and adolescents: Reanalyses of a meta-analysis. *American Journal of Clinical Nutrition*, **89**, 438–439.

Manasse, S. M., Juarascio, A. S., Forman, E. M., et al. (2014). Executive functioning in overweight individuals with and without loss-of-control eating. *European Eating Disorders Review*, **22**(5), 373–377.

Martin, A. A., Davidson, T. L. & McCrory, M. A. (2018). Deficits in episodic memory are related to uncontrolled eating in a sample of healthy adults. *Appetite*, **124**, 33–42.

Martineau, F., Tyner, E., Lorenc, T., Petticrew, M. & Lock, K. (2013). Population-level interventions to reduce alcohol-related harm: An overview of systematic reviews. *Preventive Medicine*, **57**(4), 278–296.

McElroy, S. L., Arnold, L. M., Shapira, N. A., et al. (2003). Topiramate in the treatment of binge eating disorder associated with obesity: A randomized, placebo-controlled trial. *American Journal of Psychiatry*, **160**(2), 255–261.

McElroy, S. L., Hudson, J., Ferreira-Cornwell, M. C., et al. (2016). Lisdexamfetamine dimesylate for adults with moderate to severe binge eating disorder: Results of two pivotal phase 3 randomized controlled trials. *Neuropsychopharmacology*, **41**(5), 1251.

McElroy, S. L., Hudson, J. I., Mitchell, J. E., et al. (2015). Efficacy and safety of lisdexamfetamine for treatment of adults with moderate to severe binge-eating disorder: A randomized clinical trial. *JAMA Psychiatry*, **72**(3), 235–246.

McKenna, R. A., Skinner, J. A. & Burrows, T. L. (2018) Food addiction support: Website content analysis. *JMIR Cardio*, **2**, e10.

Meadows, A., Nolan, L. J. & Higgs, S. (2017). Self-perceived food addiction: Prevalence, predictors, and prognosis. *Appetite*, **114**, 282–298.

Micha, R., Karageorgou, D., Bakogianni, I., et al. (2018). Effectiveness of school food environment policies on children's dietary behaviors: A systematic review and meta-analysis. *PLoS ONE*, March 29, journal. pone.0194555.

Monteiro, C. A., Cannon, G., Moubarac, J-C., et al. (2017). The UN decade of nutrition, the NOVA food classification and the trouble with ulta-processing. *Public Health Nutrition*, **21**, 5–17.

Moodie, R., Stuckler, D., Monteiro, C., et al., (2013). Profits and pandemics: Prevention of harmful effects of tobacco, alcohol, and ultra-processed food and drink industries. *The Lancet*, **381**, 509.

Murphy, C. M., Stojek, M. K. & MacKillop, J. (2014). Interrelationships among impulsive personality traits, food addiction, and body mass index. *Appetite*, **73**, 45–50.

Nunes-Neto, P. R., Kohler, C. A., Schuch, F. B., et al. (2018). Food addiction: Prevalence, psychopathological correlates and associations with quality of life in a large sample. *Journal of Psychiatric Research*, **96**, 145–152.

Pierce, M., Sutterland, A., Beraha, E. M., Morley, K. & van den Brink, W. (2018). Efficacy, tolerability, and safety of low-dose and high-dose baclofen in the treatment of alcohol dependence: A systematic review and meta-analysis. *European Neuropsychopharmacology*, **28**(7), 795–806.

Popkin, B. M. (2010). Patterns of beverage consumption use across the lifecycle. *Physiology & Behavior*, **100**, 4–9.

O'Callaghan, T. (2017). Sugar's mortal enemy. *New Scientist*, **235**, 42–43.

O'Neill, J., Daniel, T. O. & Epstein, L. H. (2016). Episodic future thinking reduces eating in a food court. *Eating Behaviors*, **20**, 9–13.

Oomen, D., Grol, M., Spronk, D., Booth, C. & Fox, E. (2018). Beating uncontrolled eating: Training inhibitory control to reduce food intake and food cue sensitivity. *Appetite*, **131**, 73–83.

Ouzir, M. & Errami, M. (2016). Etiological theories of addiction: A comprehensive update on neurobiological, genetic and behavioural vulnerability. *Pharmacology, Biochemistry and Behavior*, **148**, 59–68.

Panksepp, J., Knutson, B. & Burdorf, J. (2002). The role of brain emotional systems in addictions: A neuro-evolutionary perspective and new 'self-report' animal model. *Addiction*, **97**, 459–469.

Pedram, P., Wadden, D., Amini, P., et al. (2013). Food addiction: Its prevalence and significant association with obesity in the general population. *PLoS ONE*, **8**, e74832.

Pelchat, M. L., Johnson, A., Chan, R., Valdez, J. & Ragland, J. D. (2004). Images of desire: Food-craving activation during fMRI. *NeuroImage*, **23**(4), 1486–1493.

Pepino, M. Y., Bradley, D., Eagon, J. C., et al. (2014a). Changes in taste perception and eating behavior after bariatric surgery-induced weight loss in women. *Obesity*, **22**(5), E13–E20.

Pepino, M. Y., Stein, R. I., Eagon, J. C. & Klein, S. (2014b). Bariatric surgery-induced weight loss causes remission of food addiction in extreme obesity. *Obesity*, **22**(8), 1792–1798.

Primeaux, S. D., Silva, T. de, Tzeng, T. H., Chiang, M. C. & Hsia, D. S. (2016). Recent advances in the modification of taste and food preferences following bariatric surgery. *Reviews in Endocrine and Metabolic Disorders*, **17**(2), 195–207.

Reas, D. L. & Grilo, C. M. (2015). Pharmacological treatment of binge eating disorder: update review and synthesis. *Expert Opinion on Pharmacotherapy*, **16**(10), 1463–1478.

Rebello, C. J. & Greenway, F. L. (2016). Reward-induced eating: Therapeutic approaches to addressing food cravings. *Advances in Therapy*, 1–14.

Rebello, C. J., Nikonova, E. V., Zhou, S., et al. (2018). Effect of Lorcaserin alone and in combination with Phentermine on food cravings after 12-week treatment: A randomized substudy. *Obesity*, **26**(2), 332–339.

Riediger, N. D. & Bombak, A. E. (2018) Sugar-sweetened beverages as the new tobacco: Examining a proposed policy through a Canadian social justice lens. *Canadian Medical Association Journal*, **190**, E327–E330.

Robinson, S. M. & Adinoff, B. (2016). The classification of substance use disorders: Historical, contextual, and conceptual considerations. *Behavioral Sciences*, **6**, 18.

Rogers, P. J. & Smit, H. J. (2000). Food craving and food "addiction": A critical review of the evidence from a biopsychosocial perspective. *Pharmacology Biochemistry and Behavior*, **66** (1), 3–14.

Ronel, N. & Libman, G. (2003). Eating Disorders and Recovery: Lessons from Overeaters Anonymous. *Clinical Social Work Journal*, **31** (2), 155–171.

Rose, A. K. & Jones, A. (2018). Baclofen: Its effectiveness in reducing harmful drinking, craving, and negative mood. A meta-analysis. *Addiction*, **113**(8), 1396–1406.

Rosettie, K. L., Micha, R., Cudhea, F., et al. (2018). Comparative risk assessment of school food environment policies and childhood diets, childhood obesity, and future cardiometabolic mortality in the United States. *PLoS ONE*, **13**(7), e0200378.

Sanmiguel, C. P., Jacobs, J., Gupta, A., et al. (2017). Surgically induced changes in gut microbiome and hedonic eating as related to weight loss: Preliminary findings in obese women undergoing bariatric surgery. *Psychosomatic Medicine*, **79**(8), 880.

Sassi, F., Belloni, A., Mirelman, A. J., et al. (2018). Equity impacts of price policies to promote healthy behaviours. *The Lancet*, **391**, 2059–2070.

Schulte, E. M., Avena, N. M. & Gearhardt, A. N. (2015). Which foods may be addictive? The roles of processing, fat content, and glycemic load. *PLoS ONE*, **10**(2), e0117959.

Schulte, E. M., Schiestl, E. T. & Gearhardt, A. N. (2020). Food versus eating addictions. In S. Sussman (Ed.), *The Cambridge Handbook of Substance and Behavioral Addictions*. Cambridge, UK: Cambridge University Press, pp. 340–352.

Schultes, B., Ernst, B., Wilms, B., Thurnheer, M. & Hallschmid, M. (2010). Hedonic hunger is increased in severely obese patients and is reduced after gastric bypass surgery. *The American Journal of Clinical Nutrition*, **92**(2), 277–283.

Schumacher, S. E., Kemps, E. & Tiggemann, M. (2016). Bias modification training can alter approach bias and chocolate consumption. *Appetite*, **96**, 219–224.

Sevinçer, G. M., Konuk, N., Bozkurt, S. & Coşkun, H. (2016). Food addiction and the outcome of bariatric surgery at 1-year: Prospective observational study. *Psychiatry Research*, **244**, 159–164.

Shinn, A. K. & Greenfield, S. F. (2010). Topiramate in the treatment of substance related disorders: A critical review of the literature. *The Journal of Clinical Psychiatry*, **71**(5), 634–648.

Siervo, M., Montagnesse, C., Mathers, J. C., et al. (2013). Sugar consumption and global prevalence of obesity and hypertension: An ecological analysis. *Public Health Nutrition*, **17**, 587–596.

Smith, M. A., Greene-Naples, J. L., Felder, J. N., et al. (2009). The effects of repeated opioid administration on locomotor activity: II. Unidirectional cross-sensitization to cocaine. *Journal of Pharmacology and Experimental Therapeutics*, **330**, 476.

Stice, E. & Yokum, S. (2016). Neural vulnerability factors that increase risk for future weight gain. *Psychological Bulletin*, **142**(5), 447–471.

Stojek, M., Shank, L. M., Vannucci, A., et al. (2018). A systematic review of attentional biases in disorders involving binge eating. *Appetite*, **123**, 367–389.

Sussman, S. & Pakdaman, S. (2020). Appetitive needs and addiction. In S. Sussman (Ed.), *The Cambridge Handbook of Substance and Behavioral Addictions*, Cambridge, UK: Cambridge University Press, pp. 3–12.

Svaldi, J., Naumann, E., Trentowska, M. & Schmitz, F. (2014). General and food-specific inhibitory deficits in binge eating disorder. *International Journal of Eating Disorders*, **47** (5), 534–542.

Tang, D. W., Fellows, L. K., Small, D. M. & Dagher, A. (2012). Food and drug cues activate similar brain regions: A meta-analysis of functional MRI studies. *Physiology & Behavior*, **106**(3), 317–324.

Turton, R., Bruidegom, K., Cardi, V., Hirsch, C. R. & Treasure, J. (2016). Novel methods to help develop healthier eating habits for eating and weight disorders: A systematic review and meta-analysis. *Neuroscience & Biobehavioral Reviews*, **61**, 132–155.

Vainik, U., Neseliler, S., Konstabel, K., Fellows, L. K. & Dagher, A. (2015). Eating traits questionnaires as a continuum of a single construct. *Appetite*, **90**, 229–239.

Vartanian, L. R., Chen, W. H., Reily, N. M. & Castel, A. D. (2016). The parallel impact of episodic memory and episodic future thinking on food intake. *Appetite*, **101**, 31–36.

Viner, R. M. & Cole, T. J. (2006). Who changes body mass between adolescence and adulthood? Factors predicting change in BMI between 16 year and 30 years in the 1970 British Birth Cohort. *International Journal of Obesity*, **30**, 1368–1374.

Volkow, N. D., Koob, G. & McLellan, A. T. (2016). Neurobiologic advance from the brain disease model of addiction. *The New England Journal of Medicine*, **374**, 363–371.

Volkow, N. D., Wise, R. A. & Baler R. (2017). The dopamine motive system: Implications for drug and food addiction. *Nature Reviews Neuroscience*, **18**, 741–752.

Vos, M. B., Kimmon, J. E., Gillespie, C., Welsh, J. & Blanck, H. M. (2008). Dietary frustose consumption among US children and adults: The Third National Health and Nutrition Examination Survey. *Medscape Journal of Medicine*, **10**, 160.

Vreman, R. A., Goodell, A. J., Rodriguez, L. A., et al. (2017). Health and economic benefits of reducing sugar intake in the USA, including effects via non-alcoholic fatty liver disease: A microsimulation model. *BMJ Open*, **7**, e013543.

Wagenaar, A. C., Salois, M. J. & Komro, K. A. (2009). Effects of beverage alcohol price and tax levels on drinking: A meta-analysis of 1003 estimates from 112 studies. *Addiction*, **104**(2), 179–190.

Weafer, J., Mitchell, S. H. & de Wit, H. (2014). Recent translational findings on impulsivity in relation to drug abuse. *Current Addiction Reports*, **1**, 289–300.

Weinstein, A., Zlatkes, M., Gingis, A. & Lejoyeux, M. (2015). The effects of a 12-Step self-help group for compulsive eating on measures of food addiction, anxiety, depression, and self-efficacy. *Journal of Groups in Addiction & Recovery*, **10**(2), 190–200.

Werthmann, J., Jansen, A. & Roefs, A. (2015). Worry or craving? A selective review of evidence for food-related attention biases in obese individuals, eating-disorder patients, restrained eaters and healthy samples. *Proceedings of the Nutrition Society*, **74**(2), 99–114.

Wiers, R. W., Gladwin, T. E., Hofmann, W., Salemink, E. & Ridderinkhof, K. R. (2013). Cognitive bias modification and cognitive control training in addiction and related psychopathology: Mechanisms, clinical perspectives, and ways forward. *Clinical Psychological Science*, **1**(2), 192–212.

Wise, R. A. (2000). Addiction becomes a brain disease. *Neuron*, **26**, 27–33.

Wu, M., Giel, K. E., Skunde, M., et al. (2013). Inhibitory control and decision making under risk in bulimia nervosa and binge-eating disorder. *International Journal of Eating Disorders*, **46**(7), 721–728.

Yeary, J. (1987). The use of overeaters anonymous in the treatment of eating disorders. *Journal of Psychoactive Drugs*, **19** (3), 303–309.

Yoshida, Y. & Simoes, E. J. (2018). Sugar-sweetened beverage, obesity, and type 2 diabetes in children and adolescents' policies, taxation, and programs. *Current Diabetes Reports*, **18**, 31.

Yu, Z., Indelicato, N. A., Fuglestad, P., Tan, M. & Bane, L. (2018) Sex differences in disordered eating and food addiction among college students. *Appetite*, **129**, 12–18.

Zemore, S. E., Lui, C., Mericle, A., Hemberg, J. & Kaskutas, L. A. (2018). A longitudinal study of the comparative efficacy of Women for Sobriety, LifeRing, SMART Recovery, and 12-step groups for those with AUD. *Journal of Substance Abuse Treatment*, **88**, 18–26.

18 The Prevention and Treatment of Gambling Disorders: Some Art, Some Science

Jeffrey L. Derevensky, PhD

Introduction

The history of gambling is complete with colorful characters and institutions from Julius Caesar to Casanova, George Washington to Steve Wynn, from Harvard University to Las Vegas, from gunslingers in the Old West to our current governments who view gambling as a recreational activity that can generate huge tax revenues (Schwartz, 2006). Gambling operators have evolved from local bookmakers and relegated to a few international locations (Nevada – both Las Vegas and Reno – Atlantic City, Monaco, and Macau) to multinational corporations establishing a wide diversity of gambling venues across the globe. While gambling was once viewed as a sinister activity with shady characters over the past century, today's gambling opportunities are readily available and widely perceived to be a socially acceptable form of entertainment. As with other potentially high-risk behaviors, for example alcohol consumption, if done excessively without controls and limits, disordered/problematic gambling can lead to a host of adverse mental health, financial, academic, familial, judicial, and vocational negative outcomes. Once thought to be primarily a male activity, there is growing evidence that there are an increasing number of females engaged in gambling and experiencing gambling-related disorders (Bowden-Jones & Prever, 2017; Volberg, 2004). While the types of gambling activities females prefer may differ from males, the severity of problems associated with disordered gambling is pervasive independent of gender.

Originally, compulsive, problem, or pathological gambling was characterized as an impulse control disorder (see earlier versions of the *Diagnostic Statistical Manual* (DSM) developed by the American Psychiatric Association and the International Classification of Disorders (ICD) developed by the World Health Organization). The current acceptance of a Gambling Disorder can be best viewed as a Non-Substance-Related Disorder (DSM-5; American Psychiatric Association, 2013). A Gambling Disorder is conceptualized as a persistent and recurrent gambling behavior leading to clinically significant impairment or distress experienced by the individual. It is important to note that to be clinically diagnosed as a disordered gambler this behavior is not better explained by a manic episode. As such, according to the DSM-5 (American Psychiatric Association, 2013), the individual with a Gambling Disorder exhibits four or more of the following symptoms (during a twelve-month period):

(1) Needs to gamble with increasing amounts of money in order to achieve the desired level of excitement.
(2) Is restless or irritable when attempting to cut down or stop gambling.
(3) Has made repeated unsuccessful efforts to control, cut back, or stop gambling.
(4) Is often preoccupied with gambling (including persistent thoughts of reliving past gambling experiences, handicapping or planning the next gambling venture, and/or thinking of ways with which to gamble).
(5) Often gambles when feeling distress (e.g., helplessness, guilty, anxious, depressed).
(6) After losing money gambling, often returns another day to get even (chasing one's losses).
(7) Lies to conceal the extent of involvement with gambling.
(8) Has jeopardized or lost a significant relationship, job, educational, or career opportunity because of gambling.
(9) Relies on others to provide money to relieve desperate financial situations caused by gambling.

It should be noted that each of these diagnostic criteria are weighted equally in spite of differences in the severity of consequences. No single constellation of endorsements on the DSM-5 exists among disordered gamblers. However, it is not unusual for help-seeking disordered gamblers in treatment to have endorsed either eight or nine of the criteria (Derevensky, 2017).

The prevalence rates of gambling disorder have varied from jurisdiction to jurisdiction, as do the minimum age at which individuals can gamble, the types, availability, and accessibility of gambling activities, religious/cultural attitudes toward gambling, and governmental regulatory statutes. In spite of the proliferation of worldwide gambling activities, their ease of accessibility and the multitude of venues where individuals can gamble, the prevalence rates of disordered/problematic gambling have remained remarkably stable. Past-year prevalence rates of a gambling disorder typically range from 0.2 percent to 1 percent or 2 percent, with males reporting a higher incidence of problem gambling. Researchers employing screening instruments have reported significantly higher prevalence rates of adult problem or pathological gambling of between 2 percent and 5 percent of the adult population in jurisdictions with mature gambling markets (Volberg, 2007). However, prevalence rates among regular machine players (e.g., slots, VLTs) is as high as 25 percent (Productivity Commission, 1999; Schull, 2014). High prevalence estimates of between 4.3 percent and 6.9 percent among substance abusing and psychiatric inpatients have been reported (Cowlishaw & Hakes, 2015; Grant et al., 2005; Petry, Stinson & Grant, 2005). There are estimates that upwards of 96 percent of individuals with a significant gambling disorder have one or more psychiatric disorders, with 64 percent having three or more psychiatric disorders (Kessler et al., 2008). As such, Potenza et al. (2019) argue that screening for disordered gambling within mental healthcare settings remains particularly important. The question remains as to whether mental-health issues result in problem gambling, or whether problem gambling results in mental-health issues.

While gambling has been thought to be an adult activity, there is abundant international research suggesting that it remains a popular activity among adolescents, and that a growing number of adolescents are experiencing gambling disorders. In general, the results suggest that an even greater proportion of adolescents are experiencing significant gambling problems than adults – ranging anywhere from 3 percent to

12.3 percent (Blinn-Pike, Worthy & Jonkman, 2010; Calado, Alexandre & Griffiths, 2017; Derevensky, 2012; Volberg et al., 2010). If one examines international adult problem gambling prevalence data, there is clear indication that it is the eighteen- to twenty-five- year olds that have the highest incidence of problem gambling. Whether these early gambling problems are enduring remains an important question. While older adults have a lower prevalence rate, the limited number of longitudinal studies (Billi et al., 2014; Romild, Volberg & Abbott, 2014; Slutske, 2006; Williams et al., 2015) precludes a definitive answer. What we do know is that individuals with a gambling disorder, irrespective of age, gender, ethnicity, or geographical location endure a wide range of mental health, personal, social, interpersonal, financial, educational/vocational, and familial problems (some also experience significant legal problems). As such, preventative measures and treatment approaches need to be explored.

Abstinence versus Harm Minimization

Prevention approaches can be classified into two general paradigms; abstinence and harm minimization (sometimes referred to as harm reduction or responsible gambling approaches). While these two approaches are not mutually exclusive, they are predicated on different goals and processes. A harm reduction framework encompasses policies, programs or strategies that help individuals to reduce the harmful, negative consequences incurred through involvement in a potentially risky behavior without necessarily requiring abstinence (Ariyabuddhiphongs, 2013; Dickson, Derevensky & Gupta, 2004). In many jurisdictions, youth are legally prohibited access to government-regulated gambling venues, supporting an abstinence approach. It is important to note that the age at which individuals can legally gamble varies considerably and is often dependent upon the activity (e.g., lottery purchases typically have a lower minimum age than casino gambling). Nevertheless, age prohibitions imposed on government-regulated forms of gambling do not preclude underage individuals from gambling amongst peers, bookmakers, or lying about one's age to gain access to a gambling venue. The question remains as to whether or not an abstinence model is a realistic goal for youth when the majority of adolescents report having gambled in the past twelve months and report gambling amongst peers on unregulated gambling activities (see Derevensky (2012) for a comprehensive discussion of this issue). For adults, there typically exist a wide diversity of gambling activities (e.g., gambling amongst peers, lotteries, bingo, machine and casino gambling, sports wagering, online gambling activities).

Blaszczynski (2002) correctly makes the point that negative, harmful consequences are not necessarily limited to pathological or disordered gamblers but may also occasionally impact nonproblematic social, recreational, or occasional gamblers. Given this conceptualization, he suggests that an abstinence approach may not be necessary, feasible, or universally effective. There is also evidence from several longitudinal studies that pathological gambling is not a static state, with some individuals moving from recreational to pathological gambling and back during the course of their life. Still further, there is a body of literature (e.g., Ladouceur, 2005) suggesting that *controlled* gambling may be a viable alternative to abstinence even for some individuals with severe gambling problems. It is equally important to note that pathological or disordered gamblers are not a homogeneous group; they differ on their preferred game of choice, frequency of gambling, personality, cultural and ethnic factors, and more importantly on the reasons and motivations underlying their gambling. This highlights both the paradox and the confusion as to which primary prevention approach to promote: abstinence or harm reduction (Dickson et al., 2004).

In a number of seminal papers entitled *The Reno Model*, Blaszczynski, Ladouceur and Shaffer (2004) and Shaffer et al. (2016) articulated a science-based framework of responsible gambling principles for industry operators, health service providers, community and consumer groups, and government agencies. These strategic principles were developed to serve as a guide for the adoption and implementation of responsible gambling and harm minimization initiatives. In essence, this represented an approach to keep gamblers "safe" from excessive gambling and as a way of minimizing harms associated with disordered/pathological gambling, thereby ultimately reducing the prevalence and incidence of problem/disordered gamblers. They articulated a set of principles for Responsible Gambling (RG) processes (many of these RG principles have been adopted by the industry and governmental regulatory bodies). Incorporating a public health model, RG is believed to reflect a shared interest and responsibility among the gambler, the gambling operator, community, regulators, and governments (most governments regulate gambling while some are actually operators). According to the *Reno Model*, RG programs designed to reduce the prevalence and incidence of gambling-related harms should be based upon scientific, empirically validated data. However, Ladouceur and his colleagues (Ladouceur, Blaszczynski & Lalande, 2012) have argued that quite a few jurisdictions have developed, introduced, and maintained specific programs without much, if any, empirical support. A number of these programs and initiatives are gambling-activity specific. For example, some are intended for casino gambling, others for machine gambling, and still others for online gambling.

Assuming a harm minimization strategy, the goals of such programs are to reduce, minimize or eliminate the potential harmful consequences concomitant with gambling, in general, and problem gambling, in particular. While it should be noted that the Australian Productivity (Gambling) Commission (2010) reported that approximately 80 percent of adults considered that the onus for responsible gambling rested upon the individual to control their gambling, there is little doubt that accessibility and availability (the supply side) play a role in understanding problem gambling. As well, independent of the type of gambling, there is ample evidence that certain individual characteristics (e.g., gender) and cultural variables (cultural values and beliefs, effects of acculturation, and attitudes toward gambling) play an important interactive role (Abbott et al., 2013; Raylu & Oei, 2004). While it is beyond the scope of this review to examine specific culturally relevant gambling behaviors, their importance should not be underestimated. See Meyer, Hayer and Griffiths (2009) for a review of disordered gambling in European countries; also see articles on prevention and treatment of disordered gambling among Asian communities (Chim, 2011; Toyama et al., 2014; Tse et al., 2010). Loo, Raylu and Oei (2008) reviewed twenty-five studies among Chinese populations, and concluded that gambling in general among Chinese populations is widespread as it is viewed as a socially accepted form of entertainment, prevalence estimates of problem gambling have generally increased for Chinese adults and ranged from 2.5 percent to 4.0 percent, Chinese problem gamblers have difficulty admitting gambling-related issues, and those with gambling problems have difficult seeking professional help for fear of losing respect. In a recent epidemiological study of adults in New Jersey, Hispanics were found to have significantly high rates of problem gambling by Caler, Garcia and Nower (2017).

There also remains concern that several of the more visible RG strategies being used (e.g., time clocks, money limits through bill acceptors on gambling machines, the use of smartcard technology or behavioral tracking and pop-up messaging) may be misleading the general public into believing a product is safe without empirical support. While there may be a justifiable argument in not including such strategies because of the lack of empirical support, others have argued that, in the absence of research, we should be using our best judgment as to what may or may not be effective until such time as empirical evidence is available (see Griffiths, 2020).

Responsible Gambling (RG) Strategies

Setting aside the complexity and difficulties associated with determining causal attributes of problem gambling associated with different games, there is a growing body of evidence suggesting some forms of gambling may be more problematic than others. Electronic gaming machines (EGMs) (slots, VLTs) have attracted particular attention as they have been reported to be more highly problematic than other games and have been reported to have the greatest capacity to cause harm and impaired control (Dowling, Smith & Thomas, 2005; Productivity Commission, 1999; 2010; Schull, 2014). Similar concerns have been raised over online/internet/mobile wagering (Gainsbury, 2012; Gainsbury & Blaszczynski, 2012; Gainsbury & Wood, 2011; Gainsbury et al., 2014a, 2014b; Williams, West & Simpson, 2007; Wood & Williams, 2007). Griffiths and his colleagues (Griffiths, 1990, 1999; Griffiths, Parke & Derevensky, 2012; Parke & Griffiths, 2007) have similarly argued that games incorporating rapid response rates, intermittent reinforcement schedules, and technological forms of gambling, may in general, be particularly problematic. Binde (2011), after analysis of eighteen international gambling prevalence studies, reported that interactive internet, casino, EGM, and high-stakes unregulated gambling (e.g., poker, sports wagering) are the forms of gambling most likely associated with problem/disordered gambling. It is equally important to note that Davidson & Rodgers (2010) reported 87 percent of EGM players also gambled on at least one other activity (besides the lottery), with only a small percentage of individuals (5.2 percent) indicating exclusive play on EGMs. For high-frequency players across all forms of gambling, 31 percent of these individuals reported gambling on four or more different forms of gambling activities. Derevensky (2012) has suggested that if one removes a preferred form of gambling, most problem gamblers will seek alternative forms of gambling which is also likely to become problematic. Whether the onset of problem/disordered gambling may be more prevalent among EGM players remains to be verified.

In an informative study, Wood, Shorter & Griffiths (2014a) investigated the perceived effectiveness of forty-five responsible gambling features in relation to twenty distinct gambling type games. Sixty-one participants (RG experts, treatment providers, and recovered problem gamblers), from seven countries, rated forty-five RG features. Wood and his colleagues concluded that the most highly recommended RG features could be divided into three broad types: (a) player-initiated RG features designed to aid the player in controlling their behavior (e.g., self-exclusion or quick breaks, tools for establishing personal spending and time limits – personal limit setting rather than operator set limits); (b) promotions aimed at informed player choice (e.g., providing clear and concise information – winnings are presented as monetary values (versus credits), clear information on prize structures and winning percentages, the availability of self-diagnostic tools and responsible gambling literature, behavioral feedback with warnings of potentially negative changes in play patterns, pop-up reminders of time and money spent, and problem gambling referral information) (see Griffiths, 2020); and (c) gambling operator actions (e.g., delaying player reinvestment after large wins, prohibiting credit for gambling, restricting physical access to money [ATMs], controlling access to gaming areas through identification checks, and the availability of trained RG staff to identify and help individuals with gambling problems). While there was general agreement among the three groups of raters, problem gamblers were much more likely to report being skeptical of gaming operators' motives in including responsible gambling features.

Evidence-Based Player Protection and Harm Minimization Measures: What Have We Learned?

A growing number of harm minimization strategies have been suggested and implemented internationally, with some having had more research to assess their effectiveness than others. These strategies have typically been relegated to the different forms of gambling, their ease of implementation based upon the venue and/or game, and their perceived risk for inducing excessive gambling. Addressing structural and situational factors have been met with intermittent success. Understanding structural (the characteristics of the games themselves) and situational factors, however, remains crucial for both the prevention and treatment of a gambling disorder. Situational factors are often considered instrumental in influencing initial decisions to begin gambling (e.g., geographical proximity, accessibility, cultural beliefs and acceptance, and marketing and advertising/promotions) (Meyer et al., 2009; Petry, 2005), while structural characteristics are thought to be more likely facilitate the acquisition, development and maintenance of gambling behavior (e.g., Griffiths, 1993; Griffiths et al., 2012; Parke & Parke, 2013).

While many harm minimization strategies are intended to cut across all or multiple types of venues, some are more focused on the game itself, with others more dedicated exclusively to a single form of gambling. Numerous studies have described putative individual intra- and interpersonal risk factors for the development of gambling disorders (see Blaszczynski & Nower, 2002; Johansson et al., 2009; Raylu & Oei, 2002). A large number of approaches have been focused upon EGM playing because (a) the structural features of the machines themselves are thought to induce more problematic gambling, (b) clinical reports and gambling helpline calls suggest that EGM players have a higher incidence of problem gambling, and (c) RG features addressing some of the structural characteristics remain somewhat easier to implement. It should be noted that a number of these structural characteristics and RG features have been implemented on internet casino gambling sites. While there has been in general a significant absence of credible scientific research on the effectiveness of many specific harm minimization approaches, there nevertheless is a growing body of evidence suggesting at least short-term effectiveness for some strategies for certain individuals.

Understanding and treating individuals with a gambling disorder as a homogenous group may not be effective. Understanding their motivations to gamble, the types of gambling in which they engage, and the contextual issues underlying the need to gamble are important. The generalizability of such strategies for different cultural groups also requires further research. Nevertheless, in the absence of strong empirical findings, governments are mandating specific RG policies be implemented, many of which may have intuitive appeal. However, their effects may be limited at best and in some circumstances may have negative unintended consequences.

Structural Features that Might be Modified

Most evidence-based research for harm minimization-strategies has focused on EGM's and online casino type games. A number of specific structural features are thought to impact both gambling and problem gambling on EGMs and online operations including modifying (a) stake/bet size (Griffiths et al., 2012), (b) event frequency and speed of play (Blaszczynski, Sharpe & Walker, 2001; Dickerson et al., 1991; Ladouceur & Sévigny, 2006, (c) jackpot size (Griffiths et al., 2012; Parke & Parke, 2013), (d) ambient characteristics (e.g., sound, color and lighting) (Griffiths, 1990; Loba et al., 2001), (e) the use of displaying cash amounts versus credits on machines (Ladouceur & Sévigny, 2009; Loba et al., 2001), (f) the limitation of the use of note/bill acceptors on slot machines (Productivity Commission, 2010; Schottler Consulting, 2009; White et al., 2006), (g) mandatory breaks in play (Focal Research, 2002; White et al., 2006; Wood et al., 2014b), and (h) specific messaging (Argo & Main, 2004; Cloutier, Ladouceur & Sévigny, 2006; Kim et al., 2014; Monaghan & Blaszczynski, 2010; Stewart & Wohl, 2013). In general, the impact of different strategies upon individuals experiencing problem gambling has been found to vary considerably. The research concerning many of these structural characteristics is simplistic at best and it is often difficult to tease out the efficacy of one feature without examining a combination of features. As well, the impact may be limited as they treat disordered/problem gamblers as a homogenous group. Still further, there remains great variability among problem gamblers, such that while one individual perceives one harm minimization strategy as effective, others tend to diminish its importance. As an example, speed of play on EGMs may be important but identifying the optimal speed has not yet been identified for dissuading problem gamblers from wanting to play on EGMs. While the use of a visible clock or timer was helpful to some, others suggested it was ineffective in modifying their playing behavior. Manipulating/decreasing interesting sounds and lights may discourage some from playing an EGM; however, most have argued that removing these features limits the individual's right to play these machines for enjoyment.

Situational Strategies

Situational strategies also play an important role. While difficult to curtail the expansion of gambling, a potentially effective harm minimization strategy seems to be related to the removal (or limit setting) of ATMs in land-based operations (Productivity Commission, 1999, 2010; Thomas et al., 2013; White et al., 2006; Wood, Griffiths & Shorter, 2014a, 2014b), the use of behavioral tracking systems for EGMs and online operations (Auer & Griffiths, 2012; Gainsbury, 2012; Griffiths, 2013, 2020; Schellinck & Schrans, 2011), the importance in providing breaks in play, more effective messaging, self-exclusion policies and providing normative feedback (Auer & Griffiths, 2014; Neighbors et al., 2013).

Precommitment Strategies

Given the assumption that some risks are taken under a clear and rational frame of mind while others are made more impulsively, in the "heat of the moment" (Helfinstein et al., 2014), if one can get players to precommit to their playing behavior before gambling, then possibly the harms associated with excessive gambling may be limited. A small number of studies (more are currently underway in the USA, Europe, and Australia) have empirically examined the nature of card-based precommitment approaches to gambling and their impact on behaviour and problem gambling (Bernhard et al., 2006; Brevers et al., 2016; Schellinck & Schrans, 2007; Schottler Consulting, 2009, 2010). In a review of the available literature examining the effects of limit setting on EGMs, Ladouceur and his colleagues (2012) concluded that the vast majority of gamblers (approximately 80 percent) already set their own gambling limits (e.g., identifying the maximum amounts of money they were prepared to lose) without the need for an external limit setting procedure. In spite of individuals precommitting the amounts of money they were prepared to lose, we know that many gamblers ultimately wind up exceeding these limits. As such, a growing number of jurisdictions have incorporated smartcard technology to help individuals preset their limits (time and/or money). Notwithstanding methodological concerns, Ladouceur and his colleagues (2012) concluded that almost 70 percent of gamblers do not voluntarily use limit-setting options when available, and those who do use them are more likely to restrict their money limits, and an even smaller number of individuals use time limits. Many of the existing evaluation studies have methodological limitations in that individuals may have to precommit in one venue or online gambling site but may go to another venue and gamble continuously. In spite of some promising research suggesting precommitment's potential usefulness, the general public has not been keen to adopt its use. The general perception is that many of the RG/harm minimization features, in particular precommitment strategies, are designed for disordered gamblers. Since most individuals do not have a gambling problem, the perception is that there is really no need for such programs. To make matters worse, most disordered gamblers often do not recognize the severity of their symptoms (Hardoon, Derevensky & Gupta, 2003) and perceive the utility of precommitment as unnecessary for them (Derevensky, 2012).

Self-Exclusion

One of the earliest and most popular forms of harm minimization, originally thought to be best suited for casino and online gambling, is related to self-exclusion and has had worldwide acceptance (see Collins & Kelly, 2002; Gainsbury, 2014 for in-depth reviews). Self-exclusion programs are provided by the gambling operator as an option for individuals experiencing gambling problems to avoid further continued gambling (another variant is referred to as third-party exclusion, where a family member can seek to have a problem gambler placed on an exclusion list prohibiting entry into a particular gambling venue). Self-exclusion programs, to a large degree, are highly dependent on the effectiveness of the operator's monitoring systems in detecting infringements (many current lawsuits against gambling operators have centered on the fact that in spite of the individual signing a self-exclusion contract it is rarely enforced). While individuals in self-exclusion programs elect to place themselves on a list barring entry into a particular venue, it may not be inclusive of all venues. For example, excluding oneself on a particular online gambling site may not necessarily prevent you from gambling on another site. More recently, several large land-based casinos have adopted a policy whereby if an individual self-excludes from one property, they are automatically excluded from another. While there is a committee consisting of UK online gambling operators attempting to develop a national self-exclusion database (exclusion from one online gambling operator would be honored amongst all), this does not prohibit individuals from going to other venues or online sites. The fact that most gamblers who engage in online gambling hold multiple accounts with different online operators as well as gambling at a variety of land-based venues limits its potential usefulness.

Similar to other harm minimization strategies, self-exclusion programs come in many forms. Differences in time limits have been highly variable ranging from one day, one week, one month, one year, to permanent exclusion. Penalties for breaching a self-exclusion agreement range from being escorted from the venue, to being found criminally responsible for trespassing, and in some cases forfeiting winnings. A number of studies have examined the effectiveness of such programs (Croucher & Leslie, 2007; Gainsbury, 2014; Ladouceur et al., 2000; Wardle & Dobbie, 2011). The Productivity Commission (2010) concluded, after looking at the available evidence, that decreases in gambling expenditures for individuals enrolled in self-exclusion programs were common, individuals were found to have improved their financial resources, believed they had better control over their gambling, with most reporting not breaching their agreements. Gainsbury's (2014) comprehensive review of self-exclusion studies suggests that self-exclusion programs typically remain under-utilized by a vast majority of gamblers and are not completely effective in preventing individuals from gambling in the venues from which they have excluded. The Australian Productivity Commission (2010) concurred with Gainsbury and suggested that while such programs may have beneficial effects for some individuals, "many who need it do not use it." On a positive note, Blaszczynski, Ladouceur and Nower (2007) have suggested that such programs may nevertheless be a stimulus for individuals to seek treatment.

Other RG Strategies

Other RG strategies have incorporated enhanced staff training to identify and talk with patrons who appear to be experiencing a gambling problem (Delfabrro et al., 2007; Delfabbro, Borgas & King, 2012; Hancock et al., 2008; Hing, 2003; White et al., 2006), the early detection of gambling problems through self-administered screening instruments often housed within kiosks located in gambling venues (Hayer et al., 2013), providing informational materials on the risks of excessive gambling, warning of the dangers associated with a gambling addiction (Meyer & Bachmann, 2011; Meyer & Hayer, 2010; Wood et al., 2014a, 2014b), the use of pop-up messages geared to provide warning messages to the player (Monaghan & Blaszczynski, 2010; Monaghan, Blaszczynski & Nower, 2009; Stewart & Wohl, 2013), the use of cash designations versus credits on EGMs (Ladouceur & Sévigny, 2009; Loba et al., 2001), the placement of a clock on EGMS (Ladouceur & Sévigny, 2009), and mandatory breaks in play on EGMs (e.g., cashing out after either a predetermined time limit or after a certain amount of money has been reached) (Caraniche Pty Ltd, 2005). The efficacy of these RG strategies is not known.

Situational Determinants and Reduction of Risk

A number of situational factors have been tried to help minimize the risks associated with disordered/problem gambling. Wardle et al. (2014) and other researchers (e.g., Abbott, 2006; Derevensky et al., 2013; Welte et al., 2006; White et al., 2006) have all pointed to the complexities of contributory social and contextual factors including convenience of access, availability of machines, demographic characteristics, venue type including access to money and provision of alcohol, and hours of operation. All of these factors contribute to overall prevalence rates. These researchers have argued that consideration should be given to the totality of individual, social and contextual factors, taking into account participation in all forms of gambling in the aggregate (rather than an over-emphasis on single forms) in the creation of a comprehensive harm minimization policy.

In spite of the complexities of disentangling the various situational factors from structural factors, a number of studies have attempted to examine some other variables thought to impact playing behaviors and problem/disordered gambling. Such research has looked at the closing of twenty-four-hour venues for short periods of times (often referred to as a mandatory shut-down period e.g., McMillen & Pitt, 2005; Wood, Shorter & Griffiths, 2014a), the ease of access to money (either through readily available ATMs or credits) (Productivity Commission, 1999, 2010; White et al., 2006; Wood, Griffiths & Shorter, 2014a, 2014b), the use of player tracking behavior and the development of behavioral algorithms where high risk players can be identified early (Auer & Griffiths, 2012; Griffiths, 2013, 2020), and the development of personalized normative feedback approaches (Delfabbro 2004; Griffiths, 2020; Marchica & Derevensky, 2016; Neighbors et al., 2013; Wohl et al., 2010).These approaches are quite well suited for online gambling, each of which has been shown to have positive effects for some individuals. It is important to note, as aptly stated by Gainsbury et al. (2014) that, while positive effects have been found for several harm-minimization approaches, researchers would be well advised to look at the unintended consequences of some well-intentioned harm minimizations strategies and polices as well as their feasibility, effectiveness and costs. For example, slowing down slot machines may have the effect of keeping disordered gamblers on the machines for longer periods of time.

Youth Prevention Programs

In spite of our increased knowledge about the risk and protective factors, correlates associated with youth gambling, and the impact of problem gambling experienced by some adolescents, there have been very few systematic attempts at educating today's youth about the risks and warning signs associated with excessive gambling. Gambling has come to be perceived as a benign socially acceptable form of entertainment. While most individuals, including adolescents, typically gamble in a responsible manner, setting and generally maintaining both time and money limits, a considerable number of youth go on to have quite severe gambling-related problems (Calado et al., 2017).

School-based primary prevention programs are generally available concerning issues related to substance use and abuse, excessive use of alcohol (drinking and driving), sex education, bullying (including cyber-bullying), smoking, eating disorders, amongst other mental health issues, yet a limited number of programs exist for the prevention of gambling problems. School administrators, educators, and parents tend to work on a crisis model, intervening only when a significant problem arises.

As universal findings have shown that adolescents and young adults are at significantly greater risk for gambling problems (Blinn-Pike et al., 2010; Calado et al., 2017; Derevensky, 2012; Nowak, 2018; Volberg et al., 2010), a number of school-based gambling prevention programs have been developed (see Table 18.1). Such programs typically incorporate

Table 18.1 Gambling prevention programs

Youth Gambling Prevention Initiatives[a]			
Prevention program	School level	Developer	Website
Amazing Chateau	Grades 4–6	International Centre for Youth Gambling problems and High-Risk behaviors – McGill University	www.youthgambling.com
Clean Break	Grades 8–12	International Centre for Youth Gambling problems and High-Risk behaviors – McGill University	www.youthgambling.com
Deal or No Dice	Grades 6–8	Lane County Problem Gambling Prevention	https://preventionlane.org/deal-no-dice-problem-gambling-prevention-tool
Facing the Odds	Grades 5–8	Harvard Medical School – Division of Addictions	
Game Brain	Grades 9–12	Responsible Gambling Council	www.responsiblegambling.org/safer-play/youth-and-young-adults/game-brain
Hooked city	Grades 6–8	International Centre for Youth Gambling problems and High-Risk behaviors – McGill University	www.youthgambling.com
Know Limits	Grades 7–12	International Centre for Youth Gambling problems and High-Risk behaviors – McGill University	www.youthgambling.com
Stacked Deck	Grades 9–12	Robert Williams and Robert Wood	
Wanna bet?	Grades 3–8	Minnesota Council on Compulsive Gambling	www.nati.org/prevention_tools/youth.aspx
Youth Gambling: An awareness and prevention workshop – Level I	Grades 4–6	International Centre for Youth Gambling problems and High-Risk behaviors – McGill University	www.youthgambling.com
Youth Gambling: An awareness and prevention workshop – Level II	Grades 7–10	International Centre for Youth Gambling problems and High-Risk behaviors – McGill University	www.youthgambling.com
Youth Making Choices: A Curriculum-Based Gambling Prevention Program	Grades 10–12	Centre for Addiction and Mental Health (CAMH)	www.problemgambling.ca/EN/ResourcesForProfessionals/Pages/CurriculumYouthMakingChoices.aspx
Youth Gambling Problems: Practical Information for Health Practitioners	Physicians	International Centre for Youth Gambling problems and High-Risk behaviors – McGill University	www.youthgambling.com
Youth Gambling Problems – Practical Information for Professional in the Criminal Justice System	Judges, Attorneys	International Centre for Youth Gambling problems and High-Risk behaviors – McGill University	www.youthgambling.com

Adult Gambling Prevention Initiatives	
Prevention Tool Classification	Prevention Initiative
Behavioral Analytics (Online Gambling)	Standards for safe playing (e.g., BetBuddy, Mentor)
Machine-Based Gambling Tools	Pop-up Messaging
	Limit setting (time and money)
	Enforced breaks in play
	Structural modifications (e.g., displaying money vs. credits, automatic cash-outs, etc.)
Gambling Information	Promotion of responsible gambling
	Public Service Announcements
	Staff training
	Advertisements and brochures
	Identification of potential problem lottery tickets (e.g., GamGard)
User/Third-Party Initiatives	Self-exclusion/third-party exclusion
Precommitment	Preidentified time and money limits

Notes. [a]Adapted from Derevensky, J. & Gilbeau, L. (2019). Preventing adolescent gambling problems. In A. Heinz, N. Romanczuk-Seiferth & M. Potenza (Eds.). *Gambling Disorders.* Berlin: Springer International.

For more information see:

Harris, A. & Griffiths, M. D. (2017). A critical review of the harm-minimisation tools available for electronic gambling. *Journal of Gambling Studies,* 33(1), 187–221.

Robillard, C. (2017). *Responsible Gambling Programs and Tools.* Report prepared for Gambling Research Exchange Ontario (GREO).

the following harm minimization and educational objectives: (1) accentuating the differences between games of chance and games of skill, (2) educating participants about probability and the independence of events, (3) dispelling erroneous cognitions concerning the "illusion of control" regarding random events, (4) defining the signs of problem gambling, and (5) providing resources to aid those experiencing a gambling problem (Derevensky, 2012; Ladouceur, Goulet & Vitaro, 2013; Turner, Macdonald & Somerset, 2008; Williams, West & Simpson, 2012). It is important to note that while the legal age to gamble varies between jurisdictions and between games (e.g., most states permit lottery play at age eighteen, while the age for casino gambling is typically twenty-one), adolescents are involved in a wide variety of nonregulated gambling activities (e.g., sports wagering, gambling on games of personal skill, card betting).

Several more-comprehensive prevention curricula seek to encourage the development of interpersonal skills, strategies for fostering effective coping strategies, providing examples of positive decision-making, educating youth about the short-term and long-term risks associated with excessive gambling, and providing techniques to improve self-esteem and providing strategies for resisting peer pressure (Derevensky, 2012; Derevensky & Gupta, 2011; more details can be found in Derevensky & Gilbeau, 2017, and on McGill's International Centre for Youth Gambling Problems and High Risk Behavior's website www.youthgambling.com.

Other strategies have included parent, educator, and mental health workshops to help raise awareness about issues related to youth gambling and problem gambling. In a series of studies in Canada, Romania, Israel, and Finland it was found that amongst thirteen potentially adolescent risky behaviors, gambling problems was the least concern for parents, teachers, and mental health professionals (Campbell et al., 2011; Castren et al., 2017; Sansanwal et al., 2015; Sansanwal, Derevensky & Gavriel-Fried, 2016; Temcheff et al., 2014). Derevensky (2012) and his colleagues have argued for a multilevel approach addressing a number of different audiences including children and adolescents, parents, physicians, mental health professionals and attorneys (for more specific information see Derevensky & Gilbeau, 2019).

Treating Gambling Disorders: The Problem

Understanding and preventing problem gambling is complex. While harm minimization is essential for individuals with a gambling disorder, this may be too late. Unfortunately, few individuals with a gambling disorder actually seek treatment. This is not to suggest that all individuals will require professional help to stop gambling. Based on the data provided by the US Gambling Impact and Behavior Study and the National Epidemiologic Survey on Alcohol and Related Conditions, Slutske (2006) reported that, among individuals with a lifetime history of pathological gambling, 36 percent to 39 percent did not experience any gambling-related problems in the past year even though only 7 percent to 12 percent of individuals had sought help for a gambling disorder. Approximately one-third of individuals with pathological gambling disorders in these two nationally representative US samples where characterized by natural recovery. This is increasingly important given some recent findings that a large percentage of individuals with a gambling disorder have a host of other mental health disorders including anxiety and mood disorders, substance use and personality disorders, as well as psychotic spectrum disorders (Lorains, Cowlishaw & Thomas, 2011). More recently, Dowling et al. (2015) in a systematic review of treatment seeking problem gamblers estimated that 75 percent of individuals met the criteria of a current comorbid Axis I disorder, while Himelhoch et al. (2016) reported 46 percent of their sample of disordered gamblers was also opioid dependent. These substantial comorbidity occurrences introduce complexity to the treatment of individuals with a gambling disorder (Yakovenko & Hodgins, 2018). There is ample evidence that treatment (and assessment) solely for a gambling disorder cannot operate in a vacuum and must address many of the co-morbid, co-occurring behaviors (Gupta & Derevensky, 2008).

The good news is that there exist a variety of treatments for individuals with a gambling disorder. A number of outcome studies suggest that individuals who stay in treatment (a considerable number drop out) can be helped. Blaszczynski and Nower (2014) estimate that, independent of type of treatment, 70 percent to 85 percent of individuals experiencing gambling problems achieve positive outcomes at twelve-month follow-up with rates reducing to 50 percent over a longer time frame (thus necessitating continued follow through to minimize relapse rates).

Treatment Approaches to Working with Disordered Gamblers

As there remains no single identifiable cause or universally accepted theoretical model for understanding disordered gamblers, a number of psychological, psychosocial and pharmacological treatments for gambling disorder have been suggested. Individuals' motivation to gamble, their desire to gamble excessively in spite of repeated losses and negative consequences, and their comorbid disorders vary greatly. A number of reviews of these different treatment modalities have been published citing the empirical evidence in support of their approach and/or their limitations (see Choi et al., 2017; Derevensky, 2012; Hodgins, Stea & Grant, 2011; Lupi et al., 2014; Petry, 2005; Potenza et al., 2019; Rasch & Petry, 2014; Richard, Blaszczynski & Nower, 2014; Yip & Potenza, 2014). The following brief descriptions highlight some of the major approaches.

Self-Directed Interventions

Self-help interventions are typically designed to reduce the barriers (e.g., cost, stigma, difficulties with transportation, minimizing distances needed to travel for help) associated with seeking treatment for a gambling disorder. Such approaches may include teleconferencing, self-directed computer interventions and online support groups, bibliotherapy, workbooks and more traditional peer-support meetings (e.g., Gamblers Anonymous). Gamblers Anonymous (GA), similar to the Alcoholics Anonymous twelve step-programs, views disordered gambling as a lifelong affliction that requires complete abstinence. Social support from peers and family members remains an integral component of treatment. Family members can attend sister meetings (GamAnon) to learn how to help support themselves through the stresses of the disordered gambler (and possibly assist the gambler). Mutual aid is provided in a broad context. The program was designed by and for gamblers. While the efficacy of these programs has been challenged, Rash and Petry (2014) found positive results of GA attendance in conjunction with other psychological approaches. Like so many other programs, individuals who adhere to the program are generally successful

(Ferentzy, Skinner & Antze, 2014). Other approaches, such as the use of telephone support augmented by workbooks, have also met with some success (Hodgins et al., 2009).

Cognitive-Behavioral Therapy

Cognitive-behavioral therapy (CBT), one of the most widely used treatment approaches, targets maladaptive cognitions and related behaviors, with an emphasis on understanding the interrelatedness of cognitions, emotions and behavior. To best understand this model, one may make assumptions that disordered gamblers maintain distorted cognitions. Such distorted cognitions include overrating of one's skills, superstitious beliefs, interpretative biases (e.g., the belief that a win is due after a series of losses, the notion that one has to continually gamble [chasing one's losses] in order to recoup losses), temporal telescoping (the belief that wins are actually closer than further away), selective memory (gamblers tend to selectively remember wins and repress losses), illusions of control over luck, and illusory associations (for example, believing that one's lucky shirt helps them win resulting from an association of a win while previously wearing the shirt) (Hodgins, Stea & Grant, 2011). One fundamental aim of CBT is to help the individual identify and change irrational and erroneous beliefs (Blaszczynski & Nower, 2014; Petry, 2005). Petry's eight-session CBT program includes topics such as identifying and managing triggers, conducting a functional analysis of gambling episodes, increasing the client's participation in alternate activities, dealing with urges and cravings, building interpersonal conflict skills, recognizing and correcting cognitive biases, and relapse prevention (Rash & Petry, 2014).

Cognitive Therapy Focus

Given the research findings that faulty cognitions are symptomatic of a gambling disorder, some interventions have focused directly on attempting to primarily alter these cognitions. Ladouceur and his colleagues (Ladouceur et al., 1998) introduced a cognitive therapy and relapse prevention program among disordered gamblers and found that individuals receiving cognitive therapy endorsed fewer gambling diagnostic criteria, gambled less, and spent less money and less time gambling than a control group.

Imaginal Desensitization

One effective behavioral intervention, often overlooked, is the use of imaginal desensitization, which has been shown to reduce the urge, drive and motivation to continue gambling (Blaszczynski & Nower, 2014; Grant et al., 2009; McConaghy, 1988). The underlying premise is that systematic desensitization allows the individual to control their impulsive behaviors.

Motivational Interviewing

Motivational Interviewing (MI) is a client-centered therapeutic intervention aimed to resolve ambivalence toward changing a specific behavior, in this case a gambling disorder. Motivational Interviewing is primarily guided by five therapeutic principles: (a) expression of empathy (acceptance of the individual and recognition that ambivalence about desiring to change is normal), (b) development and articulation of the discrepancy between an individual's current behavior and his/her goal and self-image, (c) avoidance of arguments and confrontational situations, (d) rolling with resistance (looking for opportunities to reinforce accurate perceptions rather than correcting misperceptions), and (e) support of the individual's self-ability to change (Miller & Rollnick, 2002). A number of systematic reviews and meta-analyses examining the efficacy of MI for disordered gambling have been conducted (Hodgins et al., 2009; O'Neill, 2017; Yakovenko et al., 2015). Yakovenko and his colleagues concluded that MI was associated with a significant reduction in gambling frequency up to one-year posttreatment and significant reductions in gambling expenditures between one and three months posttreatment. Motivational Interviewing is relatively brief, easy to administer, cost effective, and seemingly reduces the treatment dropout rate; it may be a viable supplemental intervention to other evidence-based treatments as well (e.g., CBT; O'Neill, 2017). To summarize, the available evidence suggests that MI may be an efficacious therapeutic intervention for disordered gambling at least for the short term. Whether treatment effects can be maintained over long periods of time merits further investigation.

Psychopharmacological Treatment Approaches

There are a growing number of psychopharmacological treatment trials aimed at modifying disordered gamblers' impulsive behaviors and urges. At the same time, pharmacological therapies focus on clinical dimensions (e.g., impulsivity, compulsivity) or the comorbid psychiatric disorders (Lupi et al., 2014; Potenza et al., 2019). While multiple open-label drugs have shown promise, results from double-blind, placebo-controlled studies have demonstrated mixed efficacy (Bartley & Bloch, 2013). Potenza and his colleagues (2019) have argued that the best psychopharmacological efficacy of gambling disorder is the use of opioid-receptor antagonists (e.g., naltrexone or nalmefene). Although the systematic study of pharmacotherapy treatment efficacy for a gambling disorder is in its early stages, specific drug therapies may offer promise for treatment of some individuals experiencing a gambling disorder. At the very least, there are certain medications that are thought to have proven successful for treating a variety of comorbid disorders.

Conclusions

The landscape of gambling has radically changed during the past two decades with governments viewing gambling as a significant source of tax revenue and individuals viewing gambling as a socially acceptable recreational activity. No longer does one have to go to Las Vegas, Atlantic City, Monte Carlo, or Macau to find a casino or place to gamble. The thrill, excitement and enjoyment associated with gambling can ultimately lead some individuals to gamble excessively. Just as a large percentage of the population consumes alcohol and are not alcoholics, so too most adults who gamble are not problem gamblers. Most individuals can readily set time and money limits and more or less adhere to their preset limits. Yet, for some individuals, social/recreational gambling ultimately leads them to excessive gambling in spite of the myriad of negative consequences. Future empirical research is needed in the field of gambling studies to develop strong and consistent gambling policies related to harm minimization strategies and the establishment of *best practices* in the prevention and treatment of individuals with a gambling disorder. What works in one venue (or jurisdiction) may not be appropriate in another. As previously noted, disordered/problem/compulsive gamblers are not a homogenous group. They differ in their motivations to gamble, their preferred types of gambling, and their concomitant/comorbid mental health issues. Our understanding will change as new strategies, technologies, practices and policies are developed. We must keep up with technological changes in the gambling industry and new gambling opportunities (e.g., legalized sports wagering). The proliferation of gambling venues and use of smartphones and tablets as a primary platform for gambling represent some unique challenges but may similarly present some opportunities in directly reaching individuals. Some structural and situational factors are easier to manipulate and have greater credibility than others. Whether or not moderate risk and problem gamblers will avail themselves of voluntary measures remains to be seen. Researchers and clinicians may be wise to focus on getting individuals to adopt effective harm minimization strategies and to seek treatment when problems persist.

Ultimately, while governments and gambling operators can mandate or voluntarily implement responsible harm-minimization gambling strategies, individuals retain the ultimate responsibility over gambling choices and level of their participation. Optimal decision making depends on a wide number of factors. The *Reno Model* (Blaszczynski et al., 2004; Ladouceur et al., 2016), early on, formulated a framework to assist gambling operators, regulatory agencies, health and welfare workers and community members to develop a systematic coordinated approach to safe gambling. Blaszczynski and his colleagues argued for using a science-based approach to help minimize potential social harms as a strategy for protecting individuals, predicated on informed choice. While some of the specific harm minimization approaches previously discussed have great intuitive appeal, many have not been empirically tested for their effectiveness. No single strategy or program will be effective for all individuals, and one must be cognizant of cultural differences as well as availability and accessibility issues when implementing such programs. There is little doubt that specific and measurable advances have been made in the area of harm minimization and the treatment of disordered gamblers. Yet, researchers still have much to learn.

In a world of evolving technologies, research on harm minimization and treatment approaches needs to keep up with not only the activities upon which people gamble but the mode of delivery of gambling. Gambling remains one of the fastest growing industries in the world and technological advances have changed the face of the industry. Every computer, smartphone, or tablet can be a casino – open twenty-four hours per day, 365 days per year. Conversely, such devices also hold promise for delivering harm reduction and harm minimization messaging to vulnerable individuals through personalized normative feedback messages and may help those unable to travel to clinicians. Unlike educational programs for youth focused on excessive alcohol and drug use, cigarette smoking, risky sexual behaviors, and bullying, youth have not been receiving education about the warning signs associated with problem gambling. This is the first generation where individuals will spend their entire lives in an environment where gambling is prolific, legal, and viewed as a socially acceptable pastime. Legislators, regulators, gambling operators, mental health professionals, educators, and parents all have an important role to play in preventing disordered gambling.

REFERENCES

Abbott, M. (2006). Do EGMs and problem gambling go together like a horse and carriage? *Gambling Research*, **18**(1), 7–38.

Abbott, M., Binde, P., Hodgins, D., et al. (2013). *Conceptual framework of harmful gambling: An international collaboration*. Report to the Ontario Problem Gambling Research Centre (OPGRC). Guelph, Ontario.

American Psychiatric Association. (2013). *Diagnostic and Statistical Manual of Mental Disorders* (5th edition). Washington, DC: American Psychiatric Association.

Argo, J. J. & Main, K. J. (2004). Meta-analyses of the effectiveness of warning labels. *Journal of Public Policy & Marketing*, **23**(2), 193–208.

Ariyabuddhiphongs, V. (2013). Problem gambling prevention: Before, during, and after measures. *International Journal of Mental Health and Addiction*, **11**(5), 568–582.

Auer, M. & Griffiths, M. D. (2012). Voluntary limit setting and player choice in most intense online gamblers: An empirical study of gambling behaviour. *Journal of Gambling Studies*, **29**(4), 1–14.

Auer, M. & Griffiths, M. D. (2014). Personalised feedback in the promotion of responsible gambling: A brief overview. *Responsible Gambling Review*, **1**(1), 27–36.

Bartley, C. A. & Bloch, M. H. (2013). Meta-analysis: Pharmacological treatment of pathological gambling. *Expert Review of Neurotherapeutics*, **13**(8), 887–894.

Bernhard, B. J., Lucas, A. F. & Jang, D. S. (2006). *Responsible gaming device research report*. International Gaming Institute, University of Nevada, Las Vegas, pp. 1–56.

Billi, R., Stone, C. A., Marden, P. & Yeung, K. (2014). *The Victorian Gambling Study: A Longitudinal Study of Gambling and Health in Victoria, 2008–2012*. Victorian Responsible Gambling Foundation.

Binde, P. (2011). *What are the most harmful forms of gambling? Analyzing problem gambling prevalence surveys (Center for Public Sector Research), CEFOS Working Paper no. 12*. Retrieved from: www.utbildning.gu.se/digitalAssets/1327/1327132_cefos-wp12.pdf.

Blaszczynski, A. (2002). *Harm minimization strategies in gambling: An overview of International initiatives and interventions*. Report prepared for the Australian Gaming Council.

Blaszczynski, A. & Nower, L. (2002). A pathwaysmodelofproblem and pathological gambling. *Addiction*, **97**(5), 487–499.

Blaszczynski, A. & Nower, L. (2014). Cognitive-behavioral therapy: Translating research in clinical practice. In D C. Richard, A. Blaszczynski & L. Nower (Eds.), *The Wiley-Blackwell Handbook of Disordered Gambling*. West Sussex, UK: John Wiley & Sons, pp. 204–224.

Blaszczynski, A., Ladouceur, R. & Nower, L. (2007). Self-exclusion: A proposed gateway to a treatment model. *International Gambling Studies*, **7**(1), 59–71.

Blaszczynski, A., Ladouceur, R. & Shaffer, H. J. (2004). A science-based framework for responsible gambling: The Reno model. *Journal of Gambling Studies*, **20**(3), 301–317.

Blaszczynski, A., Sharpe, L. & Walker, M. (2001). *The assessment of the impact of the reconfiguration of electronic gambling machines as harm minimization strategies for problem gambling*. Sydney: The University of Sydney Gambling Research Unit.

Blinn-Pike, L., Worthy, S. L. & Jonkman, J. N. (2010). Adolescent gambling: A review of an emerging field of research. *Journal of Adolescent Health*, **47**(3), 223–236.

Bowden-Jones, H. & Prever, F. (2017). *Gambling Disorders in Women: An International Perspective on Treatment and Research*. New York: Routledge.

Brevers, D., Noel, X., Clark, L., et al. (2016). The impact of precommitment on risk-taking while gambling: A preliminary study. *Journal of Behavioral Addictions*, **5**(1), 51–58.

Calado, F., Alexandre, J. & Griffiths, M. D. (2017). Prevalence of adolescent problem gambling: A systematic review of recent research. *Journal of Gambling Studies*, **33**(2), 397–424.

Caler, K. R., Garcia, J. R.V. & Nower, L. (2017). Problem gambling among ethnic minorities: Results from an epidemiological study. *Asian Journal of Gambling Issues and Public Health*, **7**(1), 7.

Campbell, C., Derevensky, J., Meerkamper, E. & Cutajar, J. (2011). Parents' perceptions of adolescent gambling: A Canadian national study. *Journal of Gambling Issues*, **25**, 36–53.

Caraniche Pty Ltd. (2005). *Evaluation of electronic gaming machine harm minimization measures in Victoria*. Victorian Government Department of Justice. Office of Gaming and Racing.

Castren, S., Temcheff, C., Derevensky, J., et al. (2017). Teacher awareness and attitudes regarding adolescent risk behaviours: A sample of Finnish Middle and High School teachers. *International Journal of Mental Health & Addiction*, **15**(2), 295–311.

Chim, D. (2011). Gambling addiction in Asia: Need for a medical perspective? *Asian Journal of Gambling Issues and Public Health*, **2**, 68–74.

Choi, S. W., Shin, Y. C., Kim, D. J., et al. (2017). Treatment modalities for patients with gambling disorder. *Annals of General Psychiatry*, **16**(1), 23.

Collins, P. & Kelly, J. (2002). Problem gambling and self-exclusion: A report to the South African Responsible Gambling Trust. *Gaming Law Review*, **6**(6), 517–531.

Cowlishaw, S. & Hakes, J. K. (2015). Pathological and problem gambling in substance use treatment: Results from the National Epidemiologic Survey on Alcohol and Related Conditions (NESARC). *The American Journal on Addictions*, **24**(5), 467–474.

Cloutier, M., Ladouceur, R. & Sévigny, S. (2006). Responsible gambling tools: Pop-up messages and pauses on video lottery terminals. *The Journal of Psychology*, **140**(5), 434–438.

Croucher, J. & Leslie, J. (2007).Self-exclusion programs for problem gamblers in Australia. *Journal of the Academy of Business and Economics*, **5**, 61–66.

Davidson, T. & Rodgers, B. (2010). *2009 Survey of the nature and extent of gambling, and problem gambling, in the Australian Capital Territory.*

Delfabbro, P. (2004). The stubborn logic of regular gamblers: Obstacles and dilemmas in cognitive gambling research. *Journal of Gambling Studies*, **20**(1), 1–21.

Delfabbro, P., Borgas, M. & King, D. (2012). Venue staff knowledge of their patrons' gambling and problem gambling. *Journal of Gambling Studies*, **28**, 155–169.

Delfabbro, P., Osborne, A., Nevile, M., Skelt, L. & McMillen, J. (2007). *Identifying problem gamblers in gambling venues*. Final report prepared for Gambling Research Australia.

Derevensky, J. (2012). *Teen Gambling: Understanding a Growing Epidemic*. New York: Rowman & Littlefield Publishing.

Derevensky, J. (2017). *Annual Treatment Report for Problem Gambling in Florida*. Report prepared for the Florida Council on Compulsive Gambling, 27 pages.

Derevensky, J. & Gilbeau, L. (2017). *Adolescent gambling: Another risky behavior*. In D L. Evans, E.B. Foa, R.E. Gur, et al. (Eds.) *Treating and Preventing Adolescent Mental Health Disorders: What We Know and What We Don't Know. A Research Agenda for Improving the Mental Health of our Youth* (2nd edition). New York: Oxford University Press, pp. 571–584.

Derevensky, J. & Gilbeau, L. (2019). Preventing adolescent gambling problems. In A. Heinz, N. Romanczuk-Seiferth & M. Potenza (Eds.), *Gambling Disorders*. Berlin: Springer International, pp. 297–311.

Derevensky, J. & Gupta, R. (2011). Youth gambling prevention initiatives: A decade of research. In J. Derevensky, D. Shek & J. Merrick (Eds.), *Youth Gambling Problems: The Hidden Addiction*. Berlin: De Gruyter, pp. 213–230.

Derevensky, J., St-Pierre, R., Walker, D. & Gupta, R. (2013). *Availability and accessibility of gambling venues: An examination of the literature concerning: How these impact problem gambling*. Final report to Mise Sur Toi, 42 pages.

Dickerson, M. G., Cunningham, R., Legg England, S. & Hinchey, J. (1991). On the determinants of persistent gambling behaviour III: Personality prior mood and poker machine playing. *International Journal of Addictions*, **26**, 531–548.

Dickson, L., Derevensky, J. & Gupta, R. (2004). Youth gambling problems: A harm reduction prevention model. *Addiction Research & Theory*, **12**, 305–316.

Dowling, N. A., Cowlishaw, S., Jackson, A. C., et al. (2015). The prevalence of comorbid personality disorders in treatment-seeking problem gamblers: A systematic review and meta-analysis. *Journal of Personality Disorders*, **29**(6), 735–754.

Dowling, N., Smith, D. & Thomas, T. (2005). Electronic gaming machines: Are they the 'crack-cocaine' of gambling? *Addiction*, **100** (1), 33–45.

Ferentzy, P., Skinner, W. & Antze, P. (2014). Understanding Gamblers Anonymous – A practitioner's guide. In D. C. Richard, A. Blaszczynski & L. Nower (Eds.), *The Wiley-Blackwell Handbook of Disordered Gambling*. West Sussex, UK: John Wiley & Sons, pp. 251–262.

Focal Research (2002). *Atlantic Lottery Corporation video lottery responsible gaming feature research. Final report*. Nova Scotia: Focal Research Consultants Ltd.

Gainsbury. S. (2012). *Internet Gambling: Current Research Findings and Implications*. New York: Springer.

Gainsbury, S. (2014). Internet gaming and disordered gambling. In D. C. Richard, A. Blaszczynski and L. Nower (Eds.), *The Wiley-Blackwell Handbook of Disordered Gambling*. West Sussex, UK: John Wiley & Sons, pp. 361–385.

Gainsbury, S. & Blaszczynski, A. (2012). Harm minimization: Gambling. In R. Pates & D. Riley (Eds.), *Harm Reduction in Substance Use and High Risk Behaviour*. Oxford: Wiley-Blackwell.

Gainsbury, S. & Wood, R. (2011). Internet gambling policy in critical comparative perspective: The effectiveness of existing regulatory frameworks. *International Gambling Studies*, **11**(3), 309–323.

Gainsbury, S. M., Blankers, M., Wilkinson, C., Schelleman-Offermans, K. & Cousijn, J. (2014a). Recommendations for international gambling harm-minimisation guidelines: Comparison with effective public health policy. *Journal of Gambling Studies*, **30**(4), 771–788.

Gainsbury, S. M., Russell, A., Hing, N., et al. (2014b). The prevalence and determinants of problem gambling in Australia: Assessing the impact of interactive gambling and new technologies. *Psychology of Addictive Behaviors*, **28**(3), 769.

Grant, J. E., Donahue, C. B., Odlaug, B. L., et al. (2009). Imaginal desensitisation plus motivational interviewing for pathological gambling: Randomised controlled trial. *The British Journal of Psychiatry*, **195**(3), 266–267.

Grant, J. E., Levine, L., Kim, D. & Potenza, M. N. (2005). Impulse control disorders in adult psychiatric inpatients. *American Journal of Psychiatry*, **162**(11), 2184–2188.

Griffiths, M. (1990). Addiction of fruit machines: A preliminary study among males. *Journal of Gambling Studies*, **6**, 113–126.

Griffiths, M. (1993). Fruit machine gambling: The importance of structural characteristics. *Journal of Gambling Studies*, **9**(2), 101–120.

Griffiths, M. (1999). Gambling technologies: Prospects for problem gambling. *Journal of Gambling Studies*, **15**(3), 265–283.

Griffiths, M. (2013). *Behavioral tracking in gambling: New empirical data and the development of a new social responsibility tool.* Presentation at the Discovery Conference, Toronto, April.

Griffiths, M. D. (2020). Feedback models for gambling control: The use and efficacy of online responsible gambling tools. In S. Sussman (Ed.), *The Cambridge Handbook of Substance and Behavioral Addictions.* Cambridge, UK: Cambridge University Press, pp. 333–340

Griffiths, M., Parke, J. & Derevensky, J. (2012). *Structural and situational characteristics in slot machine gambling.* Report prepared for Assissa Consultancy.

Gupta, R. & Derevensky, J. (2008). A treatment approach for adolescents with gambling problems. In M. Zangeneh, A. Blaszczynski & N. Turner (Eds.), *In the Pursuit of Winning: Problem Gambling Theory, Research and Treatment.* New York: Springer Books, pp. 271–290.

Hancock, L., Schellinck, T. & Schrans, T. (2008). Gambling and corporate social responsibility (CSR): Re-defining industry and state roles on duty of care, host responsibility and risk management. *Policy and Society*, **27** (1), 55–68.

Hardoon, K., Derevensky, J. & Gupta, R. (2003). Empirical measures vs. perceived gambling severity among youth: Why adolescent problem gamblers fail to seek treatment. *Addictive Behaviors*, **28**(5), 933–946.

Harris, A. & Griffiths, M. D. (2017). A critical review of the harm-minimisation tools available for electronic gambling. *Journal of Gambling Studies*, **33**(1), 187–221.

Hayer, T., Kalke, J., Buth, S. & Meyer, G. (2013). *Die Früherkennung von Problemspielerinnen und Problemspielern in Spielhallen: Entwicklung und Validierung eines Screening-Instrumentes Abschlussbericht an die Behörde für Gesundheit und Verbraucherschutz, Hamburg.* Bremen.

Helfinstein, S. M., Schonberg, T., Congdon, E., et al. (2014). Predicting risky choices from brain activity patterns. *Proceedings of the National Academy of Sciences*, **111**(7), 2470–2475.

Himelhoch, S. S., Miles-McLean, H., Medoff, D., et al. (2016). Twelve-Month Prevalence of DSM-5 gambling disorder and associated gambling behaviors among those receiving methadone maintenance. *Journal of Gambling Studies*, **32**(1), 1–10.

Hodgins, D. C., Ching, L. E. & McEwen, J. (2009). Strength of commitment language in motivational interviewing and gambling outcomes. *Psychology of Addictive Behaviors*, **23**(1), 122–130.

Hodgins, D. C., Stea, J. N. & Grant, J. E. (2011). Gambling disorders. *The Lancet*, **378**(9806), 1874–1884.

Hing, N. (2003). *An assessment of member awareness, perceived adequacy and perceived effectiveness of responsible gambling strategies in Sydney clubs.* Retrieved from www.dgr.nsw .gov.au.

Johansson, A., Grant, J., Kim, S., Odlaug, B. & Götestam, K. (2009). Risk factors for problematic gambling: A critical literature review. *Journal of Gambling Studies*, **25**(1), 67–92.

Kessler, R., Hwang, I., LaBrie, R., et al. (2008). DSM-IV pathological gambling in the National Comorbidity Survey Replication. *Psychological Medicine*, **38**(9), 1351–1360.

Kim, H. S., Wohl, M. J., Stewart, M. J., Sztainert, T. & Gainsbury, S. M. (2014). Limit your time, gamble responsibly: Setting a time limit (via pop-up message) on an electronic gaming machine reduces time on device. *International Gambling Studies*, **14**, 266–278.

Ladouceur, R. (2005). Controlled gambling for pathological gamblers. *Journal of Gambling Studies*, **21**, 49–57.

Ladouceur, R. & Sévigny, S. (2006). The impact of video lottery game speed on gamblers. *Journal of Gambling Issues*, 17. doi:10.4309/ jgi.2006.17.12

Ladouceur, R. & Sévigny, S. (2009). Electronic gambling machines: Influence of a clock, a cash display, and a pre-commitment on gambling time. *Journal of Gambling Issues*, 23, 31–41.

Ladouceur, R., Blaszczynski, A. & Lalande, D. R. (2012). Pre-commitment in gambling: A review of the empirical evidence. *International Gambling Studies*, **12**(2), 215–230.

Ladouceur, R., Blaszczynski, A., Shaffer, H. J. & Fong, D. (2016). Extending the Reno model: Responsible gambling evaluation guidelines for gambling operators, public policymakers, and regulators. *Gaming Law Review and Economics*, **20**(7), 580–586.

Ladouceur, R., Goulet, A. & Vitaro, F. (2013). Prevention programs for youth gambling: A review of the empirical evidence. *International Gambling Studies*, **13** (2), 141–159.

Ladouceur, R., Jacques, C., Giroux, I., Ferland, F. & Leblond, J. (2000). Brief communications: Analysis of a casino's self-exclusion program. *Journal of Gambling Studies*, **16**(4), 453–460.

Ladouceur, R., Sylvain, C., Letarte, H., Giroux, I. & Jacques, C. (1998). Cognitive treatment for pathological gamblers. *Behavior Research and Therapy*, **36**, 1111–1119.

Loba, P., Stewart, S., Klein, R. & Blackburn, J. (2001). Manipulations of the features of standard video lottery terminal (VLT) games: Effects in pathological and non-pathological gamblers. *Journal of Gambling Studies*, **17**(4), 297–320.

Loo, J. M. Y., Raylu, N. & Oei, T. P. S. (2008). Gambling among the Chinese: A comprehensive review. *Clinical Psychology Review*, **28**, 1152–1166.

Lorains, F. K., Cowlishaw, S. & Thomas, S. A. (2011). Prevalence of comorbid disorders in problem and pathological gambling: Systematic review and meta-analysis of population surveys. *Addiction*, **106**(3), 490–498.

Lupi, M., Martinotti, G., Acciavatti, T., et al. (2014). Pharmacological treatments in gambling disorder: A qualitative review. *BioMed Research International*, **2014**, 1–7.

Marchica, L. & Derevensky, J. (2016). Fantasy sports: A growing concern among college student-athletes. *International Journal of Mental Health & Addiction*, **14**, 635–645.

McConaghy, N. (1988). Assessment and management of pathological gambling. *British Journal of Hospital Medicine*, **40**, 131–134.

McMillen, J. & Pitt, S. (2005). *Review of the ACT Government's Harm Minimization Measures.* Canberra: Australian Centre for Gambling Research.

Meyer, G. & Bachmann, M. (2011). *Spielsucht. Ursachen, Therapie und Prävention von glücksspielbezogenem Suchtverhalten.* Heidelberg.

Meyer, G. & Hayer, T. (2010). Problematisches und pathologisches Spielverhalten bei Glücksspielen. Epidemiologie und Prävention. *Bundesgesundheitsblatt*, **5**, 295–305.

Meyer, G., Hayer, T. & Griffiths, M. (Eds.) (2009). *Problem Gambling in Europe: Challenges, Prevention, and Interventions.* New York: Springer Science & Business Media.

Miller, W. & Rollick, S. (2002). *Motivational Interviewing: Preparing People for Change.* New York: Guilford Press.

Monaghan, S. & Blaszczynski, A. (2010). Electronic gaming machine warning messages: Information versus self-evaluation. *Journal of Psychology*, **144**(1), 83–96.

Monaghan, S., Blaszczynski, A. & Nower, L. (2009). Do warning signs on electronic gaming machines influence irrational cognitions? *Psychological Reports*, **105**(1), 173–187.

Neighbors, C., Rodriguez, L. M., Rinker, D. V., et al. (2013). *Efficacy of personalized normative feedback as a brief intervention for college student gambling: A randomized* *controlled trial.* Paper presented at the National Center for Responsible Gaming annual conference, Las Vegas.

Nowak, D. (2018). A meta-analytical synthesis and examination of pathological and problem gambling rates and associated moderators among college students, 1987–2016. *Journal of Gambling Studies*, **34**, 465–498.

O'Neill, K. (2017). Motivational Interviewing for problem gambling. In C. McIntosh & K. O'Neill (Eds.) *Evidence-Based Treatments for Problem Gambling.* Cham, Switzerland: Springer, pp. 19–25.

Parke, J. & Griffiths, M. (2007).The role of structural characteristics in gambling. In. G. Smith, D. C. Hodgins & R. J. Williams (Eds.), *Research and Measurement Issues in Gambling Studies.* Amsterdam: Elsevier.

Parke, J. & Parke, A. (2013). Does size really matter? A review of the role of stake and prize levels in relation to gambling-related harm. *The Journal of Gambling Business and Economics*, **7**(3), 77–110.

Petry, N. (2005). *Pathological Gambling: Etiology, Comorbidity, and Treatment.* Washington, DC: American Psychiatric Publishing.

Petry, N. M., Stinson, F. S. & Grant, B. F. (2005). Comorbidity of DSM-IV pathological gambling and other psychiatric disorders: Results from the National Epidemiologic Survey on Alcohol and Related Conditions. *The Journal of Clinical Psychiatry*, **66**(5), 564–574.

Potenza, M., Balodis, I., Derevensky, J., et al. (2019). Gambling disorder. *Nature Reviews Disease Primers*, **5**(1), 51.

Productivity Commission (1999). *Gambling Productivity Commission Inquiry Report.* Australian Government.

Productivity Commission (2010). *Gambling Productivity Commission Inquiry Report.* Australian Government.

Rash, C. J. & Petry, N. M. (2014). Psychological treatments for gambling disorder. *Psychology Research and Behavior Management*, **7**, 285–295.

Raylu, N. & Oei, T. (2002). Pathological gambling: A comprehensive review. *Clinical Psychology Review*, **22**(7), 1009–1061.

Raylu, N. & Oei, T. (2004). Role of culture in gambling and problem gambling. *Clinical Psychology Review*, **23**(8), 1087–1114.

Richard, D. C., Blaszczynski, A. & Nower, L. (Eds.) (2014). *The Wiley-Blackwell Handbook of Disordered Gambling.* John Wiley & Sons.

Robillard, C. (2017). *Responsible Gambling Programs and Tools.* Report prepared for Gambling Research Exchange Ontario (GREO).

Romild, U., Volberg, R. & Abbott, M. (2014). The Swedish Longitudinal Gambling Study (Swelogs): Design and methods of the epidemiological (EP) track. *International Journal of Methods in Psychiatric Research*, **23** (3), 372–386.

Sansanwal, R. M., Derevensky, J. & Gavriel-Fried, B. (2016). What mental health professionals in Israel know and think about adolescent problem gambling. *International Gambling Studies*, **16**, 67–84.

Sansanwal, R. M., Derevensky, J., Lupu, I. R. & Lupu, V. (2015). Knowledge and attitudes regarding adolescent problem gambling: A cross-cultural comparative analysis of Romanian and Canadian teachers. *International Journal of Mental Health and Addiction*, **13**, 33–48.

Schellinck, T. & Schrans, T. (2007). *VLT player tracking system: Nova Scotia Gaming Corporation Responsible Gaming Research device project.* Nova Scotia, Canada: Focal Research, 104 pages.

Schellinck, T. & Schrans, T. (2011). Intelligent design: How to model gambler risk assessment by using loyalty tracking data. *Journal of Gambling Issues*, **26**, 51–68.

Schottler Consulting (2009). *Impact of changes to EGM characteristics on play behaviour of recreational gamblers.* Report prepared for the Department of Justice (Victoria).

Schottler Consulting (2010). *Major findings and implications: Player tracking and pre-commitment trial. A program and outcome evaluation of the PlaySmart pre-commitment system.* Brisbane, Australia.

Schull, N. (2014). *Addiction by Design: Machine Gambling in Las Vegas.* New Jersey: Princeton University Press.

Schwartz, D. G. (2006). *Roll the Bones: The History of Gambling.* New York: Gotham Books.

Shaffer, H. J., Ladouceur, R., Blaszczynski, A. & Whyte, K. (2016). Extending the RENO model: Clinical and ethical applications. *American Journal of Orthopsychiatry*, **86**(3), 297.

Slutske, W. S. (2006). Natural recovery and treatment-seeking in pathological gambling: Results of two U.S. national surveys. *American Journal of Psychiatry*, **163**, 297–302.

Stewart, M. J. & Wohl, M. (2013). Pop-up messages, dissociation, and craving: How monetary limit reminders facilitate adherence in a session of slot machine gambling. *Psychology of Addictive Behaviors*, **27**(1), 268–273.

Temcheff, C., Derevensky, J., St-Pierre, R, Gupta, R. & Martin, I. (2014). Beliefs and attitudes of mental health professionals with respect to gambling and other high risk behaviors in schools. *International Journal of Mental Health and Addiction*, **12**, 716–729.

Thomas, A., Pfeifer, J., Moore, S., et al. (2013). *Evaluation of the removal of ATMs from gaming venues in Victoria, Australia.* Final Report to the Department of Justice, Victoria, Australia.

Toyama, T., Nakayama, H., Takimura, T., et al. (2014). SY17-4 prevalence of pathological gambling in Japan: Results of national surveys of the general adult population in 2008 and 2013. *Alcohol and Alcoholism*, **49**(Issue Supplement 1), i17.

Tse, S., Yu, A., Rossen, F. & Wang, C.-W. (2010). Examination of Chinese gambling problems through a socio-historical-cultural perspective. *The Scientific World Journal*, **10**, 1694–1704.

Turner, N. E., Macdonald, J. & Somerset, M. (2008). Life skills, mathematical reasoning and critical thinking: A curriculum for the prevention of problem gambling. *Journal of Gambling Studies*, **24**(3), 367–380.

Volberg, R. A. (2004). Fifteen years of prevalence research: What do we know? Where do we go? *Journal of Gambling Issues*, **10**, 1–19.

Volberg, R. (2007). Population surveys. In G. Smith, D. Hodgins & R. Williams (Eds). *Research and Measurement Issues in Gambling Studies.* Burlington, MA: Elsevier, pp. 33–55.

Volberg, R. A., Gupta, R., Griffiths, M. D., Olason, D. T. & Delfabbro, P. (2010). An international perspective on youth gambling prevalence studies. *International Journal of Adolescent Medicine and Health*, **22**(1), 3–38.

Wardle, H. & Dobbie, F. (2011). *Betfair self-exclusion project: Understanding the profile of self-excluders.* Report prepared for Betfair.

Wardle, H., Keily, R., Astbury, G. & Reith, G. (2014). 'Risky places?': Mapping gambling machine density and socio-economic deprivation. *Journal of Gambling Studies*, **30** (1), 201–212.

Welte, J. W., Wieczorek, W. F., Barnes, G. M. & Tidwell, M. C. (2006). Multiple risk factors for frequent and problem gambling: Individual, social ecological. *Journal of Applied Social Psychology*, **36**, 1548–1568.

White, M., Mun, P., Kauffman, N., et al. (2006). *Electronic gaming machines and problem gambling.* Report prepared for the Saskatchewan Liquor and Gaming Authority by the Responsible Gambling Council.

Williams, R. J., Hann, R. G., Schopflocher, D. P., et al. (2015). *Quinte Longitudinal Study of Gambling and Problem Gambling.* Ontario Problem Gambling Research Centre.

Williams, R., West, B. & Simpson, R. (2007). *Prevention of problem gambling: A comprehensive review of the evidence.* Report prepared for the Ontario Problem Gambling Research Centre, Guelph, Ontario.

Williams, R. J., West, B. L. & Simpson, R. I. (2012). *Prevention of Problem Gambling: A Comprehensive Review of the Evidence, and Identified Best Practices.* Report prepared for the Ontario Problem Gambling Research Centre and the Ontario Ministry of Health and Long Term Care.

Wohl, M., Christie, K., Matheson, K. & Anisman, H. (2010). Animation-based education as a gambling prevention tool: Correcting erroneous cognitions and reducing the frequency of exceeding limits among slots players. *Journal of Gambling Studies*, **26**(3), 469–486.

Wood, R. & Williams, R. (2007). Problem gambling on the internet: Implications for internet gambling policy in North America. *New Media & Society*, **9**(3), 520–542.

Wood, R. T., Shorter, G. W. & Griffiths, M. D. (2014a). Selecting the right responsible gambling features, according to the specific portfolio of games. *Responsible Gambling Review*, **1**(1), 51–63.

Wood, R. T., Shorter, G. W. & Griffiths, M. D. (2014b). Rating the suitability of responsible gambling features for specific game types: A resource for optimizing responsible gambling strategy. *International Journal of Mental Health and Addiction*, **12**(1), 94–112.

Yakovenko, I. & Hodgins, D. C. (2018). A scoping review of co-morbidity in individuals with disordered gambling. *International Gambling Studies*, **18**(1), 143–172.

Yakovenko, I., Quigley, L., Hemmelgarn, B. R., Hodgins, D. C. & Ronksley, P. (2015). The efficacy of motivational interviewing for disordered gambling: Systematic review and meta-analysis. *Addictive Behaviors*, **43**, 72-82.

Yip, S. W. & Potenza, M. N. (2014). Treatment of gambling disorders. *Current Treatment Options in Psychiatry*, **1**(2), 189–203.

19 Prevention and Treatment of Sex Addiction

Rory C. Reid, PhD, Joshua B. Grubbs, PhD, and Shane W. Kraus, PhD

Introduction

The past decade has brought increased attention to the phenomenon of sex addiction. Scandals involving celebrities, politicians, and prominent athletes have been a catalyst for media inquiries that often characterize sex addiction as an "excuse" to engage in sexually promiscuous behavior. Controversy has also emerged among researchers with findings both supporting and challenging the scientific merit of sex addiction (Kingston, 2015; Ley et al., 2014; Prause & Pfaus, 2015). Moreover, mental health providers have wrestled with a variety of clinical questions arising from efforts to help patients seeking treatment for chief complaints related to nonparaphilic dysregulated sexual behavior (i.e., not such disorders as pedophilia, voyeurism, exhibitionism, or transvestic eroticism). Understandably, the general public, as well as individuals who may be questioning their own patterns of behavior, report feeling confused about the concept of sex addiction. Indeed, among the many proposed behavioral addictions, sex addiction might arguably be the most controversial and challenging to understand, operationalize, study, and treat. This chapter will highlight perspectives and offer clarity on definitions, measurement, correlates, prevention, and treatment of sex addiction.

Origins, Current Terminology, and Definitions

The concept of excessive or uncontrolled sexual behavior has its historical roots in psychiatry with early references to "hyperesthesia," a condition characterized by Richard von Krafft-Ebing, involving the abuse of one's self and an abnormally increased and intense libido (Krafft-Ebing, 1886). Krafft-Ebing coined the terms "satyriasis" and "nymphomania," which remained in the sexual taxonomy of behavior in the *International Classification of Diseases*, 10th edition, under "sexual dysfunction, not caused by organic disorder or disease." Although previous versions of the DSM included references to "sexual addiction" in the category of a nonparaphilic Sexual Disorder Not Otherwise Specified (DSM-III-R), it was discontinued in subsequent manuals largely due to a lack of empirical research validating the phenomenon (Krueger, 2016; Reid et al., 2011). Carnes (2001) wrote extensively about sex addiction giving this terminology some early traction. As discussed below, DSM-5 proposed hypersexual disorder although this was ultimately not included for a variety of reasons (Kafka, 2014; Reid & Kafka, 2014). However, ICD-11 has adopted compulsive sexual behavior disorder in a section for impulse control disorders (World Health Organization, 2018).

The social science literature has characterized sex addiction by using a variety of labels such as sexual impulsivity, sexual compulsivity, sexual dependence, hypersexual disorder, unrestrained sexual desire, sexual disinhibition, hypersexual behavior, sexual torridity, sexual sensation seeking, sexual desire disorders, excessive sexual desire disorder, hyperlibido, hyperactive sexual behavior, uninhibited sexual desire, paraphilia-related disorders, nonparaphilic sexual disorders, Don Juanism, erotomania, nymphomania, and satyriasis (Reid, 2007). While this myriad of labels is secondary to the phenomenon itself, terminology such as sex addiction, sexual compulsivity, or hypersexual behavior have relevance for how one conceptualizes and potentially treats patient populations. Scientifically, labels are important for theoretical models which are sorely needed in the field, yet sadly there is a lack of rigorous research to support or refute models of this phenomenon. Many studies applying some of these labels do not attempt to test models. Rather, terms are applied interchangeably while describing the same construct – dysregulated nonparaphilic sexual behavior (Reid & Grant, 2017).

The authors' preferred terminology both clinically and in research has been hypersexual behavior or compulsive sexual behavior. *The Diagnostic and Statistical Manual of Mental Disorders* (fifth edition; DSM-5) field trial proposed *hypersexual disorder* while the *International Statistical Classification of Disease and Related Health Problems* (ICD) has decided to use *compulsive sexual behavior disorder* for the ICD-11. Elsewhere, similarities with these conceptualizations and sex addiction have been discussed in the context of an addiction classification (Kor et al., 2013; Kraus, Voon & Potenza, 2016). Thus, throughout this chapter, terminology may be used interchangeably while acknowledging that scientifically each term has its own etiological or theoretical significance (e.g., an addiction model, a compulsivity model, an impulsivity model, as examples). When the term sex addiction is used, in most instances we are discussing nonparaphilic dysregulated sexual behavior that has also been labeled hypersexual behavior or compulsive sexual behavior.

Despite the existing differences in terminology and possibly etiology, there is a generally a consensus among clinicians about the core characteristics of this phenomena. As outlined in the proposal for hypersexual disorder in the DSM-5 field trial (see Figure 19.1), sex addiction was characterized as a nonparaphilic repetitive and intense preoccupation with sexual fantasies, urges, and behaviors, leading to adverse consequences and clinically significant distress or impairment in social, occupational, or other important areas of functioning. Patients seeking help for hypersexual disorder typically experience multiple unsuccessful attempts to control or diminish the amount of time spent engaging in sexual fantasies, urges, and behaviors in response to dysphoric mood states or stressful life events; and symptoms were required for a period of at least six months. These symptoms also needed to occur independent of drug use, a general medical condition, or mania (Kafka, 2010; Reid et al., 2012a). This definition seemed to capture the essence of what most researchers and clinicians believed about this phenomenon.

Not surprising, in a similar fashion, the ICD-11 characterized compulsive sexual behavior disorder as a persistent pattern of an inability to control intense, repetitive sexual impulses or urges for an extended period of time (e.g., six months or more) causing marked distress or impairment in personal, family, social, educational, occupational or other important areas of functioning. As noted by Kraus and colleagues (2018), the pattern can be manifested in one or more of the following: (1) engagement in repetitive sexual activities becomes a central focus of life

A. Over a period of at least six months, recurrent and intense sexual fantasies, sexual urges, and sexual behavior in association with four or more of the following five criteria:
   1. Excessive time is consumed by sexual fantasies and urges, and by planning for and engaging in sexual behavior.
   2. Repetitively engaging in these sexual fantasies, urges, and behavior in response to dysphoric mood states (e.g., anxiety, depression, boredom, irritability).
   3. Repetitively engaging in sexual fantasies, urges, and behavior in response to stressful life events.
   4. Repetitive but unsuccessful efforts to control or significantly reduce these sexual fantasies, urges, and behavior.
   5. Repetitively engaging insexual behavior while disregarding the risk for physical or emotional harm to self or others.

B. There is clinically significant personal distress or impairment in social, occupational or other important areas of functioning associated with the frequency and intensity of these sexual fantasies, urges, and behavior.

C. These sexual fantasies, urges, and behavior are not due to direct physiological effects of exogenous substances (e.g., drugs of abuse or medications), a cooccurring general medical condition, or to Manic Episodes.

D. The person is at least 18 years of age.

Specify if: Masturbation, Pornography, Sexual Behavior With Consenting Adults, Cybersex, Telephone Sex, Strip Clubs

Figure 19.1 DSM-5 proposed criteria for Hypersexual Disorder

to the extent of neglecting health and personal care or other interests, activities. and responsibilities; (2) numerous unsuccessful efforts are attempted to control or significantly reduce repetitive sexual behavior; (3) continued repetitive sexual behavior occurs despite adverse consequences (e.g., repeated relationship disruption, occupational consequences, negative impact on health); or (4) continued repetitive sexual behavior occurs despite deriving little or no satisfaction from it.

Currently the authors are developing a measure, with other experts in the field, that combines the slight overlap in hypersexual disorder and compulsive sexual behavior disorder. The difference in the criteria is that hypersexual disorder addresses (1) the disregard of risks for emotional and/or physical harm to self or others, and (2) the use of sex to attenuate dysphoric moods or stressful life events. Compulsive sexual behavior disorder addresses continued engagement in sexual behavior even when deriving little or no satisfaction from it, where hypersexual disorder does not. The slight differences in the criteria for hypersexual disorder and compulsive sexual behavior disorder appear to highlight "risk" as a marker for diminished control (e.g., a lack of control leads someone to take risks they normally would not in order to have sex). The World Health Organization has not commented on why they excluded emotional dysregulation criteria despite a substantial body of research to justify its inclusion.

When the hypersexual disorder criteria were proposed in 2010, there was a paucity of research supporting the notion of individuals turning to sex despite deriving little or no satisfaction, whereas now this is commonly reported by providers working with this population. It might be mentioned that advocates for a sex addiction model would largely agree with these two definitions but might also add criteria related to symptoms of withdrawal and tolerance (although little research has been advanced to support these two symptoms). These various nuances may be resolved as further findings help elucidate understanding of this condition.

Controversy

Several controversies have challenged the legitimacy of sex addiction as a mental health disorder, cite concerns about its misuse diagnostically, or insist it will be abused in forensic applications. Critics have also suggested that sex addiction pathologizes normal variants of human sexuality. For example, individuals with high sexual desire are characterized as sex addicts because their partner with a lower sexual appetite protests about the incompatibility in their relationship (Moser, 2013). Using data drawn from a large community sample of adults, research examined the overlap between hypersexuality and high sexual desire. Cluster analysis revealed two subgroups: problematic (reflected by lack of control over sexual behaviors with negative outcomes), and high sexual and frequent sexual activity (desire and activity only) (Carvalho, 2015). Reasonable concerns have been raised about falsely labeling individuals with hypersexuality who present with high sexual desire/activity. In some cases, normative behavior is classified as a sex addiction because of incongruence with religious values or beliefs (Grubbs et al., 2019). Some researchers have suggested that there is a lack of empirical evidence identifying any dysfunction of a biological mechanism to explain the symptoms of sex addiction.

Many of these concerns have resulted in heated debates or disputes, particularly among members of the clinical community. Organizations representing different camps of healthcare providers have even released official statements about sex addiction with several opposing viewpoints (see the *American Association of Sexuality Educators, Counselors and Therapists Position on Sex Addiction* compared to the *Society for the Advancement of Sexual Health Position Paper on Sexual Addictions*). A review of such position papers reveals several valid points by opposing groups, which may diverge in part due to the emphasis on very strong sexual desire (e.g., preoccupation) versus lack of control over sexual urges. Such divergent perspectives may lead to different curative agendas.

With the newly released ICD-11 and adoption of compulsive sexual behavior disorder, there may result more banter between camps although, clinically, one may suspect that most clinicians will accept the ICD-11 criteria and begin to use this in practice and for billing insurance companies with the accompanying diagnostic codes.

In the wake of the DSM-5 proposal for hypersexual disorder, concern arose about misapplication or abuse as a diagnosis in forensic settings. Some policy makers suggested that the legal community would advance hypersexuality as a mitigating factor in the defense of hypersexual criminal defendants being prosecuted for felonies such as child sex abuse or rape. These challenges, however, did not offer any data indicating that sex offenders suffering from a paraphilia such as pedophilia, for example, secured for themselves reduced sentences. Conversely, it is widely known that criminals who use a mental disorder as a defense often receive longer incarceration sentences (Reid & Kafka, 2014). Regardless, some individuals who have gained prominent attention in the news media have attempted to self-identify as sex addicts when their alleged conduct clearly crossed the line into sex-offending behavior. Interestingly, very few news reports of these cases acknowledged the possibility that sex-offending behavior could exist *concurrently* with sex addiction but, instead, erroneously portrayed them as mutually exclusive classifications.

There has also been some evidence that "sex addiction" has been abused in divorce proceedings where it is asserted as a "diagnosis" to manipulate court rulings. In some cases, it is used as a defense to explain behavior while others attempt to use it as a rationale to restrict access to children in custody disputes (Ley, Brovko & Reid, 2015; Montgomery-Graham, 2017). Collectively, some of the concerns raised about the construct of sex addiction have been addressed (Reid & Kafka, 2014). However, much more research is required to bring scientific and clinical clarity to the concept of sex addiction.

Closely related to controversies about the legitimacy of sex addiction is the heightened debate about what model (e.g., addiction, impulsivity, compulsivity, hypersexuality) might best explain patterns of nonparaphilic dysregulated sexual behavior. Even within each of these respective constructs, there is not a consensus on the operationalization and definitions. For example, difficulties have arisen in efforts to differentiate impulsivity and compulsivity separate from understanding how such variables might be implicated in dysregulated sexual behavior (see Blum & Grant, 2020; Reid, Berlin & Kingston, 2015). Interestingly, when attempts were made to apply a widely used measure of impulsivity to sex addicts, an alternative factor structure emerged questioning if traditional conceptualizations of hypersexual behavior are appropriate (Reid et al., 2014). In essence, work is still evolving in the field around theories and, as noted elsewhere, researchers are still in search of a parsimonious model to explain hypersexual behavior (Reid & Grant, 2017).

Prevalence of Sex Addiction

There is a paucity of studies examining the prevalence of sex addiction. Although some individuals have estimated that 3 percent to 6 percent of the general population in the United States may be sexually compulsive (Carnes et al., 2012; Coleman, 1992; Sussman, Lisha & Griffiths, 2011), only one published study appears to support figures in this range (Kuzma & Black, 2008). In a Swedish study, Langstrom and Hanson (2006) reported prevalence rates of behavior in 12.1 percent of men ($n = 1{,}244$) and 7.0 percent of women ($n = 1{,}142$) based upon the frequency of masturbation, pornography consumption, and sexual infidelity. A nonclinical sample of men ($n = 474$) and women ($n = 466$) in New Zealand were asked to report "out of control" sexual fantasies and urges over a twelve-month period. Although 12.7 percent of men and 6.7 percent of women reported having a lack of control over their sexual fantasies and urges, these rates dropped to only 0.8 percent and 0.6 percent, respectively, when actual sexual behavior that disrupted daily life was analyzed (Skegg et al., 2010). An online study of men ($n = 5{,}834$) and women ($n = 7{,}251$) designed to help the researchers investigate differences between sexually dysregulated behavior and high levels of sexual desire found that 1.83 percent of men and 0.95 percent of women had significantly elevated scores on the Sexual Compulsivity Scale and a history of having sought treatment for sexual compulsivity, addiction, or impulsivity (Winters, Christoff & Gorzalka, 2010). The most recent studies or reviews suggest low prevalence rates of 1 percent to 3 percent (Klein, Rettenberger & Briken, 2014; Sussman et al., 2011). Like other forms of sexual behavior such as those among the paraphilias, obtaining accurate estimates of the prevalence of HD is a difficult task due to underreporting, differences in definitions, and other challenges commonly encountered in conducting sex research (Reid, 2010). A recent study of 2,325 adults found that 8.6 percent of the nationally representative sample (7.0 percent of women and 10.3 percent of men) endorsed clinically relevant levels of distress and/or impairment associated with difficulty controlling sexual feelings, urges, and behaviors (Dickenson et al., 2018).

Etiology and Prevention

Etiology

The etiology of sex addiction has not been clearly delineated. Research suggests multiple possible etiological pathways. One pathway includes neurobiological factors such as executive deficits or other potentially neuromechanisms that might create a vulnerability to developing sex addiction (Gola et al, 2017; Reid et al., 2010; Stark et al., 2018; Voon et al., 2014). Not surprisingly, associated features of neurobiological deficits can include poor judgment, impulsivity, and emotional dysregulation which have all be linked to sex addiction.

Some have suggested individuals develop sex addiction in response to unmet needs from maladaptive family attachments or as a way of coping with difficult affective experiences such as those associated with trauma (Efrati & Gola, 2019; Engel et al., 2019; Gilliland et al., 2015; Larsen, 2019; Weinstein et al., 2015). These variables are difficult to disentangle given so much research is done on treatment seeking samples where a patient might present with multiple issues that could implicate several of these factors in their history. Complicating matters, some cooccurring psychopathology such as adult ADHD or substance use disorders might explain, in part, why someone develops sex addiction.

Prevention

By extension, given the various perspectives on possible etiology it is difficult to ascertain what approaches might help prevent the onset of sexual addiction. Insofar as it is rare to see a patient seeking help for sex addiction who has adaptive coping skills such as the ability to respond appropriately to stress or unpleasant affective states, one might speculate that the acquisition of such skills might be a protective factor. Cultivating the ability to form a healthy secure attachment in romantic relationships might also be preventative. Many patients report coming from families where caregivers simply avoided conversations about sex or sexual health. Whether such conversations are preventative is uncertain, but it is clear in Western society with so many conflicting messages about sex, including those often promoted in pornography, that frank and candid conversations about sex are sorely needed. If nothing else, helping younger generations discuss and negotiate their sexual needs in appropriate ways might help them avoid mismatched mate selection or finding themselves in situations where their relationship needs diverge from their sexual needs leading to internal conflicts or moral incongruence. Sussman and Tsai offer some possible preventative approaches including family, community, group, and individual programming, especially in cases where children may be predisposed to engage in risky sexual behavior (Sussman & Tsai, in press).

Measurement

A number of scales have been developed to assess nonparaphilic dysregulated sexual behavior. Two prominent reviews considered seventeen and thirty-two scales respectively (Hook et al., 2010; Womack et al., 2013). Scales have also been published on specific manifestations of sex addiction such as excessive pornography problems or assessing the consequences of hypersexual behavior. A sample of popularly used measures, with both clinical and research utility, are presented next.

Sex Addiction Screening Test – Revised

The Sexual Addiction Screening Test – Revised (SAST-R; Carnes et al., 2010) is a forty-five-item measure that includes twenty core items designed to assess sexual addiction broadly, with an additional four subscales (Internet, Men's, Women's and Gay Men's) assessing sexual addiction for certain groups. While the SAST-R has gained popularity among clinicians, there have been few studies evaluating its psychometric properties or validity in assessing and treating people with sexual addiction. There may be some problems with the measure. One may wonder if it assesses all aspects of the hypersexual disorder or compulsive sexual behavior disorder criteria. Also, it includes some poorly worded items (e.g., double-barreled items such as "I have used magazines, videos or online pornography even when there was considerable risk of being caught by family members who would be upset by my behavior"). Finally, some items might create false positives such as "Were you sexually abused as a child or adolescent?" which has not been shown to be predictive of sex addiction. Clearly, more work and revision may be needed.

Hypersexual Behavior Inventory (HBI)

The HBI is a nineteen-item, three-factor, self-report measure scored on a five-point Likert format (1 = Never to 5 = Very Often) with possible scores ranging from nineteen to ninety-five (Reid, Garos & Carpenter, 2011). Subscales include Control, Consequences, and Coping reflecting diminished control, consequences for sexual behavior, and using sex to cope with unpleasant affective states or stress. Scale items reflect the DSM-5 proposed classification criteria for HD and the scale has demonstrated excellent psychometric properties (see Reid et al., 2011). The HBI was used in the DSM-5 field trial and has since gained wide acceptance among researchers and clinicians.

Sexual Compulsivity Scale (SCS)

The SCS was developed to assist in research of high-risk sexual behaviors and contains ten items that queries sexual thoughts, feelings, and behaviors (Kalichman & Rompa, 1995). Respondents endorse items on a four-point Likert-type scale (1 = Not at all like me to 4 = Very much like me). The scale has been widely used in numerous studies, especially among homosexual men and has demonstrated adequate psychometric properties. Item examples include "I have to struggle to control my sexual thoughts and behavior" or "My sexual thoughts and behaviors are causing problems in my life." The SCS is beneficial for its brevity; however, individuals with solo-sex behaviors are likely not to endorse several items that describe relational sex. A cursory, unpublished review we have completed over the past five years suggests that the SCS has been less prominent in the research arena with studies favoring the HBI or the SAST.

The Pornography Craving Questionnaire (PCQ)

The PCQ (Kraus & Rosenberg, 2014) is a self-report measure created to assess subjective reports of pornography craving. Rather than focusing on hypersexuality, this measure is intended to gauge the extent to which individuals experience a desire to view pornography. This twelve-item measure asks participants to rate their agreement with a series of statements (for example, "I want to watch porn right now") on a seven-point response format (1 = Disagree completely to 7 = Agree completely). Although this measure was only normed on young adult men, initial results indicated that craving pornography was directly related to frequency of use and time spent viewing pornography (Kraus & Rosenberg, 2014). The PCQ has been tested among international samples and found to be a robust predictor of pornography severity. The PCQ is likely a helpful tool as a general measure of hypersexuality, particularly for individuals reporting problematic use of pornography.

More About Assessment: The Issue of Severity

As with all assessment, instruments help guide a diagnosis but do not determine an actual diagnosis. The DSM-5 Field Trial for hypersexual disorder demonstrated criteria can be easy to use, reliably applied, and clinically relevant in helping clinical providers determine a diagnosis. We recommend considering both the criteria for hypersexual disorder and compulsive sexual behavior disorder to inform clinical diagnostic decisions.

Assessments should also consider the question of severity, although this has not been clearly defined (Reid, 2015). Indeed, there has been a paucity of dialogue about this topic. Some have advocated symptom count yet this approach assumes all symptoms are equal in their contribution to severity. It also ignores the magnitude of how someone might experience a given symptom. For example, the subjective experience of "distress" may vary from person to person. Time spent in pursuit of sex might constitute a proxy for severity, but this might also vary based on the specific type of sexual behavior or ease of access (e.g., daily use of pornography versus daily engaging in sex with a commercial sex worker). Similarly, the level of impairment, diminished control, and consequences might determine how severity is defined (of course, there may be some overlap; for example, diminished feelings of control may be a consequence). Multiple unsuccessful attempts to control or significantly reduce sexual fantasies, urges and behaviors might suggest a greater level of severity. Perhaps diminished control in one context might have greater consequences than others (e.g., inability to refrain from pornography on a work versus a home computer).

The number or types of consequences might also influence how severity is assigned. Consequences, however, vary depending on several other factors and some consequences might be considered more severe based on the implications, frequency, or subjective values. For example, consequences leading to interference with friendships typically have different ramifications than those leading to divorce. A consequence such as job loss might also vary in severity depending on other variables. For example, job loss might be associated with greater severity if one is financially struggling for money or if it is highly publicized in the media as with some political scandals, celebrities, or well-known sports figures. The related legal problems that can be associated with hypersexual behavior can also heighten the seriousness of a case presentation and by extension, how severity is conceptualized.

Comorbidity with Substance Use Disorders

A number of early papers on sex addiction and substance use disorders (SUDs) sought to draw comparisons between the two in what appears to have been an effort to legitimize sexual behavior as an addictive disorder. Theories purported that some individuals may turn to substance misuse to self-medicate from shame or other unpleasant affective states in the same way drug addicts used substances. The past decade as seen more empirical studies attempting to explore these relationships, with Sussman and colleagues (2011) estimating the cooccurrence of sex addiction with SUDs to be approximately 40 percent. Reid and Meyer (2016) also reviewed the literature and noted high rates of comorbid SUDs with sex addiction, particularly alcohol abuse.

Studies have also sought to determine if sex addiction is an extension of some other pathology or a separate construct, or reflects an addiction fusion of sorts, insofar as those who engage in problematic sexual behavior exclusively when intoxicated by drugs or alcohol may not exhibit symptoms of sex addiction otherwise. It's noteworthy that the DSM-5 proposal for hypersexual disorder stipulated if hypersexual behavior was primarily associated with alcohol or drug misuse that a hypersexual disorder diagnosis would not be made. The intention of the DSM-5 committee was to delineate a difference between substance-induced hypersexual behavior and a distinct condition that was independent from psychoactive substance abuse.[1]

It is also relevant that many sex addicts have characteristics highly correlated with SUDs such as sensation seeking, impulsivity, shame, and developmental histories of emotional neglect (Reid & Meyer, 2016). Thus, more research is needed to elucidate the constellation of interactions and variables that may influence relationships between sex addiction and SUDs.

Comorbidity with Psychopathology and Other Correlates

Several studies have explored comorbid psychopathology associated with sex addiction. Research findings have consistently shown sex addiction often co-occurs with mood and anxiety disorders (Kraus et al., 2015b) in addition to SUDs noted above. Given these cooccurring disorders, some have speculated that sex is being used fundamentally to tranquilize these unpleasant affective states or, alternatively, such psychopathology occurs as consequences related problematic sexual behavior. Among a sample of 103 male with hypersexuality, 71 percent met criteria for a mood disorder, 40 percent for an anxiety disorder, 41 percent for a substance use disorders (e.g., 33 percent alcohol, 10 percent cannabis), and 24percent for an impulse control disorder (e.g., 20 percent pathological gambling) (Kraus et al., 2015b).

Adult attention-deficit hyperactivity disorder has also been observed in approximately 25 percent of those seeking help for sex addiction (Reid et al., 2013). Interestingly, more than 95 percent of patients are diagnosed with predominantly inattentive subtype. Thus, while some hypothesized that the "impulsivity" facet of ADHD might be the catalyst for hypersexual behavior, patients with ADHD and sex addiction showed no more impulsivity than those assessed with sex addiction alone. On the other hand, patients with ADHD did show higher levels of shame, suggesting the important role it might have in precipitating and perpetuating hypersexual behavior.

Facets of personality have also been explored among those seeking help for sex addiction. Studies have noted elevated levels on the domain of neuroticism with mixed findings across other domains (e.g., using NEO-Personality Inventory). One study examined facets of personality between genders, noting parallels between groups including similar levels of impulsivity, emotional dysregulation, and difficulties coping with stress. Women, compared to men, tend to exhibit higher levels of distrust toward others, lower levels of self-confidence and ambition, and a greater preference for excitement and stimulation (Reid et al., 2012b).

Treatment

Treatments for sex addiction are varied. This is to be expected, given the heterogeneous presentations among those seeking help for sex addiction. Trials validating treatment approaches are in their infancy. Several treatments have been developed and piloted for hypersexuality, including problematic use of pornography. Preliminary evidence suggests that cognitive behavioral therapy (Hallberg et al., 2017), acceptance commitment therapy (Crosby & Twohig, 2016) or mindfulness-based approaches (Brem et al., 2017; Reid et al., 2014) may be efficacious. These treatment modalities focus on restructuring irrational cognitions associated with sex addiction, helping individuals reorganize their relationship with unpleasant affective states, or teach people to observe their experiences in a nonjudgmental way without overreacting to bodily felt sensations (e.g., a sexual urge). There is also growing support for the use of pharmacological interventions (Gola & Potenza, 2016; Klein, Rettenberger & Briken, 2014; Kraus et al., 2015a; Raymond, Grant & Coleman, 2010). However, there is an absence of robust clinical trials to test the efficacy of both psychotherapy and pharmacological approaches for sex addiction.

In contemplating treatment, perhaps it is helpful to consider the three challenges commonly encountered and reported in treatment seeking populations for sex addiction and then determine what interventions would be most appropriate. These three are noted below.

(1) *Emotional Dysregulation*: Most patients struggle to effectively regulate their emotions, especially in the wake of challenging experiences. Some of these may lead to psychopathology such as clinical depression or anxiety, while others are subthreshold. Research has

[1] During the DSM-5 Field Trial for HD, it was observed that several gay men abused alcohol or drugs (predominantly methamphetamine) to disconnect from internalized shame about their sexual orientation and create opportunities to engage in hypersexual behavior. Although the majority of hypersexual behavior occurred in the context of substance abuse, these were clearly cases where the predominant issue was hypersexuality, not a SUD. The recommendation was to consider a SUD secondary to HD rather than omit the HD diagnosis based on the proposed HD criteria.

consistently found high prevalence of adaptive shame arising from interpersonal sensitivity (Reid, 2010; Reid, Harper & Anderson, 2009). Providers need to determine what their theory of change is, particularly mediation of change, considering dysregulated emotions common among this population. They also need to explore what interventions might enhance emotional regulation.

(2) *Impulsivity*: Difficulties with impulse control are common. But more specifically, it should be noted this likely refers to context specific impulsivity rather than problems with generalized impulsivity (Reid et al., 2014). This impulsivity also appears independent of any impulsivity due to adult ADHD (common in ~25 percent of sex addicts). An interesting article was recently published examining facets of impulsivity among patients with gambling disorder using the UPPS-P Impulsive Behavior Scale (Reid et al., 2018). This study allowed researchers to consider what percentage of patients had clinically elevated scores across each of the facets of the UPPS-P (Figure 19.2) and provided greater specificity in understanding what types of impulsivity might be associated with problem gambling. One might likewise assume, given similarities between problem gamblers and sex addicts that similar findings would emerge for sex addicts. Thus, as providers assess impulsivity using an instrument such as the UPPS-P, they might consider what treatment interventions will attenuate such manifestations of impulsivity.

(3) *Stress Proneness*: Stress proneness is common among sex addicts who struggle to respond to everyday life challenges or feel quickly overwhelmed by experiences. Some overcommit to unattainable schedules and then feel stressed about their ability to attain unrealistic goals. Regardless, patients commonly report turning to sex as a stress-coping or stress-reduction behavior, which ultimately leads to more stress as the original problems remain unresolved. Further, the uncontrolled sexual behavior may worsen subjective stress. Thus, cultivating stress management and stress coping, to help "break" the chain of maladaptive behavior, is important in working with sex addiction.

The reasons for these three challenges may vary. For example, a patient may be depressed (emotionally dysregulated) primarily due to biological factors, suggesting a pharmacological approach would be effective, possibly combined with cognitive behavioral therapy. A patient's anxiety may arise from unresolved trauma, in which case trauma resolution might play an important role in treatment. Stress proneness may be present from lacking effective coping skills to respond to stressors. Subsequently, mindfulness approaches or acceptance and commitment therapy might empower someone to respond more adaptively to stressful experiences.

Clinicians have advanced several approaches to treatment that often integrate an eclectic strategy. These include twelve-step approaches, mindfulness-based stress reduction, cognitive-behavioral therapy, neurofeedback, pharmacological approaches, and lifestyle changes (e.g., nutrition, physical exercise, adequate sleep). In reviewing the existing

Negative Urgency: Items on this subscale measure the tendency to act rashly in response to negative affective experiences or impulsivity when experiencing unpleasant emotions (e.g., feeling bad, upset, rejected, etc.). A few items on this scale capture difficulty resisting cravings and feelings. Several items inquire about making impulsive decisions that are later regretted. Higher scores reflect greater impulsivity in the wake of cravings or uncomfortable emotions.

Positive Urgency: Several items on this subscale measures the tendency to exhibit diminished control in the wake of positive emotions (e.g., excited, happy) leading to impulsive behavior that may cause problems or negative consequences. One item queries respondents about giving into "cravings" or overindulging when they are happy. Another item reflects "going overboard" when feeling overjoyed. Higher scores reflect more impulsive behavior in response to positive emotional experiences.

Sensation Seeking: Items on this subscale measure tendencies to engage in excitement-seeking, novelty, or thrilling experiences. Many of the items on this scale tap into desires to pursue what some may consider risky/extreme sports (e.g., skydiving, speeding, scuba diving) or simply enjoyment from taking risks. Higher scores are associated with greater sensation-seeking behaviors and have been linked to greater propensity for risk-taking.

Lack of Premeditation: This subscale taps into future directed thinking about consequences prior to making decisions. Higher scores on this factor suggest individuals are careless in their choices, acting without purposefully thinking about the ramifications of decisions or weighing the advantages/disadvantages of their actions.

Lack of Perseverance: Items on this subscale capture diligence, persistence, and the ability to follow tasks through completion. One item appears to capture sustained attention "I concentrate easily." Higher scores reflect tendencies to quit prematurely, become distracted, difficulties with task completion and are positively correlated with boredom proneness and procrastination.

Figure 19.2 Facets of the UPPS-P Impulsiveness Scale

literature, Hook and colleagues (2014) noted that most drug treatments target serotonergic reuptake and most psychotherapy treatments involve cognitive restructuring. Finally, some researchers have targeted different mechanisms to directly enhance coping with cravings using naltrexone, combined with SSRI treatment, showing some potential (Raymond, Grant & Coleman, 2010).

Conclusions

Hypersexual disorder (e.g., sex addiction) was excluded from the DSM-5 but will be classified as compulsive sexual behavior disorder in the forthcoming ICD-11 under the impulse control disorders category. Interestingly, pathological gambling was once classified as an impulse control disorder and is now in the DSM-5 under the section on addictive disorders. While the ICD-11 inclusion is likely to silence some nay-sayers about the legitimacy of this phenomena, controversy will continue among researchers and clinicians for some time to come. As debates and research evolve, one might hope for clarification about the etiology and mechanisms implicated in sex addiction. This is likely to occur as different theories and models are tested using falsifiable hypotheses as a guide per the scientific method. Meanwhile, individuals will continue to seek treatment for their nonparaphilic dysregulated sexual behavior. Such individuals are likely to be less concerned with how their behavior is labeled and more interested in the practitioner's ability to alleviate their suffering and emotional distress. Like any presenting clinical problem, accurate diagnosis and assessment will be invaluable as it informs case conceptualization and treatment. Common challenges among patients include emotional dysregulation, stress proneness, and impulsivity. Subsequently, treatments targeting these problems is likely to be helpful in working with sex addiction. Finally, the field is in its infancy and there is a great need for continued research to help clarify and better understand this important clinical problem.

REFERENCES

Blum, A. W. & Grant, J. E. (2020). Considering the overlap and nonoverlap of compulsivity, impulsivity, and addiction. In S. Sussman (Ed.), *The Cambridge Handbook of Substance and Behavioral Addictions*. Cambridge, UK: Cambridge University Press, pp. 373–386.

Brem, M. J., Shorey, R. C., Anderson, S. & Stuart, G. L. (2017). Dispositional mindfulness, shame, and compulsive sexual behaviors among men in residential treatment for substance use disorders. *Mindfulness*, **8**(6), 1552–1558.

Carnes, P. (2001). *Out of the Shadows: Understanding Sexual Addiction*. Center City, MN: Hazelden Publishing.

Carnes, P., Green, B. & Carnes, S. (2010). The same yet different: Refocusing the Sexual Addiction Screening Test (SAST) to reflect orientation and gender. *Sexual Addiction & Compulsivity*, **17**(1), 7–30.

Carnes, P. J., Green, B. A., Merlo, L. J., et al. (2012). PATHOS: A brief screening application for assessing sexual addiction. *Journal of Addiction Medicine*, **6**(1), 29–34.

Carvalho, J., Štulhofer, A., Vieira, A. L. & Jurin, T. (2015). Hypersexuality and high sexual desire: Exploring the structure of problematic sexuality. *The Journal of Sexual Medicine*, **12** (6), 1356–1367.

Coleman, E. (1992). Is your patient suffering from compulsive sexual behavior? *Psychiatric Annals*, 22(6), 320–325.

Crosby, J. M. & Twohig, M. P. (2016). Acceptance and commitment therapy for problematic internet pornography use: A randomized trial. *Behavior Therapy*, **47**(3), 355–366.

Dickenson, J. A., Gleason, N., Coleman, E. & Miner, M. H. (2018). Prevalence of distress associated with difficulty controlling sexual urges, feelings, and behaviors in the United States. *JAMA Network Open*, **1**(7), e184468.

Efrati, Y. & Gola, M. (2019). The effect of early life trauma on compulsive sexual behavior among members of a 12-step group. *Journal of Sexual Medicine*, **16**(6), 803–811.

Engel, J., Veit, M., Sinke, C., et al. (2019). Same but different: A clinical characterization of men with hypersexual disorder in the sex@brain-study. *Journal of Clinical Medicine*, **8**(2), e157.

Gilliland, R., Blue, S. J., Hansen, B. & Carpenter, B. (2015). Relationship attachment styles in a sample of hypersexual patients. *Journal of Sex and Marital Therapy*, **41**(6), 581–592.

Gola, M. & Potenza, M. (2016). Paroxetine treatment of problematic pornography use: A case series. *Journal of Behavioral Addictions*, **5**(3), 529–532.

Gola, M., Wordecha, M., Sescousse, G., et al. (2017). Can pornography be addictive? An fMRI study of men seeking treatment for problematic pornography use. *Neuropsychopharmacology*, **10**, 2021–2031.

Grubbs, J. B., Perry, S. L., Wilt, J. A. & Reid, R. C. (2019). Pornography problems due to moral incongruence: An integrative model with a systematic review and meta-analysis. *Archives of Sexual Behavior*, **48**(2), 397–415.

Hallberg, J., Kaldo, V., Arver, S., Dhejne, C. & Öberg, K. G. (2017). A cognitive-behavioral therapy group intervention for hypersexual disorder: A feasibility study. *Journal of Sexual Medicine*, **14**(7), 950–958.

Hook, J. N., Hook, J. P., Davis, D. E., Worthington, E. L., Jr. & Penberthy, J. K. (2010). Measuring sexual addiction and compulsivity: A critical review of instruments. *Journal of Sex and Marital Therapy*, **36**, 227–260.

Hook, J. N., Reid, R. C., Penberthy, J. K., David, D. E. & Jennings, D. J. (2014). Methodological review of treatments for nonparaphilic hypersexual behavior. *Journal of Sex & Marital Therapy*, **40**(4), 294–308.

Kafka, M. P. (2010). Hypersexual Disorder: A proposed diagnosis for DSM-V. *Archives of Sexual Behavior*, **39**(2), 377–400.

Kafka, M. P. (2014). What happened to hypersexual disorder? *Archives of Sexual Behavior*, **43**(7), 1259–1261.

Kalichman, S. C. & Rompa, D. (1995). Sexual sensation seeking and sexual compulsivity scales: Reliability, validity, and predicting HIV risk behavior. *Journal of Personality Assessment*, **65**, 586–601.

Kingston, D. A. (2015). Debating the conceptualization of sex as an addictive disorder. *Current Addiction Reports*, **2**, 195–201.

Klein, V., Rettenberger, M. & Briken, P. (2014). Self-reported indicators of hypersexuality and its correlates in a female online sample. *Journal of Sexual Medicine*, **11**(8), 1974–1981.

Kor, A., Fogel, Y. A., Reid, R. C. & Potenza, M. N. (2013). Should hypersexual disorder be classified as an addiction? *Sexual Addiction & Compulsivity*, **20**, 27–47.

Krafft-Ebing R. (1886/1965). *Psychopathia sexualis*, translated by Rebman, F. J. New York, NY: Physicians and Surgeons Book, p. 927.

Kraus, S. & Rosenberg, H. (2014). The Pornography Craving Questionnaire: Psychometric properties. *Archives of Sexual Behavior*, **43**(3), 451–462.

Kraus, S. W., Krueger, R. B., Briken, P., et al. (2018). Compulsive sexual behaviour disorder in the ICD-11. *World Psychiatry*, **17**(1), 109–110.

Kraus, S. W., Meshberg-Cohen, S., Martino, S., Quinones, L. J. & Potenza, M. N. (2015a). Treatment of compulsive pornography use with naltrexone: A case report. *American Journal of Psychiatry*, **172**(12), 1260–1261.

Kraus, S. W., Potenza, M. N., Martino, S. & Grant, J. E. (2015b). Examining the psychometric properties of the Yale-Brown Obsessive-Compulsive Scale in a sample of compulsive pornography users. *Comprehensive Psychiatry*, **59**, 117–122.

Kraus, S. W., Voon, V. & Potenza, M. N. (2016). Should compulsive sexual behavior be considered an addiction? *Addiction*, **111**(12), 2097–2106.

Krueger, R. B. (2016). Diagnosis of hypersexual or compulsive sexual behavior can be made using ICD-10 and DSM-5 despite rejection of this diagnosis by the American Psychiatric Association. *Addiction*, **111**, 2110–2111.

Kuzma, J. M. & Black, D. W. (2008). Epidemiology, prevalence, and natural history of compulsive sexual behavior. *Psychiatric Clinics of North America*, **31**(4), 603–611.

Langstrom, N. & Hanson, R. K. (2006). Population correlates are relevant to understanding hypersexuality: A response to Giles. *Archive of Sexual Behavior*, **35**, 643–644.

Larsen, S. E. (2019). Hypersexual behavior as a symptom of PTSD: Using cognitive processing therapy in a veteran with military sexual trauma-related PTSD. *Archives of Sexual Behavior*, **48**, 987–993.

Ley, D., Brovko, J. M. & Reid, R. (2015). Forensic applications of "sex addiction" in US legal proceedings. *Current Sexual Health Report*, **7**, 108–116.

Ley, D., Prause, N. & Finn, P. (2014). The emperor has no clothes: A review of the pornography addiction model. *Current Sexual Health Reports*, **6**(2), 94–105.

Montgomery-Graham, S. (2017). Disorder in the court: The approach to sex addiction in Canadian legal proceedings. *The Canadian Journal of Human Sexuality*, **26**(3), 1–11.

Moser, C. (2013). Hypersexual disorder: Searching for clarity. *Sexual Addiction & Compulsivity*, **20**, 48–58.

Prause, N. & Pfaus, J. (2015). Viewing sexual stimuli associated with greater sexual responsiveness, not erectile dysfunction. *Sexual Medicine*, **3**(2), 90–98.

Raymond, N. C., Grant, J. E. & Coleman, E. (2010). Augmentation with naltrexone to treat compulsive sexual behavior: A case series. *Annals of Clinical Psychiatry*, **22**(1), 56–62.

Reid, R. C. (2007). Assessing readiness to change among client seeking help for hypersexual behavior. *Sexual Addiction &Compulsivity*, **14**, 167–186.

Reid, R. C. (2010). Differentiating emotions in sample men in treatment for hypersexual behavior. *Journal of Social Work Practice in the Addictions*, **10**(2), 197–213.

Reid, R. C. (2015). How should severity be determined for the DSM-5 proposed classification of Hypersexual Disorder? *Journal of Behavioral Addictions*, **4**(4), 221–225.

Reid, R. C. & Grant, J. E. (2017). In search of a parsimonious model to explain hypersexual behavior. *Archives of Sexual Behavior*, 46(8), 2275-2277.

Reid, R. C. & Kafka, M. (2014). Controversies about hypersexual disorder and DSM-V. *Current Sexual Health Report*, **6**, 259–264.

Reid, R. C. & Meyer, M. D. (2016). Substance use disorders in hypersexual adults. *Current Addiction Reports*, **3**, 400–405.

Reid, R. C., Bramen, J. E., Anderson, A. & Cohen, M. S. (2014). Mindfulness, emotional dysregulation, impulsivity, and stress proneness among hypersexual patients. *Journal of Clinical Psychology*, **70**(4), 313–321.

Reid, R. C., Berlin, H. A. & Kingston, D. A. (2015). Sexual impulsivity in hypersexual men. *Current Behavioral Neuroscience Reports*, **2**, 1–8.

Reid, R. C., Campos, M., Selochan, N. & Fong, T. W. (2018). Characteristics of treatment seeking problem gamblers with adult ADHD. *International Journal of Mental Health in the Addictions*, 1–16.

Reid, R. C., Carpenter, B. N., Hook, J. N., et al. (2012a). Report of findings in a DSM-5 field trial for hypersexual disorder. *Journal of Sexual Medicine*, **9**, 2868–2877.

Reid, R. C., Cyders, M. A., Moghaddam, J. F. & Fong, T. W. (2014). Psychometric properties of the Barratt Impulsiveness Scale in patients with gambling disorders, hypesexuality, and methamphetamine dependence. *Addictive Behaviors*, **39**, 1640–1645.

Reid, R. C., Davtian, M., Lenartowicz, A., Torrevillas, R. M. & Fong, T. W. (2013). Perspectives on the assessment and treatment of adult ADHD in hypersexual men. *Neuropsychiatry*, **3**(3), 295–308.

Reid, R. C., Dhuffar, M. K., Parhami, I. & Fong, T. W. (2012b). Exploring facets of personality in a patient sample of hypersexual women compared with hypersexual men. *Journal of Psychiatric Practice*, **18**(4), 262–268.

Reid, R. C., Garos, S. & Carpenter, B. N. (2011). Reliability, validity, and psychometric development of the Hypersexual Behavior Inventory in an outpatient sample of men. *Sexual Addiction & Compulsivity*, **18**, 30–51.

Reid, R. C., Garos, S., Carpenter, B. N. & Coleman, E. (2011). A surprising finding related to executive control in a patient sample of hypersexual men. *Journal of Sexual Medicine*, **8**(8), 2227–2236.

Reid, R. C., Harper, J. M. & Anderson, E. H. (2009). Coping strategies used by hypersexual patients to defend against the painful effects of shame. *Clinical Psychology & Psychotherapy*, **16**(2), 125–138.

Reid, R. C., Karim, R., McCrory, E. & Carpenter, B. N. (2010). Self-reported differences on measures of executive function and hypersexual behavior in a patient and community sample of men. *International Journal of Neuroscience*, **120**(2), 120–127.

Skegg, K., Nada-Raja, S. Dickson, N. & Paul, C. (2010). Perceived "out of control" sexual behavior in a cohort of young adults from the Dunedin Multidisciplinary Health and Development Study. *Archives of Sexual Behavior*, **39**(4), 968–978.

Stark, R., Klucken, T., Potenza, M. N. Brand, M. & Strahler, J. (2018). A current understanding of the behavioral neuroscience of compulsive sexual behavior disorder and problematic pornography use. *Current Behavioral Neuroscience Reports*, **5**(4), 218–231.

Sussman, S. & Tsai, J. Y. (2020). Teen sexual addiction. In C. A. Essau (Ed.), *Adolescent Addiction: Epidemiology, Assessment and Treatment* (2nd edition). Amsterdam, Netherlands: Elsevier, 241–263.

Sussman, S., Lisha, N. & Griffiths, M., (2011). Prevalence of the addictions: A problem of the majority or the minority? *Evaluation & the Health Professions*, **34**(1), 3–56.

Voon, V., Mole, T. B., Banca, P., et al. (2014). Neural correlates of sexual cue reactivity in individuals with and without compulsive sexual behaviours. *PLoS ONE*, **9**, e102419.

Weinstein, A., Katz, L., Eberhardt, H., Cohen, K. & Lejoyeux, M. (2015). Sexual compulsion-relationship with sex, attachment, and sexual orientation. *Journal of Behavioral Addiction*, **4** (1), 22–26.

Winters, J., Christoff, K. & Gorzalka, B. B. (2010). Dysregulated sexuality and high sexual desire: Distinct constructs? *Archives of Sexual Behavior*, **39**(5), 1029–1043.

Womack, S. D., Hook, J. N., Ramos, M., Davis, D. E. & Penberthy, J. K. (2013). Measuring hypersexual behavior. *Sexual Addiction & Compulsivity*, **20**, 65–78.

World Health Organization (2018). *International Classification of Diseases for Mortality and Morbidity Statistics* (11th Revision).

20 Passionate Love Addiction: An Evolutionary Survival Mechanism That Can Go Terribly Wrong

Maria Bolshakova, BS, Helen Fisher, PhD, Henri-Jean Aubin, MD, PhD, and Steve Sussman, PhD, FAAHB, FAPA, FSPR

Introduction

Feelings of intense romantic love have been documented in over 160 societies (Jankowiak & Fischer, 1992). In about 90 percent of the cultures where anthropologists have investigated this phenomenon, they have found evidence in songs, stories, myths, legends, plays, operas, ballets, poems, magazine articles, self-help books, gift cards, holidays, newspaper columns, emojis, podcasts, and other forums on the internet – all depicting romantic love. Children's fairytales and movies depict princesses and princes falling in love; and nearly every movie and TV show has some sort of romance or love interest. Around the world, people pine for love, live for love, kill for love, and die for passionate romantic love (e.g., people sometimes say "I can't live without you").

Dysregulated love, itself, has tended to be romanticized. Consider, for instance, an immensely popular teenage book series which was later adapted into a blockbuster hit movie, *Twilight* (from Summit Entertainment, 2008). The story focuses on a passionate relationship between an awkward teenage girl and an aged (forever young looking) vampire. The vampire is about eighty years older than the girl; and in the beginning of their relationship the vampire sneaks into her room to watch her sleep, a form of stalking. Moreover, the girl is so much "in love" with the vampire that she wants him to kill her and transform her into a vampire so she will be with him eternally. This tween novel series also includes a breakup, in which a girl becomes heartbroken beyond repair after a courtship that lasts less than a year. These are unhealthy representations of romantic love. Yet, the book series sold over 120 million copies and the movie grossed over 3.3 billion dollars worldwide (with follow-up novels and films in the series). There are many other forms of entertainment in which an unhealthy romantic relationship is glorified, exposing people of all ages to romantic relationships that can produce profoundly detrimental effects, as evidenced by increased suicidal ideation and suicide attempts by teens after viewing widespread media portrayals of romantic suicide (Gould, Jamieson & Romer, 2003).

Love addiction exhibits the behavioral and neurochemical characteristics of substance and behavioral addictions (Fisher et al., 2010, 2016; Reynaud et al., 2010; Sussman, 2010). Yet it is unique in that romantic love is a universal human drive that many people cross-culturally hope to feel at least once in their lives (Jankowiak & Fischer, 1992). Love addiction reflects a dysregulation of appetitive motivation processes pertaining to love-related motives (see Sussman & Pakdaman, 2020); and is associated with unhealthy emotions, behaviors, and coping mechanisms. To the extent that feelings of love involve preoccupation and loss of control that precludes other activity, and leads to undesired consequences (e.g., relationship dissatisfaction), it then reflects a negative consequential addiction (Sussman & Sussman, 2011). In this chapter, we examine the evolutionary origins and neurophysiology of love addiction, possible forms of love addiction (clinical features, personality types), and methods to prevent and treat love addiction.

Neurochemistry of Romance Addiction and the Evolutionary Origins of Passionate Love

Fisher et al. (2010) conducted a study using functional Magnetic Resonance Imaging (fMRI) on five men and ten women who had recently been rejected in love. While in the brain scanner, participants looked at two photographs, one of their departed beloved and one of a familiar neutral individual who stimulated no strong emotion when viewed. These photos were interspersed with a distraction task designed to cleanse the brain of passionate feelings after looking at the face of one's rejecting beloved and before looking at the neutral face. The distraction task consisted of counting backwards from a large number, such as 5,723, in increments of seven.

While the sample size was not large, that data were quite interesting. Results showed that rejection in love is associated with activation in several brain systems, including brain regions linked with addiction. Specifically, participants showed activity in the ventral tegmental area (VTA; associated with romantic love and the manufacture of mesolimbic dopamine), the nucleus accumbens (mesolimbic dopamine distribution point), the ventral pallidum (associated with feelings of attachment), the insular cortex (associated with craving; see Christie & Bechara, 2020), the anterior cingulate cortex (associated with executive processing), the orbitofrontal cortex (associated with implicit cognition), and the prefrontal cortex (associated with assessing one's gains and losses). These brain regions suggest a circuit pertaining to appetitive motivation and potential addiction (Burkett & Young, 2012; Di Chiara et al., 2004; Fisher et al., 2010, 2016; Kirsch et al., 2006; Sussman, 2017).

Various fMRI studies do converge on showing romantic love being associated with innervation of the VTA, associated with appetitive motives (Fisher et al., 2003; Fisher, Aron & Brown, 2005). The brain system for romantic love evolved to enable ancestral hominins to focus their mating energy on *particular* conspecifics; while the brain system for feelings of deep attachment evolved to enable early hominins to remain with a partner at least long enough to raise a single child through infancy (Fisher 1989, 1998, 2000, 2004, 2011; Fisher, Aron & Brown, 2005, 2006; Fisher et al., 2003, 2016). Thus, romantic love has been regarded as a "survival mechanism" as potent as thirst and hunger (Fisher, 2011; Sussman, 2017).

Evolution of Romantic Love

It has been proposed that the neural system associated with human romantic love evolved from mammalian antecedents (Fisher et al.,

2016). Prairie voles and rats, for example, show increased dopamine activity in related brain regions when exposed to a conspecific of potential mating interest to them (Gingrich et al., 2000; Robinson, Heien & Wightman, 2002). All birds and mammals have courting rituals during which they display, including enhanced energy, focused attention on a specific mating partner, obsessive following, and high motivation to mate with the potential partner. However, avian and mammalian species show only a brief "attraction response" when courting, whereas human romantic love can last weeks, months, or years.

Fisher proposes that romantic love began to take its human form in conjunction with the evolution of human serial social pair-bonding, perhaps among *Ardipithecus ramidus* living approximately 4.4 million years ago (Fisher, 2011). Regardless of when this occurred, with the expansion of early hominins into the woodland/savannah eco-niche, the first forebears adopted bipedalism to walk, forage, and *carry* provisions to protected locations. This development required females to shift away from carrying their offspring on their backs to carrying them in their arms. The evolutionary singularity of human nature is also tightly linked to the evolution of social cognitive abilities and large brains. The tradeoffs of large brains include complicated childbirth, which also requires prolonged afterbirth neurodevelopment, during which the offspring is highly dependent on huge investments from the parental dyad. In nomadic hunter-gatherer cultures, the average time between pregnancies is three to four years, during which paternal investment is crucial (Buss & Schmitt, 1993; Fisher, 1992, 2016; Fletcher et al., 2015). This may have pushed human forebears over a "monogamy threshold." Males could protect and provide for a single female as she carried her infant through the terrain. So, pair-bonding became essential to ancestral females and suitable to ancestral males, stimulating the evolution of social pair-bonding at least through the infancy of a single child (Fisher, 1992, 2016). Most partners may have become involved in other romantic relationships; however, once their infant had been weaned, it could join a multiage play group, and be provisioned and protected by a host of other band members.

A primitive form of divorce would have enabled dyadic partners to form a new pair-bond with yet another, thereby enabling them to bear new and genetically more varied young (Fisher, 1989, 1992, 1998, 2004, 2011, 2016; Fisher et al., 2016). Thus, during humans' long prehistoric past, social groups may have consisted largely of serially pair-bonded mates, their young, and single members of the social group. Today, approximately 84 percent of cultures allow polygyny. However, only about 5 percent to 10 percent of men in cultures that do allow polygyny take more than one wife at a time. Nevertheless, among cultures that allow polygyny, romantic love maintains a strong presence (Fletcher et al., 2015). Moreover, concomitant with the evolution of serial social monogamy (and clandestine adultery), the neural circuitry for human romantic love and attachment also evolved.

The evolution of the neural pathways associated with passionate romantic love most likely served several purposes: (1) to predispose ancestral males and females to rear their young at least through infancy as a pair; (2) to predispose ancestral hominins to engage in clandestine extra-pair copulations to acquire extra resources and/or more young; (3) to curb adultery among pair-bonded individuals, thus protecting males from cuckoldry and females from abandonment during their infant-rearing years; and (4) to become restless in long dyadic relationships, disband, and select new partners to rear more varied young.

Love and Addiction: Clinical Features

Substance and behavioral addictions have a set of characteristics that have been summarized as recurrent successful attempts to achieve an appetitive effect, which also include preoccupation, loss of control, and negative consequences (Sussman & Sussman, 2011). Specific features of these characteristics are several and may include: euphoria when the addictive love object is obtained; heightened energy to acquire the addictive object; focused attention on the love object (salience); craving for the love object; needing more and more of the love object to achieve satiation (intensification); personality changes (affect disturbance); lifestyle changes (more focused on the object of addiction to the preclusion of other activities); distortion of reality; loss of self-control resulting from involvement with the love object; doing inappropriate and/or dangerous things to acquire the addictive love object (e.g., stalking); emotional and physical dependence on the love object (separation anxiety); mood swings into despair and anhedonia, or irritability and difficulty concentrating when the love object is unavailable; and relapse when the addictive behavior is attempted after a period of abstinence (Fisher et al., 2016; Sussman, 2017).

Love addicted men and women experience these features pertaining to a love object; that is, another person or persons (Stanton, Campbell & Loving, 2014). Moreover, barriers may intensify the lover's wanting, seeking, and obsessive thinking. Rejected lovers regularly experience intense withdrawal-like symptoms, including crying, loss of appetite, insomnia, cognitive preoccupation with the love object, obsessive talking about the broken partnership, and possibly drinking, drugging and/or driving too fast, isolating oneself at home, as well as irritability, anger, depression, anxiety, and sensations of emptiness (e.g., Sussman, 2010).

External cues, including places, objects, events and/or songs can trigger memories and reactivate craving for the love object. Love addicts may go to extreme lengths to "win back" their love, from drunk dialing to stalking. Furthermore, the addict may suffer severe social consequences from friends and family due to their preoccupation with the love object, as well as legal consequences if they begin to stalk a rejecting sweetheart. Most of these behaviors mimic the withdrawal symptoms of other kinds of addicts (Fisher et al., 2010, 2016; Reynaud et al., 2010). As with some substance abusers, and possibly of higher prevalence, some rejected lovers commit suicide or homicide (Rosenthal, 2002). Over 10 percent of homicides are committed by a lover or previous partner (FBI, 2011).

Reynaud and colleagues (Reynaud et al., 2010) sum up six psychological criteria associated with love addiction. These include: (1) existence of a characterized withdrawal syndrome in the absence of the loved one, by significant suffering and a compulsive need for the other; (2) considerable amount of time spent on this relationship, in reality and/or in thought; (3) reduction in important social, professional and/or leisure activities; (4) persistent desire and/or fruitless efforts to reduce or control the relationship; (5) pursuit of the relationship despite the existence of problems created by this partnership; and (6) existence of attachment difficulties as manifested by repeated amorous relationships that fail to endure.

Personality and Love Addiction

An individual's attachment style, developed during childhood, could contribute to the development of love addiction in the future. Hazan and Shaver theorized that attachment theory, which was originally associated with infant-caregiver attachment, also extends to adult relationships (Hazan & Shaver, 1987). They proposed that three basic styles of attachment play a role in adult romantic relationships and may correspond to the ancient Greek's conceptions of love. Secure attachment, they maintain, corresponds to Eros (passionate or romantic love) and to a less extreme version of Agape (selfless, unconditional love, oftentimes associated with God). Avoidant attachment they associate with Ludus (treating love as a game – to manipulate and "play" with others' emotions). Finally, anxious-ambivalent attachment they regard as similar to mania (a possessive and jealous form of love; Shaver et al., 1988).

Supporting this hypothesis, Feeney and Noller noted that one's attachment style is predictive of their type of romantic relationship. In their study of 374 undergraduate students (Feeney & Noller, 1990), they first found that 55 percent of their subjects identified themselves as having a secure attachment style; 30 percent identified themselves as avoidant; and 15 percent identified themselves as having an anxious-ambivalent attachment style. Moreover, securely attached subjects tended to have the longest lasting and most trusting relationships. Subjects identifying as avoidant were most likely to have never been in love or to have low-intensity love experiences. Interestingly, anxious-ambivalent subjects had the *least* enduring relationships and were the most likely to idealize their partner, corresponding with the notion of a possessive type of love. In fact, the scores of anxious-ambivalent participants reflected their extreme approach to love, including dependence on others and a strong desire for relationship commitment. More important to this paper, those expressing an anxious-ambivalent attachment style were the most prone to obsessive love; that is, love addiction (Ahmadi et al., 2013; Feeney & Noller, 1990).

Other psychological phenomena may contribute to love addiction. Schaeffer (2009) proposed that some couples assume one of two roles, each of which can lead to love addiction: the role of the victim and the "grandiose" role. The "grandiose" role is played by someone who is energetic, driven, power-hungry and uses the victim as a coping mechanism onto whom they project their emotional and life problems, such as problems with their career, family and friends. Conversely, the "victim" plays the passive role, yet is skilled at manipulating the grandiose partner to take care of him or her. Schaeffer then proposes a list of signs that can lead to love addiction, including: overadapting to the other's needs (codependence), failure to build and maintain one's psychological boundaries, fear of letting go, "giving to get," needing the other to feel complete, looking to the other for affirmation of worth, and/or fear of abandonment.

A Neurobiological Hypothesis

Fisher has proposed an additional theory regarding personality and negative love addiction. She hypothesizes that each of four broad biologically based temperament dimensions (or styles of thinking and behaving) are associated with distinct neural systems, specifically the dopamine, serotonin, testosterone, and estrogen systems (Brown et al., 2013; Fisher et al., 2015, 2016). Moreover, those individuals primarily expressive of each of these four basic temperament dimensions are predisposed to express one of four broad styles of love addiction. Preliminary hypotheses are offered here.

The dopamine system is associated with a constellation of cognitive and behavioral traits. These include novelty-seeking, thrill and adventure seeking, impulsivity, susceptibility to boredom, abstract intellectual exploration, cognitive flexibility, openness to new experiences, curiosity, energy, verbal and nonlinguistic creativity, and idea generation. Fisher has labeled this suite of traits as the *Curious/Energetic* temperament dimension and those primarily expressive of this trait constellation, "The Explorer." These men and women may be predisposed to a particular form of love addiction, labeled *romance junkies*. Romance junkies may express a disproportionate inability to commit (despite feeling of intense romantic love), extreme restlessness in long-term relationships, a disproportionate tendency toward infidelity, and a tendency to abandon a partner as the relationship matures, in order to seek the "high" of new romance.

The serotonin system is associated with a different constellation of behavioral and cognitive traits. These include: observing social norms (conventionality); adherence to plans, methods, and habits; harm avoidance; orderliness; sociability; self-control; conscientiousness; managerial skills (cooperation and reduced autonomous problem solving); precision; interest in details; figural and numeric creativity; and self-transcendence (religiosity). Fisher has designated this suite of traits as the *Cautious/Social Norm Compliant* temperament dimension, and those primarily expressive of this trait constellation, "The Builder." These individuals may be predisposed to a different form of romantic addiction: *attachment junkies*. They may remain in a dysfunctional, even abusive, partnership just to keep up appearances or believe that this is the "right" thing to do, as well as be inappropriately controlling during a relationship.

The testosterone system has been associated in the academic literature with yet another a constellation of cognitive and behavioral traits. These include enhanced visual–spatial perception; mathematical/engineering/mechanical skills; music aptitude; intense focus; narrow but deep interests; less emotion recognition; less eye contact; reduced empathy; compromised verbal fluency; less social sensitivity; heightened sensitivity to social dominance; the drive for rank; emotional containment; and elevated confidence, forthrightness and assertiveness. This suite of traits has been designated the *Analytical/Tough-minded* temperament dimension and those primarily expressive of this trait constellation labeled "The Director." Individuals primarily expressive of this suite of traits, predominantly men (Fisher, 2016), may be predisposed to violence in relationships, or *violence junkies* – expressed with emotional flooding and abandonment rage, which could lead to domestic violence, narcissistic stalking, and impulsive homicide and/or rage suicide. Some data support this hypothesis: Men are two to three times more likely to commit suicide after being rejected (Hatfield & Rapson, 1996); and men are far more likely than women to stalk a rejecting partner, as well as batter or kill her (Meloy, Davis & Lovette, 2001).

The estrogen system (and interconnected oxytocin system) are associated in the literature with yet another suite of cognitive and behavioral traits. Included are contextual/holistic/synthetic thinking, linguistic and people skills, agreeableness, cooperation, theory of mind (intuition), empathy, nurturing, generosity, trust, the drive to make social attachments, heightened memory for emotional experiences, and emotional expressiveness. Oxytocin is also associated with several prosocial traits, including trust, reading emotions in others, and theory of mind. Fisher has designated this trait constellation the *Prosocial/Empathetic* temperament dimension, and those who primarily express this trait constellation labeled "The Negotiator." Individuals who primarily express this suite of traits, predominantly women (Fisher et al., 2016), may be disproportionately predisposed to becoming *Codependence junkies* – in which they obsessively analyze the partnership, as well as possess increased susceptibility to clinical depression and attempted suicide in response to romantic rejection. Some data support this hypothesis. Romantically rejected women report more severe feelings of depression than do men (Mearns, 1991), as well as more chronic strain and rumination after being rejected (Nolen-Hoeksema, Larson & Grayson, 1999). Women are also more likely to talk about their trauma, inadvertently retraumatizing themselves (Hatfield & Rapson, 1996).

Although the above hypotheses regarding four basic varieties of love addiction – romance junkies, attachment junkies, violence junkies and codependence junkies – are speculative at present, further research may find that various sorts of love addiction tendencies, including the inability to commit, constant adultery, inappropriate sexual jealousy, mate guarding, partner stalking, spouse abuse, love homicide, love suicide, and clinical depression are linked with specific biologically-based temperament dimensions. If these hypotheses hold true, they may help to inform tailored prevention and treatment options for each individual temperament-dimension.

Prevention of Love Addiction

As prevention of love addiction has rarely been studied, one must rely heavily on hypotheses of what might work for this behavioral addiction. One might suggest application of evidence-based drug abuse prevention strategies (e.g., in Sussman, 2017) to love addiction prevention. Several of the mediators of preventive effects considered in drug abuse programming (Hansen, 1992, 1996; Hansen & McNeal, 1997) may be applied. One may attempt to *lower estimates of prevalence or acceptability* of love addiction-related normative beliefs (e.g., that anything is possible through love; that stalking a loved one is normal). One may assist the participant in elaboration of how love addiction-related behaviors may be *incongruent with lifestyle* and future aspirations. Understanding and applying a rational strategy for *making decisions* may help one avoid self-defeating, impulsive situations related to love addiction. One may learn how to enjoy *alternative activities* that do not involve romance. One may assist the participant in *self-esteem enhancement* techniques. Enhanced self-esteem may help prevent entering into and accepting relationships based on power struggles, typical of love addiction (Sussman, 2010). *Stress-management skills* may assist in helping the person to cope without relying on romantic fantasy. *Social skills instruction* may assist the person to establish healthy platonic friendships, be assertive with friends, and get along with others.

These strategies may be implemented through a number of modalities including school-based classroom education, family involvement, as well as community outreach. Across modalities, to best achieve changes in beliefs and behavior, use of Socratic dialogue may be useful. That is, the participants should generate the appropriate answers through a series of carefully chosen questions so that they may identify with and internalize the answers they generate (Sussman, 2017).

Programming at a high-school level may be particularly effective, as this is the developmental period in which teens are beginning to have crushes and go on dates. Teaching adolescents *how to form and nurture healthy relationships* may be useful – specifically showing them how to set boundaries, communicate successfully, solve conflicts effectively and avoid sexual harassment, conducted in an age-appropriate manner. Education on healthy versus toxic behaviors in relationships could be beneficial, as many people, even adults, are not able to distinguish toxic relationship behavior when deep into a romantic relationship. One's attachment style can change with time (Iwaniec & Sneddon, 2001), largely by increasing an individual's self-confidence and providing them with new ways to cope with problems (Lopez & Gormley, 2002). *Correcting "myths"* about romance and love may be a useful addition to high school-based programming. Such myths may be portrayed in many plays, movies and TV shows (e.g., *Romeo and Juliet*). Use of media literacy strategies may assist. These may involve instruction of a typology of love-addiction-related "ploys" (e.g., the myth that stalking behavior shows love, the myth that relationship breakups mean that life stops, the myth that there is one true love, the myth that ideal love exists) and counteraction of such ploys as depicted in the media by dramatic portrayal or drawings of the opposite (e.g., showing that stalking shows aggression, that relationship breakup means moving on to new activities, that there may be new loves, that ideal love is a fantasy that youth may find uncomfortable when carefully considered).

Other strategies might be attempted among high school youth at the school, or in another community setting. *Mood management skills*, along with *cognitive restructuring* techniques, can aid in regulating excessive emotions that may result in unhealthy behavior and negative consequences. *Meditation* may be taught to enhance mood to counteract the motivation for love-seeking, as well as to fulfill one's own needs and "love themselves" without having to rely obsessively on a partner. *Cognitive restructuring* techniques can allow an individual to separate inner speech and form alternate speech, such as going from the thought of "Only this one person can satisfy all of my needs," to "There are many people who may be right for me." Cognitive methods can also be greatly beneficial in counteracting fantasy-based thinking, dramatization, and romanticization of situations.

Large social climate factors might be addressed. The entertainment industry might assert for more media portrayals of healthy relationships, which might lead to prosocial impacts, compared to fairy-tale romances in movies, TV shows, and novels, similar to attempts to incorporate racial and sexual diversity into many aspects of the media. *Policy* prevention measures could be useful to regulate some large social climate influences that might facilitate love addiction and be avoidable. For older movies and TV shows that feature obsessive and toxic relationship behaviors, perhaps warning labels could be added to the beginning of the programming. Just as there are warnings for "violence, graphic and/or sexual content," adding warnings about the unrealistic and unhealthy portrayals of relationships may remind viewers that what they are seeing is purely fiction, not an example of what they should strive for their relationships to look like.

Love Addiction Prevention Considered Across the Lifespan

Sussman (2013) discusses utilizing preventive strategies across the lifespan, tailoring different types of programming depending on the age range of the participants. Possibly, love addiction prevention programming could be applied at various stages of development. Prevention programming could aim to *educate new parents* on the importance of developing a secure attachment style with their toddlers. For children who are older and are exhibiting signs of an anxious-ambivalent attachment style, clinicians may wish to provide these young children and adolescents with therapy that aims to increase their self-confidence. *Cognitive-behavioral therapy* that counteracts negative cognitions about oneself, and tools to help them anticipate and avoid a love addiction in their future, may also be beneficial.

For young children, it may be wise to have children's books that encourage positive, healthy, and realistic relationship behaviors between characters in their stories. At some point in development, teens may gravitate toward romance novels. *Warning labels* or information packets on differentiating "love fiction" from "love fact" may help youth to enjoy such novels without succumbing to implicit messages in them. Also, for adolescents, interactive techniques such as *role-playing* could offer an engaging way of learning about healthy behaviors, as well as letting the teenagers have some fun. Role-playing dating scenarios and behaviors for older adolescents could foster an appreciation for healthy relationships, as well as possibly help identify dangerous situations such as harassment, assault, and violence, all of which are becoming more and more relevant. This may, in turn, help to prevent "violence junkies" from developing an association between romance and acting violent toward their objects of desire.

Emerging adults and older adults who are susceptible to toxic behaviors and addiction-like traits when it comes to relationships may benefit from *implementation intention training*. This training helps the participant identify problematic situations that may occur and sets goals and precedents for what that individual will do if that situation arises (Sussman, 2017). For example, one may be instructed to think about what they would do when they feel themselves falling in love with someone new, and immediately wanting to move in with them after only a few weeks. The individual would then develop a plan, such as waiting six months, and speaking with their partner as well as their friends and family about the consequences of this decision, before proceeding (e.g., consider the lessons instructed in *Frozen*, Walt Disney Pictures, 2013).

Treatment of Love Addiction

Assessment

Once a person develops a pattern of love addiction, treatment may be needed to arrest the addiction, permit recovery from the consequences suffered, and help establish new, healthier behaviors. Certain groups may be more at risk for the development of love addiction, as previously mentioned, such as those with anxious attachment styles. These individuals could be identified through psychological assessment, which may tap over-reliance on partner ("most alive with partner") and unfulfilled hopes ("never satisfied with partners" for long) (e.g., Feeney & Noller, 1990, twelve-item measure; Hunter, Nitschke & Hogan, 1981, twenty-item measure; Sussman, 2010). Examples of other items that may be used to identify persons who may be suffering from love addiction, identified by Sussman (2010), include: "Have you ever tried to control how often you would see someone?" "Do you get high from romance?" "Do you believe that a relationship will make your life bearable?" "Do you believe that someone can 'fix' you?" "Do you feel desperation or uneasiness when you are away from your lover?" and "Do you feel that you're not 'really alive' unless you are with your romantic partner?" (also see: https://markfalango.com/wp-content/uploads/lasa.pdf; http://centerforhealthysex.com/sex-therapy-resources/love-addiction-test/; accessed March 6, 2019). A "Love Addiction Inventory (LAI)" has recently been developed, which includes four items relating to each of the six criteria of behavioral addiction (salience, tolerance, mood modification, relapse, withdrawal, and conflict; Griffiths, 2005). The LAI showed good reliability and concurrent validity among a sample of 663 participants involved in an intimate relationship (Costa et al., 2019).

Assessments could be tailored for the aforementioned four different personality types of love addiction. Certainly, much assessment research is needed, as primarily heuristic clinical measures exist. Researchers and practitioners have suggested several strategies for alleviating a love addiction. One review of love addiction treatment found a total of twelve empirical papers detailing clinical management of this disorder, which were broken up into the following interventions: self-help groups, cognitive-behavioral therapy (CBT), psychodynamic therapy, psychodrama group therapy, and pharmacotherapy (Sanches & John, 2019).

Arresting Love Addiction and Use of Twelve-Step Program-Related Advice

First and foremost, it is important to recommend that the addict refrain from making life-changing decisions until some of this "natural elixir" becomes subdued with time – because, when in love, neural regions linked with social judgment and negative assessment become deactivated (Bartels & Zeki, 2004), rendering the lover less equipped to make well-reasoned decisions. Currently, many practitioners recommend participation in twelve-step programs, particularly *Sex and Love Addicts Anonymous*, including following the instructions of its principles and suggestions of its members (see https://slaafws.org/; accessed March 5th, 2019). For example, all twelve-step programs advise addicted men and women to remove all reasonable evidence of their addiction, in this case evidence of the abandoning sweetheart. Cards, letters, songs, photos, memorabilia, and all forms of social media contact may be advised to be deleted. One may be told to maintain a strict no-contact policy, avoiding any form of communication with the ex-partner that may trigger renewed feelings of craving and retard the healing process. Most rejecters do not know how to handle the rejected lover's grief or their own feelings about the ruptured tie (Baumeister & Dhavale, 2001); so, although the rejecter may be friendly when the disappointed lover contacts him or her, many will be perplexed, annoyed, or angry at the intrusion (Baumeister, Wotman & Stillwell, 1993).

Love addicts who have been rejected or broken up with are also advised to stay busy, preferably doing novel (healthy) activities, because novelty activates the dopamine system in the brain to create energy and optimism (Fisher, 2016; Rosenthal, 2002), as well as redirect attention away from preoccupation with the love object. Sunlight can enhance positive feelings because it stimulates the pineal gland in the brain to regulate bodily rhythms in ways that elevate mood (Rosenthal, 2002). Meditation affects several neural systems, thereby decreasing anxiety and escalating focus and sustained attention (Compson, 2014; Davidson & Begley, 2012; Grant et al., 2017). Affirmations and other repeated (positive) phrases may also affect brain pathways to redirect one's obsessive thoughts away from the love object.

Physical exercise may help love addicts elevate mood (Fisher, 2016; Rosenthal, 2002) because it triggers dopamine activity in the nucleus accumbens, bestowing pleasure as well as increasing activity of the endorphins and endocannabinoids, associated respectively with pain relief and pleasure (Dietrich and McDaniel, 2004; Goldfarb & Jamuras, 1997; Heijnen et al., 2016). Strenuous physical exercise also increases brain-derived neurotrophic factor (BDNF) in the hippocampus to protect and make new nerve cells in this part of the memory system. Some psychiatrists even believe that exercise (aerobic or anaerobic) can be as effective in healing depression (a byproduct of thwarted love addiction-related relationships) as antidepressant drugs or psychotherapy (Rosenthal, 2002).

Group and Individual Therapies for Love Addicts

Group and individual therapy are likely to help love addicts. Relevant techniques include: guided cognitive restructuring; role-playing to replace fantasy-based thinking with a more realistic perspective, and instruction in accurate and grounded portrayal of long-term relationship behavior (Fisher, 2016). One pilot study found that a convenience sample of eight love addicts who participated in eighteen psychodrama group therapy sessions showed a significant reduction of obsessive romantic craving for a partner (Lorena et al., 2008). Key material in the sessions included establishing a therapeutic contract, mood management, choosing goals, reducing myths about love, and working through inner conflict and emotional emptiness. The authors suggested that such an approach helps to provide insight, improves self-esteem, and can lead to development of more prosocial relationships. In fact, *the brain is primed to engage in talking therapy.* Research shows that rejected lovers are activating brain regions associated with assessing one's "gains and losses," indicating that these men and women are self-motivated to evaluate and learn from their situation (Fisher et al., 2010).

A cognitive-behavioral approach (CBT) can be utilized. This approach aims to help individuals monitor their behavior, provide corrective cognitive function (self-instructional training for impulsive behavior, cognitive restructuring for irrational thought), as well as instruction in how to cope effectively during stressful situations. Self-monitoring skills for love addiction could include teaching individuals to identify when they are thinking obsessively; for example, when a love addict is "stalking" their object of affection on social media or in real life. Coping skills could perhaps teach methods to manage a painful rejection or feelings of jealousy of intimate partners, as well as how to react in an appropriate way to a relationship ending or not going according to plan.

Motivational Interviewing (MI) can also be used for an individual who is currently suffering from love addiction by helping them identify toxic traits and behaviors that they wish to change. For example, features of MI such as establishing a collaborative, trusting therapeutic relationship, rolling with resistance, and use of reflective listening, may help a "codependence junkie" to see how their behavior of obsessively analyzing relationships may cause them unnecessary anxiety and depression, an outcome that they may want to change. If love-addicted individuals are able to consider what a healthy, nonaddictive love relationship entails, they may be further inclined to pursue a more moderate approach to their partners and relationships.

Use of Medication

Several neurochemicals may also serve as antidotes to some of the symptoms of romantic rejection, including prolactin agonists, norepinephrine agonists, and oxytocin agonists (see Panksepp et al., 2002). Oxytocin, for example, helps to regulate social interaction and plays a role in attachment and bonding. In a study with prairie voles, a monogamous species, an oxytocin antagonist caused them to lose preference for their partner and lose interest in securing an attachment once mating was complete (Liu & Wang, 2003). As humans exhibit a similar neural system for oxytocin, antagonists for this neurochemical may be of use in treating love addiction.

Currently, however, various serotonin-enhancing antidepressant medications are most widely used to counteract depression and love addiction. These medications help to relieve physical and psychic pain and obsession. But many of these serotonin-elevating medications have adverse sexual side effects (Fisher & Thomson, 2007) as well as produce "emotional blunting" and apathy (Frohlich & Meston, 2000; Rosenthal, 2002). These side effects may be worth enduring if the lover is highly dysfunctional. But as rejected lovers begin to heal, they need an active emotion system to accurately assess potential new mates, select an appropriate new partner and build a stable new relationship (Fisher, 2004; Fisher & Thomson, 2007). Thus, data from neuroscience suggest that antidepressant and OCD medications, particularly selective serotonin reuptake inhibitors (SSRIs) that blunt the emotions, should be used only short term, unless the individual needs these drugs long term for other medical reasons.

Earp et al. (2013) have proposed four conditions for the ethical use of any biotechnology to alleviate love addiction: (1) the love in question must be *clearly* so harmful that it must be dissolved; (2) the person must *want* to use the biomedical technology; (3) the technology must help the person follow his/her higher-level goals and commitments instead of just help their emotional state (e.g., combining use of medication with cognitive therapy); (4) and other forms of treatment have not been or are not likely to be effective for overcoming the love addiction. Nevertheless, as is commonly practiced today, a combination of talking therapy and short-term appropriate antidepressant medication may be the most effective treatment for love addiction, especially a love addiction in which the individual has been rejected.

Is Falling in Love with Someone New a Solution?

Falling in love with someone new may alleviate some of the negative behaviors of a prior love addiction situation. However, a new romantic relationship may just replace the previous addiction, initiating new pain and craving, and triggering more inappropriate and negative addictive behaviors. Thus, an individual who has just gotten out of a relationship in which either they or their partner was a love addict, may want to take some time and work on their issues with a therapist before diving into a new relationship too quickly. By engaging in novel and/or interesting activities, the addicted lover is likely to expand their sense of self, and acquire new and pleasurable rewards (Aron & Aron, 1986; Aron, Paris & Aron, 1995; Aron et al., 2000; Mattingly et al., 2012). This is a time when the individual can begin to recognize their pattern of addictive behavior, and work on reshaping their attitudes and beliefs before starting a new relationship. Entering a new love relationship can reflect the positive consequences of the therapeutic process; that is, if the new relationship is healthy. A quick gage to assess a healthy relationship is whether or not that relationship helps to bring out individual strengths and improvement in both partners.

Conclusions

Nature's primordial mechanism to heal a negative love addiction is likely to be time. Time heals. Fisher and colleagues (2010, 2016) found that as more weeks went by since an initial relationship breakup, there was decreased activity in the ventral pallidum, a brain region linked to attachment. The brain is built to heal itself – most likely so that men and women can resume their search for an appropriate breeding and parenting partner. So as disappointed lovers remove the stimuli that fan their ardor, follow some precepts of a twelve-step program, build new daily habits, meet new people, take up new interests, find the right medication and/or therapist, and wait out the long days and nights of intrusive/obsessive thinking and craving, their addiction may eventually subside.

Although we are aware of the ongoing debate regarding boundaries when defining behavioral additions, keeping in mind the risk of pathologizing common behaviors (Kardefelt-Winther et al., 2017), we nevertheless make the case that individuals in the early stage of intense romantic love exhibit many symptoms of addiction, including euphoria (intoxication), craving, loss of control, intrusive/obsessive thinking, distortion of reality, and relapse. Functional magnetic resonance imaging (fMRI) studies indicate that romantic love engages a constellation of dynamic brain systems associated with craving, reward, and motivation mediated by dopamine activity; and dopamine pathways are implicated in seemingly all substance addictions and behavioral addictions for which there is neural evidence (Nutt et al., 2015).

Sussman (2010) reports that a behavioral addiction, such as romantic love, is best defined as an *obsession* that does not require ingestion of any type of chemical, and is associated with certain activities or behaviors that produce natural rewards in the brain but also drive an individual to engage in inappropriate, unhealthy, and dangerous behaviors. We concur, proposing that a romantic love obsession only becomes love addiction when the lover's ideations and behaviors become extreme and harmful. This often includes inappropriate jealousy, misplaced attention-seeking behaviors, excessive mate-guarding, stalking and/or other unfitting, untimely, dangerous and inacceptable activities that impair the lover's ability to participate in ordinary daily activities, threaten their mental and physical health and that of others, and jeopardize their ability to build healthy relationships (Earp et al., 2017).

These above expressions of love addiction may vary according to one's attachment style, the roles one adopts when in a partnership, and the four primary biologically based temperament dimensions, each of which may play a role in specific forms of love addiction. Currently, love addiction is not classified in the DSM-5 as a disorder; nor do many clinicians and those in the legal and medical fields regard love as a possibly evolving into an addiction. Regardless, in its extreme, inappropriate, unhealthy, and dangerous form, love addiction could benefit from preventive and treatment measures. Education programs in schools, homes, and communities may help to offset the development of unhealthy relationship behaviors that could lead to love addiction. Moreover, treatment for love addiction could include: attendance in a twelve-step program (preferably Sex and Love Addicts Anonymous); group and/or individual therapy; short-term neurochemical therapy using one or more antidepressant medications; a combination of talking therapy *with* short-term neurochemical medication; and/or natural therapies such as exercise, meditation, and regularly doing novel things with friends and relatives.

People do suffer at one time or another from problems associated with romantic love, sometimes involving realistic suffering. It is imperative to distinguish love addiction from healthy love and reduce the prevalence of love addiction. The sooner the medical and legal communities appreciate the negative impact of this behavior addiction, the sooner humanity will enjoy one of life's greatest prizes – a healthy, happy, and productive partnership.

REFERENCES

Ahmadi, V., Davoudi, I., Ghazaei, M. & Mardani, M. (2013). Prevalence of obsessive love and its association with attachment styles. *Procedia-Social and Behavioral Sciences*, **84**, 696–700.

Aron, A. & Aron, E. (1986). *Love and the Expansion of Self: Understanding Attraction and Satisfaction*. New York, NY: Hemisphere.

Aron, A., Paris, M. & Aron, E. N. (1995). Falling in love: Prospective studies of self-concept change. *Journal of Personality and Social Psychology*, **69**, 1102–1112.

Aron, A., Norman, C. C., Aron, E. N., McKenna, C. & Heyman, R. (2000). Couples shared participation in novel and arousing activities and experienced relationship quality. *Journal of Personality and Social Psychology*, **78**, 273–283.

Bartels, A. & Zeki, S. (2004). The neural correlates of maternal and romantic love. *Neuroimage*, **21**, 1155–1166.

Baumeister, R. F. & Dhavale, D. A. W. N. (2001). Two sides of romantic rejection. *Interpersonal Rejection*, 55–71.

Baumeister, R. F., Wotman, S. R. & Stillwell, A. M. (1993). Unrequited love: On heartbreak, anger, guilt, scriptlessness, and humiliation. *Journal of Personality and Social Psychology*, **64**, 377.

Brown, L. L., Acevedo, B. & Fisher, H. E. (2013). Neural correlates of four broad temperament dimensions: Testing predictions for a novel construct of personality. *PLoS ONE*, **8**, e78734.

Burkett, J. P. & Young, L. J. (2012). The behavioral, anatomical and pharmacological parallels between social attachment, love and addiction. *Psychopharmacology*, **224**, 1–26.

Buss, D. M. & Schmitt, D. P. (1993). Sexual strategies theory: An evolutionary perspective on human mating. *Psychological Review*, **100**, 204.

Christie, N. & Bechara, A. (2020). Neurobiology of substance addictions. In S. Sussman (Ed.), *The Cambridge Handbook of Substance and Behavioral Addictions*. Cambridge, UK: Cambridge University Press, pp. 121–136.

Compson, J. (2014). Meditation, trauma and suffering in silence: Raising questions about how meditation is taught and practiced in Western contexts in the light of a contemporary trauma resiliency model. *Contemporary Buddhism*, **15**, 274–297.

Costa, S., Barberis, N., Griffiths, M. D., Benedetto, L. & Ingrassia, M. (2019). The love addiction inventory: Preliminary findings of the development process and psychometric characteristics. *International Journal of Mental Health and Addiction*, 1–18.

Davidson, R. J. & Begley, S. (2012). *The Emotional Life of Your Brain: How its Unique Patterns Affect the Way You Think, Feel, and Live – and How You Can Change Them*. Penguin.

Di Chiara, G., Bassareo, V., Fenu, S., et al. (2004). Dopamine and drug addiction: The nucleus accumbens shell connection. *Neuropharmacology*, **47**, 227–241.

Dietrich, A. & McDaniel, W. F. (2004). Endocannabinoids and exercise. *British Journal of Sports Medicine*, **38**, 536–541.

Earp, B. D., Wudarczyk, O. A., Sandberg, A. & Savulescu, J. (2013). If I could just stop loving you: Anti-love biotechnology and the ethics of a chemical breakup. *The American Journal of Bioethics*, **13**, 3–17.

Earp, B. D., Wudarczyk, O. A., Foddy, B. & Savulescu, J. (2017). Addicted to love: What is love addiction and when should it be treated? *Philosophy, Psychiatry, & Psychology*, 24(1), 77–92.

Federal Bureau of Investigation [FBI] (2011). *Uniform crime reports, expanded homicide data table 10*. Accessed at: www.fbi.gov/about-us/cjis/ucr/crime-in-the-u.s/2011/crime-in-the-u.s.-2011/tables/expanded-homicide-data-table-10.

Feeney, J. A. & Noller, P. (1990). Attachment style as a predictor of adult romantic relationships. *Journal of Personality and Social Psychology*, **58**, 281.

Fisher, H. E. (1989). Evolution of human serial pair-bonding. *American Journal of Physical Anthropology*, **78**, 331–354.

Fisher, H. E. (1992). *Anatomy of Love: The Natural History of Monogamy, Adultery, and Divorce*. New York: W. W. Norton & Company Incorporated.

Fisher, H. E. (1998). Lust, attraction, and attachment in mammalian reproduction. *Human Nature*, **9**, 23–52.

Fisher, H. E. (2000). Lust, attraction, attachment: Biology and evolution of the three primary emotion systems for mating, reproduction, and parenting. *Journal of Sex Education and Therapy*, **25**, 96–104.

Fisher, H. E. (2004). *Why We Love: The Nature and Chemistry of Romantic Love*. New York, NY: Henry Holt.

Fisher, H. E. (2011). Serial monogamy and clandestine adultery: Evolution and consequences of the dual human reproductive strategy. In S. C. Roberts (Ed.) *Applied Evolutionary Psychology*. New York, NY: Oxford University Press, pp. 96–111.

Fisher, H. E. (2016). *Anatomy of Love* (2nd edition). New York: W. W. Norton.

Fisher, H. E. & Thomson Jr., J. A. (2007). Lust, romance, attachment: Do the side effects of serotonin-enhancing antidepressants jeopardize romantic love, marriage, and fertility? *Evolutionary Cognitive Neuroscience*, 245–283.

Fisher, H., Aron, A., Mashek, D., et al. (2003). Early stage intense romantic love activates cortical-basal-ganglia reward/motivation, emotion and attention systems: An fMRI study of a dynamic network that varies with relationship length, passion intensity and gender. *Poster presented at the Annual Meeting of the Society for Neuroscience*, New Orleans.

Fisher, H., Aron, A. & Brown, L. L. (2005). Romantic love: An fMRI study of a neural mechanism for mate choice. *Journal of Comparative Neurology*, **493**, 58–62.

Fisher, H. E., Aron, A. & Brown, L. L. (2006). Romantic love: A mammalian brain system for mate choice. *Philosophical Transactions of the Royal Society B: Biological Sciences*, **361**, 2173–2186.

Fisher, H. E., Brown, L. L., Aron, A., Strong, G. & Mashek, D. (2010). Reward, addiction, and emotion regulation systems associated with rejection in love. *Journal of Neurophysiology*, **104**, 51–60.

Fisher, H. E., Island, H. D., Rich, J. Marchalik, D. & Brown, L. L. (2015). Four broad temperament dimensions: Description, convergent validation correlations, and comparison with the Big Five. *Frontiers in Psychology: Personality and Social Psychology*, **6**, 1098.

Fisher, H. E., Xu, X., Aron, A. & Brown, L. L. (2016). Intense, passionate, romantic love: A natural addiction? How the fields that investigate romance and substance abuse can inform each other. *Frontiers in Psychology*, **7**, 687.

Fletcher, G. J., Simpson, J. A., Campbell, L. & Overall, N. C. (2015). Pair-bonding, romantic love, and evolution: The curious case of Homo sapiens. *Perspectives on Psychological Science*, **10**, 20–36.

Frohlich, P. F. & Meston, C. M. (2000). Evidence that serotonin affects female sexual functioning via peripheral mechanisms. *Physiology & Behavior*, **71**, 383–393.

Gingrich, B., Liu, Y., Cascio, C. Z. & Insel, T. R. (2000). Dopamine D2 receptors in the nucleus accumbens are important for social attachment in female prairie voles (*Microtus ochrogaster*). *Behavioral Neuroscience*, **114**, 173–183.

Goldfarb, A. H. & Jamurtas, A. Z. (1997). Beta-endorphin response to exercise. An update. *Sports Medicine*, **24**, 8–16.

Gould, M., Jamieson, P. & Romer, D. (2003). Media contagion and suicide among the young. *American Behavioral Scientist*, **46**, 1269–1284.

Grant, S., Colaiaco, B., Motala, A., et al. (2017). Mindfulness-based relapse prevention for substance use disorders: A systematic review and meta-analysis. *Journal of Addiction Medicine*, **11**, 386.

Griffiths, M. (2005). A 'components' model of addiction within a biopsychosocial framework. Journal of Substance Use, **10**, 191–197.

Hansen, W. B. (1992). School-based substance abuse prevention: A review of the state of the art in curriculum, 1980–1990. *Health Education Research*, **7**, 403–430.

Hansen, W. B. (1996). Pilot test results comparing the All Stars program with seventh grade DARE: Program integrity and mediating variable analysis. *Substance Use & Misuse*, **31**, 1359–1377.

Hansen, W. B. & McNeal Jr, R. B. (1997). How DARE works: An examination of program effects on mediating variables. *Health Education & Behavior*, **24**, 165–176.

Hatfield, E. & Rapson, R. L. (1996). Stress and passionate love. *Stress and Emotion: Anxiety, Anger, and Curiosity*, **16**, 29–50.

Hazan, C. & Shaver, P. (1987). Romantic love conceptualized as an attachment process. *Journal of Personality and Social Psychology*, **52**, 511–524.

Heijnen, S., Hommel, B., Kibele, A. & Colzato, L. S. (2016). Neuromodulation of aerobic exercise – A review. *Frontiers in Psychology*, **6**, 1890.

Hunter, M. S., Nitschke, C. & Hogan, L. (1981). A scale to measure love addiction. *Psychological Reports*, **48**, 582–582.

Iwaniec, D. & Sneddon, H. (2001). Attachment style in adults who failed to thrive as children: Outcomes of a 20 year follow-up study of factors influencing maintenance or change in attachment style. *British Journal of Social Work*, **31**, 179–195.

Jankowiak, W. R. & Fischer, E. F. (1992). A cross-cultural perspective on romantic love. *Ethnology*, **31**, 149–155.

Kardefelt-Winther, D., Heeren, A., Schimmenti, A., et al. (2017). How can we conceptualize behavioral addiction without pathologizing common behaviors? *Addiction*, **112**, 1709–1715.

Kirsch, P., Reuter, M., Mier, D., et al. (2006). Imaging gene-substance interactions: The effect of the DRD2 TaqIA polymorphism and the dopamine agonist bromocriptine on the brain activation during the anticipation of reward. *Neuroscience Letters*, **405**, 196–201.

Liu, Y. & Wang, Z. X. (2003). Nucleus accumbens oxytocin and dopamine interact to regulate pair bond formation in female prairie voles. *Neuroscience*, **121**, 537–544.

Lopez, F. G. & Gormley, B. (2002). Stability and change in adult attachment style over the first-year college transition: Relations to self-confidence, coping, and distress patterns. *Journal of Counseling Psychology*, **49**, 355.

Lorena, A., Sophia, E. C., Mello, C., Tavares, H. & Ziberman, M. L. (2008). Group therapy for pathological love. *Review of Brasilian Psychiatry (Revista Brasileira de Psiquiatria)*, **30**, 292–293.

Mattingly, B. A., Mcintyre, K. P. & Lewandowski Jr, G. W. (2012). Approach motivation and the expansion of self in close relationships. *Personal Relationships*, **19**, 113–127.

Mearns, J. (1991). Coping with a breakup: Negative mood regulation expectancies and depression following the end of a romantic relationship. *Journal of Personality and Social Psychology*, **60**, 327.

Meloy, J. R., Davis, B. & Lovette, J. (2001). Risk factors for violence among stalkers. *Journal of Threat Assessment*, **1**(1), 3–16.

Nolen-Hoeksema, S., Larson, J. & Grayson, C. (1999). Explaining the gender difference in depressive symptoms. *Journal of Personality and Social Psychology*, **77**, 1061.

Nutt, D. J., Lingford-Hughes, A., Erritzoe, D. & Stokes, P. R. (2015). The dopamine theory of addiction: 40 years of highs and lows. *Nature Reviews Neuroscience*, **16**, 305.

Panksepp, J., Knutson, B. & Burgdorf, J. (2002). The role of brain emotional systems in addictions: A neuro-evolutionary perspective and new 'self-report' animal model. *Addiction*, **97**, 459–469.

Reynaud, M., Karila, L., Blecha, L. & Benyamina, A. (2010). Is love passion an addictive disorder? *The American Journal of Drug and Alcohol Abuse*, **36**, 261–267.

Robinson, D. L., Heien, M. L. & Wightman, R. M. (2002). Frequency of dopamine concentration transients increases in dorsal and ventral striatum of male rats during introduction of conspecifics. *Journal of Neuroscience*, **22**, 10477–10486.

Rosenthal, N. E. (2002). *The Emotional Revolution: How the New Science of Feelings can Transform Your Life.* New York: Citadel Press Books.

Sanches, M. & John, V. P. (2019). Treatment of love addiction: Current status and perspectives. *The European Journal of Psychiatry*, 33(1), 38–44.

Schaeffer, B. (2009). *Is it Love or is it Addiction: The Book that Changed the Way We Think About Romance and Intimacy*. Simon and Schuster.

Shaver, P., Hazan, C. & Bradshaw, D. (1988). Love as attachment: The integration of three behavioral systems. In R. J. Sternberg & M. L. Barnes (Eds.), *The Psychology of Love.* New Haven, CT: Yale University Press, pp. 68–99.

Stanton, S. C., Campbell, L. & Loving, T. J. (2014). Energized by love: Thinking about romantic relationships increases positive affect and blood glucose levels. *Psychophysiology*, **51**, 990–995.

Sussman, S. (2010). Love addiction: Definition, etiology, treatment. *Sexual Addiction & Compulsivity*, **17**, 31–45.

Sussman, S. (2013). A lifespan developmental-stage approach to tobacco and other drug abuse prevention. *ISRN Addiction*, article ID 745783, 19 pages.

Sussman, S. (2017). *Substance and Behavioral Addictions: Concepts, Causes, and Cures.* Cambridge: Cambridge University Press.

Sussman, S. & Pakdaman, S. (2020). Appetitive needs and addiction. In S. Sussman (Ed.), *The Cambridge Handbook of Substance and Behavioral Addictions.* Cambridge, UK: Cambridge University Press, pp. 3–12.

Sussman, S. & Sussman, A. N. (2011). Considering the definition of addiction. *International Journal of Environmental Research and Public Health*, **8**, 4025–4038.

21 Prevention and Treatment of Compulsive Buying Disorder

Artur Galimov, MD, and Donald W. Black, MD

Introduction

Shopping is an activity that is part of daily life and contributes to the world economy; yet, for some, shopping can become excessive and problematic. Purchases may be sudden and unplanned, or associated with excessive or poorly controlled preoccupations and urges that lead to subjective distress or impaired quality of life (Black, 2007a; Black et al., 2012). Problematic shopping behavior, now recognized as *compulsive buying disorder* (CBD), was first described by Bluer and Kraepelin (Bleuler, 1924; Kraepelin, 1915) in the early twentieth century in their respective textbooks. They placed CBD ("oniomania") alongside kleptomania and pyromania, and viewed it as an example of a reactive impulse or impulsive insanity (Bleuler, 1924). Professional interest was limited in subsequent years, except for rare clinical case reports in the psychoanalytic literature (Krueger, 1988; Lawrence, 1990; Winestine, 1985), or reports by researchers interested in consumer behavior (Faber & O'Guinn, 1989, 1992; O'Guinn & Faber, 1989; Scherhorn, Reisch & Raab, 1990; Valence, d'Astous & Fortier, 1988). In the early 1990s, clinical interest was revived after McElroy and colleagues (McElroy et al., 1991) described the improvement in three individuals with compulsive buying disorder who were administered antidepressants, followed by three independent case series involving ninety individuals (Christenson, Faber & Mitchell, 1994; McElroy et al., 1994; Schlosser et al., 1994).

In this chapter, we review compulsive shopping, including its classification, epidemiology, etiology, course, and psychiatric comorbidity. Next, we provide a thorough discussion of assessment, followed by an overview of treatment and prevention strategies. The terms compulsive shopping and compulsive buying disorder will be used interchangeably.

Definition and Classification

McElroy and colleagues proposed an operational definition of CBD for clinical and research use (Table 21.1), suggesting that the disorder has cognitive (i.e., buying preoccupation) and behavioral (i.e., buying impulses) components, that potentially lead to personal distress, social, marital, or occupational dysfunction, and financial or legal problems (McElroy et al., 1994). While the reliability and validity of this definition are not established, these criteria have achieved wide acceptance in the research community (Black, 2007a).

The appropriate classification of CBD has led to ongoing debate. Some researchers have placed it alongside alcohol and drug use disorders (Krych, 1989), while others have linked it to mood disorders (Lejoyeux et al., 1996), or to obsessive-compulsive disorders (OCD) (Hollander, 1993). Some have argued that it is not an independent disorder, but rather overlaps with other psychiatric disorders such as obsessive-compulsive, anxiety, and depressive disorders (Weinstein et al., 2015). CBD is not included in DSM-5 (American Psychiatric Association, 2013), although WHO *International Classification of Diseases*, 11th revision, has classified it as an "other specified impulse control disorder." There was some discussion regarding its inclusion in the addictive disorders as "shopping addiction," but the research base was not considered sufficient to justify its inclusion (American Psychiatric Association, 2013).

Epidemiology

Prevalence

In a meta-analysis, Maraz et al. estimated the pooled prevalence of CBD. They identified forty studies reporting forty-nine different estimates of CBD in the general population among more than 32,000 participants (Maraz, Griffiths & Demetrovics, 2016). The estimated prevalence rate of compulsive buying in the adult representative population (i.e., general population) was 4.9 percent, whereas in an adult nonrepresentative population (i.e., university staff members, internet forum users) it was 12.3 percent. Prevalence rates were also higher in university students and among shopper-specific samples compared to representative ones: 8.3 percent and 16.2 percent respectively.

Prevalence rates vary across different countries but appear to range overall from 2 percent to 8 percent. For instance, Faber and O'Guinn (Faber & O'Guinn, 1989) surveyed 292 subjects in Illinois (United States) and reported the prevalence of compulsive buying disorder to fall between 2 percent and 8 percent. Meanwhile, Koran and colleagues, in a random telephone survey of 2,513 US adults, estimated the point prevalence of compulsive buying disorder at 5.8 percent (Koran et al., 2006). The estimated prevalence rates reported in other countries were 1.85 percent in Hungary (Maraz et al., 2016), 7.1 percent in Spain (Otero-López & Villardefrancos, 2014), 1 percent to 8 percent in Germany (Mueller et al., 2010b; Neuner, Raab & Reisch, 2005), 10.9 percent in Brazil (Leite et al., 2013), and 7.1 percent in Italy (Tommasi & Busonera, 2012).

Age of Onset and Demographic Features

Mean age of onset reported in most of the literature ranges from eighteen to twenty-two years (Christenson et al., 1994; Koran et al., 2003; Miltenberger et al., 2003; Schlosser et al., 1994). An exception, McElroy et al. reported a mean age of onset of thirty years (McElroy et al., 1994). The observed variation may reflect the difference in way the subjects were enrolled into the studies. McElroy and colleagues recruited persons with CBD who had received psychotherapy treatment (McElroy et al., 1994), and perhaps were emancipated from home at older ages, while Christenson et al. enrolled subjects through advertisements (Christenson et al., 1994). According to Black (2007b) age of onset typically coincides

Table 21.1 McElroy et al.'s diagnostic criteria for compulsive buying

Inappropriate preoccupations with buying or shopping, or inappropriate buying or shopping impulses or behavior, as indicated by at least one of the following:
• Frequent preoccupations with buying or impulses to buy that are experienced as irresistible, intrusive, and/or senseless.
• Frequent buying of more than can be afforded, frequent buying of items that are not needed, or shopping for longer periods of time than intended.
• The buying preoccupations, impulses, or behaviors cause marked distress, are time-consuming, significantly interfere with social or occupational functioning, or result in financial problems (e.g., indebtedness or bankruptcy).
• The excessive buying or shopping behavior does not occur exclusively during periods of hypomania or mania

Note: Adapted from McElroy et al. (1994).

with the age at which people first establish credit accounts and with emancipation from home.

Most clinical studies report that women (80 percent to 94 percent) are more likely to become compulsive buyers compared to men (Christenson et al., 1994; McElroy et al., 1994; Miltenberger et al., 2003; Schlosser et al., 1994). However, two general population surveys failed to find significant differences between men and women (Koran et al., 2006; Mueller et al., 2010b). Black concluded that observed gender difference could be artifactual, and suggested that it may be because of the fact that women appear to readily acknowledge that they enjoy shopping, whereas men are more likely to report that they "collect" things (Black, 2007a).

Among other predictors, Black and colleagues showed that lower gross income and having little ability to control or to delay urges to make impulsive purchases are associated with the greater CBD severity. Of course, the presence of a market-based economy, the availability of a wide variety of goods, disposable income, and significant leisure time appear necessary for the development of CBD (Black, 2001). Finally, it was shown that CBD occurs mainly in developed countries. Cultural and social factors have been proposed as either causing, or promoting the disorder (Black, 2001). Elements that appear necessary for the development of compulsive buying disorder include the presence of a market-based economy, the availability of a wide variety of goods, easily abstained credit, disposable income, and significant leisure time (Lee & Mysyk, 2004). For these reasons, Black (2007b) concluded that CBD is unlikely to occur in poorly developed countries, except among the wealthy elite.

Etiology

Neurobiological

Etiology of CBD involves a combination of developmental, neurobiologic, and cultural factors. In some studies, early childhood adversity, such as sexual abuse, have been proposed as causative factors. Nonetheless, no special or unique family constellation or pattern of early life events have been identified in persons with compulsive buying disorder (Black, 2007a).

Knudson et al. examined purchasing decisions in twenty-six healthy consumers using functional Magnetic Resonance Imaging (fMRI) (Knutson et al., 2007). They showed that buying behavior was associated with an increased activity in the nucleus accumbens (as with substance addictions) and the medial prefrontal cortex. It was also hypothesized that the insula might play an important role in the decision-making process, since it was activated prior to the purchasing decision (Christie & Bechara, 2020). In the other study, Raab et al. compared compulsive shoppers (n = 23) with healthy individuals (n = 26) on a multiphase purchasing task by using fMRI (Raab et al., 2011). Women with CBD had greater nucleus accumbens activity during product presentation and lower insula and anterior cingulate cortex (ACC) activation during the presentation of prices than those without CBD. Observed differences could serve as a potential explanation for the fact that compulsive buyers lose control over their buying behavior (Müller, Mitchell & de Zwaan, 2015). Conversely, greater ACC activity has been found to occur with gambling and gaming disorder (Vaccaro & Potenza, 2020). The role of the ACC in loss of control is not yet clear. Possibly, presentation of prices, as an inhibitory signal, might reflect part of a sequence of relatively greater fluctuation in neurobiological activity among through with CBD.

Little is known about pharmacogenetics and neural mechanisms underlying shopping addiction. In a molecular genetics study, Devor et al. failed to find an association between frequencies of two serotonin transporter gene polymorphism and compulsive buying disorder (Devor et al., 1999). In another study, Comings observed an association of the D1 (dopamine) receptor gene with compulsive shopping and pathological gambling (Comings, 1998).

Other neurobiological theories have suggested disturbed neurotransmission as causative, particularly involving the serotonergic, dopaminergic, or opioid systems. A few researchers have noted similarities between CBD and obsessive-compulsive disorder and have used selective serotonin reuptake inhibitors (SSRIs) to treat compulsive buying disorder (Black et al., 2000; Black, Monahan & Gabel, 1997; Koran, 2005; Koran et al., 2003; Ninan et al., 2000). It has been theorized that dopamine plays an important role in "reward dependence," which has been claimed to foster behavioral addictions (CBD and gambling disorder) (Holden, 2001). After two case reports suggesting benefit from the opiate antagonist naltrexone, others have speculated about the role of opiate receptors in CBD development (Grant, 2003; Kim, 1998). Further research in this field is warranted.

Family History

There is some evidence that CBD runs in families. McElroy et al. observed the family history on eighteen individuals with CBD (McElroy et al., 1994). They reported that seventeen had one or more first-degree relatives with a mood disorder, eleven with alcohol or substance abuse, and three with an anxiety disorder. In addition, three individuals had relatives who were also diagnosed with CBD.

In another study, Black et al. used the family history method to assess 137 first-degree relatives of thirty-one individuals diagnosed with CBD (Black et al., 1998). Relatives of individuals with CBD were more likely to experience depression, suffer from alcoholism or drug abuse, and were more likely to have "any" or "more than one" psychiatric disorder compared to relatives of comparison group individuals. In addition, compulsive buying was diagnosed in 9.5 percent of the first-degree relatives of individuals with CBD, but the disorder was not assessed in the comparison group relatives.

Clinical Symptoms

Compulsive buying disorder (CBD) shares similar clinical characteristics with the addictive disorders including obtaining an appetitive effect, preoccupation, craving, loss of control, and negative consequences of shopping (Sussman & Sussman, 2011). Experienced subjective feeling states are similar to alcohol or drug intoxication effects, and many compulsive buyers describe their shopping experiences as inducing "a high," "a buzz," or "a rush." They may describe an increasing level of anxiety that can only be relieved when a purchase is made (McElroy et al., 1994). Koran et al. found that compulsive shoppers experience a depressed affect after shopping (remorse), make senseless and impulsive purchases, experience uncontrollable buying binges, and engage in "problem shopping" more frequently and for longer period of time than other respondents (Koran et al., 2006). Persons with CBD are preoccupied with shopping and spending, and they devote significant time to these behaviors.

Based on his personal observations, Black (Black, 2007a) has identified four phases of compulsive buying disorder: anticipation, preparation, shopping, and spending. In the first phase, the person with compulsive buying disorder develops a preoccupation with either having a specific item or in the act of shopping itself. This leads to the second phase, when the individual prepares for the shopping. During this phase, the compulsive buyer decides on when and where to go, the clothes to wear, and even which credit cards to take. In the third phase, the actual shopping occurs. Many compulsive shoppers describe this event as intensely exciting, while others report experiencing a sexual feeling (Schlosser et al., 1994). Finally, the act is completed with the purchase (i.e., spending), often followed by a sense of letdown, or disappointment with oneself. In the studies by Miltenberger et al. (2003) and Müller et al. (2012), it was shown that negative affect increased prior to shopping episodes and decreased immediately after spending. Anger, anxiety, depression, boredom, and self-critical thoughts were the most commonly cited antecedents to CBD, while euphoria or relief of the negative emotions were the most common immediate consequences while making a purchase, followed by decreasing affect thereafter. Müller et al. concluded that CBD might be less reward driven or positively reinforcing than originally anticipated in previous studies (Müller et al., 2012).

Some persons with CBD describe their behavior as episodic with "free of buying" periods. Typically, one to five hours pass between initially experiencing their urge to buy and the eventual purchase (Schlosser et al., 1994). The buying episodes occur year round, though the symptoms tend to be more severe during key socially accepted or promoted buying periods such as Christmas and other holidays, as well as around the birthdays of family members and friends (Black, 2007a).

In a recent study, Black and colleagues assessed clinical symptoms and self-reported shopping and spending behavior in seventeen people diagnosed with CBD at a five-year follow-up interview (Black, Shaw & Allen, 2016). Fourteen subjects (82 percent) had continued to spend excessively or to report being preoccupied with shopping urges. Eleven subjects (65 percent) attempted to quit their compulsive shopping; however, only three respondents were successful. The median length of abstinence was ten weeks, while feelings of build-up tension to shop, negative feelings (i.e., boredom, sadness, depression, frustration, anger), and desire for positive feelings (i.e., happiness, power, or elation) were the most commonly cited triggers associated with relapse. Nonetheless, subjects showed significant improvement in compulsive shopping symptoms severity and were less impulsive. Thus, the authors concluded that CBD symptoms might gradually diminish over time (Black et al., 2016).

A few studies have identified that clothing, jewelry, make-up, shoes, and collectibles are the most popular items purchased by compulsive shoppers (Duroy, Gorse & Lejoyeux, 2014; McElroy et al., 1994; Schlosser et al., 1994). Black noted that many shoppers report buying an item based on its attractiveness or because it was a bargain (Black, 2007a). Often compulsive buyers report the need to buy clothes from famous designers and top of the line items in order to impress other people, demonstrate social-financial prowess, and match their subjective perceptions of socially desirable appearance (Roberts James & Jones, 2005). The average amount of money spent by subjects per buying episode was $92 in a study by Schlosser et al. (1994), compared with $110 reported in the study by Christenson et al. (1994). (This is equivalent to a $160 value in 2018.) The items purchased by compulsive shoppers tend not to be particularly expensive, but many will buy in quantity so that spending tends to get out of hand. With regards to gender-specific buying patterns, men often times buy larger items such as cars, furniture, computers, hardware goods, and stereo equipment compared to women (Black, 2007a). Women are relatively likely to buy smaller items such as clothes and jewelry. Compulsive shoppers show a range of behavior regarding the items they buy. For instance, Schlosser et al. have reported that many subjects fail to remove the items from the packaging and return them, others give them away or put them to the storage, while others sell them or even throw them out (Schlosser et al., 1994).

Compulsive shopping tends to be a private pleasure; individuals with CBD prefer to shop alone (Schlosser et al., 1994). Today, many prefer to shop online, where they are free from social constraints (Dittmar, Long & Bond, 2007; Dittmar, Long & Meek, 2004). Kukar-Kinney et al. reported that persons with CBD shop online more frequently than the controls subjects (Kukar-Kinney, Ridgway & Monroe, 2009). In fact, Lejoyeux et al. showed that compulsive buyers spend four times more time on the internet than noncompulsive buyers, but only if they have an opportunity to buy (Lejoyeux et al., 2007). Still many prefer to shop at high-end department stores, boutiques or consignment shops, and garage sales. Black suggested that income has a relatively small impact on the presence of compulsive buying disorder (Black, 2007b). For instance, a person with a low income may still fulfill his shopping and spending preoccupation at a consignment shop rather than at a department store. Great wealth does not protect against compulsive buying disorder either, since the presence of compulsive buying disorder may lead to interpersonal problems, even when it does not cause financial problems.

Indeed, like other addictions, CBD is associated with a number of negative consequences, such as substantial debts, legal problems, personal distress, and marital conflict (McElroy, Keck & Phillips, 1995). Koran et al. found that compulsive shoppers are more likely to report an income <$50,000, and are less likely to pay off credit card balances in full compared to other respondents (Koran et al., 2006). Christenson et al. reported that 58.3 percent of compulsive purchases entailed going into debt; meanwhile 41.7 percent of compulsive buyers were unable to pay for the purchased items (Christenson et al., 1994).

Compulsive buying disorder sufferers also experience notable interpersonal problems. For instance, one-third of compulsive buyers suffer negative comments from relatives and friends, 8.3 percent face criminal or legal complications, while 45.8 percent are exposed to feelings of guilt. Subjects generally are willing to admit that CBD is problematic for them. Christenson et al. reported that 92 percent CBD subjects described attempts to resist urges to buy, yet in 74 percent cases these attempts were unsuccessful (Christenson et al., 1994).

Compulsive buying disorder has been examined in terms of severity. Black et al. recruited forty-four subjects with a compulsive buying problem and divided them into quartiles from most to least severe based on the Compulsive Buying Scale (CBS) score (Black et al., 2001). Subjects with greater severity of CBD reported lower gross income, were less likely to have an income above the median, were more likely to spend a higher percentage of income compulsively buying, while spending less on sale items. Subjects with more severe compulsive buying disorder were also more likely to have Axis I or Axis II comorbidity (e.g., major depressive or anxiety disorders, or personality disorders). Thus, Black concluded that the most severe buying disorders are found in psychologically distressed persons with low incomes who have little ability to control or to delay their urges to make inappropriate purchases (Black, 2007b).

Differential Diagnosis

Normal Buying Behavior

Compulsive buying disorder should be distinguished from normal buying behavior. Although the distinctions are sometimes arbitrary, frequent shopping on its own does not constitute evidence in support of a diagnosis of CBD. Normal buying can also sometimes take on a compulsive quality, especially around holidays or birthdays or if individual receives an inheritance or wins a lottery (Black, 2007a). Buying to achieve a high, preoccupation with buying, loss of control of buying behavior, and negative consequences defines CBD as an addiction (Sussman & Sussman, 2011).

Collectors

Even though collectors also spend a lot of time and money in their hunt for desired goods, their attitudes toward the purchases is different than in persons with CBD (Belk, 1999). Collectors focus on the item itself, which they often show to others with considerable pride. On the other hand, compulsive buyers focus on the buying process and often are disappointed with a purchase. Many subjects fail to remove the items from the packaging and return them; others give them away or put them into storage (Schlosser et al., 1994).

Buying During Manic Episodes

Bipolar disorder can also cause excessive shopping and spending. This behavior is driven by euphoric mood, grandiosity, and unrealistic plans. This behavior is only present during manic episodes and disappears when the emotional state becomes normal. The pattern of shopping and spending in the person with compulsive buying disorder lacks the periodicity seen in bipolar patients (Kuzma & Black, 2006).

Buying Related to Psychosis

Excessive buying can also be observed in patients diagnosed with schizophrenia. The buying behavior observed in these patients is discordant or bizarre and may reflect delusional thinking. For instance, they may buy high-tech electronics to contact aliens from another planet. Excessive shopping of the typical compulsive buyer is not associated with delusions (Christenson et al., 1994).

Psychiatric Comorbidity

Mood Disorders, OCD, and Personality Disorders

Compulsive buying disorder is usually associated with comorbid psychiatric disorders. In a study of persons suffering from CBD, it was shown that nearly 90 percent of the total sample (n = 170) had at least one Axis I disorder in their lifetime, while 51 percent met criteria for a current Axis I disorder (Mueller et al., 2010a). The most prevalent were mood disorders (70.3 percent) and anxiety disorders (57.3 percent); followed by substance dependence (20.5 percent), impulse control (20.5 percent), and eating disorders (19.9 percent). It was also shown that more severe or frequent occurrences of psychiatric comorbidity (especially with mood and anxiety disorders) was associated with more severe compulsive buying problems.

Muller et al. reported that *major depressive disorder (MDD)* was the most common (62.6 percent) mood disorder associated with CBD (Mueller et al., 2010a). This finding is in line with an earlier study by McElroy et al., who found that nineteen out of twenty patients with CBD met DSM-III-R criteria for lifetime diagnosis of a MDD (McElroy et al., 1994). They also reported that the onset of mood disorder preceded the onset of compulsive buying by at least one year in fourteen patients. In the other study, Black et al. compared twenty-six compulsive buyers with controls. CBD subjects had higher prevalence of lifetime mood (62 percent versus 5 percent), anxiety (50 percent versus 9 percent), and impulse control (69 percent versus 6 percent) disorders compared to controls (Black et al., 2012). They also had higher prevalence of trait impulsivity (46 percent versus 16 percent) and ADHD symptoms (65 percent versus 34 percent) than controls.

Compulsive buying was also found to be prevalent in patients with *obsessive-compulsive disorder (OCD)*, particularly among compulsive hoarders (Torres et al., 2012). Compulsive hoarders are those persons that acquire, and failure to discard, possessions that are of limited use or value (Frost et al., 1998). Muller et al. reported 18.7 percent lifetime prevalence of OCD in CBD patients (Mueller et al., 2010a). These results are comparable with those reported by Lejoyeux et al., who reported 23 percent prevalence of OCD in compulsive shoppers (Lejoyeux et al., 2005). Weinstein et al. have examined compulsive buying, state and trait anxiety, and general obsessive-compulsive measures among 120 habitual internet shoppers (Weinstein et al., 2015). The results of this study showed a positive association between Edward's compulsive buying scale measures (Edwards, 1993) and Spielberger's trait anxiety measures (Spielberger et al., 1983). In addition, they also found an association between Spielberger trait anxiety measures and the Yale-Brown Obsessive-Compulsive Scale (Goodman et al., 1989), which supports the connection between compulsive buying and OCD. Finally, among other anxiety disorders, panic disorder (24.6 percent) and social phobia (28.1 percent) were commonly prevalent among those suffering from CBD (Mueller et al., 2010a).

Several studies have shown an association of CBD with *personality disorders*. Schlosser et al. reported that 60 percent of subjects with CBD met criteria for at least one personality disorder (Schlosser et al., 1994). Even though there was no special "shopping" personality, the most commonly identified personality disorders were the obsessive-compulsive (22 percent), avoidant (15 percent), and borderline (15 percent) types. In another report, four patients with CBD were described by psychoanalyst Krueger (1988). He demonstrated that these patients carried the aspects of narcissistic character pathology.

Substance Use Disorders

Black et al. showed that the relatives of compulsive shoppers had higher prevalence of *alcohol dependence* (20 percent) than relatives of control subjects (Black et al., 1998). Sansone et al. reported a significant association between CBD and self-reported alcohol and drug problems in consecutive female patients who were examined at an obstetrics/gynecology outpatient clinic (Sansone et al., 2012). Lejoyeux et al. observed that 45.6 percent of women with *nicotine* dependence had CBD (Lejoyeux et al., 2006). Muller et al. reported 14 percent lifetime prevalence of alcohol dependence in subjects with CBD (Mueller et al., 2010a).

Compulsive buying disorder often cooccurs with *eating disorders*. Black et al. reported that 17.6 percent of subjects with eating disorders were diagnosed with CBD, conversely 20 percent of compulsive buyers suffered from eating disorders (Black et al., 1998). Muller et al. showed that 14.0 percent of compulsive buyers experienced binge-eating disorder (a proxy for food addiction) in their lifetime, whereas only 3.7 percent and 2.3 percent of subjects reported bulimia and anorexia nervosa, respectively (Mueller et al., 2010a). Another study by Fernadez-Aranda et al. found that CBD commonly developed before the onset of eating disorders (Fernández-Aranda et al., 2006).

Behavioral Addictions

With regard to other behavioral addictions, a few studies indicate an overlap between CBD and *pathological internet use* (Mazhari, 2012), *exercise* dependence (Lejoyeux et al., 2008), and pathological *gambling* (PG) (Grant & Kim, 2003). In a recent study, Black et al. reported that 17 percent of probands with pathological gambling were diagnosed with CBD (Black et al., 2015). They also observed a strong familial association between pathological gambling and CBD and concluded that the latter falls within a PG spectrum of disorders.

Assessment

Several instruments have been developed to identify CBD or to rate its severity (Black, 2007a; Müller et al., 2015). The *Compulsive Buying Scale (CBS)* is a widely used seven-item screening instrument. Developed by Faber and O'Guinn, the scale is a reliable and valid measure of CBD severity, including of symptoms such as lack of impulse control, irrational use of credit cards, and use of shopping and buying to feel better (Faber & O'Guinn, 1992).

Monahan et al. modified the Yale-Brown Obsessive-Compulsive Scale (Y-BOCS) (Goodman et al., 1989) to create the ten-item *Yale-Brown Obsessive-Compulsive Scale - Shopping Version (Y-BOCS-SV)* (Monahan, Black & Gabel, 1996). The Y-BOCS-SV explores thoughts and behaviors associated with buying episodes, resistance to them, interference in other daily tasks due to preoccupation with buying, and the degree of control over the shopping and buying cognitions and behaviors (Müller et al., 2015). This scale has shown good inter-rater reliability and is recommended in assessing the severity and clinical change of CBD.

Lejoyeux et al. developed the *Questionnaire about Buying Behavior (QABB)* (Lejoyeux et al., 1997), which is based on the criteria of McElroy and colleagues (McElroy et al., 1994). This measurement consists of nineteen yes-no items, and measures the basic features of compulsive buying, for instance: the frequency of purchases, urges to shop and buy, the impact of the buying behavior in the individual's social life, and postpurchase guilt.

Christenson et al. developed the *Minnesota Impulsive Disorders Interview (MIDI)* (Christenson et al., 1994). This thirty-six-item semistructured interview is aimed to explore CBD among other impulse controls disorders, such as kleptomania, trichotillomania, intermittent explosive disorder, compulsive sexual behavior, pathological gambling, and compulsive exercise. This instrument showed 100 percent sensitivity, and 96.2 percent specificity when it was compared with McElroy and colleagues' criteria (McElroy et al., 1994).

Other clinical instruments include the *Canadian Compulsive Buying Measurement Scale* (Valence et al., 1988), the *Edwards Compulsive Buying Scale* (Edwards, 1993), and the *Ridgway's Compulsive Buying Scale* (Ridgway, Kukar-Kinney & Monroe, 2008). Self-reported ratings and semistructured interviews cannot replace clinical evaluation. CBD should be assessed using a detailed clinical interview to tap a person's attitudes and feelings toward shopping and spending, interference with social, financial, and occupational functioning, and the extent of preoccupation with buying and shopping, as well as account for the influence of other disorders on CBD. A history of physical illness, surgical procedures, drug allergies, or medical treatment is also important to note, because it may help rule out medical explanations as a cause of the compulsive buying disorder (e.g., neurological disorders, brain tumors) (Black, 2007b; Lejoyeux & Weinstein, 2010; Müller et al., 2015).

Treatment

There are no standard treatments for CBD. Because of relatively small sample sizes and their inconsistent results it is hard to establish recommendations based on published clinical trials. Nevertheless, some studies show that psychopharmacological or psychotherapeutic interventions may be beneficial (Aboujaoude, 2014; Black, 2007b; Lejoyeux & Weinstein, 2010). Psychiatric comorbidity itself may help guide pharmacotherapy.

Psychotherapy

Cognitive-behavioral therapy (CBT) is an evidence-based treatment for CBD. The therapy is aimed at interrupting and controlling the problematic buying behavior, establishing healthy purchasing patterns, as well as developing healthy coping, stress-management, and problem-solving skills. CBT is provided both as an individual therapy regimen and as a guiding aspect of group therapy. A recent systematic review, with a retained sample of twenty-nine articles that evaluated quality and effectiveness of CBD treatments ($n = 17$, psychotherapy; $n = 12$, pharmacotherapy), suggested that CBT therapy was efficacious although only five of the studies were of high methodological quality (Hague, Hall & Kellett, 2016). The authors of this review concluded that long-term treatment was associated with improved outcome with pharmacotherapy, but not for psychotherapy and that group psychotherapy (generally involving CBT) appeared the most promising option for CBD.

In an early study, Mitchell et al. assigned twenty-eight subjects to a CBT group that received twelve 1.5-hour intervention sessions over ten weeks, while eleven subjects were assigned to a waitlist control group (Mitchell et al., 2006). The authors reported that 57 percent of twenty-one CBT group patients that completed the study showed significant improvement in the number of compulsive buying episodes and time spent buying, and reduction in CBS and Y-BOCS-SV scores was observed, while there was no effect in the waitlist group. (Certainly, though, an intent-to-treat analysis would conservatively indicate less-successful results.) In another study, Mueller et al. assigned thirty-one subjects to a twelve-week CBT session, and twenty-nine were in the waitlist control group (Mueller et al., 2008). The results were comparable to those of Mitchell and colleagues. In both studies, outcome measures remained improved at the six-month follow-up point.

More recently, Müeller et al. randomly assigned fifty-six subjects to one of the three treatment conditions: CBT group (twelve sessions), telephone-guided self-help (a self-help book, complemented with five twenty-minute telephone sessions), or a waitlist control (Müller et al., 2013). Subjects assigned to the treatment groups improved more than subjects in the waitlist group. Patients receiving CBT reported better outcomes (CBS scores) than the less intensive telephone-guided self-help approach. Improvement in CBS scores was maintained at the six-month follow-up period in both treatment groups.

Finally, Benson et al. evaluated the efficacy of the group treatment "Stopping Overshopping" model (includes aspects of CBT and dialectical behavior therapy, psychodynamic psychotherapy, psychoeducation, motivational interviewing, acceptance and commitment therapy, and mindfulness) by comparing this model ($n = 12$) with a waiting-list control group, which received the treatment after a twelve-week waiting period (Benson et al., 2014). Subjects receiving "overshopping" treatment showed a significant drop in the reported severity and frequency of compulsive buying symptoms and behavior, which were well maintained at six-month follow-up.

Pharmacotherapy

Medication studies have produced equivocal results. Early studies suggested that SSRIs had great promise in treating CBD due to its presumed connection with obsessive-compulsive disorders. For example, Black et al. conducted a nine-week open-label trial (Black et al., 1997). They observed that nine of ten nondepressed subjects with CBD showed benefit after treatment with fluvoxamine. In another seven-week open label trial, Koran et al. reported significant improvement in seventeen of twenty-four subjects who received citalopram (Koran et al., 2002). At six-month follow-up, those subjects who continued to use the medication were less likely to experience a relapse compared to those who discontinued.

Two subsequent randomized controlled trials showed inconsistent results. In the first, Black et al. randomized twelve subjects with CBD to receive fluvoxamine and eleven to receive a placebo (Black et al., 2000). Subjects in both groups showed improvement as early as the second week of the nine-week study, yet the response rate in the placebo group (64 percent) was higher than in the fluvoxamine group (50 percent). In the second study, Ninan et al. randomized twenty compulsive buyers to fluvoxamine and seventeen to a placebo (Ninan et al., 2000). Similarly, the intent-to-treat analysis at the end of the twelve-week trial failed to detect differences between groups.

Despite the fact that citalopram and escitalopram share the same active compound, discontinuation studies (active to placebo switch protocols) show very different results. For instance, in an open-label trial, twenty-four subjects received citalopram for seven weeks (Koran et al., 2003). Subjects who responded to treatment (fifteen subjects) were enrolled in a nine-week randomized, placebo-controlled trial. At the end of the double-blind period, five of eight placebo-assigned subjects (62.5 percent) relapsed, compared with none of seven in the citalopram group. A nearly identical study of twenty-six subjects with CBD that employed escitalopram, failed to show any drug-placebo difference (Koran et al., 2007).

Another consideration pertains to the mu-receptor antagonist, naltrexone. Based on case reports, Kim and Grant suggested that naltrexone may be effective and well tolerated (Grant, 2003; Kim, 1998), yet there are no carefully conducted trials. Similarly, use of the glutamate antagonist memantine has produced encouraging results in the treatment of OCD. Results of a smaller preliminary open-label trial with memantine showed significant reduction in the frequency of compulsive buying behaviors in eight of nine subjects (Grant et al., 2012).

Other Treatment Approaches

Other approaches may be beneficial. *Self-help* books can be helpful (Arenson, 1991; Catalano & Sonenberg, 1993; Wesson, 1990), as can *Debtors Anonymous*, modeled on Alcoholics Anonymous (Andrews, 2000). *Financial counseling*, (Benson, 2000), couples or *family* counseling (Mellan & Benson, 2000), and *Motivational Interviewing* are other approaches that could help (Donahue, Odlaug & Grant, 2011). Additional research studies are needed to evaluate their effectiveness.

Prevention

Several strategies mentioned below could be helpful in preventing CBD (Sussman, 2017). First, some compulsive shoppers may not be aware that their behavior is abnormal, which makes it critical to educate those whose shopping or spending is uncontrolled. *Knowledge* is power, and some individuals may only need to know about CBD to better self-monitor their shopping and spending behavior.

Given that CBD is associated with mood and anxiety disorders that appear to promote shopping and spending behavior, some individuals may benefit by learning new *coping skills*, an essential element of CBT. Coping may exert a proactive effect on compulsive buyer's life circumstances, or may serve a reactive function (e.g., buffering stressful events). For example, rather than going to a shopping mall to cope with painful affects, they might instead go to a gym.

The media tend to glamorize and, hence, encourage shopping. This may negatively affect individuals with CBD, for whom an advertisement is a trigger. Thus, instruction in *media literacy* (i.e., making individuals aware of advertising influences) – which has shown great potential in tobacco-prevention research – could be beneficial to those with CBD

(Sussman et al., 1995). People could learn to ignore advertisements, or at least encourage advertisers to create ads that promote the opposite message (i.e., uncontrolled shopping might cause serious problems in your life).

Parental *modeling* of appropriate buying behavior could be helpful in preventing CBD. Alternatively, parents could learn to avoid rewarding their children with "things" which might potentially facilitate uncontrolled materialism as a goal. If one's compulsive shopping behavior is established and known, friends or relatives could accompany the shopper to help curb that person's buying behavior, as a means of indicated prevention. While it is unclear that store employees could be trained to spot compulsive shoppers, providing flyers with antishopping messages and placing posters in stores with the *warning signs* of CBD could also be helpful.

Finally, public *policy* initiatives could help. For instance, more rigorous oversight of consumer credit agencies could be helpful in limiting predatory practices, because credit cards are known to fuel compulsive spending. Encouraging public health campaigns that promote awareness about compulsive shopping, as well as offering financial literacy and other courses at schools or colleges that focus on teaching students about media influences and predatory marketing could also help.

Conclusions

Compulsive buying disorder (CBD) is relatively common and can be highly problematic to those affected by the disorder. CBD shares similar clinical characteristics with classical addictive disorders including compulsive preoccupation, craving, loss of control, and negative consequences of shopping. For some, CBD is associated with relief of depressed mood, rather than enhanced pleasure or positive reinforcement. CBD is also associated with excessive or poorly controlled preoccupations, urges that lead to subjective distress, and result eventually in impaired quality of life. Compulsive shoppers often are disappointed with the purchase they made and fail to remove the items from the packaging, try to return the items, or give them away.

The classification of compulsive buying disorder remains elusive. Some researchers suggest that it should be grouped with behavioral addictions, while others have linked it to mood and to obsessive-compulsive disorders. Little is known about the neurobiological and genetic mechanisms underlying CBD, nor is there standard treatment. Cognitive-behavioral therapy is promising, while medication studies have been disappointing. Future research on CBD should target etiologic mechanisms and both psychological and pharmacological treatments.

REFERENCES

Aboujaoude, E. (2014). Compulsive buying disorder: A review and update. *Current Pharmaceutical Design*, **20**(25), 4021–4025. doi:10.2174/13816128113199990618

American Psychiatric Association (2013). *Diagnostic and Statistical Manual of Mental Disorders (DSM-5®)*. Arlington, VA: American Psychiatric Publishing.

Andrews, C. (2000). Simplicity circles and the compulsive shopper. In A. L. Benson (Ed.), *I Shop, Therefore I Am – Compulsive Buying and the Search for Self.* New York: Jason Aronson, pp. 484–496.

Arenson, G. (1991). *Born to Spend: How to Overcome Compulsive Spending.* Human Services Institute.

Belk, R. W. (1999). Leaping luxuries and transitional consumers. In R. Batra (Ed.), *Marketing Issues in Transitional Economies.* Boston, MA: Springer US, pp. 39–54.

Benson, A. L. (Ed.) (2000). *I Shop, Therefore I Am – Compulsive Buying and the Search for Self.* New York: Aronson.

Benson, A. L., Eisenach, D., Abrams, L. & van Stolk-Cooke, K. (2014). Stopping Overshopping: A preliminary randomized controlled trial of group therapy for compulsive buying disorder. *Journal of Groups in Addiction & Recovery*, **9**(2), 97–125. doi:10.1080/1556035X.2014.868725

Black, D. W. (2001). Compulsive buying disorder. *CNS Drugs*, **15**(1), 17–27. doi:10.2165/00023210-200115010-00003

Black, D. W. (2007a). Compulsive buying disorder: A review of the evidence. *CNS Spectrums*, **12**(2), 124–132. doi:10.1017/S1092852900020630

Black, D. W. (2007b). A review of compulsive buying disorder. *World Psychiatry*, **6**(1), 14–18.

Black, D. W., Coryell, W., Crowe, R., et al. (2015). The relationship of DSM-IV pathological gambling to compulsive buying and other possible spectrum disorders: Results from the Iowa PG family study. *Psychiatry Research*, **226**(1), 273–276. doi:10.1016/j.psychres.2014.12.061

Black, D. W., Gabel, J., Hansen, J. & Schlosser, S. (2000). A double-blind comparison of fluvoxamine versus placebo in the treatment of compulsive buying disorder. *Annals of Clinical Psychiatry*, **12**(4), 205–211. doi:10.1023/a:1009030425631

Black, D. W., Monahan, P. & Gabel, J. (1997). Fluvoxamine in the treatment of compulsive buying. *Journal of Clinical Psychiatry*, **58**(4), 159–163.

Black, D. W., Monahan, P., Schlosser, S. & Repertinger, S. (2001). Compulsive buying severity: An analysis of Compulsive Buying Scale results in 44 subjects. *The Journal of Nervous and Mental Disease*, **189**(2), 123–126.

Black, D. W., Repertinger, S., Gaffney, G. R. & Gabel, J. (1998). Family history and psychiatric comorbidity in persons with compulsive buying: Preliminary findings. *American Journal of Psychiatry*, **155**(7), 960–963. doi:10.1176/ajp.155.7.960

Black, D. W., Shaw, M. & Allen, J. (2016). Five-year follow-up of people diagnosed with compulsive shopping disorder. *Comprehensive Psychiatry*, **68**, 97–102. doi:10.1016/j.comppsych.2016.03.004

Black, D. W., Shaw, M., McCormick, B., Bayless, J. D. & Allen, J. (2012). Neuropsychological performance, impulsivity, ADHD symptoms, and novelty seeking in compulsive buying disorder. *Psychiatry Research*, **200**(2), 581–587. doi:10.1016/j.psychres.2012.06.003

Bleuler, E. (1924). *Textbook of Psychiatry.* New York: Macmillan.

Catalano, E. M. & Sonenberg, N. (1993). *Consuming Passion: Help for Compulsive Shoppers.* Oakland, CA: New Harbinger Publications.

Christenson, G. A., Faber, R. J. & Mitchell, J. E. (1994). "Compulsive buying: Descriptive characteristics and psychiatric comorbidity": Dr. Christenson and colleagues reply. *The Journal of Clinical Psychiatry*, **55**(12), 545–546.

Christie, N. & Bechara, A. Neurobiology of substance addictions. In S. Sussman (Ed.), The Cambridge Handbook of Substance and Behavioral Addictions. Cambridge, UK: Cambridge University Press, pp. 121–136.

Comings, D. E. (1998). The molecular genetics of pathological gambling. *CNS Spectrums*, **3**(6), 20–37.

Devor, E. J., Magee, H. J., Dill-Devor, R. M., Gabel, J. & Black, D. W. (1999). Serotonin transporter gene (5-HTT) polymorphisms and compulsive buying. *American Journal of Medical Genetics*, **88**(2), 123–125. doi:10.1002/

(SICI)1096-8628(19990416)88:2<123::AID-AJMG5>3.0.CO;2-S

Dittmar, H., Long, K. & Bond, R. (2007). When a better self is only a button click away: Associations between materialistic values, emotional and identity-related buying motives, and compulsive buying tendency online. *Journal of Social and Clinical Psychology*, **26**(3), 334–361. doi:10.1521/jscp.2007.26.3.334

Dittmar, H., Long, K. & Meek, R. (2004). Buying on the internet: Gender differences in on-line and conventional buying motivations. *Sex Roles*, **50**(5), 423–444. doi:10.1023/B:SERS.0000018896.35251.c7

Donahue, C. B., Odlaug, B. L. & Grant, J. E. (2011). Compulsive buying treated with motivational interviewing and imaginal desensitization. *Annals of Clinical Psychiatry*, **23**(3), 226–227.

Duroy, D., Gorse, P. & Lejoyeux, M. (2014). Characteristics of online compulsive buying in Parisian students. *Addictive Behaviors*, **39**(12), 1827–1830. doi:https://doi.org/10.1016/j.addbeh.2014.07.028

Edwards, E. A. (1993). Development of a new scale for measuring compulsive buying behavior. *Financial Counseling and Planning*, **4**(1), 67–84.

Faber, R. J. & O'Guinn, T. C. (1989). *Classifying Compulsive Consumers: Advances in the Development of a Diagnostic Tool.* ACR North American Advances.

Faber, R. J. & O'Guinn, T. C. (1992). A clinical screener for compulsive buying. *Journal of Consumer Research*, **19**(3), 459-469. doi:10.1086/209315

Fernández-Aranda, F., Jiménez-Murcia, S., Álvarez-Moya, E. M., Granero, R., Vallejo, J. & Bulik, C. M. (2006). Impulse control disorders in eating disorders: Clinical and therapeutic implications. *Comprehensive Psychiatry*, **47**(6), 482–488. doi:10.1016/j.comppsych.2006.03.002

Frost, R. O., Kim, H.-J., Morris, C., et al. (1998). Hoarding, compulsive buying and reasons for saving. *Behaviour Research and Therapy*, **36**(7), 657–664. doi:10.1016/S0005-7967(98)00056-4

Goodman, W., Price, L., Rasmussen, S., et al. (1989). Yale-Brown obsessive compulsive scale (Y-BOCS). *Archives of General Psychiatry*, **46**, 1006–1011.

Grant, J. E. (2003). Three cases of compulsive buying treated with naltrexone. *International Journal of Psychiatry in Clinical Practice*, **7**(3), 223–225.

Grant, J. E. & Kim, S. W. (2003). Comorbidity of impulse control disorders in pathological gamblers. *Acta Psychiatrica Scandinavica*, **108**(3), 203–207. doi:10.1034/j.1600-0447.2003.00162.x

Grant, J. E., Odlaug, B. L., Mooney, M., O'Brien, R. & Kim, S. W. (2012). Open-label pilot study of memantine in the treatment of compulsive buying. *Annals of Clinical Psychiatry: Official Journal of the American Academy of Clinical Psychiatrists*, **24**(2), 119–126.

Hague, B., Hall, J. & Kellett, S. (2016). Treatments for compulsive buying: A systematic review of the quality, effectiveness and progression of the outcome evidence. *Journal of Behavioral Addictions*, **5**(3), 379–394. doi:10.1556/2006.5.2016.064

Holden, C. (2001). 'Behavioral' addictions: Do they exist? *Science*, **294**(5544), 980–982. doi:10.1126/science.294.5544.980

Hollander, E. (1993). *Obsessive-Compulsive-Related Disorders.* Arlington, VA: American Psychiatric Publishing.

Kim, S. W. (1998). Opioid antagonists in the treatment of impulse-control disorders. *Journal of Clinical Psychiatry*, **59**(4), 159–164.

Knutson, B., Rick, S., Wimmer, G. E., Prelec, D. & Loewenstein, G. (2007). Neural predictors of purchases. *Neuron*, **53**(1), 147–156. doi:10.1016/j.neuron.2006.11.010

Koran, L. (2005). Escitalopram treatment evaluated in patients with compulsive shopping disorder. *Primary Psychiatry*, **12**(12), 13.

Koran, L. M., Aboujaoude, E. N., Solvason, B., Gamel, N. N. & Smith, E. H. (2007). Escitalopram for compulsive buying disorder: A double-blind discontinuation study. *Journal of Clinical Psychopharmacology*, **27**(2), 225–227. doi:10.1097/01.jcp.0000264975.79367.f4

Koran, L. M., Bullock, K. D., Hartston, H. J., Elliott, M. A. & D'Andrea, V. (2002). Citalopram treatment of compulsive shopping: An open-label study. *Journal of Clinical Psychiatry*, **63**(8), 704–708. doi:10.4088/JCP.v63n0808

Koran, L. M., Chuong, H. W., Bullock, K. D. & Smith, S. C. (2003). Citalopram for compulsive shopping disorder: An open-label study followed by double-blind discontinuation. *Journal of Clinical Psychiatry*, **64**(7), 793–798.

Koran, L. M., Faber, R. J., Aboujaoude, E., Large, M. D. & Serpe, R. T. (2006). Estimated prevalence of compulsive buying behavior in the United States. *American Journal of Psychiatry*, **163**(10), 1806–1812. doi:10.1176/ajp.2006.163.10.1806

Kraepelin, E. (1915). *Psychiatrie; ein Lehrbuch für Studierende und Aerzte.* Leipzig: Barth.

Krueger, D. W. (1988). On compulsive shopping and spending: A psychodynamic inquiry. *American Journal of Psychotherapy*, **42**(4), 574–584. doi:10.1176/appi.psychotherapy.1988.42.4.574

Krych, R. (1989). *Abnormal Consumer Behavior: a Model of Addictive Behaviors.* ACR North American Advances.

Kukar-Kinney, M., Ridgway, N. M. & Monroe, K. B. (2009). The relationship between consumers' tendencies to buy compulsively and their motivations to shop and buy on the internet. *Journal of Retailing*, **85**(3), 298–307. doi:10.1016/j.jretai.2009.05.002

Kuzma, J. M. & Black, D. W. (2006). Compulsive shopping. *Current Psychiatry*, **5**(7), 26.

Lawrence, L. (1990). The psychodynamics of the compulsive female shopper. *The American Journal of Psychoanalysis*, **50**(1), 67–70. doi:10.1007/bf01253458

Lee, S. & Mysyk, A. (2004). The medicalization of compulsive buying. *Social Science & Medicine*, **58**(9), 1709–1718. doi:10.1016/S0277-9536(03)00340-X

Leite, P., Rangé, B., Kukar-Kiney, M., et al. (2013). Cross-cultural adaptation, validation and reliability of the Brazilian version of the Richmond Compulsive Buying Scale. *Revista Brasileira de Psiquiatria*, **35**(1), 38–43.

Lejoyeux, M. & Weinstein, A. (2010). Compulsive buying. *The American Journal of Drug and Alcohol Abuse*, **36**(5), 248–253. doi:10.3109/00952990.2010.493590

Lejoyeux, M., Ades, J., Tassain, V. & Solomon, J. (1996). Phenomenology and psychopathology of uncontrolled buying. *The American Journal of Psychiatry*, **153**(12), 1524.

Lejoyeux, M., Avril, M., Richoux, C., Embouazza, H. & Nivoli, F. (2008). Prevalence of exercise dependence and other behavioral addictions among clients of a Parisian fitness room. *Comprehensive Psychiatry*, **49**(4), 353–358. doi:10.1016/j.comppsych.2007.12.005

Lejoyeux, M., Bailly, F., Moula, H., Loi, S. & Adès, J. (2005). Study of compulsive buying in patients presenting obsessive-compulsive disorder. *Comprehensive Psychiatry*, **46**(2), 105–110. doi:10.1016/j.comppsych.2004.07.027

Lejoyeux, M., Kerner, L., Thauvin, I. & Loi, S. (2006). Study of impulse control disorders among women presenting nicotine dependence. *International Journal of Psychiatry in Clinical Practice*, **10**(4), 241–246. doi:10.1080/13651500600650000

Lejoyeux, M., Mathieu, K., Embouazza, H., Huet, F. & Lequen, V. (2007). Prevalence of compulsive buying among customers of a Parisian general store. *Comprehensive Psychiatry*, **48**(1), 42–46. doi:10.1016/j.comppsych.2006.05.005

Lejoyeux, M., Tassain, V., Solomon, J. & Adès, J. (1997). Study of compulsive buying in depressed patients. *Journal of Clinical Psychiatry*, **58**(4), 169–173. doi:10.4088/JCP.v58n0406

Maraz, A., Griffiths, M. D. & Demetrovics, Z. (2016). The prevalence of compulsive buying: A meta-analysis. *Addiction*, **111**(3), 408–419. doi:10.1111/add.13223

Mazhari, S. (2012). Association between problematic internet use and impulse control disorders among Iranian university students. *Cyberpsychology, Behavior, and Social Networking*, **15**(5), 270–273. doi:10.1089/cyber.2011.0548

McElroy, S. L., Keck, P. E., Jr., Pope, H. G., Jr., Smith, J. M. & Strakowski, S. M. (1994). Compulsive buying: a report of 20 cases. *J ournal of Clinical Psychiatry*, **55**(6), 242–248.

McElroy, S. L., Keck, P. E. & Phillips, K. A. (1995). Kleptomania, compulsive buying, and binge-eating disorder. *Journal of Clinical Psychiatry*, **56** (Supplement 4), 14–26; discussion 27.

McElroy, S. L., Satlin, A., Pope, H. G., Keck, P. E. & Hudson, J. I. (1991). Treatment of compulsive shopping with antidepressants: A report of three cases. *Annals of Clinical Psychiatry*, **3**(3), 199–204. doi:10.3109/10401239109147991

Mellan, O. & Benson, A. L. (2000). Overcoming overspending in couples. In A. L. Benson (Ed.), *I Shop, Therefore I Am – Compulsive Buying and the Search for Self.* New York: Aronson, pp. 341–366.

Miltenberger, R. G., Redlin, J., Crosby, R., et al. (2003). Direct and retrospective assessment of factors contributing to compulsive buying. *Journal of Behavior Therapy and Experimental Psychiatry*, **34**(1), 1–9. doi:10.1016/S0005-7916(03)00002-8

Mitchell, J. E., Burgard, M., Faber, R., Crosby, R. D. & de Zwaan, M. (2006). Cognitive behavioral therapy for compulsive buying disorder. *Behaviour Research and Therapy*, **44**(12), 1859–1865. doi:10.1016/j.brat.2005.12.009

Monahan, P., Black, D. W. & Gabel, J. (1996). Reliability and validity of a scale to measure change in persons with compulsive buying. *Psychiatry Research*, **64**(1), 59–67. doi:10.1016/0165-1781(96)02908-3

Mueller, A., Mitchell, J. E., Black, D. W., et al. (2010a). Latent profile analysis and comorbidity in a sample of individuals with compulsive buying disorder. *Psychiatry Research*, **178**(2), 348–353. doi:10.1016/j.psychres.2010.04.021

Mueller, A., Mitchell, J. E., Crosby, R. D., et al. (2010b). Estimated prevalence of compulsive buying in Germany and its association with sociodemographic characteristics and depressive symptoms. *Psychiatry Research*, **180**(2), 137–142. doi:10.1016/j.psychres.2009.12.001

Mueller, A., Mueller, U., Silbermann, A., et al. (2008). A randomized, controlled trial of group cognitive-behavioral therapy for compulsive buying disorder: Posttreatment and 6-month follow-up results. *Journal of Clinical Psychiatry*, **69**(7), 1131–1138. doi:10.4088/JCP.v69n0713

Müller, A., Arikian, A., Zwaan, M. & Mitchell, J. E. (2013). Cognitive-behavioural group therapy versus guided self-help for compulsive buying disorder: A preliminary study. *Clinical Psychology and Psychotherapy*, **20**(1), 28–35. doi:10.1002/cpp.773

Müller, A., Mitchell, J. E., Crosby, R. D., et al. (2012). Mood states preceding and following compulsive buying episodes: an ecological momentary assessment study. *Psychiatry Research*, **200**(2), 575–580. doi:10.1016/j.psychres.2012.04.015

Müller, A., Mitchell, J. E. & de Zwaan, M. (2015). Compulsive buying. *The American Journal on Addictions*, **24**(2), 132–137. doi:doi:10.1111/ajad.12111

Neuner, M., Raab, G. & Reisch, L. A. (2005). Compulsive buying in maturing consumer societies: An empirical re-inquiry. *Journal of Economic Psychology*, **26**(4), 509–522. doi:10.1016/j.joep.2004.08.002

Ninan, P. T., McElroy, S. L., Kane, C. P., et al. (2000). Placebo-controlled study of fluvoxamine in the treatment of patients with compulsive buying. *Journal of Clinical Psychopharmacology*, **20**(3), 362–366.

O'Guinn, T. C. & Faber, R. J. (1989). Compulsive buying: A phenomenological exploration. *Journal of Consumer Research*, **16**(2), 147–157. doi:10.1086/209204

Otero-López, J. M. & Villardefrancos, E. (2014). Prevalence, sociodemographic factors, psychological distress, and coping strategies related to compulsive buying: a cross sectional study in Galicia, Spain. *BMC Psychiatry*, **14**(1), 101. doi:10.1186/1471-244x-14-101

Raab, G., Elger, C. E., Neuner, M. & Weber, B. (2011). A neurological study of compulsive buying behaviour. *Journal of Consumer Policy*, **34**(4), 401. doi:10.1007/s10603-011-9168-3

Ridgway, N. M., Kukar-Kinney, M. & Monroe, K. B. (2008). An expanded conceptualization and a new measure of compulsive buying. *Journal of Consumer Research*, **35**(4), 622–639. doi:10.1086/591108

Roberts James, A. & Jones, E. L. I. (2005). Money attitudes, credit card use, and compulsive buying among American college students. *Journal of Consumer Affairs*, **35**(2), 213–240. doi:10.1111/j.1745-6606.2001.tb00111.x

Sansone, R. A., Chang, J., Jewell, B. & Sellbom, M. (2012). Compulsive buying: Associations with self-reported alcohol and drug problems. *The American Journal on Addictions*, **21**(2), 178–179. doi:10.1111/j.1521-0391.2011.00211.x

Scherhorn, G., Reisch, L. A. & Raab, G. (1990). Addictive buying in West Germany: An empirical study. *Journal of Consumer Policy*, **13**(4), 355–387. doi:10.1007/bf00412336

Schlosser, S., Black, D. W., Repertinger, S. & Freet, D. (1994). Compulsive buying: Demography, phenomenology, and comorbidity in 46 subjects. *General Hospital Psychiatry*, **16**(3), 205–212.

Spielberger, C. D., Gorsuch, R. L., Lushene, R., Vagg, P. & Jacobs, G. (1983). *Manual for the State-Trait Anxiety Inventory*. Palo Alto, CA: Consulting Psychologists Press.

Sussman, S. (2017). *Substance and Behavioral Addictions: Concepts, Causes, and Cures.* Cambridge: Cambridge University Press.

Sussman, S. & Sussman, A. N. (2011). Considering the definition of addiction. *International Journal of Environmental Research and Public Health*, **8**(10), 4025–4038.

Sussman, S., Dent, C. W., Burton, D., Stacy, A. W. & Flay, B. R. (1995). *Developing School-Based Tobacco Use Prevention and Cessation Programs*. Sage Publications, Inc.

Tommasi, M. & Busonera, A. (2012). Validation of three compulsive buying scales on an Italian sample. *Psychological Reports*, **111**(3), 831–844. doi:10.2466/03.15.20.pr0.111.6.831-844

Torres, A. R., Fontenelle, L. F., Ferrão, Y. A., et al. (2012). Clinical features of obsessive-compulsive disorder with hoarding symptoms: A multicenter study. *Journal of Psychiatric Research*, **46**(6), 724–732. doi:10.1016/j.jpsychires.2012.03.005

Vaccaro, A. G. & Potenza, M. N. (2020). Neurobiological Foundations of Behavioral Addictions. In S. Sussman (Ed.), *The Cambridge Handbook of Substance and Behavioral Addictions*. Cambridge, UK: Cambridge University Press, pp. 136–152.

Valence, G., d'Astous, A. & Fortier, L. (1988). Compulsive buying: Concept and measurement. *Journal of Consumer Policy*, **11**(4), 419–433. doi:10.1007/bf00411854

Weinstein, A., Mezig, H., Mizrachi, S. & Lejoyeux, M. (2015). A study investigating the association between compulsive buying with measures of anxiety and obsessive-compulsive behavior among internet shoppers. *Comprehensive Psychiatry*, **57**, 46–50. doi:https://doi.org/10.1016/j.comppsych.2014.11.003

Wesson, C. (1990). *Women Who Shop Too Much: Overcoming the Urge to Splurge.* New York: St. Martin's Press.

Winestine, M. C. (1985). Compulsive shopping as a derivative of a childhood deduction. *The Psychoanalytic Quarterly*, **54**(1), 70–72. doi:10.1080/21674086.1985.11927095

22 Prevention and Treatment of Work Addiction

Cristina Quinones, PhD, CPsychol, and Mark D. Griffiths, PhD

Introduction: What Workaholism Is (And Is Not)

Oates (1971) was the first person to conceptualize workaholism as an addiction, building on the observed cognitive-behavioral pattern that resembled that of alcohol addiction and defined it a workaholic as:

> ...a person whose need for work has become so excessive that it creates noticeable disturbance or interference with his bodily health, personal happiness, and interpersonal relations, and with his smooth social functioning
>
> (Oates, 1971; p. 4).

This neat conceptualization became gradually blurred in the literature as researchers sought to identify the dimensions that made up this multifaceted construct, often by including variables that were correlated with such compulsive behavior rather than based on sound theoretical justifications (Andreassen, 2014; Ng, Sorensen & Feldman, 2007). The present authors review some of these explanations and discuss why some of these personality traits, affective components, and attitudes are not "workaholism."

Criteria for Inclusion in This Review

The most comprehensive meta-analysis studies were examined, and searches were made between 2011 and 2018 in PsycINFO, MedLine, and the Google Scholar search engine with the terms "workaholism," "work addiction," and "compulsive work." The start date of 2011 was used to follow up from Sussman's (2012) meta-analysis that reviewed all studies up to 2011. Sussman's study was chosen not only for its relevance but also for the transparency in terms of how the searches were conducted. Sussman's review included definition, prevalence, etiology, measurement, prevention, and treatment. This chapter briefly examines how the conceptualization has changed since Sussman's review and includes a more-recent conceptual review by the present authors (Quinones & Griffiths, 2015), but also expands on these by also examining prevention and treatment. Also building on the work by Clarke et al. (2016), the chapter focuses on studies that conceptualize workaholism as addiction, not merely as working excessively (DeLíbano et al., 2012). Consequently, studies focusing on excessive work rather than addiction to work were omitted from the present review. Furthermore, although the chapter briefly examines cross-sectional studies identifying single personality factors (e.g., narcissism and workaholism; Andreassen et al., 2012a), these were (on the whole) not reviewed, as the aim of this chapter was to ascertain those factors that were present across a large number of studies and/or those showing stronger research designs (e.g., including more than one wave, not just a typical cross-sectional design).

Workaholism Is Not the "High Involvement-Low Enjoyment" Combination

Spence and Robbins (1992) conceptualized workaholism as a trait-based multidimensional construct comprising enjoyment, drive, and work involvement, and developed one of the most influential instruments to assess workaholism, namely the Workaholism Battery (WorkBat). The authors distinguished between real workaholics from the enjoyment workaholic type because although they shared high levels of involvement and drive, real workaholics reported low enjoyment from the work they did. Affective dimensions have since been included in subsequent work by others (Ng et al., 2007). However, the enjoyment dimension as a key component of workaholism is problematic. First, the idea of being affectively attached to one's work was never psychometrically nor theoretically strong (McMillan et al., 2002). In fact, accumulated evidence suggests that over-engagement with enjoyment (negatively or positively) is a separate construct from workaholism and is better represented by the construct of "work engagement" (DeCarlo et al., 2014; Taris et al., 2010; Van Beek et al., 2012).

Unlike what was initially thought, workaholism and work engagement are in fact associated with very different outcomes. For instance, one of longest follow-up studies with a seven-year gap between measurements confirmed that work engagement boosted positive work to family interaction and decreased the negative side of this interference in the long term, as opposed to workaholism which led to lower satisfaction and poorer health outcomes (Hakanen & Peeters, 2015). Furthermore, work engagement and workaholism appear to be only weakly related, with longitudinal studies reporting less than 7 percent shared variance (Shimazu et al., 2012). In short, enjoyment of work is relevant when it comes to work engagement, but it is not a central feature of workaholism (Clarke et al., 2016; Mudrack, 2006; Schaufeli, Taris & Bakker, 2006; Taris et al., 2010).

Workaholism Is Not a Stable Individual Characteristic

Workaholism has been conceptualized as a stable individual characteristic by a number of scholars, either because of the need to exhibit specific personality traits, or as a symptom of compulsive-obsessive personality disorder (American Psychiatric Association: APA, 2013). Within this compulsive-obsessive conceptualization, workaholism is characterized by "perfectionism, inflexibility, and preoccupation with work, and by an excessive devotion to work and productivity to the exclusion of leisure activities and friendships" (Molino, Bakker & Ghislieri, 2016, p. 401).

The idea of a stable trait within the obsessive-compulsive realm has been operationalized by the work of Schaufeli and colleagues, who defined workaholism as a two-dimensional construct comprising of working excessively (i.e., working too hard) and working compulsively (i.e., the inner drive to work incessantly), and they developed an instrument to assess these subdimensions (Dutch Work Addiction Scale; Schaufeli et al., 2009a; Schaufeli, Shimazu & Taris, 2009b). Current thinking in this field rejects the notion that excessive behavior is necessarily a key component of addiction, although strong correlations exist (Griffiths, 2011). Furthermore, studies examining the motivational dispositions of workaholism have found that working excessively is not related to controlled motivation, which is a commonly cited antecedent of the key compulsive element of workaholism (Van den Broeck et al., 2011). In addition to the conceptual issues, the operationalization is also problematic because the excessive work subscale developed by Schaufeli et al. (2009a, 2009b) shows poor psychometric qualities (Sussman, 2012). Robinson (1999) also conceptualized workaholism as the combination of compulsive tendencies and control along with other abilities and personality traits (e.g., impaired communication/self-absorption, inability to delegate, and self-worth). This multidimensional view was operationalized in the widely used diagnostic tool, the Work Addiction Risk Test (WART). However, factor analysis failed to confirm the five dimensions. This and the high correlations with general anxiety and Type A personality have either deterred researchers from using the WART model to assess workaholism or to only use the first two subscales (Andreassen, 2014).

In short, although the various multidimensional approaches (typically taking a trait view) have been useful in fostering discussion on what drives individuals to work excessively, there has not been strong empirical support concerning the number and type of dimensions proposed. As discussed earlier, enjoying work is a key dimension of work engagement, which is a separate (although related) construct from workaholism. Similarly, excessive behavior does not qualify as a key dimension of addiction on its own (Griffiths, 2011). Additionally, many of the personality variables that were once thought to be defining dimensions have now been shown to be weakly related, with only two variables (i.e., "compulsive tendencies" and "control") showing consistent antecedent value across studies (Clarke et al., 2016). More specifically, the compulsive tendencies (i.e., the compelling need to work) and control dimensions (i.e., the experience of negative emotions such as anger and impatience as a result of not having full control over work) appear to discriminate between workaholics and nonworkaholics (Flowers & Robinson, 2002). Recent meta-analysis and previous theoretical reviews have led many to agree that an addiction-based explanation of workaholism appears the most sensible approach to understand this phenomenon (Clarke et al., 2016; Griffiths, 2011; Griffiths, Demetrovics & Atrosko, 2018; Schimazu et al., 2015).

The Biopsychosocial Perspective of Workaholism

A robust theoretically driven conceptualization of workaholism is possible by building upon the strong body of knowledge concerning behavioral addictions more generally to conceptualize workaholism (Andreassen et al., 2014; Sussman, Lisha & Griffiths, 2011). In this section, key theoretical contributions are drawn upon to examine (i) key dimensions of workaholism and the (ii) vulnerability factors.

Theorizing on the Dimensions of Workaholism: The Component Model of Addiction

The components model of addiction draws upon Brown's (1993) *hedonic management model* and has been largely inspired by the diagnostic classification of pathological gambling in the DSM-IV (Griffiths, 2011). According to this framework, an addict displays symptoms that represent each of the following components: *cognitive and/or behavioral salience* (i.e., the activity dominates one's thoughts and/or behavior), *mood modification* (i.e., the behavior is used as a way to modify mood), *tolerance* (i.e., the increasing amount of time required to obtain the same experience with the activity), *withdrawal symptoms* (i.e., feeling negative emotions when the activity is stopped or diminished), *relapse and reinstatement/loss of control* (i.e., the need to return to the same level of use after trying to stop, and losing control over the use), and *conflict* (i.e., the behavior conflicts with everything in the person's life such as relationships, job, and/or education) (Brown, 1993; Griffiths, 2005).

This model has been validated in a variety of substance and nonsubstance based addictions and has been widely used to develop tools to understand and assess prevalence across a number of different addictions such as gaming addiction (e.g., Griffiths, 2002), exercise addiction (e.g., Allegre et al., 2006), internet addiction (Widyanto & Griffiths, 2006), and more recently social networking addiction (Andreassen et al., 2012a). Building on these findings, Andreassen et al., (2012b) developed the Bergen Work Addiction Scale (BWAS). The scale comprises seven items tapping into each of the aforementioned components, and each item is scored on a Likert scale from "never" to "always." Individuals are operationally classified as workaholics if they endorse four or more out of seven items (i.e., scoring "often" or "always"). Although still in relative infancy, it has already been validated in Norwegian samples of over 12,000 people with high Cronbach's alphas in the range of 0.80–0.85. Convergent and discriminant validity analysis suggests that the BWAS converges well with existing workaholism scales tapping the compulsive element (r = 0.50–0.84). Given the strong conceptual foundation, the brevity of the scale (favoring its use for prevalence studies or for screening within the workplace), and considering that its operationalization enables the integration of this behavior with potential cooccurring addictions, the BWAS is a promising tool in advancing the understanding of workaholism.

Examining Vulnerability Factors

The syndrome-based model of addiction has been most helpful in understanding antecedents and vulnerability in behavioral addictions and helps integrate current understanding of antecedents of workaholism. This model suggests that similar underlying mechanisms operate regardless of the object of addiction, and that manifestations of the syndrome are both generic and unique to the specific addiction (e.g., see Sussman & Pakdaman, 2020). Similar underlying vulnerabilities may be operating along with more unique psychosocial variables that predispose the individual to interact with a particular object of addiction and no other. Increasing research evidence in the field is supportive of such a model. For instance, self-report multiaddiction survey studies have found strong correlations among different behavioral and substance addictions (Villella et al., 2011). Furthermore, an increasing number of studies report both chemical and behavioral addictions share similar course, history, and neurobiological correlates (Grant et al., 2010; Griffiths, 2005; Orford, 2001). Perhaps the most compelling evidence comes from neurological studies, as these support the hypothesis that reward circuits in the brain are involved in both substance- and nonsubstance-based addictions, both share similar genetic vulnerability and clinical features, and that they develop following a similar pattern, which adheres to the components model of addiction (i.e., initial arousal before the act, pleasure/high relief linked to the act, lowered arousal afterwards along with guilt, withdrawal, and potential tolerance) (Grant et al., 2010;

Villella et al., 2011). Many studies in this field have traditionally been cross-sectional, which interferes in the ability to distinguish between antecedents and simple correlates (Quinones & Griffiths, 2015; Quinones, Griffiths & Kakabadse, 2016). Nonetheless, empirical evidence accumulated to date can be used to identify what appear to be the most salient individual, familial, and sociocultural factors favor the development of workaholism (Griffiths & Karanika-Murray, 2012).

Individual Factors

Clarke et al.'s (2016) meta-analysis suggested that, aside from mere correlations, it is only the achievement-oriented personality traits (perfectionism and Type A personality) that are strong antecedents of workaholism across empirical studies. In contrast, there is no (or at best weak) support with other personality traits (e.g., conscientiousness, self-esteem, positive affect). Equally, demographic factors such as gender, parental status, and marital status appear to have mixed relationships with workaholism. Consequently, these are not unequivocal antecedents of workaholism. With regards to psychopathological factors, a largescale study by Andreassen et al. (2016) showed that anxiety and ADHD were strong contributors to the variability of workaholism, more so than obsessive-compulsive symptoms, which is at odds with the compulsive-based conceptualizations of workaholism discussed earlier in this chapter.

Familial Factors

The family therapist and academic Robinson (2013; p. ix) – who called workaholism the "best dressed problem of the twenty-first century" (p. ix) – drew on his clinical practice to explain how specific family dynamics, such as over-responsibility, contribute to the development of workaholism in adulthood. Considering the strong association between managerial roles and high responsibility, and the complex dynamics between that and gender, it is unsurprising that Andreassen et al. (2016) found these participants most likely to be classified as workaholics. Over-responsibility is also more significantly found in children of workaholic parents. For instance, Carrol and Robinson's (2000) study found that adult children of workaholics show greater levels of parentification (i.e., role reversal whereby children act as parent to their own parent) than those of nonworkaholic parents.

Sociocultural Factors

Workaholic behaviors are often socially acceptable and even rewarded in society. Sussman et al. (2014) argued that workaholism is a "nurturance-type" addiction. Consequently, although like other addictions it causes interpersonal conflict, the behaviors are also socially associated with the achievement of financial resources and in that way adheres to social expectations about adulthood. In contrast to this nurturance-type of addiction, other behaviors such as gambling, are viewed negatively because they are perceived to be pleasure-seeking driven, often to the detriment of nurturance because gambling addiction is associated with economic losses (Schwartz, 2010).

The socioeconomic context characterized by job insecurity and uncertainty (Molino et al., 2016; Quinones, 2016) may also contribute to the increasing trend concerning maladaptive work behavior that could potentially trigger workaholism among vulnerable individuals. For instance, Kanai and Mitsuru's (2004) study of Japanese workers during the times of economic downturn showed how work overload increased as enjoyment decreased, and that the "drive to work" component of workaholism remained high. Studies suggest that workaholism also depends on work culture. At a broad level, work investment appears to be higher in societies that emphasize economic security than in those which emphasize subjective wellbeing and quality of life (Snir & Harpaz, 2012). Arguably, it also fits within a wider capitalist system which tends to favor instrumental gains over relationships (Clark et al., 2016). It is also shaped by organizational culture, in particular, those that favor role-modeling workaholic behavior, and spread what has been termed "unhealthy heroism" (Hakanen & Peeters, 2015). Professional culture is also an important factor to consider, and workaholism is less likely in blue collar employees. Where the professional culture is one of excellence, and workers have freedom to work at their own pace, such as high-tech industry, there is a much higher tendency to work more hours. Although the externally imposed pressure to work harder cannot cause workaholism on its own, it can lead to maladaptive work habits which coupled with individual vulnerabilities may develop in workaholism (Sharone, 2004).

In short, considering the social acceptance, the reward of overwork in western societies, and the ability to connect to work 24/7, strategies and tools are needed to help individuals engage with work in a more sustainably healthy way and prevent workaholism (Quinones, 2017). Before exploring prevention and treatment, the importance of broadening our understanding of addictions is discussed to further the understanding of what it means to be addicted to work.

Critical Perspectives on Addiction

The components model of addiction (Griffiths, 2005) is sometimes characterized as the "diagnostic" or "symptomatic" model. The model (and variations upon it) helps in understanding the extent to which specific behaviors (e.g., work) fit a pattern of addiction by stressing the importance of loss of control over the activity, impulsivity, and conflict (Van der Linden, 2015). The BWAS diagnostic tool (derived from such a model) was inspired by the DMS IV-TR criteria on pathological gambling justified by the fact that work addiction, like other behavioral addictions, share phenomenological and neurobiological commonalities. The present authors believe the greater value of this model is for self-assessment and monitoring of behavior at the individual level, and also as one of the tools that clinicians will consider when examining the underlying psychological process behind those symptoms. Most research on workaholism tends to focus on the individual addiction aspects (and the implications this have for prevention and treatment). However, the problem (and its symptoms) have deeper psychological, socioeconomic, and even historical and cultural roots. If these are ignored in favor of implementing addiction-based treatments, one is not only risking the social condition that reinforces the behavior at a macro-level, but also more likely to be applying generic addiction treatments that may temporarily fix the problem while leaving the underlying dysfunctional psychological processes untouched (Billieux et al., 2015).

Critical psychologists have longed argued for complementing the disease model of addiction with a thorough consideration of the social determinants of addiction (e.g., poverty, weak social support, exclusion, unemployment, hyper-individualism) (Reinarman & Granfield, 2015; Suissa, 2014). Critical psychologists argue that the excessive emphasis on the individual aspects removes the social, cultural, and political triggers from the etiology and maintenance of the problem, thereby eliminating key components in the prevention and treatment of addiction. Instead, the focus and responsibility are now on "addicts" and their support networks (Reinarman & Granfield, 2015; Van der Linden, 2015). Any addiction, including substance-based addictions, benefit from this contextualization. As Reinarman and Granfield (2015) state, Andean peasants rarely become cocaine addicts regardless of their regular coca chewing because the habit is deeply integrated in that culture. Workaholism is a strong example of an addiction that could not be understood without the socioeconomic context in which it emerges, and it is difficult to find a work addict in a noncapitalist society.

The acknowledgement of social factors is not new, and some authors have emphasized its importance. Sussman et al. (2011) argued that lifestyle and the type of social learning from the environment have as much explanatory value or more in workaholism than personal vulnerabilities. Nonetheless, a more varied multidisciplinary approach may help to actually examine ways in which these factors can be more seriously included in the academic debate particularly when talking about prevention and treatment. For example, the concept of "loss of control" is central to disease theories of addiction (Reinerman & Granfield, 2015) and is one of the core symptoms in the components model of addiction (and related biological models). A historically contextualized approach to work addiction stresses the conflict inherent in a society that both pushes and punishes pleasure-seeking through consumption. Individuals are surrounded by easy access, fast, frequent (though often short-lived) sources of pleasure, and gratification enveloped in well-designed marketing strategies. Yet society also bombards individuals with the idea of taking responsibility for their pleasure-seeking and to exert self-control. This is worsened by the fact that western societies are becoming more individualistic in spite of the strong support for the health promotion effects of strong social ties. In short, widening the focus to the cultural and contextual factors enabling work addiction, will complement the brain disease approach to provide a more-balanced understanding of the multiple factors contributing to these problem (Reinaman & Granfield, 2015; Sussman, 2017; Sussman & Pakdaman, 2020; Van der Linden, 2015).

An Integrative View on Prevention and Treatment

Although full-on workaholism only affects a minority of the population, working compulsively, even for a short period of time, or for a longer period but not to the point of work addiction, can still harm interpersonal relationships and health, and therefore prevention is important. It is important to bear in mind that the lack of conceptual clarity discussed earlier in this chapter, and the limited power of many empirical studies that exist in the work addiction field, limit the extent to which interventions have been extensively validated (Andreassen, 2014). In this section, existing strategies from a multilevel interdisciplinary approach are discussed according to two main organizing principles: (i) the target population and the stage they are in relation to the problem, and (ii) the stakeholder involved in the intervention (this is, who is responsible for leading the intervention: individuals, clinicians, and/or organizations).

With regards to the target population, using the classic intervention typology, it needs to be determined whether the aim is (i) educating healthy populations to reduce any risk of work addiction by promoting healthy habits and preventing ill-health (i.e., *primary intervention*), (ii) supporting people to develop adaptive coping mechanisms against triggers to those who are at risk of work addiction (i.e., *secondary intervention*), or (iii) minimizing the consequences of work addiction (i.e., *tertiary intervention*). When examining secondary and tertiary interventions it is also important to identify the stage at which the individual is at because workaholism is at the extreme end of a continuum which develops over time. Piotrowski and Vodanovich's (2008) development process model is a useful framework to evaluate the stage at which the individual is at. The model comprises two stages. (i) *The initial stage:* This is where individuals begin to exhibit patterns of compulsive work that result from the interaction between traits, family values/roles, and stressors. During this time, there is no significant interference with an individual's life or their meaningful others (primary and secondary prevention are relevant). (ii) *Full-on workaholism:* Here, the behaviors increase in intensity and frequency as a learned mechanism to deal with the demands resulting from the combination of personal and work-related stressors (tertiary prevention is relevant). These behaviors lead to problems both at work and outside of work, and the experience of loss of control resembles the key components of a behavioral addiction (Griffiths, 2005). The vast majority of individuals will never cross to the second stage, and even if they do, they might only stay there for a limited period of time owing to particular economic or personal circumstances. Building upon the two organizing principles discussed, what is known about prevention and treatment is reviewed in the following subsections in relation to the leading stakeholder involved, and examples are included in Table 22.1.

Table 22.1 Level of intervention in work addiction by type of stakeholder

Level of intervention	Stakeholder involvement		
	Individual	Clinician	Organization
Prevention: primary intervention	- Monitor time spent at work vs. objectives met - Engage in off-work fun, learning and/or exercise	- Disseminate through all meaningful channels - Raise awareness	- Reward relevant role models - Support organizational culture that values psychological recovery outside work
Reducing early signs: secondary intervention	- Practice some relaxation strategy. For instance, ten minute of mindfulness meditation has been found to reduce early symptoms (Quinones & Griffiths, 2019)	- Help develop adaptive coping strategies	- Training workshops, importance of switching off
Treatment: tertiary intervention	- Seek professional help	- Diagnose and treat accordingly	- Employee Assistance Program (EAP) - Support for external counseling/therapy

For Clinicians, Therapists, and Scholars

According to Van Wijhe and colleagues (2010, 2014), successful prevention and treatment strategies for this particular problem should address four inherent complexities, which set it apart from other behavioral and substance-based addictions:

(1) Abstinence is not an option. Hence, interventions must set realistic goals.
(2) Unlike with other addictions, workaholism is the extreme of an otherwise socially valued behavior. Thus, an effective intervention should enhance clients' awareness about the triggers and consequences that working in such a way has on them.
(3) Derived from the previous two points, individuals are more likely to seek medical help for problems associated with workaholism (e.g., poor sleep, stress). Thus, effective interventions should tackle the compulsive behavior but also address the associated damage of work addiction.
(4) Workaholics will, by definition, struggle to find time to do other things than work. Hence, feasible interventions should be designed bearing in mind, where possible, that briefness is crucial.

Points (1)–(3) are particularly relevant when it comes to primary and secondary interventions. Therapists, clinicians, and scholars in the field should use the different means at their disposal to communicate widely and clearly about the extent to which work addiction can become a problem for some individuals in contemporary society. This is likely to involve helping people to articulate implicit assumptions about the nature of work, and whether or not there is such a thing as an unhealthy work pattern. If these assumptions are not articulated, they cannot be challenged, and individuals are more likely to end up needing tertiary interventions rather than being more effectively supported through primary and secondary efforts. Also, building on the literature on healthy psychological recovery activities (e.g., de Jonge et al., 2018; Quinones, 2017), these professionals can help workers and students to develop healthy and adaptive habits of coping with stress, working on self-esteem, and developing interests and hobbies outside work.

Diagnosis to Inform Treatment. When it comes to secondary and tertiary interventions (i.e., clients at risk or already addicted to work), the first step is to ensure the problem is properly diagnosed. Clinicians should use specific addiction-related screening instruments coupled with a broader examination of the underlying psychological processes to be addressed. An assessment that is based only on the addiction symptoms may leave the underlying psychological dysfunctional processes untouched. The danger of doing so is illustrated by Billieux et al. (2015), who reported the case of a client who was diagnosed with mobile-phone addiction using a symptoms-based approach (i.e., adopting the DSM-IV-TR substance abuse criteria according to which symptoms must be present for at least twelve months). Then the authors followed a broader psychological processes approach to analyze the same client via the use of screening instruments and different clinical methods such functional analyses. This approach led them to identify irrational beliefs, dependent relationship maintenance, and low impulse control, targeted for treatment. The therapeutic strategy that followed would then be aimed at addressing the psychopathological processes, and problematic mobile-phone use (here used as a maladaptive coping strategy) that would diminish as a function of the effectiveness of the treatment. In short, clinical treatment was tailored to the individual's needs depending upon the psychopathological processes involved and the extent to which the compulsive behavior is just a means to temporarily cope with events or a more fundamental and stable way of coping with pain or anxiety. This may be a good protocol to use when considering treatment of work addicts. Some of these specific techniques are now discussed.

Treatment Techniques. Mindfulness training and gradual muscle relaxation techniques have been proved effective in reducing the physiological arousal associated with the stress response which may otherwise trigger maladaptive coping strategies (Quinones & Griffiths, 2019). Meditation is particularly effective in preventing individuals going into the automatic pilot reaction associated with behavioral addictions, even if it is practiced for a short period of time a day (Quinones, 2017; Shonin et al., 2014). The positive psychology approach that focuses on supporting individuals to engage in healthy living includes developing a guiding meaningful vision, and then applying it to associated behaviors, thoughts about strengths, and self-care rather than focusing on problems per se (Andreassen et al., 2014). For instance, helping individuals to reflect on and develop meaningful life goals, and learning to examine how work and other areas of life are contributing toward that goal, may facilitate a more positive life trajectory.

Cognitive-behavioral therapy (CBT) is a robust tool for therapists in many areas, including behavioral addictions. It helps tackle the irrational rigid beliefs that trigger workaholic behaviors (Andreassen et al., 2016). One type of CBT, *emotive behavioral therapy* (Ellis, 1957; cited in Chen, 2006) is an example of approach that can be helpful. Going from working compulsively to working more adaptively is a process that can be mapped onto different stages (from unawareness, to awareness to being treated and preventing relapse), which at the very least involves some level of ambivalence; strong reasons are needed to change the behavior (e.g., "I cannot see my kids awake when I get home"). However, other reasons for carrying on the behavior are likely to arise (e.g., "I need the promotion," "I might get fired if I don't work at the same level").

This Ellis approach involves confrontative statements. However, for many ambivalent and/or resistant patients, an approach to roll with resistance may be needed. In this type of case, CBT may be particularly effective if combined with *Motivational Interviewing.* This technique helps the client develop stronger awareness about their work behavior, and the discrepancy between values and behaviors, thereby increasing motivation for change. This addresses what Suissa (2014) believes to be central to developing addiction – the motives to work. More specifically, he argues that workaholism operates if individuals engage on this behavior as means to escape from psychological pain. That is, engaging in compulsive work will initially be a strategy to evade pain or psychological dysfunction (e.g., feelings of loneliness, rigid perfectionism, need for achievement). This lessens the negative emotions associated with such underlying problems and, in turn, becomes a more salient way of coping with these emotions in the future. Motivational Interviewing has been successfully applied to treat other substance and behavioral addictions (Andreassen et al., 2016; Sussman, 2017; Van Whije et al., 2010).

As this is a problem often associated with interpersonal consequences or triggers, *family therapy* has also been suggested as crucial (Robinson, Carrol & Flowres, 2001). Analyzing and developing better communication channels and more effective family dynamics in relation to work-life balance can be unpacked to help draw boundaries and achieve a better balance for all. Some therapists may find that self-help groups are useful for their clients. *Workaholics Anonymous,* based on the twelve-step tradition developed from Alcoholics Anonymous is by far the most established of its type (Sussman, 2012).

For Organizations: Line Managers, Executives, Human Resources Professionals

It is very important for employers to understand what work addiction is, and that, although this is a problem that affects a minority, the consequences of compulsive working patterns can be devastating for individuals' health and organizational objectives. While supporting employees through counseling is positive and welcomed, it only addresses one part of the problem. The problem involves multiple levels that produces and maintains the problematic behavior (individual, familial, sociocultural) and these need to be addressed. Workaholism is maintained via a system of unhealthy work practices and more deeply ingrained societal values such as presenteeism (even if this means being virtually present by engaging in sending emails when working off-site).

Unsurprisingly, workaholics tend to work in job sites that are less supportive about employees' work–life balance. This is likely the combination of both self-selection and organizational rewards (Van Whije et al., 2010). For instance, some organizational cultures nurture long working hours applied to workers that do not switch off, by providing rewards such as promotions or pay raises or, indirectly, by using them as role models and mentors for new employees.

Diagnosis: How Workaholic-Friendly is the Culture? This diagnosis can be done by undertaking an organizational culture analysis collecting data from different stakeholders. This may include asking questions such as:

- Are we incentivizing overwork through promotions, stronger status, etc.?
- Are we encouraging an "always-on" culture explicitly or implicitly, perhaps through the ways in which we send our emails during weekends or outside of office hours?

It is important to monitor implicit connectivity rules, particularly ways in which the more powerful members of organizations communicate with junior employees or members of minority groups. These may be setting unwritten rules of connectivity that may favor unnecessary rules of "always-on" connectivity for the less advantageous group.

Prevention and Intervention Strategies. Employers need to offer support and develop policies that help individuals to work more healthily and to alleviate the pressure experienced by increased work intensification, working remotely, and/or achieving better work–life balance, which ultimately lead to a less "workaholic-friendly" organizational culture. These include:

- Ensuring that workaholic behaviors are not incentivized (e.g., delayed promotions; Hamermesh & Slemrod, 2008) and instead, encouraging models of sustainable long-term productivity (Yaniv, 2011).
- Ensuring that promotions and status are not associated with a particular "heroic" workaholic role model. This is particularly relevant for managers because studies show a higher prevalence of workaholics amongst managers (Taris et al., 2010).
- Telling stories of individuals who achieve success through working smart rather than hard or all the time, celebrate families and employees' lives outside work, and promoting a reasonable work–life balance (Hakanen & Peeters, 2015).
- Hosting leadership development programs that address the aforementioned issues and encourage the development of boundaries (studies show that flexible working may increase excessive working; e.g., Kelliher & Anderson, 2010), and providing healthy role models.
- Hosting specific training programs on time management, assertiveness, and adaptive stress coping techniques. These are particularly important for people with early signs of work addiction as they struggle to say "no" to work requests (Van Whije et al., 2010).
- Encouraging off-work recovery activities that seem to be most effective in helping people restore the psychological resources spent at work such as mindfulness meditation and gradual relaxation techniques (e.g., Quinones, 2017).

Finally, in those cases where employees seek direct support for their excessive work patterns, organizations should offer confidential employee wellbeing support, either directly or indirectly related to this issue. Both family and work lives are intertwined and impact on each other, and more often than not, employees may not seek support directly for the work addiction problem but for related issues.

For the Self

The increasing interest in healthy habits, along with the growing dissemination about the risks of excessive engagement with technology and accessing "work on the go" (to a great extent related to the rise of mobile technology), is planting the seeds for more conscious self-monitoring and self-care activities. Here, freely available tools could be used to monitor how an individual's suspected over work may be problematic using the brief seven-item Bergen Work Addiction Scale (Andreassen et al., 2012a). Alternatively, or in combination with this, individuals may monitor the way they work, their motivation to do so, and the impact this has on their lives and others over a period of one or two weeks in order to decide whether any behavioral change in their work pattern is needed. Some of the strategies to regulate excessive behavior and preventing it from escalating were highlighted by Quinones (2017). If the individual feels either unable to change a behavior that they feel is problematic, or they feel they need further support from experts and peers, then they need to seek professional help.

Conclusions

In this chapter different conceptualizations of workaholism were explored and evaluated in relation to the existing empirical data accumulated over the past few decades with a view to establishing what workaholism is (and what it is not) – in other words, the key dimensions as opposed to just correlates. It was argued that the addiction-based explanations of workaholism appear the most sensible approach in understanding the manifestation of this problem particularly at the individual level. Additionally, it was argued that this needs to be complemented by a cultural, a historical, social, and cultural analysis of the circumstances that sustain the lifestyle enabling workaholism in a society that both pushes and punishes pleasure-seeking through consumption. Without this broader understanding, efforts and individual prevention and treatment are likely to be futile. To further a broader gage of workaholism causes and sustaining variables, as well as prevention and treatment possibilities, academics and practitioners from different disciplines including psychology, sociology, and anthropology should work collaboratively. This type of collaboration can occur in parallel to the different individual efforts by challenging the status quo and developing different ways of organizing work in a more balanced and sustainable way. Finally, existing prevention and treatment strategies were reviewed at different levels (i.e., primary, secondary, and tertiary). Interventions need to set realistic goals, and not be too lengthy. There is also a crucial need to develop a strong awareness of the client about how and why work addiction has or will cause problems in different areas of individuals' lives.

REFERENCES

Allegre, B., Souville, M., Therme, P. & Griffiths, M. (2006). Definitions and measures of exercise dependence. *Addiction Research & Theory*, 14(6), 631–646.

American Psychiatric Association [APA] (2013). *Diagnostic and Statistical Manual of Mental Disorders* (5th edition). Washington, DC: American Psychiatric Association.

Andreassen, C. S. (2014). Workaholism: an overview and current status of the research. *Journal of Behavioral Addictions*, **3**, 1–11.

Andreassen, C. S., Griffiths, M. D., Hetland, J., et al. (2014). The prevalence of workaholism: A survey study in a nationally representative sample of Norwegian employees. *PLoS ONE*, 9, e102446. doi:10.1371/journal.pone.0102446

Andreassen, C. S., Griffiths, M. D., Hetland, J. & Pallesen, S. (2012a). Development of a work addiction scale. *Scandinavian Journal of Psychology*, **53**(3), 265–272.

Andreassen, C. S., Griffiths, M. D., Sinha, R., Hetland, J. & Pallesen, S. (2016). The relationships between workaholism and symptoms of psychiatric disorders: A large-scale cross-sectional study. *PLoS ONE*, **11**(5), e0152978.

Andreassen, C. S., Tosheim, T., BrunBerg, G. S. & Pallesen, S. (2012b). Development of a Facebook Addiction Scale. *Psychological Reports*, **110**, 501–517.

Billieux, J., Philippot, P., Schmid, C., et al. M. (2015). Is dysfunctional use of the mobile phone a behavioural addiction? Confronting symptom-based versus process-based approaches. *Clinical Psychology and Psychotherapy*, **22**, 460–468.

Brown, R. I. F. (1993). Some contributions of the study of gambling to the study of other addictions. In W. R. Eadington & J. Cornelius (Eds.), *Gambling Behavior and Problem Gambling*. Reno, NV: University of Nevada Press, pp. 241–272.

Carroll, J. J. & Robinson, B. E. (2000). Parentification and depression among adult children of workaholics and adult children of alcoholics. *The Family Journal*, **8**, 360–367.

Chen, C. P. (2006). Improving work-life balance: REBT for workaholic treatment. Research companion to working time and work addiction. In R. J. Burke (Ed.), *Research Companion to Working Time and Work Addiction*. Cheltenham, UK: Edward Elgar, pp. 310–329.

Clark, M. A., Michel, J. S., Zhdanova, L., Pui, S. Y. & Baltes, B. B. (2016). All work and no play? A meta-analytic examination of the correlates and outcomes of workaholism. *Journal of Management*, **42**(7), 1836–1873.

De Carlo, N. A., Falco, A., Pierro, A., et al. (2014). Regulatory mode orientations and well-being in an organizational setting: the differential mediating roles of workaholism and work engagement. *Journal of Applied Social Psychology*, **44**, 725–738.

de Jonge, J., Shimazu, A. & Dollard, M. (2018). Short-term and long-term effects of off-job activities on recovery and sleep: A two-wave panel study among health care employees. *International Journal of Environmental Research and Public Health*, **15** (9), 2044.

Del Líbano, M., Llorens, S., Salanova, M. & Schaufeli, W. B. (2012). About the dark and bright sides of self-efficacy: Workaholism and work engagement. *Spanish Journal of Psychology*, **15**(2), 688–701.

Flowers, C. P. & Robinson, B. (2002). A structural and discriminant analysis of the work addiction risk test. *Educational and Psychological Measurement*, **62**, 517–526.

Grant, J. E., Potenza, M. N., Weinstein, A. & Gorelick, D. A. (2010). Introduction to behavioral addictions. *American Journal of Drug and Alcohol Abuse*, **36**, 233–241.

Griffiths, M. D. (2002). *Gambling and Gaming Addictions in Adolescence*. Leicester: BPS Blackwell.

Griffiths, M. D. (2005). A components model of addiction within a biopsychological framework. *Journal of Substance Use*, **10**, 191–197.

Griffiths, M. D. (2011). Workaholism: A 21st century addiction. *The Psychologist: Bulletin of the British Psychological Society*, **24**, 740–744.

Griffiths, M. D. & Karanika-Murray, M. (2012). Contextualising over-engagement in work: Towards a more global understanding of workaholism as an addiction. *Journal of Behavioral Addictions*, **1**(3), 87–95.

Griffiths, M. D., Demetrovics, Z. & Atroszko, P. A. (2018). Ten myths about work addiction. *Journal of Behavioral Addictions*, **7**(4), 845–857.

Hakanen, J. & Peeters, M. (2015). How do work engagement, workaholism, and the work-to-family interface affect each other? A 7-year follow-up study. *Journal of Occupational and Environmental Medicine*, **57**(6), 601–609.

Hamermesh, D. S. & Slemrod, J. B. (2008). The economics of workaholism: We should not have worked on this paper. *The BE Journal of Economic Analysis & Policy*, **8**(1). doi:10.2202/1935-1682.1793

Kanai, A. & Mitsuru, M. (2004). Effects of economic environmental changes on job demands and workaholism in Japan. *Journal of Organizational Change Management*, **17**, 537–548.

Kelliher, C. & Anderson, D. (2010). Doing more with less? Flexible working practices and the intensification of work. *Human Relations*, **63** (1), 83–106.

McMillan, L. H. W., Brady, E. C., O'Driscoll, M. P. & Marsh, N. V. (2002). A multifaceted validation study of Spence and Robbins' (1992) workaholism battery. *Journal of Occupational and Organisational Psychology*, **75**, 357–368.

Molino, M., Bakker, A. B. & Ghislieri, C. (2016). The role of workaholism in the job demands-resources model. *Anxiety, Stress, & Coping*, **29**, 400–414.

Mudrack, P. E. (2006). Understanding workaholism: The case for behavioral tendencies. In R. J. Burke (Ed.), *Research Companion to Working Time and Work Addiction*. Northampton, MA: Edward Elgar Publishing, pp. 108–128.

Ng, T. W. H., Sorensen, K. L. & Feldman, D. C. (2007). Dimensions, antecedents, and consequences of workaholism: A conceptual integration and extension. *Journal of Organizational Behavior*, **28**, 111–136.

Oates, W. (1971). *Confessions of a Workaholic: The Facts about Work Addiction*. New York: World.

Orford, J. (2001). Conceptualizing addiction: Addiction as excessive appetite. *Addiction*, **96**, 15–31.

Piotrowski, C. & Vodanovich, S. J. (2008). The Workaholism Syndrome: An emerging issue in the psychological literature. *Journal of Instructional Psychology*, **35**(1), 103–105.

Quinones, C. (2016). The 'always on' workplace: Risks, opportunities and how to make it work. *HR Magazine*, February 16. Available at: www.hrmagazine.co.uk/article-details/the-always-on-workplace-risks-opportunities-and-how-to-make-it-work

Quinones, C. (2017). Does intense ICT use after work help or hinder psychological recovery? The shifting landscape of work and working lives. Conference paper number: CIPD/ARC/ 2016/1 retrieved November 1, 2018, from: www.cipd.co.uk/learn/events-networks/ applied-research-conference

Quinones, C. & Griffiths, M. (2015). Addiction to work: A critical review of the workaholism construct and recommendations for assessment. *Journal of Psychiatric Nursing*, **53** (10), 48–59.

Quinones, C. & Griffiths, M. D. (2019). Reducing compulsive Internet use and anxiety symptoms via two brief interventions: A comparison between mindfulness and gradual muscle relaxation. *Journal of Behavioral Addictions*, **8**(3), 530–536.

Quinones. C., Griffiths, M. & Kakabadse, N. (2016). Compulsive Internet use and workaholism: An exploratory two-wave longitudinal study. *Computers in Human Behaviour*, **60**, 492–499.

Reinarman, C. & Granfield, R. (2015). Addiction is not just a brain disease: Critical studies of addiction. In R. Granfield & C. Reinarman (Eds.), *Expanding Addictions. Critical Essays*. New York: Routledge, pp. 1–21.

Robinson, B. E. (1999). The Work Addiction Risk Test: Development of a tentative measure of workaholism. *Perceptual and Motor Skills*, **88**, 199–210.

Robinson B. E. (2013). *Chained to the Desk: A Guidebook for Workaholics, their Partners and Children, and the Clinicians who Treat Them* (3rd edition). New York: New York University Press

Robinson, B. E., Carroll, J. J. & Flowers, C. (2001). Marital estrangement, positive affect, and locus of control among spouses of workaholics and spouses of nonworkaholics: A national study. *American Journal of Family Therapy*, **29**, 397–410.

Sharone, O. (2004). Engineering overwork: Bell-curve management at a high-tech firm. In C. Fuchs Epstein, & A. L. Kalleberg (Eds.), *Fighting for Time: Shifting Boundaries of Work and Social Life*. New York: Russell Sage Foundation, pp. 191–218.

Schaufeli, W. B., Bakker, A. B., van der Heijden, F. M. M. A. & Prins, J. T. (2009a). Workaholism among medical residents: It is the combination of working excessively and compulsively that counts. *International Journal of Stress Management*, **16**, 249–272.

Schaufeli, W. B., Shimazu, A. & Taris, T. W. (2009b). Being driven to work excessively hard: The evaluation of a two-factor measure of workaholism in the Netherlands and Japan. *Cross-Cultural Research*, **43**, 320–348.

Schaufeli, W. B., Taris, T. W. & Bakker, A. (2006). Dr. Jekyll and Mr. Hide: On the differences between work engagement and workaholism. In R. J. Burke (Ed.), *Research Companion to Working Time and Work Addiction*. Northampton, MA: Edward Elgar, pp. 193–217.

Schwartz, S. H. (2010). Basic values: How they motivate and inhibit prosocial behavior. In M. Mikulincer & P. R. Shaver (Eds.), *Prosocial Motives, Emotions, and Behavior: The Better Angels of our Nature*. Washington, DC: American Psychological Association, pp. 221–241.

Shimazu, A., Schaufeli, W. B., Kubota, K. & Kawakam, N. (2012). Do workaholism and work engagement predict employee well-being and performance in opposite directions? *Industrial Health*, **50**, 316–321.

Shimazu, A., Schaufeli, W. B., Kamiyama, K. & Kawakami, N. (2015). Workaholism vs. work engagement: The two different predictors of future well-being and performance. *International Journal of Behavioral Medicine*, **22**(1),18–23.

Shonin, E., Van Gordon, W. & Griffiths, M. D. (2014). The treatment of workaholism with meditation awareness training: A case study. *Explore: The Journal of Science and Healing*, **10**(3), 193–195.

Snir R. & Harpaz I. (2012). Beyond workaholism: Towards a general model of heavy work investment. *Human Resource Management Review*, **22**, 232–243.

Spence, J. T. & Robbins, A. S. (1992). Workaholism: Definition, measurement, and preliminary results. *Journal of Personality Assessment*, **58**, 160–178.

Suissa A. J. (2014). Cyberaddictions: Toward a psychosocial perspective. *Addictive Behaviors*, **39**, 1914–1918.

Sussman, S. (2012). Workaholism: A review. *Journal of Addiction Research and Therapy*, **S6**, 1–10. doi:10.4172/2155-6105.S6-001

Sussman S. (2017). *Substance and Behavioral Addictions: Concepts, Causes, and Cures*. Cambridge: Cambridge University Press.

Sussman, S. & Pakdaman, S. (2020). Appetitive needs and addiction. In S. Sussman (Ed.), *The Cambridge Handbook of Substance and Behavioral Addictions*. Cambridge, UK: Cambridge University Press, pp. 3–12.

Sussman, S., Arpawong, T. E. M., Sun, P., et al. (2014). Prevalence and co-occurrence of addictive behaviors among former alternative high school youth. *Journal of Behavioral Addictions*, **3**(1), 33–40.

Sussman, S., Lisha, N. & Griffiths, M. (2011). Prevalence of the addictions: A problem of the majority or the minority? *Evaluation and the Health Professions*, **34**(1), 3–56.

Van Wijhe, C. I., Peeters, M. C. & Schaufeli, W. B. (2014). Enough is enough: Cognitive antecedents of workaholism and its aftermath. *Human Resource Management*, **53** (1), 157–177.

Van Wijhe, C. I., Schaufeli, W. & Peeters, M. C. W. (2010). Understanding and treating workaholism: Setting the stage for successful interventions. In C. L. Cooper & R. J. Burke (Eds.), *Psychological and Behavioural Risks at Work*. Farham: Ashgate, pp. 107–134.

Van Beek, I., Hu, Q., Schaufeli, W. B., Taris, T. W. & Schreurs, B. H. J. (2012). For fun, love, or money: What drives workaholic, engaged, and burned-out employees at work? *Applied Psychology*, **61**, 30–55.

Van den Broeck, A., Schreurs, B., De Witte, H., et al. (2011). Understanding workaholics' motivations: A self-determination perspective. *Applied Psychology*, **60**, 600–621.

Van Der Linden, M. (2015). Commentary on: Are we overpathologizing everyday life? A tenable blueprint for behavioral addiction research: Addictions as a psychosocial and cultural construction. *Journal of Behavioral Addictions*, **4**(3), 145–147.

Villella, C., Martinotti, G., Di Nicola, M., et al. (2011). Behavioural addictions in adolescents and young adults: Results from a prevalence study. *Journal of Gambling Studies*, **27**, 203–214.

Widyanto, L. & Griffiths, M. D. (2006). Internet addiction: A critical review. *International Journal of Mental Health and Addiction*, **4**, 31–51.

Yaniv, G. (2011). Workaholism and marital estrangement: A rational-choice perspective. *Mathematical Social Sciences*, **61**, 104–108.

23 Gaming Disorder and Its Treatment

Mark D. Griffiths, PhD, Daria J. Kuss, PhD, and Halley M. Pontes, PhD

Introduction

Research into online addictions has grown considerably over the past two decades (Kuss et al., 2014), and much of it has concentrated on Gaming Disorder (GD). In the latest (fifth) edition of the *Diagnostic and Statistical Manual of Mental Disorders* (DSM-5; American Psychiatric Association [APA], 2013), *Internet Gaming Disorder* (IGD) (also commonly referred to in the literature as problematic gaming and gaming addiction) was included in Section 3 ("Emerging Measures and Models") as a promising area that needed future research before being formally included in the next revision of the DSM. More recently, the World Health Organization (WHO) proposed the introduction of GD in the eleventh revision of the *International Classification of Diseases* (ICD-11; Reed et al., 2019).

The DSM-5 defined IGD by nine clinical criteria (of which five or more need to be endorsed over the period of twelve months and result in clinically significant impairment to be diagnosed as experiencing IGD). More specifically, the criteria develop by the APA include: (1) preoccupation with games; (2) withdrawal symptoms when gaming is taken away; (3) the need to spend increasing amounts of time engaged in gaming; (4) unsuccessful attempts to control participation in gaming; (5) loss of interest in hobbies and entertainment as a result of, and with the exception of, gaming; (6) continued excessive use of games despite knowledge of psychosocial problems; (7) deception of family members, therapists, or others regarding the amount of gaming; (8) use of gaming to escape or relieve a negative mood; and (9) loss of a significant relationship, job, or educational or career opportunity because of participation in games.

In the proposed ICD-11, Gaming Disorder (GD) is defined as "a pattern of gaming behavior ("digital-gaming" or "video-gaming") characterized by impaired control over gaming, increasing priority given to gaming over other activities to the extent that gaming takes precedence over other interests and daily activities, and continuation or escalation of gaming despite the occurrence of negative consequences" (WHO, 2018). The decision to include GD in ICD-11 was based on extensive reviews of available empirical and clinical evidence on the phenomenon and reflected a general consensus among experts from different disciplines and geographical regions that were involved in the process of technical consultations undertaken by WHO in the revision and development process of the ICD-11. Despite making progress toward formally recognizing GD and attempting to define it clinically, the proposed inclusion in both the DSM-5 and ICD-11 has led to many debates among scholars in the literature, further generating controversies regarding the clinical status and merits accepting GD as a bona fide addictive disorder (e.g., Aarseth et al., 2017; Griffiths et al., 2016; Petry et al., 2014; Saunders et al., 2017).

Prevalence of Gaming Disorder

Currently there is no agreement on the prevalence rates of GD as the vast majority of studies have used self-selected samples (King et al., 2013; Pontes & Griffiths, 2015a). A review of GD prevalence studies conducted by Griffiths et al. (2015) reported a large variation in the prevalence rates (from 0.2 percent up to 34 percent). However, the authors noted that there were many factors that could have accounted for the wide variation in prevalence rates including the type of gaming examined (i.e., some studies just examined online gaming, whereas others examined console gaming or a mixture of both), sample size, participants' age range, participant type (i.e., some surveyed the general population while others assessed gamers only, the latter which would inflate estimates), and instruments used to assess gaming.

There have been a handful of studies that have reported the prevalence of GD using nationally representative samples. The prevalence rates reported in these studies were 8.5 percent of American youth aged eight to eighteen years (Gentile, 2009), 1.2 percent of German adolescents aged thirteen to eighteen years (Rehbein et al., 2015), 5.5 percent among Dutch adolescents aged thirteen to twenty, and 5.4 percent among Dutch adults (Lemmens, Valkenburg & Gentile, 2015), 4.3 percent of Hungarian adolescents aged fifteen to sixteen years (Király et al., 2014), 1.4 percent of Norwegian gamers (Wittek et al., 2016), 2.5 percent among Slovenian adolescents aged twelve to sixteen years (Pontes, Macur & Griffiths, 2016), and 1.6 percent of European youth from seven countries aged fourteen to seventeen years (Müller et al., 2015). More recent epidemiological findings from robust studies using large and nationally representative samples reported comparable prevalence rates according to geographical regions and age of gamers. More specifically, GD has been found to affect 2 percent of adults in Macao, China (Wu et al., 2018), and 1.2 percent of Norwegian adolescents (Myrseth & Notelaers, 2018). One may speculate that prevalence is relatively high among American youth, and that, otherwise, prevalence is between 1 percent and 5 percent. However, it is premature to suggest a consistent pattern of prevalence estimates by age or location based on the studies completed to date.

Assessment and Neurobiology of Gaming Disorder

Assessment

There are now over twenty-five different screening instruments including a number of new ones specifically incorporating the DSM-5 IGD criteria (e.g., Király et al., 2017; Lemmens et al., 2015; Pontes & Griffiths, 2015b; van Rooij, Schoenmakers & van de Mheen, 2017). A comprehensive review by King et al. (2013) examined the criteria of eighteen problematic gaming screens. The eighteen screens had been utilized in sixty-three quantitative studies (N = 58,415 participants). The main weaknesses identified were (i) inconsistency of core addiction indicators across studies, (ii) a general lack of any temporal dimension, (iii) inconsistent cutoff scores relating to clinical status, (iv) poor and/or inadequate inter-rater reliability and predictive validity, and (v) inconsistent and/or untested dimensionality. King et al. (2013) also questioned the appropriateness of certain screens for certain settings, because those used in

Table 23.1 Clinical interview screening questions for the assessment of problematic video-game use

Area of assessment	Screening questions
Presenting problem	1. When did you begin to notice problems with your gaming? 2. How long have you been gaming? 3. How much time do you spend on gaming each day? Week? Month? 4. What was going on in your life when you began gaming? 5. What was going on in your life when you began to have difficulties with your gaming?
Biological areas	1. Are you experiencing or previously experienced any health concerns? If so, please describe. 2. How have these health concerns been impacted by your gaming? 3. What treatment you have received for these health concerns? 4. Does your gaming interfere with your sleep/meal schedule? 5. What exercise patterns do you engage in? 6. What drugs and/or medications do you take? How much? How often? In the past?
Psychological areas	1. What types of gaming do you engage in? 2. What do you like/dislike about gaming? 3. How do you feel before, during, and after gaming? 4. What are your thoughts before, during, and after gaming? 5. Have you ever used gaming to help improve your mood or change your thoughts? 6. In what places at home or elsewhere do you usually engage in gaming 7. Have you ever felt anxious, depressed or isolated when not gaming?
Social areas	1. Has your gaming caused concerns with your family? 2. Has your gaming caused concerns with your significant other? 3. Has gaming caused concerns with your social activities and friendships? 4. Has gaming interfered with your performance at school or work? 5. What are your social/leisure/hobby activities?
Relapse prevention areas	1. Do you believe that you have a problem with your level of gaming? 2. What do you see as the benefits and costs of continued gaming? 3. What is your level of commitment to change your current gaming patterns? 4. What plans have you implemented in the past to deal with your level of gaming? 5. Have these plans worked?

Adapted from Beard (2005) and King et al. (2012).

clinical practice may require a different emphasis than those used in epidemiological, experimental, or neurobiological research settings (King et al., 2013; Koronczai et al., 2011).

For assessing clients with GD (but not necessarily intending to diagnose), King, Delfabbro and Griffiths (2012) noted that clinicians could use Beard's (2005) assessment protocol (which was designed for internet-related problems, but can be used for GD). The protocol (see Table 23.1) was originally designed to be used as a structured clinical interview but may be of practical utility for clinicians. The screening protocol may be particularly useful in cases where the clinician is aware of concurrent issues of GD, but is unsure of its relevance to the overall clinical conceptualization (King et al., 2012). The clinical assessment tool (C-VAT 2.0; by van Rooij et al., 2017) has been developed using a clinical sample of thirty-two Dutch adolescents (ages between thirteen and twenty-three years) and may be a potentially useful tool to be used by clinicians and practitioners in the future since it is based on the DSM-5 framework. However, more robust testing with large sample sizes and cross-cultural studies supporting the initial findings is warranted before definite conclusions can be made regarding the general validity of this tool. Finally, a recent study (Ko et al., 2014) has found that using the nine IGD criteria as in the DSM-5 (i.e., endorsement of five or more out of the nine criteria) may also be a valid procedure for clinical diagnosis of IGD.

Neurobiology

Further research into GD is needed to uncover key clinical, epidemiological, and neurobiological aspects associate to the phenomenon. More recently, several empirical reports and review studies with broad coverage of neurocognitive, neurophysiological, neurochemical, and neuroimaging research techniques have been published on GD and other behavioral addictions (Choi, King & Jung, 2019). Furthermore, a meta-analysis (Meng et al., 2014) of ten neuroimaging studies investigating the functional brain response to cognitive tasks from GD found reliable clusters of abnormal activation in GD within the regions comprising the bilateral medial frontal gyrus/cingulate gyrus, the left middle temporal gyrus, and fusiform gyrus when compared to healthy controls. Moreover, Meng and colleagues (2014) also found that greater amounts of time spent per week playing was associated with hyperactivity in the left medial frontal gyrus and the right cingulate gyrus. However, one of the major limitations of this meta-analysis was that 90 percent of the studies reviewed were conducted in Asian countries or regions, which might be problematic since prevalence rates of GD in these populations are usually inflated compared to prevalence rates reported in Western countries (Pontes & Griffiths, 2015a).

More recently, a systematic review by Kuss, Pontes and Griffiths (2018) on neuroimaging studies concluded that there appeared to be significant neurobiological differences between healthy controls and individuals with GD. The included studies suggest that disordered gamers present with worse response inhibition and emotion regulation, impaired prefrontal cortex functioning and cognitive control, worse working memory and decision-making capabilities, decreased visual and auditory functioning, and a deficiency in their neuronal reward system. These deficiencies are similar to those found in individuals with substance-related addictions, suggesting that both substance-related and behavioral addictions share common predisposing factors and may be part of an addiction syndrome (Shaffer et al., 2004; Spechler et al., 2016).

Despite the invaluable contributions offered by neuroimaging studies on GD, several limitations potentially compromising the generalizability of the results of these studies need to be highlighted. As the majority of these studies are cross-sectional, it is not possible to ascertain the causal relationships between GD and the altered structures in the brain reported across these studies. Further prospective studies are necessary to understand the roles of altered brain structures in the mechanism of GD. In addition to this, further studies would benefit from larger sample sizes, as the studies reviewed by Kuss et al. (2018) were limited with regards to the number of participants. Another well-known problem in these studies is the use of generalized Internet addiction assessment tools to assess GD (see Pontes, Kuss & Griffiths [2017] for a review on the topic). Still, the emerging body of research on the neurobiology of GD demonstrate that the study of GD from a neurobiological perspective is continuing to flourish (Choi et al., 2019).

Etiology of Gaming Disorder

Over the past decade, a number of studies have investigated the association between GD (and its derivatives) and various personality and comorbidity factors. A review by Griffiths et al. (2015) summarized the research examining the relationship between personality traits and GD. Empirical studies have shown GD to be associated with (i) neuroticism, (ii) aggression and hostility, (iii) avoidant and schizoid tendencies, loneliness and introversion, (iv) social inhibition, (v) boredom inclination, (vi) sensation-seeking, (vii) diminished agreeableness, (viii) diminished self-control and narcissistic personality traits, (ix) low self-esteem, (x) state and trait anxiety, and (xi) low emotional intelligence. However, Griffiths and colleagues (2015) noted that it was difficult to assess the etiological significance of such associations because these personality factors are not unique to GD. The same review also reported that GD had been associated with various comorbid disorders, including (i) attention deficit hyperactivity disorder, (ii) symptoms of generalized anxiety disorder, panic disorder, depression, and social phobia, and (iii) various psychosomatic symptoms (Griffiths et al., 2015).

A recent empirical study investigating the potential etiology of GD and its implication with personality traits found that the relationship between GD and maladaptive personality traits (i.e., negative affectivity, detachment, and psychoticism) was mediated by avoidance expectancies (i.e., that gaming can help one to escape from reality or avoid negative feelings; Laier, Wegmann & Brand, 2018). Furthermore, the same study reported that negative affectivity, detachment, antagonism, disinhibition, psychoticism and gaming-related positive and avoidance expectancies were strongly associated to symptoms of GD (Laier et al., 2018). In sum, recent studies suggest that maladaptive personality traits and gaming-related positive expectancies and avoidance expectancies are key risk factors for the development of GD, and that positive expectancies and avoidance expectancies play a distinct role in relation to their mediating role between general personality characteristics and symptoms of GD (Laier et al., 2018).

Internet Gaming Disorder versus Internet Addiction

Before IGD appeared in Section 3 of the DSM-5, there had been debates about whether internet addiction (IA) or its derivatives (e.g., Internet Use Disorder, Internet Addiction Disorder) should have also been included as a separate disorder (Block, 2008; Christakis, 2010; Griffiths, King & Demetrovics, 2014; Petry & O'Brien, 2013; Pies, 2009). This mirrored debates among scholars as to whether excessive problematic Internet use can be considered a genuine addiction. Some scholars differentiate between generalized IA (i.e., the totality of all online activities) and specific addictions on the internet, such as internet gambling, internet gaming and internet sex (Davis, 2001; Griffiths, 2000; Griffiths & Pontes, 2014; Griffiths & Szabo, 2014; Pontes & Patrão, 2014; Pontes, Szabo & Griffiths, 2015). Since the late 1990s, Griffiths (1999, 2000) has constantly argued that there is a fundamental difference between addictions *on* the internet, and addictions *to* the internet. Griffiths argued that the overwhelming majority of individuals that were allegedly addicted to the internet were not internet addicts; these were individuals that used the medium of the internet as a vehicle for other addictions. More specifically, he argued that internet gaming addicts were not internet addicts but were gaming addicts using the convenience and ubiquity of the internet to play video games (Griffiths, 2000).

An empirical survey using a nationally representative population of adolescents clearly showed that IA and internet gaming addiction are not the same. More specifically, Király et al. (2014) examined the interrelationship and the overlap between IA and IGD in as a function of variables including gender, time spent using the internet and/or online gaming, and preferred online activities. They collected their data from a nationally representative sample of over 2,000 adolescents. They found that IGD was much more strongly associated with being male, and that IA was positively associated with online chatting, online gaming, and social networking, while IGD was only associated with online gaming. Similar to previous studies (Griffiths & Pontes, 2014; Montag et al., 2014; Rehbein & Mößle, 2013), the authors argued that IGD was a conceptually different behavior than IA and that their data supported the notion that IA and IGD are separate nosological entities.

Treatment of Gaming Disorder

There have been over twenty treatment studies published (e.g., Graham, 2014; Han, Kim & Renshaw, 2015; Jiménez-Murcia et al., 2015; Pallesen et al., 2015; Poddar, Sayeed & Mitra, 2015; Sachdeva & Verma, 2015; Torres-Rodríguez & Carbonell, 2015). However, many of the treatment studies do not distinguish between Internet Use Disorder (IUD; sometimes referred to as IA) and GD. For instance, a meta-analysis by Winkler and colleagues (2013) evaluated the short-term and long-term efficacy of both pharmacological and psychological treatments for IUD in sixteen studies (N = 670 patients) that also included treatment of IGD. The authors concluded that both types of treatment were effective in treating and reducing symptoms of IUD, time spent online, anxiety, and depression. For psychological treatments, the short-term efficacy was reported as large and robust (and maintained over follow-up).

Przepiórka et al. (2014) recommended that clinicians should combine both cognitive-behavioral therapy (CBT) and pharmacological treatments, including use of opioid receptor antagonists (e.g., naltrexone combined with sertraline), antidepressants (e.g., escitalopram, bupropion), antipsychotics (e.g., olanzapine, quetiapine), and psychostimulants (e.g., methylphenidate). On the other hand, recent reviews have suggested that multimodal treatments were most effective in combatting online addictions (Pontes et al., 2017). Multimodal interventions typically include group CBT for students with Internet addiction, psychoeducation for teachers on the recognition and psychological treatment of internet addiction, and simultaneous group cognitive behavioral parent training (Du, Jiang & Vance, 2010).

In terms of psychological treatments for GD, CBT appears to be the most widely used. A number of review papers have noted that this model has been used to treat GD (King et al., 2011; Pontes, Kuss & Griffiths, 2015; Winkler et al., 2013). The first stage of treatment is typically focused on the behavioral aspects of the gaming addict, so that at subsequent stages the focus of treatment is gradually shifted toward the development of positive cognitive assumptions. During therapy, gaming addicts identify false beliefs and learn how to modify them into more adaptive ones (cognitive restructuring). Additionally, the cognitive-behavioral approach also advocates that the addict should monitor their thoughts in order to identify affective and situational triggers associated with their addictive gaming behavior (self-instructional training).

A recent systematic review of clinical research included forty-six studies with clinical samples (Kuss & Lopez-Fernandez, 2016). Studies were selected based on the following inclusion criteria. Studies had to (i) contain quantitative empirical data; (ii) have been published after 2000; (iii) include clinical samples and/or clinical interventions for Internet and/or gaming addiction; (iv) provide a full text paper (rather than a conference abstract) published in a peer-reviewed journal; and (v) be published in English, German, Polish, Spanish, Portuguese, or French as the authors spoke these languages. The included studies used clinical samples and outlined characteristics of individuals seeking treatment and the different treatment approaches used. Four main types of clinical research studies were identified, namely research involving: (i) treatment seeker characteristics; (ii) psychopharmacotherapy; (iii) psychological therapy; and (iv) combined treatment. Regarding the treatment, both psychological as well as psychopharmacological treatments appear efficacious in treating Internet and gaming addiction. Psychopharmacological treatment often included prescribing selective serotonin reuptake inhibitors (SSRIs), such as escitalopram, anxiolytics, often used to treat anxiety disorders, including Obsessive-Compulsive Disorder (OCD); stimulants often used for Attention Deficit Hyperactivity Disorder (ADHD); and atypical antipsychotics often administered for schizophrenia spectrum disorders (such as psychosis and schizotypal personality disorder). Overall, the studies using psychopharmacological therapy to treat internet and gaming addiction lead to decreasing internet addiction symptoms and the time spent on the internet and gaming. Antidepressants were used most often, indicating that mood disorders have a relatively high comorbidity with internet and gaming addiction. In addition to this, Kuss & Lopez-Fernandez (2016) suggested that if other (primary or secondary) disorders are comorbid conditions (such as OCD and ADHD), pharmaceutical medication often used for these conditions may be useful in decreasing problems associated with internet addiction.

Furthermore, Kuss & Lopez-Fernandez (2016) reported that ten studies used individual and group therapy to treat Internet and gaming addiction and associated symptoms. Based on their analysis, CBT was the type of psychological therapy most often used to treat internet and gaming addiction. Generally, CBT included eight to twenty-eight sessions that incorporated the following elements: psychoeducation, problem identification, teaching healthy communication, increasing internet awareness, and teaching cessation techniques, such as response inhibition. Moreover, a comparable short-term treatment for internet and video-game addiction was applied, as well as group therapy, including systemic therapy with parents/teachers/peer support and/or multilevel interventions, that incorporated Motivational Interviewing, often used to treat substance-related addictions.

In their review, Kuss and Lopez-Fernandez (2016) identified six studies that combined psychological treatment (primarily CBT) with other psychological therapies, such as Motivational Enhancement Therapy, a Lifestyle Training Programme, psychopharmacotherapy (such as antidepressants and anxiolytics), or with electroacupuncture therapy. Poddar and colleagues (2015) used Motivational Enhancement Therapy together with CBT (METCB). METCBT included various stages: (i) a contemplation stage (i.e., initial sessions of rapport building including a detailed interview and case formulation; (ii) a preparation stage (i.e., sessions delivered in an empathetic atmosphere to emphasize psychoeducation, including managing physiological and emotional arousal through relaxation techniques, and a cost-benefit analysis of gaming addiction); and (iii) a contract stage with the patient, a parent, and the therapist (i.e., behavior modification of gaming, reducing time spent online and promoting healthy activities). Using METCBT resulted in symptom decrease, and the young patients improved their school performance (Poddar et al., 2015). Electroacupuncture was also used as an adjunct to CBT by Zhu and colleagues (2008), and was applied at acupoints Baihui (GV20), Sishencong (EX-HN1), Hegu (LI4), Neiguan (PC6), Taichong (LR3), and Sanyinjiao (SP6), and retained for thirty minutes every other day with successful results (Kuss & Lopez-Fernandez, 2016).

Taken together, therapy that combined different approaches was beneficial for all groups because internet addiction symptomatology decreased at all measurement time points. For instance, applying electroacupuncture in combination with a psychological treatment enhanced treatment outcomes for Internet addiction above CBT alone, providing evidence for the effectiveness of this approach (Zhu et al., 2008). In addition to this, psychopharmacological therapy is not always as efficacious for cooccurring conditions, such as major depressive disorder, relative to its effectiveness for internet and gaming addiction, suggesting that medication may work better for gaming addiction relative to a comorbid disorder. This is noteworthy because it appears that internet addiction commonly cooccurs with other psychological disorders. This review also indicated that psychopharmacotherapy added to psychological treatment may not always be beneficial in alleviating problems of comorbidity (such as depressive symptoms which often accompany internet and gaming addiction), and therefore the appropriate treatment should be chosen based on the individual client's needs (Kuss & Lopez-Fernandez, 2016).

More recently, Torres-Rodriguez and colleagues have published a number of studies concerning a new treatment for adolescent GD developed in Spain – the Programa Individualizado Psicoterapéutico para la Adicción a las Tecnologías de la Información y la Comunicación" [PIPATIC] program (Torres-Rodriguez et al., 2017, 2018a, 2018b, 2018c). The primary goal of the PIPATIC program (see Torres-Rodríguez et al. [2017] for an in-depth description) is to offer specialized psychotherapy for adolescents with symptoms of GD and comorbid disorders. The program comprises six therapeutic work modules, in turn made up of more specific subobjectives. The program has an integrative focus (including the GD, the comorbid symptoms, intrapersonal and interpersonal abilities, and family psychotherapy). Their study involved a small sample of thirty-one adolescents (aged twelve to eighteen years) from two public mental health centers who were assigned to either the (i) PIPATIC intervention experimental group or (ii) standard CBT. Significant differences were found at pre-test and post-test on various variables (comorbid disorders, intrapersonal and interpersonal abilities, family relationships and therapists' measures). Both groups experienced a significant reduction of GD symptoms, although the PIPATIC group experienced higher significant improvements in the remainder of the variables examined.

A systematic review (Pontes & Griffiths, 2015c) of seventeen empirical studies that analyzed GD and its associated cognitions and cognitive-related impairments found that several types of cognitive impairments were frequently reported by empirical studies meeting the inclusion criteria. More specifically, the set of cognitive-related factors and specific cognitive impairments associated with GD were the following: deficient self-regulation; preference for a virtual life; cognitive bias; impaired cognitive control ability; cognitive deficits; poor cognitive error processing; decision-making deficits; maladaptive cognitions; and cognitive distortions. Given the prominence of the cognitive-related variables in GD, Pontes and Griffiths (2015c) noted that the CBT approach could benefit from taking into account the different sets of cognitions present in disordered gamers.

Early intervention approaches by Young (1999) proposed strategies for treatment of online addiction (including gaming), including: (i) practicing the opposite (i.e., identifying patients' patterns of gaming use and then helping them disrupt their normal routine of gaming usage and readapting new time patterns of use to break the online gaming habits), (ii) using external stoppers (i.e., real events or activities that prompt addicts to disconnect from the their gaming), (iii) setting goals with regard to the amount of time spent gaming online, (iv) using reminder cards that serve as cues to remind addicts of the costs of excessive gaming and benefits of breaking free from it, (v) developing a personal inventory of activities the addicts can engage in instead of engaging in excessive gaming, (vi) entering a support group to compensate for the lack of social support (if applicable), and (vii) engaging in family therapy to address relational problems between addicts and their family. As far as the present authors are aware, the effectiveness of such an approach has not yet been evaluated in a randomized controlled trial. Although the CBT model for treating GD appears to be effective, there do not appear to be significant differences between CBT and other psychological treatments that treat GD (Winkler et al., 2013). For this reason, other treatment approaches might be useful to treat this condition, such as multifamily group therapy (Liu et al., 2015).

A systematic review of online addiction treatment studies using the Consolidating Standards of Reporting Trials (CONSORT) guidelines by King et al. (2011) noted that almost all of them had severe methodological problems and several key limitations. The review found that there was a lack of adequate controls or other comparison groups; randomization and blinding techniques; information concerning recruitment dates, sample characteristics, and treatment effect sizes.

Conclusions

According to Petry and O'Brien (2013), IGD will not be included as a separate mental disorder in future editions of the DSM until the (i) defining features of IGD have been identified, (ii) reliability and validity of specific IGD criteria have been obtained cross-culturally, (iii) prevalence rates have been determined in representative epidemiological samples across the world, and (iv) etiology and associated biological features have been evaluated. Standardized and comprehensive methods of diagnosis are at present lacking. As noted above, almost all IGD treatment studies have methodological shortcomings and none have assessed long-term efficacy of the interventions. To determine posttreatment outcomes, diagnostic assessment should include gaming frequency, IGD symptoms (e.g., tolerance, withdrawal, relapse), functioning at work/school/college, participation in leisure time activities and hobbies, and quality of interpersonal relationships, among other criteria (Király, Griffiths & Demetrovics, 2015). Additionally, factors that prevent relapse should also be investigated, such as the influence of social context (Kuss & Pontes, 2019). Previous research (Kuss & Griffiths, 2015) has also investigated perceptions and experiences of psychotherapists who are treating individuals presenting with the problem of Internet and gaming addiction, yielding relevant results with regards to diagnosis, problem experience, and risk factors. This research should be extended by specifically addressing issues of relapse risk and prevention from the perspective of both the clients seeking help as well as the trained experts providing it.

Griffiths et al. (2016) have also made recommendations about how consensus concerning GD in studying gaming behaviors can be achieved. These included: (a) carrying out further studies from treatment seeking individuals in the clinical population (i.e., live field testing) rather than further epidemiological studies in countries that have already carried out such studies (because epidemiological studies are not the best place to identify and examine new disorders); (b) carrying out studies on heavy use of gaming among those without any problems (i.e., high engagement players); (c) forming an international alliance of GD researchers to generate an item pool of GD items for use in multinational collaborative studies; (d) forming working parties that comprise multistakeholders rather than just academics (e.g., gaming industry, gamers, psychiatrists, therapists); and (e) reevaluating already existing data on GD more effectively and critically to help develop consensus (as this might be helpful for understanding the nature of some aspects, such as withdrawal. Given the potentially detrimental social, psychological and physiological health consequences of excessive gaming and gaming addiction, there is a collective responsibility as researchers, health care providers, parents, teachers, governments and gaming developers to prevent gaming addiction from developing in the first place, to raise awareness of possible negative consequences, and to provide treatments for those who need them (Kuss et al., 2019).

REFERENCES

Aarseth, E., Bean, A. M., Boonen, H., et al. (2017). Scholars' open debate paper on the World Health Organization ICD-11 Gaming Disorder proposal. *Journal of Behavioral Addiction*, **6**(3), 267–270.

American Psychiatric Association [APA] (2013). *Diagnostic and Statistical Manual of Mental Disorders - Text Revision* (5th edition). Arlington, VA: American Psychiatric Publishing.

Beard, K. W. (2005). Internet Addiction: A review of current assessment techniques and potential assessment questions. *CyberPsychology & Behavior*, **8**(1), 7–14.

Block, J. (2008). Issues for DSM-V: Internet addiction. *American Journal of Psychiatry*, **165**(3), 306–307.

Choi, J. S., King, D. L. & Jung, Y. C. (2019). Editorial: Neurobiological perspectives in behavioral addiction. *Frontiers in Psychiatry*, **10**(3). https://doi.org/10.3389/fpsyt.2019.00003

Christakis, D. (2010). Internet addiction: A 21st century epidemic? *BMC Medicine*, **8**(1), 61.

Davis, R. A. (2001). A cognitive-behavioral model of pathological Internet use. *Computers in Human Behavior*, **17**(2), 187–195.

Du, Y. S., Jiang, W. Q. & Vance, A. (2010). Longer term effect of randomized, controlled group cognitive behavioural therapy for Internet addiction in adolescent students in Shanghai. *Australian and New Zealand Journal of Psychiatry*, **44**(2), 129–134.

Gentile, D. (2009). Pathological video-game use among youth ages 8–18: A national study. *Psychological Science*, **20**(5), 594–602.

Graham Jr., J. M. (2014). Narrative therapy for treating video game addiction. *International Journal of Mental Health and Addiction*, **12**, 701–707.

Griffiths, M.D. (1999). Internet addiction: Internet fuels other addictions. *Student British Medical Journal*, **7**, 428–429.

Griffiths, M. D. (2000). Internet addiction – Time to be taken seriously? *Addiction Research*, **8**(5), 413–418.

Griffiths, M. D. & Pontes, H. M. (2014). Internet Addiction Disorder and Internet Gaming Disorder are not the same. *Journal of Addiction Research & Therapy*, **5**(4), e124.

Griffiths, M. D. & Szabo, A. (2014). Is excessive online usage a function of medium or activity? An empirical pilot study. *Journal of Behavioral Addictions*, **3**(1), 74–77.

Griffiths, M. D., King, D. L. & Demetrovics, Z. (2014). DSM-5 Internet Gaming Disorder needs a unified approach to assessment. *Neuropsychiatry*, **4**(1), 1–4.

Griffiths, M. D., Király, O., Pontes, H. M. & Demetrovics, Z. (2015). An overview of problematic gaming. In E. Aboujaoude & V. Starcevic (Eds.), *Mental Health in the Digital Age: Grave Dangers, Great Promise*. Oxford: Oxford University Press, pp. 27–45.

Griffiths, M. D., Van Rooij, A., Kardefelt-Winther, D., et al. (2016). Working towards an international consensus on criteria for assessing Internet gaming disorder: A critical commentary on Petry et al. (2014). *Addiction*, **111**, 167–175.

Han, D. H., Kim, S. M. & Renshaw, P. F. (2015). Functional brain changes in response to treatment of Internet Gaming Disorder. In C. Montag & M. Reuter (Eds.), *Internet Addiction*. Springer International Publishing, pp. 77–91.

Jiménez-Murcia, S., Fernández-Aranda, F., Granero, R., et al. (2015). Nuevas tecnologías como estrategia terapéutica complementaria para el Transtorno de Juego [New technologies as a complimentary therapeutic strategy for the treatment of Internet Gaming Disorder]. *Aloma: Revista de Psicologia, Ciències de l'Educació i de l'Esport*, **33**(2), 59–66.

King, D. L., Delfabbro, P. H. & Griffiths, M. D. (2012). Clinical interventions for technology-based problems: Excessive Internet and video game use. *Journal of Cognitive Psychotherapy: An International Quarterly*, **26**(1), 43–56.

King, D. L., Delfabbro, P. H., Griffiths, M. D. & Gradisar, M. (2011). Assessing clinical trials of Internet addiction treatment: A systematic review and CONSORT evaluation. *Clinical Psychology Review*, **31**(7), 1110–1116.

King, D. L., Haagsma, M. C., Delfabbro, P. H., Gradisar, M. S. & Griffiths, M. D. (2013). Toward a consensus definition of pathological video-gaming: A systematic review of psychometric assessment tools. *Clinical Psychology Review*, **33**(3), 331–342.

Király, O., Griffiths, M. D. & Demetrovics, Z. (2015). Internet Gaming Disorder and the DSM-5: Conceptualization, debates, and controversies. *Current Addiction Reports*, **2**(3), 254–262.

Király, O., Griffiths, M. D., Urbán, R., et al. (2014). Problematic internet use and problematic online gaming are not the same: Findings from a large nationally representative adolescent sample. *Cyberpsychology, Behavior, and Social Networking*, **17**(12), 749–754.

Király, O., Sleczka, P., Pontes, H. M., et al. (2017). Validation of the ten-item Internet Gaming Disorder Test (IGDT-10) and evaluation of the nine DSM-5 Internet Gaming Disorder criteria. *Addictive Behaviors*, **64**, 253–260.

Ko, C. H., Yen, J. Y., Chen, S. H., et al. (2014). Evaluation of the diagnostic criteria of Internet Gaming Disorder in the DSM-5 among young adults in Taiwan. *Journal of Psychiatric Research*, **53**(6), 103–110.

Koronczai, B., Urbán, R., Kökönyei, G., et al. (2011). Confirmation of the three-factor model of problematic internet use on off-line adolescent and adult samples. *Cyberpsychology, Behavior, and Social Networking*, **14**(11), 657–664.

Kuss, D. J. & Griffiths, M. D. (2015). *Internet Addiction in Psychotherapy*. London: Palgrave.

Kuss, D. J. & Lopez-Fernandez, O. (2016). Internet addiction and problematic Internet use: A systematic review of clinical research. *World Journal of Psychiatry*, **6**(1), 143–176.

Kuss, D. J. & Pontes, H. M. (2019). *Internet Addiction. Advances in Psychotherapy – Evidence-Based Practice (Volume 47)*. Hogrefe.

Kuss, D. J., Griffiths, M. D., Karila, L. & Billieux, J. (2014). Internet addiction: A systematic review of epidemiological research for the last decade. *Current Pharmaceutical Design*, ***20***(25), 4026–4052.

Kuss, D. J., Pontes, H. M. & Griffiths, M. D. (2018). Neurobiological correlates in Internet Gaming Disorder: A systematic review. *Frontiers in Psychiatry*, **9**, 166.

Kuss, D. J., Throuvala, M., Pontes, H. M., et al. (2019). *Tackling digital and gaming addiction: A challenge for the 21st Century*. Report submitted to the UK Parliament's Select Committee on Digital, Culture, Media and Sport relating to Immersive and Addictive Technologies. Nottingham: Nottingham Trent University.

Laier, C., Wegmann, E. & Brand, M. (2018). Personality and cognition in gamers: Avoidance expectancies mediate the relationship between maladaptive personality traits and symptoms of Internet-Gaming Disorder. *Frontiers in Psychiatry*, **9**, 304.

Lemmens, J. S., Valkenburg, P. M. & Gentile, D.A. (2015). The Internet Gaming Disorder Scale. *Psychological Assessment*, **27**(2), 567–582.

Liu, Q-X., Fang, X-Y., Yan, N., et al. (2015). Multi-family group therapy for adolescent Internet addiction: Exploring the underlying mechanisms. *Addictive Behaviors*, **42**, 1–8.

Meng, Y., Deng, W., Wang, H., Guo, W. & Li, T. (2014). The prefrontal dysfunction in individuals with Internet Gaming Disorder: A meta-analysis of functional magnetic resonance imaging studies. *Addiction Biology*, **20**(4), 799–808.

Montag, C., Bey, K., Sha, P., et al. (2014). Is it meaningful to distinguish between generalized and specific internet addiction? Evidence from a cross-cultural study from Germany, Sweden, Taiwan and China. *Asia-Pacific Psychiatry*, **7**(1), 20–26.

Müller, K. W., Janikian, M., Dreier, M., et al. (2015). Regular gaming behavior and internet gaming disorder in European adolescents: Results from a cross-national representative survey of prevalence, predictors, and psychopathological correlates. *European Child and Adolescent Psychiatry*, **24**(5), 565–574.

Myrseth, H. & Notelaers, G. (2018). A latent class approach for classifying the problem and disordered gamers in a group of adolescence. *Frontiers in Psychology*, **9**(2273). doi: 10.3389/fpsyg.2018.02273

Pallesen, S., Lorvik, I. M., Bu, E. H. & Molde, H. (2015). An exploratory study investigating the effects of a treatment manual for video game addiction. *Psychological Reports*, **117**(2), 490–495.

Petry, N. M. & O'Brien, C. P. (2013). Internet gaming disorder and the DSM-5. *Addiction*, **108**(7), 1186–1187.

Petry, N. M., Rehbein, F., Gentile, D. A., et al. (2014). An international consensus for assessing internet gaming disorder using the new DSM-5 approach. *Addiction*, **109**(9), 1399–1406.

Pies, R. (2009). Should DSM-V Designate "Internet Addiction" a Mental Disorder? *Psychiatry (Edgmont)*, **6**(2), 31–37.

Poddar, S., Sayeed, N. & Mitra, S. (2015). Internet Gaming Disorder: Application of motivational enhancement therapy principles in treatment. *Indian Journal of Psychiatry*, **57** (1), 100–101.

Pontes, H. M. & Griffiths, M. D. (2015a). New concepts, old known issues: The DSM-5 and Internet Gaming Disorder and its assessment. In J. Bishop (Ed.), *Psychological and Social Implications Surrounding Internet and Gaming Addiction*. Hershey, PA: Information Science Reference, pp. 16–30.

Pontes, H. & Griffiths, M.D. (2015b). Measuring DSM-5 Internet Gaming Disorder: Development and validation of a short psychometric scale. *Computers in Human Behavior*, **45**, 137–143.

Pontes, H. M. & Griffiths, M. D. (2015c). Internet Gaming Disorder and its associated cognitions and cognitive-related impairments: A systematic review using PRISMA guidelines. *Revista Argentina de Ciencias del Comportamiento*, **7**(3), 102–118.

Pontes, H. M. & Patrão, I. M. (2014). Estudo exploratório sobre as motivações percebidas no uso excessivo da Internet em adolescentes e jovens adultos [An exploratory study on the perceived motivations underpinning excessive Internet use among adolescents and young adults]. *Psychology, Community & Health*, **3**(2), 90–102.

Pontes, H. M., Kuss, D. J. & Griffiths, M. D. (2015). Clinical psychology of Internet addiction: A review of its conceptualization, prevalence, neuronal processes, and implications for treatment. *Neuroscience and Neuroeconomics*, **4**, 11–23.

Pontes, H. M., Kuss, D. J. & Griffiths, M. D. (2017). Psychometric assessment of Internet Gaming Disorder in neuroimaging studies: A systematic review. In C. Montag & M. Reuter (Eds.), *Internet Addiction: Neuroscientific Approaches and Therapeutical Implications Including Smartphone Addiction*. Cham: Springer International Publishing, pp. 181–208.

Pontes, H. M., Macur, M. & Griffiths, M. D. (2016). Internet Gaming Disorder among Slovenian primary schoolchildren: Findings from a nationally representative sample of adolescents. *Journal of Behavioral Addictions*, **5**, 304–310.

Pontes, H. M., Szabo, A. & Griffiths, M. D. (2015). The impact of Internet-based specific activities on the perceptions of Internet addiction, quality of life, and excessive usage: A cross-sectional study. *Addictive Behaviors Reports*, **1**, 19–25.

Przepiórka, A. M., Blachnio, A., Miziak, B. & Czuczwar, S. J. (2014). Clinical approaches to treatment of Internet addiction. *Pharmacological Reports*, **66**(2), 187–191.

Reed, G. M., First, M. B., Kogan, C. S., et al. (2019). Innovations and changes in the ICD-11 classification of mental, behavioural and neurodevelopmental disorders. *World Psychiatry*, **18**(1), 3–19.

Rehbein, F. & Mößle, T. (2013). Video game and internet addiction: Is there a need for differentiation? *SUCHT-Zeitschrift für Wissenschaft und Praxis/Journal of Addiction Research and Practice*, **59**(3), 129–142.

Rehbein, F., Kliem, S., Baier, D., Mößle, T. & Petry, N. M. (2015). Prevalence of Internet Gaming Disorder in German adolescents: Diagnostic contribution of the nine DSM-5 criteria in a state-wide representative sample. *Addiction*, **110**(5), 842–851.

Sachdeva, A. & Verma, R. (2015). Internet gaming addiction: A technological hazard. *International Journal of High Risk Behaviors and Addiction*, **4**(4), e26359.

Saunders, J. B., Hao, W., Long, J., et al. (2017). Gaming disorder: Its delineation as an important condition for diagnosis, management and prevention. *Journal of Behavioral Addictions*, **6**, 271–279.

Shaffer, H. J., LaPlante, D. A., LaBrie, R. A., et al. (2004). Toward a syndrome model of addiction: Multiple expressions, common etiology. *Harvard Review of Psychiatry*, **12**(6), 367–374.

Spechler, P. A., Chaarani, B., Hudson, K. E., et al. (2016). Response inhibition and addiction medicine: From use to abstinence. *Progress in Brain Research*, **223**, 143–164.

Torres-Rodríguez, A. & Carbonell, X. (2015). Adicción a los videjuegos en línea: tratamiento mediante el programa PIPATIC [Online Gaming Addiction: The PIPATIC treatement program]. *Aloma: Revista de Psicologia, Ciències de l'Educació i de l'Esport*, **33**(2), 67–75.

Torres-Rodriguez, A., Griffiths, M. D. & Carbonell, X. (2018a). The treatment of Internet Gaming Disorder: A brief overview of the PIPATIC program. *International Journal of Mental Health and Addiction*, **16**, 1000–1015.

Torres-Rodriguez, A., Griffiths, M. D., Carbonell, X. Farriols-Hernando, N. & Torres-Jimenez, E. (2017). Internet gaming disorder treatment: A case study evaluation of four adolescent problematic gamers. *International Journal of Mental Health and Addiction*. Epub ahead of print. https://doi.org/10.1007/s11469-017-9845-9

Torres-Rodriguez, A., Griffiths, M. D., Carbonell, X. & Oberst, U. (2018b). Psychological characteristics of an adolescent clinical sample with Internet Gaming Disorder. *Journal of Behavioral Addictions*, **7**, 707–718.

Torres-Rodriguez, A., Griffiths, M. D., Carbonell, X. & Oberst, U. (2018c). Treatment effectiveness of a specialized psychotherapy program for Internet Gaming Disorder. *Journal of Behavioral Addictions*, **7**, 939–952.

van Rooij, A. J., Schoenmakers, T. M. & van de Mheen, D. (2017). Clinical validation of the C-VAT 2.0 assessment tool for gaming disorder: A sensitivity analysis of the proposed DSM-5 criteria and the clinical characteristics of young patients with 'video game addiction'. *Addictive Behaviors*, **64**, 269–274.

Winkler, A., Dörsing, B., Rief, W., Shen, Y. & Glombiewski, J. A. (2013). Treatment of Internet addiction: A meta-analysis. *Clinical Psychology Review*, **33**(2), 317–329.

Wittek, C. T., Finserås, T. R., Pallesen, S., et al. (2016). Prevalence and predictors of video game addiction: A study based on a national representative sample of gamers. *International Journal of Mental Health and Addiction*, **14**, 672–686.

World Health Organization (2018). Gaming disorder. Retrieved from http://id.who.int/icd/entity/1448597234. Accessed by February 15, 2019. (Archived by WebCite at www.webcitation.org/6m0iJOU1Q)

Wu, A. M. S., Chen, J. H., Tong, K. K., Yu, S. & Lau, J. T. F. (2018). Prevalence and associated factors of Internet gaming disorder among community dwelling adults in Macao, China. *Journal of Behavioral Addictions*, **7**(1), 62–69.

Young, K.S. (1999). *Internet Addiction: Symptoms, Evaluation and Treatment. Innovations in Clinical Practice: A Source Book (Volume 17)*. Sarasota, FL: Professional Resource Press, pp. 19–31.

Zhu, T.-M., Jin, R.-J., Zhong, X.-M., Chen, J. & Li, H. (2008). Paper in Chinese [Effects of electroacupuncture combined with psychologic interference on anxiety state and serum NE content in the patient of internet addiction disorder]. *Zhongguo Zhen Jiu*, **28**(8), 561–564.

Part V

Ongoing and Future Research Directions

24 Precision Behavioral Management (PBM): A Novel Genetically Guided Therapy to Combat Reward Deficiency Syndrome (RDS) Relevant to the Opiate Crisis

Kenneth Blum, PhD, DHL, Alphonse Kenison Roy III, MD, DFASAM, DLFAPA, Arwen Podesta, MD, Edward J. Modestino, PhD, Bruce Steinberg, PhD, Marjorie C. Gondré-Lewis, PhD, David Baron, DO, Panayotis K. Thanos, PhD, Lisa Lott, PhD, Sampada Badgaiyan, MD, Jessica Valdez Ponce, MS, Brent Boyett, DMD, DO, David Siwicki, MD, Mark Moran, MD, Drew Edwards, PhD, Thomas McLaughlin, MD, Eric R. Braverman, MD, Thomas A. Simpatico, MD, Mary Hauser, MA, Bernard William Downs, BS, and Rajendra D. Badgaiyan, MD

Introduction

The primary use of opioids, as analgesic pain treatment, is a momentous public health problem. Overdose deaths from prescription opioids increased significantly in parallel with increased opioid prescribing between 1999 and 2010 (Pergolizzi et al., 2018). Of the 33,091 deaths from drug overdoses in 2015, approximately half involved prescription opioids (Rudd et al., 2016). In the USA, an estimated two million individuals have opioid use disorder (OUD) with an estimated $78.5 billion in economic costs annually (Florence et al., 2016). Understanding the neurogenetic and neurobiological correlates of this addictive behavior can assist in changing prescribing practices, one step toward addressing the opioid overdose epidemic and its adverse effects on the US and global populations (Blum et al. 2015a, 2018h).

The interaction of neurotransmitters and second messengers that control the release of dopamine is known as the Brain Reward Cascade (BRC) (Blum et al., 2014a; Volkow, Wise & Baler, 2017; Willuhn et al., 2014). Opiate prescription medications impact the operations of the BRC. The BRC plays a central role in the modulation of nociception; the sensory nervous system's response to certain harmful stimuli, such as pain. Adaptations may impact several sensory and affective components of chronic pain syndromes in dopaminergic circuitry (Chen et al., 2009). The neurochemical impact of chronic opioids on the BRC is the down regulation of several neurotransmitters, including dopamine, mainly, at the reward site of the brain located in the Nucleus Accumbens (NAc) (see Figure 24.1).

Despite the well-known risk for opioid-induced hyperalgesia (OIH), which commonly results from long-term use of opioids, the medical establishment has encouraged the expanded use of opioids for the treatment of chronic pain. The process of OIH involves an alteration of pain salience, determined in the periaqueductal gray matter and the rostroventral medulla through hypodopaminergia, potentially via glutaminergic attenuation, resulting in increased pain sensitivity (Chen et al., 2009).

The challenge is to identify nonaddicting and nonpharmacological alternatives to assist in pain and addiction attenuation (Blum et al., 2018c; Salling & Martinez, 2016). Notably, a recent JAMA report provides strong evidence that nonopioid treatment like nonsteroidal anti-inflammatory drugs (NSAIDs) may be more effective than chronic opioids (Krebs et al., 2018; Smith et al., 2016). Several additional proven strategies have been developed to manage chronic pain effectively without opioids (Severino et al., 2018). They include "Reward Deficiency Solution System" (RDSS) and "Precision Behavioral Management" (PBM) based on analytic evidence, as presented in this chapter.

Assessment: Analytics of Genetic Addiction Risk Score (GARS)

In the mid 1990s, Blum coined the term, "Reward Deficiency Syndrome" (RDS) to portray behaviors found to have a gene-based association with hypo-dopaminergic function (Blum et al., 1990, 2017a, b; Smith, 2012). RDS has been embraced in many subsequent studies to increase the understanding of addictions and other obsessive, compulsive, and impulsive behaviors. Also, over the past thirty years, Blum's group has developed a ten-gene panel with several polymorphic variants of the functional genes that govern the brain reward circuit. This panel is called the Genetic Addiction Risk Score (GARS).

Knowing the result of the patient's GARS test can provide an in-depth assessment of a patient's brain reward functioning and assist in prophylaxis and early intervention for those at high risk for addiction (Blum et al., 2018a); Blum's group and others (Barh et al., 2017; Blum et al., 2012, 2014c), have published extensively on the genes related to dopaminergic function and reward (Berridge & Robinson, 2016). Interestingly, in one published study, Blum's group was able to describe lifetime RDS behaviors in a recovering addict (seventeen years sober) by assessing only the resultant Genetic Addiction Risk Score (GARS) data (Blum et al., 2013a). Based on early genetic testing it is possible that an effective strategy, like environmental manipulation, might prevent, reduce, or eliminate pathological substance and behavioral seeking activity (Loth et al., 2011).

RDS-Free Controls

Counting several risk alleles in an individual's GARS panel, as a measure of addiction risk severity seems quite acceptable as has been verified by

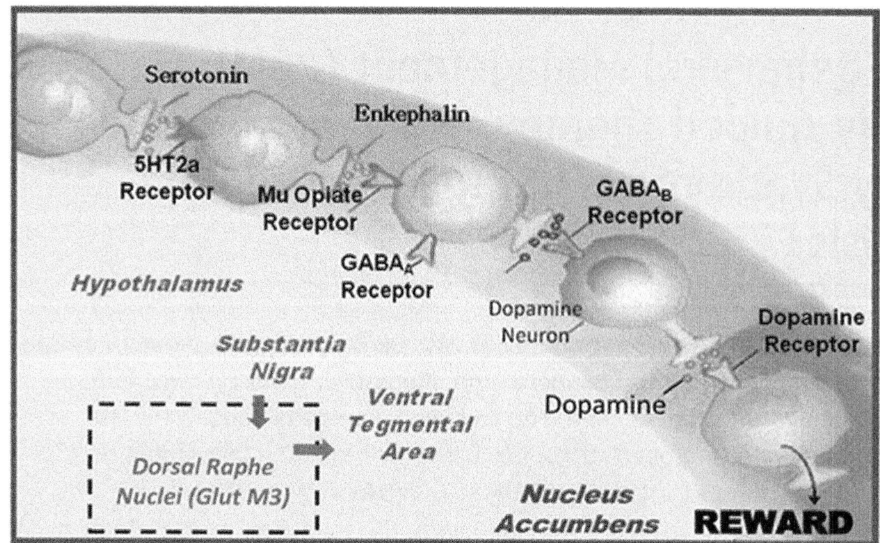

Figure 24.1 The Brain Reward Cascade
Note. Figure 24.1 illustrates the interaction of neurotransmitters within the mesolimbic reward system. (Modified from Erickson, 2007)

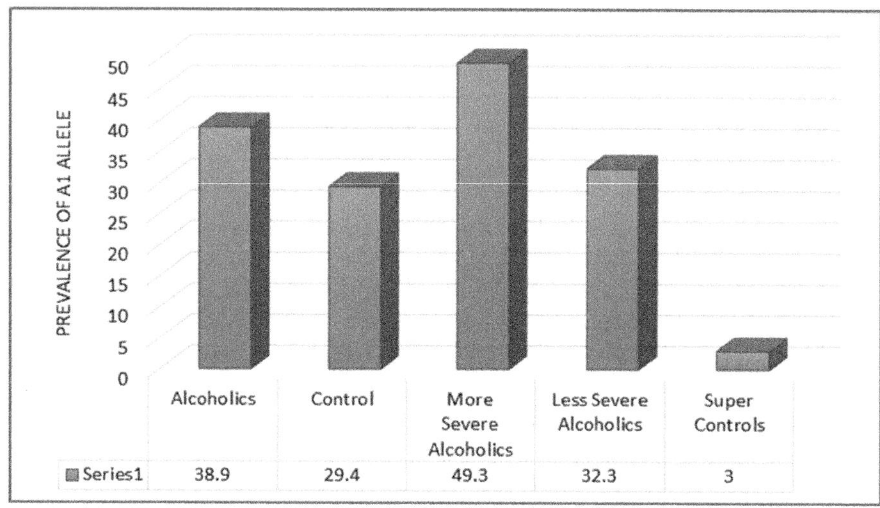

Figure 24.2 Prevalence of DRD2 A1 allele in unscreened AUD controls and screened RDS-free controls

other investigators with nonaddicting gene panels (Chen et al., 2005). However, the development of RDS free "super controls" would make it possible, instead, to weigh the effect of each gene based on Level of Detection (LOD) scores. Statistical analysis between RDS-free controls and cases (RDS behaviors) will enable the accurate development of weighing the effect of each gene (LOD score provides statistical power) and as such provide a "true" measurement of risk rather than a diagnostic assessment (Blum et al., 2018d).

Follow-up genetic research in this area, resulting in confirmation of positive correlations with dopaminergic polymorphisms, and utilizing highly screened controls (eliminating any addictive, compulsive, and impulsive behaviors in both proband and family), may have pertinent ramifications such as reducing spurious results and, thus, confusion. In this regard, the importance of using non-RDS controls has been demonstrated in earlier studies from Blum's group (Chen et al., 2005).

While there may be concerns about many of the so-called controls, for example, blood donors, it is remarkable that there is a plethora of case-controlled studies, indicating a selective association of these risk alleles (measured in GARS), for the most part, indicating hypodopaminergia (except for D3 polymorphisms). Interestingly, a neurology and family practice clinic in Princeton, NJ, using a computerized program, eliminated every possible RDS behavior in 183 patients and family members of the proband, and found only thirty patients were free of any RDS behavior. When genotyped for the A1 allele (known to cause a 30 percent to 40 percent reduction in the number of DRD2 receptors), the A1 allele was found in about 33% of the unscreened patient population. However, in the highly screened, non-RDS controls, the A1 allele was found in only one patient, 3.3 percent (Chen et al., 2005, 2012) (see Figure 24.2).

The systematic elimination of hidden RDS behaviors from control groups is required to avoid spurious study results. For example, a disputed study was published in JAMA by Yale scientists concerning the role of DRD2 allele and alcoholism, whereby controls came from a French cohort of Tourette's syndrome (Gelernter et al., 1991), an RDS subset. Over the years, following this negative report, there have been many studies including meta-analyses showing a positive association of the DRD2 A1 allele with alcohol and opioid dependence and other addictions (Chen et al., 2011).

RDS as Endophenotype

The proposition that RDS is the "true" phenotype may indeed change the recovery landscape (Blum et al., 2011). The pathology of RDS is a dysfunction in the brain reward cascade (Blum et al., 2016b). A family history of substance abuse may indicate individuals who are born with a reduced ability to produce or use these neurotransmitters. In an ancient environment, this reduced ability may have provided a superior survival advantage, driving more aggressive and intense survival-induced, reward-seeking behaviors. However, in modern industrialized societies of chronically overfed but undernourished people (the suboptimal availability of nutritional resources necessary to fund reward satisfaction and survival), exposure to prolonged periods of stress and alcohol or other substances can induce a corruption or highjacking of the brain reward cascade function (Elston et al., 1982) notably, attenuation of endorphinergic synthesis (also see Sussman & Pakdaman, 2020). Persons with RDS may be relatively vulnerable to the effects of opiates.

The Benefits of GARS Testing in Substance Use Disorder (SUD)

There are several benefits of GARS™ testing in known addicts already in treatment programs (Blum et al., 2016a, 2018e). These benefits are listed next.

Denial

It is well-known that many patients in treatment programs deny that they have a problem and believe that they can control their addiction. The GARS test predicts risk for both substance and nonsubstance severity; this helps to remove denial by providing evidence of hereditary biological disease and helps to promote recovery-oriented approaches to reduce misconceptions, labeling, and stigmatization (Corrigan et al., 2017). The twelve-step recovery movement has been the leading approach to SUDs, emphasizing first confession/admission (to remove denial), abstinence, and spiritual connection with a higher power (Blum et al., 2015a).

Guilt/Shame

A widespread response from people already addicted is a profound sense of shame and guilt (Matthews, Dwyer & Snoek, 2017). Addiction is a lonely person-level phenomenon. Guilt and shame are part of the nature of addiction, part of the standard phenomenology of addiction and often motivate the healing process. Recently, addiction literature has attempted to return to normative concepts, including choice and drinking goal responsibility, in understanding how to treat addiction (Dunn & Strain, 2013).

In many cases, people with RDS behaviors are unable to exert self-control and feel ashamed of their lack of self-control capacity and of failing to live a good human life (Vonasch et al., 2017). Many with RDS addictions experience their behaviors as ego-dystonic (Joseph, Victor & Rimona, 2011). It is conceivable that providing biological and genetic (GARS) evidence to predict risk for both substance and nonsubstance addiction severity may help remove both guilt and shame in patients (Blum et al., 2015c).

Genogram Confirmation

Patients enrolled in treatment programs are usually asked to provide a Genogram; a family history of all kinds of RDS behaviors, including addictions, in the form of a family tree (Raheb et al., 2016). A genogram allows the treatment professionals and families to visualize hereditary patterns and psychological factors that highlight relationships. This approach is a simple way to view various relationship dynamics and to review and identify a variety of trends and developmental influences. Within the genogram, representation of individuals and relationships illustrated by the unique placement of each symbol, and the lines illuminate dynamic patterns and individual qualities. Health professionals, including doctors, researchers, psychiatrists, counselors, and psychologists, use genograms. Multiple genograms are conglomerated by medical and behavioral researchers to uncover recurring patterns in the data, such as violence and aberrant sexual behaviors within family groups. Multigenerational interviewing and subsequent coding of multilevel data may suggest causal elements, such as generational learning, genetics, and how factors, such as the environment and socioeconomic status, influence family functioning and personal development. Offering the GARS test to persons in treatment and their family may be the best way to confirm addiction risk (i.e., alcoholism and opioid use disorder) within the family and identify the genetic basis of the Genogram.

Medication-Assisted Treatment (MAT) Dosing

The amount of scientific research that shows successful treatment of opioid dependence with buprenorphine or the buprenorphine–naloxone combination (Suboxone®) is overwhelming. However, the use of these agents for long-term maintenance requires caution. There may often be severe withdrawal symptoms that are often the consequence of tapering the dosage. Additionally, Hill et al. (2013) have shown a long-term flat affect with chronic Suboxone® use, and other unwanted side effects, including diversion and anhedonia-related suicide attempts. Comprehending the interaction of reward circuitry and genotypes in treatment to augment a patient's clinical experience, such as with buprenorphine, provides a novel framework and benefits during opioid replacement therapy.

The first reported association between the TaqI A1 allele and a substantially increased relapse rate in Alcohol Use Disorder (AUD) patients was from Dahlgren et al. (2011). Along similar lines, Ritchie and Noble (1996) measured post-mortem (3H) Naloxone binding in AUD and non-AUD brain tissue. They found that (3H) naloxone binding was less in all brain regions examined of subjects with the A1 allele rather than in those without this allele; however, the difference was significant in the caudate nucleus. They suggested that in subjects with the A1 allele, the decreased (3H) naloxone binding might be compensation for decreased dopaminergic modulation of opiate receptor activity. This result is crucial for Vivitrol® (naltrexone) therapy for the treatment of opioid use disorder (OUD).

Interestingly, Gerra et al. (2014) provided clear evidence that buprenorphine treatment response in heroin-addicted humans has an influential relationship to the dopaminergic system. Unexpectedly, the frequency of the kappa opioid receptor (OPRK1), 36G>T SNP was not significantly different between responders and non-responders to buprenorphine. However, for the dopamine transporter (DAT) in "nonresponders," the frequency polymorphism (SLC6A3/DAT1), allele 10 was slightly higher (64 percent) than in "responder" individuals (55.93 percent), and frequencies in other alleles category was higher in "responder" (11.02 percent) than in nonresponder individuals (2.13 percent). It appears that hypodopaminergic traits mediate a better response during treatment. It is noted that the 9 allele transports dopamine out of the synapse back to the presynaptic neuron four times faster than the 10 allele, supporting the view that response is a function of need. One may hypothesize that the 9 allele of the DAT1 carriers would have a hypodopaminergic trait due to its faster transport activity, and better treatment response with buprenorphine. Finally, Barratt, Coller and Somogyi (2006) while not showing significant differences in methadone or buprenorphine maintenance outcomes regarding ***TaqI A1 allele*** carriers, did show in successful methadone patients that significantly fewer A(1) allele carriers had withdrawal than A2 carriers ($P = 0.04$).

Moreover, Blum et al. (2013b) found in a patient with genetically determined hypodopaminergic trait at 432 days post-Suboxone® withdrawal, abstinence was maintained on the dopamine agonist KB220Z, as verified by opiate-free urine testing. Genotype data revealed a moderate risk of addiction with a hypodopaminergic trait. Another case of buprenorphine withdrawal syndrome was observed and treated by Makhinson and Gomez-Makhinson (2014). The symptoms, including restlessness, had been resistant to benzodiazepines and clonidine but were treated successfully with a D2 agonist, pramipexole.

As proposed previously by Blum et al. (2008a), activation rather than blocking mesolimbic dopaminergic reward circuitry is the preferred modality in the long-term treatment of RDS. Acute treatment consisting of antagonism of postsynaptic NAc dopamine receptors (D1–D5), in long-term treatment should consist of activation of the DA system, by the release and activation of DA in the NAc. This hypothesis attributes excessive craving behavior to the effect of the DRD2 A1 allele; a reduced number of D2 receptors, in contrast to a sufficient density of D2 receptors, which results in reducing craving. A primary goal of treatment and prevention of opiate misuse (Blum et al., 2018g) might be to restore neuroplasticity and induce proliferation of D2 receptors in individuals with the A1 genotype making them genetically less vulnerable. Experiments in vivo used a typical D2 receptor agonist to induce down-regulation; however, in vitro experimental results have shown that, genetic antecedents notwithstanding, constant stimulation by a D2 agonist, for example, bromocriptine, results in significant acute D2 receptors proliferation in the dopamine system (Boundy et al., 1995). However, down-regulation, instead of up-regulation is the product of chronic treatment. That effect is a reason for failure in treatment with potent D2 agonists like bromocriptine. Dopaminergic balance is the goal of proposed treatment with the neuronutrient KB220Z (Febo et al., 2017a).

Treatment Compliance

Blum et al. (2008b) underscored the feasibility of treating RDS based upon pharmacogenetics. Pearson correlation with the days within treatment ($r = 0.42$) was significant for the DRD2 gene variant (A1 allele versus A2 allele). The number of days within treatment for the DRD2 A1 negative carriers, with the dopamine-promoting compound KB220, was 51.9 ± 9.9 SE (95 percent CI, 30.8–73.0) versus 110.6 ± 31.1 (95 percent CI, 38.9–182.3) days within treatment for the DRD2 A1 positive carriers. As expected, the attrition rate was highest in the A1 negative genotype group. Thus, the suggestion was that genotype might predict compliance and treatment persistence and that a relapse might depend upon treatment response effected by the DRD2 A1 allele.

Resource Allocation

Stepped-care models focus on matching treatment defined by the needs of the patient. Avoiding misplacements may be a way to make the best use of available treatment resources. Stepped-care models introduced in the medical field, including psychiatry, start with the least intensive care, progressing to more intensive regimes for nonresponders. Stepwise patient placement models within addiction treatment are well known from North America (Andrews et al., 2015) and employed in both adolescent and adult settings, and with patients experiencing dual diagnoses (Schoenthaler et al., 2017). Another model developed in Europe is the Dutch model 'Measurements in the Addictions for Triage and Evaluation' (MATE), a model ideal for judicial patients (Simpatico, 2015). Placement decisions about placement intensity require feasibility, validity, reliability, effectiveness, and cost-effectiveness. GARS testing will provide a genetically based method to support effective resource allocation methodology.

Opioid Pain Compound Avoidance

The role of neurogenetics of opioids and pain mechanisms has indicated that both sensitivity and tolerance to morphine are dependent on genotype, with inheritance characterized by dominance or partial dominance as seen in many published works (Gold et al., 2018). For example, individuals respond better to a particular type of opioids. There are differences in individual responses to analgesic and other effects, toxicities, side effects, and interactions. Some of the differences unraveled by research into various genetic receptor interactions, and biochemical differences of opioid responses in humans, may be exploited to provide better care. Genetic testing has become more readily available and cost-effective instead of relying solely on patient feedback and trial and error. Individualized selection and dosing for opioid analgesic therapy and optimal opioid rotation strategies can be devised and supported by genetic information available to clinicians.

Although not obvious at present, candidate genes for gene-directed opioid therapy have been studied. Associations have been found of specific candidate genes, including some genes in the GARS test with pain sensitivity and analgesic requirements for both acute and chronic pain (Blum et al., 2014b). Stamer and Stüber (2007) found an association with analgesia for chronic pain and variants of the mu-opioid receptor, guanosine triphosphate glycohydrolase, melanocortin-1 receptor catechol-O-methyl-transferase, candidate genes.

In contrast, the genetic variants of drug-metabolizing enzymes that influence the effect of pharmacotherapies are well-known. Polymorphisms of the cytochrome P450 enzymes influence responses to tramadol, nonsteroidal anti-inflammatory drugs, codeine, and tricyclic antidepressants. An example is the cytochrome P450 (CYP) 2D6. It results in inactivity that decreases the clearance of methadone slightly, decreases the efficacy of tramadol by lack of formation of the active O-desmethyl-tramadol, and it also renders codeine ineffective due to lack of morphine formation (Lötsch et al., 2004). In an animal genetic experiment, Mogil and Wilson (1997), found that sensitivity and tolerance to morphine were dependent on genotype. They used two strains of mice BALB/cByand C57BL/6By, as well as seven recombinant inbred strains of their reciprocal F1 hybrids, and measured sensitivity using a locomotive activity; the "hot plate" method, and tolerance following administration of single or repeated of 20 mg/kg of morphine hydrochloride or saline.

The primary legal gateway to opioid addiction and abuse starts in many cases with iatrogenic prescribing of potent analgesics (e.g., OxyContin®). The GARS test prevents this legal dilemma by revealing opioid dependence risk and supporting the use of other non-opioid pain relievers like electrotherapies (Johnson et al., 2015) and nonsteroid analgesics (Bershad et al., 2018) or, possibly, customized neuronutrients (Blum et al., 2007b).

Pro-Dopamine Regulation and Precision Personalized Therapy

Gene-guided precision neuronutrients, KB220 variants, are a complex mixture of amino acids, herbals, and trace metals, and are pioneers and standard-bearers for state-of-the-art DNA customization (Blum et al., 2007b, 2018f). KB220 variants may be able to influence, based on genetics, amelioration of extreme cravings. This possibility may be the cornerstone of the practical applications of neurogenetics/nutrigenomics (Blum et al., 2015c).

Neuronutrigenomics is now a vital field of scientific investigation that offers great promise to improve the human condition. Individual customization of neuronutrients has now been commercialized for RDS behaviors, known as "Precision Addiction Management" (PAM) and "Precision Behavioral Management" (PBM) and is already having impact on addiction treatment programs and modalities (Blum et al., 2018g). These benefits of the GARS test in SUD are carefully reviewed in a recent paper (Blum et al., 2018a).

Reductionist versus Systems Biology Therapeutic Interventions

Up to this point, the discussion has been about different types of interventions that have been used to reduce RDS behaviors. An essential distinction of therapeutic interventions is that most of them employ a reductionist approach, whether as dopamine antagonists or agonist therapies. In general, a reductionist approach (or "paradigm") is an intervention: reduced to a single active substance; relies on a single mechanism of action; targets a single biological site; and has the objective of achieving a single beneficial outcome. There are some creative mechanistic exceptions like with Suboxone and Wellbutrin, for example, but even these are employing a targeted pharmacological effect. However, with pharmaceuticals, the outcome can be accompanied by a plethora of undesirable side effects from the pharmacological imposition. These and other consequences, like the development of tolerance from feedback signaling and compensatory homeostatic "adjustments" are characteristic of biphasic actions; the drug exerts its pharmacological effect (phase 1), and the body mounts a retaliatory/adversarial response to the pharmacological effect (phase 2). An example of a biphasic action is with Bromocriptine, which results in down-regulation, instead of up-regulation or balance as is proposed for KB220Z (Febo et al., 2017a). That effect is a reason for failure in treatment with potent D2 agonists.

The other paradigm is a "systems biology" therapeutic approach. In this approach, the objective is to positively influence the functional relationships and mechanistic interactions of an entire "suite" (or "system") of biomolecules; in this case, targeting the neurotransmitters in the brain reward cascade (BRC) from serotonin down to dopamine (Figure 24.1). The goal is to epigenetically optimize the expression of genes involved in regulating the synthesis, transport, reception, and degradation/reuptake of each of the BRC neurotransmitters. It involves optimizing the interconnective signaling of neurotransmitters downstream, upstream (via feedback), and cross-stream (collateral effects). This effect is achieved through nutrigenomic mechanisms whereby a selection of vitamins, minerals, and botanicals, have been shown to restore BRC normalization and functional competence. The restoration of functional competence is analogous to the "orchestra of nutrition going in and enabling the symphony of neurochemistry." The KB220 variants have been shown in over 44 published clinical studies to promote BRC neurotransmitter function; interconnectivity; and brain reward processing and satisfaction (Blum et al., 2018f).

Based on animal research and clinical trials to date, the pro-dopamine regulator known as KB220 and variants show promise in treating addiction and pain. Other neurobiological and genetic studies are required to help understand the mechanism of action of this neuronutrient formulation. The evidence to date, however, points to induction of "dopamine homeostasis" enabling an asymptotic approach for epigenetic induced "normalization" of brain neurotransmitter signaling and associated improved function in the face of either genetic or epigenetic impairment of the BRC (Blum et al., 2007a).

The KB220 complex may provide substantial clinical benefit to the victims of RDS and assist in recovery from iatrogenically induced addiction to unwanted opioids and other addictive behaviors. Inducing "dopamine homeostasis" (balance) across the brain reward circuitry has been the best way to treat all addictive-like behaviors. Moreover, utilizing fMRI in abstinent heroin addicts in China (see Figure 24.3), one hour after

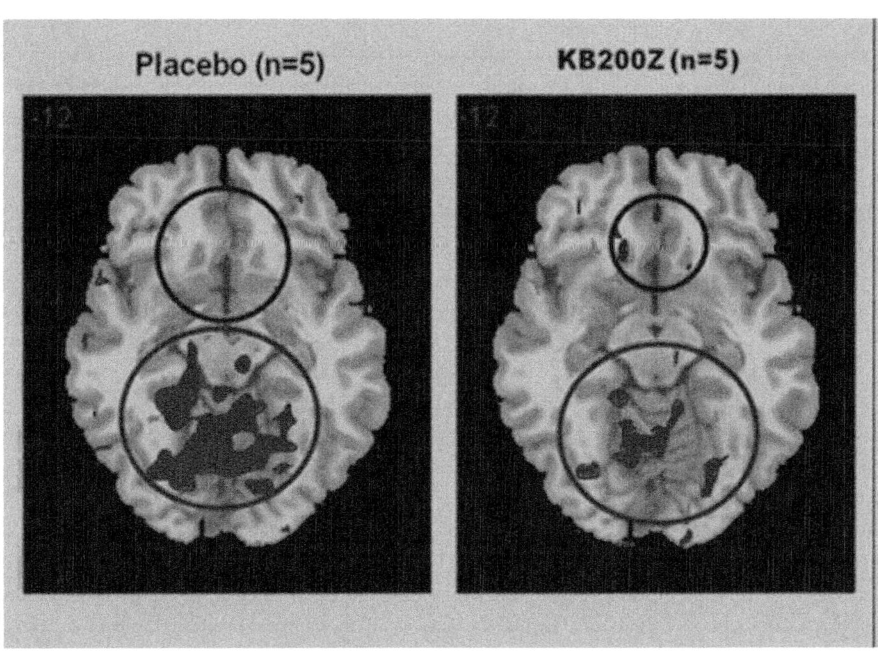

Figure 24.3 fMRI in abstinent heroin addicts one hour after administration of KB220Z

administration of KB220Z (the "Z" represents the addition of some botanicals rich in various saccharides), compared to placebo, showed profound activation of dopamine pathways of the caudate-accumbens region of the brain and reduction in dopaminergic activation of cerebellum (Blum et al., 2015b). This experiment demonstrates that through this mechanism, activation of dopamine pathways, craving behavior, as well as stress, will be reduced.

Figure 24.3 is resting state fMRI data analysis in the heroin users (n = 5) one hour after placebo and KB220Z. Significant increases in BOLD rsfMRI response with KB220Z versus placebo were observed. The small circles indicate caudate-accumbens region the larger circles indicate the cerebellum. BOLD activation is illustrated with blackened areas in this modified figure from a review article by Blum et al. (2015b).

Understanding Precision Addiction or Behavioral Management (PAM/PBM)

GARS testing of dependent persons in treatment provides a map of the brain's chemical messenger function (receptor number and neurotransmitter production) and can lead to personalized addiction medicine, based on pro-dopamine regulation. The Genetic Addiction Risk Score (GARS) test for reward genes, such as DRD2, for risk for narcotic addiction predisposition, together with P450 genotyping for narcotic metabolism, can identify patients in the early stages of treatment with a predisposition to addiction (Blum et al., 2017a–d, 2018a; Bousman, Maruf & Müller, 2019). These unique identified gene polymorphisms can provide therapeutic targets for nonnarcotic pharmacogenomic solutions and other nonaddictive alternative treatment that can be used to treat pain.

One such alternative is a natural dopaminergic agonist KB220Z that was tested utilizing neuroimaging tools including fMRI, and QEEG in both humans and, most recently, rodent models. The rodent fMRI's showed blood oxygen level dependent (BOLD) regulation of PFC-cingulate gyrus activity and activation of dopaminergic pathways (Febo et al., 2017b), and in abstinent heroin (Blum et al., 2015b) and psychostimulant abusers using qEEG (Blum et al., 2010). Finally, the Comprehensive Analysis of Reported Drugs (CARD) analysis on thousands of specimens reveals a significant difference in both compliance and abstinence rates. Opioid substitution programs show the best compliance with a range of 88 percent to 92 percent with methadone and buprenorphine/naloxone, respectively, but also show high drug-abuse rates during treatment; approximately 47 percent (Blum et al., 2014b, 2018f, 2018b).

We continue to propose the use of "Precision Behavioral Management," which includes genetic testing, assessing both metabolism and narcotic risk before opioid prescription; electrotherapy, a nonaddicting alternative to opioid prescription; dopaminergic activation with KB220PBM; medical monitoring with CARD; and twelve-step self-help programs (Blum et al., 2015c).

Genetic Testing and Screening and Ethical Issues

Genetic screening differs from genetic testing. Although the terms are interchangeable, genetic screening is carried out on a defined (by age, sex, or other risk factors) section or a subgroup of the population, in which specific disabilities may be the result of genetic factors. On the other hand, genetic testing involves the analysis of a specific gene, its product or function, or other DNA and chromosome analysis, to detect or exclude an alteration likely to be associated with a genetic disorder, and results in a definitive assessment that measures the potential risk to develop a disorder for the individual involved.

There are some concerns that genetic testing of the human population could slide into eugenics. However, this is far from the case for genetic screening or testing for the RDS-phenotype, suggested in order to facilitate early and accurate genetic assessments and preventive treatments. Nonetheless, it is noteworthy that the negative impact of genetic screenings has ethical implications, both personal and societal categories of harm.

Challenges of genetic testing include the impact that such knowledge can have on the individual, on one's sense of self; misunderstanding of the consequences of genetic predisposition and discrimination; and using genetic information to deny a person access to, for example, employment and insurance. Most American states have some legislation aimed at preventing discrimination. However, coverage by most state law is spotty. Now with the US Genetic Information Non-Discrimination Act (GINA) of 2008 in place, individuals are protected by federal law. Physicians may find that they have new duties created by reports of genetic test results, including addressing common misunderstandings of the consequences of possessing an affected allele and alerting third parties, who may share the patient's genetic endowment.

Ethical concerns arise over the genetic testing of children, such as disclosure to the child and informed consent. Even if future research confirms the need to test preschoolers for RDS-ADHD risk behaviors, specific laws now in place will govern the subsequent testing in children. If the provider's view is that the potential for harm would outweigh the potential benefit of the test, or if no benefit from medical intervention would be possible until adulthood, the test would be deferred until adulthood. Only when it is in the child's best interest can the test be conducted, the justification being that the test should be timely and medically beneficial to the child.

Future Perspectives

Blum et al. (2012) proposed that any disturbances along the reward cascade that might be due to either gene variations (polymorphisms) and environmental influences (epigenetics) can result in various SUD (RDS) including alcoholism. Despite a continued globe-wide search to find specific candidate genes or clusters characterized from high-density SNP arrays, many attempts have failed to replicate and have been inconclusive. However, Palmer et al. (2015) demonstrated that between 25 percent and 36 percent of the genetic variance might be attributable to common single nucleotide polymorphisms in the generalized vulnerability to substance dependence. Also, common single nucleotide polymorphisms share the additive effect across principal indicators of various comorbidities. Also, as a result of such research studies, even more, recent evidence has shown that specific gene variants may account for risk-prediction.

Importantly, the Bayesian study by Blum et al. (1995) concluded that the DRD2 A1 allele appeared to be an indication that if a child is born with this polymorphism, they will have a much higher risk for engaging in excessive potentially unhealthy reward-seeking behaviors. The study demonstrated a Positive Predictive Value (PPV) of 74 percent for future RDS behaviors. Since the 1990 finding of the association of the DRD2 gene Taq A1 allele with severe alcoholism, laboratories across the world including NIDA and NIAAA have done work that confirmed and extended on the importance of various candidate genes, specifically, genes for secondary messengers in the reward system (Reilly et al., 2017).

An example is Moeller et al. (2013), whose neurogenetic results identified the DAT1R 9R allele as a risk allele for relapse, especially during detoxification and early abstinence. They also suggested that drug cues contribute to relapse. As mentioned earlier, the DAT1R 9R allele influences the fast-acting transport of dopamine, sequestered from the synapse, leading to a hypodopaminergic trait.

The use of genetic testing to uncover reward circuitry gene polymorphisms is essential, as a method of obtaining better treatment results, mainly, those linked to dopaminergic pathways, including opioid receptors. Knowing the relationship between buprenorphine and the reward circuitry is a model that can enhance a patient's clinical experience and prevent relapse during opioid substitution therapy. The utilization of GARS testing provides important and clinically relevant application to alcohol abuse as well. Certainly, GARS testing will play a role in the judicial system through drug courts and probation monitoring.

Finally, we propose that PBM, a genetically based approach to achieving required dopamine homeostasis via customized dopamine regulation, should be considered. In addition to early identification of genetic risk for RDS and early intervention, this new dopaminergic regulatory approach seems more prudent than continuing to "lock people into an addiction to potent opioid-like molecules" rather than finding ways to ameliorate a potential hypodopaminergia (a root cause of all addictive behaviors). Dopaminergic regulation combats not only the opioid /alcohol crisis but all RDS nonsubstance addictive-type behaviors as well. The implementation of this approach now is indeed a laudable positively forward-thinking goal, especially while being cognizant of the complexity of the brain.

One must keep in mind that while childhood behavioral addictions such as internet gaming or even smartphone addiction may seem innocuous, it warrants serious consideration within the family. If the gravity of this behavior is unrecognized as an RDS behavior, it could indeed contribute to future fatality of a loved one, due to, for example, an unwanted fentanyl overdose as they move from internet gaming to opioid abuse. Epigenetic studies have found that nurture or deprivation, as practiced by maternal rodents, can have an effect on the dopamine homeostasis for up to two generations (Szutorisz & Hurd, 2016). It is imperative to recognize that addictive disease, including pathologically rewarding behaviors, are increasing for most countries. As scientific and clinically experienced authors, we are compelled to fix our gaze on the most recent and probably the most lethal manifestation of our evolving drug epidemic; specifically, the mortality associated with opioid use disorder. In this sense, we are indirectly bolstering our belief in "reward deficiency" as the most viable determinant of the etiology and pathophysiology of not only addictive disease but also of the statistically significant concordant psychopathology, e.g., depression, anxiety disorders, PTSD, and ADHD. Accordingly, recent breakthroughs in neuroscience, brain imaging, and neuropharmacology have not only shed much-needed light on the skyrocketing worldwide psychopathology it is also a beacon of hope for those suffering from this debilitating condition (Gressler et al., 2018).

While there are several proven strategies available to manage chronic pain without opioids, there remain millions of nonaddicted, but opioid-dependent patients with chronic or intractable pain syndromes (Schreiber, 2014). Chronic pain, like so many other chronic conditions, is phenotypical and widely diverse. The novel, analytically derived, evidence based PBM presented herein, provides a diagnostic tool for understanding the neurogenetic and neurobiological correlates of the many iterations of reward deficiency. This integrated technology can tip the balance in favor of patient-centered care or contingency management plans, in which clinical practice guidelines of assessment and treatment modalities, including prescribing practices are based on data never before available on this scale. Indeed, this is an essential step in addressing the current opioid overdose epidemic and the devastating toll on individuals, families, and communities across the USA and the world (Blum et al., 2015a, 2018h).

Conclusions

While there are several proven strategies available to manage chronic pain effectively without opioids, such as Transcranial Magnetic Stimulation (TMS)and H-Wave therapy, the principal agencies agree that we are being challenged to provide alternative nonaddicting and nonpharmacological alternatives to treat pain and attenuate addiction (Johnson et al., 2015) . The medical establishment is now encouraging alternatives with no risk of side-effects. Moderate-quality evidence supports the use of nonsteroidal anti-inflammatory drugs (NSAIDs) in chronic pain patients. Knowing a patient's GARS result could help provide an in-depth map of a patient's brain and assist in prophylaxis, especially by early genetic identification of high addiction risk.

In this chapter, we argued that if key opinion leaders continue to promote opioids to treat opioid use disorder (similar in some ways like prescribing doughnuts for serious cake addicts) except as a harm reducing agent (Blum & Baron, 2019), without actually developing epigenetic manipulation of brain neurochemistry to induce homeostasis across brain circuitry, we are setting up patients and care providers for dismal failure. We also ask the addiction medicine research community to perform needed research and embrace "Precision Behavioral Management" (PBM) or "Precision Addiction Management" (PAM). Following continued preclinical research, this approach couples genetic testing with pro-dopamine regulation as a frontline gene-guided therapy to provide early identification of RDS behaviors (Baron et al., 2018; Gardner, 2011; Hyman, 2007)

REFERENCES

Andrews, C., Abraham, A., Grogan, C. M., et al. (2015). Despite resources from the ACA, Most states do little to help addiction treatment programs implement health care reform. *Health Affairs (Millwood)*, **5**, 828–835.

Barh, D., García-Solano, M. E., Tiwari, S., et al. (2017). BARHL1 is downregulated in Alzheimer's disease and may regulate cognitive functions through ESR1 and multiple pathways. *Genes (Basel)*, **10**, 245.

Baron, D., Blum, K., Chen, A., Gold, M. & Badgaiyan, R. D. (2018). Conceptualizing addiction from an osteopathic perspective: Dopamine homeostasis. *Journal of the American Osteopathic Association*, **118**, 115–118.

Barratt, D. T., Coller, J. K. & Somogyi, A. A. (2006). Association between the DRD2 A1 allele and response to methadone and buprenorphine maintenance treatments. *American Journal of Medical Genetics Part B Neuropsychiatric Genetics*, **141**, 323–331.

Berridge, K. C. & Robinson, T. E. (2016). Liking, wanting, and the incentive-sensitization theory of addiction. *American Psychologist Journal*, **71**, 670–679.

Bershad, A. K., Miller, M. A., Norman, G. J. & de Wit, H. (2018). Effects of opioid- and non-opioid analgesics on responses to psychosocial stress in humans. *Hormones and Behavior*, **102**, 41–47.

Blum, K. (2017). *Reward Deficiency Syndrome. The Sage Encyclopedia of Abnormal Clinical Psychology*, A. Wenzel (Ed.). Pennsylvania: Sage Publications.

Blum, K. & Baron, D. (2019). Opioid substitution therapy: Achieving harm reduction while searching for a prophylactic solution. *Current Pharmaceutical Biotechnology*, **20**, 180–182.

Blum, K., Badgaiyan, R. D., Braverman, E. R., et al. (2016a). Hypothesizing that, a pro-dopamine regulator (KB220Z) should optimize, but not hyper-activate the activity of Trace Amine-Associated Receptor 1 (TAAR-1) and induce anti-craving of psychostimulants in the long-term. *Journal of Reward Deficiency Syndrome Addiction Science*, **2**, 14–21.

Blum, K., Chen, A. L., Chen, T. J., et al. (2008a). Activation instead of blocking mesolimbic dopaminergic reward circuitry is a preferred modality in the long-term treatment of reward deficiency syndrome (RDS): A commentary. *Theoretical Biology Medical Modelling*, **12**(5), 24.

Blum, K., Chen, T. J., Meshkin, B., et al. (2007a) Genotrim, a DNA-customized nutrigenomic product, targets genetic factors of obesity: Hypothesizing a dopamine-glucose correlation demonstrating reward deficiency syndrome (RDS). *Medical Hypotheses*, **68**, 844–852.

Blum, K., Chen, A. L., Oscar-Berman, M., et al. (2011). Generational association studies of dopaminergic genes in reward deficiency syndrome (RDS) subjects: Selecting appropriate phenotypes for reward dependence behaviors. *International Journal of Environmental Research and Public Health*, **8**, 4425–4459.

Blum, K., Chen, A. L. C., Thanos, P. K., et al. (2018a). Genetic addiction risk score (GARS) ™, a predictor of vulnerability to opioid dependence. *Frontiers in Bioscience (Elite Edition)*, **10**, 175–196.

Blum, K., Chen, T. J., Meshkin, B., et al. (2007b). Genotrim, a DNA-customized nutrigenomic product, targets genetic factors of obesity: Hypothesizing a dopamine-glucose correlation demonstrating reward deficiency syndrome (RDS). *Medical Hypotheses*, **68**, 844–852.

Blum, K., Chen, T. J., Morse, S., et al. (2010). Overcoming qEEG abnormalities and reward gene deficits during protracted abstinence in male psychostimulant and polydrug abusers utilizing putative dopamine D2 agonist therapy: Part 2. *Postgraduate Medical Journal*, **122**, 214–226.

Blum, K., Chen, T. J. H., Chen, A. L. C., et al. (2008b). Dopamine D2 receptor Taq A1 allele predicts treatment compliance of LG839 in a subset analysis of pilot study in the Netherlands. *Gene Therapy & Molecular Biology*, **12**, 129–140.

Blum, K., Febo, M. & Badgaiyan, R. D. (2016b). Fifty years in the development of a glutaminergic-dopaminergic optimization complex (KB220) to balance brain reward circuitry in Reward Deficiency Syndrome: A pictorial. *Austin Addiction Sciences*, **1**, 1006.

Blum, K., Febo, M., Badgaiyan, R. D., et al. (2017a). Common neurogenetic diagnosis and meso-limbic manipulation of hypodopaminergic function in Reward Deficiency Syndrome (RDS): Changing the recovery landscape. *Current Neuropharmacology*, **15**, 184–194.

Blum, K., Febo, M., Fried, L., et al. (2017b). Hypothesizing that neuropharmacological and neuroimaging studies of glutaminergic-dopaminergic optimization complex (KB220Z) are associated with "dopamine homeostasis" in Reward Deficiency Syndrome (RDS). *Substance Use and Misuse*, **52**, 535–547.

Blum, K., Febo, M., McLaughlin, T., et al. (2014a). Hatching the behavioral addiction egg: Reward Deficiency Solution System (RDSS)™ as a function of dopaminergic neurogenetics and brain functional connectivity linking all addictions under a common rubric. *Journal of Behavioral Addictions*, **3**, 149–156.

Blum, K., Febo, M., Thanos, P. K., et al. (2015a). Clinically combating Reward Deficiency Syndrome (RDS) with dopamine agonist therapy as a paradigm shift: Dopamine for dinner? *Molecular Neurobiology*, **52**, 1862–1869.

Blum, K., Gardner, E., Oscar-Berman, M. & Gold, M. (2012). "Liking" and "wanting" linked to Reward Deficiency Syndrome (RDS): Hypothesizing differential responsivity in brain reward circuitry. *Current Pharmaceutical Design*, **18**, 113–118.

Blum, K., Han, D., Hauser, M., et al. (2013a). Neurogenetic impairments of brain reward circuitry links to Reward Deficiency Syndrome (RDS) as evidenced by Genetic Addiction Risk Score (GARS): A case study. *The Institute of Integrative Omics and Applied Biotechnology Journal*, **4**, 4–9.

Blum, K., Han, D., Modestino, E. J., et al. (2018b). A systematic, intensive statistical investigation of data from the Comprehensive Analysis of Reported Drugs (CARD) for compliance and illicit opioid abstinence in substance addiction treatment with buprenorphine/naloxone. *Substance Use and Misuse*, **53**, 220–229.

Blum, K., Han. D., Femino, J., et al. (2014b). Systematic evaluation of "compliance" to prescribed treatment medications and "abstinence" from psychoactive drug abuse in chemical dependence programs: Data from the comprehensive analysis of reported drugs. *PLoS ONE*, **9**, e104275.

Blum, K., Jacobs, W., Modestino, E. J., et al. (2018c). Insurance companies fighting the peer review empire without any validity: The case for addiction and pain modalities in the face of an American drug epidemic. *SEJ Surgery and Pain*, **1**, 1–11.

Blum, K., Liu, Y., Wang, W., et al. (2015b). rsfMRI effects of KB220Z™ on neural pathways in reward circuitry of abstinent genotyped heroin addicts. *Postgraduate Medical Journal*, **127**, 232–241.

Blum, K., Lott, L. Siwicki, D., et al. (2018d). Genetic Addiction Risk Score (GARS) as a predictor of substance use disorder: Identifying predisposition not diagnosis. *Current Trends in Medical Diagnostic Methods*, **1**, 1–3.

Blum, K., Madigan, M. A., Fried, L., et al. (2017c). Coupling Genetic Addiction Risk Score (GARS) and pro dopamine regulation (KB220) to combat substance use disorder (SUD). *Global Journal of Addiction and Rehabilitation Medicine*, **1**.

Blum, K., Modestino, E. J., Gondre-Lewis, M., et al. (2018e). The benefits of Genetic Addiction Risk Score (GARS™) testing in Substance Use Disorder (SUD). *International Journal of Genomics and Data Mining*, **1**, 115.

Blum, K., Modestino, E. J., Gondré-Lewis, M. C., et al. (2017d). Global opioid epidemic: Doomed to fail without genetically based precision addiction medicine (PAMTM): Lessons learned from America. *Journal of Laboratory and Precision Medicine (Bangalore)*, **2**, 17–22.

Blum, K., Modestino, J. E., Gondre Lewis, C. M., et al. (2018f). Pro-dopamine regulator (KB220) a fifty year sojourn to combat Reward Deficiency Syndrome (RDS): Evidence based bibliography (annotated). *CPQ Journal of Neurology and Psychology*, **1**.

Blum, K., Modestino, E. J., Lott, L., et al. (2018g). Introducing "Precision Addiction Management (PAM®)" as an adjunctive genetic guided therapy for abusable drugs in America. *Open Access Journal of Psychology and Behavioral Science*, **1**, 1–4.

Blum, K., Modestino, E. J., Neary, J., et al. (2018h). Promoting Precision Addiction

Management (PAM) to combat the global opioid crisis. *Biomedical Journal of Scientific and Technical Research*, **2**, 1–4.

Blum, K., Noble, E. P., Sheridan, P. J., et al. (1990). Allelic association of human dopamine D2 receptor gene in alcoholism. *The Journal of American Medical Association*, **263**(15), 2055–2060.

Blum, K., Oscar-Berman, M., Demetrovics, Z., Barh, D. & Gold, M. S. (2014c). Genetic Addiction Risk Score (GARS): Molecular neurogenetic evidence for predisposition to Reward Deficiency Syndrome (RDS). *Molecular Neurobiology*, **50**, 765–796.

Blum, K., Oscar-Berman, M., Femino, J., et al. (2013b). Withdrawal from buprenorphine/naloxone and maintenance with a natural dopaminergic agonist: A cautionary note. *Journal of Addiction Research and Therapy*, **4**.

Blum, K., Thompson, B., Demotrovics, Z., et al. (2015c). The molecular neurobiology of twelve steps program & fellowship: Connecting the dots for recovery. *Journal of Reward Deficiency Syndrome*, **1**, 46–64.

Blum, K., Wood, R. C., Braverman, E. P., Chen, T. J. H. & Sheridan, P. J. (1995). D2 dopamine receptor gene as a predictor of compulsive disease: Bayes' theorem. *Functional Neurology*, **10**, 37–44.

Bousman, C., Maruf, A. A. & Müller, D. J. (2019). Towards the integration of pharmacogenetics in psychiatry: a minimum, evidence-based genetic testing panel. *Current Opinion in Psychiatry*, **32**, 7–15.

Casey, B. J., Craddock, N., Cuthbert, B. N., Hyman, S. E., Lee, F. S. & Ressler, K. J. (2013). DSM-5 and RDoC: progress in psychiatry research? Nature reviews. *Neuroscience*, **14**, 810–814.

Chen, A. L., Blum, K., Chen, T. J., et al. (2012). Correlation of the Taq1 dopamine D2 receptor gene and percent body fat in obese and screened control subjects: a preliminary report. *Food and Function*, **3**, 40–48.

Chen, A. L., Chen, T. J., Waite, R. L., et al. (2009). Hypothesizing that brain reward circuitry genes are genetic antecedents of pain sensitivity and critical diagnostic and pharmacogenomic treatment targets for chronic pain conditions. *Medical Hypotheses*, **72**, 14–22.

Chen, D., Liu, F., Shang, Q., et al. (2011). Association between polymorphisms of DRD2 and DRD4 and opioid dependence: evidence from the current studies. *American Journal of Medical Genetics*, **156**, 661–670.

Chen, T. J., Blum, K., Mathews, D., et al. (2005). Are dopaminergic genes involved in a predisposition to pathological aggression? Hypothesizing the importance of "super normal controls" in psychiatricgenetic research of complex behavioral disorders. *Medical Hypotheses*, **65**, 703–707.

Comings, D. E., MacMurray, J., Johnson, P., Dietz, G. & Muhleman, D. (1995). Dopamine D2 receptor gene (DRD2) haplotypes and the defense style questionnaire in substance abuse, Tourette syndrome, and controls. *Biological Psychiatry*, **37**, 798–805.

Corrigan, P. W., Schomerus, G., Shuman, V., et al. (2017). Developing a research agenda for reducing the stigma of addictions, part II: lessons from the mental health stigma literature. *American Journal on Addictions*, **1**, 67–74.

Dahlgren, A., Wargelius, H. L., Berglund, K. J., et al. (2011). Do alcohol-dependent individuals with DRD2 A1 allele have an increased risk of relapse? *Alcohol and Alcoholism*, **46**, 509–513.

Dunn, K E. & Strain, E. C. (2013). Pretreatment alcohol drinking goals are associated with treatment outcomes. *Alcoholism: Clinical and Experimental Research*, **37**, 1745–1752.

Elston, S. F., Blum, K., DeLallo, L. & Briggs, A. H. (1982). Ethanol intoxication as a function of genotype dependent responses in three inbred mice strains. *Pharmacology Biochemistry and Behavior*, **16**, 13–15.

Erickson, C. (2007). *The Science of Addiction.* New York: W. W. Norton & Co.

Febo, M., Blum, K., Badgaiyan, R. D., et al. (2017a). Enhanced functional connectivity and volume between cognitive and reward centers of naïve rodent brain produced by pro-dopaminergic agent KB220Z. *PLoS ONE*, **12**, e0174774.

Febo, M., Blum, K., Badgaiyan, R. D., et al. (2017b). Dopamine homeostasis: brain functional connectivity in reward deficiency syndrome. *Frontiers Bioscience (Landmark Edition)*, **22**, 669–691.

Florence, C. S., Zhou, C., Luo, F. & Xu, L. (2016). The economic burden of prescription opioid overdose, abuse, and dependence in the United States. *Medical Care*, **54**, 901–906.

Gardner, E. L. (2011). Addiction and brain reward and antireward pathways. *Advances in Psychosomatic Medicine*, **30**, 22–60.

Gelernter, J., O'Malley, S., Risch, N., et al. (1991). No association between an allele at the D2 dopamine receptor gene (DRD2) and alcoholism. *The Journal of American Medical Association*, **266**, 1801–1807.

Gerra, G., Somaini, L., Leonardi, C., et al. (2014). Association between gene variants and response to buprenorphine maintenance treatment. *Psychiatry Research*, **215**, 202–207.

Gold, M. S., Blum, K., Febo, M., et al. (2018). Molecular role of dopamine in anhedonia linked to reward deficiency syndrome (RDS) and anti-reward systems. *Frontiers in Bioscience (Scholar Edition)*, **10**, 309–325.

Gressler, L. E., Martin, B. C., Hudson, T. J. & Painter, J. T. (2018) Relationship between concomitant benzodiazepine-opioid use and adverse outcomes among US veterans. *Pain*, **159**, 451–459.

Hill, E., Han, D., Dumouchel, P., et al. (2013). Long term Suboxone™ emotional reactivity as measured by automatic detection in speech. *PLoS ONE*, **8**, e69043.

Hyman, S. E. (2007). Can neuroscience be integrated into the DSM-V? *Nature Reviews Neuroscience*, **8**(9), 725–732.

Johnson, M. I., Paley, C. A., Howe, T. E. & Sluka, K. A. (2015). Transcutaneous electrical nerve stimulation for acute pain. *Cochrane Database Systematic Review*, CD006142.

Joseph, Z., Victor, K. & Rimona, D. (2011). "Ego-dystonic" delusions as a predictor of dangerous behavior. *Psychiatric Quaterly*, **82**, 113–120.

Kandel, D. & Kandel, E. (2015). The Gateway Hypothesis of substance abuse: developmental, biological and societal perspectives. *Acta Paediatrica*, **104**, 130–137.

Krebs, E. E., Gravely, A., Nugent, S., et al. (2018). Effect of opioid vs nonopioid medications on pain-related function in patients with chronic back pain or hip or knee osteoarthritis pain: The SPACE randomized clinical trial. *The Journal of American Medical Association*, **319**, 872–882.

Loth, E., Carvalho, F. & Schumann, G. (2011). The contribution of imaging genetics to the development of predictive markers for addictions. *Trends in Cognitive Sciences*, **15**, 436–446.

Lötsch, J., Skarke, C., Liefhold, J. & Geisslinger, G. (2004). Genetic predictors of the clinical response to opioid analgesics: clinical utility and future perspectives. *Clinical Pharmacokinetics*, **43**, 983–1013.

Makhinson, M. & Gomez-Makhinson, J. (2014). A successful treatment of buprenorphine withdrawal with the dopamine receptor agonist pramipexole. *The American Journal on Addictions*, **23**, 475–477.

Matthews, S., Dwyer, R. & Snoek, A. (2017). Stigma and self-stigma in addiction. *Journal of Bioethical Inquiry*, **14**, 275–286.

Moeller, S. J., Parvaz, M. A., Shumay, E., et al. (2013). Gene x abstinence effects on drug cue reactivity in addiction: multimodal evidence. *Journal of Neuroscience*, **33**, 10027–10036.

Mogil, J. S. & Wilson, S. G. (1997). Nociceptive and morphine antinociceptive sensitivity of 129 and C57BL/6 inbred mouse strains: implications for transgenic knock-out studies. *European Journal of Pain*, **1**, 293–297.

Palmer, R. H., Brick, L., Nugent, N. R., et al. (2015). Examining the role of common genetic variants on alcohol, tobacco, cannabis and illicit drug dependence: genetics of vulnerability to drug dependence. *Addiction*, **110**, 530–537.

Pergolizzi, J. V. Jr, LeQuang, J. A., Taylor, R. Jr. & Raffa, R. B. (2018) Going beyond prescription pain relievers to understand the opioid epidemic: the role of illicit fentanyl, new psychoactive substances, and street heroin. *Postgraduate Medicine Journal*, **130**, 1–8.

Raheb, G., Khaleghi, E., Moghanibashi-Mansourieh, A., Farhoudian, A. & Teymouri, R. (2016). Effectiveness of social work intervention with a systematic approach to improve general health in opioid addicts in addiction treatment centers. *Psychology Research and Behavior Management*, **9**, 309–315.

Reilly, M. T., Noronha, A., Goldman, D. & Koob, G. F. (2017). Genetic studies of alcohol dependence in the context of the addiction cycle. *Neuropharmacology*, **122**, 3–21.

Ritchie, T. & Noble, E. P. (1996). (3H) naloxone binding in the human brain: alcoholism and the TaqI A D2 dopamine receptor polymorphism. *Brain Research*, **718**, 193–197.

Rudd, R. A., Seth, P., David, F. & Scholl, L. (2016). Increases in drug and opioid-involved overdose deaths – United States, 2010–2015. *Morbidity and Mortality Weekly Report*, **65**, 1445–1452.

Salling, M. C. & Martinez, D. (2016). Brain stimulation in addiction. *Neuropsychopharmacology*, **41**, 2798–2809.

Schoenthaler, S. J., Blum, K., Fried, L., et al. (2017). The effects of residential dual diagnosis treatment on alcohol abuse. *Journal of Systems and Integrative Neuroscience*, **3**.

Schreiber, A. L. (2014). Challenging pain syndromes. *Physical Medicine and Rehabilitation Clinics of North America*, **2**, xv–xvi.

Severino, A. L., Shadfar, A., Hakimian, J. K., et al. (2018). Pain therapy guided by purpose and perspective in light of the opioid epidemic. *Frontiers in Psychiatry*, **9**, 119.

Simpatico, T. A. (2015). Vermont responds to its opioid crisis. *Preventive Medicine*, **80**, 10–11.

Smith, D. E. (2012). The process addictions and the new ASAM definition of addiction. *Journal of Psychoactive Drugs*, **44**, 1–4.

Smith, S. R., Deshpande, B. R., Collins, J. E., Katz, J. N. & Losina, E. (2016). Comparative pain reduction of oral non-steroidal anti-inflammatory drugs and opioids for knee osteoarthritis: systematic analytic review. *Osteoarthritis Cartilage*, **24**, 962–972.

Stamer, U. M. & Stüber, F. (2007). Genetic factors in pain and its treatment. *Current Opinion in Anaesthesiology*, **20**, 478–484.

Sussman, S. & Pakdaman, S. (2020). Appetitive needs and addiction. In S. Sussman (Ed.) *The Cambridge Handbook of Substance and Behavioral Addictions*. Cambridge, UK: Cambridge University Press, pp. 3–11.

Szutorisz, H. & Hurd, Y. L. (2016). Epigenetic effects of cannabis exposure. *Biological Psychiatry*, **79**, 586–594.

Volkow, N. D., Wise, R. A. & Baler, R. (2017). The dopamine motive system: implications for drug and food addiction. *Nature Reviews Neuroscience*, **18**, 741–752.

Vonasch, A. J., Clark, C. J., Lau, S., Vohs, K. D. & Baumeister, R. F. (2017). Ordinary people associate addiction with loss of free will. *Addictive Behaviors Reports*, **5**, 56–66.

Willuhn, I., Burgeno, L. M., Groblewski, P. A. & Phillips, P. E. (2014). Excessive cocaine use results from decreased phasic dopamine signaling in the striatum. *Nature Neuroscience*, **17**, 704–709.

25 Novel Psychoactive Substances: A New Challenge for Prevention and Treatment

Máté Kapitány-Fövény, PhD, Ornella Corazza, PhD, Shanna Marrinan, PhD, and Zsolt Demetrovics, DSc, PhD

Epidemiology of NPS

The widespread emergence of Novel Psychoactive Substances (NPS) was initally explained by their legal status and availability on the internet. Most countries have since implemented some form of control legislations though these vary broadly in breath, type and depth (Corazza & Roman-Urrestarazu, 2017, 2018). Novel detection methods (e.g. Cannaert et al., 2016; Griswold et al., 2017) have also been developed and the public dissemination of research findings, dealing with both the desired and adverse effects of these substances, have helped to lower curiosity regarding their effects (Vidourek, King & Burbage, 2013). According to the qualitative study of Van Hout and Brennan (2012, p. 158), regular users of mephedrone (a stimulant NPS legal in the United Kingdom until 2010) attributed their choice to "street availability, favourable pricing and pleasurable drug effects." Once mephedrone became a class B drug, many users reported reverting back to traditional illicit drugs such as ecstasy (MDMA) or cocaine (Van Hout & Brennan, 2012). The UK Psychoactive Substances Act of 2016 formed a "blanket ban" on NPS, but its efficacy, or potential to reduce drugs harms, has been heavily criticized (e.g., Nutt, 2015; Reuter & Pardo, 2017).

Despite the changes in regulatory frameworks in various countries, easy availability of NPS is still supported by online trafficking (EMCDDA, 2016a), providing relative anonymity and convenience for the users (Dick & Torrance, 2010). This newer format of drug sales also removed a lot of the "middle man" adulturation ("cutting") that often previously occurred with traditional illicit drugs. As a result, purity of synthetic cathinones and SCRAs (synthetic cannabinoids) was often very high (Ginsburg et al., 2012). Below we present a brief summary of the available epidemiological data based on general population studies and further subpopulation research as presented in Table 25.1.

As can be seen from Table 25.1, lifetime use of NPS is highly variable according to the specific subpopulation, the assessment methods, the location of data collection and the category of NPS. Members of certain subpopulations (e.g., patients with psychiatric comorbidity, MSM, clubgoers, prisoners) may be substantially more likely to use NPS. Furthermore, the majority of the studies presented rely upon self-reported data, carrying potential for either over- or underestimated prevalences. Importantly, there is a lack of cross-national studies with comparable methodology which would enable us to draw reliable conclusions about the country-level variability of NPS use. In the abscence of this, a variety of proxy markers can be considered. In the case of NSO epidemiology, trends in availability and consumption rates is mainly estimated from seizures, emergency department visits and overdose cases (Prekupec, Mansky & Baumann, 2017) as prevalence of their use remained un(der)studied.

Acknowledgments Máté Kapitány-Fövény acknowledges the support by the János Bolyai Research Scholarship of the Hungarian Academy of Sciences and the support by the ÚNKP-19 New National Excellence Program of the Hungarian Ministry for Innovation and Technology. This study was supported by the Hungarian National Research, Development and Innovation Office (Grant numbers: KKP126835, NKFIH-1157-8/2019-DT).

User and Consumption Characteristics

It is important to differentiate between the user groups of various NPS as their characteristics may vary vastly. For example users of NSO, such as U-47700 (Armenian et al., 2017) or U-49900 (Alzghari et al., 2017), typically derive from the subpopulation of active or former opioid users, some of whom began using synthetic cathinones as a substitute for heroin and other opioids (Kapitány-Fövény et al., 2017). A common consequence for users of NSO (to a greater extent than for other types of NPS) are acute intoxications or fatal overdoses (Prekupec et al., 2017). NPS-consuming opiate users, as compared to those clients without a history of NPS use, have been found to show more severe psychiatric symptoms and an increased emotional reactivity to interpersonal conflicts (Kapitány-Fövény et al., 2017).

Considering adolescent NPS users, characteristics such as male gender, truancy, concomitant or preceding use of cigarettes, alcohol, and cannabis, have been found to be associated with higher frequencies of both synthetic cannabinoid and cathinone use (Patrick et al., 2016). Champion and colleagues (2016b) similarly described adolescents using NPS as showing higher odds of having a binge drinking episode in the past six months, more likely to try tobacco, and characterized by higher levels of psychological distress, and reported lower perceived self-efficacy to resist peer pressure than nonusers and illegal substance users. Similarly, Vreeker and colleagues (2017) compared NPS users with users of illicit drugs, legal substances and nonusers, in terms of risk-related behavior and personality traits, including sensation seeking and impulsivity. NPS users showed higher level of sensation seeking and impulsivity compared to both illicit drug users and nonusers. Furthermore, NPS users had more substance-using peers and reported a lower risk perception for most psychoactive substances. Regarding associated symptomatology of NPS use, Acciavatti and colleagues (2017) found bipolar disorder to be the most inherent comorbid psychopatology (23.1 percent) in case of young adult psychiatric patients with NPS use history.

One study, which recruited young adults via social media and Bluelight, a drug information-sharing website favoured by "pychonauts" (Deligianni et al., 2017), noted increased awareness about NPS among bisexual and homosexual individuals and those in employment, while

Table 25.1 Lifetime use of various NPS classes in different populations

		Assessed population			
NPS class[a]	Specific substance	General population	Nonprobability adult subpopulation	Representative adolescent samples	Nonprobability adolescent subsamples
		Lifetime prevalence rates: percent (%) with year and location of data collection (publication source)			
Piperazines	Benzylpiperazine (BZP)	13.5% in 2007/2008, New Zealand (Ministry of Health – New Zealand, 2012)	-	-	-
Arylcyclo-hexylamines	Ketamine	1% in 2004, Australia (Degenhardt & Dunn, 2008) 0.6% in 2010/2011, England and Wales (Smith & Flatley, 2011)	6.7% of Czech, 10.8% of Italian, 16.4% of French, 17% of British and 20.9% of Hungarian club-goers in 2005 (EMCDDA, 2006)	2.2% in 2009, respondents of the OSDUHS study in Canada (Paglia-Boak et al., 2009)	-
Synthetic cathinones	Mephedrone	1.4% in 2010/2011, England and Wales (Smith & Flatley, 2011) 0.6% in 2015, Hungary (Paksi et al., 2016)	63.8% in 2011, South London's MSM[b] gay club-goers (Wood et al., 2012) 1.1% in 2012, US patrons of nightlife scenes (Kelly et al., 2013) 19%–23% in 2012, Australian psychostimulant users (Sindicich & Burns, 2012) 1.9% in 2017, respondents of the Global Drug Survey (Winstock et al., 2017)	-	20.3% in 2010, mixed sample of high-school, college and university students in the Tayside area of Scotland (Dargan et al., 2010) 3.3% between 2012 and 2013, mixed Italian sample of adolescents and young adults (Martinotti et al., 2015)
	2C-I, 2C-B or 2C-E	-	7%–24% in 2012, Australian psychostimulant users (Sindicich & Burns, 2012) 8%–14% in 2013, Australian ecstasy users (Burns et al., 2014) 5.1% in 2017, respondents of the Global Drug Survey (Winstock et al., 2017)	-	-
	Methylone	-	10% in 2012, Australian psychostimulant users (Sindicich & Burns, 2012)	-	-
	MDPV	-	5% in 2012, Australian psychostimulant users (Sindicich & Burns, 2012)	-	-
	Merged category of synthetic cathinones and designer stimulants	0.5% between 2009 and 2013, United States (Palamar et al., 2015) 1.3% in 2015, Hungary (Paksi et al., 2016)	-	0.4% in 2014, Australian high-school students (Champion et al., 2016b)	-

Tryptamines	Psychedelic tryptamines	1.06% between 2009 and 2013, United States (Palamar et al., 2015)	-	-	-
	N,N-Dimethyltryptamine (DMT)	-	3.7% in 2017, respondents of the Global Drug Survey (Winstock et al., 2017)	-	
Syntetic cannabinoids		0.05% between 2009 and 2013, United States (Palamar et al., 2015)	8.2% in 2012, US patrons of nightlife scenes (Kelly et al., 2013)	2.4% in 2014, Australian high-school students (Champion et al., 2016a)	1.2% between 2012 and 2013, mixed Italian sample of adolescents and young adults (Martinotti et al., 2015)
		1.3% in 2015, Hungary (Paksi et al., 2016)	5.8% in 2017, respondents of the Global Drug Survey (Winstock et al., 2017)		
Any NPS (as merged category)		2.3% in 2015, Germany (EMCDDA, 2017)	44% in 2013, Australian ecstasy users (Burns et al., 2014) 22.2% in 2014, inpatients of a Scottish general psychiatric ward (Stanley et al., 2016) 9.8% between 2013 and 2014, Italian psychiatric patients (Martinotti et al., 2014) 8.2% between 2013 and 2015, Italian psychiatric patients (Acciavatti et al., 2017)	3% in 2014, Australian high-school students (Champion et al., 2016b) 5% in 2015, respondents of the SALSUS study (Black et al., 2016) 4% in 2015, respondents of the ESPAD study (ESPAD Group, 2016)	79% between 2009-2011, clients of the Youth Drug & Alcohol (YoDA) service in Dublin (Smyth et al., 2015) 4.7% between 2012-2013, mixed Italian sample of adolescents and young adults (Martinotti et al., 2015) 1.1% in 2015, London high-school students (Penney et al., 2016)

Notes. [a]There were no available or adequate data on synthetic opioids' prevalence; [b]MSM = men who have sex with men.

NPS awareness and use seemed to be unaffected by the level of education. However, users in this study were members of a highly self-selected and well-educated population. Considering age, gender distribution and level of education, the majority of NPS users – either assessed in a clinical or nonclinical setting – are reported to be males (e.g., Barratt, Cakic & Lenton, 2013; Carhart-Harris, King & Nutt, 2011; Castaneto et al., 2014; Caudevilla-Gálligo et al., 2012; Palamar, Su & Hoffman, 2016; Romanek et al., 2017; Winstock, Marsden & Mitcheson, 2010) in their twenties (e.g., Caviness et al., 2015; Gunderson et al., 2014; Lea, Reynolds & De Wit, 2011; Sanders et al., 2008), with a relatively high educational background (i.e., high school or even college/university degree) (e.g., Castaneto et al., 2014; Caudevilla-Gálligo et al., 2012; Dargan et al., 2010; Lea et al., 2011). Nonetheless, it needs mentioning that other studies have described NPS users as often marginalized individuals (e.g., Joseph et al., 2017; Sanders et al., 2008) (e.g., due to homelessness or mental illness), with criminal records (Nurmedov et al., 2015). These differences are largely explained by the type of NPS being used, and highlight the need to make sustained distinctions between substances, or at the very least, categories of substance. Although criminal activites were linked to the use of synthetic cannabinoids (Nurmedov et al., 2015) and synthetic cathinones (Addison et al., 2018), such deviant behavior might be explained by the setting of NPS consumption, rather than the specific NPS compounds being used. Users self-identifying as "psychonauts" or those engaging in chemsex have higher than average education levels, whereas use of SCRAs became restricted to highly marginalized populations such as people in prison, and the homeless (Blackman & Bradley, 2017), primarily due to their lower price and easy availability. These particular substances have been largely deemed undesirable by other NPS-using populations due to their significant side effects.

The motives behind NPS consumption also show high variability. As Soussan and Kjellgren (2016) highlighted, NPS are typically sought for pleasure and enjoyment. However, the consumption of hallucinogenic NPSs (e.g., 25i-NBOMe, 4-AcO-DMT or 2C-B) are often driven by the needs of self-exploration and spiritual development, while SCRAs are mainly chosen for pragmatic and external reasons, such as their easy availability compared with other drugs, legality in some countries, and their low toxicological detectability (Marrinan et al., 2017).

Still, desired psychopharmacological effects of distinct NPS also contribute to their popularity. Synthetic cathinones' preferred effects consist of increased energy, self-esteem, sociability, empathy, reduced fear, disinhibition, and enhanced sexual urge and stimulation (Karila et al., 2015; Shimizu et al., 2007; Winstock et al., 2011). The use of cathinones is sometimes linked to "chemsex" parties, mostly among men who have sex with men, utilizing the sexual enhancing effects of these NPS (McCall et al., 2015). Desired effects of synthetic cannabinoids include a 'new kind of high' (Gunderson et al., 2014), euphoria, relaxation, increased creativity, and well-being (Spaderna, Addy & D'Souza, 2013), but more usual motivations of SCRA use are associated with the strength of their effects or their capability to make time pass more quickly (Ralphs et al., 2017). Users of NSO usually seek an anesthetic effect, pain management, euphoria, relaxation, and pleasant mood (Katselou et al., 2015) as most desirable outcomes of NSO use.

Tryptamines – such as DMT (N,N-dimethyltryptamine), DPT (N,N-dipropyltryptamine) or 5-MeO-DiPT (1-methyl-5-methoxy-diisopropyl-tryptamine) – are mainly chosen for their ability to induce psychedelic experiences, including ego loss, enhanced intensity of music and colors, visuals and new perspectives and insights (Tittarelli et al., 2015). Piperazines – e.g., mCPP (m-chlorophenylpiperazine), BZP (n-benzylpiperazine) or TFMPP (1-(3-trifluoromethylphenylpiperazine) – primarily induce amphetamine-like effects (Schifano et al., 2015), such as increased energy, euphoria or mild hallucinations at higher doses.

The set and setting of NPS use usually depend on both the user group characteristics (i.e., subcultural factors) and the type of NPS being administered. For instance, stimulant-type NPS (e.g., phenethylamines), functioning as effective entactogens (Miliano et al., 2016), are most likely used within the recreational scene (e.g., Moore et al., 2013; Vento et al., 2014), mainly by snorting or sniffing (e.g., Dargan et al., 2010; Winstock et al., 2011), by users seeking increased energy and enhanced sociability. At the same time, high rates of synthetic cathinone injectors were observed among clients of needle exchange programs (Csák, Demetrovics & Rácz, 2013; Péterfi et al., 2014), indicating that cathinones became the drug of choice for a subpopulation of injecting drug users (IDU) as well, seeking alternatives for banned or sparsely available substances.

Many of the observed reasons for NPS use (and substance use in general) overlap with those of novel behavioral addictions, including accessibility, social enhancement, a preference for immediate rewards, or mood modification (in the case of excessive smartphone use) (e.g., Cha & Seo, 2018; Lee, Kim & Choi, 2017). They are also used for recreational purposes, and coping, escapism or enhancing cognition in a simlar way to the stimuli used by online/offline video gamers (e.g., Demetrovics et al., 2011; Oei & Patterson, 2013). Parellels may also be drawn between the avoidance and excitment-seeking behaviors of NPS users and those engaged in pathological gambling (e.g., Lee et al., 2007).

Pharmacokinetics and Toxicology of NPS

Although a substainal amount of research is now available on the risks and adverse consequences related to the use of various NPS, understanding and knowledge of these is still limited among health and other professionals. A study by Guirguis et al. (2015) highlighted, for example, that the majority of pharmacists in their sample had poor knowledge of NPS and considered these substances to be irrelevant to their work, similar results have been found among physicians (Simonato et al., 2013). Wood and colleagues (2016) also observed that health professionals (physicians, nurses) are less confident about managing NPS-related acute toxicity as compared to that of classical recreational drugs, as well as showing lower knowledge about NPS. These findings reveal the need of further and more effective dissemination regarding the epidemiology and toxicity of these substances. In the following paragraphs, pharmacokinetic and toxicological properties of the most popular NPS (i.e., synthetic cathinones, SCRAs, novel synthetic opioids, tryptamines and piperazines) are briefly presented.

Synthetic Cathinones

Cathinone, as the main psychoactive compound of the khat (catha edulis) leaves, has been used during social and cultural events for centuries in certain areas of Saudi Arabia and East Africa. Its synthetic derivatives (synthetic cathinones) were initially developed for therapeutic purposes, but in the mid 2000s, they became popular substitutes of amphetamine derivatives, as they produce similar psychopharmacological effects (Valente et al., 2014). In accordance with the opinion of Weinstein and colleagues (2017), the class of synthetic cathinones include substances with such diverse psychoactive compounds and different action mechanisms, that it is not reasonable to present synthetic cathinone toxicity in general terms. Considering the pharmacokinetics of specific types of cathinones and derivatives, a number of studies – primarily utilizing in-vivo animal models – are available that have explored these properties. *Mephedrone* was found to induce a dose-dependent increase in locomotor activity in male Sprague-Dawley rats lasting for about two hours, reaching peak concentration between half an hour and one hour after oral administration (Martinez-Clemente et al., 2013), reducing body temperature as a result of its thermoregulatory characteristics (Miller et al., 2013), increasing both dopamine and 5-HT levels in the nucleus accumbens (Kehr et al., 2011), striatum and frontal cortex (Gołembiowska et al., 2016), and producing behavioral sensitization (Gregg et al., 2013). Papaseit and colleagues (2016) were the first who published a paper on mephedrone's in-vivo pharmacological effects in humans (n = 12), implementing an experimental design.

As compared to the pharmacokinetic parameters of MDMA, mephedrone's main stimulant-like effects (i.e., euphoria, well-being, changes in perception) peaked earlier and were shorter in duration, with a half-life elimination of 2.15 hours. These properties might contribute to the fact that mephedrone users often show a more compulsive pattern of consumption. Several human studies confirmed that all types of synthetic cathinones have the potential of inducing lethal overdoses due to various complications. Papaseit and colleagues (2017) reviewed the literature of both lethal and nonfatal mephedrone-induced clinical intoxication cases and described the mean blood concentration of mephedrone to be 2,663 ng/ml in fatal cases. Nevertheless, a wide range (between 51 and 22,000 ng/ml) was identified, which might encumber the establishment of a generalizable cut-off value regarding lethal toxicity. Among the leading causes of mephedrone-related lethal fatalities, excited delirium (Lusthof et al., 2011), cerebral edema, cardiac arrest, hyponatremia, and brain death (Gustavsson & Escher, 2009; Wood et al., 2010) have been mentioned, although poly drug use is a common factor in these deaths, and mephedrone is less risky than other substances in this category.

Pentedrone (2-(methylamino)-1-phenylpentan-1-one) and *pentylone* (β-keto-methylbenzodioxolylpentanamine) both increase locomotion and body temperature in Wistar rats, with the longest effects observed after the administration of pentedrone as compared to pentylone and mephedrone (Javadi-Paydar et al., 2018). These are commonly falsely sold as being MDMA, due to their cheaper production costs and lower risk of criminal repurcussions associated with their import. Initial user experiences are quite similar to MDMA, but unpleasant (and dangerous) side effects are far more common and sustained in duration.

Similarly to mephedrone, *methylone* (3,4-methylenedioxy-N-methylcathinone) – with a thirty-minute peak effect concentration after administration in rats – produces increased overall locomotion and hyperthermic effects (Štefková et al., 2017), and might also cause fatality in case of human users due to hyperthermia (Pearson et al., 2012). MDPV (3,4-methylenedioxypyrovalerone) meanwhile can be defined as a dopamine transporter blocker, and as a locomotor stimulant, almost ten-fold more potent than cocaine in case of rats (Anizan et al., 2016). It is characterized by rapid pharmacokinetics, especially when administered intravenously, reaching peak plasma concentrations in ten to twenty minutes (Baumann et al., 2017). Both MDPV and second-generation "bath salts" α-PVP are considered to have low affinity and potency as serotonin transporters (Meltzer et al., 2006), but may act as powerful inhibitors of norepinephrine as well as dopamine transporters (Stanciu et al., 2017).

Main reasons for methylone-induced death include the aforementioned hyperthermia (Kesha et al., 2013), anoxia (Barrios et al., 2016), sudden cardiac death (Carbone et al., 2013), steatosis of the heart muscle, congenital heart disease, bronchial asthma (Kovács, Tóth & Kereszty, 2012) and serotonin syndrome (Warrick et al., 2012). MDPV as a cardiotoxic substance may cause cardiomyopathy and acute coronary syndrome (Schindler et al., 2016; Sivagnanam et al., 2013) and its use might lead to death by producing rhabdomyolysis, coagulopathy, acidosis, or anoxic brain injury (Murray, Murphy & Beuhler, 2012). Deaths associated with either sole α-PVP consumption or α-PVP combined with pentedrone intake were caused by cardiac arrest (Potocka-Banaś et al., 2017), pulmonary edema, atherosclerotic lesions of the arteries (Sykutera, Cychowska & Bloch-Boguslawska, 2015) or as a result of heart failure after a sustained restraint of substance use (Nagai et al., 2014).

Synthetic Cannabinoid Receptor Agonists (SCRAs)

Just like synthetic cathinones, SCRAs were primarily developed for therapeutic and research purposes by possessing some of the properties of Δ^9-tetrahydrocannabinol (THC), the psychoactive compound of cannabis. And just like many other drugs that started as a medication, SCRAs were soon misused as recreational drugs (Wiley et al., 2011). SCRAs are pharmacologically very distinct from natural cannabis, acting on the same receptors (hence the name) but in very different ways, with different subjective user experiences and vastly diverse risk profiles. Most SCRAs act as a full agonist at the CB_1 receptor, and their binding affinity is much higher than that of natural cannabis (Spaderna et al., 2013), which is linked to their enhanced toxicity (Fantegrossi et al., 2014). Main causes of synthetic cannabinoid-induced fatalities have included excited delirium, trauma or accidents (Labay et al., 2016), sudden cardiac death (Westin et al., 2016), diabetic ketoacidosis (Hess et al., 2015), rhabdomyolysis, and anoxic brain injury (Katz et al., 2016). Further severe adverse effects of synthetic cannabinoid use include kidney injury (Srisung, Jamal & Prabhakar, 2015), cardiotoxic effects (Trecki, Gerona & Schwartz, 2015), hyperthermia (Katz et al., 2016) or psychosis (Van Amsterdam, Brunt & van den Brink, 2015). Regarding SCRAs' toxicity and adverse effects, Pintori and colleagues (2017) refer to the main synthetic cannabinoid-induced states as the "synthetic cannabinoid tetrad effects," consisting of hypothermia, analgesia, hypolocomotion and catalepsy.

SCRAs carry significant potential for overdose: the use of various synthetic cannabinoid compounds have been linked to fatalities, including *5F-AMB* (methyl 2-(1-(5-fluoropentyl)-1H-INdazole-3-carboxamide)-3-methylbutanoate), *ADB-FUBINACA* (N-1-amino-3,3-dimethyl-1-oxobutan-2-yl)-1-(4-fluorobenzyl) 1H indazole 3 carboxamide), *MDMB-CHMICA* (methyl 2 - [[1-(cyclohexylmethyl)-1H-indole-3-carbonyl]amino]-3,3-dimethylbutanoate), and *MAB-CHMINACA* (N-(1-amino 3,3-dimethyl-1-oxobutan-2-yl)-1-(cyclohexylmethyl)-1H-indazole-3-carboxamide) (e.g., Katz et al., 2016; Shanks & Behonick, 2016; Shanks, Clark & Behonick, 2016; Westin et al., 2016). The consumption of natural cannabis is not considered to cause lethal overdoses.

A recent study assessed the pharmacokinetic properties of one of the most frequently used synthetic cannabinoid compounds, *JWH-018*, in human subjects (Toennes et al., 2017), and found that serum concentration reaches its maximum within the first one and a half hours after inhalation (2.9–9.9 ng/ml). The authors also described that partly due to the fast multiexponential decline that follows the peak concentration, the detection of JWH-018 requires high analytical sensitivity. Teske and colleagues (2010) also reported fast (within three hours after administration) increase and drop of JWH-018 concentration in human volunteers.

Synthetic Opioids

In the case of Novel Synthetic Opioids (NSO), it is mainly the source of manufacturing, the route of purchase, and the setting of their consumption that make them NPS, since these compounds and substances are generally available as prescription drugs as well. Some authors (e.g., Prekupec et al., 2017) therefore distinguish prescription opioids from illicitly manufactured opioids and NSO. The class of NSO - just like that of synthetic cathinones and cannabinoids - contains numerous different highly potent substances. Reports (e.g., Armenian et al., 2018; Zawilska, 2017) suggest that mostly fentanyl-types and some new generation opioids (e.g., AH-7921, U-47700, MT-45) should be highlighted as the most dangerous NSO, which pose significant higher life-threatening risk of medical and psychiatric comorbidities compared to classical opioids, including overdose, respiratory arrest and risk of infectious diseases (HIV, or hepatitis C) when injected.

As compared to formerly scheduled opioids, NSO-like *acetylfentanyls* are usually much more potent (i.e., fifteen times more potent than heroin) and their use may lead to severe adverse consequences, including fatal overdoses (e.g., Lozier et al., 2015; McIntyre et al., 2015; Takase et al., 2016). Lethal cases were explained by congestion and edema of the lungs or the brain (McIntyre et al., 2016; Poklis et al., 2016), suffocation due to froth in the airways and generalized visceral congestion (Guerrieri et al., 2017), or hyperemia of the internal organs (Fels et al., 2017).

To date, none of the NSO has been studied in a controlled clinical context among human subjects. Therefore, their pharmacokinetic properties in humans are unkown and may vary greatly between specific types of NSO. For instance, self-reported experiences posted online suggest that the intensity of the effects of substances such as U-47700 rapidly decreases after administration, which might facilitate re-dosing (Elliott, Brandt & Smith, 2016), while slower onset of action (one to two hours after oral intake) is reported (Helander, Bäckberg & Beck, 2014) in cases of MT-45 (1-cyclohexyl-4-(1,2-diphenylethyl)piperazine).

Tryptamines

Unregulated, substituted tryptamines - as NPS-type substances - mimic the effects of controlled tryptamines (e.g., psilocybin, DMT) and are marketed as nonillegal alternatives of psychedelic drugs (Palma-Conesa et al., 2017). *5-MeO-DiPT*, a lesser-known psychedelic, is mainly sought by "psychonauts" for its tendancy to induce sensory hallucinations rather than visual effects. Fantegrossi and colleagues (2006) explored in-vivo properties of 5-MeO-DiPT in mice and rats. Their finding that 5-MeO-DiPT shows affinity at receptors relevant to hallucinogen effects might explain human users' psychedelic experiences with 5-MeO-DiPT and tryptamine-type NSOs. Users further reported that the effects of specific tryptamines (e.g., *5-MEO-DALT*: 5-methoxy-N,N-diallyltryptamine) might appear within fifteen minutes and reach the peak in thirty minutes (Tittarelli et al., 2015).

DMT is possibly the most popular tryptamine, generally consumed via heating crystals in a glass pipe. Users report powerful, immediate effects with strong imagery, and it is considered to one of the most intense psychedelic experiences. The action mechanism and effects of this was tested in a sample of experienced hallucinogen users (Strassman, 1996), indicating that a 5-HT1A agonist has a buffering effect on the 5-HT2-mediated hallucinogen effects of DMT. Tryptamines are usually characterized by rapid onset and short duration of effects, but some substances from this class, especially when possessing a monoamine oxidase inhibiting action, (e.g., *5-MeO-AMT*: 5-methoxy-α-methyltryptamine) may produce long lasting effects of up to twelve to eighteen hours (Tittarelli et al., 2015).

While tryptamines are comparatively safer than many other classes of psychoactive substances, adverse consequences of tryptamine (e.g., 5-MeO-DMT, 5-MeO-DiPT, 5-MeO-DALT) consumption have been found to include agitation, prolonged hallucination, paranoid symptoms, mydriasis, tachycardia, hyperpyrexia, diaphoresis, catalepsy, rhabdomyolisis, or acute renal failure (Brush, Bird & Boyer, 2004; Jovel, Felthous & Bhattacharyya, 2014; Smolinske, Ragosti & Schenkel, 2005; Wilson et al., 2005). Fatal overdoses due to tryptamine intake are rare but not unknown. In these cases, leading causes of death were reported as malignant hyperthermia (Daldrup et al., 1986), pulmonary edema, generalized visceral congestion (Morano et al., 1993), periarteritis nodosa, myocardial ischaemia, or periprostatic bleeding (Tanaka et al., 2006). Furthermore, the hallucinogenic effects of tryptamines may also lead to life-threatening situations or even lethal accidents, through the alteration of perception (Araújo et al., 2015).

Piperazines

Since the early 2000s, piperazine derivatives, such as *N-benzylpiperazine* (BZP) and *1-[3-(trifluoro-methyl)-phenyl]piperazine* (TFMPP) have become drugs of abuse (de Boer et al., 2001). Antia and colleagues (2009b) studied in-vivo interactions of BZP (N-benzylpiperazine) and TFMPP (1-[3-(trifluoro-methyl)-phenyl]piperazine) and found that metabolic profiles of these piperazines are altered when coingested. In mice, the combination of BZP and TFMPP produces MDMA-like effects with the release of both dopamine (DA) and serotonin (5-HT; Baumann et al., 2005). BZP pharmacokinetics were also explored in human participants (Antia et al., 2009a). Plasma concentrations of BZP peaked within seventy-five minutes (262 ng/ml), with an elimination half-life of 5.5 hours. A randomised double-blind, placebo-controlled trial examined the effects and outcomes of the use of BZP/TFMPP in human volunteers (Thompson et al., 2010). Severe adverse events - i.e., agitation, anxiety, hallucinations, insomnia, migraine and vomiting - occured in some respondents, with increased heart rate and blood pressure. Decreased body temperature was observed by Lin and colleagues (2009) after the administration of BZP in human female subjects. Mild stimulant and hallucinogenic effects were reported by *pMeOPP* (1-(4-methoxyphenyl) piperazine) and *mCPP* (meta-chlorophenylpiperazine) users (Elliott, 2011).

Kersten and McLaughlin (2015) listed hyponatremia, serotonin syndrome and renal failure as potential risks of piperazine toxicity. Further unwanted effects of piperazines consist of palpitations, seizures, tremor, chest pain, urinary retention, or nausea (Gee et al., 2005; Wilkins, Sweetsur & Girling, 2008). Additionally, some studies linked fatal cases to the overuse of piperazines as well (e.g., Elliott & Smith, 2008). Table 25.2 summarizes main desired effects, intoxication symptoms and adverse consequences of NPS consumption per various NPS classes and highlighted compounds, based on the available human studies.

Table 25.2 NPS use-related desired effects, toxicity, and further adverse outcomes in humans

Desired effects[a]	NPS class: Synthetic cathinones					SCRAs[b]	Synthetic opioids						Tryptamines			Piperazines			
	Mephedrone	Methylone	MDPV	α-PVP	4-MEC		MT-45	Butyryl-fentanyl	Acetyl-fentanyl	AH-7921	Furanyl-fentanyl	U-47700	5-MeO-DMT	5-MeO-DiPT	5-MeO-DALT	BZP	mCPP	MeOPP	TFMPP
Euphoria	✓	✓	✓	✓	✓	✓	✓	✓	✓	✓	✓	✓	✓	n.d.	✓	✓	✓	✓	n.d.
Well-being	✓	✓	n.d.	n.d.	n.d.	✓	✓	n.d.	n.d.	n.d.	n.d.	n.d.	n.d.	n.d.	n.d.	n.d.	n.d.	n.d.	n.d.
Perceptual changes	✓	n.d.	n.d.	n.d.	n.d.	n.d.	n.d.	n.d.	n.d.	n.d.	n.d.	n.d.	n.d.	n.d.	n.d.	n.d.	n.d.	n.d.	n.d.
Elevated mood	✓	✓	✓	n.d.	✓	✓	✓	n.d.	n.d.	✓	n.d.	✓	n.d.	n.d.	n.d.	n.d.	n.d.	n.d.	n.d.
Increased self-esteem	✓	n.d.	✓	n.d.	n.d.	n.d.	n.d.	n.d.	n.d.	n.d.	n.d.	n.d.	n.d.	n.d.	n.d.	✓	n.d.	n.d.	n.d.
Motor excitation	✓	✓	✓	✓	n.d.	n.d.	n.d.	n.d.	n.d.	n.d.	n.d.	n.d.	n.d.	n.d.	n.d.	n.d.	n.d.	n.d.	n.d.
Reduced fatigue	✓	✓	n.d.	✓	n.d.	✓	n.d.	n.d.	n.d.	n.d.	n.d.	n.d.	n.d.	n.d.	n.d.	✓	n.d.	✓	✓
Increased concentration	✓	n.d.	n.d.	n.d.	n.d.	n.d.	n.d.	n.d.	n.d.	n.d.	n.d.	n.d.	n.d.	n.d.	n.d.	n.d.	n.d.	n.d.	n.d.
Talkativeness and sociability	✓	n.d.	✓	n.d.	✓	✓	n.d.	n.d.	n.d.	n.d.	n.d.	n.d.	n.d.	n.d.	n.d.	✓	n.d.	n.d.	n.d.
Empathy	✓	✓	✓	✓	✓	n.d.	n.d.	n.d.	n.d.	n.d.	n.d.	n.d.	n.d.	n.d.	✓	n.d.	✓	n.d.	n.d.
Disinhibition	✓	n.d.		n.d.	n.d.	n.d.	n.d.	n.d.	n.d.	n.d.	n.d.	n.d.	n.d.	n.d.	n.d.	n.d.	n.d.	n.d.	n.d.
Mild sexual stimulation or enhanced sexual desire	✓	n.d.	✓	✓	n.d.	n.d.	n.d.	n.d.	n.d.	n.d.	n.d.	n.d.	n.d.	✓	n.d.	n.d.	n.d.	n.d.	n.d.
Thought accelaration	n.d.	✓	✓	n.d.	n.d.	n.d.	n.d.	n.d.	n.d.	n.d.	n.d.	n.d.	n.d.	n.d.	n.d.	n.d.	n.d.	n.d.	n.d.
Reduced fear	n.d.	✓	n.d.	n.d.	n.d.	n.d.	n.d.	n.d.	n.d.	n.d.	n.d.	n.d.	n.d.	n.d.	n.d.	n.d.	n.d.	n.d.	n.d.
Increased productivity	n.d.	n.d.	✓	n.d.	n.d.	n.d.	n.d.	n.d.	n.d.	n.d.	n.d.	n.d.	n.d.	n.d.	n.d.	n.d.	n.d.	n.d.	n.d.
Relaxed feeling	n.d.	n.d.	n.d.	n.d.	✓	✓	✓	n.d.	n.d.	✓	✓	✓	n.d.	n.d.	n.d.	n.d.	n.d.	✓	n.d.
Appreciation of music	n.d.	n.d.	n.d.	n.d.	✓	n.d.	n.d.	n.d.	n.d.	n.d.	n.d.	n.d.	n.d.	n.d.	n.d.	n.d.	✓	✓	n.d.
Intense high	n.d.	n.d.	n.d.	n.d.	n.d.	✓	✓	✓	✓	n.d.	n.d.	n.d.	n.d.	n.d.	n.d.	n.d.	✓	n.d.	✓
Sedation	n.d.	n.d.	n.d.	n.d.	n.d.	n.d.	✓	n.d.	n.d.	✓	n.d.	✓	n.d.	n.d.	n.d.	n.d.	n.d.	n.d.	n.d.
Feeling of warmth	n.d.	n.d.	n.d.	n.d.	n.d.	n.d.	✓	n.d.	n.d.	✓	n.d.	n.d.	n.d.	n.d.	n.d.	n.d.	n.d.	n.d.	n.d.
Quietness of the mind	n.d.	n.d.	n.d.	n.d.	n.d.	n.d.	✓	n.d.	n.d.	n.d.	n.d.	n.d.	n.d.	n.d.	n.d.	n.d.	n.d.	n.d.	n.d.
Pain relief	n.d.	n.d.	n.d.	n.d.	n.d.	n.d.	n.d.	n.d.	n.d.	✓	n.d.	✓	n.d.	n.d.	n.d.	n.d.	n.d.	n.d.	n.d.
Dreamy and inattentive state	n.d.	n.d.	n.d.	n.d.	n.d.	n.d.	n.d.	n.d.	n.d.	✓	n.d.	n.d.	✓	n.d.	✓	n.d.	n.d.	n.d.	n.d.
Anxiolytic effect	n.d.	n.d.	n.d.	n.d.	n.d.	n.d.	n.d.	n.d.	n.d.	n.d.	n.d.	✓	n.d.	n.d.	n.d.	n.d.	n.d.	✓	n.d.
Visual and/or auditory hallucinations	n.d.	n.d.	n.d.	n.d.	n.d.	n.d.	n.d.	n.d.	n.d.	n.d.	n.d.	n.d.	n.d.	✓	n.d.	n.d.	n.d.	✓	n.d.

Adverse effects and outcomes[a]	Synthetic cathinones					SCRAs[b]	Synthetic opioids						Tryptamines			Piperazines			
	Mephedrone	Methylone	MDPV	α-PVP	4-MEC		MT-45	Butyryl-fentanyl	Acetyl-fentanyl	AH-7921	Furanyl-fentanyl	U-47700	5-MeO-DMT	5-MeO-DiPT	5-MeO-DALT	BZP	mCPP	MeOPP	TFMPP
Tachycardia	✓	✓	✓	✓	✓	n.d.	n.d.	✓	n.d.	✓	n.d.	✓	✓	✓	✓	✓	✓	n.d.	n.d.
Tachypsychia	✓	n.d.	n.d.	n.d.	n.d.	n.d.	n.d.	n.d.	n.d.	n.d.	n.d.	n.d.	n.d.	n.d.	n.d.	n.d.	n.d.	n.d.	n.d.
Anorexia	✓	✓	n.d.	n.d.	n.d.	n.d.	n.d.	n.d.	n.d.	n.d.	n.d.	n.d.	n.d.	n.d.	n.d.	n.d.	n.d.	✓	n.d.
Hyperthermia and/or dehydration	✓	✓	✓	n.d.	n.d.	✓	✓	n.d.	n.d.	n.d.	n.d.	n.d.	n.d.	✓	✓	n.d.	✓	✓	n.d.
Sweating	✓	✓	n.d.	n.d.	n.d.	n.d.	✓	n.d.	n.d.	n.d.	n.d.	n.d.	n.d.	n.d.	n.d.	n.d.	✓	n.d.	n.d.
Headache	✓	n.d.	n.d.	n.d.	n.d.	n.d.	n.d.	n.d.	n.d.	n.d.	n.d.	n.d.	n.d.	n.d.	n.d.	n.d.	✓	✓	n.d.
Hypertension	✓	✓	n.d.	✓	n.d.	n.d.	n.d.	n.d.	n.d.	✓	n.d.	n.d.	n.d.	✓	n.d.	n.d.	n.d.	n.d.	n.d.
Arrhythmias	✓	n.d.	n.d.	n.d.	n.d.	n.d.	n.d.	n.d.	n.d.	n.d.	n.d.	n.d.	n.d.	n.d.	n.d.	n.d.	n.d.	n.d.	n.d.
Chest pain	✓	n.d.	n.d.	n.d.	n.d.	n.d.	n.d.	n.d.	n.d.	n.d.	n.d.	n.d.	n.d.	n.d.	n.d.	n.d.	n.d.	n.d.	n.d.
Seizures	✓	✓	n.d.	n.d.	n.d.	✓	n.d.	n.d.	n.d.	✓	n.d.	n.d.	n.d.	n.d.	n.d.	n.d.	n.d.	n.d.	n.d.
Nausea and/or vomiting	✓	✓	n.d.	n.d.	✓	✓	✓	n.d.	n.d.	✓	n.d.	✓	n.d.	✓	n.d.	✓	✓	✓	n.d.
Bruxism and/or jaw clenching	✓	✓	n.d.	n.d.	✓	n.d.	n.d.	n.d.	n.d.	n.d.	n.d.	n.d.	n.d.	n.d.	n.d.	n.d.	n.d.	n.d.	n.d.
Mydriasis	n.d.	✓	✓	n.d.	n.d.	n.d.	n.d.	n.d.	n.d.	n.d.	n.d.	n.d.	n.d.	✓	n.d.	n.d.	n.d.	n.d.	n.d.
Nystagmus	n.d.	✓	n.d.	n.d.	✓	n.d.	n.d.	n.d.	n.d.	n.d.	n.d.	n.d.	n.d.	n.d.	n.d.	n.d.	n.d.	n.d.	n.d.
Tremors	n.d.	✓	n.d.	n.d.	n.d.	n.d.	n.d.	n.d.	n.d.	n.d.	n.d.	✓	n.d.	n.d.	n.d.	n.d.	n.d.	n.d.	n.d.
Dry mouth	n.d.	✓	n.d.	n.d.	n.d.	n.d.	n.d.	n.d.	n.d.	n.d.	n.d.	n.d.	n.d.	n.d.	n.d.	n.d.	n.d.	n.d.	n.d.
Difficulty urinating	n.d.	✓	n.d.	n.d.	n.d.	n.d.	n.d.	n.d.	n.d.	n.d.	n.d.	n.d.	n.d.	n.d.	n.d.	n.d.	n.d.	n.d.	n.d.
Anxiety	n.d.	✓	n.d.	n.d.	n.d.	✓	✓	✓	✓	n.d.	n.d.	✓	n.d.	✓	n.d.	✓	✓	n.d.	✓
Derealization or depersonalization	n.d.	✓	n.d.	n.d.	n.d.	n.d.	n.d.	n.d.	n.d.	n.d.	n.d.	n.d.	n.d.	n.d.	n.d.	n.d.	n.d.	n.d.	n.d.
Suicidal ideation	n.d.	✓	n.d.	n.d.	n.d.	n.d.	n.d.	n.d.	n.d.	n.d.	n.d.	n.d.	n.d.	n.d.	n.d.	n.d.	n.d.	n.d.	n.d.
Agitation	n.d.	n.d.	✓	✓	n.d.	✓	n.d.	n.d.	n.d.	n.d.	n.d.	n.d.	✓	n.d.	✓	✓	n.d.	n.d.	n.d.
Paranoia	n.d.	n.d.	✓	n.d.	n.d.	✓	n.d.	n.d.	n.d.	n.d.	n.d.	n.d.	n.d.	✓	✓	✓	n.d.	n.d.	n.d.
Hypokalemia	n.d.	n.d.	✓	n.d.	n.d.	n.d.	n.d.	n.d.	n.d.	n.d.	n.d.	n.d.	n.d.	n.d.	n.d.	n.d.	n.d.	n.d.	n.d.
Excited delirium	✓	n.d.	✓	✓	n.d.	n.d.	n.d.	n.d.	n.d.	n.d.	n.d.	n.d.	n.d.	n.d.	n.d.	n.d.	n.d.	n.d.	n.d.
Hallucinations and/or psychosis	n.d.	n.d.	n.d.	✓	n.d.	✓	n.d.	n.d.	n.d.	n.d.	n.d.	n.d.	n.d.	n.d.	n.d.	✓	✓	n.d.	n.d.

Table 25.2 (*cont.*)

Adverse effects and outcomes[a]	Synthetic cathinones					SCRAs[b]	Synthetic opioids						Tryptamines			Piperazines			
	Mephedrone	Methylone	MDPV	α-PVP	4-MEC		MT-45	Butyryl-fentanyl	Acetyl-fentanyl	AH-7921	Furanyl-fentanyl	U-47700	5-MeO-DMT	5-MeO-DiPT	5-MeO-DALT	BZP	mCPP	MeOPP	TFMPP
Palpitations	n.d.	n.d.	n.d.	n.d.	✓	n.d.	n.d.	n.d.	n.d.	n.d.	n.d.	n.d.	n.d.	n.d.	n.d.	n.d.	n.d.	n.d.	n.d.
Insomnia	n.d.	n.d.	n.d.	n.d.	✓	n.d.	✓	✓	n.d.	✓	n.d.	n.d.	n.d.	✓	n.d.	✓	✓	n.d.	n.d.
Mood swings	n.d.	n.d.	n.d.	n.d.	n.d.	✓	n.d.	n.d.	n.d.	n.d.	n.d.	n.d.	n.d.	n.d.	n.d.	n.d.	n.d.	n.d.	✓
Myoclonia	n.d.	n.d.	n.d.	n.d.	n.d.	✓	n.d.	n.d.	n.d.	n.d.	n.d.	n.d.	n.d.	✓	✓	n.d.	n.d.	n.d.	n.d.
Respiratory depression and/or cyanosis	n.d.	n.d.	n.d.	n.d.	n.d.	n.d.	✓	✓	✓	✓	✓	✓	n.d.	n.d.	n.d.	n.d.	n.d.	n.d.	n.d.
Hearing loss	n.d.	n.d.	n.d.	n.d.	n.d.	n.d.	✓	n.d.	n.d.	n.d.	n.d.	n.d.	n.d.	n.d.	n.d.	n.d.	n.d.	n.d.	n.d.
Hair depigmentation and/or hair loss	n.d.	n.d.	n.d.	n.d.	n.d.	n.d.	✓	n.d.	n.d.	n.d.	n.d.	n.d.	n.d.	n.d.	n.d.	n.d.	n.d.	n.d.	n.d.
Folliculitis and dermatitis	n.d.	n.d.	n.d.	n.d.	n.d.	n.d.	✓	n.d.	n.d.	n.d.	n.d.	n.d.	n.d.	n.d.	n.d.	n.d.	n.d.	n.d.	n.d.
Apnea	n.d.	n.d.	n.d.	n.d.	n.d.	n.d.	n.d.	✓	n.d.	n.d.	✓	n.d.	n.d.	n.d.	n.d.	n.d.	n.d.	n.d.	n.d.
Diffuse alveolar hemorrhage	n.d.	n.d.	n.d.	n.d.	n.d.	n.d.	n.d.	✓	n.d.	n.d.	n.d.	n.d.	n.d.	n.d.	n.d.	n.d.	n.d.	n.d.	n.d.
Miosis	n.d.	n.d.	n.d.	n.d.	n.d.	n.d.	n.d.	n.d.	✓	n.d.	✓	n.d.	n.d.	n.d.	n.d.	n.d.	n.d.	n.d.	n.d.
Constipation	n.d.	n.d.	n.d.	n.d.	n.d.	n.d.	n.d.	n.d.	✓	n.d.	n.d.	n.d.	n.d.	n.d.	n.d.	n.d.	n.d.	n.d.	n.d.
Bradycardia	n.d.	n.d.	n.d.	n.d.	n.d.	n.d.	n.d.	n.d.	✓	n.d.	n.d.	n.d.	n.d.	n.d.	n.d.	n.d.	n.d.	n.d.	n.d.
Hypotension	n.d.	n.d.	n.d.	n.d.	n.d.	n.d.	n.d.	n.d.	✓	n.d.	n.d.	n.d.	n.d.	n.d.	n.d.	n.d.	n.d.	n.d.	n.d.
Hypothermia	n.d.	n.d.	n.d.	n.d.	n.d.	n.d.	n.d.	n.d.	n.d.	✓	n.d.	n.d.	n.d.	n.d.	n.d.	✓	n.d.	n.d.	n.d.
Bradypnea	n.d.	n.d.	n.d.	n.d.	n.d.	n.d.	n.d.	n.d.	n.d.	n.d.	n.d.	✓	n.d.	n.d.	n.d.	n.d.	n.d.	n.d.	n.d.
Rhabdomyolysis	n.d.	n.d.	n.d.	n.d.	n.d.	n.d.	n.d.	n.d.	n.d.	n.d.	n.d.	n.d.	✓	✓	✓	n.d.	n.d.	n.d.	n.d.
Catalepsy	n.d.	n.d.	n.d.	n.d.	n.d.	n.d.	n.d.	n.d.	n.d.	n.d.	n.d.	n.d.	n.d.	✓	n.d.	n.d.	n.d.	n.d.	n.d.
Formication	n.d.	n.d.	n.d.	n.d.	n.d.	n.d.	n.d.	n.d.	n.d.	n.d.	n.d.	n.d.	n.d.	✓	n.d.	n.d.	n.d.	n.d.	n.d.
Echolalia	n.d.	n.d.	n.d.	n.d.	n.d.	n.d.	n.d.	n.d.	n.d.	n.d.	n.d.	n.d.	n.d.	✓	n.d.	n.d.	n.d.	n.d.	n.d.
Diaphoresis	n.d.	n.d.	n.d.	n.d.	n.d.	n.d.	n.d.	n.d.	n.d.	n.d.	n.d.	n.d.	n.d.	n.d.	✓	n.d.	n.d.	n.d.	n.d.
Panic attacks	n.d.	n.d.	n.d.	n.d.	n.d.	n.d.	n.d.	n.d.	n.d.	n.d.	n.d.	n.d.	n.d.	n.d.	n.d.	n.d.	✓	n.d.	n.d.
Fatal outcome	✓	✓	✓	✓	n.d.	✓	✓	✓	✓	✓	✓	✓	n.d.	✓	n.d.	n.d.	n.d.	n.d.	n.d.

Notes. n.d.: no data.

[a] NPS-specific desired effects and adverse outcomes are listed based on the following scientific literature:

- *Synthetic cathinones* (incl. mephedrone, methylone, MDPV, α-PVP and 4-MEC): Barrios et al., 2016; Borek and Holstede, 2012; Carbone et al., 2012; EMCDDA, 2016b; German et al., 2014; Gustavsson & Escher, 2009; Kapitány-Fövény et al., 2013b; Karila et al., 2015, 2016, 2018; Kovács et al., 2012; Larabi et al., 2018; Lusthof et al., 2011; Murray et al., 2012; Nagai et al., 2014; Papaseit et al., 2016; Pearson et al., 2012; Penders et al., 2012; Potocka-Banaś et al., 2017; Shimizu et al., 2007; Spiller et al., 2011; Stanciu et al., 2017; Sykutera et al., 2015; VanHout, 2014; Warrick et al., 2012; Winstock et al., 2010, 2011; Wood et al., 2010; Wyman et al., 2013; Zawilska & Wojcieszak, 2017
- *SCRAs* (incl. JWH-018, 5F-AMB, ADB-FUBINACA, MDMB-CHMICA and MAB-CHMINACA): Barratt et al., 2013; Bonar et al., 2014; Cohen et al., 2017; Cooper & Haney, 2008; Every-Palmer, 2011; Fattore & Fratta, 2011; Gunderson et al., 2014; Hermanns-Clausen et al., 2013; Hess et al., 2015; Kapitány-Fövény et al., 2013a; Katz et al., 2016; Labay et al., 2016; Spaderna et al., 2013; Srisung et al., 2015; Trecki et al., 2015; Ustundag et al., 2015; van Amsterdam et al., 2015; Westin et al., 2016; Winstock & Barratt, 2013
- *Synthetic opioids* (incl. MT-45, butyrylfentanyl, acetylfentanyl, AH-7921, Furanylfentanyl and U-47700): Bäckberg et al., 2015; Cole et al., 2015; Cunningham et al., 2016; Domanski et al., 2017; Elliott et al., 2016; EMCDDA-Europol, 2017; Fels et al., 2017; Guerrieri et al., 2017; Helander et al., 2014, 2016, 2017; Jones et al., 2017; Katselou et al., 2015; Kjellgren et al., 2016; McIntyre et al., 2015, 2016; Miller et al., 2018; Papsun et al., 2016; Poklis et al., 2016; Rambaran et al., 2017; Schneir et al., 2017; Siddiqi et al., 2015; Stogner, 2014; Vorce et al., 2014; Reddit user report: www.reddit.com/r/researchchemicals/comments/35dmg3/butyrfentanyl_got_some_recently_and_it_was_great/
- *Tryptamines* (incl. 5-Meo-DMT, 5-MeO-DiPT and 5-MeO-DALT): Alatrash et al., 2006; Brush et al., 2004; Corkery et al., 2012; Ikeda et al., 2005; Itowaka et al., 2007; Jebadurai, 2012; Jovel et al., 2014; Kalasho and Vibe Nielsen, 2016; Ott, 2001; Smolinske et al., 2005; Tanaka et al., 2006; Thammongkolchai et al., 2015; Wilson et al., 2005
- *Piperazines* (incl. BZP, mCPP, MeOPP – pMeOPP and TFMPP): Butler and Sheridan, 2007; Jan et al., 2010; Jebadurai, 2012; Kovaleva et al., 2008; Lin et al., 2009, 2011; Murphy et al., 1991; Tancer and Johanson, 2001; Thompson et al., 2010

[b] In the case of SCRAs, the majority of the human studies either explored synthetic cannabinoid effects in general or presented toxicological cases with multiple synthetic cannabinoid compounds identified. The current table therefore overviews available data in an aggregated way for SCRAs, instead of listing compound-specific effects and outcomes.

Proposed Treatment

Pharmacological Treatment

Despite the emerging knowledge about the dangers of NPS use, only a few studies considered potentially effective treatment of NPS-related problems, including both somatic and psychological harms. Regarding synthetic cathinones, Prosser and Nelson (2012) described that patients exposed to synthetic cathinones may experience adverse outcomes of a sympathomimetic toxidrome including agitation, seizures, psychosis, tachycardia, or hypertension. These presentations are mainly treated with benzodiazepines in order to counteract the release and reuptake inhibition of epinephrine and norepinephrine (Prosser & Nelson, 2012). If hyperthermia occurs, aggressive cooling is suggested, whereas hyponatremia should be treated similarly to MDMA-induced hyponatremia: i.e., the application of water restriction or hypertonic saline is recommended. Banks and colleagues (2014) further emphasized that in addition to the reduction of agitation and psychosis, the support of renal perfusion might become necessary as well. The authors concur with Prosser and Nelson to suggest the use of benzodiazepines and antipsychotics in specific cases, alongside general supportive care. The utilization of physical restraints in cases of excited delirium has been known to provoke sudden death among patients with stimulant-induced psychosis (Stratton et al., 2001). As such, the application of chemical restraints is advised to be a better option (Banks et al., 2014).

Cooper (2016) provided a substantial review on the treatment options of synthetic cannabinoid-related intoxication and detoxification. Based on the presented findings (e.g., Hermanns-Clausen et al., 2013; Rodgman et al., 2014; Schep et al., 2015; Ukaigwe et al., 2014), acute intoxication in these cases necessitates supportive care and intravenous fluids in order to manage electrolyte and fluid disturbances. Adverse intoxication effects may similarly be treated with benzodiazepines (or Quetiapine for patients who are not responding to benzodiazepines), but psychotic states and mania may indicate the use of neuroleptics. In some cases where hyperemesis occurs, antiemetics are suggested by some clinicians. Throughout the process of detoxification, strong cravings might be counteracted with the administration of Naltrexone.

First-line treatment of NSO-induced intoxication, similarly to that of other opioids, includes the application of Naloxone (Zawilska, 2017), with an initial dose between 0.4 mg and 2 mg (adults) or 0.01 mg/kg (children). Dose repetition should be carried out in every two to three minutes, until the patient's breathing reaches a rate greater than ten breaths per minute. As Armenian and colleagues (2017) pointed out, many of the NSOs have high affinity for μ-opioid receptors, which often indicates larger doses of naloxone than usually applied. Some authors (e.g., Hawk, Vaca & D'Onofrio, 2015) highlighted the importance of effective use reduction/prevention to cope with the NSO epidemic and resulting overdose risks and fatalities. These proposed strategies are comprised of targeted education, widespread access to treatment options, availability of naloxone or the support of harm reduction programs. Dean and colleagues (2013) described focused, symptom-based supportive care as the recommended management of acute phenethylamine intoxication, with an initial phase of maintaining the airway, breathing, and circulation. Excited delirium can be prevented with sedation, fluid resuscitation, and the reduction of hyperthermia (e.g., with rapid cooling).

Tryptamine (i.e., 5-MeO-DiPT)-induced intoxication symptoms were reported to be treated effectively with the administration of Lorazepam (Smolinske et al., 2005) or providing supportive care in less severe cases (Wilson et al., 2005). Araújo and colleagues (2015) further stressed the relevance of supportive care and sedation and considered the application of activated charcoal useful in cases of oral exposure. Tryptamine-induced agitation, hypertension and hallucinations might be managed with benzodiazepines, while the disturbance of vital signs may necessitate the appliance of β-adrenergic antagonists or nitroprusside.

The treatment of serotonin toxicity – as one of the adverse outcomes of piperazine (i.e., BZP) intoxication – can be accomplished by the administration of benzodazepines, cyproheptadine and chlorpromazine (Schep et al., 2011). Piperazine toxicity might be associated with sympathomimetic toxidrome (Kersten & McLaughlin, 2015), which is usually treated with cooling measures and antihypertensives respectively, in cases where benzodiazepines fail to act as first-line treatment agents. Antipsychotics are not suggested for the management of severe agitation due to their extrapyramidal side effects and their ability to cause hypotension and arrhythmias (Arbo, Bastos & Carmo, 2012). Hypertension can be treated with intravenously administered antihypertensives and Clonidine, whereas Labetalol is suggested in patients with refractory hypertension (Schep et al., 2011).

Psychosocial Treatment

Applied psychotherapy in case of NPS-related problems does not differ significantly from that of formerly scheduled substances. However, a routine screening for NPS use on admission to either psychiatric wards or emergency units is of high relevance, as NPS – even more than traditional controlled substances – increases the occurence and severity of comorbid psychiatric pathologies (Anderson, Morrell & Marchevsky, 2015). The NEPTUNE guidelines propose a thorough assessment of the severity of NPS use, based on which the most appropriate response should be offered (Abdulrahim & Bowden-Jones, 2015). For instance, clients showing low risk NPS use might benefit from either general or tailored advice or self-support approaches, while those individuals with more harmful patterns of NPS consumption may need individual or group-based psychosocial interventions (EMCDDA, 2016c).

While some authors (e.g., Tracy, Wood & Baumeister, 2017) argue that the same interventions (such as harm reduction programs, motivational interviewing, counseling) should be applied regardless of the substance in question, others (e.g., Ralphs & Gray, 2017) suggest NPS-type specific strategies in health care. Ralphs and Gray (2017) stress the relevance of (1) a holistic approach regarding the treatment of coexisting mental health and NPS use problems; (2) the integration of sexual health and substance use services, especially in case of MSM clients involving in chemsex events; (3) clearer referral pathways; and (4) the development of service user engagement strategies. The authors also point out that many NPS users consider existing health and addiction care services to be created specifically for heroin users but not for them. This may act as a barrier to treatment engagement among these users. Furthermore, some clients think that practicioners do not possess enough knowledge and expertise about NPS-type substances and as a consequence, are not prepared to properly treat them. In order to increase user engagement, Ralphs and Gray propose the need for more targeted outreach and in-reach, alongside with the revision of marketing strategies and the review of the location of service provision.

Novel Prevention Strategies for NPS

Preventing NPS Use

Considering the theoretical framework of potential prevention programs that specifically target NPS use, some authors have suggested adapting existing prevention models – e.g., the ecology of human development, social learning, theories of social norms and health beliefs, theory of planned behavior (Kempf et al., 2017) – and apply or adopt them for addressing NPS users (Mdege et al., 2017). Based on the extensive literature review of Catalano and colleagues (2012), effective prevention efforts might follow a multilevel approach, incorporating policy, community, family and individual-focused interventions, thus creating complex "prevention systems." These interventions may target school, family and individual risk factors among adolescents, improving social competencies, strenghtening parenting skills (Catalano et al., 2012) or providing evidence-based knowledge about the realistic risks of NPS consumption (Mdege et al., 2017). It is also worth mentioning that a recent scoping review (Meader, Mdege & McCambridge, 2018) emphasized the lack of available data on the effectiveness of legislative efforts on the reduction of NPS use incidences. The most recent policy intervention in the United Kingdom, in the form of the Psychoactive Substances Act, may arguably increase NPS harms due to unintended, although not unanticipated, secondary impacts (Stevens et al., 2015). Some other existing international examples (e.g., Portugal's or the Czech Republic's current drug policy) suggest that responses to NPS use should be based on a public health approach rather than a criminal justice one. These approaches replace former prohibitionist approaches with a decriminalization perspective, leading to a more cost-effective policy with less custodial sentencing and relevant public health benefits (Csete et al., 2016).

The spread of NPS-related evidence-based knowledge was supported by organizations and programs, such as the Drugs Early Warning System offering access to health and law enforcement agencies, while sharing data from the European Union's Early Warning System) (The New Psychoactive Substances Review Expert Panel, 2014). The New Psychoactive Substances Review Expert Panel (2014) further expressed some recommendations on how to improve the efficacy of NPS use prevention. These suggestions include the development of evidence-based public health campaigns, the identification of harm reduction tools or interventions and the shedding of inefficient prevention and education programs.

The implemetation of school-based NPS prevention programs is advised as part of a generic prevention effort (EMCDDA, 2016c), following evidence-based guidelines or resources such as the European Drug Prevention Quality Standards (Brotherhood & Sumnall, 2011). As an example for NPS-related harm reduction, on- and off-site drug testing services (e.g., the Loop, that offers festival and city-centre testing in the United Kingdom) support users to make informed choices about their substances and, in many cases, those submitting samples decide not to take the substances based on the testing results, or take a lesser amount as a result of the specific concerns highlighted (TEDI, 2013). Various front-line projects deal directly and specifically with NPS users, such as Ai Laket!!, Check !n, Checkit!, DIMS, Energy Control, Jellinek, Modus Vivendi, Saferparty.ch or Techno plus. Needle exchange programs distributing sterile equipment may reduce harms among those injecting NPS (EMCDDA, 2016c). Further projects (e.g., Euro-DEN project) aim to improve the efficacy of prehospital care of unwell drug consumers (including of NPS), by disseminating professional guidelines (Euro-DEN, 2015; Wood et al., 2014) on when to call the emergency service (e.g., in case of seizures, unconsciousness, significant agitation, signs of tachycardia, etc.).

The motivations of NPS users – e.g., curiosity, self-exploration, inducing enhanced performance or increased sociability, coping with everyday problems, etc. – also need to be understood to improve the efficacy of prevention programs or to reduce NPS-related harms (Soussan, Andersson & Kjellgren, 2018). These might best be considered in user-specific terms, rather than substance-specific reasons; therefore, tailored interventions should refer to the need of the individual itself and the function of his/her NPS consumption.

Piloting Web-Based Projects and Applications

The setting of NPS consumption is broadly affected by rapid technological development and changing lifestyles. Increasing speeds of transportation and communication combined with the unprecedented use of digital tools influence our daily lives to an increasing extent, and this is reflected in the drug market. Digital spaces – e.g., online forums, blog entries, web markets – play a relevant role in NPS-related information gathering as well as a novel form of drug trafficking and purchase. Web-based drug markets increased the availability and decreased the price of NPS (Gilani, 2016). They also made it more challenging to properly monitor the spread of these psychoactive substances. People who consume drugs and those who sell them have gained considerable knowledge via online platforms (Deluca et al., 2012; Smith & Garlich, 2013). Networking populated by the so-called psychonauts, individuals experimenting with mind-altering psychoactive substances (Corazza et al., 2013; Móró & Rácz, 2013; Smith & Garlich, 2013), further facilitate the dissemination of such knowledge in ways which may prove protective at times and harmful at others. Such users on occasion act as willing "human guinea pigs" for previously untested substances and demonstrate greater impulsivity compared with traditional drug users (e.g., Vreeker et al., 2017).

The darknet drug market relies on sophisticated technologies to provide anonymity for users when they purchase. The use of specific or customised internet browsers, passwords specific to each e-market, secured routing protocols, virtual private networks (VPN), Internet Protocol Masking (IP masking), and Bitcoin payment systems (RAND, 2016), have showed a continous growth in the past few years (RAND, 2016; Winstock & Barratt, 2016). Digital spaces, however, may also be utilized in prevention research or even drug user-led harm reduction (e.g., Evenepoel, 2015; Móró & Rácz, 2013). Web search queries – identified by for instance Google Trends – have been used to explore the fluctuation in public interest toward various NPS as a result of sales restrictions (Zheluk, Quinn & Meylakhs, 2014), legislation (Bright et al., 2013; Kapitány-Fövény & Demetrovics, 2017), due to news reports about fatal NPS overdoses (Forsyth, 2012), or as a potential indicator of toxicological cases (Yin & Ho, 2012). Various international research projects (e.g., the Psychonaut Web Mapping Project; the ReDNet Project) monitored the web (e.g., social network sites, video sharing sites, blogs or online user reports) in order to identify trends and provide knowledge related to the use or distribution of NPS and develop innovative technology-based prevention tools (e.g., Corazza et al., 2013, 2014; Deluca et al., 2012).

In recent years, drug prevention projects have also started to develop smartphone applications on NPS as new tools of prevention and information sharing among professionals working in the field (Simonato et al., 2017). The anonymity and accessibility of these programs may help facilitate self-disclosure regarding sensitive subjects (e.g., illegal substance use, sexual dysfunctions), and may provide opportunity to reach substance users who otherwise do not seek professional help (e.g., Majeed-Ariss et al., 2015; Turner et al., 1998). There are a few partially successful examples of internet-based prevention programs which reduce adolescents' intentions to consume NPS (Champion et al., 2016a) or smartphone applications (Kapitány-Fövény et al., 2018) using "gamification" elements (e.g., quiz-games and role-play games), or combinations of the two mediums as in the case of the EU-funded project "Click for Support." These interventions, however, were mainly effective in changing attitudes or increasing knowledge about NPS but were not proven to be successful in decreasing the frequency of NPS consumption.

"Talk to Frank," a UK drug education service established by the Department of Health and Home Office of the British government in 2003, provides confidential advice to adolescents about the potential risks of drug use (including NPS) via phone talk, email, or online live chat. Furthermore, the project's website is one of the main information source of British teachers who prepare lessons on psychoactive substances (Health and Social Care Information Centre, 2015). Information from the same website was lately utilized and delivered by adapting the peer-led prevention intervention, ASSIST (White et al., 2017) as well, that was primarily developed for preventing adolescent smoking (Campbell et al., 2008). Nevertheless, it is also important to mention that the literature of well-established efficacy studies regarding NPS-specific web- or smartphone-based prevention programs is still lacking and needs future research.

Conclusions

The significant shift on how drugs are now manufactured, marketed, sold and consumed, driven by technological development and by globalization, has raised major challenges in terms of regulatory responses, questioning policy governance, and whether the existing domestic and international drug control systems are capable of responding in a timely and effective way. While some authors (e.g., Negrei et al., 2017; Reuter & Pardo, 2017) describe the challenges and burdens of restrictive regulatory approaches, others (e.g., Kikura-Hanajiri, Kawamura & Goda, 2014; Smyth, Lyons & Cullen, 2017) emphasize that a significant decline in NPS use prevalences can be associated with legislative efforts. However, these changes are hard to reliably measure due to hidden/undergroud substance use or the phenomenon of shifting to other drugs. Further, reduced consumption does not necessarily equate to reduced drug harms as it is often the socioeconomic-political factors surrounding drug use, as opposed to the pharmacology of the substances themselves, which causes the greatest negative impacts on users.

As was highlighted in the chapter, still little is known about pharmacological and toxicological aspects of NPS and risk assessments are often based on poor or sparse evidence. At the same time there appears to be little justification for a criminal justice-oriented approach, which often criminalizes a new cohort of users who subsequently incur all the consequences attached to entry into the justice system, and are often exposed to much greater risk of problematic drug use in the process (Corazza & Roman-Urrestarazu, 2017). Drugs are also increasingly used to enhance performance and help persons cope with hectic lifestyle rather than solely for recreational purposes as in the past. This emphasizes the need for innovative responses and prevention activities able to encompass such as the newly emerging drug trends.

Evidence-based knowledge about NPS is growing, but there is a serious gap between such knowledge and the policy responses. Research itself still contains several blind spots. As Mdege and colleagues (2017) indicated as a result of their scoping review, studies (1) dealing with the simultaneous use of multiple NPS (in terms of pharmacological and toxicological outcomes), (2) exploring cohorts and subgroups of NPS users (in terms of epidemiology and assessment methodology), (3) research regarding the development and evaluation of prevention and intervention programs targeting NPS consumption (in terms of efficacy), and (4) more effective dissemination of NPS-related knowledge to increase public understanding and awareness or to strengthen the contribution of social sciences would be welcomed in the near future. However, progress on this front relies on more effective, sustained collaboration between research and policy-making.

In order to "stay on top of the flood of novel psychoactive substances" (Baumeister, Tojo & Tracy, 2015), a strong international collaboration is also necessary from the sides of health care providers, policy-makers, representatives from the social sector or professionals from the education system. It is important to diminish false perceptions about NPS (e.g., some users tend to consider "herbal drugs" to be completely natural and harmless) by providing open access to evidence-based findings not just to experts but to lay individuals as well. It is also timely for health professionals to recognize that NPS, while ever-evolving in composition, are not a transient phenomena, but are likely to remain firmly ensconced in society as widespread alternates of formerly scheduled substances and will subsequently be around for the long-haul.

REFERENCES

Abdulrahim, D. & Bowden-Jones, O., on behalf of the NEPTUNE Expert Group (2015). *Guidance on the Management of Acute and Chronic Harms of Club Drugs and Novel Psychoactive Substances.* London: Novel Psychoactive Treatment UK Network (NEPTUNE).

Acciavatti, T., Lupi, M., Santacroce, R., et al. (2017). Novel psychoactive substance consumption is more represented in bipolar disorder than in psychotic disorders: A multicenter-observational study. *Human Psychopharmacology*, **32**(3), doi: 10.1002/hup.2578.

Addison, M., Stockdale, K., McGovern, R., et al. (2018). Exploring intersections between Novel Psychoactive Substances (NPS) and other substance use in a police custody suite setting in the North East of England. *Drugs: Education, Prevention & Policy*, **25**(4), 313–319.

Alatrash, G., Majhail, N. S. & Pile, J.C. (2006). Rhabdomyolysis after ingestion of "foxy," a hallucinogenic tryptamine derivative. *Mayo Clinic Proceedings*, **81**(4), 550–551.

Alzghari, S. K., Amin, Z. M., Chau, S., et al. (2017). On the horizon: The synthetic opioid U-49900. *Cureus*, **9**(9), e1679. http://doi.org/10.7759/cureus.1679

Anderson, C. Morrell, C. & Marchevsky, D. (2015). A novel psychoactive substance poses a new challenge in the management of paranoid schizophrenia. *BMJ Case Reports*, bcr2015209573 http://doi.org/10.1136/bcr-2015-209573

Anizan, S., Concheiro, M., Lehner, K. R., et al. (2016). Linear pharmacokinetics of 3,4-methylenedioxypyrovalerone (MDPV) and its metabolites in the rat: relationship to pharmacodynamic effects. *Addiction Biology*, **21**(2), 339–347.

Antia, U., Lee, H. S., Kydd, R. R., Tingle, M. D. & Russell, B. R. (2009a). Pharmacokinetics of 'party pill' drug N-benzylpiperazine (BZP) in healthy human participants. *Forensic Science International*, **186**(1–3), 63–67.

Antia, U., Tingle, M. D. & Russell, B. R. (2009b). In vivo interactions between BZP and TFMPP (party pill drugs). *The New Zealand Medical Journal*, **122**(1303), 29–38.

Araújo, A. M., Carvalho, F., Bastos Mde, L., Guedes de Pinho, P. & Carvalho, M. (2015). The hallucinogenic world of tryptamines: An updated review. *Archives of Toxicology*, **89**(8), 1151–1173.

Arbo, M. D., Bastos, M. L. & Carmo, H. F. (2012). Piperazine compounds as drugs of abuse. *Drug and Alcohol Dependence*, **122**(3), 174–185.

Armenian, P., Olson, A., Anaya, A., et al. (2017). Fentanyl and a novel synthetic opioid U-47700 masquerading as street "Norco" in central California: a case report. *Annals of Emergency Medicine*, **69**(1), 87–90.

Armenian, P., Vo, K. T., Barr-Walker, J. & Lynch, K. L. (2018). Fentanyl, fentanyl analogs and novel synthetic opioids: A comprehensive review. *Neuropharmacology*, **134**(Part A), 121–132. doi: 10.1016/j.neuropharm.2017.10.016

Bäckberg, M., Beck, O., Jönsson, K. H. & Helander, A. (2015). Opioid intoxications involving butyrfentanyl, 4-fluorobutyrfentanyl, and fentanyl from the Swedish STRIDA project. *Clinical Toxicology (Philadelphia, Pa.)*, **53**(7), 609–617.

Banks, M. L., Worst, T. J. & Sprague, J. E. (2014). Synthetic Cathinones and amphetamine analogues: What's the rave about? *The Journal of Emergency Medicine*, **46** (5), 632–642.

Barratt, M. J., Cakic, V. & Lenton, S. (2013). Patterns of synthetic cannabinoid use in Australia. *Drug and Alcohol Review*, **32**(2), 141–146.

Barrios, L., Grison-Hernando, H., Boels, D., et al. (2016). Death following ingestion of methylone. *International Journal of Legal Medicine*, **130**(2), 381–385.

Baumann, M. H., Bukhari, M. O., Lehner, K. R., et al. (2017). Neuropharmacology of 3,4-methylenedioxypyrovalerone (MDPV), its metabolites, and related analogs. *Current Topics in Behavioral Neurosciences*, **32**, 93–117.

Baumann, M. H., Clark, R. D., Budzynski, A. G., et al. (2005). N-substituted piperazines abused by humans mimic the molecular mechanism of 3,4-methylenedioxymethamphetamine (MDMA, or 'Ecstasy'). *Neuropsychopharmacology*, **30**(3), 550–560.

Baumeister, D., Tojo, L. M. & Tracy, D. K. (2015). Legal highs: Staying on top of the flood of novel psychoactive substances. *Therapeutic Advances in Psychopharmacology*, **5**(2), 97–132.

Black, C., Setterfield, L. & Murray, L. (2016). *Scottish Schools Adolescent Lifestyle and Substance Use Survey (SALSUS): Drug Use Report (2015)*. Scotland: Scottish Government, National Statistics publication for Scotland.

Blackman, S. & Bradley, R. (2017). From niche to stigma – Headshops to prison: Exploring the rise and fall of synthetic cannabinoid use among young adults. *The International Journal on Drug Policy*, **40**, 70–77.

Bonar, E. E., Ashrafioun, L. & Ilgen, M. A. (2014). Synthetic cannabinoid use among patients in residential substance use disorder treatment: Prevalence, motives, and correlates. *Drug and Alcohol Dependence*, **143**, 268–271.

Borek, H. A. & Holstege, C. P. (2012). Hyperthermia and multiorgan failure after abuse of "bath salts" containing 3,4-methylenedioxypyrovalerone. *Annals of Emergency Medicine*, **60**(1), 103–105.

Bright, S. J., Bishop, B., Kane, R., Marsh, A. & Barratt, M. J. (2013). Kronic hysteria: Exploring the intersection between Australian synthetic cannabis legislation, the media, and drug-related harm. *The International Journal on Drug Policy*, **24**(3), 231–237.

Brotherhood, A. & Sumnall, H. R. (2011). *European Drug Prevention Quality Standards, Manual No 7*. Lisbon: EMCDDA.

Brush, D. E., Bird, S. B. & Boyer, E. W. (2004). Monoamine oxidase inhibitor poisoning resulting from Internet misinformation on illicit substances. *Journal of Toxicology. Clinical Toxicology*, **42**(2), 191–195.

Burns, L., Roxburgh, A., Matthews, A., et al. (2014). The rise of new psychoactive substance use in Australia. *Drug Testing and Analysis*, **6**(7–8), 846–849.

Butler, R. A. & Sheridan, J. L. (2007). Highs and lows: patterns of use, positive and negative effects of benzylpiperazine-containing party pills (BZP-party pills) amongst young people in New Zealand. *Harm Reduction Journal*, **4**, 18. doi:10.1186/1477-7517-4-18

Campbell, R., Starkey, F., Holliday, J., et al. (2008). An informal school-based peer-led intervention for smoking prevention in adolescence (ASSIST): A cluster randomised trial. *The Lancet*, **371**(9624), 1595–1602.

Cannaert, A., Storme, J., Franz, F., Auwärter, V. & Stove, C. P. (2016). Detection and activity profiling of synthetic cannabinoids and their metabolites with a newly developed bioassay. *Analytical Chemistry*, **88**(23), 11476–11485.

Carbone, P. N., Carbone, D. L., Carstairs, S. D. & Luzi, S. A. (2013). Sudden cardiac death associated with methylone use. *The American Journal of Forensic Medicine and Pathology*, **34**(1), 26–28.

Carhart-Harris, R. L., King, L. A. & Nutt, D. J. (2011). A web-based survey on mephedrone. *Drug and Alcohol Dependence*, **118**(1), 19–22.

Castaneto, M. S., Gorelick, D. A., Desrosiers, N. A., et al. (2014). Synthetic cannabinoids: Epidemiology, pharmacodynamics, and clinical implications. *Drug and Alcohol Dependence*, **144**, 12–41.

Catalano, R. F., Fagan, A. A., Gavin, L. E., et al. (2012). Worldwide application of prevention science in adolescent health. *The Lancet*, **379** (9826), 1653–1664.

Caudevilla-Gálligo, F., Riba, J., Ventura, M., et al. (2012). 4-Bromo-2,5-dimethoxyphenethylamine (2C-B): Presence in the recreational drug market in Spain, pattern of use and subjective effects. *Journal of Psychopharmacology*, **26**(7), 1026–1035.

Caviness, C. M., Tzilos, G., Anderson, B. J. & Stein, M. D. (2015). Synthetic cannabinoids: Use and predictors in a community sample of young adults. *Substance Abuse*, **36**(3), 368–373.

Cha, S.-S. & Seo, B.-K. (2018). Smartphone use and smartphone addiction in middle school students in Korea: Prevalence, social networking service, and game use. *Health Psychology Open*, **5**(1), 2055102918755046. doi:10.1177/2055102918755046.

Champion, K. E., Newton, N. C., Stapinski, L. A. & Teesson, M. (2016a). Effectiveness of a universal internet-based prevention program for ecstasy and new psychoactive substances: A cluster randomized controlled trial. *Addiction*, **111**(8), 1396–1405.

Champion, K. E., Teeson, M. & Newton N. C. (2016b). Patterns and correlates of new psychoactive substance use in a sample of Australian high school students. *Drug and Alcohol Review*, **35**(3), 338–344.

Cohen, K., Kapitány-Fövény, M., Mama, Y., et al. (2017). The effects of synthetic cannabinoids on executive function. *Psychopharmacology (Berlin)*, **234**(7), 1121–1134.

Cole, J. B., Dunbar, J. F., McIntire, S. A., Regelmann, W. E. & Slusher, T. M. (2015). Butyrfentanyl overdose resulting in diffuse alveolar hemorrhage. *Pediatrics*, **135**(3), e740–743.

Cooper, Z. D. (2016). Adverse effects of synthetic cannabinoids: Management of acute toxicity and withdrawal. *Current Psychiatry Reports*, **18**(5), 52. http://doi.org/10.1007/s11920-016-0694-1

Cooper, Z. D. & Haney, M. (2008). Cannabis reinforcement and dependence: role of the cannabinoid CB1 receptor. *Addiction Biology*, **13**(2), 188–195.

Corazza, O., Assi, S., Malekianragheb, S., et al. (2014). Monitoring novel psychoactive substances allegedly offered online for sale in Persian and Arabic languages. *The*

International Journal on Drug Policy, **25**(4), 724–726.

Corazza, O., Assi, S., Simonato, P., et al. (2013). Promoting innovation and excellence to face the rapid diffusion of novel psychoactive substances in the EU: The outcomes of the ReDNet project. *Human Psychopharmacology*, **28**(4), 317–323.

Corazza, O. & Roman-Urrestarazu, A. (Eds.) (2017). *Novel Psychoactive Substances: Policy, Economics and Drug Regulation.* Berlin: Springer.

Corazza, O. & Roman-Urrestarazu, A. (Eds.) (2018). *Handbook on Novel Psychoactive Substances. What Clinicians Should Know about NPS.* New York: Routledge.

Corkery, J. M., Durkin, E., Elliott, S., Schifano, F. & Ghodse, A. H. (2012). The recreational tryptamine 5-MeO-DALT (N,N-diallyl-5-methoxytryptamine): A brief review. *Progress in Neuropsychopharmacology & Biological Psychiatry*, **39**(2), 259–262.

Csák, R., Demetrovics, Zs. & Rácz, J. (2013). Transition to injecting 3,4-methylene-dioxy-pyrovalerone (MDPV) among needle exchange program participants in Hungary. *Journal of Psychopharmacology*, **27**(6), 559–563.

Csete, J., Kamarulzaman, A., Kazatchkine, M., et al. (2016). Public Health and International Drug Policy: Report of the Johns Hopkins – Lancet Commission on Drug Policy and Health. *Lancet (London, England)*, **387** (10026), 1427–1480.

Cunningham, S. M., Haikal, N. A. & Kraner, J. C. (2016). Fatal intoxication with acetyl fentanyl. *Journal of Forensic Sciences*, **61** (Supplement 1), S276–280.

Daldrup, T., Heller, C., Matthiesen, U., et al. (1986). [Etryptamine, a new designer drug with a fatal effect]. *Zeitschrift für Rechtsmedizin*, **97**(1), 61–68.

Dargan, P. I., Albert, S. & Wood, D. M. (2010). Mephedrone use and associated adverse effects in school and college/university students before the UK legislation change. *QJM: An International Journal of Medicine*, **103**(11), 875–879.

de Boer, D., Bosman, I. J., Hidvégi, E., et al. (2001). Piperazine-like compounds: A new group of designer drugs-of-abuse on the European market. *Forensic Science International*, **121**(1–2), 47–56.

Dean, B. V., Stellpflug, S. J., Burnett, A. M. & Engebretsen, K. M. (2013). 2C or not 2C: Phenethylamine designer drug review. *Journal of Medical Toxicology*, **9**(2), 172–178.

Degenhardt, L. & Dunn, M. (2008). The epidemiology of GHB and ketamine use in an Australian household survey. *The International Journal on Drug Policy*, **19**(4), 311–316.

Deligianni, E., Corkery, J. M., Schifano, F. & Lione, L. A. (2017). An international survey on the awareness, use, preference, and health perception of novel psychoactive substances (NPS). *Human Psychopharmacology*, **32**(3), doi: 10.1002/hup.2581.

Deluca, P., Davey, Z., Corazza, O., et al. (2012). Identifying emerging trends in recreational drug use; outcomes from the Psychonaut Web Mapping Project. *Progress in Neuropsychopharmacology & Biological Psychiatry*, **39**(2), 221–226.

Demetrovics, Z., Urbán, R., Nagygyörgy, K., et al. (2011). Why do you play? The development of the motives for online gaming questionnaire (MOGQ). *Behavioral Research Methods*, **43**(3), 814–825.

Dick, D. & Torrance, C. (2010). Mixmag drug survey. *Mixmag*, **225**, 44–53.

Domanski, K., Kleinschmidt, K. C., Schulte, J. M., et al. (2017). Two cases of intoxication with new synthetic opioid, U-47700. *Clinical Toxicology (Philadelphia, Pa.)*, **55**(1), 46–50.

Elliott, S. (2011). Current awareness of piperazines: Pharmacology and toxicology. *Drug Testing and Analysis*, **3**(7–8), 430–438.

Elliott, S. & Smith, C. (2008). Investigation of the first deaths in the United Kingdom involving the detection and quantitation of the piperazines BZP and 3-TFMPP. *Journal of Analytical Toxicology*, **32**(2), 172–177.

Elliott, S. P., Brandt, S. D. & Smith, C. (2016). The first reported fatality associated with the synthetic opioid 3,4-dichloro-N-[2-(dimethylamino)cyclohexyl]-N-methylbenzamide (U-47700) and implications for forensic analysis. *Drug Testing and Analysis*, **8**(8), 875–879.

EMCDDA (2006). *Selected Issue 3: Developments in Drug Use Within Recreational Settings.* Luxembourg: Publications Office of the European Union. Available at: www.emcdda.europa.eu/system/files/publications/424/sel2006_3-en_69713.pdf [Accessed June 10, 2018]

EMCDDA (2016a). *The Internet and Drug Markets.* Luxembourg: Publications Office of the European Union. Available at: www.emcdda.europa.eu/publications/insights/internet-drug-markets [Accessed November 2, 2017]

EMCDDA (2016b). *Report on the risk assessment of 1-phenyl-2-(pyrrolidin-1-yl)pentan-1-one (α-pyrrolidinovalerophenone, α-PVP) in the framework of the Council Decision on newpsychoactive substances).* Luxembourg: Publications Office of the European Union. Available at: www.emcdda.europa.eu/system/files/publications/2934/TDAK16001ENN.pdf [Accessed May 25, 2018]

EMCDDA (2016c). *Perspectives on drugs: Health Responses to New Psychoactive Substances.* Luxembourg: Publications Office of the European Union. Available at:www.emcdda.europa.eu/system/files/publications/2933/NPS%20health%20responses_POD2016.pdf [Accessed June 05, 2018]

EMCDDA (2017). *Germany – Country Drug Report 2017.* Luxembourg: Publications Office of the European Union, Available at: www.emcdda.europa.eu/system/files/publications/4528/TD0416906ENN.pdf [Accessed December 10, 2017]

EMCDDA-Europol (2017). *Joint Report on a New Psychoactive Substance: N-phenyl-N-[1-(2-Phenylethyl)piperidin-4-yl]-furan-2-carboxamide (furanylfentanyl).* Luxembourg: Publications Office of the European Union, Available at: www.emcdda.europa.eu/system/files/publications/4682/JOINT_REPORT_furanylfentanyl_web.pdf [Accessed June 1, 2018]

ESPAD Group (2016). *ESPAD Report 2015 – Results from the European School Survey Project on Alcohol and Other Drugs.* Luxembourg: Publications Office of the European Union. Available at: www.espad.org/sites/espad.org/files/ESPAD_report_2015.pdf [Accessed October 17, 2017]

Euro-DEN (2015). *Guidelines on when to call the Emergency Services 112 for unwell recreational drug users.* Lisbon: EMCDDA.

Evenepoel, T. (2015). Drug helplines, online health and NPS. Presentation at the *Health responses to NPS* EMCDDA expert meeting, October 28–29, 2015, EMCDDA, Lisbon. Available at: www.emcdda.europa.eu/events/meetings/2015/nps-health-responses [Accessed December 20, 2017]

Every-Palmer, S. (2011). Synthetic cannabinoid JWH-018 and psychosis: An explorative study. *Drug and Alcohol Dependence*, **117**(2–3), 152–157.

Fantegrossi, W. E., Harrington, A. W., Kiessel, C. L., et al. (2006). Hallucinogen-like actions of 5-methoxy N,N diisopropyltryptamine in mice and rats. *Pharmacology, Biochemistry and Behavior*, **83**(1), 122–129.

Fantegrossi, W. E., Moran, J. H., Radominska-Pandya, A. & Prather, P. L. (2014). Distinct pharmacology and metabolism of K2 synthetic cannabinoids compared to Δ9-THC: Mechanism underlying greater toxicity? *Life Sciences*, **97**(1), 45–54.

Fattore, L. & Fratta, W. (2011). Beyond THC: The new generation of cannabinoid designer drugs. *Frontiers in Behavioral Neuroscience*, **5**, 60. doi: 10.3389/fnbeh.2011.00060.

Fels, H., Krueger, J., Sachs, H., et al. (2017). Two fatalities associated with synthetic opioids: AH-7921 and MT-45. *Forensic Science International*, e30–e35. doi: 10.1016/j.forsciint.2017.04.003.

Forsyth, A. J. M. (2012). Virtually a drug scare: Mephedrone and the impact of the Internet on drug news transmission. *The International Journal on Drug Policy*, **23**(3), 198–209.

Gee, P., Richardson, S., Woltersdorf, W. & Moore, G. (2005). Toxic effects of BZP-based herbal party pills in humans: A prospective study in Christchurch, New Zealand. *The New Zealand Medical Journal*, **118**(1227), U1784.

German, C. L., Fleckenstein, A. E. & Hanson, G. R. (2014). Bath salts and synthetic cathinones: An emerging designer drug phenomenon. *Life Sciences*, **97**(1), 2–8.

Gilani, F. (2016). Novel psychoactive substances: The rising wave of "legal highs". *The British Journal of General Practice*, **66** (642), 8–9.

Ginsburg, B. C., McMahon, L. R., Sanchez, J. J. & Javors, M. A. (2012). Purity of synthetic cannabinoids sold online for recreational use. *Journal of Analytical Toxicology*, **36**(1), 66–68.

Golembiowska, K., Jurczak, A., Kamińska, K., Noworyta-Sokołowska, K. & Górska, A. (2016). Effect of some psychoactive drugs used as "legal highs" on brain neurotransmitters. *Neurotoxicity Research*, **29**, 394–407.

Gregg, R. A., Tallarida, C. S., Reitz, A., McCurdy, C. & Rawls, S. M. (2013). Mephedrone (4-methylmethcathinone), a principal constituent of psychoactive bath salts, produces behavioral sensitization in rats. *Drug and Alcohol Dependence*, **133**(2), 746–750.

Griswold, M. K., Chai, P. R., Krotulski, A. J., et al. (2017). A novel oral fluid assay (LC-QTOF-MS) for the detection of fentanyl and clandestine opioids in oral fluid after reported heroin overdose. *Journal of Medical Toxicology*, **13**(4), 287–292.

Guerrieri, D., Rapp, E., Roman, M., Druid, H. & Kronstrand, R. (2017). Postmortem and toxicological findings in a series of furanylfentanyl-related deaths. *Journal of Analytical Toxicology*, **41**(3), 242–249.

Guirguis, A., Corkery, J., Stair, J., et al. (2015). Survey of knowledge of legal highs (novel psychoactivesubstances) amongst London pharmacists. *Drugs and Alcohol Today*, **15**(2), 93–99.

Gunderson, E. W., Haughey, H. M., Ait-Daoud, N., Joshi, A. S. & Hart, C. L. (2014). A Survey of synthetic cannabinoid consumption by current cannabis users. *Substance Abuse*, **35** (2), 184–189.

Gustavsson, D. & Escher, C. (2009). [Mephedrone-Internet drug which seems to have come and stay. Fatal cases in Sweden have drawn attention to previously unknown substance]. *Lakartidningen*, **106**(43), 2769–2771.

Hawk, K. F., Vaca, F. E. & D'Onofrio, G. (2015). Reducing fatal opioid overdose: Prevention, treatment and harm reduction strategies. *The Yale Journal of Biology and Medicine*, **88**(3), 235–245.

Health and Social Care Information Centre (2015). *Smoking, Drinking and Drug Use among Young People in England – 2013.* London: Health and Social Care Information Centre.

Helander, A., Bäckberg, M. & Beck, O. (2014). MT-45, a new psychoactive substance associated with hearing loss and unconsciousness. *Clinical Toxicology (Philadelphia, Pa.)*, **52**(8), 901–904.

Helander, A., Bäckberg, M. & Beck, O. (2016). Intoxications involving the fentanyl analogs acetylfentanyl, 4-methoxybutyrfentanyl and furanylfentanyl: Results from the Swedish STRIDA project. *Clinical Toxicology (Philadelphia, Pa.)*, **54**(4), 324–332.

Helander, A., Bradley, M., Hasselblad, A., et al. (2017). Acute skin and hair symptoms followed by severe, delayed eye complications in subjects using the synthetic opioid MT-45. *The British Journal of Dermatology*, **176**(4), 1021–1027.

Hermanns-Clausen, M., Kneisel, S., Szabo, B. & Auwärter, V. (2013). Acute toxicity due to the confirmed consumption of synthetic cannabinoids: Clinical and laboratory findings. *Addiction*, **108**(3), 534–544.

Hess, C., Stockhausen, S., Kernbach-Wighton, G. & Madea, B. (2015). Death due to diabetic ketoacidosis: Induction by the consumption of synthetic cannabinoids? *Forensic Science International*, **257**, e6–11. doi: 10.1016/j.forsciint.2015.08.012.

Ikeda, A., Sekiguchi, K., Fujita, K., Yamadera, H. & Koga, Y. (2005). 5-methoxy-N,N-diisopropyltryptamine-induced flashbacks. *The American Journal of Psychiatry*, **162**(4), 815.

Itokawa, M., Iwata, K., Takahashi, M., et al. (2007). Acute confusional state after designer tryptamine abuse. *Psychiatry and Clinical Neurosciences*, **61**(2), 196–199.

Jan, R. K., Lin, J. C., Lee, H., et al. (2010). Determining the subjective effects of TFMPP in human males. *Psychopharmacology (Berlin)*, **211**(3), 347–353.

Javadi-Paydar, M., Nguyen, J. D., Vandewater, S. A., Dickerson, T. J. & Taffe, M. A. (2018). Locomotor and reinforcing effects of pentedrone, pentylone and methylone in rats. *Neuropharmacology*, **134**(Part A), 57–64. doi: 10.1016/j.neuropharm.2017.09.002.

Jebadurai, J. K. (2012). *Qualitative research of online drug misuse communities with reference to the novel psychoactive substances.* Doctoral Thesis at the University of Hertfordshire.

Jones, M. J., Hernandez, B. S., Janis, G. C. & Stellpflug, S. J. (2017). A case of U-47700 overdose with laboratory confirmation and metabolite identification. *Clinical Toxicology (Philadelphia, Pa.)*, **55**(1), 55–59.

Joseph, A. M., Manseau, M. W., Lalane, M., Rajparia, A. & Lewis, C. F. (2017). Characteristics associated with synthetic cannabinoid use among patients treated in a public psychiatric emergency setting. *The American Journal of Drug and Alcohol Abuse*, **43**(1), 117–122.

Jovel, A., Felthous, A. & Bhattacharyya, A. (2014). Delirium due to intoxication from the novel synthetic tryptamine 5-MeO-DALT. *Journal of Forensic Sciences*, **59**(3), 844–846.

Kalasho, A. & Vibe Nielsen, S. (2016). 5-MeO-DALT; a novel designer drug on the market causing acute delirium and rhabdomyolysis. *Acta Anaesthesiologica Scandinavica*, **60**(9), 1332–1336.

Kapitány-Fövény, M. & Demetrovics, Z. (2017). Utility of Web search query data in testing theoretical assumptions about mephedrone. *Human Psychopharmacology*, **32**(3). doi: 10.1002/hup.2620

Kapitány-Fövény, M., Farkas, J., Csorba, J., Szabó, T. & Demetrovics, Z. (2013a). *Különbségek a szintetikus kannabinoidok és a kannabisz szubjektív hatásaiban, a használati mintázatban és a használat okaiban.* Magyar Addiktológiai Társaság IX. Országos Kongresszus, Siófok, 2013.11.21-2013.11.23, p. 25.

Kapitány-Fövény, M., Farkas, J., Pataki, P. A., et al. (2017). Novel psychoactive substance use among treatment-seeking opiate users: The role of life events and psychiatric symptoms. *Human Psychopharmacology*, **32** (3), doi: 10.1002/hup.2602

Kapitány-Fövény, M., Kertész, M., Winstock, A., et al. (2013b). Substitutional potential of mephedrone: An analysis of the subjective effects. *Human Psychopharmacology*, **28**(4), 308–316.

Kapitány-Fövény, M., Vagdalt, E., Ruttkay, Z., et al. (2018). Potential of an interactive drug prevention mobile phone app (Once Upon a High): Questionnaire study among students.. *JMIR Serious Games*, **6**(4), e19. doi: 10.2196/games.9944

Karila, L., Billieux, J., Benyamina, A., Lançon, C. & Cottencin, O. (2016). The effects and risks associated to mephedrone and methylone in humans: A review of the preliminary evidences. *Brain Research Bulletin*, **126**(Part 1), 61–67.

Karila, L., Lafaye, G., Scocard, A., Cottencin, O. & Benyamina, A. (2018). MDPV and α-PVP use in humans: The twisted sisters. *Neuropharmacology*, **134**(Part A), 65–72.

Karila, L., Megarbane, B., Cottencin, O. & Lejoyeux, M. (2015). Synthetic cathinones: A new public health problem. *Current Neuropharmacology*, **13**(1), 12–20.

Katselou, M., Papoutsis, I., Nikolaou, P., Spiliopoulou, C. & Athanaselis, S. (2015). AH-7921: The list of new psychoactive opioids is expanded. *Forensic Toxicology*, **33**(2), 195–201.

Katz, K. D., Leonetti, A. L., Bailey, B. C., et al. (2016). Case series of synthetic cannabinoid intoxication from one toxicology center. *Western Journal of Emergency Medicine*, **17**(3), 290–294.

Kehr, J., Ichinose, F., Yoshitake, S., et al. (2011). Mephedrone, compared with MDMA (ecstasy) and amphetamine, rapidly increases both dopamine and 5-HT levels in nucleus accumbens of awake rats. *British Journal of Pharmacology*, **164**(8), 1949–1958.

Kelly, B. C., Wells, B. E., Pawson, M., et al. (2013). Novel psychoactive drug use among younger adults involved in US nightlife scenes. *Drug and Alcohol Review*, **32**(6), 10.1111/dar.12058. http://doi.org/10.1111/dar.12058

Kempf, C., Llorca, P-M., Pizon, F., Brousse, G. & Flaudias, V. (2017). What's new in addiction prevention in young people: A literature review of the last years of research. *Frontiers in Psychology*, **8**, 1131. doi:10.3389/fpsyg.2017.01131.

Kersten, B. P. & McLaughlin, M. E. (2015). Toxicology and management of novel psychoactive drugs. *Journal of Pharmacy Practice*, **28**(1), 50–65.

Kesha, K., Boggs, C. L., Ripple, M. G., et al. (2013). Methylenedioxypyrovalerone ("bath salts"), related death: Case report and review of the literature. *Journal of Forensic Sciences*, **58**(6), 1654–1659.

Kikura-Hanajiri, R., Kawamura, N. U. & Goda, Y. (2014). Changes in the prevalence of new psychoactive substances before and after the introduction of the generic scheduling of synthetic cannabinoids in Japan. *Drug Testing and Analysis*, **6**(7–8), 832–839.

Kjellgren, A., Jacobsson, K. & Soussan, C. (2016). The quest for well-being and pleasure: Experiences of the novel synthetic opioids AH-7921 and MT-45, as reported by anonymous users online. *Journal of Addiction Research & Therapy*, **7**, 287. doi: 10.4172/2155-6105.1000287

Kovács, K., Tóth, A. R. & Kereszty, E. M. (2012). [A new designer drug: methylone related death]. *Orvosi Hetilap*, **153**(7), 271–276.

Kovaleva, J., Devuyst, E., De Paepe, P. & Verstraete, A. (2008). Acute chlorophenylpiperazine overdose: A case report and review of the literature. *Therapeutic Drug Monitoring*, **30**(3), 394–398.

Labay, L. M., Caruso, J. L., Gilson, T. P., et al. (2016). Synthetic cannabinoid drug use as a cause or contributory cause of death. *Forensic Science International*, **260**, 31–39.

Larabi, I. A., Martin, M., Etting, I., et al. (2018). Drug-facilitated sexual assault (DFSA) involving 4-methylethcathinone (4-MEC), 3,4-Methylenedioxypyrovalerone (MDPV), and doxylamine highlighted by hair analysis. *Drug Testing and Analysis*. doi: 10.1002/dta.2377.

Lea, T., Reynolds, R. & De Wit, J. (2011). Mephedrone use among same-sex attracted young people in Sydney, Australia. *Drug and Alcohol Review*, **30**(4), 438–440.

Lee, H. P., Chae, P. K., Lee, H. S. & Kim, Y. K. (2007). The five-factor gambling motivation model. *Psychiatry Research*, **150**(1), 21–32.

Lee, H., Kim, J. W. & Choi, T. Y. (2017). Risk factors for smartphone addiction in Korean adolescents: Smartphone use patterns. *Journal of Korean Medical Science*, **32**(10), 1674–1679.

Lin, J. C., Bangs, N., Lee, H., Kydd, R. R. & Russell, B. R. (2009). Determining the subjective and physiological effects of BZP on human females. *Psychopharmacology*, **207**(3), 439–446.

Lin, J. C., Jan, R. K., Kydd, R. R. & Russell, B. R. (2011). Subjective effects in humans following administration of party pill drugs BZP and TFMPP alone and in combination. *Drug Testing and Analysis*, **3**(9), 582–585.

Lozier, M. J., Boyd, M., Stanley, C., et al. (2015). Acetyl fentanyl, a novel fentanyl analog, causes 14 overdose deaths in Rhode Island, March–May 2013. *Journal of Medical Toxicology*, **11**(2), 208–217.

Lusthof, K. J., Oosting, R., Maes, A., et al. (2011). A case of extreme agitation and death after the use of mephedrone in The Netherlands. *Forensic Science International*, **206**(1–3), e93–95. doi: 10.1016/j.forsciint.2010.12.014.

Majeed-Ariss, R., Baildam, E., Campbell, M., et al. (2015). Apps and adolescents: A systematic review of adolescents' use of mobile phone and tablet apps that support personal management of their chronic or long-term physical conditions. *Journal of Medical Internet Research*, **17**(12), e287. doi: 10.2196/jmir.5043

Marrinan, S., Roman-Urrestarazu, A., Naughton, D., et al. (2017). Hair analysis for the detection of drug use-is there potential for evasion? *Human Psychopharmacology*, **32**(3), doi: 10.1002/hup.2587.

Martínez-Clemente, J., López-Arnau, R., Carbó, M., et al. (2013). Mephedrone pharmacokinetics after intravenous and oral administration in rats: Relation to pharmacodynamics. *Psychopharmacology*, **229**(2), 295–306.

Martinotti, G., Lupi, M., Acciavatti, T., et al. (2014). Novel psychoactive substances in young adults with and without psychiatric comorbidities. *BioMed Research International*, **2014**, 815424. doi: 10.1155/2014/815424.

Martinotti, G., Lupi, M., Carlucci, L., et al. (2015). Novel psychoactive substances: Use and knowledge among adolescents and young adults in urban and rural areas. *Human Psychopharmacology*, **30**(4), 295–301.

McCall, H., Adams, N., Mason, D. & Willis, J. (2015). What is chemsex and why does it matter? *BMJ*, **351**, h5790. doi: 10.1136/bmj.h5790

McIntyre, I. M., Trochta, A., Gary, R. D., Malamatos, M. & Lucas, J. R. (2015). acute acetyl fentanyl fatality: A case report with postmortem concentrations. *Journal of Analytical Toxicology*, **39**(6), 490–494.

McIntyre, I. M., Trochta, A., Gary, R. D., Wright, J. & Mena, O. (2016). An acute butyr-fentanyl fatality: A case report with postmortem concentrations. *Journal of Analytical Toxicology*, **40**(2), 162–166.

Mdege, N. D., Meader, N., Lloyd, C., Parrott, S. & McCambridge, J. (2017). *The Novel Psychoactive Substances in the UK Project: Empirical and Conceptual Review Work to Produce Research Recommendations.* Southampton (UK): NIHR Journals Library. Available at: www.ncbi.nlm.nih.gov/pubmedhealth/PMH0095704/ [Accessed December 20, 2017]

Meader, N., Mdege, N. & McCambridge, J. (2018). The public health evidence-base on novel psychoactive substance use: Scoping review with narrative synthesis of selected bodies of evidence. *Journal of Public Health (Oxford, England)*. doi: 10.1093/pubmed/fdy016

Meltzer, P. C., Butler, D., Deschamps, J. R. & Madras, B. K. (2006). 1-(4-Methylphenyl)-2-pyrrolidin-1-yl-pentan-1-one (Pyrovalerone) analogs. A promising class of monoamine uptake inhibitors. *Journal of Medicinal Chemistry*, **49**(4), 1420–1432.

Miliano, C., Serpelloni, G., Rimondo, C., et al. (2016). Neuropharmacology of New Psychoactive Substances (NPS): Focus on the rewarding and reinforcing properties of cannabimimetics and amphetamine-like stimulants. *Frontiers in Neuroscience*, **10**, 153. http://doi.org/10.3389/fnins.2016.00153

Miller, M. L., Creehan, K. M., Angrish, D., et al. (2013). Changes in ambient temperature differentially alter the thermoregulatory, cardiac and locomotor stimulant effects of 4-methylmethcathinone (mephedrone). *Drug and Alcohol Dependence*, **127**(1–3), 248–253.

Miller, J. M., Stogner, J. M., Miller, B. L. & Blough, S. (2018). Exploring synthetic heroin: Accounts of acetyl fentanyl use from a sample of dually diagnosed drug offenders. *Drug and Alcohol Review*, **37**(1), 121–127.

Ministry of Health – New Zealand (2012). *Regulatory impact statement, new regulatory regime for psychoactive substances.* Wellington, New Zealand: The Treasury. Available at: www.health.govt.nz/about-ministry/legislation-and-regulation/regulatory-impact-statements/new-regulatory-regime-psychoactive-substances. [Accessed October 16, 2017]

Moore, K., Dargan, P. I., Wood, D. M. & Measham, F. (2013). Do novel psychoactive substances displace established club drugs, supplement them or act as drugs of initiation? The relationship between mephedrone, ecstasy and cocaine. *European Addiction Research*, **19**(5), 276–282.

Morano, R. A., Spies, C., Walker, F. B. & Plank, S. M. (1993). Fatal intoxication involving etryptamine. *Journal of Forensic Sciences*, **38** (3), 721–725.

Móró, L. & Rácz, J. (2013). Online drug user-led harm reduction in Hungary: A review of "Daath". *Harm Reduction Journal*, **10**, 18. doi: 10.1186/1477-7517-10-18.

Murphy, D. L., Lesch, K. P., Aulakh, C. S. & Pigott, T. A. (1991). Serotonin-selective arylpiperazines with neuroendocrine, behavioral, temperature, and cardiovascular effects in humans. *Pharmacological Reviews*, **43**(4), 527–552.

Murray, B. L., Murphy, C. M. & Beuhler, M. C. (2012). Death following recreational use of designer drug "bath salts" containing 3,4-methylenedioxypyrovalerone (MDPV). *Journal of Medical Toxicology*, **8**(1), 69–75.

Nagai, H., Saka, K., Nakajima, M., et al. (2014). Sudden death after sustained restraint following self-administration of the designer drug α-pyrrolidinovalerophenone. *International Journal of Cardiology*, **172**(1), 263–265.

Negrei, C., Galateanu, B., Stan, M., et al. (2017). Worldwide legislative challenges related to psychoactive drugs. *DARU Journal of Pharmaceutical Sciences*, **25**, 14. http://doi .org/10.1186/s40199-017-0180-2

Nurmedov, S., Yilmaz, O., Darcin, A. E., Noyan, O. C. & Dilbaz, N. (2015). Frequency of synthetic cannabinoid use and its relationship with socio-demographic characteristics and treatment outcomes in alcohol- and substance-dependent inpatients: A retrospective study. *Klinik Psikofarmakoloji Bulteni – Bulletin of Clinical Psychopharmacology*, **25**(4), 348–354.

Nutt, D. (2015). Open letter to David Cameron, Prime Minister. www.independent.co.uk/news/uk/home-news/former-government-drugs-adviser-professor-david-nutt-writes-to-pm-arguing-against-banning-legal-10374433 .html

Oei, A. C. & Patterson, M. D. (2013). Enhancing cognition with video games: A multiple game training study, J. J. Geng (Ed.). *PLoS ONE*, **8**(3), e58546. doi:10.1371/journal.pone .0058546.

Ott, J. (2001). Pharmepéna-Psychonautics: Human intranasal, sublingual and oral pharmacology of 5-methoxy-N,N-dimethyl-tryptamine. *Journal of Psychoactive Drugs*, **33** (4), 403–407.

Paglia-Boak, A., Mann, R. E., Adlaf, E. M. & Rehm, J. (2009). *Drug Use among Ontario Students, 1977–2009: Detailed OSDUHS Findings*. Toronto, Ontario: Centre for Addiction and Mental Health. Available at: http://odesi1.scholarsportal.info/documentation/PHIRN/OSDUHS/Highlights_DrugReport_2009OSDUHS_Final_Web.pdf [Accessed: May 15, 2018]

Paksi, B., Magi, A., Felvinczi, K. & Demetrovics, Zs. (2016). The prevalence of new psychoactive substances in Hungary – Based on a general population survey dealing with addiction related problems (OLAAP 2015). IV. International Conference on Novel Psychoactive Substances (NPS). Budapest, May 30-31, 2016.

Palamar, J. J., Martins, S. S., Su, M. K. & Ompad, D.C. (2015). Self-reported use of novel psychoactive substances in a US nationally representative survey: Prevalence, correlates, and a call for new survey methods to prevent underreporting. *Drug and Alcohol Dependence*, **156**, 112–119.

Palamar, J. J., Su, M. K. & Hoffman, R. S. (2016). Characteristics of novel psychoactive substance exposures reported to New York City Poison Center, 2011–2014. *The American Journal of Drug and Alcohol Abuse*, **42**(1), 39–47.

Palma-Conesa, Á. J., Ventura, M., Galindo, L., et al. (2017). Something new about something old: A 10-year follow-up on classical and new psychoactive tryptamines and results of analysis. *Journal of Psychoactive Drugs*, **49**(4), 297–305.

Papaseit, E., Olesti, E., de la Torre, R., Torrens, M. & Farré, M. (2017). Mephedrone concentrations in cases of clinical intoxication. *Current Pharmaceutical Design*. doi: 10.2174/1381612823666170704130213.

Papaseit, E., Pérez-Mañá, C., Mateus, J.-A., et al. (2016). Human pharmacology of mephedrone in comparison with MDMA. *Neuropsychopharmacology*, **41**(11), 2704–2713.

Papsun, D., Krywanczyk, A., Vose, J. C., Bundock, E. A. & Logan, B. K. (2016). Analysis of MT-45, a novel synthetic opioid, in human whole blood by LC-MS-MS and its identification in a drug-related death. *Journal of Analytical Toxicology*, **40**(4), 313–317.

Patrick, M. E., O'Malley, P. M., Kloska, D. D., et al. (2016). Novel psychoactive substance use by US adolescents: Characteristics associated with use of synthetic cannabinoids and synthetic cathinones. *Drug and Alcohol Review*, **35**(5), 586–590.

Pearson, J. M., Hargraves, T. L., Hair, L. S., et al. (2012). Three fatal intoxications due to methylone. *Journal of Analytical Toxicology*, **36**(6), 444–451.

Penders, T. M., Gestring, R. E. & Vilensky, D. A. (2012). Intoxication delirium following use of synthetic cathinone derivatives. *The American Journal of Drug and Alcohol Abuse*, **38**(6), 616–617.

Penney, J., Dargan, P. I., Padmore, J., Wood, D. M. & Norman, I. J. (2016). Epidemiology of adolescent substance use in London schools. *QJM: An International Journal of Medicine*, **109**(6), 405–409.

Péterfi, A., Tarján, A., Horváth, G. C., Csesztregi, T. & Nyírády, A. (2014). Changes in patterns of injecting drug use in Hungary: A shift to synthetic cathinones. *Drug Testing and Analysis*, **6**(7–8), 825–831.

Pintori, N., Loi, B. & Mereu, M. (2017). Synthetic cannabinoids: The hidden side of Spice drugs. *Behavioral Pharmacology*, **28**(6), 409–419.

Poklis, J., Poklis, A., Wolf, C., et al. (2016). Two fatal intoxications involving butyryl fentanyl. *Journal of Analytical Toxicology*, **40**(8), 703–708.

Potocka-Banaś, B., Janus, T., Majdanik, S., et al. (2017). Fatal intoxication with α-PVP, a synthetic cathinone derivative. *Journal of Forensic Sciences*, **62**(2), 553–556.

Prekupec, M. P., Mansky, P. A. & Baumann, M. H. (2017). Misuse of novel synthetic opioids: A deadly new trend. *Journal of Addiction Medicine*, **11**(4), 256–265.

Prosser, J. M. & Nelson, L. S. (2012). The toxicology of bath salts: A review of synthetic cathinones. *Journal of Medical Toxicology*, **8** (1), 33–42.

Ralphs, R. & Gray, P. (2017). New psychoactive substances: New service provider challenges.

Drugs: Education, Prevention and Policy, **25** (4), 301–312.

Ralphs, R., Williams, L., Askew, R. & Norton, A. (2017). Adding Spice to the Porridge: The development of a synthetic cannabinoid market in an English prison. *The International Journal on Drug Policy*, **40**, 57–69.

Rambaran, K. A., Fleming, S. W., An, J., et al. (2017). U-47700: A clinical review of the literature. *The Journal of Emergency Medicine*, **53**(4), 509–519.

RAND (EUROPE) (2016). *The role of the 'dark' web in the trade of illicit drugs. Research brief.* Available at: www.rand.org/content/dam/rand/pubs/research_briefs/RB9900/RB9925/RAND_RB9925.pdf [Accessed: June 06, 2018]

Reuter, P. & Pardo, B. (2017). Can new psychoactive substances be regulated effectively? An assessment of the British Psychoactive Substances Bill. *Addiction*, **112** (1), 25–31.

Rodgman, C. J. C., Verrico, C. D., Worthy, R. B. & Lewis, E. E. (2014). Inpatient detoxification from a synthetic cannabinoid and control of postdetoxification cravings with naltrexone. *The Primary Care Companion for CNS Disorders*, **16**(4), 10.4088/PCC.13l01594. http://doi.org/10.4088/PCC.13l01594

Romanek, K., Stenzel, J., Schmoll, S., et al. (2017). Synthetic cathinones in Southern Germany – Characteristics of users, substance-patterns, co-ingestions, and complications. *Clinical Toxicology (Philadelphia, Pa.)*, **55**(6), 573–578.

Sanders, B., Lankenau, S. E., Bloom, J. J. & Hathazi, D. (2008). "Research Chemicals": Tryptamine and phenethylamine use among high-risk youth. *Substance Use & Misuse*, **43** (3–4), 389–402.

Schep, L. J., Slaughter, R. J., Hudson, S., Place, R. & Watts, M. (2015). Delayed seizure-like activity following analytically confirmed use of previously unreported synthetic cannabinoid analogues. *Human & Experimental Toxicology*, **34**(5), 557–560.

Schep, L. J., Slaughter, R. J., Vale, J. A., Beasley, D. M. & Gee, P. (2011). The clinical toxicology of the designer party pills benzylpiperazine and trifluoromethylphenylpiperazine. *Clinical Toxicology (Philadelphia, Pa.)*, **49**(3), 131–141.

Schifano, F., Orsolini, L., Duccio Papanti, G. & Corkery, J. M. (2015). Novel psychoactive substances of interest for psychiatry. *World Psychiatry*, **14**(1), 15–26.

Schindler, C. W., Thorndike, E. B., Suzuki, M., Rice, K. C. & Baumann, M. H. (2016). Pharmacological mechanisms underlying the cardiovascular effects of the "bath salt" constituent 3,4-methylenedioxypyrovalerone (MDPV). *British Journal of Pharmacology*, **173** (24), 3492–3501.

Schneir, A., Metushi, I. G., Sloane, C., Benaron, D. J. & Fitzgerald, R. L. (2017). Near death from a novel synthetic opioid labeled U-47700: Emergence of a new opioid class. *Clinical Toxicology (Philadelphia, Pa.)*, **55**(1), 51–54.

Shanks, K. G. & Behonick, G. S. (2016). Death after use of the synthetic cannabinoid 5F-AMB. *Forensic Science International*, **262**, e21–24, doi: 10.1016/j.forsciint.2016.03.004.

Shanks, K. G., Clark, W. & Behonick, G. (2016). Death associated with the use of the synthetic cannabinoid ADB-FUBINACA. *Journal of Analytical Toxicology*, **40**(3), 236–239.

Shimizu, E., Watanabe, H., Kojima, T., et al. (2007). Combined intoxication with methylone and 5-MeO-MIPT. *Progress in Neuropsychopharmacology & Biological Psychiatry*, **31**(1), 288–291.

Siddiqi, S., Verney, C., Dargan, P. & Wood, D. M. (2015). Understanding the availability, prevalence of use, desired effects, acute toxicity and dependence potential of the novel opioid MT-45. *Clinical Toxicology (Philadelphia, Pa.)*, **53**(1), 54–59.

Simonato, P., Bersani, F. S., Santacroce, R., et al. (2017). Can mobile phone technology support a rapid sharing of information on novel psychoactive substances among health and other professionals internationally? *Human Psychopharmacology*, **32**(3). doi: 10.1002/hup.2580

Simonato, P., Corazza, O., Santonastaso, P., et al. (2013). Novel psychoactive substances as a novel challenge for health professionals; results from an Italian survey. *Human Psychopharmacology*, **28**(4), 324–331.

Sindicich, N. & Burns, L. (2012). *Australian trends in ecstasy and related drug markets 2012: Findings from the Ecstasy and Related Drugs Reporting System (EDRS). Australian Drug Trends Series No.100.* National Drug and Alcohol Research Centre, University of New South Wales. Available at: https://ndarc.med.unsw.edu.au/sites/default/files/ndarc/resources/EDRS%202012%20national%20report%20FINAL.pdf [Accessed: October 16, 2017]

Sivagnanam, K., Chaudari, D., Lopez, P., Sutherland, M. E. & Ramu, V. K. (2013). "Bath salts" induced severe reversible cardiomyopathy. *The American Journal of Case Reports*, **14**, 288–291.

Smith, K. & Flatley, J. (2011). *Drug Misuse Declared: Findings from the 2010/2011 British Crime Survey England and Wales.* UK: Home Office.

Smith, S. W. & Garlich, F. M. (2013). Availability and supply of novel psy-choactive substances. In P. I. Dargan & D. M. Wood (Eds.), *Novelpsychoactive Substances: Classification, Pharmacology and Toxicology*. Elsevier, UK: Academic Press, pp. 55–86.

Smolinske, S. C., Rastogi, R. & Schenkel, S. (2005). Foxy methoxy: A new drug of abuse. *Journal of Medical Toxicology*, **1**(1), 22–25.

Smyth, B. P., James, P., Cullen, W. & Darker, C. (2015). "So prohibition can work?" Changes in use of novel psychoactive substances among adolescents attending a drug and alcohol treatment service following a legislative ban. *The International Journal on Drug Policy*, **26**(9), 887–889.

Smyth, B. P., Lyons, S. & Cullen, W. (2017). Decline in new psychoactive substance use disorders following legislation targeting headshops: Evidence from national addiction treatment data. *Drug and Alcohol Review*, **36**(5), 609–617.

Soussan, C. & Kjellgren, A. (2016). The users of Novel Psychoactive Substances: Online survey about their characteristics, attitudes and motivations. *The International Journal of Drug Policy*, **32**, 77–84.

Soussan, C., Andersson, M. & Kjellgren, A. (2018). The diverse reasons for using Novel Psychoactive Substances – A qualitative study of the users' own perspectives. *The International Journal on Drug Policy*, **52**, 71–78.

Spaderna, M., Addy, P. H. & D'Souza, D. C. (2013). Spicing thing up: Synthetic cannabinoids. *Psychopharmacology*, **228**(4), 525–540.

Spiller, H. A., Ryan, M. L., Weston, R. G. & Jansen, J. (2011). Clinical experience with and analytical confirmation of "bath salts" and "legal highs" (synthetic cathinones) in the United States. *Clinical Toxicology (Philadelphia, Pa.)*, **49**(6), 499–505.

Srisung, W., Jamal, F. & Prabhakar, S. (2015). Synthetic cannabinoids and acute kidney injury. *Proceedings (Baylor University Medical Center)*, **28**(4), 475–477.

Stanciu, C. N., Penders, T. M., Gnanasegaram, S. A., et al. (2017). The behavioral profile of methylenedioxypyrovalerone (MDPV) and α-pyrrolidinopentiophenone (PVP) – A systematic review. *Current Drug Abuse Reviews*. doi: 10.2174/1874473710666170321122226.

Stanley, J. L., Mogford, D. V., Lawrence, R. J. & Lawrie, S. M. (2016). Use of novel psychoactive substances by inpatients on general adult psychiatric wards. *BMJ Open*, **6** (5), e009430. http://doi.org/10.1136/bmjopen-2015-009430

Štefková, K., Židková, M., Horsley, R. R., et al. (2017). Pharmacokinetic, ambulatory, and hyperthermic effects of 3,4-methylenedioxy-N-methylcathinone (methylone) in rats. *Frontiers in Psychiatry*, **8**, 232. http://doi.org/10.3389/fpsyt.2017.00232

Stevens, A., Fortson, R., Measham, F. & Sumnall, H. (2015). 'Legally flawed, scientifically problematic, potentially harmful: The UK Psychoactive Substance Bill'. *International Journal of Drug Policy*, **26**(12), 1167–1170.

Stogner, J. M. (2014). The potential threat of acetyl fentanyl: Legal issues, contaminated heroin, and acetyl fentanyl "disguised" as other opioids. *Annals of Emergency Medicine*, **64**(6), 637–639.

Strassman, R. J. (1996). Human psychopharmacology of N,N-dimethyltryptamine. *Behavioural Brain Research*, **73**(1–2), 121–124.

Stratton, S. J., Rogers, C., Brickett, K. & Gruzinski, G. (2001). Factors associated with sudden death of individuals requiring restraint for excited delirium. *The American Journal of Emergency Medicine*, **19**(3), 187–191.

Sykutera, M., Cychowska, M. & Bloch-Boguslawska, E. (2015). A fatal case of pentedrone and α-pyrrolidinovalerophenone poisoning. *Journal of Analytical Toxicology*, **39** (4), 324–329.

Takase, I., Koizumi, T., Fujimoto, I., Yanai, A. & Fujimiya, T. (2016). An autopsy case of acetyl fentanyl intoxication caused by insufflation of 'designer drugs'. *Legal Medicine (Tokyo)*, **21**, 38–44.

Tanaka, E., Kamata, T., Katagi, M., Tsuchihashi, H. & Honda, K. (2006). A fatal poisoning with 5-methoxy-N,N-diisopropyltryptamine, Foxy. *Forensic Science International*, **163**(1–2), 152–154.

Tancer, M. E. & Johanson, C. E. (2001). The subjective effects of MDMA and mCPP in moderate MDMA users. *Drug and Alcohol Dependence*, **65**(1), 97–101.

TEDI (Trans European Drug Information) (2013). *2nd TEDI Trend Report, Nightlife Empowerment and Well-Being Information Project (NEWIP)*. Available at: http://fileserver.idpc.net/library/Tedi_trend_report_feb2013.pdf [Accessed June 05, 2018]

Teske, J., Weller, J. P., Fieguth, A., et al. (2010). Sensitive and rapid quantification of the cannabinoid receptor agonist naphthalen-1-yl-(1-pentylindol-3-yl)methanone (JWH-018) in human serum by liquid chromatography-tandem mass spectrometry. *Journal of Chromatography, B. Analytical Technologies in the Biomedical and Life Sciences*, **878**(27), 2659–2663.

Thammongkolchai, T., Termsarasab, P., Alkhachroum, A., et al. (2015). 5-Meo-DALT-induced cyclic myoclonus (P3.013). *Neurology*, **84** (14 Supplement), P3.013.

The New Psychoactive Substances Review Expert Panel (2014). *New Psychoactive Substances: Report of the Expert Panel*. Available at: https://assets.publishing.service.gov.uk/government/uploads/system/uploads/attachment_data/file/368583/NPSexpertReviewPanelReport.pdf [Accessed: June 06, 2018]

Thompson, I., Williams, G., Caldwell, B., et al. (2010). Randomised double-blind, placebo-controlled trial of the effects of the 'party pills' BZP/TFMPP alone and in combination with alcohol. *Journal of Psychopharmacology*, **24** (9), 1299–1308.

Tittarelli, R., Mannocchi, G., Pantano, F. & Romolo, F. S. (2015). Recreational use, analysis and toxicity of tryptamines. *Current Neuropharmacology*, **13**(1), 26–46.

Toennes, S. W., Geraths, A., Pogoda, W., et al. (2017). Pharmacokinetic properties of the synthetic cannabinoid JWH-018 and of its metabolites in serum after inhalation. *Journal of Pharmaceutical and Biomedical Analysis*, **140**, 215–222.

Tracy, D. K., Wood, D. M. & Baumeister, D. (2017). Novel psychoactive substances: Identifying and managing acute and chronic harmful use. *BMJ*, **356**. doi: 10.1136/bmj.i6814.

Trecki, J., Gerona, R. R. & Schwartz, M.D. (2015). Perspective: synthetic cannabinoid-related illnesses and deaths. *The New England Journal of Medicine*, **373**(2), 103–107.

Turner, C. F., Ku, L., Rogers, S. M., et al. (1998). Adolescent sexual behavior, drug use, and violence. *Science*, **280**(5365), 867–873.

United Nation Office on Drugs and Crime (UNODC) (2015). *Special Segment, Legal responses to NPS: multiple approaches to a multi-faceted problem*. Global Smart Update, Vol 14. Available at: www.unodc.org/documents/scientific/Global_SMART_Update_14-web.pdf [Accessed: June 06, 2018]

Ukaigwe, A., Karmacharya, P. & Donato, A. (2014). A gut gone to pot: A case of cannabinoid hyperemesis syndrome due to K2, a synthetic cannabinoid. *Case Reports in Emergency Medicine*, 167098. http://doi.org/10.1155/2014/167098

Ustundag, M. F., Ozhan Ibis, E., Yucel, A. & Ozcan, H. (2015). Synthetic cannabis-induced mania. *Case Reports in Psychiatry*. doi: 10.1155/2015/310930.

Valente, M. J., Guedes de Pinho, P., de Lourdes Bastos, M., Carvalho, F. & Carvalho, M. (2014). Khat and synthetic cathinones: A review. *Archives of Toxicology*, **88**(1), 15–45.

Van Amsterdam, J., Brunt, T. & van den Brink, W. (2015). The adverse health effects of synthetic cannabinoids with emphasis on psychosis-like effects. *Journal of Psychopharmacology*, **29**(3), 254–263.

Van Hout, M. C. (2014). An internet study of user's experiences of the synthetic cathinone 4-methylethcathinone (4-MEC). *Journal of Psychoactive Drugs*, **46**(4), 273–286.

Van Hout, M. C. & Brennan, R. (2012). Curiosity killed M-Cat: A post-legislative study on mephedrone use in Ireland. *Drugs: Education Prevention and Policy*, **19**(2), 156–162.

Vento, A. E., Martinotti, G., Cinosi, E., et al. (2014). Substance use in the club scene of Rome: A pilot study. *BioMed Research International*, **2014**, 617546. http://doi.org/10.1155/2014/617546

Vidourek, R. A., King, K. A. & Burbage, M.L. (2013). Reasons for synthetic THC use among college students. *Journal of Drug Education*, **43**(4), 353–363.

Vorce, S. P., Knittel, J. L., Holler, J. M., et al. (2014). A fatality involving AH-7921. *Journal of Analytical Toxicology*, **38**(4), 226–230.

Vreeker, A., van der Burg, B. G., van Laar, M. & Brunt, T.M. (2017). Characterizing users of new psychoactive substances using psychometric scales for risk-related behavior. *Addictive Behaviors*, **70**, 72–78.

Warrick, B. J., Wilson, J., Hedge, M., et al. (2012). Lethal serotonin syndrome after methylone and butylone ingestion. *Journal of Medical Toxicology*, **8**(1), 65–68.

Weinstein, A. M., Rosca, P., Fattore, L. & London, E. D. (2017). Synthetic cathinone and cannabinoid designer drugs pose a major risk for public health. *Frontiers in Psychiatry*, **8**, 156. http://doi.org/10.3389/fpsyt.2017.00156

Westin, A. A., Frost, J., Brede, W. R., et al. (2016). Sudden cardiac death following use of the synthetic cannabinoid MDMB-CHMICA. *Journal of Analytical Toxicology*, **40**(1), 86–87.

White, J., Hawkins, J., Madden, K., et al. (2017). *Adapting the ASSIST model of informal peer-led intervention delivery to the Talk to FRANK drug prevention programme in UK secondary schools (ASSIST + FRANK): intervention development, refinement and a pilot cluster randomised controlled trial.* Public Health Research, No. 5.7. Southampton (UK): NIHR Journals Library.

Wiley, J. L., Marusich, J. A., Huffman, J. W., Balster, R. L. & Thomas, B. F. (2011). Hijacking of basic research: The case of synthetic cannabinoids. *Methods Report (RTI Press)*, **2011**, 17971.

Wilkins, C., Sweetsur, P. & Girling, M. (2008). Patterns of benzylpiperazine/trifluoromethylphenylpiperazine party pill use and adverse effects in a population sample in New Zealand. *Drug and Alcohol Review*, **27**(6), 633–639.

Wilson, J. M., McGeorge, F., Smolinske, S. & Meatherall, R. (2005). A foxy intoxication. *Forensic Science International*, **148**(1), 31–36.

Winstock, A. R. & Barratt, M. J. (2013). Synthetic cannabis: A comparison of patterns of use and effect profile with natural cannabis in a large global sample. *Drug and Alcohol Depend*, **131**(1–2), 106–111.

Winstock, A. R. & Barratt, M. (2016). *Dark-net markets: the good, the bad and ugly?* Available at: www.globaldrugsurvey.com/gds2017-launch/dark-net-markets-the-good-the-bad-and-ugly/ [Accessed: December 20, 2017]

Winstock, A., Barratt, M., Ferris, J. & Maier, L. (2017). *Global Drug Survey 2017 – Global Overview and Highlights.* Available at: www.globaldrugsurvey.com/wp-content/themes/globaldrugsurvey/results/GDS2017_key-findings-report_final.pdf [Accessed: October 17, 2017]

Winstock, A. R., Marsden, J. & Mitcheson, L. (2010). What should be done about mephedrone? *BMJ*, **340**, c1605. doi: 10.1136/bmj.c1605.

Winstock, A. R., Mitcheson, L. R., Deluca, P., et al. (2011). Mephedrone, new kid for the chop? *Addiction*, **106**(1), 154–161.

Wood, D. M., Ceronie, B. & Dargan, P. I. (2016). Healthcare professionals are less confident in managing acute toxicity related to the use of new psychoactive substances (NPS) compared with classical recreational drugs. *QJM: An International Journal of Medicine*, **109**(8), 527–529.

Wood, D. M., Davies, S., Greene, S. L., et al. (2010). Case series of individuals with analytically confirmed acute mephedrone toxicity. *Clinical Toxicology (Philadelphia, Pa)*, **48**(9), 924–927.

Wood, D. M., Heyerdahl, F., Yates, C. B., et al. (2014). The European Drug Emergencies Network (Euro-DEN). *Clinical Toxicology (Philadelphia, Pa.)*, **52**(4), 239–241.

Wood, D. M., Measham, F. & Dargan, P. I. (2012). 'Our favourite drug': prevalence of use and preference for mephedrone in the London night-time economy 1 year after control. *Journal of Substance Use*, **17**(2), 91–97.

Wyman, J. F., Lavins, E. S., Engelhart, D., et al. (2013). Postmortem tissue distribution of MDPV following lethal intoxication by "bath salts". *Journal of Analytical Toxicology*, **37**(3), 182–185.

Yin, S. & Ho, M. (2012). Monitoring a toxicological outbreak using Internet search query data. *Clinical Toxicology (Philadelphia, Pa.)*, **50**(9), 818–822.

Zawilska, J. B. (2017). An expanding world of novel psychoactive substances: Opioids. *Frontiers in Psychiatry*, **8**, 110. http://doi.org/10.3389/fpsyt.2017.00110

Zawilska, J. B. & Wojcieszak, J. (2017). α-Pyrrolidinophenones: A new wave of designer cathinones. *Forensic Toxicology*, **35**(2), 201–216.

Zheluk, A., Quinn, C. &, Meylakhs, P. (2014). Internet search and krokodil in the Russian Federation: An infoveillance study. *Journal of Medical Internet Research*, **16**(9), e212. doi: 10.2196/jmir.3203

26 Impaired Physicians

A. Benjamin Srivastava, MD, and Mark S. Gold, MD

Men, who follow professions, which require constant exercise of the faculties of their minds, are very apt to seek relief, by the use of ardent spirits, from the fatigue which succeeds great mental exertions.

- Benjamin Rush, *An Inquiry into the Effect of Ardent Spirits upon the Human Body and Mind, with an Account of the Means of Preventing and of the Remedies for Curing Them* (Rush, 1823)

Introduction

In 1784, Benjamin Rush, a physician and one of the Founding Fathers of the United States who is rightly considered the "Father of American Psychiatry" first published *An Inquiry into the Effect of Ardent Spirits upon the Human Body and Mind, with an Account of the Means of Preventing and of the Remedies for Curing Them,* one of the first treatises on alcoholism in the United States. This influential report was likewise one of the first to make references to professions of a cerebral disposition. Rush's observation was prescient, particularly regarding the study of impaired physicians (White, 1998).

Perhaps the two most well-known physicians with well-documented histories of substance use disorders were Sigmund Freud and William Halstead. Freud began experimenting (including self-experimenting) with cocaine in the 1880s while he was a house officer at the University of Vienna (Markel, 2012; Shaffer, 1984). In 1884 he published *Über Coca,* at that time a definitive treatise on cocaine, and to this day holds its place as one of the most vivid descriptions of the cocaine toxidrome (Markel, 2012; Shaffer, 1984). Freud writes, "a few minutes after taking cocaine, one experiences a sudden exhilaration and feeling of lightness...One senses an increase of self-control and feels more vigorous and more capable of work..." (Freud, 1884; Shaffer, 1984). From this description as well as extensive historical documentation, it is clear that Freud became addicted to cocaine. However, Freud's use of cocaine is thought to have influenced his professional transition from a neurologist and neuropathologist into the father of psychoanalysis for which he gained worldwide prominence (Markel, 2012). Similarly, the use of cocaine was thought to be paramount in the transition of William Halstead from a cavalier, dynamic surgeon into the figure known for meticulous suturing, aggressive monitoring of hemostasis, and the development of paradigm shifting surgical innovations that immortalized him as one of the greatest surgeons to ever live (Markel, 2012). As renowned physician and historian Howard Markel describes in *Anatomy of Addiction: Sigmund Freud, William Halstead, and the Miracle Drug Cocaine,* the professional acclaim of Freud and Halstead notwithstanding, their addictions to cocaine led to immense interpersonal conflict, physical harm, and personal anguish (Markel, 2012). Freud and Halsted are two prime examples of a common, underappreciated, and seemingly paradoxical phenomenon, the impaired physician. In this chapter, we will give an overview of impaired physicians in terms of prevalence, characteristics and qualities, and treatment strategies, as applied primarily to substance addictions. We will also discuss how some of the treatment strategies that have proven efficacy for impaired physicians may be extended to the general population. Further we will comment on related topics including burnout, pathological gambling, and inappropriate sexual behavior in the workplace.

Epidemiology

While the exact prevalence of substance use disorders tends to vary between studies, most literature suggests that it approximates that of the general population (Brewster, 1986; Hughes et al., 1992; Oreskovich et al., 2015; Vaillant, Brighton & McArthur, 1970). In 1970, Harvard psychiatrist George Vaillant and colleagues published a now-famous twenty-year longitudinal study in the *New England Journal of Medicine* in which sample of undergraduate students were followed longitudinally, and those who became physicians tended to use sedatives, tranquilizers, and stimulants more than nonphysician subjects, while use of alcohol and tobacco remained the same as others (Vaillant et al., 1970). More recently, in 2015, Oreskovich and colleagues surveyed over 27,000 physicians and found the prevalence of substance use disorders to be 15.4 percent, compared to a lifetime prevalence of 14.6 percent in the general population in the United States (Oreskovich et al., 2015; US Department of Health and Human Services (HHS) & Office of the Surgeon General, 2016). When Cottler et al. compared physicians with substance use disorders with a substance treatment seeking, aged-matched cohort from the general population, physicians demonstrated higher life prevalence of alcohol, cocaine, cannabis, and opioid use disorders (Cottler et al., 2013).

Characteristics of Impaired Physicians

Addiction among physicians shares similarities with addiction in the general population; however, the two populations likewise differ in several important ways. Regarding similarities, in both physicians and the general population, experimentation with substances at a young age and a family history of addiction may contribute to the development of addiction (Merlo & Gold, 2008). Both impaired physicians and their counterparts in the general population give similar reasons for initiating drug and/or alcohol use including curiosity, peer pressure, and availability of a given substance (Merlo et al., 2013b) Some predictors of use among physicians seem of unique interest. First, some of the same factors that drive physicians to achieve success (persistence, ability to set aside personal problems) may contribute to the development of substance use disorders (SUDs) (Boisaubin & Levine, 2001). Second, physician burnout rates are high, and thus initiation of substance use may help them cope with psychiatric distress (Hughes et al., 1992; Shanafelt, Sloan & Habermann, 2003). Because many drugs of abuse indeed have clinical indications, physicians may attempt to self-treat their own physical pain or other ailments (Hughes et al., 1992; Merlo et al., 2013a). The drugs themselves are often more readily available to physicians, who may have a sense of over-confidence when self-prescribing and thus quickly, yet unknowingly develop tolerance leading to addiction (Merlo & Gold, 2008).

Use by Specialty

Research suggests differential patterns of substance use disorders among different medical specialties; however, the specific specialties that are found to be over-represented vary among different studies. For example, in 1987, Talbott and colleagues surveyed the first 1,000 physicians in the state of Georgia referred for evaluation and/or treatment for substance use disorders and found that anesthesiology and family medicine were overrepresented. When examining five-year data from physicians enrolled in state Physician Health Programs, the most common specialties represented were family medicine (20 percent), internal medicine (13 percent), anesthesiology (11 percent), emergency medicine (7 percent), and psychiatry (7 percent) (DuPont et al., 2009b). When Hughes et al. surveyed over 5,000 physicians examining particular substances used by individual specialty, emergency medicine physicians reported higher rates of marijuana use, psychiatrists reported higher rates of benzodiazepine use, and anesthesiologists reported higher rates of opioid use (Hughes et al., 1999). More recently, in 2015, Oreskovich et al. surveyed over 27,000 physicians and found that compared with internal medicine physicians, dermatologists and orthopedic surgeons were more likely to misuse alcohol. Further, anesthesiologists were more likely to misuse alcohol rather than opioids (Oreskovich et al., 2015). Differences between studies may reflect the patient population (e.g., physicians sent for evaluation and treatment versus anonymous surveys sent to a community sample of physicians), as well as the methods used (comprehensive interviews versus self-report questionnaires) (Oreskovich et al., 2015). These results notwithstanding, anecdotal data and relative ease of access suggests that anesthesiologists may be relatively likely to be addicted to intravenous opioids, surgeons may experience alcoholism, and psychiatrists and family medicine physicians may be addicted to alcohol and prescription opioids.

Anesthesiology in particular has garnered significant attention, given the high prevalence of addiction generally as well as abuse of opioids and intravenous propofol specifically. Access to these medications, which are some of the most common medications used for general anesthesia, enables use (Warner et al., 2013). Gold et al. surveyed physicians enrolled in the Florida state physician's health program and found that, of physicians who abused fentanyl, anesthesiologists represented 80 percent (Gold et al., 2006). These findings are of significant import given that, when compared with other physicians, anesthesiologists have higher rates of relapse, overdose, and suicide (Alexander et al., 2000; Merlo & Gold, 2008; Warner et al., 2013). Contributing factors to such high prevalence of drug abuse in anesthesiologists may similarly include easy access and "treatment" of psychiatric distress.

The "secondhand exposure hypothesis" also posits an explanation for the alarming prevalence of disease severity, recidivism, and mortality in anesthesiologists with SUDs. In a series experiments, Gold and colleagues, using liquid-chromatography mass spectroscopy methods, measured fentanyl particles in the air of an operating room, finding the highest concentration of aerosolized particles near the patient's expiratory circuit, near where the anesthesiologist is positioned during an operation (Gold et al., 2006). Further work by Merlo et al. demonstrated that fentanyl is detectable on surfaces in the operating room (Merlo et al., 2008). Collectively, along with evidence that physicians with family histories of opioid addiction have higher rates of opioid addiction, these studies suggest that incidental inhalation or transdermal absorption of fentanyl particles during an operation may prime a genetically high-risk anesthesiologist by altering reward circuitry resulting in cravings, drug seeking behavior, and, ultimately, addiction (Gold et al., 2006; Merlo & Gold, 2008; Merlo et al., 2008).

Related Issues: Burnout, Workaholism, Gambling, and Compulsive Sexual Behavior

Burnout and Workaholism

Inextricably linked to addiction among physicians is burnout. While a comprehensive discussion of burnout is beyond the scope of this chapter, we will briefly discuss its relationship to addiction among physicians. Over 50 percent of all physicians report feelings of burnout at some point during their careers, and it can often be the harbinger of addiction and/or suicide (Shanafelt et al., 2015). Further, burnout can lead to medical errors, decreased job satisfaction, and physician turnover, all of which can be a consequence of addiction itself, among other factors (Dewa et al., 2017; Xiong, 2017). Among the causes of burnout include increasing workloads with limited patient interaction time, increased paperwork (e.g., electronic medical records, prior authorizations), and physician's loss of leadership roles (e.g., due to healthcare management bureaucracies) (Drummond, 2015). Further, burnout may drive physicians to work reduced hours or leave medicine altogether, possibly further accelerating the projected physician shortage (Sinsky et al., 2017). On the other hand, despite burnout and perhaps somewhat paradoxically, some physicians do become "addicted" to work (working excessive hours to the detriment of their personal lives), and in the context of a burnout inducing work environment creates a perfect storm for the initiation of substance use and progression to a substance use disorder (Rezvani et al., 2014).

A host of other behavioral addictions may be experienced among physicians as well, defined as impulsive turned compulsive behaviors that result in subjective effects of reward and continue despite negative consequences. These include gambling, food, sex, and internet addictions (Grant, Potenza, Weinstein & Gorelick, 2010). While the topic is not without controversy (to what extent are these "addictions" valid entities?) the behaviors can cause significant impairment, and treaters of physicians have seen and treated a number of physicians with problematic gambling and sexual behavior over the years.

Gambling Disorder

Because of evidence documenting similarity in symptomatology to substance use disorders, Gambling Disorder (GD) was included as a "Substance Related and Addictive Disorder" in the fifth edition of the *Diagnostic and Statistical Manual for Mental Disorders* (DSM-5), whereas in DSM-IV-TR it was classified as an Impulse Control Disorder Not Otherwise Specified (NOS) (American Psychiatric Association, 2000, 2013). While no existing literature on the prevalence of problematic gambling in physicians exists (1 percent in the general population) (Kessler et al., 2008), GD presenting with other substance use is not an unrecognized phenomenon. Absent any hard data, it is difficult to characterize which physician phenotypes demonstrate a proclivity toward GD and should be the subject of future studies.

Deviant Sexual Behavior

Whether sexual addiction (or "Compulsive Sexual Behavior") is a valid disease entity is still an active debate (Kraus, Voon & Potenza, 2016); however, it is not uncommon see physicians with SUDs also presenting with significant psychosocial problems due to sexual behavior (e.g., adultery, multiple partners resulting in sexually transmitted diseases, sex with patients). The Federation for State Medical Boards (FSMB) has adopted a "zero tolerance" toward physician-patient sexual interactions, and almost invariably an instance of sexual encounters with patients, if discovered, will result in license suspension and/or revocation (Federation of State Medical Boards, 2006). Often times these behaviors are best explained by a maladaptive personality structure and can be addressed in the context of treatment, as will be discussed later in this chapter. Certainly, one may speculate that having disposable income along with opportunity are facilitating factors as well.

Intervention and Treatment

Impaired physicians are difficult to identify for a variety of reasons. Physicians often have ready access to controlled substances, circumventing the need for an unscrupulous supplier (DuPont et al., 2009b). Physicians may also be more adept at hiding substance use from colleagues and may develop complex, sophisticated denial strategies (DuPont et al., 2009b). For example, an anesthesiologist may rationalize to himself or herself that, because of his or her expertise in pharmacology, what he or she is doing (e.g., using opioids) is safe and of minimal harm, particularly if he or she is able to perform clinical duties without incident. Further, a surgeon may rationalize morning drinking in order to suppress alcohol withdrawal or alleviate a hangover to ensure he or she is able to perform an operation without incident (allegedly a frequent practice of the founders of Alcoholics Anonymous, Dr. Bob Smith). This scenario is not uncommon, and often only with an adverse outcome or threat of discipline will the physician agree to treatment (DuPont et al., 2009a, 2009b).

Additionally, physicians are less likely to report substance abuse among colleagues because of profession implications, stigma, and lack of education about the addictions (DuPont et al., 2009b) Thus, similar to the general population albeit for different reasons, most impaired physicians do not receive adequate treatment, and of those who do, nearly 75 percent are referred from an external source (e.g., colleague, loved one, state board of medicine) (DuPont et al., 2009a; US Department of Health and Human Services (HHS) & Office of the Surgeon General, 2016) For physicians who do enter treatment, the usual mechanism involves a state Physician Health Program (PHP).

History of the PHP

The origins of the PHPs can be traced back to the founding of Alcoholics Anonymous, as one of its cofounders, Dr. Robert Holbrook Smith ("Dr. Bob"), was a colorectal surgeon. Later, Dr. Clarence Pearson founded the International Doctors of Alcoholics Anonymous (IDAA), a mutual support society that has had yearly meetings since 1949. The endeavors of both Dr. Smith and Dr. Pearson raised awareness about treating the impaired physician, and in 1953 the Federation of State Medical Boards (FSMB) called for the development of programs to assist physicians with addictive disorders (White, 1998; White, DuPont & Skipper, 2007). This call to action was accelerated by (1) the American Medical Association's (AMA) 1973 report on "The Sick Physician," (2) the 1974 AMA Council of Mental Health report that addressed physician impairment, (3) the United States Disabled Doctors Act of 1974 that exhorted mandatory reporting of impaired physicians, and (4) the 1975 and 1977 AMA conferences on impaired physicians (White, 1998; White et al., 2007). Formal PHPs were established in the years thereafter and in 1990 became organized into the Federation of State Physician Health Programs (White, 1998; White et al., 2007).

Structure of the PHP

PHPs exist in forty-seven states("Federation of State Physician Health Programs State Programs,") and are entities that work with the state board of medicine to arrange treatment and subsequent monitoring of the impaired physicians. Following an evaluation by a qualified physician with expertise in addiction (either addiction psychiatry or addiction medicine), with a diagnostic focus on both addiction and psychiatric histories (using the DSM-5 SCID interview; APA, 2013), recommendations are made to the state PHP regarding treatment and future monitoring. In general, the focus is on identifying substance use disorders but may include behavioral addictions as well. The state PHP uses the evaluation to draft a contract detailing the requisite treatment, monitoring, and longitudinal care requirements with which the impaired physician must comply before returning to work (DuPont et al., 2009a, 2009b). Generally the physician is offered to consent to treatment voluntarily; however, uncooperative physicians deemed at risk to themselves or others may be involuntarily committed to attend treatment, depending on state law (Merlo & Gold, 2008; Nace et al., 2007; Nelson et al., 1996).

PHPs designate treatment centers that have outstanding reputations in terms of delivering effective, state-of-the-art treatment, usually with specific programs or "tracks" for impaired physicians. Though some contracts may allow for intensive outpatient treatment, residential treatment for approximately ninety days (following acute, medical detoxification) is recommended. Treatment is almost exclusively abstinence focused, and participants receive individual, group, and family-oriented therapy with required attendance at Alcoholics Anonymous (AA), Narcotics Anonymous (NA), and/or Caduceus (twelve-step-based Fellowship for physicians) meetings. If impaired physicians do not feel comfortable in twelve-step meetings, the PHPs will attempt to be accommodating (either through use of intensive, individual therapy or alternative mutual support groups) insofar as the physician displays a commitment to recovery and is compliant with all other aspects of the monitoring contract. Additionally, psychiatric comorbidities are closely evaluated and treated. Further, treatment is provided for some behavioral addictions, particularly gambling disorder, includingnaltrexone, Motivational Interviewing, cognitive-behavioral therapy (CBT) and/or Gambler's Anonymous (Hloch et al., 2017; Yip & Potenza, 2014). Often times, treatment centers can provide resources for addressing outstanding addiction related legal issues (DuPont et al., 2009a, 2009b). Neuropsychological testing is frequently employed because of its utility in assessing cognitive deficits that may impact job performance and provide guidance for a remediation strategy (Williams et al., 2018).

Increasingly, a person-centered approach focus has become a paradigm shift both in mental healthcare generally and addiction treatment specifically. Famed psychiatrist C. Robert Cloninger, MD, of the Department of Psychiatry at Washington University in St. Louis School of Medicine has been one of the foremost thinkers in this area. Rather than strictly focusing on psychopathology, Cloninger, using the putative concepts of Temperament (innate, heritable traits that can be either adaptive or maladaptive depending on the situation) and Character (modifiable traits that can be enhanced in a therapeutic setting), posits that personality change and well-being should be an area of prime focus (Cloninger, Svrakic & Przybeck, 1993; Cloninger, Zohar & Cloninger, 2010). Noted addiction psychiatrist Dr. Daniel Angres of Northwestern University has adopted this model of care for addiction treatment at the Positive Sobriety Institute in Chicago, IL, with fruitful results (Angres, 2010). Angres notes that for physicians specifically, an individualized treatment plan focused on enhancing the character dimensions of Self-Directedness, Cooperativeness, and Self-Transcendence, which is complimentary to mindfulness and twelve-step engagement, provides a person centered approach that can lend itself to a roadmap for long-term Recovery (Angres & Nielsen, 2007). Additionally, the Minnesota Multiphasic Personality Inventory (MMPI), which has utility in assessing personality pathology or tendency toward deviant behavior, has been used in evaluation of impaired physicians (Dorr, 1981).

Following successful completion of residential treatment, the impaired physician begins the monitoring phase of the contract, which uses a contingency management paradigm, one of the oldest and most effective behavioral treatments of addiction (Rash, Stitzer & Weinstock, 2017). One of the central components to monitoring is frequent (at first, weekly) testing using a variety of modalities including urine, hair, and nail clippings. During this period, which typically lasts five years, the physician is usually required to attend monitored, group meetings with an experienced group facilitator and regular mutual support (e.g., AA, NA) meetings. Additionally, the contract usually requires the physician to establish care with a primary care physician as well as a psychiatrist and/or therapist (if necessary). For noncompliance with contract obligations (missed appointments/meetings, lying, relapse), consequences are typically based on severity of offense, and include, but are not limited to, warnings, increase in intensity/frequency of monitoring, mandated return to residential treatment, and/or referral to the state board of medicine for punitive measures (DuPont et al., 2009a, 2009b).

Pharmacotherapy

The role of pharmacotherapy in treating the impaired physician is somewhat of a contested issue. When examining a cohort of physicians enrolled in PHPs, addiction-specific pharmacotherapy was rarely utilized, which likely reflects, when compared to the general population, a near absence of prescribing of opioid maintenance therapy (OMT), specifically buprenorphine or methadone (DuPont et al., 2009a; Merlo et al., 2016). Many PHPs have informal policies prohibiting the use of OMT, and in treating the impaired physician the principle reason for not prescribing OMT is safety: buprenorphine and methadone have the potential to cause CNS side effects and are themselves abusable, and no rigorous literature exists demonstrating that physicians, whose work requires intact cognitive and technical abilities, can practice medicine safely while on OMT (Merlo et al., 2016).

Conversely, non-OMT pharmacotherapy (e.g., naltrexone) may have considerable benefit based on extant literature. In 1984, Washton and colleagues demonstrated that oral naltrexone could be successfully utilized in the treatment of opioid-addicted physicians (Washton, Gold & Pottash, 1984). Similarly, Merlo et al. retrospectively studied the utility of either oral or injectable naltrexone treatment in a sample of eleven anesthesiologists enrolled in the PHP in Florida, which, in 2005, implemented a mandatory naltrexone policy for anesthesiologists treated for opioid use disorder. In the cohort treated with naltrexone (i.e., who enrolled just after the 2005 mandate), eight (over 90 percent) remained relapse free through the duration of their monitoring contracts and successfully returned to work. For anesthesiologists not treated with naltrexone (i.e., enrolled just before the 2005 naltrexone mandate) over 70 percent relapsed at least once during treatment, with only 9 percent returning to work in anesthesiology (Merlo, Greene & Pomm, 2011). Obviously prospective studies with larger sample sizes are needed to further validate these findings, yet these results are nonetheless promising.

Outcomes of PHP Engagement

In a landmark study by McLellan et al., a single cohort of over 900 physicians from sixteen PHPs was followed longitudinally for the entire five-year duration of their monitoring contracts; 78 percent maintained drug-screen confirmed abstinence from alcohol and/or drugs, and 72 percent were working without restrictions (DuPont et al., 2009b; McLellan et al., 2008). Of those who had a relapsed (19 percent of the total population surveyed), only 22 percent had a second relapse, indicating that treatment, contract, and monitoring modifications were in general successful (DuPont et al., 2009b). Outcomes were consistent across physicians surveyed, irrespective of substance type or number of substances used (DuPont et al., 2009b). While this was a single cohort design with no control group, the rather high success rate amongst a fairly large sample size is promising. As mentioned previously, most PHPs prohibit OMT, and thus opioid addicted physicians were monitored under abstinence-only contracts (e.g., without OMT). Interestingly, these opioid-addicted physicians had similar rates of five-year abstinence, relapse, and return to work as those physicians addicted to other substances (Merlo et al., 2016). Additionally, despite existing evidence of naltrexone in treating opioid-addicted physicians, only 5.7 percent of the enrolled patients (of whom 87.5 percent were in treatment for opioids, 5 percent for alcohol, 7.5 percent for other substances) were prescribed naltrexone. While physicians who were prescribed naltrexone had slightly higher relapse rates than other physicians in the study, the temporal sequence of positive drug tests and naltrexone initiation is unknown, i.e., if the naltrexone prescription preceded or followed the relapse (Merlo et al., 2016). Clearly, more data on use of naltrexone in the PHP setting are needed to determine its appropriate role in the treatment of impaired physicians (Merlo et al., 2016).

Controversies about PHPs

While PHPs have been successful, they have not been without controversy. One of the commonest criticisms of PHPs is that of coercion: PHPs often have agreements with state boards of medicine that allow the state board to revoke medical licensure if the physician is noncompliant with the PHP contract dictates, with lack of due process (Boyd, 2015a, 2015b; Boyd & Knight, 2012; Lenzer, 2016). Further complaints include the prohibitive nature of costs (evaluations can cost in excess of $4,500 and residential treatment can cost in excess of $10,000 per month), arbitrary treatment lengths of stay, financial relationships between the PHPs and treatment centers, and exclusive focus on twelve-step recovery (Boyd, 2015a, 2015b; Boyd & Knight, 2012; Lenzer, 2016). Multiple lawsuits have been filed in several different states including Oregon, Michigan, Massachusetts, and Florida, with a $1.3 million verdict awarded to a Florida physician in 1999 for "false imprisonment" following a purported incomplete evaluation with insufficient collateral (all of whom corroborated that the patient had never shown signs of impairment) resulting in mandated treatment (Lenzer, 2016). In 2014, North Carolina published an audit of its PHP following the complaints of several physicians. The report noted lack of due process and oversight precluding any systematic reporting of abuse, conflicts of interest between the PHP and treatment centers, lack of standardized criteria for evaluating physicians and determining treatment disposition, and an abundance of referrals to out of state treatment centers, creating undue hardships for many of the physicians (Wood, 2014).

Clearly, PHP program operations have raised some ethical questions, but one can readily address each point of contention raised above. First, the threat of loss of licensure and other "punitive" measures may be viewed in a different light. For adhering to treatment recommendations, the physician is awarded with the ability to stay in practice and retain licensure, a form of contingency management that is supported by an extensive literature in the treatment of substance use disorders (Higgins, Heil & Lussier, 2004) and appears particularly effective in the impaired physician population (DuPont et al., 2009b). Certainly, voluntary engagement is preferable because the process is viewed as "treatment" rather than "punishment" (as in involuntary or "coerced" treatment) (Merlo & Gold, 2008). Nevertheless existing literature suggests that outcomes (negative drug screens, return to work) among physicians are similar irrespective of their treatment-entry status (McLellan et al., 2008; Merlo & Gold, 2008; Nace et al., 2007; Nelson et al., 1996).

Second, the claims of "lack of due process" are somewhat spurious, as physicians are able to utilize a number of sources including hospital bylaws, employment contracts, board regulations, and employment attorneys (Candilis, 2016). Though the above-mentioned North Carolina audit and other literature suggested a lack of scrutiny or quality control and possible conflicts of interest with the relationships between PHPs and state boards of medicine, the State Boards of Medicine regularly evaluate PHPs, which in turn evaluate treatment centers, ensuring only skilled physicians conduct evaluations and that treatment centers provide evidenced-based care (DuPont et al., 2009a, 2009b).

The strongest argument in support of the PHP model of care is grounded in Social Contract Theory. Physicians enter a reciprocal relationship with the state licensure board in which they are granted the privilege of practising medicine while agreeing to adhere to a certain set of board mandated regulations, and thus, the citizens of an individual state can entrust that the medical care they will receive will be of a high standard (Candilis, 2016) Indeed, the physician gives up some of his or her individual rights, but doing so ensures a higher standard of care and benefit to society. For the social contract to be sustained, an enforcement mechanism must be put into place (the Board of Medicine and its dictates). The PHP, however, offers a security measure for the physician who may become afflicted with addiction and thus become at risk for violating the social contract: the physician, through completing prespecified requirements, is again able to practice when it is determined that he or she can with "reasonable skill and safety", and thus society continues to benefit (Candilis, 2016). Overall satisfaction with PHPs remain high. Merlo and Greene found that of physicians who completed a five-year monitoring contract, over 90 percent reported a satisfactory experience and would recommend the PHP to others, and nearly 85 percent reported continued attendance at twelve-step and other mutual support meetings (Merlo & Greene, 2010).

Implications beyond the Treatment of Addiction

The PHP model has implications in addiction treatment that extend beyond the treatment of impaired physicians. Because of the success of PHPs, professional licensing boards that govern commercial pilots, attorneys, and other healthcare workers (including nurses and pharmacists) have adopted this model of care. Though literature comparing different groups of professionals is scant, compared with nurses, physicians who present for treatment have been more often referred by a PHP level organization, have been generally more impaired and have shown more personality pathology; however, they also have been judged to have a greater capacity for treatment. Thus, some of the traits unique to physicians that might predispose them to addiction might in fact be predictive of their success with treatment. More specifically, persistence, a dimension of Temperament described by Cloninger and measured on the TCI, may both in part drive addictive behavior and engagement in treatment/sustained recovery (Angres, 2010; Cloninger et al., 1993, 2010).

Despite issues and circumstances unique to impaired physicians (as well as other professionals with licenses), certain components of PHPs may be extended to addiction treatment for the general public, with the potential to improve outcomes. Currently, most addiction treatment available to the general public focuses on standard sets of treatment services (e.g., medication and/or counseling) in time-limited settings (DuPont, Compton & McLellan, 2015). In contrast, the PHP model focuses on five-year outcomes with frequent monitoring, accountability, contingency management, and continued support, which may become the standard of care in mainstream addiction treatment (DuPont et al., 2009b, 2015).

Conclusions

Physician impairment is an under-recognized problem that is inextricably linked to high rates of burnout and suicide. However, the advent of PHPs has produced unparalleled success in the realm of addiction treatment. The PHP model will likely be expanded in the near-future to address any number of addictive behaviors that physicians may suffer (e.g., gambling, sex), and randomized controlled trials should be conducted to determine the most efficacious treatments. In addition, given the utility of buprenorphine treatment in the general public, more data is needed to assess the safety (especially vis-à-vis job performance) of buprenorphine treatment in opioid-addicted physicians as an option for severely impaired physicians that are refractory to nonpharmacologic treatment and/or naltrexone. The PHP model represents a paradigm shift in addiction treatment, whereby addiction treatment is viewed as chronic disease management with ongoing treatment, monitoring, and support (similar to hypertension or diabetes) and a focus on five-year outcomes (in the model of cancer) (DuPont et al., 2015). Thus, the study of impaired physicians has broad implications: efforts should be made to disseminate and implement core elements from the PHP model to the general public in order to better address America's most significant public health crisis.

REFERENCES

Alexander, B. H., Checkoway, H., Nagahama, S. I. & Domino, K. B. (2000). Cause-specific mortality risks of anesthesiologists. *Anesthesiology*, **93**(4), 922–930.

American Psychiatric Association (2000). *Diagnostic and Statistical Manual of Mental Disorders: DSM-IV-TR*. Arlington, VA: American Psychiatric Publishing.

American Psychiatric Association (2013). *Diagnostic and Statistical Manual of Mental Disorders* (5th edition). Arlington, VA: American Psychiatric Publishing.

Angres D. H. (2010). The temperament and character inventory in addiction treatment. *Focus*, **8**(2), 187–198. doi:10.1176/foc.8.2.foc187

Angres, D. H. & Nielsen, A. K. (2007). The role of the TCI-R (Temperament Character Inventory) in individualized treatment plannning in a population of addicted professionals. *Journal of Addictive Diseases*, **26** (Supplement 1), 51–64. doi:10.1300/J069v26S01_06

Boisaubin, E. V. & Levine, R. E. (2001). Identifying and assisting the impaired physician. *American Journal of Medical Sciences*, **322**(1), 31–36.

Boyd, J. W. (2015a). A call for national standards and oversight of state physician health programs. *Journal of Addiction Medicine*, **9**(6), 431–432. doi:10.1097/adm.0000000000000174

Boyd, J. W. (2015b). Deciding whether to refer a colleague to a physician health program. *AMA Journal of Ethics*, **17**(10), 888–893. doi:10.1001/journalofethics.2015.17.10.specl-1510

Boyd, J. W. & Knight, J. R. (2012). Ethical and managerial considerations regarding state physician health programs. *Journal of Addiction Medicine*, **6**(4), 243–246. doi:10.1097/ADM.0b013e318262ab09

Brewster, J. M. (1986). Prevalence of alcohol and other drug problems among physicians. *JAMA*, **255**(14), 1913–1920. doi:10.1001/jama.1986.03370140111034

Candilis, P. J. (2016). Physician health programs and the social contract. *AMA Journal of Ethics*, **18**(1), 77–81. doi:10.1001/journalofethics.2016.18.1.corr1-1601

Cloninger, C. R., Svrakic, D. M. & Przybeck, T. R. (1993). A psychobiological model of temperament and character. *Archives of General Psychiatry*, **50**(12), 975–990.

Cloninger, C. R., Zohar, A. H. & Cloninger, K. M. (2010). Promotion of well-being in person-centered mental health care. *Focus*, **8** (2), 165–179. doi:10.1176/foc.8.2.foc165

Cottler, L. B., Ajinkya, S., Merlo, L. J., et al. (2013). Lifetime psychiatric and substance use disorders among impaired physicians in a physicians health program: Comparison to a general treatment population: Psychopathology of impaired physicians. *Journal of Addiction Medicine*, **7**(2), 108–112. doi:10.1097/ADM.0b013e31827fadc9

Dewa, C. S., Loong, D., Bonato, S. & Trojanowski, L. (2017). The relationship between physician burnout and quality of healthcare in terms of safety and acceptability: A systematic review. *BMJ Open*, **7**.

Dorr, D. (1981). MMPI profiles of emotionally impaired physicians. *Journal of Clinical Psychology*, **37**(2), 451–455.

Drummond, D. (2015). Physician burnout: Its origin, symptoms, and five main causes. *Family Practice Management*, **22**(5), 42–47.

DuPont, R. L., Compton, W. M. & McLellan, A. T. (2015). Five-year recovery: A new standard for assessing effectiveness of substance use disorder treatment. *Journal of Substance Abuse Treatment*, **58**, 1–5. doi:10.1016/j.jsat.2015.06.024

DuPont, R. L., McLellan, A. T., Carr, G., Gendel, M. & Skipper, G. E. (2009a). How are addicted physicians treated? A national survey of Physician Health Programs. *Journal of Substance Abuse Treatment*, **37**(1), 1–7. doi:10.1016/j.jsat.2009.03.010

DuPont, R. L., McLellan, A. T., White, W. L., Merlo, L. J. & Gold, M. S. (2009b). Setting the standard for recovery: Physicians' Health Programs. *Journal of Substance Abuse Treatment*, **36**(2), 159–171. doi:10.1016/j.jsat.2008.01.004

Federation of State Medical Boards (2006). *Addressing Sexual Boundaries: Guidelines for State Medical Boards*. Retrieved from Federation of State Physician Health Programs State Programs. Retrieved from www.fsphp.org/state-programs

Freud, S. (1884). Über Coca. *Centralblatt für die gesamte Therapie*, **2**, 289–314.

Gold, M. S., Melker, R. J., Dennis, D. M., et al. (2006). Fentanyl abuse and dependence: Further evidence for second hand exposure hypothesis. *Journal of Addictive Diseases*, **25** (1), 15–21. doi:10.1300/J069v25n01_04

Grant, J. E., Potenza, M. N., Weinstein, A. & Gorelick, D. A. (2010). Introduction to behavioral addictions. *The American Journal of Drug and Alcohol Abuse*, **36**(5), 233–241. doi:10.3109/00952990.2010.491884

Higgins, S. T., Heil, S. H. & Lussier, J. P. (2004). Clinical implications of reinforcement as a determinant of substance use disorders. *Annual Review of Psychology*, **55**, 431–461. doi:10.1146/annurev.psych.55.090902.142033

Hloch, K., Mladenka, P., Dosedel, M., Adriani, W. & Zoratto, F. (2017). The current clinical knowledge on the treatment of gambling disorder: A summary. *Synapse*, **71**(8). doi:10.1002/syn.21976

Hughes, P. H., Brandenburg, N., Baldwin, D. C., Jr., et al. (1992). Prevalence of substance use among US physicians. *JAMA*, **267**(17), 2333–2339.

Hughes, P. H., Storr, C. L., Brandenburg, N. A., et al. (1999). Physician substance use by medical specialty. *Journal of Addictive Diseases*, **18**(2), 23–37. doi:10.1300/J069v18n02_03

Kessler, R. C., Hwang, I., LaBrie, R., et al. (2008). DSM-IV pathological gambling in the National Comorbidity Survey Replication. *Psychological Medicine*, **38**(9), 1351–1360. doi:10.1017/s0033291708002900

Kraus, S. W., Voon, V. & Potenza, M. N. (2016). Should compulsive sexual behavior be considered an addiction? *Addiction*, **111**(12), 2097–2106. doi:10.1111/add.13297

Lenzer, J. (2016). Physician health programs under fire. *BMJ*, **353**, i3568. doi:10.1136/bmj.i3568

Markel, H. (2012). *An Anatomy of Addiction: Sigmund Freud, William Halsted, and the Miracle Drug Cocaine*. New York, NY: Vintage Books, Random House, Inc.

McLellan, A. T., Skipper, G. S., Campbell, M. & DuPont, R. L. (2008). Five year outcomes in a cohort study of physicians treated for substance use disorders in the United States. *BMJ*, **337**, a2038. doi:10.1136/bmj.a2038

Merlo, L. J. & Gold, M. S. (2008). Prescription opioid abuse and dependence among physicians: Hypotheses and treatment. *Harvard Review of Psychiatry*, **16**(3), 181–194. doi:10.1080/10673220802160316

Merlo, L. J. & Greene, W. M. (2010). Physician views regarding substance use-related participation in a state physician health program. *American Journal on Addictions,* **19** (6), 529–533. doi:10.1111/j.1521-0391.2010.00088.x

Merlo, L. J., Campbell, M. D., Skipper, G. E., Shea, C. L. & DuPont, R. L. (2016). Outcomes for physicians with opioid dependence treated without agonist pharmacotherapy in physician health programs. *Journal of Substance Abuse Treatment,* **64**, 47–54. doi:10.1016/j.jsat.2016.02.004

Merlo, L. J., Goldberger, B. A., Kolodner, D., Fitzgerald, K. & Gold, M. S. (2008). Fentanyl and propofol exposure in the operating room: Sensitization hypotheses and further data. *Journal of Addictive Diseases,* **27**(3), 67–76. doi:10.1080/10550880802122661

Merlo, L. J., Greene, W. M. & Pomm, R. (2011). Mandatory naltrexone treatment prevents relapse among opiate-dependent anesthesiologists returning to practice. *Journal of Addiction Medicine,* **5**(4), 279–283. doi:10.1097/ADM.0b013e31821852a0

Merlo, L. J., Singhakant, S., Cummings, S. M. & Cottler, L. B. (2013a). Reasons for misuse of prescription medication among physicians undergoing monitoring by a physician health program. *Journal of Addiction Medicine,* **7**(5), 349–353. doi:10.1097/ADM.0b013e31829da074

Merlo, L. J., Trejo-Lopez, J., Conwell, T. & Rivenbark, J. (2013b). Patterns of substance use initiation among healthcare professionals in recovery. *American Journal on Addictions,* **22**(6), 605–612. doi:10.1111/j.1521-0391.2013.12017.x

Nace, E. P., Birkmayer, F., Sullivan, M. A., et al. (2007). Socially sanctioned coercion mechanisms for addiction treatment. *American Journal on Addictions,* **16**(1), 15–23. doi:10.1080/10550490601077783

Nelson, H. D., Matthews, A. M., Girard, D. E. & Bloom, J. D. (1996). Substance-impaired physicians probationary and voluntary treatment programs compared. *Western Journal of Medicine,* **165**(1–2), 31–36.

Oreskovich, M. R., Shanafelt, T., Dyrbye, L. N., et al. (2015). The prevalence of substance use disorders in American physicians. *American Journal on Addictions,* **24**(1), 30–38. doi:10.1111/ajad.12173

Rash, C. J., Stitzer, M. & Weinstock, J. (2017). Contingency management: New directions and remaining challenges for an evidence-based intervention. *Journal of Substance Abuse Treatment,* **72**, 10–18. doi:10.1016/j.jsat.2016.09.008

Rezvani, A., Bouju, G., Keriven-Dessomme, B., Moret, L. & Grall-Bronnec, M. (2014). Workaholism: Are physicians at risk? *Occupational Medicine (London),* **64**(6), 410–416. doi:10.1093/occmed/kqu081

Rush, B. (1823). *An Inquiry into the Effect of Ardent Spirits upon the Human Body and Mind, with an Account of the Means of Preventing and of the Remedies for Curing Them* (8th edition). Boston: James Loring.

Shaffer, H. (1984). Uber coca: Freud's cocaine discoveries. *Journal of Substance Abuse Treatment,* **1**(3), 205–217. doi:http://dx.doi.org/10.1016/0740-5472(84)90023-0

Shanafelt, T. D., Hasan, O., Dyrbye, L. N., et al. (2015). Changes in burnout and satisfaction with work-life balance in physicians and the general US working population between 2011 and 2014. *Mayo Clinic Proceedings,* **90** (12), 1600–1613. doi:10.1016/j.mayocp.2015.08.023

Shanafelt, T. D., Sloan, J. A. & Habermann, T. M. (2003). The well-being of physicians. *American Journal of Medicine,* **114**(6), 513–519.

Sinsky, C. A., Dyrbye, L. N., West, C. P., et al. (2017). Professional satisfaction and the career plans of US physicians. *Mayo Clinic Proceedings,* **92**(11), 1625–1635. doi:10.1016/j.mayocp.2017.08.017

US Department of Health and Human Services (HHS) & Office of the Surgeon General. (November 2016). *Facing Addiction in America: The Surgeon General's Report on Alcohol, Drugs, and Health.* Washington, DC: HHS.

Vaillant, G. E., Brighton, J. R. & McArthur, C. (1970). Physicians' use of mood-altering drugs. A 20-year follow-up report. *New England Journal of Medicine,* **282**(7), 365–370. doi:10.1056/nejm197002122820705

Warner, D. O., Berge, K., Sun, H., et al. (2013). Substance use disorder among anesthesiology residents, 1975-2009. *JAMA,* **310**(21), 2289–2296. doi:10.1001/jama.2013.281954

Washton, A. M., Gold, M. S. & Pottash, A. C. (1984). Naltrexone in addicted physicians and business executives. *NIDA Research Monographs,* **55**, 185–190.

White, W. L. (1998). *Slaying the Dragon: The History of Addiction Treatment and Recovery in America.* Normal, IL: Chestnut Health Systems/Lighthouse Institute.

White, W. L., DuPont, R. L. & Skipper, G.E. (2007). Physicians health programs: What counselors can learn from these remarkable programs. *Counselor,* **8**(2), 42–47.

Xiong, W. (2017). Physician burnout: An epidemic or the new norm? *American Journal of Psychiatry Residents' Journal,* **12**(4), 2. doi:10.1176/appi.ajp-rj.2017.120401

Williams, B. W., Flanders, P., Welindt, D. & Williams, M. V. (2018). Importance of neuropsychological screening in physicians referred for performance concerns. *PloS ONE,* **13**(11), e0207874–e0207874. doi:10.1371/journal.pone.0207874

Wood, B. A. (2014). *Performance audit: North Carolina physicians health program. North Carolina Office of the State Health Auditor.*

Yip, S. W. & Potenza, M. N. (2014). Treatment of gambling disorders. *Current Treatment Options in Psychiatry,* **1**(2), 189–203. doi:10.1007/s40501-014-0014-5

27 Feedback Models for Gambling Control: The Use and Efficacy of Online Responsible Gambling Tools

Mark D. Griffiths, PhD

Introduction

Online gambling is a psychological and sociological phenomenon that is becoming a focus of interest for an increasing number of researchers in the social sciences. As the internet offers a new venue for gambling, the risks for engaging in pathological behaviors are potentially increased (Griffiths, 2003). This has resulted in a large increase of empirical research into online gambling (Gainsbury, 2015; Kuss & Griffiths, 2012). At present, there are numerous different methodologies in which data about online gambling can be collected (e.g., online surveys, online experiments, online interviews and focus groups, online ethnographic methods) (Griffiths, 2010). However, this chapter briefly examines one of the newer methodologies that have been utilized in the past few years by those in the gambling studies field (i.e., behavioral tracking), and briefly reviews the advantages, disadvantages, and uses, as well as examining how such data have been used to evaluate the effectiveness of various online pathological gambling protection tools such as limit setting, pop-up messaging, and personalized feedback.

The Use of Online Methodologies to Study Gambling

Over the past decade, researchers in the gambling studies field have started to use online methods to gather their data, rather than traditional offline research approaches (Griffiths, 2010; Wood & Griffiths, 2007). Psychological research that can be done online includes experimental, self-report, and/or observational research. A methodological review paper by Griffiths (2010) examined seven different online data collection methods used for collecting gambling and gaming data including (i) online questionnaires, (ii) online forums, (iii) online participant observation, (iv) online secondary data, (v) online interviews, (vi) online exemplar websites, and (vii) online evaluations (including online "mystery shopping"). He also argued in the same paper that the internet can be a very useful medium for eliciting rich and detailed data in sensitive areas such as problem gambling because the online medium is nonface-to-face, nonthreatening, nonalienating, and nonstigmatizing, and that individuals were more likely to give honest and truthful answers compared to face-to-face data collection methods.

There are a number of reasons why the online medium is a good place to conduct research with online gamblers. This is because the internet: (i) is usually accessible to these gamblers, and they are usually proficient in using it (Wood & Griffiths, 2007); (ii) allows for studies to be administered to potentially large-scale samples quickly and efficiently (Buchanan, 2000, 2007; Wood, Griffiths & Eatough, 2004); (iii) can facilitate automated data inputting, allowing large-scale samples to be administered at a fraction of the cost and time of "pen and paper" equivalents (Buchanan, 2007); (iv) has a disinhibiting effect on users and reduces social desirability, leading to increased levels of honesty (and therefore higher validity in the case of self-report) (Joinson et al., 2008); (v) has a potentially global pool of participants, therefore researchers are able to study extreme and uncommon behaviors as well as make cross-cultural comparisons (Buchanan, 2000); (vi) provides access to "socially unskilled" individuals who may not have taken part in the research if it was offline (Wood & Griffiths, 2007; Wood et al., 2004); (vii) can aid participant recruitment through advertising on various bulletin boards and websites (Wysocki, 1998); and (viii) can aid researchers because they do not have to be in the same geographical location as either the participants or fellow research colleagues (e.g., Whitty, 2004; Wood et al., 2004). It should also be added that in contemporary society very few people live their lives completely offline.

Online Behavioral Tracking in Gambling

Over fifteen years ago, Griffiths and Parke (2002) noted that one of the most potentially worrying concerns about online gambling was the way online gambling website operators could collect data about their players (i.e., those who gamble on their websites). Customer data is the lifeblood of any company and online gamblers provide tracking data that can be used to compile customer profiles. Such data can tell commercial enterprises (such as those in the gambling industry) exactly how customers are spending their time in any given financial transaction (i.e., in the case of online gambling, which games their customers are gambling on, for how long, how much money they are spending, what games are profitable). This information can help in the retention of customers, and can also link up with existing customer databases and operating loyalty schemes. Companies who have one central repository for all their customer data have an advantage. It can also be accessed by different parts of the business. Many consumers are unknowingly passing on information about themselves, and are being profiled according to how they transact with service providers. Linked loyalty schemes can then track the account from the opening established date.

The technology to sift and assess vast amounts of customer information has developed substantially over the past decade. Using the latest sophisticated software, gaming companies can tailor their service to the customer's known interests. When it comes to gambling, there is a very fine line between providing what the customer wants and exploitation. The gaming industry sells products in much the same way that any other business sells things. They are now in the business of brand marketing, direct marketing (via mail with personalized and customized offers), and loyalty schemes (that create the illusion of awareness, recognition, and loyalty).

On joining loyalty schemes, players supply lots of information including name, address, telephone number, date of birth, and gender.

Those who operate online gambling sites are no different. They know the gambler's favorite game and the amounts they have wagered. Basically, gambling operators can track the playing patterns of any gambler. They arguably know more about the gambler's playing behavior than the gamblers themselves. They are able to send the gambler offers and redemption vouchers, complimentary accounts, and other "incentives." These are done to enhance customer experience (Griffiths & Wood, 2008a). Benefits and rewards to the customer can include cash, food and beverages, entertainment, and general retail. However, more unscrupulous operators have the means to entice known problem gamblers back onto their premises with tailored freebies (such as the inducement of "free" bets in the case of internet gambling). However, later papers by Griffiths and colleagues began to argue that behavioral tracking data could potentially be used to help identify problem gamblers rather than exploit them, and to use behavioral tracking data for research purposes (Griffiths & Wood, 2008b; Griffiths et al., 2007).

The Advantages and Disadvantages of Behavioral Tracking Methods in Gambling Research

There have been several different approaches to collecting data from, and about, gamblers. This has traditionally included self-report methods (e.g., surveys, focus groups, interviews), experiments (in the laboratory or in gambling venues), and participant and/or nonparticipant observation. More recently (i.e., since around 2005), a number of researchers in the gambling studies field have been given direct access to gambling data collected by gaming companies from their commercial online gambling sites. These types of data (i.e., behavioral tracking data) are providing insights into gamblers' behavior that are helping to better understand how such people act and behave online and over long periods of time.

There has been a very recent debate in the gambling studies field as to whether online gambling is more dangerous and harmful than offline gambling. Much of the debate has relied on the data collected by either behavioral tracking or survey methodologies. Griffiths and colleagues (Auer & Griffiths, 2013, 2014a; Delfabbro, King & Griffiths, 2012; Griffiths & Auer, 2011; Griffiths & Whitty, 2010; Griffiths, Wood & Parke, 2009) have written a number of papers outlining the key differences between these two methods. These can be summarized as follows (the first four points suggest a data collection of behavioral tracking over self-report, whereas the remaining points favour the converse):

- Behavioral tracking data provide a totally objective record of an individual's gambling behavior on a particular online gambling website (whereas gamblers in self-report studies may be prone to social desirability factors, unreliable memory).
- Behavioral tracking data overcome the problem of finding suitable online gambling participants as they provide an immediate data set (if access is granted by the gaming company). Participants do not even have to travel to participate in the study.
- Behavioral tracking data provide a record of events and can be revisited after the event itself has finished (whereas in general self-report studies cannot).
- Behavioral tracking data usually comprise very large sample sizes (e.g., studies by Auer and Griffiths [2013, 2014b, 2015a, 2015b, 2016, 2017a, 2017b; Auer, Malischnig & Griffiths, 2014] have used databases with access to over 50,000–100,000 online gamblers) whereas self-report studies are based on much smaller sample sizes (e.g., the national *British Gambling Prevalence Surveys* typically comprise samples of around 8,000–9,000 people [e.g., Wardle et al., 2007]).
- Behavioral tracking data collects data from only one gambling site and tells us nothing about the person's internet gambling in general as Internet gamblers typically gamble on more than one site (Wardle et al., 2007).
- Behavioral tracking data always come from unrepresentative samples (i.e., the players that use one particular internet gambling site) whereas the very best self-report studies (e.g., the *British Gambling Prevalence Surveys* in Great Britain) use random and nationally representative samples (e.g., Wardle et al., 2007).
- Behavioral tracking data do not account for the fact that more than one person can use a particular account.
- Behavioral tracking data tell us nothing about *why* people gamble (whereas self-report data can provide greater insight into motivation to gamble).
- Behavioral tracking data cannot be used for comparing online and offline gambling or for making comparisons about whether online gambling is safer or more dangerous than offline gambling as data are only collected on one group of people (i.e., online gamblers).
- Self-report methods can be used to compare two (or more) groups of gamblers and these are the only methods we currently have to infer to what extent one medium of gambling may or may not be more or less safe.
- Some self-report studies have the potential to use nationally representative samples of gamblers whereas behavioral tracking studies rely on self-selected samples of gamblers who use one specific online gambling website.
- Behavioral tracking data tell us nothing about the relationships between gambling and other behaviors (e.g., the relationship between gambling and alcohol or the relationship between gambling and tobacco use).
- Behavioral tracking data cannot examine problem gambling using current diagnostic criteria (whereas self-report studies can). In fact, behavioral tracking data studies cannot tell us anything about problem gambling as this is not a variable that has been examined in any of the published studies to date (except by using proxy measures of problem gamblers, such as those people who exclude themselves from the site to prevent further gambling on it).

Research using actual gambling data began when one team of researchers affiliated with Harvard University were given access to a large behavioral tracking data set of over 47,000 online gamblers by the Austrian gaming company *bwin*. This has led to many papers examining the actual behavior of online gamblers based on behavioral tracking data (e.g., Broda et al., 2008; LaBrie et al., 2007, 2008; LaPlante et al., 2008, 2009; Xuan & Shaffer, 2009). These data have been used to make claims along the lines that online gambling is no more problematic than offline gambling.

However, comparative statements relating to whether one medium of gambling is more problematic than another can only be made if actual gambling behavior between modalities is studied across different forms of gambling (e.g., direct comparison of internet gambling with land-based casino gambling among the same individuals). None of the various publications by the Harvard-affiliated research team has empirically compared different forms of gambling. Nor have they examined "problem gambling," as no problem gambling screens were given to any online gambler included in their studies. Therefore, conclusions about the harmfulness of online gambling in comparison to other forms of gambling cannot be drawn from these particular studies using these types of behavioral tracking data. Furthermore, none of the publications focusing on online gambling examines overall gambling behavior. All the publications have tended to examine a single type of game (e.g., sports betting, casino games, poker).

Behavioral tracking has also been used in other innovative ways. For instance, Leino et al. (2015) used online behavioral tracking data from Norwegian video lottery terminal (VLT) players (*N* = 31,109) who had gambled in January 2010. The results show that the number of bets made was positively associated with payback percentage, win frequency, being female, and age, and negatively associated with size of wins and range of available betting options. In summary, the results show that the reward characteristics and betting options explained 27 percent and 15 percent of the variance in the number of bets made, respectively. The same team also used Norwegian gambler tracking data to compare the relationship between gambling behavior in alcohol-serving venues (ASVs) and nonalcohol-serving venues (NASVs) over a one-month period (*N* = 726). Findings showed that gamblers appeared to be more willing to take more risk and spend more money in ASVs compared to NASVs (Leino et al., 2017).

Studies by Auer and Griffiths (2014b, 2015c) used tracking data to develop a stable and reliable measure for "gambling intensity" called "theoretical loss" (a product of total bet size multiplied by house advantage). Even for single bets, the theoretical loss reflects the amount a player is willing to risk. Using behavioral tracking data of 100,000 players who played online casino, lottery, and poker games, the study demonstrated that bet size does not equate to or explain theoretical loss as it does not take into account the house advantage. This lack of accuracy was shown to be even more pronounced for gamblers who play a variety of games.

Other studies have used tracking data to demonstrate that what money individuals say they have spent gambling is different from their actual gambling behavior with all studies showing that the more someone gambles, the less reliable they are about estimating what they have financially spent gambling (Auer & Griffiths, 2017a; Braverman, Tom & Shaffer, 2014; Wohl, Davis & Hollingshead, 2017). For instance, Auer and Griffiths compared the self-reported gambling expenditure data of 1,335 Norwegian gamblers with their actual gambling account data (supplied by the Government-owned gambling operator *Norsk Tipping*). The study found that the estimated loss self-reported by gamblers was correlated with the actual objective loss but that players with higher losses tended to have more difficulty estimating their gambling expenditure (i.e., players who spent more money gambling also appeared to have more trouble estimating their expenses accurately).

Braverman et al. (2013) used tracking data to develop behavioral markers that operators that predict the development of gambling-related problems (*N* = 4,056 online gamblers who played with *bwin.party*). Using daily aggregated online betting transactions over a one-month period, they identified two subgroups of high-risk online gamblers that were different from the rest of the sample. The first group engaged in three or more gambling activities and displayed high betting variability on casino-type games. The second group engaged in two different gambling activities and displayed high betting variability on live action sports events. Similar studies by the same research team have used tracking data to identify other behavioral markers of high-risk online gambling (Braverman & Shaffer, 2012; Gray, LaPlante & Shaffer, 2012), while others have used tracking data to demonstrate that online gamblers who self-exclude display different characteristics than those that do not (Dragicevic et al., 2015).

Auer and Griffiths (2017b) used tracking data to test classic psychological theory in the form of cognitive dissonance. The argued that providing personalized feedback about the amount of money that gamblers had actually spent may – in some cases – result in cognitive dissonance due to the mismatch between what gamblers actually spent and what they thought they had spent. Using a participant sample (*N* = 11,829) drawn from Norwegian gamblers that had played at the *Norsk Tipping* online gambling website, players were told that they could retrieve personalized information about the amount of money they had lost over the previous six-month period. Out of the 11,829 players, 4,045 players accessed this information and were asked whether they thought the amount they lost gambling was (i) more than expected, (ii) about as much as expected, or (iii) less than expected. Auer and Griffiths hypothesized that players who claimed that the amount of money lost gambling was more than they had expected were more likely to experience a state of cognitive dissonance and would attempt to reduce their gambling expenditure more than other players who claimed that the amount of money lost was as much as they expected. Overall, the results contradicted the hypothesis because players without any cognitive dissonance decreased their gambling expenditure more than players experiencing cognitive dissonance. However, a more detailed analysis of the tracking data supported the hypothesis because specific playing patterns of six different types of gambler using a learning tree algorithm explained the paradoxical overall result.

Behavioral Tracking Tools

Over the past few decades, innovative social responsibility tools that track player behavior with the aim of preventing problem gambling have been developed, including *PlayScan* – developed by the Swedish gaming company *Svenska Spel*, *Observer* – developed by Israeli gaming company *888.com*, and *mentor* – developed by *neccton Ltd* (Griffiths et al., 2007, 2009). These tracking tools are providing insights about problematic gambling behavior that in turn may lead to new avenues for future research in the area. The companies who have developed these tools claim that they can detect problematic gambling behavior through analysis of behavioral tracking data (Delfabbro et al., 2012; Griffiths et al., 2009). If problem gambling can be detected online via observational tracking data, it suggests that there are identifiable behaviors associated with online problem gambling. Given that almost all of the current validated problem gambling screens diagnose problem gambling based on many of the consequences of problem gambling (e.g., compromising job, education, hobbies and/or relationship because of gambling; committing criminal acts to fund gambling behavior; lying to family and friends about the extent of gambling), behavioral tracking data appears to suggest that problem gambling can be identified without the need to assess the negative psychosocial consequences of problem gambling.

Behavioral tracking tools generally use a combination of behavioral science, psychology, mathematics, and artificial intelligence. Some tools (such as *PlayScan*) claim to detect players at risk of developing gambling problems, and offer the gamblers ways to help change their behavior (e.g., tools that help gamblers set time and money limits on what they are prepared to lose over predetermined time periods) – although it should be noted that these claims have not been verified because the developers of these commercial products have not published their internal research in externally peer-reviewed journals. Unlike the conventional purpose of customer databases (i.e., to increase sales), the objective of these new tools is the opposite. They are designed to detect and help those who would benefit from playing less. Such tools have been compared to a safety belt (i.e., something you use without intending to actually make use of). The use of these systems is voluntary, but the gaming operator strongly recommends its customers to use it (Griffiths et al., 2009). These tools use many parameters of the player's behavior from the preceding year that are then matched against a model based on behavioral characteristics for problem players. If it predicts players' behavior as risky, they get an advance warning together with advice on how they can change their patterns in order to avoid future unhealthy and/or risky gambling. Behavioral tracking data can also be used to evaluate whether the tools and advice given to gamblers can actually change (i.e., reduce) potentially problematic behavior. These studies are briefly reviewed in the next section.

Evaluation of Responsible Gambling Tools Using Tracking Data

Responsible gambling tools (e.g., limit-setting tools, pop-up messages, personalized feedback, temporary self-exclusions) are a way of facilitating players to gamble in a more responsible manner (Harris & Griffiths, 2017). However, very few of these tools have been evaluated empirically in real gambling environments. Broda et al. (2008) examined the effects of player deposit limits on internet sports betting by customers of *bwin Interactive Entertainment*. Their study examined 47,000 subscribers to *bwin* over a period of two years and compared the behavior of players who tried to exceed their deposit limit with all other players. Deposit limit referred to the amount of money deposited into a player's spend account excluding any accumulated winnings. At the time of initial data collection in 2005, *bwin* set a mandatory deposit limit of no more than €1,000 per day or €5,000 per 30 days. Players could also set their own deposit limits (per 30 days) below the mandatory limits. Overall, the study found that less than 1 percent of the players (0.3 percent) attempted to exceed their deposit limit. However, Wood and Griffiths (2010) argued that the large mandatory limit may be the main reason for this finding as LaPlante et al. (2008) noted that the majority of online gamblers never reached the maximum deposit limit. In fact, 95 percent of the players never deposited more than €1,050 per 30 days (i.e., one-fifth of the €5,000 maximum). Furthermore, LaPlante and colleagues did not distinguish between those who attempted to exceed either their own personally set deposit limits or mandatory limits. Using the same dataset, Nelson et al. (2008) examined online gamblers that voluntarily set limits on the *bwin* gambling website over an eighteen-month period. A total of 567 online gamblers (out of more than 47,000) used the voluntary limit-setting feature, and the findings demonstrated that limit-setting gamblers bet more heavily and played a wider variety of games prior to setting limits. After setting voluntary limits, these online gamblers reduced their gambling activity, but not the amount wagered per bet.

A study by Auer and Griffiths (2013a) used behavioral tracking data to evaluate whether the setting of voluntary time and money limits helped players who gambled the most (i.e., the most gambling intense individuals using "theoretical loss" [Auer, Schneeberger & Griffiths, 2012; Auer & Griffiths, 2014a]). Data were collected from a representative random sample of 100,000 online players who gambled on the *win2day* gambling website during a three-month test period. This sample comprised 5,000 registered gamblers who chose to set themselves limits while playing on *win2day*. During the registration process, there was a mandatory requirement for all players to set time and cash-in limits. For instance, the player could limit the daily, weekly and/or monthly cash-in amount and the playing duration. The latter could be limited per playing session and/or per day. In the three-month test period, all voluntary limit setting behavior by online gamblers was tracked and recorded for subsequent data analysis. Changes in gambling behavior were analyzed overall and separately for casino, lottery, and poker gambling.

The results of this study clearly showed that voluntary limit setting had a specific and statistically significant effect on high-intensity gamblers (i.e., voluntary limit setting had the largest effect on the most gaming intense players). More specifically, the analysis showed that (in general) gaming intense players specifically changed their behavior in a positive way after they limited themselves with respect to both time and money spent. Voluntary spending limits had the highest significant effect on subsequent monetary spending among casino and lottery gamblers. Monetary spending among poker players significantly decreased after setting a voluntary time limit. Studies such as this highlight the advantageous way in which behavioral tracking methodologies can be used to provide results and insights that would be highly difficult to show using other more traditional methodologies, and no control groups are needed in studies that compare groups that are differentiated by gambling intensity and/or gambling type.

Auer et al. (2014) investigated the effect of a pop-up message that appeared after 1,000 consecutive online slot machine games had been played by individuals during a single gambling session (i.e., *"You have now played 1,000 slot games. Do you want to continue? [yes/no]"*). The study analyzed 800,000 gambling sessions (400,000 sessions before the pop-up had been introduced and 400,000 after the pop-up had been introduced, comprising around 50,000 online gamblers). The study found that the pop-up message had a limited effect on a small percentage of players. More specifically, prior to the pop-up message being introduced, five gamblers ceased playing after 1,000 consecutive spins of the online slot machine within a single playing session (out of approximately 10,000 playing sessions). Following the introduction of the pop-up message, forty-five gamblers ceased playing after 1,000 consecutive spins (i.e., a nine-fold increase in session cessations). In the latter case, the number of gamblers ceasing play was less than 1 percent of the gamblers who played 1,000 games consecutively.

In a follow-up study, Auer and Griffiths (2015a) argued that the original pop-up message was very basic and that re-designing the message using normative feedback and self-appraisal feedback may increase the efficacy of gamblers ceasing play. The new enhanced pop-up message read: *"We would like to inform you, that you have just played 1,000 slot games. Only a few people play more than 1,000 slot games. The chance of winning does not increase with the duration of the session. Taking a break often helps, and you can choose the duration of the break"*. The reasoning behind the messaging is as follows.

- *"We would like to inform you, that you have just played 1,000 slot games":* This part of the message objectively informs players about the behavior they engaged in.
- *"Only a few people play more than 1,000 slot games":* This part of the message provides normative feedback that very few other gamblers play 1000 consecutive slots games.
- *"The chance of winning does not increase with the duration of the session":* This part of the message addresses a common misbelief among gamblers (i.e., the gamblers' fallacy).

- *"Taking a break often helps, and you can choose the duration of the break":* This part of the message provides advice (to aid self-efficacy) and leaves the decision up to the player and is in line with the techniques of motivational interviewing (Miller & Rollnick, 1991)

As in the previous study, the new enhanced pop-up message that appeared within a single session after a gambler had played 1,000 consecutive slot games. In the follow-up study, Auer and Griffiths (2015a) examined 1.6 million playing sessions comprising two conditions (i.e., simple pop-up message [800,000 slot machine sessions] versus an enhanced pop-up message [800,000 slot machine sessions]) with approximately 70,000 online gamblers. The study found that the message with enhanced content more than doubled the number of players who ceased playing (1.39 percent who received the enhanced pop-up compared to 0.67 percent who received the simple pop-up). However, as in Auer et al.'s (2014) previous study, the enhanced pop-up only influenced a small number of gamblers to cease playing after a long continuous playing session.

Auer and Griffiths (2016), in a study of the efficacy of personalised feedback, examined whether the use of three types of information (i.e., personalized feedback, normative feedback, and/or a recommendation) could enable players to gamble more responsibly as assessed using three measures of gambling behavior, i.e., theoretical loss, amount of money wagered, and gross gaming revenue (i.e., net win/loss). By manipulating the three forms of information, data from six different groups of players were analyzed. The participant sample drawn from the population were those that had played at least one game for money on the *Norsk Tipping* online platform (*Instaspill*) during April 2015. A total of 17,452 players were randomly selected from 69,631 players that fulfilled the selection criteria. Gambling activity among the control group (who received no personalized feedback, normative feedback or no recommendation) was also compared with the other five groups that received information of some kind (personalized feedback, normative feedback, and/or a recommendation). Compared to the control group, all groups that received some kind of messaging significantly reduced their gambling behavior as assessed by theoretical loss, amount of money wagered, and gross gaming revenue. The results supported the hypothesis that personalized behavioral feedback can enable behavioral change in gambling. However, normative feedback did not appear to change behavior significantly more than personalized feedback (although the effect sizes was not reported).

Forsström, Hesser and Carlbring (2016) carried out a study on the use of the behavioral tracking tool *PlayScan*. The data from a total of 9,528 players who voluntarily used the system were analyzed. They found that the initial usage of the tool was high, but that repeated usage was low. Two groups of users – "self-testers" (those who made use of the self-diagnostic problem gambling test) and "multifunction users" (those who used two or more of the responsible gambling tools in the *PlayScan* tool portfolio) – utilized the tool to a much greater extent than other groups. However, the study did not analyze changes in behavior as a consequence of using the tool.

Wood and Wohl (2015) obtained data from 779 *Svenska Spel* online players who received behavioral feedback using *PlayScan*. Feedback to players took the form of a "traffic-light" risk rating that was created via a proprietary algorithm (red = problematic gambling, yellow = at-risk gambling, and green = no gambling issues). In addition, expenditure data (i.e., amounts deposited and gambled) were collected at three time points: the week of *PlayScan* enrolment, the week following *PlayScan* enrolment, and twenty-four weeks after *PlayScan* enrolment. The findings indicated that those players at-risk (yellow gamblers) who used *PlayScan* significantly reduced the amounts of money both deposited and gambled compared to those who did not use *PlayScan*. This effect was also found the week following *PlayScan* enrolment as well as the twenty-four-week mark. Overall, the authors concluded that informing at-risk gamblers about their gambling behavior appeared to have a desired impact on their subsequent monetary spending (although the effect sizes using eta partial squared were generally small).

Conclusions

This chapter highlighted that when it comes to studying online gambling behavior, behavioral tracking methodologies offer a number of advantages for researchers. However, it should also be noted that there are a number of disadvantages of using tracking data only when compared to other more traditional research methods (i.e., surveys), and that no single methodology is better than another in the collection of data concerning online gamblers. However, when evaluating the results of studies that make statements about whether one medium of gambling is more problematic to gamblers than another, the inherent strengths and weaknesses of the methodology used must be taken into consideration. In relation to the efficacy of online responsible gambling tools, there are some types of study (e.g., the evaluation of whether social responsibility tools actually have an effect on subsequent player behavior) where behavioral tracking methodologies appear to be the only reliable way of collecting data to show that specific interventions have a direct effect on player behavior. Findings to date suggest that limit setting and personalized feedback appear to be responsible gambling tools with high efficacy but that further replication studies are needed. The studies evaluating pop-up messaging are far from conclusive and suggest that on their own, pop-up messages only help a very small percentage of within-session intense gamblers.

REFERENCES

Auer, M. & Griffiths, M. D. (2013). Voluntary limit setting and player choice in most intense online gamblers: An empirical study of gambling behaviour. *Journal of Gambling Studies*, 29, 647–660.

Auer, M. & Griffiths, M. D. (2014a). Personalised feedback in the promotion of responsible gambling: A brief overview. *Responsible Gambling Review*, 1, 27–36.

Auer, M. & Griffiths, M. D. (2014b). An empirical investigation of theoretical loss and gambling intensity. *Journal of Gambling Studies*, 30, 879–887.

Auer, M. & Griffiths, M. D. (2015a). Testing normative and self-appraisal feedback in an online slot-machine pop-up message in a real-world setting. *Frontiers in Psychology*, 6, 339. doi: 10.3389/fpsyg.2015.00339

Auer, M. & Griffiths, M. D. (2015b). The use of personalized behavioral feedback for problematic online gamblers: An empirical study. *Frontiers in Psychology*, 6, 1406. doi: 10.3389/fpsyg.2015.01406.

Auer, M. & Griffiths, M. D. (2015c). Theoretical loss and gambling intensity (revisited): A response to Braverman et al. (2013). *Journal of Gambling Studies*, 31, 921–931.

Auer, M. & Griffiths, M. D. (2016). Personalized behavioral feedback for online gamblers: A real world empirical study. *Frontiers in Psychology*, 7, 1875. doi: 10.3389/fpsyg.2016.01875

Auer, M. & Griffiths, M. D. (2017a). Self-reported losses versus actual losses in online gambling: An empirical study. *Journal of Gambling Studies*, 33, 795–806.

Auer, M. & Griffiths, M. D. (2017b). Cognitive dissonance, personalized feedback, and online gambling behavior: An exploratory study using objective tracking data and subjective self-report. *International Journal of Mental Health and Addiction.* Epub ahead of print. doi: 10.1007/s11469-017-9808-1

Auer, M., Malischnig, D. & Griffiths, M. D. (2014). Is 'pop-up' messaging in online slot machine gambling effective? An empirical research note. *Journal of Gambling Issues*, 29, 1–10.

Auer, M., Schneeberger, A. & Griffiths, M. D. (2012). Theoretical loss and gambling intensity: A simulation study. *Gaming Law Review and Economics*, 16, 269–273.

Braverman, J., LaPlante, D. A., Nelson, S. E. & Shaffer, H. J. (2013). Using crossgame behavioral markers for early identification of high-risk Internet gamblers. *Psychology of Addictive Behaviors*, 27, 868–877.

Braverman, J. & Shaffer, H. J. (2012). How do gamblers start gambling: Identifying behavioral markers for high-risk Internet gambling. *European Journal of Public Health*, 22, 273–278.

Braverman, J., Tom, M. A. & Shaffer, H. J. (2014). Accuracy of self-reported versus actual online-gambling wins and losses. *Psychological Assessment*, 26, 865–877.

Broda, A., LaPlante, D. A., Nelson, S. E., et al. (2008). Virtual harm reduction efforts for Internet gambling: Effects of deposit limits on actual Internet sports gambling behaviour. *Harm Reduction Journal*, 5, 27.

Buchanan, T. (2000). Potential of the Internet for personality research. In M. H. Birnbaum (Ed.), *Psychological Experiments on the Internet.* San Diego: Academic Press, pp.121–140.

Buchanan, T. (2007). Personality testing on the Internet: What we know, and what we do not. In A. N. Joinson, K. Y. A. McKenna, T. Postmes & U. R. Reips (Eds.), *Oxford Handbook of Internet Psychology.* Oxford: Oxford University Press, pp. 447–459.

Delfabbro, P. H., King, D. L. & Griffiths, M. D. (2012). Behavioural profiling of problem gamblers: A critical review. *International Gambling Studies*, 12, 349–366.

Dragicevic, S., Percy, C., Kudic, A. & Parke J. (2015). A descriptive analysis of demographic and behavioral data from internet gamblers and those who self-exclude from online gambling platforms. *Journal of Gambling Studies*, 31, 105–132.

Forsström, D., Hesser, H. & Carlbring, P. (2016). Usage of a responsible gambling tool: A descriptive analysis of latent class analysis of user behavior. *Journal of Gambling Studies*, 32, 889–904.

Gainsbury, S. M. (2015). Online gambling addiction: The relationship between Internet gambling and disordered gambling. *Current Addiction Reports*, 2(2), 185–193.

Gray, H. M., LaPlante, D. A. & Shaffer, H. J. (2012). Behavioral characteristics of Internet gamblers who trigger corporate responsible gambling interventions. *Psychology of Addictive Behaviors*, 26, 527–535.

Griffiths, M. D. (2003). Internet gambling: Issues, concerns and recommendations. *CyberPsychology and Behavior*, 6, 557–568.

Griffiths, M. D. (2010). The use of online methodologies in data collection for gambling and gaming addictions. *International Journal of Mental Health and Addiction*, 8, 8–20.

Griffiths, M. D. & Auer, M. (2011). Approaches to understanding online versus offline gaming impacts. *Casino and Gaming International*, 7 (3), 45–48.

Griffiths, M. D. & Parke, J. (2002). The social impact of Internet gambling. *Social Science Computer Review*, 20, 312–320.

Griffiths, M. D. & Whitty, M. W. (2010). Online behavioural tracking in Internet gambling research: Ethical and methodological issues. *International Journal of Internet Research Ethics*, 3, 104–117.

Griffiths, M. D. & Wood, R. T. A. (2008a). Gambling loyalty schemes: Treading a fine line? *Casino and Gaming International*, 4(2), 105–108.

Griffiths, M. D. & Wood, R. T. A. (2008b). Responsible gaming and best practice: How can academics help? *Casino and Gaming International*, 4(1), 107–112.

Griffiths, M. D., Wood, R. T. A. & Parke, J. (2009). Social responsibility tools in online gambling: A survey of attitudes and behaviour among Internet gamblers. *CyberPsychology and Behavior*, 12, 413–421.

Griffiths, M. D., Wood, R. T. A., Parke, J. & Parke, A. (2007). Gaming research and best practice: Gaming industry, social responsibility and academia. *Casino and Gaming International*, 3, 97–103.

Harris, A. & Griffiths, M. D. (2017). A critical review of the harm-minimisation tools available for electronic gambling. *Journal of Gambling Studies*, 33, 187–221.

Joinson, A. N., Paine, C., Buchanan, T. & Reips, U-D. (2008). Measuring self-disclosure online: Blurring and non-response to sensitive items in web-based surveys. *Computers in Human Behavior*, 24, 2158–2171.

Kuss, D. J. & Griffiths, M. D. (2012). Internet gambling behavior. In Z. Yan (Ed.), *Encyclopedia of Cyber Behavior.* Pennsylvania: IGI Global, pp. 735–753.

LaBrie, R. A., Kaplan, S., LaPlante, D. A., Nelson, S. E. & Shaffer, H. J. (2008). Inside the virtual casino: A prospective longitudinal study of Internet casino gambling. *European Journal of Public Health*, 18(4), 410–416.

LaBrie, R. A., LaPlante, D. A., Nelson, S.E., Schumann, A. & Shaffer, H. J. (2007). Assessing the playing field: A prospective longitudinal study of internet sports gambling behavior. *Journal of Gambling Studies*, 23, 347–363.

LaPlante, D. A., Kleschinsky, J. H., LaBrie, R. A., Nelson, S. E. & Shaffer, H. J. (2009). Sitting at the virtual poker table: A prospective epidemiological study of actual Internet poker gambling behavior. *Computers in Human Behavior*, 25, 711–717.

LaPlante, D. A., Schumann, A., LaBrie, R. A. & Shaffer, H. J. (2008). Population trends in Internet sports gambling. *Computers in Human Behavior*, 24(5), 2399–2414.

Leino, T., Sagoe, D., Griffiths, M. D., et al. (2017). Gambling behavior in alcohol-serving and non-alcohol-serving venues: A study of electronic gaming machine players using account records. *Addiction Research and Theory*, 25, 201–207.

Leino, T., Torsheim, T., Blaszczynski, A., et al. (2015). The relationship between structural characteristics and gambling behavior: A population based study. *Journal of Gambling Studies*, 31, 1297–1315.

Miller, W. R. & Rollnick, S. (1991). *Motivational Interviewing: Preparing People to Change Addictive Behavior.* New York: Guilford Press.

Nelson, S. E., LaPlante, D. A., Peller, A. J., et al. (2008). Real limits in the virtual world: Self-limiting behavior of Internet gamblers. *Journal of Gambling Studies*, 24(4), 463–477.

Wardle, H., Sproston, K., Orford, J., et al. (2007). *The British Gambling Prevalence Survey 2007.* London: The Stationery Office.

Whitty, M. T. (2004). Peering into online bedroom windows: Considering the ethical implications of investigating Internet relationships and sexuality. In E. Buchanan (Ed.), *Readings in Virtual Research Ethics: Issues and Controversies.* Hershey, USA: Idea Group Inc., pp. 203–218.

Wohl, M. J. A., Davis, C. G. & Hollingshead, S. J. (2017). How much have you won or lost? Personalized behavioral feedback about gambling expenditures regulates play. *Computers in Human Behavior*, 70, 437–455.

Wood, R. T. A. & Griffiths, M. D. (2007). Online data collection from gamblers: Methodological issues. *International Journal of Mental Health and Addiction*, 5, 151–163.

Wood, R. T. A. & Griffiths, M. D. (2010). Social responsibility in online gambling: Voluntary limit setting. *World Online Gambling Law Report*, 9(11), 10–11.

Wood, R. T. A. & Wohl, M. J. (2015). Assessing the effectiveness of a responsible gambling behavioural feedback tool for reducing the gambling expenditure of at-risk players. *International Gambling Studies*, 15(2), 1–16.

Wood, R. T. A., Griffiths, M. D. & Eatough, V. (2004). Online data collection from videogame players: Methodological issues. *Cyberpsychology and Behavior*, 7, 511–518.

Wysocki, D. K. (1998). Let your fingers to do the talking: Sex on an adult chat-line. *Sexualities*, 1, 425–452.

Xuan, Z. M. & Shaffer, H. J. (2009). How do gamblers end gambling: Longitudinal analysis of internet gambling behaviors prior to account closure due to gambling related problems. *Journal of Gambling Studies*, 25, 239–252.

28 Food versus Eating Addictions

Erica M. Schulte, PhD, Emma. T. Schiestl, MS, and Ashley N. Gearhardt, PhD

Introduction

Obesity continues to be a global health epidemic associated with numerous preventable illnesses (e.g., Type 2 diabetes) and significant financial burden (Seidell & Halberstadt, 2015). Behavioral weight-loss interventions focused on a caloric deficit have had limited long-term success (Wadden et al., 2004), which has prompted researchers to explore causal mechanisms driving the development and maintenance of elevated body weight. In the past decade, studies have focused on biological and behavioral overlaps between obesity and addictive disorders (Volkow & Wise, 2005; Volkow et al., 2012; Wang et al., 2004), and evaluating the hypothesis that some individuals may experience an addictive-like response to certain foods (Ahmed et al., 2013; Davis & Carter, 2009; Davis et al., 2011; Gearhardt et al., 2011a; Gold, Frost-Pineda & Jacobs, 2003; Ifland et al., 2009), particularly highly processed foods with added fat and/or refined carbohydrates (pizza, chocolate, chips) (Schulte, Avena & Gearhardt, 2015). However, a debate in this area currently exists as to whether addictive-like eating is better conceptualized as a substance use disorder, marked by an addiction to specific foods (e.g., highly processed foods), or a behavioral eating addiction, as an addiction to the act of eating (Hebebrand et al., 2014; Schulte, Potenza & Gearhardt, 2017a).

While these ideas seem similar, a substance use disorder framework posits that the physiological reward from addictive substance (e.g., alcohol) interacts with individual susceptibility for addiction and behavioral patterns of engagement (e.g., binge consumption) to result in an addiction. In contrast, existing behavioral addictions do not involve the consumption of a substance and instead reflect the interaction between an addictive behavior (e.g., gambling) with individual susceptibility for addiction and behavioral patterns of engagement (e.g., frequent participation). Notably, rewarding behaviors are relevant to elevating the addictive nature of both substance use disorders and behavioral addictions (e.g., intermittent consumption of alcohol or intermittent wins in gambling), and substance use disorder perspectives acknowledge the importance of behavioral context in motivating drug use (e.g., cue-rich contexts enhancing craving). As such, the substance-based food addiction versus behavioral eating addiction debate has artificially separated the physiological addictive potential of certain foods (e.g., highly processed foods), the problematic ways in which they are consumed (e.g., binge eating), and the contexts that may motivate consumption (e.g., cue-rich fast food restaurants). Since food is consumed, akin to substances, a behavioral addiction to the act of eating would only be supported if the food played no direct role in driving the addictive eating. This chapter argues that a substance-based food addiction framework most appropriately reflects existing research in this area and the comprehensive factors that may elevate the addictive potential of highly processed foods in a similar manner as drugs of abuse.

Specifically, several theoretical debates between the food versus eating addiction perspectives are first discussed. Second, this work details why assumptions made by researchers supporting the behavioral, eating addiction explanation do not parallel existing knowledge of behavioral addictions. Third, a critical review of measurement tools for food and eating addiction is presented. Fourth, implications of each perspective on perceptions of individuals with addictive-like eating and intervention approaches are discussed. Fifth, future research directions needed to validate the food versus eating addiction frameworks are outlined.

Debate #1: The Role of the Food

Food addiction mirrors theoretical perspectives of substance use disorders; that is, food directly contributes to an addictive-like response in vulnerable persons (Ahmed et al., 2013; Davis & Carter, 2009; Davis et al., 2011; Gearhardt, Corbin & Brownell, 2009; Gearhardt, Davis, et al., 2011a; Gold et al., 2003; Schulte et al., 2015). In contrast, an eating addiction framework posits that the behavioral act of eating may become addictive to some individuals, with the attributes of the food (e.g., added sugar) not directly triggering addictive-like eating (Hebebrand et al., 2014). As such, the central debate between the two theories is whether certain foods may be addictive, akin to drugs of abuse, and drive forward an addictive-like process in susceptive individuals. If certain foods are uniquely implicated in addictive-like eating and produce addictive-like responses, then this would be evidence for food addiction. In contrast, if all foods have the potential to be associated with problematic eating given the right behavioral conditions, then this would support eating addiction.

Evidence in Animal Models

Notably, prior work in animals appears to support the food addiction theory. Despite the implementation of behavioral circumstances that increase addictive potential, such as intermittent access (Berridge, 1996; Corwin, 2006), binge-prone rats have exhibited indicators of addictive-like eating to highly processed foods but not to nutritionally balanced chow (Avena, Rada & Hoebel, 2008b; Hoebel et al., 2009; Johnson & Kenny, 2010). For example, repeated bingeing of highly processed foods (e.g., cheesecake) has been associated with diminished dopamine receptor availability, as seen with prolonged drug abuse (Johnson & Kenny, 2010; Robinson et al., 2015). Rats have also exhibited elevated motivation to obtain highly processed foods, but not nutritionally balanced chow, even despite negative consequences (e.g., foot shock) (Oswald et al., 2011), and have shown signs of withdrawal (e.g., teeth chattering) when sugar is removed from their diet (Avena et al., 2008a; Kim et al., 2017). These observations contrast the eating addiction assumption that development of an addiction-like presentation is dependent on the act of eating, regardless of the nutritional composition of the food. Rather, biological and behavioral indicators of addiction seem to occur uniquely with highly processed foods, which may suggest that these foods directly contribute to the addictive-like process.

Supporters of the eating addiction theory point to prior animal studies that have observed overeating with nutritionally balanced chow (Hebebrand et al., 2014). However, in these cases, highly processed foods have still played an important role in the onset of the overeating. For instance, rats have overeaten chow after consuming a preload of a highly processed food (Hagan et al., 2003), but not if presented alone. Further, rats have overeaten chow in environments containing cues previously associated with highly processed food consumption (Boggiano et al., 2009). Importantly, rats have not overeaten chow when it was presented in the absence of a highly processed food preload or environment with cues signaling receipt of these foods. Thus, while rats have overconsumed nutritionally balanced chow, the conditions under which this has occurred suggest an important role of highly processed foods in triggering the overeating.

While animal models offer evidence that the type of food may play a central role in addictive-like eating behavior, proponents of an eating addiction framework have expressed caution in interpreting these findings with respect to humans, as rats are often given nutrients in isolation (e.g., sucrose, vegetable oil), which does not model a typical human diet (Hebebrand et al., 2014). However, there have been numerous studies that integrate more parallel food items like double-stuf Oreo cookies (seventy calories per cookie), cheesecake, and chocolate, with consistent findings that these foods are closely associated with addictive-like eating (Boggiano et al., 2007; Johnson & Kenny, 2010; Oswald et al., 2011). Importantly, the ability to isolate food nutrients (e.g., sugar, fat) in animal research has been essential for learning how specific food attributes may differentially contribute to addictive-like eating. For example, these studies have provided evidence that sugar, but not fat, may trigger withdrawal symptoms when removed from the diet (Avena, Rada & Hoebel, 2009; Bocarsly et al., 2011). Notably, the isolation of nutrients (e.g., administering pure sucrose or vegetable oil) to humans would be less feasible, as these ingredients presented alone may not be palatable or rewarding to humans given the complex taste profiles of highly processed foods widely available in the modern food environment. Further, animal studies of other addictive disorders have successfully translated to humans, as the substances abused by humans are similarly self-administered by animals (Balster, 1991; Haney, 2009; Lile & Nader, 2003; O'Brien & Gardner, 2005). Thus, animal studies have been valuable for discerning processes in addictive-like eating and the foods/ingredients most implicated. Collectively, animal models support a food addiction approach, where certain food types are uniquely associated with addictive-like eating behaviors.

Evidence in Humans

Importantly, previous research in humans has paralleled findings in animals to support a substance-based, food addiction framework. Schulte and colleagues (2015) observed that highly processed foods (e.g., pizza, chocolate, chips) may be uniquely associated with indicators of addictive-like eating, measured by the Yale Food Addiction Scale (YFAS), whereas foods in a natural state (e.g., fruits, vegetables, meats, nuts) seem minimally implicated. Further, persons endorsing numerous symptoms of food addiction on the YFAS (e.g., loss of control, use despite consequences) have reported more frequent consumption of highly processed foods compared to individuals without addictive-like eating behavior (Pursey et al., 2015). Highly processed foods, but not minimally processed foods, have also been associated with facets of subjective experience (e.g., craving, enjoyment) in a similar manner as drugs of abuse (Schulte, Smeal & Gearhardt, 2017), which may indicate an elevated addictive potential of highly processed foods. Further, individuals who exhibit symptoms of food addiction, according to the YFAS, have demonstrated neural reward responses during the anticipation and consumption of a highly processed food (chocolate milkshake) that paralleled findings in persons with substance use disorders with respect to drugs of abuse (Gearhardt et al., 2011b).

Highly processed foods have also been closely associated with numerous responses observed in substance-use disorders, such as craving (Gilhooly et al., 2007; Ifland et al., 2009; Polk et al., 2017; Weingarten & Elston, 1991; White & Grilo, 2005; Yanovski, 2003), binge consumption (Rosen et al., 1986; Vanderlinden et al., 2001; Yanovski et al., 1992) and consumption in greater quantities or over longer periods of time than intended (Arnow, Kenardy & Agras, 1992; Vanderlinden et al., 2001; Waters, Hill & Waller, 2001). Akin to drugs of abuse, highly processed foods have been reported to be consumed for the purpose of coping with negative affect (Epel et al., 2001; Oliver & Wardle, 1999; Oliver, Wardle & Gibson, 2000; Zellner et al., 2006). Further, neuroimaging studies have concluded that highly processed foods activate the reward system more intensely than minimally processed foods and may be capable of altering reward responses in a similar manner as drugs of abuse (Smith & Robbins, 2013; Tryon et al., 2015; Volkow & Wise, 2005; Volkow et al., 2008, 2012; Wang et al., 2004).

Similar to findings in animal models, proponents of the eating addiction perspective have noted that there may be circumstances that increase the likelihood of individuals overeating a wider range of foods (Hebebrand et al., 2014). However, the conditions where this has been observed in prior research have been extreme, such as prolonged, severe caloric deprivation (e.g., Minnesota Starvation Experiment; Keys et al., 1950) or lacking in external validity (e.g., instructed binge eating in laboratory (Goldfein et al., 1993; Guss et al., 2002; Hadigan, Kissileff & Walsh, 1989; Walsh et al., 1989; Yanovski et al., 1992). Yet, even in these studies where overeating occurs with a nutritionally diverse range of foods, highly processed foods are most implicated in problematic eating (Hadigan et al., 1989; Yanovski et al., 1992). Importantly, no previous work has investigated whether overeating behavior can occur with minimally processed foods in the absence of highly processed foods. It may be that the presence of highly processed foods or cues previously signaling their availability are necessary for overeating episodes to also include minimally processed foods, as has been observed in animal studies (Boggiano et al., 2009; Hagan et al., 2003).

Summary

Overall, animal and human studies support a substance-based, food addiction perspective, as highly processed foods appear to be uniquely associated with addictive-like responses. If the behavioral, eating addiction framework was more appropriate, then prior research would have demonstrated that all foods are relatively equally capable of triggering addictive-like food consumption across a range of circumstances (e.g., not only following severe caloric restriction). Considering substance use disorders, one would not consider alcohol-use disorder a behavioral addiction to drinking, as the alcohol is a necessary substance to produce the addictive-like response. Similarly, given that highly processed foods seem most closely implicated in addictive-like food consumption, conceptualization of this phenotype as a behavioral, eating addiction seems inappropriate. However, there has been little research into why highly processed foods may have elevated addictive potential, such as whether a specific ingredient (e.g., sugar) may be the addictive agent in these foods, akin to addictive substances (e.g., ethanol in alcohol).

Debate #2: No Specific Ingredient Has Been Deemed Addictive

Supporters of the eating addiction framework have argued that there is insufficient evidence to label any common food or ingredient as addictive (Hebebrand et al., 2014). Further, these researchers have stated that the lack of clinical case studies on addictive-like eating of specific ingredients or foods suggests that food addiction is rare or does not exist (Hebebrand et al., 2014). These two claims imply the hypothesis that certain foods or food attributes may be addictive has been extensively tested with null findings. However, this research domain is in its infancy, as the first tool to examine symptoms of addictive-like eating, the YFAS, emerged only eight years ago (Gearhardt et al., 2009). Though interest in the topic has recently grown (Corsica & Pelchat, 2010; Davis et al., 2011; Gearhardt, Murray & Avena, 2015), the study by Schulte and colleagues (2015) that observed highly processed foods to be most related to YFAS indicators of food addiction has been the only to systematically examine which foods may be addictive. While these findings represent an initial step in exploring the potential abuse liability of these foods and determining the possible addictive ingredient(s), extensive future research is needed. Thus, researchers supporting the eating addiction framework reason that the lack of evidence and studies disproves the validity of food addiction, though this more appropriately reflects a gap in the literature that warrants examination.

Debate #3: Behaviors Are Not Relevant to Substance Use Disorders

Role of Behaviors in Diagnosing Addictive Disorders

Proponents of the eating addiction framework have noted that addictive-like eating may be best conceptualized as a behavioral addiction because indicators on the YFAS represent behaviors (e.g., continued use despite negative consequences) (Hebebrand et al., 2014). However, this reflects a fundamental misunderstanding about how all addictive disorders are diagnosed. In the DSM-5, both substance use disorders (e.g., alcohol use disorder) and the one existing behavioral addiction, gambling disorder, are diagnosed using behavioral symptoms, such as consumption/use in greater quantities and/or over longer periods of time than intended (American Psychiatric Association, 2013a). While these symptoms are relatively shared across addictive disorders, adaptations are made to fit the specific phenotypes. For example, continued use despite negative consequences may reflect continued alcohol abuse despite experiencing physical health complications (e.g., liver dysfunction); this symptom may translate to continued gambling despite significant monetary loss. However, the core behavioral symptom of use despite negative consequences may be observed across substance use disorders and gambling disorder. Notably, the YFAS operationalizes food addiction based on DSM diagnostic indicators for substance use disorders (Gearhardt et al., 2009), in order to closely parallel current diagnostic practices.

Role of Behaviors in the Development and Maintenance of Addictive Disorders

Key behavioral features are present in all addictive disorders and appear to contribute to and maintain abuse and dependence. Bingeing and intermittent access are behavioral contexts that increase the addictive potential of a substance or behavior (gambling) (Hwa et al., 2011; Koob & Kreek, 2007; Sinha, 2001). Further, social learning and learned expectancies through problematic behavioral patterns of engagement (e.g., use/engagement to cope with negative affect) have been identified as factors that similarly motivate compulsive drug use or engagement in addictive behaviors (Cooper, Russell & George, 1988; Eiser, 1985; Niaura, 2000). With respect to addictive-like food consumption, researchers have posited that the behavioral, eating addiction framework is more appropriate than the food addiction perspective due to the integral role of behavioral circumstances (e.g., intermittent access, eating to cope) in perpetuating addictive-like food consumption (Hebebrand et al., 2014). However, this artificial separation of problematic eating behaviors from the possible role of highly processed foods is inconsistent with existing models of addictive disorders.

With respect to substance use disorders, certain behaviors are integral components of the addiction. For example, binge drinking is a behavior that has been shown to elevate the addictiveness of ethanol (alcohol) by increasing the amount the substance in the body (Herz, 1997; Klatsky, Armstrong & Kipp, 1990). However, the behavior of binge drinking would not produce problematic drinking behavior in beverages without alcohol like water. As such, it would be inappropriate to isolate behavioral components of drinking (e.g., bingeing, losing control over consumption) and categorize this presentation as a behavioral drinking addiction because the phenotype only emerges upon interaction with ethanol. Additionally, behaviors associated with consuming a substance may also be rewarding in nature. For example, individuals with tobacco use disorder will smoke denicotinized cigarettes and report reduced craving and reinforcement from engaging in this behavior, despite the absence of nicotine, the addictive agent (Carter et al., 2009; Donny, Houtsmuller & Stitzer, 2007). This may be driven by the rewarding effects of seeing and utilizing smoking paraphernalia and the learned expectancies of smoking a cigarette (e.g., reduced craving). However, while the behavioral component of smoking a cigarette may be a rewarding component of the addictive disorder, smoking is not considered a behavioral addiction because an addictive process is not triggered without nicotine.

Similarly, the food addiction framework supports that behavioral context is an essential component of addictive-like food consumption. Akin to other addictive disorders, the food addiction theory posits an interaction of certain foods with abuse potential (e.g., physiological reward from highly processed foods), behavioral patterns of engagement (e.g., eating to cope with negative affect, pleasure from the act of eating, learned expectancies about the effects of eating highly processed foods), and individual risk factors for addiction (e.g., impulsivity). Given that highly processed foods seem directly implicated in addictive-like eating (Boggiano et al., 2007; Johnson & Kenny, 2010; Schulte et al., 2015), it seems unsuitable to classify eating as a behavioral addiction, as this categorization would ignore the attributes of these foods that may problematically interact with rewarding behavioral contexts (e.g., intermittent access).

Inconsistencies between the Eating Addiction Perspective and Gambling Disorder

One method of exploring the suitability of applying a behavioral addiction framework to the act of eating may be to compare the existing behavioral addiction, gambling disorder, to the proposed eating addiction theory. Gambling is a behavior that is highly rewarding, reinforcing, and capable of altering the reward system in a similar manner as drugs of abuse to directly drive forward compulsive engagement in the behavior (Blaszczynski & Nower, 2002; Potenza, 2008). Gambling artificially elevates the reinforcing nature of money by through intermittency, rapid trials of winning and losing, and a cue-rich setting (Griffiths, 1999; Welte et al., 2004). While money is rewarding, it has little or no addictive potential outside the context of gambling. For example, an individual does not become addicted to earning a biweekly paycheck. Thus, the addictive nature of gambling disorder is rooted in the behavioral circumstances that are designed to be particularly reinforcing and does not involve a direct addictive potential of money.

This significantly contrasts food and eating. One of the critical comments regarding food addiction has been that all individuals need to consume food to survive, and thus food cannot be addictive (Corwin & Grigson, 2009). However, the food addiction theory posits that foods in their natural state (e.g., fruits, vegetables, nuts) do not likely have an addictive potential (Gearhardt et al., 2011a; Schulte et al., 2015). Rather, preliminary evidence has supported that highly processed foods (e.g., pizza, chocolate, chips) may uniquely exhibit an addictive potential, perhaps because these foods have been manipulated by to be particularly rewarding through the addition of added fat and refined carbohydrates (Schulte et al., 2015). While food is a physiological need, highly processed foods are created by an industry, are not found in nature, and do not offer necessary or valuable contributions to the diet (Gearhardt et al., 2011a; Ifland et al., 2015). In contrast, the act of eating is essential, and labeling eating as a behavioral addiction would mean that susceptible individuals develop an addiction to a behavior that sustains life, rather than differentiating problems with the type of food consumed. This does not parallel to gambling disorder, as eating is not a process purposefully designed to intensely activate the reward system and overwhelm inhibitory control. However, highly processed foods may be constructed in this manner (Gearhardt et al., 2011a; Ifland et al., 2015; Schulte et al., 2015), which further suggests food addiction is a more appropriate conceptualization for addictive-like eating.

Review of Measurement Tools for Food versus Eating Addictions

Operationalizing Food Addiction

To date, the YFAS is the only self-report measure validated to operationalize indicators of a substance-based, food addiction phenotype (Gearhardt et al., 2009; Gearhardt, Corbin & Brownell, 2016). As mentioned, the YFAS is directly based on the DSM criteria for diagnosing substance use disorders (American Psychiatric Association, 2013b) and captures the role of both the food and behavior in nearly every question by referencing "certain foods" in association with behavioral symptoms. For example, "I find that when I start eating certain foods, I end up eating much more than planned" is asking about whether individuals have experienced a loss of control (behavior) in response to certain foods (potentially addictive substance). As there are several questions that reflect problems associated with overeating generally, one improvement may be to add in "certain foods" to every question on the YFAS to consistently reflect the interaction of potentially addictive foods and behavioral symptoms.

Proponents of an eating addiction framework have raised the important point of whether food addiction can be diagnosed as a substance-based addiction when "certain foods" may reflect a multitude of substances (Hebebrand et al., 2014). Notably, the purpose of the YFAS is to operationalize addictive eating based on symptoms of existing substance use disorders and to examine associations with individual characteristics that may reveal which groups may be particularly prone to exhibit a food addiction phenotype. As such, this measure was not designed to be sufficient for diagnosing a clinical addiction and does not fully capture the phenomenological features of addictive-like eating. Rather, it functions as a useful measure to examine whether parallels may exist between the phenotypes of substance use disorders and problematic eating behavior, and for whom this perspective may be applicable to or useful.

Researchers have presented a gap in the specificity of the YFAS, as the phrase "certain foods" does not reflect a specific substance. While the YFAS was not designed to identify potentially addictive agents in food, evidence has grown for the role of highly processed foods (e.g., ice cream, French fries, cake) in addictive-like eating behavior since its development (Avena et al., 2009; Gearhardt et al., 2011a; Pursey et al., 2015; Schulte et al., 2015; Stice, Burger & Yokum, 2013). Importantly, the YFAS was integral in narrowing down which foods are implicated in these symptoms (Pursey et al., 2015; Schulte et al., 2015). While the addictive potential of specific ingredients (e.g., glucose, fructose) has not yet been examined scientifically, this is an essential, immediate next step in this line of research. However, it may be more appropriate to ask individuals about their addictive-like eating behaviors specific to highly processed foods, rather than the current broad categories (sweets, starches, salty snacks, fatty foods, and sugary drinks), to better present the existing state of the literature on this topic.

Measuring Eating Addiction

The Addiction-Like Eating Behaviour Scale (AEBS) was recently validated and aims to measure addictive-like eating as a behavioral, eating addiction (Ruddock et al., 2017). The authors presented this measure as an improvement over the YFAS because the AEBS assesses observable eating behaviors, which they suggest is novel to a behavioral, eating addiction perspective (Ruddock et al., 2017). As mentioned, this appears to represent a misconception: as all addictive disorders are diagnosed using observable behavioral criteria. Further, paralleling diagnostic indicators of substance use disorders, the YFAS does in fact assess addictive-like eating based on observable, measureable behavioral criteria (Gearhardt et al., 2016). Rather, the most significant feature distinguishing between substance use disorders and gambling disorder, a behavioral addiction, is that substance use disorders all involve consumption of a rewarding substance. Thus, as addictive-like eating requires consumption of food, an eating addiction perspective would only be supported if the type of food was found to have no role in the addictive-like responses.

Notably, the AEBS acknowledges that "unhealthy," "processed," and "high fat-sugar foods," all which can be considered highly processed, are most closely implicated in the assessed eating behaviors (Ruddock et al., 2017). Indeed, questions on the measure specifically evaluate problematic eating behavior with highly processed foods, such as "Despite trying to eat healthily, I end up eating 'naughty' foods" and "I tend not to buy processed foods that are high in fat and/or sugar." This approach actually mirrors a substance-based, food addiction framework, as it considers not only the eating symptom but also the important interaction with highly processed foods. If the AEBS intends to parallel assessment methods of behavioral addictions, then the measure should focus on the act of eating, irrespective of the food being consumed.

Numerous diagnostic criteria for gambling disorder may be applicable to a behavioral, eating addiction framework and may warrant consideration in measures evaluating addictive-like food consumption from this perspective. For instance, needing to gamble with increasing amounts of money to achieve the desired excitement could translate to needing to eat increasing amounts of nutritionally diverse foods to achieve the desired excitement. Additionally, preoccupation with gambling could be adapted to preoccupation with eating nutritionally diverse foods. Notably, if respondents reported exhibiting these symptoms, but only with highly processed foods, then this would support a substance-based, food addiction perspective, as the type of food would be an important contributor to the observed behavioral symptoms.

However, the AEBS was designed to move away from the DSM diagnostic criteria for substance use disorders in favor of evaluating problematic eating behaviors due to differences between drugs and food. Importantly, though variation in symptoms are largely observed across substance use disorders. For example, there are intoxication effects associated with alcohol use, whereas no intoxication occurs with tobacco use. The shared diagnostic criteria are interpreted in a way that is thoughtful of these differences, such that interference with daily functioning may pertain to intoxication in alcohol use disorder whereas this may stem from significant amounts of time being devoted to smoking cigarettes in tobacco use disorder. Thus, while addictive-like food consumption does differ from substance use disorders in important ways, this may be most appropriately addressed by adapting the substance use disorder (or behavioral addiction, from an eating addiction perspective) criteria to account for the unique considerations of food addiction. Interestingly, impairment in functioning resulting from addictive-like consumption of highly processed foods may present more similar to tobacco use disorder (e.g., spending significant amounts of time consuming highly processed foods or avoiding responsibilities due to whether highly processed foods will be accessible) and less like alcohol use disorder since intoxication effects are not relevant. Notably, these differences occur across existing substance use disorders and the unique facets of addictive-like eating would be similarly considered in applying the diagnostic criteria to food addiction.

Further, not adapting the symptoms of gambling disorder, an established behavioral addiction, to the assessment of eating as a behavioral addiction has raised concerns about the construct validity of the AEBS (Schulte, Potenza & Gearhardt, 2017b). Rather than assessing a behavioral, eating addiction, the measure seems to evaluate broad tendencies to overeat (e.g., "I serve myself overly large portions") and dietary control (of highly processed food consumption specifically) (e.g., "Despite trying to eat healthily, I end up eating 'naughty' foods"). An argument could be made that assessment of overeating parallels the behavioral addiction symptom of frequent engagement in the behavior (e.g., gambling). Additionally, the dietary control questions may assess an inability to cut down despite a desire to do so. Importantly, the dietary control questions reflect highly processed food consumption, which is more consistent with a substance-based, food addiction perspective, as the items acknowledge the importance of highly processed foods in triggering the behavioral symptom.

Conversely, there are important diagnostic indicators of behavioral addiction that are not assessed by the AEBS, namely tolerance (e.g., needing to eat more of a range of foods over time to get the desired excitement), psychological withdrawal (e.g., becoming restless or irritable when attempting to cut down on overeating nutritionally diverse foods), inability to cut down despite a desire to do so, psychological preoccupation, and clinically significant impairment and/or distress resulting from the behavior (which might be expressed behaviorally).

Overall, while the intention of the AEBS is to measure of addictive-like eating from a behavioral, eating addiction perspective, the AEBS seems to lack construct validity, as it is an incomplete survey of the symptoms implicated in behavioral addictions. Further, half of the questions reference highly processed foods specifically, which is inconsistent with a behavioral addiction to the act of eating, irrespective of the foods consumed. Thus, the usefulness of this questionnaire in operationalizing a behavioral, eating addiction and assessing its prevalence and psychological associations may be limited.

Implications of a Food versus Eating Addiction Perspective

Effects on Stigma

Researchers supporting an eating addiction perspective have suggested that the food addiction framework may offer an excuse for problematic eating behavior and reflect a passive process that befalls an individual, whereas eating addiction presents a more active explanation by focusing on the eating behaviors (Hebebrand et al., 2014). However, as discussed, behavioral contexts are similarly integral in substance use disorders and thus also the food addiction perspective, and the artificial separation of problematic behaviors from the potential role of the food is not congruent with existing models of addiction.

In all addictive disorders, including gambling disorder, a person develops an addiction due to multiple, multilevel risk factors (e.g., personal-level factors nested within contexts with elevated abuse potential). While some individuals are more prone to addiction, an addictive disorder would not develop if the individual never consumed or engaged in an addictive substance/behavior and risk would be minimized if the circumstances were low risk. For example, an individual susceptible to alcohol use disorder may not develop problems by consuming a glass of wine at dinner with friends. In contrast, certain contexts could elevate risk, such as binge drinking, consuming large quantities of liquor while alone or drinking with other heavy drinkers, and drinking to cope with negative emotions. For food addiction, the food would similarly be expected to importantly contribute to the development of addictive-like symptoms. Unlike eating, which all persons must do to survive, risk for food addiction could be mitigated by minimizing consumption of highly processed foods in situations where abuse potential is high (e.g., bingeing, in response to emotion). Thus, addiction is not a passive process, but rather a set of specific factors that interact to produce the phenotype.

Additionally, several recent studies have provided insight about the implications of applying a food addiction framework to problematic eating behavior on stigma and food consumption. Broadly, psychoeducation about the food addiction theory has been associated with decreased stigma for persons with obesity (Latner et al., 2014) but has not influenced food consumption (Hardman et al., 2015). Additionally, an individual's self-identification as a "food addict" has not been significantly related to reported weight stigma (Lee et al., 2014). Notably, these findings contrast eating addiction supporters' claims that food addiction is an excuse for an individual's problematic eating behavior (Hebebrand et al., 2014).

Treatment Implications

One common misunderstanding in the addiction literature is the assumption that behavioral addictions and traditional substance use disorders are treated using different psychotherapeutic techniques. Thus, it is assumed that the classification of addictive-like eating as either food addiction or eating addiction will impact which treatments will be most effective. However, as discussed, traditional substance use disorders and behavioral addictions are mechanistically similar (see Davis & Mason, 2020; Schulte et al., 2015), thus requiring similar treatment interventions.

Specifically, twelve-step programs, cognitive-behavioral therapy (CBT), Motivational Interviewing, harm reduction, and even pharmacological interventions have all resulted in significant symptom reduction for individuals with traditional substance use disorders and those with behavioral addictions (Sussman, 2017). The treatments most commonly associated with addiction are abstinence-based twelve-step programs, like Alcoholics Anonymous, which require individuals to completely abstain from substance use. In twelve-step programs, individuals engage in a group setting where they share their experiences and support each other in obtaining and maintaining sobriety. Individuals are taught to recognize their addiction as problematic, identify the problems arising from their substance use, and admit to powerlessness over their addiction (Emrick et al., 1993; Humphreys, 2003). In addition, participants attempt to take on a pathfinder (sponsor) to guide them through making amends and living a sober lifestyle. Twelve-step programs have been adapted to treat a variety of addictions, including both substance use disorders and behavioral addictions (Chappel & DuPont, 1999). While there are variations in the focus of twelve step programs depending on the addiction (e.g., Gamblers Anonymous requires abstinence from all forms of betting, Alcoholics Anonymous requires abstinence from all forms of alcohol), regardless of treating a substance use disorder or a behavioral addiction, the ultimate goal of any twelve-step program is abstinence from the problematic substance or behavior. Although twelve-step programs do not work for everyone, there is empirical evidence that these approaches work for individuals with both substance use disorders and behavioral addictions (Emrick et al., 1993; Toneatto & Dragonetti, 2008).

Twelve-step models like Food Addicts Anonymous (FAA) and Overeaters Anonymous (OA) have been created to treat overeating and binge eating symptoms, although there has been limited empirical evaluation of these approaches. FAA is more in alignment with a substance use disorder perspective, encouraging individuals to recognize that certain, addictive-like foods, have significant power over them. This model requires people to abstain from foods that include sugar, flour, and wheat (Food Addicts Anonymous, 2020). Alternatively, rather than focusing on the food itself, OA focuses on the behavior of compulsive eating, and is thus is more in alignment with the eating addiction perspective. OA encourages individuals to abstain from compulsively eating food but does not discriminate between which foods should and should not be consumed (Russell-Mayhew, von Ranson & Masson, 2010). The abstinence-based focus of both FAA and OA has raised concerns that this treatment approach may result in adverse outcomes, specifically increases in disordered eating (Wilson, 2000). Although these models have been adapted to treat addictive-like eating behaviors, further research assessing the utility of abstinence-based approaches for additive-like eating is necessary to determine if these approaches are safe and effective.

CBT has also proven to be an effective treatment approach for both substance use disorders and behavioral addictions (see Davis & Mason, 2019; Magill & Ray, 2009; Petry et al., 2006) While not required, the ultimate goal of CBT is often abstinence. However, CBT normalizes the occurrence of relapses in the recovery process and aids people in reestablishing their cognitive, behavioral and emotional strategies when a relapse occurs (Sylvain, Ladouceur & Boisvert, 1997). Additionally, CBT also focuses heavily on the role of environmental triggers to substance use and includes behavioral skills like thought monitoring and emotional regulation to aid in the recovery process (Kadden, 1995). For example, individuals are taught to recognize the situations and people that trigger their urge to use a substance or gamble, develop adaptive coping mechanisms in place of substance use or gambling to deal with daily stressors and negative emotion, and identify and adapt their thoughts about the utility of their addiction (i.e., self-management strategies). Thus, regardless of whether an individual is struggling with a substance use disorder or a behavioral addiction, behavioral strategies are used to aid individuals in their recovery.

Similar CBT approaches are also used to treat maladaptive eating patterns, particularly in the context of Binge Eating Disorder (BED) (Brownley et al., 2007). Like in the treatment of addiction, CBT for BED encourages individuals to recognize environmental triggers that lead to binge eating and to develop more adaptive coping skills handle daily stressors and negative emotions. Unlike twelve-step programs for maladaptive eating behaviors, CBT for BED has significant empirical support in reducing the frequency and intensity of binge eating behaviors (Brownley et al., 2007). As CBT for BED and CBT for (both substance and behavioral) addictions use similar approaches (e.g., identifying triggers, developing alternative coping strategies) these interventions are largely compatible. However, there are important differences to consider as well. Addiction perspectives place a greater emphasis on the contribution of the addictive behavior/substance, and this is integrated into treatment through approaches like psychoeducation about the addictiveness of these behaviors/substances. In contrast, CBT for BED does not consider the specific types or properties of the food consumed (merely the amount). This distinction between CBT for addiction and BED would be a particularly relevant for a food addiction approach, which highlights the contribution of highly rewarding foods to problematic overeating. Additionally, CBT for addictions do typically focus on abstinence as a goal, whereas BED focuses on reducing restraint (Brownley et al., 2007). The focus on abstinence in CBT for addictions (as with twelve-step programs) raises concerns that it may result in disordered eating and requires further study.

Another important component to address in the treatment of addictive disorders are experiences of ambivalence in the desire to change (Oser et al., 2010). Because substances are highly rewarding, many individuals maintain some desire to continue using substances maladaptively. For example, an individual with alcohol use disorder may wish to alter their drinking habits because it is interfering with her ability to excel at work. However, she may be hesitant to change because many of her social experiences include alcohol, and decreasing her drinking may lead to social isolation. Similarly, individuals with behavioral addictions, such as gambling disorder, also show ambivalence in changing their behaviors. Specifically, an individual with gambling disorder may recognize the financial strain caused by his gambling behaviors. However, because of the rewarding nature of gambling, he may be unwilling to cut down. These experiences of ambivalence can make it difficult to fully engage in treatment because, in order to be successful, an individual must commit to giving up the positive experiences associated with their addictive behaviors. Motivational Interviewing (MI) has been developed to address experiences of ambivalence in the treatment of substance use disorders and behavioral addictions to bolster an individual's desire to change (Miller & Rollnick, 2012). MI encourages an individual to focus on the problems, consequences, and risks associated with their addictive behaviors and to consider the benefits of change. Importantly, the client is encouraged to argue in favor of changing their behaviors based on their own intrinsic motivation, rather than on external pressures. While typically not used as an isolated treatment, MI has been found to greatly improve engagement in the treatment of addiction and to reduce the rate of treatment drop-out (Carroll et al., 2006).

Like individuals with substance use disorders and behavioral addictions, individuals with eating disorders and other forms of maladaptive eating also demonstrate ambivalence in altering their behaviors. For example, individuals with BED may recognize the health-related consequences of binge eating, but also still enjoy the pleasure they derive from eating highly palatable foods. As a result, MI has also adapted to address maladaptive eating behaviors, including binge eating, purging behaviors, and dietary restriction. For example, MI that has been adapted for BED encourages individuals to consider the consequences of their bingeing (e.g., weight gain, emotional distress, health problems associated with purging, etc.) and to identify personal benefits of altering their eating behaviors. In one study, women assigned to receive modified MI interventions reported greater reductions in binge eating frequency at the end of sixteen weeks of psychotherapy suggesting that MI is an effective additional treatment in conjunction with CBT and interpersonal psychotherapy (Cassin et al., 2008).

Motivational Interviewing could also be adapted to fit within either a food addiction perspective or an eating addiction perspective. Ultimately, MI would look similar across these perspectives, encouraging individuals to identify the problems associated with their eating patterns (e.g., emotional distress in response to eating, health consequences of bingeing behaviors, etc.) and to envision the benefits of change. However, like the above treatment modalities, MI for food addiction as opposed to eating addiction would involve encouraging individuals to think explicitly about the consequences associated with specific, highly processed foods while an eating addiction perspective would focus on eating behaviors more broadly. Because MI has not been adapted to treat addictive-like eating behaviors, future research is warranted to determine if MI can increase treatment adherence and improve treatment outcomes in addictive-like eaters, and to identify any potential risks this treatment modality might confer.

Another evidence-based treatment approach for substance use disorders is harm reduction. Harm reduction is a substance-focused intervention that does not require abstinence but is designed to reduce the risks associated with problematic substance use. In this treatment, individuals are taught to assess the relative riskiness of an addictive substance as well as the riskiness of the context in which they are planning to use it (Carey, 1996). For example, beverages with a lower alcohol content, such as beer, are relatively less risky in comparison to hard liquor, and social isolation may be more risky than being in the presence of supportive (sober) friends. By pairing higher-risk substances with lower-risk situations, many of the negative consequences of substance use can be reduced (Marlatt & Witkiewitz, 2002). Harm reduction has not only been found to be effective in reducing substance use at an individual level; it also results in greater societal benefit, like reduced drunk driving (Anderson, Chisholm & Fuhr, 2009). While harm-reduction approaches are successful in treating substance use disorder, they have not yet been applied in the context of behavioral addictions, like gambling disorder. Further research is needed to determine if it is possible to adapt a harm-reduction approach to the treatment of behavioral addictions and to examine if this technique is effective and appropriate for treating behavioral addictions.

Harm-reduction approaches have not been evaluated in the context of addictive-like eating. From a food addiction framework, harm-reduction approaches could be adapted by analyzing the relative risk profile of different foods and the situations in which an individual is most likely to binge eat. For example, according to the food addiction perspective, highly processed foods like candy or fast foods would be considered higher risk while complex carbohydrates and fruits and vegetables would be less risky. Individuals could practice consuming low-risk foods in the situations in which they are most likely to binge (e.g., highly emotional states) and save higher risk foods for safer situations (e.g., being with supportive friends) in order to reduce addictive-like eating behaviors (Schulte et al., 2017a). Because the eating addiction perspective does not maintain that characteristics of the food itself leads to addictive-like eating, a harm reduction approach would likely not be appropriate as all foods would be thought to generate the same level of risk.

Finally, pharmacological interventions such as naltrexone have been shown to dramatically reduce cravings and other symptomatology common to both behavioral addictions like gambling disorder (Kim et al., 2017) and traditional substance use disorders (Krystal et al., 2001). Interestingly, naltrexone has also been shown to reduce cravings for highly palatable, high-fat foods implicated in addictive-like eating, further suggesting that addictive mechanisms may contribute to excess food consumption (Carter et al., 2003). Thus, regardless of whether addictive-like eating is classified as food addiction or eating addiction, pharmacological treatment options will likely remain the same.

Despite these similarities, the treatment of a behavioral addiction like gambling disorder does require modification. Because problematic gambling can result in significant financial harm, such as bankruptcy, treatments often include interventions that focus specifically on this aspect (Sylvain et al., 1997). However, there is specificity in treatment approaches even when comparing across substance use disorders. For example, in comparison to the treatment of a legal substance like cigarettes, the treatment of an illegal substance like cocaine may require additional attention paid to legality concerns and the judicial system (Higgins et al., 1994). Alternatively, the development of an opioid addiction may be triggered by use of medication for pain management. As a result, treatment may include generating alternative coping strategies to deal with pain (Scherbaum et al., 2005). Thus, regardless of whether a behavioral or substance focus perspective is taken, tailoring treatments to address the specific substance- or behavior-related concerns is standard. In the context of addictive-like eating, whether a behavioral or substance focus is adopted, it would be appropriate to tailor treatments to address issues like the stigma facing individuals with obesity, extreme societal pressures to be thin, and the increased risk of diet-related disease.

Although food addiction and eating addiction may indicate similar treatment approaches, this distinction may be important for other reasons. Specifically, while the development and availability of empirically supported interventions for individuals with addiction is key, thus far, the largest public health gains in reducing the negative impact of addiction have been derived from wide sweeping public policy changes. For example, in the context of cigarettes, rates of smoking and the prevalence of diseases associated with smoking began to dramatically decrease when policy interventions like raising prices, clean air acts, and advertising restrictions were put into place (Levy, Chaloupka & Gitchell, 2004). Because the food addiction model recognizes the role of specific foods as driving addictive-like eating behaviors, similar approaches could be adopted to alter the food environment by using policy approaches to encourage healthy eating (e.g., restricting advertising, zoning regulations to reduce the density of fast food restaurants). Further, some accountability for addictive-like eating behaviors could be placed on corporations who manufacture and distribute highly rewarding, potentially addictive foods, increasing the need for the industry to play a major role in changing the food environment and potentially reformulating their riskiest food options. Alternatively, because all foods are considered equally risky from the eating addiction perspective, responsibility remains solely on the individual to regulate their food intake. Thus, while individual approaches to recovery may be similar regardless of the adoption of an eating or a food addition perspective, an emphasis on public policy and corporate responsibility would be more strongly indicated by the food addiction approach.

Future Research Directions

Table 28.1 provides an overview of the empirical questions that warrant investigation for determining the validity of the food and eating addiction frameworks. This table contrasts food versus eating addiction.

Food Addiction

The area that requires most attention in determining whether some individuals may experience a substance-based, food addiction pertains to which foods and food attributes may have addictive potential. While preliminary evidence has demonstrated that highly processed foods seem most closely implicated in addictive-like eating in humans (Pursey et al., 2015; Schulte et al., 2015), evaluation of the addictive ingredient in these foods is needed, akin to identification of the addictive agent in drugs of abuse (e.g., ethanol in alcohol). This has been raised as a significant criticism of the food addiction theory (Ziauddeen, Farooqi & Fletcher, 2012; Ziauddeen & Fletcher, 2013) and needs to be resolved before food addiction can be acknowledged as a substance use disorder.

Another important research question is how the unique considerations of addictive-like food consumption may be integrated into the diagnostic criteria, as has been done for all addictive disorders. For instance, certain symptoms, such as use in physically hazardous situations, may be less relevant to food addiction and thus may be changed to more appropriately reflect overconsumption of highly processed foods (e.g., excessive consumption leading to diminished physical health). Further, research is needed to translate findings from animal models to humans, such as whether removal of highly processed foods can cause physical and/or psychological withdrawal symptoms. Lastly, future studies should explore whether prolonged consumption of highly processed foods may trigger neuroplastic changes in the reward system to motivate compulsive consumption of these foods in vulnerable individuals. If these patterns are observed for highly processed foods in a similar manner as drugs of abuse, this may contribute to a deeper understanding of the public health consequences of these foods being easily accessible in the modern food environment.

Eating Addiction

As discussed, the key research question for validating the eating addiction perspective is to demonstrate that all foods are equally likely to be implicated in the addictive-like response to the act of eating. That is, to be considered a true behavioral addiction, the type of food consumed should not play a role in motivating addictive-like eating. A second topic that warrants attention is the development of a measure that operationalizes addictive-like eating from a behavioral addiction perspective, which should parallel the assessment of existing behavioral addictions.

Table 28.1 Future research directions for validating the food versus eating addiction perspectives

Theoretical evidence	Next steps to validate food addiction	Next steps to validate eating addiction
Determining the role of the food	1. Identification of the addictive ingredient(s) in highly processed foods	1. Demonstration that all foods are relatively equally implicated in addictive-like eating behavior
Refinement of assessment tools	2. Adaptation of the diagnostic criteria for substance use disorders based on the unique considerations of addictive-like food consumption	2. Development of a measure that evaluates symptoms of addictive-like eating from a behavioral addiction perspective and mirrors the assessment of existing behavioral addictions
Investigation of specific symptoms of addiction	3. Investigation into whether observations in animal models translate to human studies, such as the experience of withdrawal after highly processed foods are removed from the diet	3. Examination into whether core features of behavioral addictions (e.g., efforts to cut down or abstain) appropriately translate to an addiction to the act of eating
Longitudinal investigation of addictive potential	4. Evaluation of whether prolonged consumption of highly processed foods may alter the reward system to motivate compulsive use, akin to drugs of abuse	4. Analysis of how repeated addictive-like eating, irrespective of the type of food consumed, may alter the reward system to motivate continued compulsive engagement, akin to gambling

Further, given that eating is a required act to sustain life, proponents of the eating addiction framework should consider exploring whether certain diagnostic criteria implicated in behavioral addictions (e.g., psychological preoccupation, efforts to cut down or abstain, tolerance) appropriately translate for an addiction to the act of eating. Finally, researchers may consider whether repeated addictive-like eating, irrespective of the type of food consumed, may sensitize the reward system and motivate continued compulsive engagement in the act of eating in a similar manner as gambling.

Conclusions

While interest in whether addictive-like eating is best conceptualized as a substance-based food addiction or as a behavioral addiction to the act of eating, existing evidence seems to support the food addiction perspective for three key reasons. First, animal and human studies have observed that not all foods are associated with addictive-like eating. In order to conceptualize eating as a behavioral addiction, empirical studies would need to demonstrate that all foods have relatively equal potential to be implicated in the addictive process. Though this research is in its nascent stages, current evidence suggests a central role of highly processed foods in the development of addictive-like food consumption. Second, the lack of existing evidence for a specified addictive agent in these foods does not necessarily warrant reclassification of the food addiction construct, but rather research on this topic that has not yet been explored. Third, an eating addiction perspective artificially separates behavioral symptoms in a way that does not generalize to existing addictive disorders. Behavioral aspects of engagement (e.g., intermittency) and symptoms (e.g., loss of control) are key components in all addictions and would also be expected to contribute to food addiction. Importantly, the conceptualization of a food versus eating addiction would have different implications for individuals exhibiting addictive-like eating, with the food addiction perspective seeming more promising for reducing stigma and opening avenues for novel intervention approaches. Although future research is needed, food addiction, rather than eating addiction, seems to more appropriately mirror existing theories of addictive disorders by considering the interaction between behavioral symptoms (e.g., use despite consequences), context that elevates abuse potential (e.g., intermittent use), and the potential direct role of highly processed foods in producing the addictive-like phenotype in susceptible individuals.

REFERENCES

Ahmed, S. H., Avena, N. M., Berridge, K. C., Gearhardt, A. N. & Guillem, K. (2013). Food addiction. In *Neuroscience in the 21st Century*. Springer, pp. 2833–2857.

American Psychiatric Association (2013a). *Diagnostic and Statistical Manual of Mental Disorders*. Arlington, VA: American Psychiatric Publishing.

American Psychiatric Association (2013b). *Diagnostic and Statistical Manual of Mental Disorders* (DSM-5). Retrieved from http://dsm.psychiatryonline.org/book.aspx?bookid=556

Anderson, P., Chisholm, D. & Fuhr, D. C. (2009). Effectiveness and cost-effectiveness of policies and programmes to reduce the harm caused by alcohol. *The Lancet*, **373**(9682), 2234–2246.

Arnow, B., Kenardy, J. & Agras, W. S. (1992). Binge eating among the obese: A descriptive study. *Journal of Behavioral Medicine*, **15**(2), 155–170. doi:10.1007/bf00848323

Avena, N. M., Bocarsly, M. E., Rada, P., Kim, A. & Hoebel, B. G. (2008a). After daily bingeing on a sucrose solution, food deprivation induces anxiety and accumbens dopamine/acetylcholine imbalance. *Physiology & Behavior*, **94**(3), 309–315.

Avena, N. M., Rada, P. & Hoebel, B. G. (2008b). Evidence for sugar addiction: Behavioral and neurochemical effects of intermittent, excessive sugar intake. *Neuroscience & Biobehavioral Reviews*, **32**(1), 20–39. doi:10.1016/j.neubiorev.2007.04.019

Avena, N. M., Rada, P. & Hoebel, B. G. (2009). Sugar and fat bingeing have notable differences in addictive-like behavior. *The Journal of Nutrition*, **139**(3), 623–628.

Balster, R. L. (1991). Drug abuse potential evaluation in animals. *British Journal of Addiction*, **86**(12), 1549–1558.

Berridge, K. C. (1996). Food reward: Brain substrates of wanting and liking. *Neuroscience & Biobehavioral Reviews*, **20**(1), 1–25.

Blaszczynski, A. & Nower, L. (2002). A pathways model of problem and pathological gambling. *Addiction*, **97**(5), 487–499.

Bocarsly, M. E., Berner, L. A., Hoebel, B. G. & Avena, N. M. (2011). Rats that binge eat fat-rich food do not show somatic signs or anxiety associated with opiate-like withdrawal: Implications for nutrient-specific food addiction behaviors. *Physiology & Behavior*, **104**(5), 865–872.

Boggiano, M. M., Artiga, A. I., Pritchett, C. E., et al. (2007). High intake of palatable food predicts binge-eating independent of susceptibility to obesity: An animal model of lean vs obese binge-eating and obesity with and without binge-eating. *International Journal of Obesity*, **31**(9), 1357–1367.

Boggiano, M. M., Dorsey, J. R., Thomas, J. M. & Murdaugh, D. L. (2009). The Pavlovian power of palatable food: Lessons for weight-loss adherence from a new rodent model of cue-induced overeating. *International Journal of Obesity (London)*, **33**(6), 693–701. doi:10.1038/ijo.2009.57

Brownley, K. A., Berkman, N. D., Sedway, J. A., Lohr, K. N. & Bulik, C. M. (2007). Binge eating disorder treatment: A systematic review of randomized controlled trials. *International Journal of Eating Disorders*, **40**(4), 337–348.

Carey, K. B. (1996). Substance use reduction in the context of outpatient psychiatric treatment: A collaborative, motivational, harm reduction approach. *Community Mental Health Journal*, **32**(3), 291–306.

Carroll, K. M., Ball, S. A., Nich, C., et al. (2006). Motivational interviewing to improve treatment engagement and outcome in individuals seeking treatment for substance abuse: A multisite effectiveness study. *Drug & Alcohol Dependence*, **81**(3), 301–312.

Carter, L. P., Stitzer, M. L., Henningfield, J. E., et al. (2009). Abuse liability assessment of tobacco products including potential reduced exposure products. *Cancer Epidemiology, Biomarkers & Prevention*, **18**(12), 3241–3262. doi:10.1158/1055-9965.EPI-09-0948

Carter, W. P., Hudson, J. I., Lalonde, J. K., et al. (2003). Pharmacologic treatment of binge eating disorder. *International Journal of Eating Disorders*, **34**(S1), S74–88.

Cassin, S. E., von Ranson, K. M., Heng, K., Brar, J. & Wojtowicz, A. E. (2008). Adapted motivational interviewing for women with binge eating disorder: A randomized controlled trial. *Psychology of Addictive Behaviors*, **22**(3), 417.

Chappel, J. N. & DuPont, R. L. (1999). Twelve-step and mutual-help programs for addictive disorders. *Psychiatric Clinics*, **22**(2), 425–446.

Cooper, M. L., Russell, M. & George, W. H. (1988). Coping, expectancies, and alcohol abuse: A test of social learning formulations. *Journal of Abnormal Psychology*, **97**(2), 218.

Corsica, J. A. & Pelchat, M. L. (2010). Food addiction: True or false? *Current Opinion in Gastroenterology*, **26**(2), 165–169. doi:10.1097/MOG.0b013e328336528d

Corwin, R. L. (2006). Bingeing rats: A model of intermittent excessive behavior? *Appetite*, **46** (1), 11–15. doi:10.1016/j.appet.2004.09.002

Corwin, R. L. & Grigson, P. S. (2009). Symposium overview – Food addiction: Fact or fiction? *Journal of Nutrition*, **139**(3), 617–619. doi:10.3945/jn.108.097691

Davis, C. & Carter, J. C. (2009). Compulsive overeating as an addiction disorder. A review of theory and evidence. *Appetite*, **53**(1), 1–8. doi:10.1016/j.appet.2009.05.018

Davis, C., Curtis, C., Levitan, R. D., et al. (2011). Evidence that 'food addiction' is a valid phenotype of obesity. *Appetite*, **57**(3), 711–717. doi:10.1016/j.appet.2011.08.017

Davis, C. & Mason, A. (2020). Prevention and treatment of "food addiction" In S. Sussman (Ed.) *The Cambridge Handbook of Substance and Behavioral Addictions*. Cambridge, UK: Cambridge University Press, pp. 230–240.

Donny, E. C., Houtsmuller, E. & Stitzer, M. L. (2007). Smoking in the absence of nicotine: Behavioral, subjective and physiological effects over 11 days. *Addiction*, **102**(2), 324–334. doi:10.1111/j.1360-0443.2006.01670.x

Eiser, J. R. (1985). Smoking: The social learning of an addiction. *Journal of Social and Clinical Psychology*, **3**(4), 446.

Emrick, C. D., Tonigan, J. S., Montgomery, H. & Little, L. (1993). Alcoholics anonymous: What is currently known? In B. S. McCrady & W. R. Miller (Eds.), *Research on Alcoholics Anonymous: Opportunities and Alternatives*. Rutgers Center of Alcohol Studies, pp. 41–76.

Epel, E., Lapidus, R., McEwen, B. & Brownell, K. (2001). Stress may add bite to appetite in women: A laboratory study of stress-induced cortisol and eating behavior. *Psychoneuroendocrinology*, **26**(1), 37–9.

"**Food Addicts Anonymous.**" FAA. Accessed January 23, 2020. http://www.foodaddictsanonymous.org/faa-food-plan

Gearhardt, A. N., Corbin, W. R. & Brownell, K. D. (2009). Preliminary validation of the Yale Food Addiction Scale. *Appetite*, **52**(2), 430–436. doi:10.1016/j.appet.2008.12.003

Gearhardt, A. N., Corbin, W. R. & Brownell, K. D. (2016). Development of the Yale Food Addiction Scale Version 2.0. *Psychology of Addictive Behaviors*, **30**(1), 113.

Gearhardt, A. N., Davis, C., Kuschner, R. & Brownell, K. D. (2011a). The addiction potential of hyperpalatable foods. *Current Drug Abuse Reviews*, **4**(3), 140–145.

Gearhardt, A. N., Murray, S. & Avena, N. M. (2015). Emerging evidence of addiction in problematic eating behavior. *Emerging Trends in the Social and Behavioral Sciences: An Interdisciplinary, Searchable, and Linkable Resource*. John Wiley & Sons, Inc.

Gearhardt, A. N., Yokum, S., Orr, P. T., et al. (2011b). Neural correlates of food addiction. *Archives of General Psychiatry*, **68**(8), 808–816. doi:10.1001/archgenpsychiatry.2011.32

Gilhooly, C., Das, S., Golden, J., et al. (2007). Food cravings and energy regulation: The characteristics of craved foods and their relationship with eating behaviors and weight change during 6 months of dietary energy restriction. *International Journal of Obesity*, **31** (12), 1849–1858.

Gold, M. S., Frost-Pineda, K. & Jacobs, W. S. (2003). Overeating, binge eating, and eating disorders as addictions. *Psychiatric Annals*, **33** (2), 117–122.

Goldfein, J. A., Walsh, B. T., LaChaussee, J. L., Kissileff, H. R. & Devlin, M. J. (1993). Eating behavior in binge eating disorder. *International Journal of Eating Disordorders*, **14**(4), 427–431.

Griffiths, M. (1999). Gambling technologies: Prospects for problem gambling. *Journal of Gambling Studies*, **15**(3), 265–283.

Guss, J. L., Kissileff, H. R., Devlin, M. J., Zimmerli E. & Walsh, B. T. (2002). Binge size increases with body mass index in women with binge-eating disorder. *Obesity Research*, **10**(10), 1021–1029. doi:10.1038/oby.2002.139

Hadigan, C. M., Kissileff, H. R. & Walsh, B. T. (1989). Patterns of food selection during meals in women with bulimia. *American Journal of Clinical Nutrition*, **50**(4), 759–766.

Hagan, M. M., Chandler, P. C., Wauford, P. K., Rybak, R. J. & Oswald, K. D. (2003). The role of palatable food and hunger as trigger factors in an animal model of stress induced binge eating. *International Journal of Eating Disorders*, **34**(2), 183–197. doi:10.1002/eat.10168

Haney, M. (2009). Self-administration of cocaine, cannabis and heroin in the human laboratory: Benefits and pitfalls. *Addiction Biology*, **14**(1), 9–21. doi:10.1111/j.1369-1600.2008.00121.x

Hardman, C. A., Rogers, P. J., Dallas, R., et al. (2015). "Food addiction is real". The effects of exposure to this message on self-diagnosed food addiction and eating behaviour. *Appetite*, **91**, 179–184.

Hebebrand, J., Albayrak, Ö., Adan, R., et al. (2014). "Eating addiction", rather than "food addiction", better captures addictive-like eating behavior. *Neuroscience & Biobehavioral Reviews*, **47**, 295–306.

Herz, A. (1997). Endogenous opioid systems and alcohol addiction. *Psychopharmacology (Berlin)*, **129**(2), 99–111.

Higgins, S. T., Budney, A. J., Bickel, W. K., et al. (1994). Incentives improve outcome in outpatient behavioral treatment of cocaine dependence. *Archives of General Psychiatry*, **51**(7), 568–576.

Hoebel, B. G., Avena, N. M., Bocarsly, M. E. & Rada, P. (2009). Natural addiction: A behavioral and circuit model based on sugar addiction in rats. *Journal of Addiction Medicine*, **3**(1), 33–41. doi:10.1097/ADM.0b013e31819aa621

Humphreys, K. (2003). *Circles of Recovery: Self-Help Organizations for Addictions*. Cambridge: Cambridge University Press.

Hwa, L. S., Chu, A., Levinson, S. A., et al. (2011). Persistent escalation of alcohol drinking in C57BL/6J mice with intermittent access to 20% ethanol. *Alcoholism: Clinical and Experimental Research*, **35**(11), 1938–1947. doi:10.1111/j.1530-0277.2011.01545.x

Ifland, J. R., Preuss, H. G., Marcus, M. T., et al. (2009). Refined food addiction: A classic substance use disorder. *Medical Hypotheses*, **72**(5), 518–526. doi:10.1016/j.mehy.2008.11.035

Ifland, J. R., Preuss, H. G., Marcus, M. T., et al. (2015). Clearing the confusion around processed food addiction. *Journal of the American College of Nutrition*, **34**(3), 240–243. doi:10.1080/07315724.2015.1022466

Johnson, P. M. & Kenny, P. J. (2010). Dopamine D2 receptors in addiction-like reward dysfunction and compulsive eating in obese rats. *Nature Neuroscience*, **13**(5), 635–641.

Kadden, R. (1995). *Cognitive-Behavioral Coping Skills Therapy Manual: A Clinical Research Guide for therapists treating Individuals with Alcohol Abuse and Dependence*. DIANE Publishing.

Keys, A., Brožek, J., Henschel, A., Mickelsen, O. & Taylor, H. L. (1950). *The Biology of Human Starvation*. (Two volumes.) University of Minnesota Press.

Kim, S., Shou, J., Abera, S. & Ziff, E. B. (2017). Sucrose withdrawal induces depression and anxiety-like behavior by Kir2.1 upregulation in the nucleus accumbens. *Neuropharmacology*, **130**, 10–17. doi:10.1016/j.neuropharm.2017.11.041

Klatsky, A. L., Armstrong, M. A. & Kipp, H. (1990). Correlates of alcoholic beverage preference: Traits of persons who choose wine, liquor or beer. *British Journal of Addiction*, **85**(10), 1279–1289.

Koob, G. F. & Kreek, M. J. (2007). Stress, dysregulation of drug reward pathways, and the transition to drug dependence. *American Journal of Psychiatry*, **164**(8), 1149–1159. doi:10.1176/appi.ajp.2007.05030503

Krystal, J. H., Cramer, J. A., Krol, W. F., Kirk, G. F. & Rosenheck, R. A. (2001). Naltrexone in the treatment of alcohol dependence. *New*

England Journal of Medicine, **345**(24), 1734–1739.

Latner, J. D., Puhl, R. M., Murakami, J. M. & O'Brien, K. S. (2014). Food addiction as a causal model of obesity. Effects on stigma, blame, and perceived psychopathology. *Appetite*, **77**, 77–82. doi:10.1016/j.appet.2014.03.004

Lee, N. M., Hall, W. D., Lucke, J., Forlini, C. & Carter, A. (2014). Food addiction and its impact on weight-based stigma and the treatment of obese individuals in the U.S. and Australia. *Nutrients*, **6**(11), 5312–5326. doi:10.3390/nu6115312

Levy, D. T., Chaloupka, F. & Gitchell, J. (2004). The effects of tobacco control policies on smoking rates: A tobacco control scorecard. *Journal of Public Health Management and Practice*, **10**(4), 338–353.

Lile, J. A. & Nader, M. A. (2003). The abuse liability and therapeutic potential of drugs evaluated for cocaine addiction as predicted by animal models. *Current Neuropharmacology*, **1**(1), 21–46.

Magill, M. & Ray, L. A. (2009). Cognitive-behavioral treatment with adult alcohol and illicit drug users: A meta-analysis of randomized controlled trials. *Journal of Studies on Alcohol and Drugs*, **70**(4), 516–527.

Marlatt, G. A. & Witkiewitz, K. (2002). Harm reduction approaches to alcohol use: Health promotion, prevention, and treatment. *Addictive Behaviors*, **27**(6), 867–886.

Miller, W. R. & Rollnick, S. (2012). *Motivational Interviewing: Helping People Change*. Guilford Press.

Niaura, R. (2000). Cognitive social learning and related perspectives on drug craving. *Addiction*, **95**(8s2), 155–163.

O'Brien, C. P. & Gardner, E. L. (2005). Critical assessment of how to study addiction and its treatment: human and non-human animal models. *Pharmacology & Therapeutics*, **108**(1), 18–58.

Oliver, G. & Wardle, J. (1999). Perceived effects of stress on food choice. *Physiology & Behavoir*, **66**(3), 511–515.

Oliver, G., Wardle, J. & Gibson, E. L. (2000). Stress and food choice: A laboratory study. *Psychosomatic Medicine*, **62**(6), 853–865.

Oser, M. L., McKellar, J., Moos, B. S. & Moos, R. H. (2010). Changes in ambivalence mediate the relation between entering treatment and change in alcohol use and problems. *Addictive Behaviors*, **35**(4), 367–369.

Oswald, K. D., Murdaugh, D. L., King, V. L. & Boggiano, M. M. (2011). Motivation for palatable food despite consequences in an animal model of binge eating. *International Journal of Eating Disorders*, **44**(3), 203–211.

Petry, N. M., Ammerman, Y., Bohl, J., et al. (2006). Cognitive-behavioral therapy for pathological gamblers. *Journal of Consulting and Clinical Psychology*, **74**(3), 555.

Polk, S. E., Schulte, E. M., Furman, C. R. & Gearhardt, A. N. (2017). Wanting and liking: Separable components in problematic eating behavior? *Appetite*, **115**, 45–53. doi:10.1016/j.appet.2016.11.015

Potenza, M. N. (2008). Review. The neurobiology of pathological gambling and drug addiction: an overview and new findings. *Philosophical Transactions of the Royal Society, London B*, **363**(1507), 3181–3189. doi:10.1098/rstb.2008.0100

Pursey, K. M., Collins, C. E., Stanwell, P. & Burrows, T. L. (2015). Foods and dietary profiles associated with 'food addiction' in young adults. *Addictive Behaviors Reports*, **2**, 41–48.

Robinson, M. J., Burghardt, P. R., Patterson, C. M., et al. (2015). Individual differences in cue-induced motivation and striatal systems in rats susceptible to diet-induced obesity. *Neuropsychopharmacology*, **40**(9), 2113–2123. doi:10.1038/npp.2015.71

Rosen, J. C., Leitenberg, H., Fisher, C. & Khazam, C. (1986). Binge-eating episodes in bulimia nervosa: The amount and type of food consumed. *International Journal of Eating Disorders*, **5**(2), 255–267.

Ruddock, H. K., Christiansen, P., Halford, J. C. G. & Hardman, C. A. (2017). The development and validation of the Addiction-like Eating Behaviour Scale. *International Journal of Obesity (London)*, **41**(11), 1710–1717. doi:10.1038/ijo.2017.158

Russell-Mayhew, S., von Ranson, K. M. & Masson, P. C. (2010). How does overeaters anonymous help its members? A qualitative analysis. *European Eating Disorders Review*, **18**(1), 33–42.

Scherbaum, N., Kluwig, J., Specka, M., et al. (2005). Group psychotherapy for opiate addicts in methadone maintenance treatment – A controlled trial. *European Addiction Research*, **11**(4), 163–171.

Schulte, E. M., Avena, N. M. & Gearhardt, A. N. (2015). Which foods may be addictive? The roles of processing, fat content, and glycemic load. *PLoS ONE*, **10**(2), e0117959.

Schulte, E. M., Potenza, M. N. & Gearhardt, A. N. (2017a). A commentary on the "eating addiction" versus "food addiction" perspectives on addictive-like food consumption. *Appetite*, **115**, 9–15. doi:10.1016/j.appet.2016.10.033

Schulte, E. M., Potenza, M. N. & Gearhardt, A. N. (2017b). How much does the addiction-like eating behaviour scale add to the debate regarding food versus eating addictions? *International Journal of Obesity*, **42**(4), 946.

Schulte, E. M., Smeal, J. K. & Gearhardt, A. N. (2017). Foods are differentially associated with subjective effect report questions of abuse liability. *PLoS ONE*, **12**(8), e0184220. doi:10.1371/journal.pone.0184220

Seidell, J. C. & Halberstadt, J. (2015). The global burden of obesity and the challenges of prevention. *Annals of Nutrition and Metabolism*, **66** (Supplement 2), 7–12. doi:10.1159/000375143

Sinha, R. (2001). How does stress increase risk of drug abuse and relapse? *Psychopharmacology (Berlin)*, **158**(4), 343–359. doi:10.1007/s002130100917

Smith, D. G. & Robbins, T. W. (2013). The neurobiological underpinnings of obesity and binge eating: A rationale for adopting the food addiction model. *Biological Psychiatry*, **73**(9), 804–810. doi:10.1016/j.biopsych.2012.08.026

Sorenson, M. (2014). *Food Addiction: Current Understanding and Implications for Regulation and Research*. https://dash.harvard.edu/handle/1/11938740

Stice, E., Burger, K. S. & Yokum, S. (2013). Relative ability of fat and sugar tastes to activate reward, gustatory, and somatosensory regions. *American Journal of Clinical Nutrition*, **98**(6), 1377–1384. doi:10.3945/ajcn.113.069443

Sussman, S. (2017). *Substance and Behavioral Addictions: Concepts, Causes, and Cures*. Cambridge: Cambridge University Press.

Sylvain, C., Ladouceur, R. & Boisvert, J.-M. (1997). Cognitive and behavioral treatment of pathological gambling: A controlled study. *Journal of Consulting and Clinical Psychology*, **65**(5), 727.

Toneatto, T. & Dragonetti, R. (2008). Effectiveness of community-based treatment for problem gambling: A quasi-experimental evaluation of cognitive-behavioral vs. twelve-step therapy. *American Journal on Addictions*, **17**(4), 298–303.

Tryon, M. S., Stanhope, K. L., Epel, E. S., et al. (2015). Excessive sugar consumption may be a difficult habit to break: A view from the brain and body. *Journal of Clinical Endocrinology and Metabolism*, **100**(6), 2239–2247. doi:10.1210/jc.2014-4353

Vanderlinden, J., Dalle Grave, R., Vandereycken, W. & Noorduin, C. (2001). Which factors do provoke binge-eating? An exploratory study in female students. *Eating Behaviors*, **2**(1), 79–83.

Volkow, N. D. & Wise, R. A. (2005). How can drug addiction help us understand obesity? *Nature Neuroscience*, **8**(5), 555–560. doi:10.1038/nn1452

Volkow, N. D., Wang, G. J., Fowler, J. S. & Telang, F. (2008). Overlapping neuronal circuits in addiction and obesity: Evidence of systems pathology. *Philosophical Transactions of the Royal Society, London B*, **363**(1507), 3191–3200. doi:10.1098/rstb.2008.0107

Volkow, N. D., Wang, G. J., Fowler, J. S., Tomasi, D. & Baler, R. (2012). Food and drug reward: Overlapping circuits in human obesity and addiction. *Current Topics in Behavioral Neurosciences*, **11**, 1–24. doi:10.1007/7854_2011_169

Wadden, T. A., Foster, G. D., Sarwer, D. B., et al. (2004). Dieting and the development of eating disorders in obese women: Results of a randomized controlled trial. *American Journal of Clinical Nutrition*, **80**(3), 560–568.

Walsh, B. T., Kissileff, H. R., Cassidy, S. M. & Dantzic, S. (1989). Eating behavior of women with bulimia. *Archives of General Psychiatry*, **46**(1), 54–58.

Wang, G. J., Volkow, N. D., Thanos, P. K. & Fowler, J. S. (2004). Similarity between obesity and drug addiction as assessed by neurofunctional imaging: A concept review. *Journal of Addictive Diseases*, **23**(3), 39–53. doi:10.1300/J069v23n03_04

Waters, A., Hill, A. & Waller, G. (2001). Internal and external antecedents of binge eating episodes in a group of women with bulimia nervosa. *International Journal of Eating Disorders*, **29**(1), 17–22.

Weingarten, H. P. & Elston, D. (1991). Food cravings in a college population. *Appetite*, **17** (3), 167–175.

Welte, J. W., Barnes, G. M., Wieczorek, W. F., Tidwell, M. C. & Parker, J. C. (2004). Risk factors for pathological gambling. *Addictive Behaviors*, **29**(2), 323–335.

White, M. A. & Grilo, C. M. (2005). Psychometric properties of the Food Craving Inventory among obese patients with binge eating disorder. *Eating Behaviors*, **6**(3), 239–245. doi:10.1016/j.eatbeh.2005.01.001

Wilson, G. T. (2000). Eating disorders and addiction. *Drugs & Society*, **15**(1–2), 87–101.

Yanovski, S. Z. (2003). Sugar and fat: Cravings and aversions. *Journal of Nutrition*, **133**(3), 835S–837S.

Yanovski, S. Z., Leet, M., Yanovski, J. A., et al. (1992). Food selection and intake of obese women with binge-eating disorder. *American Journal of Clinical Nutrition*, **56**(6), 975–980.

Zellner, D. A., Loaiza, S., Gonzalez, Z., et al. (2006). Food selection changes under stress. *Physiology & Behavior*, **87**(4), 789–793. doi:10.1016/j.physbeh.2006.01.014

Ziauddeen, H. & Fletcher, P. C. (2013). Is food addiction a valid and useful concept? *Obesity Reviews*, **14**(1), 19–28. doi:10.1111/j.1467-789X.2012.01046.x

Ziauddeen, H., Farooqi, I. S. & Fletcher, P. C. (2012). Obesity and the brain: How convincing is the addiction model? *Nature Reviews Neuroscience*, **13**(4), 279–286.

29 Measurement, Prevention, and Treatment of Exercise Addiction

Heather A. Hausenblas, PhD, Derek T. Y. Mann, PhD, and Danielle Symons Downs, PhD

Introduction

Behavioral addictions is a topic of increasing interest in light of the addition of a new category on behavioral addictions in the *Diagnostic and Statistical Manual of Mental Disorders* (DSM-5), which provides a classification system for mental disorders (American Psychological Association [APA], 2013). While the DSM-5 identifies only gambling as a behavioral addiction, emerging research is revealing that other behaviors such as sex, shopping, work, internet use, video gaming, and exercise may have addictive potential. In this chapter, we will provide an overview of the origin of the concept that people may become addicted to exercise and explain the controversy regarding how to define it. We will also provide a review of the exercise addiction literature with an emphasis on the measurement, correlates, prevention, and treatment of exercise addiction.

Origins of Exercise Addiction

Similar to most other behavioral addictions, exercise addiction is a controversial concept. The notion that people may become addicted to exercise was introduced to the scientific community by a sleep researcher named Frederick Baekeland about fifty years ago. Baekeland (1970) designed a study to examine the common belief that exercise promotes deep sleep by conducting a one-month longitudinal study on the effects of exercise deprivation (i.e., no physical activity) on sleep. Two key study findings led him to the conclusion that some people may become addicted to exercise. First, he was unable to recruit habitual male exercisers (i.e., individuals who exercised five to six days a week) who were willing to abstain from physical activity for one month. He finally was able to recruit men who regularly exercised three to four days a week. Second, during the one-month deprivation period, the participants began to disclose decreased psychological well-being.

Baekeland (1970) realized the importance of these complaints and designed a self-report questionnaire to retrospectively assess the participants' distress sensations. He observed that the participants retrospectively reported their one-month deprivation from exercise caused increased anxiety and decreased sleep quality and sexual drive. In short, he found that habitual runners refused to abstain from exercise for a one-month period, whereas regular runners reported withdrawal symptoms during exercise deprivation.

Subsequent early researchers debated the differences between positive versus negative addiction and whether excessive exercise could be harmful (Glasser, 1976; Morgan, 1979). Glasser (1976) argued that excessive exercise is a positive addiction because of its many beneficial effects on self-esteem, mood, and anxiety. In contrast, Morgan (1979) pointed to the increasing number of overuse injuries and the social and occupational problems present in individuals who ran "excessively." He concluded that, for some runners, the benefits of physical activity may be offset by a negative addiction.

The debate of exercise being either a positive or negative addiction led to confusion regarding its definition and measurement. This resulted in a variety of terms being used to describe pathological patterns of excessive exercise such as: exercise dependence, obsessive exercise, compulsive exercise, exercise abuse, and obligatory exercise. The use of several terms to describe one singular phenomenon hampered the early research progress in this area. Exercise addiction has since emerged as the umbrella term currently used to describe pathological excessive exercise.

Defining Exercise Addiction

Exercise addiction is defined as a craving for leisure-time physical activity that results in uncontrollably excessive exercise behavior that manifests itself in physiological (e.g., tolerance) and/or psychological (e.g., withdrawal) symptoms; Hausenblas & Symons Downs, 2002). Characteristics of exercise addiction include exercising despite either injury or illness; experiencing withdrawal effects; and giving up social, occupational, and family obligations to exercise (Hausenblas & Symons Downs, 2002). Exercise addiction may also play a pivotal role in explaining the function of exercise behavior in the development and maintenance of body-image disturbance and eating disorders. The operational definition that has received the most recognition was presented by David DeCoverely Veale (1987, 1995). He advocated the adoption of a set of standards for diagnosing exercise dependence that are based on the American Psychiatric Association's DSM-IV criteria for substance dependence.

Expanding upon Veale's suggestion, Heather Hausenblas and Danielle Symons Downs (2002) defined exercise dependence as a multidimensional and maladaptive pattern of physical activity, leading to significant impairment or distress, as manifested by *three or more* criteria from a list of seven (APA, 2000). The seven criteria for exercise dependence are listed in Table 29.1. For example, if a person reports having feelings of anxiety and depression when unable to exercise, spends little to no time with family or friends because of physical activity involvement, and continues to exercise despite a doctor's advice to allow an overuse injury to heal, he or she could potentially be classified as exercise dependent.

It is important to note that exercise addicts are distinguished from other high-volume exercisers, like elite athletes, whose intrinsic desire to exercise is under control and does not regularly result in emotional, social, or occupational disruptions. The incidence of high risk for exercise addiction is 0.3 percent to 0.5 percent in the general population, while among regular exercisers it ranges between 1.9 percent to 3.2 percent. Convenient sample studies reveal that prevalence rates of

Table 29.1 Exercise dependence Criteria

Criteria	Description	Example
Tolerance	Need for increased exercise levels to achieve the desired effect, or diminished effects experienced from the same exercise level.	Running five miles no longer results in improved mood.
Withdrawal	Negative symptoms are evidenced with cessation of exercise, or exercise is used to relieve or forestall the onset of these symptoms.	Anxiety, depression, and/or fatigue experienced when unable to exercise.
Intention	Exercise is undertaken with greater intensity, frequency, or duration than was intended.	Intended to run for five miles, but ran for seven miles instead.
Lack of control	Exercise is maintained despite a persistent desire to cut down or control it.	Ran during lunch break despite trying to not exercise during work hours.
Time	Considerable time is spent in activities essential to exercise maintenance.	Vacations are exercise related, such as skiing or hiking.
Reduction in other activities	Social, occupational, or recreational pursuits are reduced or dropped because of exercise.	Running rather than going out with friends for dinner.
Continuance	Exercise is maintained despite the awareness of a persistent physical or psychological problem.	Running despite shin splints.

exercise addiction may vary by physical activity and gender (Monok et al., 2012). It is a commonly held belief that men are at greater risk for primary exercise dependence while women are reported to have higher rates of secondary exercise dependence, suggesting that other psychological comorbidities underlie the drive for excessive exercise (Bamber, Cockerill & Carroll, 2000; Cunningham, Pearman & Brewerton, 2016; Meulemans et al., 2014; Szabo et al., 2015). Furthermore, the prevalence of exercise dependence reportedly varies by activity/sport. For example, triathletes report the greatest rates at 64 percent (Blaydon & Lindner, 2002) followed by runners with reports ranging from 22 percent (Anderson, Basson & Geils, 1997) to 77 percent (Thornton & Scott, 1995) and gym goers reporting exercise addiction rates upwards of 42 percent (Lejoyeux et al., 2008). Those who suffer from eating disorders or disordered eating report rates ranging from 32 percent to 93 percent (Bamber et al., 2000).

Primary and Secondary Exercise Addiction

Adding further confusion to the definition of exercise addiction is the distinction between primary and secondary addiction. Primary exercise addiction is different from excessive exercise present in eating disorder patients (also known as secondary exercise addiction), in which the exercise represents a means to control weight (Veale, 1987). In these eating disorders, excessive exercise is a means for caloric control and weight loss rather than as an escape from a psychological hardship. Secondary exercise addiction is more compulsive (an attempt at over-control, reduction of anxiety, egodystonic) while primary exercise addiction is more addictive in nature. Thus, individuals suspected of exercise addiction should undergo further evaluation to determine if it is either primary or secondary to ensure that the underlying symptoms reflecting other behavioral issues are properly addressed.

The relationship between exercise and eating disorders is far from clear. This distinction is not always easy because individuals with primary exercise addiction are often preoccupied with their weight, dieting, and body image. *Primary exercise addiction* is defined as meeting the criteria for exercise addiction and continually exercising solely for the psychological gratification resulting from the exercise behavior itself. *Secondary exercise addiction* is defined as meeting the criteria for exercise addiction but using excessive exercise *primarily* to accomplish some other end (e.g., weight loss or body composition changes) that is related to the eating disorder. Thus, for secondary exercise addiction, the excessive exercise is secondary to an eating disorder and the main motivation for physical activity is the control and manipulation of body composition. Veale (1987, 1995) suggested that a diagnostic hierarchy must occur to validly identify exercise addiction. He argued that the diagnosis of an eating disorder (i.e., secondary dependence) must first be excluded before a diagnosis of primary exercise addiction can be made; that is, primary exercise addiction can be differentiated from an eating disorder by clarifying the ultimate objective of the exerciser.

Despite a lack of compelling empirical evidence, a misconception exists that excessive exercise leads to the development of an eating disorder. In their review of the literature, Patrick O'Connor and J. Carson Smith (1999) stated that "logic and empirical evidence dictate that excessive exercise cannot be a sole cause of anorexia nervosa" (p. 1010). To illustrate their point, O'Connor and Smith pointed out that about 12 percent of the adult population participates in regular vigorous physical activity; however, most of these people never develop anorexia nervosa. Also, increased exercise with anorexia nervosa is paradoxical because starvation results in reduced physical activity and fatigue. Finally, emerging research is revealing that regular exercise may be a viable treatment for eating disorders (Hausenblas, Cook & Chittester, 2008).

In an attempt to understand the relationship between exercise and eating disorders, Heather Hausenblas and her colleagues (2008) developed the exercise and eating disorders model (see Figure 29.1). The exercise and eating disorders model states that regular exercise is associated with improvements in several physiological (i.e., cardiovascular health, metabolism, adiposity, and bone density), psychological (i.e., body image, depression, anxiety, stress reactivity, and self-esteem), and social outcomes. Hence, the exercise and eating disorders model has consolidated and supported several narrative and meta-analytic reviews that have shown exercise's ability to impart positive improvements on eating disorder risk, development, and protective factors.

The model also extends our current understanding of the relationship between exercise and health status by including exercise addiction. Exercise addiction may explain why the development of eating disorders may supersede the expected benefits of exercise. Simply stated, this model posits that in the absence of pathological psychological factors such as exercise addiction, the benefits conveyed by regular exercise (e.g., improvements in depression, anxiety, stress reactivity, self-esteem, and body composition) may counteract the risk factors for eating disorders (e.g., body dissatisfaction, depression, anxiety, increased body mass).

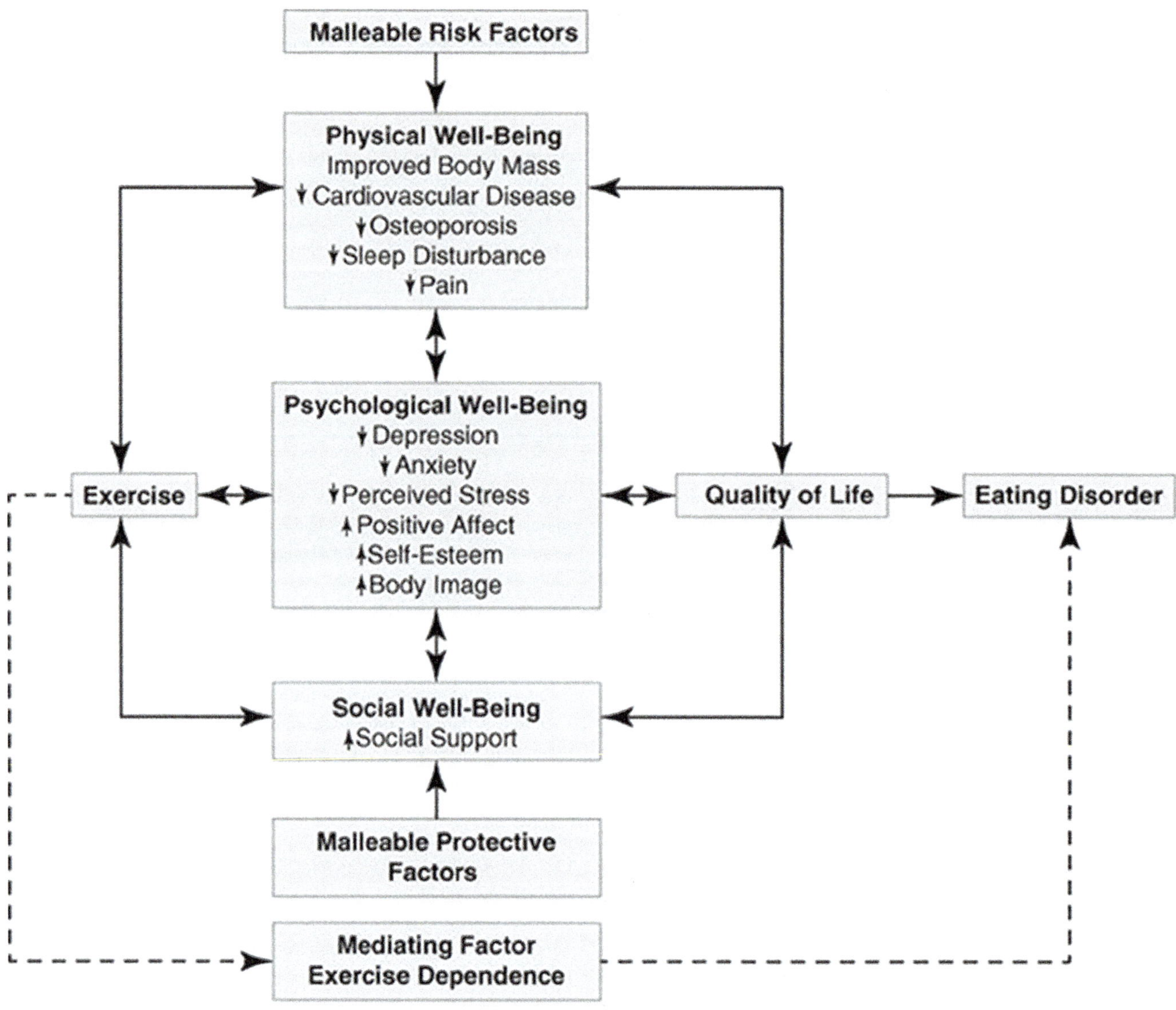

Figure 29.1 Exercise and eating disorders model
Note. From Hausenblas, H. A., Cook, B. J. & Chittester, N. I. (2008). Can exercise treat eating disorders? *Exercise and Sport Sciences Reviews*, **36**, 43–47.

Researchers have found initial support for the exercise and eating disorder model. For example, Brian Cook and his colleagues (Cook et al., 2011) had 539 university students complete self-report measures of physical and psychological quality of life, exercise behavior, eating disorder risk, and exercise dependence symptoms. Structural equation modeling analysis found support for the mediation effect of exercise dependence on eating disorders, as well as the effect of psychological well-being on eating disorders. Together, exercise behavior, psychological well-being, and exercise dependence symptoms predicted 23 percent of the variation in eating disorders. Specifically, these results indicated that the psychological health benefits conveyed by exercise reduced eating disorder risk (Cook et al., 2011). These results were replicated in a more diverse sample of college students (Cook & Hausenblas, 2011).

Initial tests of the exercise and eating disorders model suggest that the model may combine two divergent lines of research (Cook et al., 2015); that is, exercise may play a role in the development of eating disorders when exercise addiction is simultaneously present. Similarly, the psychological health benefits of exercise may also reduce eating disorder risk for individuals without exercise dependence.

Comorbidity with Other Addictions and Disorders

Researchers have also sought to determine the prevalence of exercise addiction with other forms of addictions. In other words, do people who are addicted to exercise also have a higher chance of being addicted to other behaviors (e.g., shopping, internet use, gambling, gaming, smartphone use) or substances (e.g., nicotine, alcohol)? Emerging research is revealing that there may be a high cooccurrence of exercise addiction with other types of behavioral addictions (Di Nicola et al., 2015) but not substances such as alcohol and illicit drugs (Szabo et al., 2018). Furthermore, individuals at risk for exercise addiction may exhibit the healthiest profile related to the prevalence of smoking (Szabo et al., 2018).

In a sample of 125 members of a fitness club in Paris, Michael Lejoyeux and his colleagues (Lejoyeux et al., 2008) found that exercise addiction was associated with compulsive buying. And in a larger sample of 2,853 Italian high school students, Villella and colleagues (2010) found that exercise addiction, compulsive buying, internet addiction, and work addiction were positively correlated. The authors concluded that the strong relationship among these different addictions is in line with the hypothesis of a common psychopathological dimension underlying them.

Researchers have also found a relationship between attention deficit hyperactivity disorder (ADHD) and exercise addiction. ADHD is one of the most common childhood disorders and can continue through adolescence and into adulthood. Symptoms include difficulty staying focused and paying attention, difficulty controlling behavior, and hyperactivity (also known as overactivity). The symptoms of ADHD usually cause functional impairment in social, occupational, and academic activities.

Using a retrospective design, Nikolas Berger and his colleagues (Berger et al., 2014) examined the associations of ADHD with exercise addiction symptoms in 1,615 German adults. The adults completed a retrospective assessment of childhood ADHD and adult ADHD. Adults with childhood-only ADHD had a significantly higher frequency of exercise addiction symptoms than adults without ADHD. More specifically, 9 percent of the adults with childhood-only ADHD displayed exercise addiction symptoms, compared to only 3 percent of adults without childhood ADHD. These results reveal that excessive exercising is overrepresented in people in which ADHD symptoms in childhood have not persisted into adulthood. It is plausible that some adults may suppress ADHD symptoms by excessive exercise.

Measurement of Exercise Addiction

Inconsistencies in defining and explaining exercise addiction as well as a lack of formally recognized diagnostic criteria have led to challenges in measuring this construct. Measuring exercise addiction is not simply based on exercise volume (i.e., frequency, duration, and intensity); but rather it involves assessment of multidimensional characteristics that also consider symptoms of addiction. A primary issue in the literature is the existence of many scales that assess different aspects of exercise addiction. For example, there are several unidimensional scales available to measure excessive exercise cognitions and/or behavior such as the Commitment to Running Scale (Carmack & Martens, 1979), the Negative Addiction Scale (Hailey & Bailey, 1982), and the Running Addiction Scale (Chapman & DeCastro, 1990).

There are also several multidimensional scales aiming to assess the physiological, behavioral, and cognitive dimensions of exercise dependence. For example, the Exercise Addiction Inventory (EAI; Griffiths, Szabo & Terry, 2005; Terry, Szabo & Griffiths, 2004) has been widely used in the literature. This six-item measure is based on components of addictive behavior (Griffiths, 1996) and it is useful as a brief screening tool. The Exercise Dependence Scale (EDS and EDS-Revised; Hausenblas & Symons Downs, 2002; Symons Downs, Hausenblas & Nigg, 2004) has also been frequently used in the literature because of its solid conceptual framework (i.e., based on the substance dependence criteria from the DSM-IV; APA, 2000), multidimensional criteria (i.e., there are twenty-one items based on seven subscales including tolerance, withdrawal, and lack of control; see Table 29.1 for the criteria), and clinical utility (e.g., it provides an overall score for exercise dependence symptoms as well as categorizes people as nondependent asymptomatic, nondependent symptomatic, and at-risk for exercise addiction symptoms). The EDS-R has been translated into multiple languages (e.g., Chinese, French, German, Italian, Korean, Spanish, and Turkish) illustrating its ability for broad dissemination and allowing for assessment of exercise addiction across many populations. The EAI and EDS-R both have good psychometric properties and are highly correlated with each other (e.g., $r = 0.79$; Monok et al., 2012).

From a measurement perspective, it is important to assess the presence of secondary exercise addiction – such as screening for the presence of eating disorder symptomatology – when examining exercise addiction. Common measures that have been used in the exercise addiction literature to screen for secondary exercise dependence include the Eating Disorder Examination Questionnaire (Fairburn & Beglin, 1994), the Drive for Thinness Scale of the Eating Disorders Inventory (Garner, Olmstead & Polivy, 1983), the Social physique Anxiety Scale (Hart, Leary & Rejeski, 1998), and the Body Building Dependence Scale (Smith, Hale & Collins, 1998).

More recently, Freimuth and colleagues (Freimuth, 2008; Freimuth, Moniz & Kim, 2011) used the criteria for exercise dependence developed by Hausenblas and Symons Downs (2002) to discriminate symptoms of exercise addiction from normal exercise behavior. They proposed four phases by which normal exercise behavior can transcend into symptoms of exercise addiction. The first phase is recreational exercise, whereby the individual engages in activities of enjoyment to improve one's quality of life. The second phase, at-risk exercise, is when the person starts to experience the mood-changing effects of exercise and may start to increase exercise intensity, frequency, and duration, and can experience negative effects such as exhaustion from over-exercising. The third phase is problematic exercise, when the negative symptoms of exercise (e.g., withdrawal, illness, injury) start to outweigh the positive benefits. The fourth phase, exercise addiction, is when the person's primary motivation is to exercise and the negative consequences have serious social and occupational consequences (e.g., social isolation, impairment in job performance). From a measurement perspective, it is important that the level of exercise is not the sole indicator of exercise dependence (e.g., using an activity monitor to assess minutes or miles of performance) as volume alone is not indicative of elevated negative physical/psychological consequences.

Correlates of Exercise Addiction

Alongside the growing interest in exercise addiction, both clinically and empirically, researchers have begun to dig deeper into the etiology of this behavioral addiction. Although one can resort back to the basic components of addiction outlined earlier in this chapter, researchers, clinicians, and those facing the daily challenges concomitant with exercise addiction can benefit from a deeper understanding of the various risk factors believed to be associated with exercise addiction. Of particular importance are physical self-concept, exercise identity, and perfectionism.

Physical Self-Concept and Exercise Identity

Physical self-perception is closely linked to positive and productive physical activity (Cooke, Liardi & Hall, 2011; Costa & Oliva, 2011). That is, persons who tend to be more physically active also report higher physical self-perception scores, meanwhile those who identify with lower physical self-perception tend to engage in less physical activity and report a higher prevalence of obesity, eating disorders, and depression

(Stice, Presnell & Spangler, 2002). Researchers have also supported a strong connection between lower physical self-perception and self-esteem (Hall et al., 2009), and increased body dissatisfaction (Hausenblas & Fallon, 2002) with exercise addiction.

To this point, A. L. Murray et al. (2013) proposed the relationship between exercise identity and exercise dependence. According to identity theory, role and identity become intertwined with people becoming preoccupied with the behaviors most closely related to their perceived role (Cook et al., 2015; Stets & Burke, 2000). As a result, physical self-perception, or self-concept, becomes the catalyst for future exercise behavior in an effort to maintain one's self-perception (Egorov & Szabo, 2013). Unfortunately, those with a high exercise identity or physical self-perception are likely to engage in exercise behavior despite negative consequences such as injury, excessive time commitment, or interpersonal loss (Murray et al., 2013).

Despite the natural and intuitive theoretical connections linking exercise identity to exercise dependence, the research examining associations between these constructs is equivocal. In an investigation of physical self-concept and its relationship with exercise dependence, Oliva, Costa and Rosalba (2013) reported a strong positive relationship between exercise dependence symptoms and physical self-concept. Yet, Murray et al. (2013) reported that only exercise beliefs (i.e., vision for what is possible) were related to increase risk of exercise dependence, while exercise role identity (i.e., "how others see me") was not. Meanwhile, Cook et al. (2015) reported that social physique anxiety among those who strongly identify as an exerciser are at increased risk for developing exercise dependence. Although the research isn't clear cut, there does appear to be an increased risk among those who strongly identify with exercise and it is likely a confluence of self-perception/image factors such as social physique anxiety that may combine to increase one's risk for exercise addiction (Costa et al., 2013; Hall et al., 2009; Hausenblas & Fallon, 2002; Lu et al., 2012; Murray et al., 2013).

Big-Five Model of Personality

Personality can be defined as individual differences in characteristic patterns of thinking, feeling, and behaving (APA, 2017). Although there are two distinct approaches toward advancing the measurement and understanding of personality (i.e., type and trait), the trait-based approach is characterized by the five-factor model of personality. The Big-Five factor model is affectionately known as the prevailing framework for assessing personality. Although there are several derivatives of the five-factor model along with several assessments, there is a universal acceptance of factors that comprise the model. The five factors include neuroticism (e.g., proneness to stress, anxiety, and emotional instability), extraversion (e.g., individual's energy directed toward the external, social world), openness to experience (e.g., one's willingness and eagerness to seek out new things and experiences), agreeableness (e.g., one's orientation toward others, concern for cooperation, and social harmony), and conscientiousness (e.g., one's actions and attitudes toward organization, persistence, control and goal-directed behavior).

Researchers have sought to unveil the specific personality characteristics, particularly among the Big-Five, that separate adaptive exercise behavior from the excessive, compulsive behaviors associated with exercise addiction. The relationship between personality and exercise addiction has been explored using a variety of research designs often yielding a common result with the exception of the tenuous relationship between neuroticism and exercise addiction. The early work of Jibaja-Rusth (1989) found a positive relationship between exercise addiction and neuroticism that was later supported by Andreassen et al. (2013). However, several authors have reported a negative relationship (Davis & Fox, 1993; Hausenblas & Giacobbi, 2004) between exercise dependence and neuroticism, while some have reported no relationship at all (Spano, 2001). However, a positive relationship between extraversion, facets of conscientiousness, and neuroticism (Miller & Mesagno, 2014), and a negative relationship with agreeableness have been more consistently reported with exercise addiction (Hausenblas & Giacobbi, 2004; Lichtenstien et al., 2014).

Perfectionism

Early research conducted by Coen and Ogles (1993) reported a positive relationship between perfectionism, trait anxiety and exercise addiction. Researchers have also found a positive relationship between anxiety, social physique anxiety, and exercise addiction and a negative relationship between self-esteem and exercise addiction (Cook et al., 2015; Rudy & Estok, 1989). Perfectionism is a multidimensional personality trait that necessitates the actual or perceived need to perform perfectly (Besser, Flett & Hewitt, 2004). Exercise addiction, not unlike other behavioral outlets, is often used as a means of escape from the unpleasant psychological experience the exerciser is trying to avoid (Egorov & Szabo, 2013; Korolenko, 1991). However, for those with perfectionistic tendencies, one might consider the interactive effects of the individual and the environment/situational factors. In the case of the perfectionist, one must consider the specific perfectionist belief that is held. According to the multidimensional perfectionism framework (Hewitt & Flett, 1996), perfectionism is comprised of perfectionistic self-expectations and perfectionistic interpersonal dynamics that result in three distinct personality traits (Flett & Hewitt, 2002; Hewitt, Flett & Ediger, 1996). These traits include: self-oriented perfectionism (considered to require perfection of oneself), other-oriented perfectionism (involving unrealistic expectations or judgements of others), or socially prescribed perfectionism (maintaining the perception that others are demanding perfection of oneself). In line with multidimensional perfectionism, perfectionism not only includes an embedded personal belief and self-perception (e.g., failure is not an option), it also involves personal motives or drives (e.g., pursuit of perfection) and the resultant actions or behaviors that are the manifestation of the beliefs and motives (e.g., expecting others to strive for perfection; Sherry et al., 2003).

The fact that some individuals engage in exercise behaviors beyond what is customary for health benefits, or even beyond that of what might be expected of one with a mastery orientation, is the result of a shift in belief or perception of self that results in a maladaptive pattern of exercise behavior to overcome or suppress the psychological distress being experienced (Egorov & Szabo, 2013). As a result, maladaptive coping strategies are likely and in exercisers this may result in excessive or even compulsive exercise (Flett & Hewitt, 2005). For example, Coen and Ogles (1993) identified a clear link between neurotic perfectionists and obligatory runners, while Hagan and Hausenblas (2003) reported that those in the high exercise dependence group reported higher need to excel and be the best; a belief aligned with self-oriented perfectionism.

Individuals who are exceedingly absorbed in their perfectionist tendencies are more inclined to worry about public perception and body image and tend to be more self-conscious and with greater levels of trait anxiety (Flett & Hewitt, 2005; Hausenblas & Fallon, 2002). In fact, the seminal work of Flett, Pole-Langdon and Hewitt (2003) with regular exercisers supports the contention that self-oriented perfectionism and socially prescribed perfectionism are intimately connected with compulsive exercise. Most recently, Miller and Mesagno (2014) reported that exercise addiction was positively related to self-orientated perfectionism and socially prescribed perfectionism as well as the personality trait of narcissism. In fact, the combination of narcissism and self-orientated perfectionism proved to be a unique and powerful predictor of exercise addiction. Although self-oriented perfectionism is highly motivating and even rewarding, it may also increase one's susceptibility to other psychological difficulties, especially when under stress (Flett & Hewitt, 2006). The real challenge however lies with socially prescribed perfectionism, which has been linked to various clinical outcomes, including depression and even suicidal ideation (O'Connor, 2007).

Prevention and Treatment of Exercise Addiction

Because there is substantial evidence that exercise has numerous health benefits, patients and healthcare providers may not readily recognize signs that one's exercise routine is having harmful effects (Hausenblas, Schreiber & Smoliga, 2017). Given the lack of awareness in professional and lay communities about exercise addiction symptoms, coupled with the belief by some that more exercise results in improved health, healthcare professionals may not recognize signs of exercise addiction even when its adverse health consequences are apparent (i.e., overuse injury, interpersonal dysfunction) or when it is comorbid with other conditions (i.e., eating disorders, other addictions).

One potential sign of exercise dependence is an increased rate of injury and/or repeat injury. As a result, physical therapists and athletic trainers are often the first professionals to diagnosis and then attempt to treat exercise addicted individuals. For example, Adams and Kirkby (2002) interviewed twenty-four sports physiotherapists about problems and strategies in treating patients with exercise addiction. They found that 71 percent of the respondents reported compliance problems with their patients reducing the amount that they exercised. The common treatment strategies that were recommended were: (1) education, such as warning about physical consequences if exercise was continued at the same level; (2) prescribing alternative training activities; and/or (3) referral for psychological treatment. Of the three treatment strategies psychological treatments was the most commonly implemented.

However, given the issues and challenges noted earlier in this chapter about defining exercise addiction and the lack of clinical criteria for diagnosing symptoms, physical therapists, athletic trainers, and other healthcare professionals are often at a loss with how to make decisions about treatment recommendations. For example, the care and prevention of exercise addiction should take precedence over either the treatment or cessation of excessive exercise behavior. For many afflicted with the compulsion to exercise the positive benefits (e.g., endorphin rush, decreased stress, and depression) associated with exercise may initially out shine the negative consequences associated with excessive participation making prevention and even diagnosis difficult. However, paying attention to the behavioral warning signs of exercise addiction may allow for the early recognition and intervention, permitting more effective treatment. The following list is not meant to diagnose exercise addiction but may be indicative of the onset of a maladaptive relationship with exercise while potentially providing insight on associated mental and behavioral health concerns such as anorexia, bulimia, and binge eating disorders (Gayton, Loignon & Porta, 2016).

(1) Continuing to exercise despite being injured or sick.
(2) Exercising following a binge.
(3) Using exercise as a way to escape from the days challenges.
(4) Strict adherence to workout schedules that regularly interfere with personal or professional responsibilities.
(5) Exercising to allow for the consumption of extra calories.
(6) Experiencing stress or guilt after missing a workout.
(7) Missing a workout results in negative affect and irritability.
(8) Mood or happiness is the result of one's performance during a workout.
(9) Exercise becomes a responsibility/burden and the joy is lost.
(10) The frequency, intensity, and duration of exercise continues to increase.
(11) Increased attention and effort to training regimens, supplemental resources for training, and secondary efforts to maintain training.

In the event that an individual displays either one or more of the above warning signs, early action should be taken. Of particular importance is the use of social support and education. According to the guidelines and recommendations put forth by William Gayton and his colleagues, prevention for individuals at risk for developing exercise addiction should include a thorough discussion of the negative biopsychosocial consequences of excessive exercise ensuring a thorough understanding that the deleterious effects of excessive exercise extend beyond physical hurt (Gayton et al., 2016). Equally, the individual should be aware of the potential strain that excessive training may have on one's relationships often resulting in the neglect of one's partner and responsibilities.

Psychotherapeutic interventions should focus on cognitive processing, behavioral management with respect to the fear of losing control related to compulsions (Adams, Miller & Kraus, 2003), and developing and/or rebuilding of adequate coping skills. The intervention should consist of identifying the compulsive exercise and the triggers, understanding the health benefits of exercise moderation, empowering the patient to develop adequate self-management/monitoring and coping strategies, and reframing the concept of healthy levels of exercise.

In addition to counseling on the psychosocial aspects of training, emphasis should also be placed on the management of the biological implications of training. In other words, encouraging the exerciser to pay attention to his/her body, that more is not always better, and the application of the principles of periodization, in which the frequency, intensity, time, and type of exercise is varied, should be emphasized to allow the mind and body an opportunity to adapt to the training stress, optimizing both mental and physical recovery and performance.

Exercise reprogramming is an important part of the treatment plan whereby compulsive exercisers relearn what exercising in a healthier way feels like. A goal is to work with exercisers to practice moderate amounts of exercise ranging from low-impact routines like yoga and pilates to more strenuous activities. The goal is to retrain people to exercise in ways that feel good to them both mentally and physically rather than in ways that stem from either anxiety or compulsion.

Unfortunately, there is scant literature on the actual treatment of exercise addiction and randomized controlled trials are needed (Lichtenstein et al., 2017). Exercise addicts may want to explore a range of treatment options such as cognitive behavioral therapy, acceptance and commitment therapy, medication, and alternative approaches such as nutraceuticals and mindfulness practices. Although further research needs to be conducted to validate whether such approaches are effective, these approaches have proven effective in reducing a range of mood and behavioral issues such as depression, anxiety, eating disorders, and substance dependence; rendering them as promising treatments for exercise addiction.

Like most behavioral addictions, usually some form of cognitive-behavioral therapy is recommended to help manage the underlying mood, emotional, and cognitive dysregulation that give rise to, fuel, and become exacerbated by, exercise addiction. The goal of cognitive-behavioral therapy in the context of exercise addiction is not to prevent the exerciser from exercising, but instead to learn how to recognize from where the negative thoughts arise that fuel the addictive behavior (as well as how to stop them before they consume the exercise addict). A common assignment for cognitive behavior therapy patients is the keep a "thought record" that accounts for situations, connects automatic thoughts, emotions, and moods to behaviors, looks for evidence to support as well as disprove those thoughts, and seek alternative (i.e., more logical and rational) thoughts. Exercise addicts may also be asked to keep track of automatic behaviors, antecedents to those behaviors, and the long- and short-term consequences of their reaction to stress. Identifying exercise addiction in its early stages can direct people toward behavioral treatments that help them manage symptoms before excessive and/or irreversible injury ensues (i.e., prevent interpersonal or professional damage).

Since regular exercise is a desired behavior of health promotion and maintenance, efforts should be redirected to maintaining an active lifestyle while rebalancing the role that exercise plays in one's life. Because exercise is often recommended as a desirable substitute for many compulsive acts, it can become compulsive for those inclined to addictive behavior. Therefore, treating the exercise addict necessitates a multipronged approach, and it is likely that professional approaches to its treatment will be effective. Initially, an exercise specialist should determine the person's state of health, including physical and emotional well-being. Further analyses from nutritionists and psychologists should focus on the patient's dietary habits, motivation for recovery, redirection of exercise goals, and capacity for implementing coping strategies.

The data on pharmacological approaches to reducing exercise addiction are scarce. A case study suggests antipsychotics may help lower symptom severity (Di Nicola et al., 2010). Specifically, the patient presented was a forty-seven-year-old male, diagnosed with bipolar disorder and compulsive exercise despite injuries, illness, and social isolation. He was treated with up to 600 mg/daily of the antipsychotic quetiapine, and after twelve weeks his symptoms improved. Within twenty-four weeks, his compulsive exercise behavior was almost nonexistent. The researchers concluded that quetiapine may be an effective treatment for a patient with bipolar disorder and compulsive exercise behavior. However, it is important to note that the quetiapine directly impacted the biopolar symptoms, which in turn, likely reduced the presence of the excessive exercise behaviors (which were secondary to the bipolar symptoms). Given this case report is the only located publication report on pharmacological treatment related to excessive exercise symptoms, it should not be concluded that antipsychotic drugs have a direct impact on exercise addiction. Further research is needed in this area to understand the role - if any - of pharmacological therapy for treating exercise addiction symptoms.

Another preliminary case study was recently reported by Anandkumar et al. (2018) regarding a multipronged treatment approached for exercise addiction. Two adults with exercise addiction symptoms who presented with chronic nonspecific low-back pain received treatment consisting of physical therapy management of the pain, pain education, mindfulness, breathing, quota-based reduction in exercises and modification of exercises into social participation, pleasure activities, and hobbies. This treatment approach was successful in treating both the pain and exercise addiction symptoms. When the patients were discharged at eight weeks, they were pain-free and fully functional, which was maintained at a six-month follow-up.

Treatment therapies for exercise addicts should also include the development of healthy eating habits, strategies for improving and maintaining a healthy self-esteem and body image, gradual incorporation of healthy alternative recreational pursuits, and the monitoring of progress over time. It is likely that recovery from exercise addiction may take months or even years, so it must address any underlying issues or other conditions (Jee, 2016).

Recovering exercise addicts may also want to reevaluate the kind of gym to which they belong. Many health/fitness clubs promote pushing past pain or striving toward lower weight by emphasizing calories burned. People who are already prone to body image and self-esteem issues tend to be sensitive to these campaigns and are more likely to incorporate such messages into their lives in negative ways. Even as the research into treatment efficacy progresses, individual counseling and monitoring will remain critical to achieving recovery from exercise addiction.

In summary, the prevention and treatment of exercise addiction is at its infancy and research is needed to examine the efficacy of the various potential approaches. As with most interventions, a main issue is likely to be compliance. The ultimate goal of treatment is to reduce the amount of exercise and provide healthier coping strategies. Effective and successful treatment interventions need to prevent overuse injuries, and ensure that physical, social, and psychological health of the exercise addict.

Conclusions

It is important to note that exercise addiction is not yet included in the DSM-5 as a mental disorder (APA, 2013). The substance-related disorders section of the DSM-5 includes only gambling as a form of addiction that does not involve ingestion of a substance, reflecting evidence that this repetitive behavior activates the brain's reward system in a way similar to that seen with drugs of abuse. According to the APA, all other potentially addictive behaviors - not just exercise, but also sex, internet browsing, and shopping - require further research before unequivocally being denoted as uniquely diagnosable pathologies. In other words, more research is need before exercise addiction/dependence is considered a mental disorder in the DSM.

Since Baekland's (1970) seminar study, researchers have continued to examine factors related to exercise addiction thereby shedding light on this often-overlooked behavioral addiction. Standard terminology, operational definitions, and multidimensional measures of exercise addiction have enabled this field of inquiry to systematically evolve. Further research with varied designs (e.g., prospective, experimental) will provide the scientific research required for exercise addiction to be a diagnosable disorder.

REFERENCES

Adams, J. & Kirkby, R. J. (2002). Excessive exercise as an addiction: A review. *Addiction Research and Theory*, **10**, 415–437.

Adams, J. M., Miller, T. W. & Kraus, R. F. (2003). Exercise dependence: Diagnostic and therapeutic issues for patients in psychotherapy. *Journal of Contemporary Psychotherapy*, **33**, 93–107.

American Psychiatric Association [APA] (2000). *Diagnostic and Statistical Manual of Mental Disorders* (4th edition, text revision). Washington, DC: American Psychiatric Publishing.

American Psychiatric Association [APA] (2013). *Diagnostic and Statistical Manual of Mental Disorders* (5th edition). Washington, DC: American Psychiatric Publishing.

American Psychological Association [APA] (2017). *Personality*. www.apa.org/topics/personality/

Anandkumar, S., Manivasagam, K., Kee, T. V. S. & Meyding-Lamade U. (2018). Effect of physical therapy management of nonspecific low back pain with exercise addiction behaviors: A case series. *Physiotherapy Theory and Practice*, **34**, 316–328. doi: 10.1080/09593985.2017.1394410

Andreassen, C. S., Griffiths, M. D., Gjertsen, S. R., et al. (2013). The relationship between behavioral addictions and the five-factor model of personality. *Journal of Behavioral Addictions*, **2**, 90–99. doi: 10.1556/JBA.2.2013.003

Anderson, S. J., Basson, C. J. & Geils, C. (1997). Personality style and mood states associated with a negative addiction to running. *Sports Medicine*, **4**, 6–11.

Baekeland, F. (1970). Exercise deprivation. Sleep and psychological reactions. *Archives of General Psychiatry*, **22**, 365–369. doi: 10.1001/archpsyc.1970.01740280077014

Bamber, D., Cockerill, I. M. & Carroll, D. (2000). The pathological status of exercise dependence *British Journal of Sports Medicine*, **34**, 125–132. doi: dx.doi.org/10.1136/bjsm.34.2.125

Berger, N., Muller, A., Brahler, E., Philipsen, A. & de Zwaan, M. (2014). Association of symptoms of attention-deficit/hyperactivity disorder with symptoms of excessive exercising in an adult general population sample. *BMC Psychiatry*, **14**, 250. doi:10.1186/s12888-014-0250-7

Besser, A., Flett, G. L. & Hewitt, P. L. (2004). Perfectionism, cognition, and affect in response to performance failure vs. success. *Journal of Rational-Emotive & Cognitive-Behavior Therapy*, **22**, 297–324. doi:10.1023/b:jore.0000047313.35872.5c

Blaydon, M. J. & Lindner, K. J. (2002). Eating disorders and exercise dependence in triathletes. *Eating Disorder*, **10**(1), 49–60. doi: 10.1080/106402602753573559

Carmack, M. A. & Martens, R. (1979). Measuring commitment to running: A survey of runners' attitudes and mental states. *Journal of Sport Psychology*, **1**, 25–42. doi:10.1123/jsp.1.1.25

Chapman, C. L. & DeCastro, J. M. (1990). Running addiction: Measurement and associated psychological characteristics. *The Journal of Sports Medicine and Physical Fitness*, **30**, 283–290.

Coen, S. P. & Ogles, B. M. (1993). Psychological characteristics of the obligatory runner: A critical examination of the anorexia analogue hypothesis. *Journal of Sport & Exercise Psychology*, **15**, 338–354. doi:10.1123/jsep.15.3.338

Cook, B. J. & Hausenblas, H. A. (2011). Eating disorder specific health-related quality of life and exercise in college females. *Quality of Life Research*, **20**, 1385–1390. doi:10.1007/s11136-011-9879-6

Cook, B. J., Hausenblas, H. A., Crosby, R. D., Cao, L. & Wonderlich, S. A. (2015). Exercise dependence as a mediator of the exercise and eating disorders relationship: A pilot study. *Eating Behaviors*, **16**, 9–12. doi: 10.1016/j.eatbeh.2014.10.012

Cook, B. J., Hausenblas, H. A., Tuccitto, D. & Giacobbi, P. (2011). Eating disorders and exercise: A structural equation modeling analysis of a conceptual model. *European Eating Disorders Review*, **19**, 216–225. doi: 10.1002/erv.1111

Cooke, L. M., Liardi, V. L. & Hall, C. R. (2011). Does the shoe FIT? An examination of the relationship of exercise identity with exercise frequency, intensity, and duration. *Journal of Sport & Exercise Psychology*, **33**, 138–148.

Costa, S. & Oliva, P. (2011). Attività fisica e benessere: percezione del sé fisico e motivazione all'esercizio. [Physical activity and well-being: Physical self-perception and exercise motivation]". *GIPS*, **12**, 3–7.

Costa, S., Hausenblas, H. A., Oliva, P., Cuzzocrea, F. & Larcan, R. (2013). The role of age, gender, mood states and exercise frequency on exercise dependence. *Journal of Behavioral Addictions*, **2**, 216–223. doi:10.1556/jba.2.2013.014

Cunningham, H. E., Pearman, S. & Brewerton, T. D. (2016). Conceptualizing primary and secondary pathological exercise using available measures of excessive exercise. *International Journal of Eating Disorders*, **49** (8), 778–792. doi: 10.1002/eat.22551

Davis, C. & Fox, J. (1993). Excessive exercise and weight preoccupation in women. *Addictive Behaviors*, **18**, 201–211. doi:10.1016/0306-4603(93)90050-j

Di Nicola, M., Martinotti, G., Mazza, M., et al. (2010). Quetiapine as add-on treatment for bipolar I disorder with comorbid compulsive buying and physical exercise addiction. *Progress in Neuropsychopharmacology and Biological Psychiatry*, **34**, 713–714.

Di Nicola, M., Tedeschi, D., De Risio, L., et al. (2015). Co-occurrence of alcohol use disorder and behavioral addictions: Relevance of impulsivity and craving. *Drug and Alcohol Dependence*, **148**, 118–125. doi:10.1016/j.drugalcdep.2014.12.028

Egorov, A. Y. & Szabo, A. (2013). The exercise paradox: An interactional model for a clearer conceptualization of exercise addiction. *Journal of Behavioral Addictions*, **2**, 199–208. doi:10.1556/jba.2.2013.4.2

Flett, G. L. & Hewitt, P. L. (2005). The perils of perfectionism in sports and exercise. *Current Directions in Psychological Science*, **14**, 14–18. doi:10.1111/j.0963-7214.2005.00326.x

Flett, G. L. & Hewitt, P. L. (2002). Perfectionism and maladjustment: An overview of theoretical, definitional, and treatment issues. In G. L. Flett & P. L. Hewitt (Eds.), *Perfectionism: Theory, Research, and Treatment*. American Psychological Association, pp. 5–31. https://doi.org/10.1037/10458-001

Flett, G. L. & Hewitt, P. L. (2006). Positive versus negative perfectionism in psychopathology. *Behavior Modification*, **30**, 472–495. doi:10.1177/0145445506288026

Flett, G. L., Pole-Langdon, L. & Hewitt, P. L. (2003). *Trait perfectionism and perfectionistic self-presentation in compulsive exercise.* Unpublished manuscript. York University, Toronto, Ontario, Canada.

Fairburn, C. G. & Beglin, S. J. (1994). Assessment of eating disorders: Interview or self-report questionnaire? *International Journal of Eating Disorders*, **16**, 363–370. doi:10.1037/t03974-000

Freimuth, M. (2008). *Addicted? Recognizing Destructive Behavior Before It's Too Late.* Lanham, MD: Rowman & Littlefield Publishers.

Freimuth, M., Moniz, S. & Kim, S. R. (2011). Clarifying exercise addiction: Differential diagnosis, co-occurring disorders, and phases of addiction. *International Journal of Environmental Research and Public Health*, **8**, 4069–4081.

Garner, D. M., Olmstead, M.P. & Polivy, J. (1983). Development and validation of a multidimensional eating disorder inventory for anorexia nervosa and bulimia. *International Journal of Eating Disorders*, **2**, 15–34. doi:10.1002/1098-108x(198321)2:2<15::aid-eat2260020203>3.0.co;2-6

Gayton, W. F., Loignon, A. C. & Porta, W. (2016). Exercise dependence: The dark side of exercise. *Annals of Sports Medicine and Research*, **3**(7), 1085.

Glasser, W. (1976). *Positive Addiction*. New York, NY: Harper & Row.

Griffiths, M. (1996). Behavioural addiction: An issue for everybody? *Employee Counselling Today*, **8**, 19–25. doi: 10.1108/13665629610116872

Griffiths, M., Szabo, A. & Terry, A. (2005). The exercise addiction inventory: A quick and easy screening tool for health practitioners. *British Journal of Sports Medicine*, **39**, 346–347. doi: 10.1136/bjsm.2004.017020

Hagan, A. L. & Hausenblas, H. A. (2003). The relationship between exercise dependence symptoms and perfectionism. *American Journal of Health Studies*, **18**, 133–137.

Hailey, B. J. & Bailey, L. A. (1982). Negative addiction in runners: A quantitative approach. *Journal of Sport Behavior*, **5**, 150–154.

Hall, H. K., Hill, A. P., Appleton, P. R. & Kozub, S. A. (2009). The mediating influence of unconditional self-acceptance and labile self-esteem on the relationship between multidimensional perfectionism and exercise dependence. *Psychology of Sport and Exercise*,**10**, 35–44. doi:10.1016/j.psychsport.2008.05.003

Hart, E. A., Leary, M. R. & Rejeski, W. J. (1989). The measurement of social physique anxiety. *Journal of Sport and Exercise Psychology*, **11**, 94–104.

Hausenblas, H. A. & Fallon, E. A. (2002). Relationship among body image, exercise behavior, and exercise dependence symptoms. *International Journal of Eating Disorders*, **32**, 179–185. doi:10.1002/eat.10071

Hausenblas, H. A. & Giacobbi, P. R. Jr. (2004). Relationship between exercise dependence symptoms and personality. *Personality and Individual Differences*, **36**, 1265–1273. doi:10.1016/s0191-8869(03)00214-9

Hausenblas, H. A. & Symons Downs, D. (2002). Exercise dependence: A systematic review. *Psychology of Sport and Exercise*, **3**, 89–23. doi: 10.1016/s1469-0292(00)00015-7

Hausenblas, H. A., Cook, B. J. & Chittester, N. I. (2008). Can exercise treat eating disorders? *Exercise and Sport Sciences Reviews*, **36**, 43–47. doi: 10.1097/jes.0b013e31815e4040

Hausenblas, H. A., Schreiber, K. & Smoliga, J. M. (2017). Practice pointer: Exercise addiction. *BMJ*, **26**, 357. doi: 10.1136/bmj.j1745

Hewitt, P. L. & Flett, G. L. (1996). Personality traits and the coping process. In M. Zeidner & N. S. Endler (Eds.), *Handbook of Coping: Theory, Research, Applications*. Oxford, England: John Wiley & Sons, pp. 410–433.

Hewitt, P. L., Flett, G. L. & Ediger, E. (1996). Perfectionism and depression: Longitudinal assessment of a specific vulnerability hypothesis. *Journal of Abnormal Psychology*, **105**, 276–280. doi:10.1037//0021-843x.105.2.276

Jee, Y.-S. (2016). Exercise addiction and rehabilitation. *Journal of Exercise Rehabilitation*, 12, 67–68.

Jibaja-Rusth, M. L. (1989). *The development of a psycho-social risk profile for becoming an obligatory runner*. Unpublished doctoral dissertation, University of Houston, Houston.

Korolenko, T. P. (1991). Addictive behavior: Its general traits and regular development. *The Bekhterev Review of Psychiatry and Medical Psychology*, **1**, 8–15.

Lejoyeux, M., Avril, M., Embouazza, H. & Nivoli, F. (2008). Prevalence of exercise dependence and other behavioral addictions among clients of a Parisian fitness room. *Comprehensive Psychiatry*, **49**, 353–358. doi: 10.1016/j.comppsych.2007.12.005

Lichtenstein, M. B., Christiansen, E., Elklit, A., Bilenberg, N. & Støving, R. K. (2014). Exercise addiction: A study of eating disorder symptoms, quality of life, personality traits and attachment styles. *Psychiatry Research*, **215**, 410–416. doi:10.1016/j.psychres.2013.11.010

Lichtenstein, M. B., Hinze, C. J., Emborg, B., Thomsen, F. & Hemmingsen, S. D. (2017). Compulsive exercise: Links, risks and challenges faced. *Psychology Research and Behavior Management*, **30**, 85–95. doi: 10.2147/PRBM.S113093.

Lu, F. J., Hsu, E. Y., Wang, J. M., et al. (2012). Exercisers' identities and exercise dependence: The mediating effect of exercise commitment. *Perceptual and Motor Skills*, **115**, 618–631. doi:10.2466/06.13.21.pms.115.5.618-631

Meulemans, S., Pribis, P., Grajales, T. & Krivak, G. (2014). Gender differences in exercise dependence and eating disorders in young adults: A path analysis of a conceptual model. *Nutrients*, **6**, 4895–4905. doi: 10.3390/nu6114895

Miller, K. J. & Mesagno, C. (2014). Personality traits and exercise dependence: Exploring the role of narcissism and perfectionism. *International Journal of Sport and Exercise Psychology*, **12**, 368–381. doi:10.1080/1612197x.2014.932821

Monok, K., Berczik, K., Urban, R., et al. (2012). Psychometric properties and concurrent validity of two exercise addiction measures: A population wide study. *Psychology of Sport and Exercise*, **13**, 387–404. doi:10.1016/j.psychsport.2012.06.003

Morgan, W. P. (1979). Negative addiction in runners. *The Physician and Sportsmedicine*, **7**, 57–77. doi:10.1080/00913847.1979.11948436

Murray, A. L., McKenzie, K., Newman, E. & Brown, E. (2013). Exercise identity as a risk factor for exercise dependence. *British Journal of Health Psychology*, **18**, 369–382. doi: 10.1111/j.2044-8287.2012.02091

O'Connor, R. C. (2007). The relations between perfectionism and suicidality: A systematic review. *Suicide and Life-Threatening Behavior*, **37**, 698–714. doi:10.1521/suli.2007.37.6.698

O'Connor, P. J. & Smith, J. C. (1999). *Physical activity and eating disorders*. In J. M. Rippe (Ed.), *Lifestyle Medicine*. Cambridge, MA: Blackwell Science, pp. 1005–1015.

Oliva, P., Costa, S. & Rosalba, L. (2013). Physical self-concept and its relationship to exercise dependence symptoms in young regular physical exercisers. *American Journal of Sports Science and Medicine*, **1**, 1–6.

Rudy, E. B. & Estok, P. J. (1989). Measurement and significance of negative addiction in runners. *Western Journal of Nursing Research*, **11**, 548–558. doi:10.1177/019394598901100504

Sherry, S. B., Hewitt, P. L., Flett, G. L. & Harvey, M. (2003). Perfectionism dimensions, perfectionistic attitudes, dependent attitudes, and depression in psychiatric patients and university students. *Journal of Counseling Psychology*, **50**, 373–386. doi:10.1037/0022-0167.50.3.373

Smith, D., Hale, B. D. & Collins, D. J. (1998). Measurement of exercise dependence in bodybuilders. *Journal of Sports Medicine and Physical Fitness*, **8**, 1–9.

Spano, L. (2001). The relationship between exercise and anxiety, obsessive-compulsiveness, and narcissism. *Personality and Individual Differences*, **30**, 87–93. doi:10.1016/s0191-8869(00)00012-x

Stets, J. E. & Burke, P. J. (2000). Identity theory and social identity theory. *Social Psychology Quarterly*, **63**, 224. doi:10.2307/2695870

Stice, E., Presnell, K. & Spangler, D. (2002). Risk factors for binge eating onset in adolescent girls: A 2-year prospective investigation. *Health Psychology*, **21**, 131–138. doi:10.1037//0278-6133.21.2.131

Symons Downs, D., Hausenblas, H. A. & Nigg, C. R. (2004). Factorial validity and psychometric examination of the exercise dependence scale-revised. *Measurement in Physical Education and Exercise Science*, 8 (4), 183–201. doi: 10.1207/s15327841mpee0804_1

Szabo, A., Griffiths, M. D., de la Vega Marcos, R., Mervó, B. & Demetrovics, Z. (2015). Methodological and conceptual limitations in exercise addiction research. *Yale Journal of Biology and Medicine*, **88**, 303–308.

Szabo, A., Griffiths, M. D., Høglid, R. A. & Demetrovics, Z. (2018). Drug, nicotine, and alcohol use among exercisers: Does substance addiction co-occur with exercise addiction? *Addictive Behaviors Reports*, **7**, 26–31. doi:10.1016/j.abrep.2017.12.001

Terry, A., Szabo, A. & Griffiths, M. (2004). The exercise addiction inventory: A new brief screening tool. *Addiction Research and Theory*, **12**, 489–499. doi:10.1080/16066350310001637363

Thornton, E. W. & Scott, S. E. (1995). Motivation in the committed runner: Correlations between self-report scales and behaviour. *Health Promotion International*, **10**, 177–184.

Veale, D. (1987). Exercise dependence. *British Journal of Addiction*, **82**, 735–740. doi:10.1111/j.1360-0443.1987.tb01539.x

Veale, D. (1995). Does primary exercise dependence really exist? In J. Annett, B. Cripps & H. Steinberg (Eds.), *Exercise Addiction: Motivation for Participation in Sport and Exercise*. Leicester, UK: British Psychological Society, pp. 1–5.

Villella, C., et al. (2010). Behavioural addictions in adolescents and young adults: Results from a prevalence study. *Journal of Gambling Studies*, **27**, 203–214. doi: 10.1007/s10899-010-9206-0

30 Tanning as an Addiction: The State of the Research and Implications for Intervention

Kimberly A. Miller, PhD, MPH, and Darren Mays, PhD, MPH

Introduction

Skin cancer is a major public health issue, with global rates of disease steadily on the rise (World Health Organization, 2018). In the United States, nearly five million people in are treated for all skin cancers annually, making it the most common cancer type (US Department of Health and Human Services, 2014). Intentional tanning behaviors, including sunbathing and indoor tanning, are high-risk practices strongly associated with the increased risk of skin cancer (Fisher & James, 2010). Sunbed use or indoor tanning is a major risk factor for melanoma, the most lethal form of skin cancer, and initial tanning bed use is associated with a 75 percent increased risk of the disease (Boniol et al., 2012).

Policy efforts such as a 10 percent federal excise tax on indoor tanning services passed in 2010 (US Congress, 2010) and increasing state legislation to ban minors from indoor tanning have resulted in recent decreases in indoor tanning among both youth and adults (Guy et al., 2017). However, despite the known health risks, indoor tanning remains popular, particularly among young adult women, as nearly one-third of non-Hispanic white (NHW) females aged sixteen to twenty-five use tanning beds every year (Guy et al., 2013).

In this chapter, we review the concept of tanning as an addiction. We first focus on the definition and measurement of tanning addiction, and its prevalence in the population. We then review the empirical evidence for tanning addiction, including the behavioral and biological aspects that drive this behavior. Finally, we address the implications of these findings for interventions to prevent and treat this emerging addiction and directions for future research.

Tanning as an Addiction

Recent research has focused on the emerging concept of tanning addiction, i.e., frequent and compulsive tanning exhibited by a subset of those who tan (Kourosh, Harrington & Adinoff, 2010). Among these individuals, tanning is associated with the hallmark characteristics of addiction: a maladaptive pattern of behavior characterized by preoccupation or craving for the behavior; a reinforcing or appetitive effect after performing the behavior; an inability to quit the behavior or loss of control; and negative health consequences resulting from the behavior (Kourosh et al., 2010; Poorsattar & Hornung, 2010; Sussman & Sussman, 2011).

While all intentional tanning (both indoor tanning bed use and outdoor tanning) is associated with an increased risk of skin cancer, a pattern of repeated tanning that escalates despite adverse consequences similar to substance abuse disorders has been deemed "addictive" (Heckman & Manne, 2012). As we will describe, motivations driving tanning addiction may stem from psychological factors such as aesthetic and appearance norms (wanting to look tanned) and/or from physiologic effects of exposure to ultraviolet (UV) light on brain reward pathways, influencing mood similar to opioid use.

Increasingly over the past decade, studies have identified the addiction-like properties of tanning and its relationship to other addictive behaviors. However, the precise underlying mechanisms that drive tanning addiction remain unclear. Nevertheless, a growing body of evidence has documented that for some individuals tanning becomes repetitive and uncontrollable, resulting in an array of negative sequelae including significant personal and societal financial and health impacts (Kourosh et al., 2010; Petit et al., 2014).

Measurement of Tanning Addiction

To date tanning addiction has been primarily measured with two scales developed by Warthan and colleagues (Warthan, Uchida & Wagner, 2005): the modified (m)CAGE criteria and the tanning modified DSM-IV-TR substance use disorder criteria (mDSM-IV-TR) (American Psychiatric Association, 2000). The mCAGE was adapted from the CAGE questionnaire, a brief validated measure to assess problem drinking and potential alcoholism. The mCAGE measure uses four items to assess tanning addiction: "Do you try to cut down on the time you spend tanning but find yourself still tanning?", "Do you ever get annoyed when people tell you not to tan?", "Do you ever feel guilty that you are tanning too much?", and "When you wake up in the morning, do you want to tan?" [*eye-opener*]. While the first three items of the mCAGE maps closely to the original alcohol screener substituting "tanning" for "drinking," the fourth "eye-opener" item does not directly translate from the alcohol assessment (which queries whether the respondent "ever needed a drink first thing in the morning to steady their nerves or to get rid of a hangover") modifying this question instead to "wanting to tan" first thing in the morning.

Endorsement of two or more items of the mCAGE is indicative of tanning dependence. The mDSM-IV-TR adapts eight diagnostic criteria outlined by the *Diagnostic and Statistical Manual for Mental Disorders-IV-TR* for a substance abuse disorder to tanning, with endorsement of three or more items indicative of tanning dependence. An updated version which is tailored for the DSM-5 substance use disorder category (American Psychiatric Association, 2013) has not yet been employed.

Despite being the most widely used measures of tanning addiction, extensive psychometric validation of both screening scales has not been conducted. In studies that report psychometric properties, internal consistency for both scales has been relatively low, with Cronbach's alpha ranging from 0.56 to 0.58 (Heckman et al., 2014b). At least one study has suggested that the mCAGE may overestimate the prevalence of tanning dependence in the population (Schneider et al., 2015); however, other studies have not observed an overestimation and have found comparable rates between the mCAGE and the mDSM-IV-TR (Mays et al., 2017). Since neither measure has established psychometric qualities, however, it is unclear what the meaningful of prevalence estimates is based on either measure.

In addition to the mCAGE and mDSM-IV-TR, several other tanning addiction scales have been developed, although these measures have been less widely used. Hillhouse et al. developed both The Tanning Pathology Scale (TAPS) (Hillhouse et al., 2010) and the Structured Interview for Tanning Abuse and Dependence (SITAD) (Hillhouse et al., 2012). The TAPS was adapted from a questionnaire originally developed to identify motives of pathological tanning rather than as a measure of tanning addiction (Rozin & Stoess, 1993); nevertheless, the TAPS assesses addiction-like components in its four subscales: perceiving tanning as a problem, opiate-like reactions to tanning, tolerance to tanning, and dissatisfaction with skin tone. Responses are continuous, with Cronbach's alphas ranging from 0.62 to 0.90 for the subscales (Heckman et al., 2014b; Hillhouse et al., 2010).

The SITAD was adapted from items used for opioid dependency from the *Structured Clinical Interview for DSM-IV Axis I Disorders* (First et al., 1995) and developed as a measure of tanning dependence to correct for perceived overestimation of the prevalence of tanning addiction by the mCAGE and mDSM-IV-TR. To be categorized as tanning dependent on the SITAD, three or more specific criteria must be endorsed: loss of control; persistent unsuccessful efforts to control tanning; time spent tanning; social problems resulting from tanning; physical or psychological problems resulting from tanning; tolerance; and withdrawal. The SITAD also assesses tanning abuse if one or more of the following criteria are met: recurrent tanning resulting in failure to fulfill work, school, or home obligation; recurrent tanning that is physically hazardous or that incurs tanning-related legal problems; and continued tanning despite or recurrent social/interpersonal problems caused by the behavior (i.e., it is another adaptation of DSM-IV substance abuse disorder criteria).

Additional measures developed to assess tanning addiction include the Craving to Tan Questionnaire (CTQ) (Ashrafioun & Bonar, 2015) adapted from the Penn Alcohol Craving Scale (PACS) (Flannery, Volpicelli & Pettinati, 1999) which measures the frequency, intensity, and duration of craving to tan within the past week. The Tanning Problems Index (TPI) (Ashrafioun & Bonar, 2014a) was adapted from the Short-Rutgers Alcohol Problem Index (S-RAPI) (Earleywine, LaBrie & Pedersen, 2008) and characterizes problems associated with past-year tanning. The Behavioral Addiction Indoor Tanning Screener (BAITS) (Stapleton et al., 2016), was developed based on the behavioral addiction model described in the DSM-5 (American Psychiatric Association, 2013) and assesses symptoms of addictive behavior related to tanning such as appetitive desire and diminished control in accordance with a behavioral addictions framework.

In the few studies that compare psychometric properties between measures, one study found poor internal validity for the mCAGE and mDSM-IV-TR unless used in combination (Heckman et al., 2014b). In subsequently comparing both measures to the TAPS, the study found only fair convergent validity between the three measures, suggesting that they measure somewhat different aspects of addictive tanning. Because of only fair convergent validity on various measures being obtained, current recommendations include the use of mCAGE and mDSM-IV-TR cut-points in combination, or a cut-point on the TAPS of 54 (Heckman et al., 2014b) for greater measurement validity. Thus, while several measures exist to assess tanning addiction have been developed, further evaluation of their psychometric properties is required.

Prevalence of Tanning Addiction

No prevalence estimates for tanning addiction have been drawn from nationally representative samples. Thus, the prevalence varies depending on the psychometric instrument used to measure the behavior as well as the target population (e.g., general population, those who have ever tanned, or those who tan frequently). Estimates of the prevalence of tanning addiction also primarily refer to indoor tanning, the behavior most associated with addictive tanning, although some studies have included outdoor sunbathing. In addition, a majority of studies from which estimates are drawn have been from studies conducted among the highest at-risk population, predominantly female non-Hispanic white college-aged or young adult samples, and therefore prevalence estimates are limited primarily to this population.

Among US samples, the prevalence of tanning addiction ranges between 4 percent and 23 percent in general populations (Heckman et al., 2008; Hillhouse et al., 2012; Poorsattar & Hornung, 2007). Among populations who report ever practising intentional tanning, prevalence estimates range from 9 percent to 39 percent (Ashrafioun & Bonar, 2014b; Banerjee, Hay & Greene, 2013; Mosher & Danoff-Burg, 2010a; Poorsattar & Hornung, 2007; Stapleton et al., 2016). Among those practicing frequent indoor tanning (more than three times a week), tanning addiction prevalence has been estimated at 41 percent (Harrington et al., 2011). A recent study that used both the mCAGE and the mDSM-IV-TR to categorize tanning addiction found that among community-dwelling young adult NHW females who reported ever tanning, approximately 22 percent met both criteria (Mays et al., 2017).

In summary, despite varying instruments across populations with differing risk profiles, the evidence illustrates an appreciable prevalence of tanning addiction, particularly among young NHW females. Overall, the current research suggests that between 22 percent and 44 percent report "current addiction" to tanning among those who practice indoor tanning in this highest-risk population.

Behavioral Aspects of Tanning Addiction

Recent studies have identified tanning addiction as a behavioral addiction, namely a compulsive and rewarding nondrug behavior defined by the characteristic elements of addiction: affective or appetitive effects; preoccupation with the behavior or craving; loss of control/ inability to stop the behavior; and negative consequences as a result of the behavior (Heckman et al., 2015; Sussman & Sussman, 2011). In this section, we identify behavioral aspects of tanning addiction, including cognitive motivations and the cooccurrence of tanning addiction with other behavioral addictions and risk behaviors.

Cognitive Motivations and Tanning

Indoor tanning has been found to be consistently associated with appearance-based cognitive motives including body image, appearance orientation, and pro-tanning attitudes (Gillen & Markey, 2012; Hillhouse, Turrisi & Shields, 2007; Leary, Saltzman & Georgeson, 1997). As a result, most interventions to decrease indoor tanning have focused on appearance to curb the behavior; e.g., by emphasizing photoaging (Gibbons et al., 2005; Hillhouse et al., 2008). In the case of addictive tanning, appearance motivation has also been identified as an important factor in motivating excessive tanning. Studies conducted among young adults females have found that appearance orientation and greater perceived benefits of tanning are strongly associated with tanning dependence (Mays et al., 2017). Another study found that "resistant" tanners, e.g., those knowledgeable about the adverse health effects of tanning but who continued to tan or were unable to quit tanning, were more likely to rationalize their tanning in terms of gaining immediate benefits in terms of appearance versus the long-term health effects as compared to former or nontanning dependent tanners (Banerjee et al., 2013).

Tanning Addiction, Substance Use, and Psychological Conditions

Similar to other behavioral addictions, tanning addiction has been found to cooccur with both substance use and psychological symptomology. The use of tobacco, alcohol, marijuana, and other drugs have all been positively associated with tanning addiction (Ashrafioun & Bonar, 2014b; Heckman et al., 2008; Mays et al., 2017). However, specific substances linked to addictive tanning have been inconsistent across studies. While problem alcohol and drug use have been found to be independently associated with tanning addiction in at least one study, these relationships were not sustained in others once controlling for sociodemographic and psychological variables (Ashrafioun & Bonar, 2014b). Additionally, a recent study found no relationship between tanning addiction and alcohol use among NHW females (Mays et al., 2017). However, other studies have observed a persistent relationship between frequent alcohol use or alcohol use disorder and tanning addiction in multivariable models (Heckman et al., 2014a; Mosher & Danoff-Burg, 2010a).

While tanning addiction has been studied primarily as a female addiction, indoor tanning rates among males, while lower than females, are not negligible: in a national sample, prevalence of indoor tanning among high-school male students was 5.3 percent, while 2.0 percent practiced frequent indoor tanning (Guy et al., 2015). Notably, the relationship between tanning addiction and *substance use* may be moderated by gender, though with equivocal results on cooccurrence. For example, Mosher and Danoff-Burg found that among women, while frequent indoor tanning was associated with substance use and most strongly with alcohol use and binge drinking, this association was not observed among males who frequently tanned (Mosher & Danoff-Burg, 2010b). However, Feng et al. (2017) in a study examining male tanning behavior, found that despite similar rates of frequent tanning, males in the sample were more likely to screen positively for tanning dependence and had higher comorbid risk behaviors including binge drinking and smoking. Additionally, males had higher rates of tanning in private residences (as compared to tanning salons), and more ethnic minority males tanned than minority females (Feng et al., 2017). However, few if any other studies have focused on male tanning behaviors and tanning addiction among men, and more research is needed on gender differences regarding tanning addiction and differential associations with cooccurring behavioral health risks.

A number of studies have examined the relationship between tanning addiction and a wide spectrum of *psychological conditions*, including depressive symptoms, anxiety disorders, obsessive-compulsive disorder (OCD), body dysmorphic disorder (BDD), and seasonal affective disorder (SAD). Tanning addition has been associated with generalized anxiety (Heckman et al., 2014a; Mosher & Danoff-Burg, 2010a), OCD, and BDD (Ashrafioun & Bonar, 2014b). Tanning addiction has been associated inconsistently with depressive symptoms, with one study finding high rates of depression among indoor tanners but no significant association between addictive tanning and depression among university students (Mosher & Danoff-Burg, 2010a), in contrast to a recent study that found a significant association between tanning dependence and depressive symptoms among young females (Mays et al., 2017).

However, Heckman et al. (2016) in administering a comprehensive psychiatric interview with 139 non-Hispanic white (NHW) female indoor tanners aged eighteen to twenty-five found high rates of psychiatric and addictive symptomology, with 40 percent meeting the criteria for tanning dependence, more than 50 percent meeting criteria for SAD, and over 70 percent meeting the criteria for risky alcohol use. Further, the study found decreases in negative mood states (e.g., irritability and anxiety) after indoor tanning, and found that women whose negative mood decreased after indoor tanning were more likely to be more frequent indoor tanners (Heckman et al., 2016).

Tanning addiction has also been studied in the context of seasonal affective disorder (SAD), characterized as a type of depressive disorder in the DSM-5 (American Psychiatric Association, 2013). Seasonal affective disorder may be related to inadequate serotonin regulation and Vitamin D production during winter months and is more highly prevalent in females than males (NIMH, 2018). In a study conducted among female undergraduates, Hillhouse et al. (2002) found that 80 percent of those who identified as frequent tanners also reported symptoms of SAD (Hillhouse, Stapleton & Turrisi, 2005). Similarly, Heckman et al. (2014b) found a trend toward an association between SAD and excessive tanning among young adult women (Heckman et al., 2014a).

Behavioral Aspects of Tanning Addiction: Summary

Differences in measures used for both psychological conditions, use of substance, and tanning addiction may contribute to the wide variability found in the association of tanning addiction with specific substance use and mental health conditions, and as moderated by gender or ethnicity. However, despite lack of consensus on the precise substances and psychopathological frameworks that predominate in tanning addiction, the evidence to date suggests that tanning addiction may be motivated both by cognitive attitudes toward body image and appearance and/or as comorbid to mental health or substance use disorders, with habitual practice of the behavior strengthening reward pathways. The evidence therefore points to an interplay of cognitive, psychological, and physiological factors driving the addiction. To address potential physiological factors, we turn to the evidence for biological pathways of tanning as an addiction.

Biological Aspects of Tanning Addiction

Hypothesized Neurocutaneous Model of Tanning Addiction

Fisher and James (Fisher & James, 2010) recently summarized the hypothesized biological basis for how UV exposure through indoor tanning can become an addiction, later termed a neurocutaneous model by Aubert and colleagues (Aubert et al., 2016). Fisher and James proposed a biological explanation of tanning addiction that stems directly from the process by which UV exposure leads to tanned skin. UV light exposure produces DNA damage in keratinocytes, which activates tumor protein p53; p53 is processed to proopiomelanocortin (POMC), the precursor peptide to melanocyte stimulating hormone (MSH, which induces pigmentation) and β-endorphin release. β-Endorphin is an endogenous opioid that interacts with mu-opioid receptors to produce effects similar to, but less intense than, exogenous opioids (e.g., heroin, prescription opioids) such as enhanced mood and decreased pain. The endogenous release of β-endorphin in response to UV exposure may stimulate physical dependence and addiction to UV light, particularly at high frequencies of use and with the high doses of UV exposure that can be delivered through indoor tanning. The maintenance of tanning addiction may be mediated by dopamine (Berridge & Robinson, 2016), and there is some emerging evidence, described below, supporting this mechanism. Plausibly, the addictive properties of indoor tanning may be more pronounced in groups with preexisting vulnerabilities (e.g., mental health comorbidities, those with chronic pain) similar to other forms of substance abuse and addiction. A growing body of preclinical and clinical research supports this neurocutaneous model of indoor tanning addiction and is summarized below.

Animal Studies

Fell and colleagues (Fell et al., 2014) developed a preclinical animal model to test the neurocutaneous mechanism of tanning addiction described by Fisher and James (Fisher & James, 2010). In a series of experiments involving manipulation of UV exposures and pharmacologic and genetic blockades of the hypothesized opioid pathway, this study provided evidence establishing that in rodents: (1) UV radiation exposure leads to elevated β-endorphin in plasma; (2) pain thresholds decrease with UV exposure, an indicator of opioid analgesic effect and an effect that is reversed with pharmacologic opioid antagonism; (3) pharmacologic opioid blockade triggers opioid withdrawal symptoms in animals that are chronically exposed to artificial UV light; (4) removal of prolonged exposure leads to conditioned choice behavior akin to drug-seeking where animals preferentially seek out light environments over dark environments; and (4) in β-endorphin knockout mice and those lacking the POMC gene, a peptide precursor to the release of β-endorphin in response to UV light exposure, the effects of UV exposure on pain tolerance, choice behavior, and withdrawal are absent. This model provides mechanistic support for the hypothesis that tanning can become a behavioral addiction through endogenous opioid response.

Human Clinical Studies

Clinical studies investigating variations in levels of β-endorphin in response to UV exposure in vivo in human participants emerged as early as the 1980s (Levins et al., 1983; Spiro et al., 1987). Although relatively small in number, more recent clinical studies testing whether β-endorphin and its precursor peptides are elevated in response to UV exposure have demonstrated mixed findings. A study by Wintzen and colleagues (Wintzen et al., 2001a) included eight non-Hispanic white participants with unspecified indoor or outdoor tanning history. Minimum erythemal dose (MED) of UV exposure was determined based on participants' skin phototype (i.e., the skin's inclination to tan or burn in response to UV exposure) and participants were exposed to whole body UV radiation three times a week for three weeks at escalating doses (0.5 MED, 1 MED, and increases by 20 percent MED for each subsequent exposure). The UV source was designed to stimulate the spectrum produced by natural sunlight. Skin biopsies were taken immediately before the first exposure and following the final exposure and levels of β-endorphin and precursor peptides were measured by immunohistochemistry. The findings demonstrated that β-endorphin was detectable in keratinocytes of the follicular matrix (i.e., hair) and cells of sweat ducts but was not detectable in epidermal keratinocytes. These data suggest there may be little systemic circulation of β-endorphin following repeated UV exposure, however, the findings should be interpreted in light of study limitations. This includes the relatively small sample, limited information on study participants' UV exposure history, and the non-experimental, single group design.

In a subsequent study, Wintzen and colleagues (Wintzen et al., 2001b) assessed the presence of circulating POMC-derived peptides including *β* endorphin and precursors β-lipotropin and adrenocorticotropic hormone (ACTH) following UV exposure. The study included twenty-six non-Hispanic white young adults with unspecified history of indoor tanning. Exposure consisted of a weighted dose of 15 J/cm^2 UVA, less than an average MED of 25 J/cm^2. Blood samples were taken before, immediately after, and up to four times in the hour following the UV exposure. These were compared to samples taken from thirty-five patients during the course of receiving UV therapy delivered at varying wavelengths (UVB, UVA, UVA-1) for conditions such as psoriasis and dermatitis and two unexposed control patients. Overall there were no observed increases in β-endorphin or ACTH following exposure for any of the groups, and no observed differences with the two healthy control participants included in the study. These findings should also be considered in light of limitations to the study including the relatively small convenience sample, nonrandomized design, and lack of controls for important confounding variables such as indoor and outdoor tanning behavior. The repeated exposure was assessed in a heterogeneous sample of patients undergoing UV therapy, the dose and source varied, and the study did not account for potential confounding variables across the groups compared. It is also unclear to what degree the exposures assessed correspond to those achieved through indoor tanning in retail (e.g., salons, fitness centers) and private (e.g., homes) settings. Likely, the dose and frequency of exposure tested was lower than what would be obtained in real-world settings.

Another study by Gambichler and colleagues (Gambichler et al., 2002) examined plasma β-endorphin levels in thirty-five UVA exposed and nine unexposed participants. Study participants were adults with Fitzpatrick skin types II and III (light skin that typically burns before tanning) and excluded those with photosensitivity, a history of regular indoor tanning, psychiatric disorder, drug use, and UV exposure for two months prior to the study. Participants were randomized in unequal numbers to a UV exposure or a control group. Control participants were not exposed and were instructed to rest in the tanning bed. Blood samples were taken on day 1, UV exposure delivered, and samples taken again after twenty minutes of exposure. Participants had five additional exposures over a three-week period. The exposures consisted of UVA radiation standardized to 16 J/cm^2 for skin type II and 21 J/cm^2 for skin type III. Final blood samples were taken after the last exposure. There were no statistically significant differences between exposed and unexposed participants in plasma β-endorphin. The study has limitations similar to those described above but is strengthened by the randomized design that provides better control over potential confounding variables.

In the most recent study of this kind, Jussila and colleagues (Jussila et al., 2016) enrolled a sample of twelve participants. Participants were excluded if they reported any intentional UV exposure in the preceding two months (e.g., indoor tanning), active drug use, or psychiatric disorder. All participants were skin phototypes II and III (light skin that typically burns before tanning) in order to standardize the UV dose. Participants were randomly assigned to varying doses of UV exposure: seven received one standard erythemal dose (SED; defined as 10 mJ/cm^2) whole body narrow band UVB, and five received a cumulative thee SEDs delivered over two days. Skin biopsies were collected preexposure and twenty-four hours following the last exposure. Exposure increased β-endorphin in eleven of twelve participants, with no differences by UV dose. Increase in β-endorphin was greatest in keratinocytes, and more so in basal cells.

In summary, in-vivo studies with human participants conducted to date provide somewhat mixed evidence on whether artificial UV exposure increases β-endorphin in a manner that would support addiction as indicated in animal research described above. Notably, it is challenging to synthesize findings of these studies due to differences in study participants and characteristics, differences in UV exposure protocols (wavelength, dose, timing and frequency of delivery), and differences in how and when biospecimens were collected and analyzed relative to the UV exposure across the studies. Prior research demonstrates that stimulation of POMC genes, and therefore β-endorphin or precursor peptide products, is dependent on UV wavelength (greater for more intense UVB radiation) and dose (Skobowiat et al., 2011) and is likely a critical factor influencing study findings. Commercially available, high-pressure tanning devices available for retail and private use have been observed to emit upwards of four times the level of UVA and two times the level of UVB than the midday summer sunlight at a northern latitude (e.g., Washington, DC) (Lim et al., 2011), although recent evidence suggests UVB emittance in some commercial devices may be lower. Moreover, the levels of exposure and UVA:UVB ratios may change with recent reclassification of commercial tanning devices from class I medical devices (lowest risk with little to no regulatory controls) to class II medical devices (devices with potential risks and premarket regulatory controls) by the Food and Drug Administration (FDA, 2014). Finally, individual level exposure is also likely variable based on enforcement of factors such as time and frequency of exposure, dose standardization, and access to tanning in unsupervised private settings such as fitness centers and home residences (Nilsen, Hannevik & Veierod, 2016). This implies that few, if any, of the studies conducted to date to assess the association between tanning exposure and levels of β-endorphin or precursor peptides likely replicates the dose and frequency of exposure that occurs from indoor tanning in the real world.

Studies of Tanning Reward and Withdrawal

The reinforcing effect of many addictive drugs occurs through neurobiological reward pathways and is directly or indirectly mediated by dopamine (Baler & Volkow, 2006). A hallmark feature of the physiological dependence that develops in response to chronic drug exposure is the emergence of withdrawal symptoms such as agitation, irritability, and discomfort when the reinforcing drug is removed. Several studies have assessed these aspects of tanning addiction either together or independently.

Feldman and colleagues (Feldman et al., 2004) examined the reinforcing effects of UV light in a series of within-subject controlled, blinded, repeated-choice trials. Participants were fourteen young adults who were regular indoor tanners (tanned between eight and fifteen times per month). The study excluded participants with dark skin (e.g., skin phototype V), those with skin phototypes I and II that are inclined to burn, those with current or past skin cancer, those using photosensitizing medication, those using illicit drugs, and those with major psychiatric disorders. Those reporting greater than twenty minutes per day of weekday sun exposure between the hours of 10:00 AM and 2:00 pm or greater than sixty minutes per day of weekday sun exposure at all daytime hours were also excluded. Participants were randomly exposed in a blinded within-subjects trial to UV or non-UV emitting tanning beds that were physically identical and delivered the same heat load for two days per week for six weeks. The only difference between the beds was the "sham" UV beds were equipped with an imperceptible UV light filter. On the last day of each week, participants were given the option to choose additional tanning sessions and their preferred tanning bed, and choices were recorded. Subjective preferences of the UV and sham-UV bed were also assessed. Twelve of the seventeen participants (71 percent) chose to receive additional tanning exposure, and eleven (65 percent) chose to use the UV bed instead of the sham-UV bed. In total, 95 percent of all chosen exposures were for UV emitting devices. Participants endorsed a strong subjective preference for UV versus sham-UV beds. Subjective reports also indicated that participants reported a significantly more relaxed and less tense mood after exposure to the UV versus non-UV tanning. Limitations of the study include the relatively small sample size and unclear generalizability given study exclusions such as other substance use and presence of psychiatric comorbidities.

Members of the same research team also investigated opioid withdrawal symptoms in a small randomized controlled trial with frequent indoor tanners (Kaur et al., 2006). Among eight frequent indoor tanners (eight to fifteen tanning exposures per month) and eight infrequent indoor tanners (no more than twelve times per year), the study tested whether pharmacologic opioid antagonism blocks the subjective reinforcing properties of UV light exposure observed previously, and if withdrawal symptoms occur. Study participants received either naltrexone or placebo in randomized order of dosing escalated over a two-week period (5 mg, 15 mg, 25 mg). After dosing, participants were assigned in random order to use either a UV or sham-UV tanning bed. Subjective preferences were assessed after each exposure. Findings demonstrated that opioid antagonism reduced preference for UV light in frequent tanners. With placebo and low (5 mg) naltrexone doses, frequent tanners endorsed strong preferences for the UV versus the sham-UV beds, whereas infrequent tanners did not. At the 25 mg dose, the preference for UV beds versus sham-UV beds in frequent tanners was no different. In 50 percent of frequent tanners, but none of the infrequent tanners, opioid antagonism produced withdrawal like symptoms such as nausea and jitteriness.

Harrington and colleagues assessed hypothesized central nervous system effects of indoor tanning guided by evidence on the neurobiology of drug reward (Harrington et al., 2012). The study used the experimental paradigm similar to that of Feldman and colleagues (Feldman et al., 2004) and Kaur and colleagues (Kaur et al., 2006) to test the hypothesis that neural activation in striatal brain regions associated with reward including the nucleus accumbens, caudate, and putamen would be greater in response to UV tanning than sham-UV tanning. In the study, seven frequent indoor tanners (reported tanning at least twice per week for the prior three-month period and endorsing tanning dependence criteria) were exposed to either UV tanning or sham-UV tanning in two sessions. Session order was randomized, and as with studies described above, the sham UV was identical to the UV tanning bed in all ways except for the imperceptible UV light filter, so participants were blinded to the source. Single photon emission computerized tomography (SPECT) was used to measure brain activity. Compared to the sham UV session, there was a significant increase in regional cerebral blood flow of the dorsal striatum, anterior insula, and medial orbitofrontal cortex. These changes in regional cerebral blood flow in reward-associated brain regions were associated with a decrease in participant-reported subjective desire to tan.

Aubert and colleagues (Aubert et al., 2016) tested the hypothesis that dopamine efflux, a measure of dopamine receptor binding, changes in response to indoor tanning in a manner similar to other addictive drugs and consistent with evidence regarding the neurobiological reward mechanisms of drug addiction (Baler & Volkow, 2006). This hypothesis is based on evidence that basal striatal D2/D3 dopamine receptors are relatively lower in drug addiction due to preexisting risk factors, down-regulation due to chronic drug-induced dopaminergic effects, or some combination of these processes (Aubert et al., 2016). The study was a double-blind cross-over trial that included adult (ages eighteen to forty-five) non-Hispanic white or Hispanic men and women with skin phototype II–IV. Participants were considered to be addicted tanners ($n = 10$) if they reported indoor tanning at least twice per week in the prior year and endorsed dependence criteria including inability to cut down or stop tanning. Nonaddicted tanners ($n = 10$) were sex, age, ethnicity, and skin phototype matched and had a minimum of ten lifetime tanning exposures, no more than four exposures in the prior ninety days and did not endorse dependence criteria. Participants were exposed to a UV tanning bed or a sham UV bed while undergoing neuroimaging using SPECT. UV and sham-UV exposures were delivered on two separate visits approximately one week apart with the order balanced by participants' tanning status (addicted or infrequent). SPECT examined basal/striatal D2/D3 binding potential as a measure of UVR induced striatal dopamine efflux. Results revealed a nonsignificant increase in dopamine efflux in the bilateral caudate in addicted tanners upon exposure to UV tanning beds that returned to baseline levels after exposure. Consistent with the findings of Harrington and colleagues (Harrington et al., 2012), post-hoc analyses also revealed that left caudate basal striatal dopamine binding potential significantly decreased (reflecting increased dopamine efflux) in addicted tanners but not infrequent tanners during the UV sessions but not the sham-UV sessions. Bilateral dopamine efflux was also correlated with severity of tanning (i.e., frequency) in addicted tanners but not nonaddicted tanners.

Results of these studies provide preliminary evidence supporting the reinforcing effects of indoor tanning and indicate neurobiological reward mechanisms may underlie indoor tanning addiction, similar to addictive drugs. Within the hypothesized neurocutaneous model of tanning addiction, β-endorphin may act peripherally to deliver cutaneous pain relief from acute UV exposure (Aubert et al., 2016). Centrally, addiction may transpire through opioid-like rewarding effects including relaxation and improved mood (Aubert et al., 2016). This model is consistent with other evidence indicating that while some substances are not potent euphorigenics, they are highly addictive due to their reward reinforcement (e.g., nicotine) that is mediated by dopamine (Volkow et al., 2004). This model is also consistent with evidence indicating dopamine's role in enhancing salience of substance-related cues to maintain addiction and promote relapse (Berridge & Robinson, 2016). (See also Warlow et al., 2020) The studies by Aubert and colleagues (Aubert et al., 2016) and Harrington and colleagues (Harrington et al., 2012) provide preliminary evidence that neurobiological reward mechanisms mediated by dopamine that are broadly implicated in drug abuse and addiction (Volkow et al., 2004) may underlie the rewarding properties of indoor tanning that serve to maintain addiction over time (Berridge & Robinson, 2016). Notably, the studies above demonstrate these effects are more pronounced in those who indoor tan frequently, and those endorsing symptoms of tanning dependence. Kaur and colleagues also provide evidence that the rewarding effects of UV exposure through indoor tanning are less pronounced with opioid antagonism and demonstrate that withdrawal symptoms occur in frequent indoor tanners (Kaur et al., 2006). Although these studies, collectively, provide important insights, they should be interpreted cautiously due to important limitations. Most studies involved relatively small samples with limited generalizability and lacked appropriate control or comparison groups. Research to replicate and build from their findings is critical to advance understanding of the neurobiological basis of tanning addiction.

Studies of Genetic Risks

Addictive behaviors are affected by complex factors ranging from biological to interpersonal (e.g., peer norms) and environmental (e.g., advertising, marketing, policy) influences (Sussman, 2017). At the biological level, the research on addiction genetics is vast and a review is beyond the scope of this chapter. There is abundant evidence that opioid receptor genes influence addiction to opioids, cocaine, alcohol, and methamphetamines (Levran, Yuferov & Kreek, 2012) and genes regulating dopamine pathways are involved in many forms of drug abuse and addiction as well (Le Foll et al., 2009). These dopamine pathways may be more fundamental to the maintenance of addiction behavior than opioid receptors ("wanting" versus "liking"; see (Berridge & Robinson, 2016). Research has begun to investigate potential genetic risks associated with indoor tanning.

Cartmel and colleagues (Cartmel et al., 2014) analyzed genetic associations with tanning dependence using data from a case-control study of basal cell carcinoma. They conducted exome-wide screening of a panel of approximately 319,000 single nucleotide polymorphisms and candidate genes previously associated with addiction including opioid receptor genes, genes involved in nicotine dependence, and others. The parent study was a case-control investigation of early-onset basal cell carcinoma (prior to age forty). Indoor tanning addiction was assessed in a subset of 548 cases and controls by retrospective report. Those reporting no volitional sunbathing or indoor tanning were excluded, resulting in an analytic sample of 292 participants. In the exome wide analyses, after adjustment for multiple comparisons an association was observed between tanning dependence and *PTCHD2*, a gene that has not yet been functionally characterized. Significantly fewer individuals who were addicted to tanning had minor alleles in this gene compared with individuals classified as not tanning addicted. Although none of the candidate genes that passed quality control checks evidenced significant associations with tanning addiction after adjustment for multiple comparisons, SNPs in two genes including the opioid receptor gene *OPRM1* and dopamine receptor gene *ANKK1* were associated with tanning addiction before adjustment. These preliminary data highlight that genetics may influence tanning addiction as with other forms of drug addiction and highlight novel gene *PTCHD2* that may be uniquely associated with tanning addiction but that has not yet been functionally characterized. However, the results should be interpreted cautiously relative to study limitations including potential self-report bias due to retrospective assessment of tanning behavior and dependence, and the fact that tanning may be more salient issue for those diagnosed with skin cancer.

Flores and colleagues used data from another skin cancer case control study to examine associations between genes involved in dopamine receptor regulation and drug metabolism and indoor tanning behavior (Flores et al., 2013). The parent study was a case-control investigation of melanoma in individuals twenty-five to fifty-nine years of age. A total of 1,746 individuals had complete genotype and self-report data on indoor tanning behavior for analyses. A total of sixty-seven single nucleotide polymorphisms (SNPs) from five genes previously associated with addiction to alcohol, nicotine, and other drugs were examined (*ANKK1*, *CYP2A6*, *CYP2A7*, *DRD2*, *SLCA3*). Results of candidate and haplotype gene analyses indicated that SNPs in the *DRD2* dopamine receptor and *ANKK1* signaling genes were associated with having ever tanned indoors among controls, but only associations for *ANKK1* remained statistically significant after adjustment for demographic covariates. Notably, two SNPs in *ANKK1* and three SNPs in *DRD2* that were associated with ever indoor tanning among controls were also found to be associated with increased risk of melanoma when examining differences between cases and controls. When the data were stratified by indoor tanning status, one *ANKK1* SNP was associated with melanoma among those who had never tanned indoors and three *DRD2* SNPS were associated with melanoma among ever indoor tanners or never indoor tanners, depending on the SNP. Although this study did not investigate indoor tanning addiction as a phenotype, it provides initial evidence that genes involved in hypothesized addiction reward pathways are related to indoor tanning behavior (see Blum et al., 2020). The results require replication and additional study to determine associations with tanning addiction. Notable limitations should also be considered, such as the reliance on ever indoor tanning as a behavioral phenotype.

Other Emerging Evidence

Chronic exposure to addictive drugs produces neuroplastic changes, such as changes in neurotransmitter receptor quantity and function, which may accelerate and maintain addiction (Volkow et al., 2004). Some researchers ponder whether or not exposure to UV light leads to similar changes that may facilitate addiction to indoor tanning. An intriguing line of research suggests this possibility but requires additional investigation.

In an animal model, Dulcis and colleagues demonstrated a novel phenomenon called "neurotransmitter switching" in response to environmental sensory stimuli in adult rodents (Dulcis et al., 2013). The study demonstrated that neurons in the hypothalamus switch between dopamine and somatostatin in response to exposure to short- and long-day photoperiods, respectively, in rodents. Specifically, relative to rodents in a balanced control condition (i.e., equivalent exposures to short and long photoperiods), exposure to short-day photoperiods for one week increased the number of hypothalamic dopamine neurons and increased the release of dopamine; the opposite pattern was observed with exposure to long-day photoperiods. An inverse pattern was observed for hypothalamic somatostatin neurons, which increased with long-day photoperiod exposure and decreased with short-day photoperiod exposure. The effects were specific to neurons with retinal sensory input, the varying photoperiod exposures affected animals' behavior, and pharmacologic blockade of dopaminergic neurons produced anxiety and depression, indicators of withdrawal. This study was significant because it has been widely thought that neurotransmitter identity was fixed in adulthood (Flight, 2013); however, the study also provide suggestive evidence that exposure to external stimuli such as UV light may lead to neuroplastic changes in the dopaminergic system.

Following this study, Aumann and colleagues tested the hypothesis that dopamine neurons are affected by environmental UV exposure in humans due to up- or down-regulation of expression genes that are central to dopamine synthesis (Aumann et al., 2016). The researchers examined if there are differences in tyrosine hydroxylase (TH; an enzyme central to dopamine synthesis) and dopamine transporter (DAT) neurons in the midbrain postmortem in adults who died at times of long photoperiod (summer, $n = 5$) and short photoperiod (winter, $n = 5$). Factors such as age, gender, time since death, were similar by these two groups and were included as controls in analyses. The results showed the density of TH+ neurons was increased six-fold in those who died in summer, whereas density of TH– neurons was 2.5-fold lower in those who died in winter. Density of DAT neurons was approximately two-fold higher in those who died in summer, versus approximately two-fold lower in those who died in winter; however, the differences in DAT neuron density did not reach statistical significance. Owing to the design, this study cannot rule out potential confounding processes (e.g., seasonal variation other exposures like temperature, diet, physical activity) and does not specifically investigate the direct effect of UV exposure on neuron density. However, findings of this study provide preliminary evidence that higher levels of UV exposure may lead to adaptive changes in the brain that facilitate addiction by increasing density of dopamine receptors and in turn stimulating individuals to seek repeated tanning exposure.

Biological Aspects of Tanning Addiction: Summary

Research to date provides some support for a hypothesized neurocutaneous model of tanning addiction. Preclinical evidence from animal models supports the hypothesized mechanism involving release of the endogenous opioid β-endorphin as the putative mechanism of tanning as an addictive behavior. In-vivo studies with human participants provide mixed evidence on whether artificial UV exposure increases β-endorphin in a manner that would support addiction as indicated in animal models, but studies have varied methodologically making their findings difficult to synthesize. Notably, clinical studies support the idea that tanning produces drug-like reward including evidence demonstrating a neurobiological basis for the rewarding aspects of tanning. However, these studies are limited methodologically as well. An additional emerging line of research provides preliminary evidence that exposure to UV light may lead to adaptive changes in the brain that support the hypothesized reward-based neurocutaneous model of tanning addiction.

Implications for Interventions to Prevent and Treat Tanning Addiction

Similar to other addictive behaviors (such as tobacco use, for example), experts have advocated for a comprehensive approach to prevent and reduce indoor tanning that involves deploying interventions at multiple levels of socioecological influence, including both cognitive and behavioral interventions to address excessive tanning in individuals (Stapleton et al., 2017) as well as public health policy measures (Holman et al., 2013; Seidenberg et al., 2015).

In a comprehensive review of interventions to mitigate addictive tanning, Stapleton et al. (2017) found twenty-four behavioral interventions targeting indoor tanning between the years of 2001 to 2016. Of these twenty-four, however, only three used criteria to target repeat tanners, and none used tanning addiction criteria (Chait, Thompson & Jacobsen, 2015; Hillhouse & Turrisi, 2002; Turrisi et al., 2008).

Hillhouse and colleagues conducted a randomized controlled trial using an appearance-based approach to reduce frequent tanning. Study participants were female university students who reported at least monthly indoor tanning. Participants in the treatment group were provided an eleven-page workbook that provided information on the appearance-damaging effects of indoor tanning, including tanning effects on the skin, tanning and skin aging, and appearance alternatives to tanning (e.g., sunless tanning, exercise). The control group received no intervention.

Outcomes were measured at two weeks following receipt of the workbook and were assessed on intentions to indoor tan in the future, attitudes and beliefs toward indoor tanning and alternatives, and indoor tanning knowledge. Participants were then assessed at two months post intervention and queried about indoor tanning usage over the prior two months. At short-term follow-up, those in the treatment group had significantly greater negative attitudes toward indoor tanning and fewer intentions to tan compared to controls. At two-month follow-up, those in the treatment group indoor tanned significantly less (one-half as much) as those in the control group in the prior two months.

Turrisi and colleagues in a randomized controlled trial compared two brief interventions to reduce tanning in young women with a history of very frequent tanning. Female undergraduates who reported indoor tanning more than ten times in the past year were randomized to one of two treatment conditions, a personalized Motivational Interview (MI) or receipt of a personalized graphic feedback sheet, or to a no intervention control. The personalized MI session comprised a one-on-one, thirty-minute counseling session to provide cognitive-behavioral skills information and to help participants evaluate the effects of indoor tanning to reduce the behavior. The personalized graphic feedback sheet provided similar content to the MI session (e.g., information on the participants' indoor tanning behaviors, normative beliefs about tanning and its effects, financial costs, risk of skin cancers, and protective behaviors) but delivered with no personal contact via Web site.

Participants were followed up at three months postintervention during winter months (i.e., times of highest indoor tanning). Participants in the MI group significantly decreased their mean number of indoor tanning sessions versus the nonintervention control (4.40 versus 11.78, respectively). Although mean indoor tanning sessions differed from the graphic feedback group (who had a mean number of indoor tanning sessions of 9.03), this was not statistically significant, nor was the difference between the the feedback group and the non-intervention group significant.

Chait and colleagues conducted a randomized controlled trial comparing an appearance-based dissonance intervention and an appearance-based psychoeducational intervention to a healthy lifestyle education control condition. Study participants were female undergraduate students aged eighteen to twenty-five years who engaged in indoor or outdoor tanning at least six times in the past twelve months. The appearance-based dissonance condition consisted of a single ninety-minute group session where participants completed several tasks. First, they identified what defines an ideal tan, with probing questions to formulate this concept by the group leader. Then, participants identified ways in which an ideal tan negatively affected one's appearance. Participants then identified two times in their own lives when people promoted an ideal tan and instances where they personally encouraged tanning. Following this, participants described a response or challenge to these promotions, and shared these with the group. Lastly, group participants engaged in role play activities where they were tasked with encouraging the group leader to avoid pursuing the ideal tan. The appearance-based psychoeducation condition consisted of a sixty-minute PowerPoint presentation on the health consequences of UV exposure, negative appearance-related effects, and ways to reduce risk of these outcomes. The control condition used strategies similar to the dissonance condition, but focused on healthy eating.

Outcomes were measured at one-month postintervention. At follow-up, compared with the control condition participants in the dissonance condition significantly reduced daily time spent tanning. In addition, while those in the control condition reduced their use of sunscreen, no such reduction was observed among participants in the dissonance group. Finally, the participants in the psychoeducation condition did not differ significantly from those in the control condition on follow-up outcomes.

Thus, these tanning interventions focused on frequent tanners used approaches common in addiction interventions, including Motivational Interviewing (MI), cognitive-behavioral therapy, and promotion of alternatives to/substitutions for tanning (e.g., use of sunless tanning products to replace the risk of UV exposure) (Stapleton et al., 2017). Despite these approaches, the authors conclude that intervention work that draws more precisely from the science of addiction is needed to effectively intervene for tanners who meet addiction criteria versus interventions that simply target indoor tanning regardless of addiction criteria.

In addition, evidence is mounting that tanning addiction is a phenomenon of cooccurrence or multiple addictions; that is, those who meet criteria for tanning addiction often also display problem substance use, mental health symptomology (or both), or other behavioral conditions (Miller et al., 2018). Because nearly if not all evidence to date on tanning addiction has been cross-sectional, no studies currently provide causal evidence of how tanning addiction relates to other addiction-like behaviors (e.g., as a precursor or symptom); therefore, our understanding of how tanning addiction initiates, and its temporal pattern in relation to other mental health conditions and substance use behaviors, is limited. Prospective research is important in understanding the causal patterns of tanning addiction in relation to other addiction-like behaviors and mental health conditions. Equally important to intervention development, however, is an understanding of the role or function that these co-occurring behaviors may play in addictive tanning. For example, Sussman (2017) describes how addictions may change or "transfer" over time, may be experienced concurrently, or may be a replacement after the termination of a prior addiction (Sussman, 2017). Addictions may vary with social context and developmental stage; thus, the concurrent nature of tanning addiction with problem substance use in college-aged females, for example, may reflect a specific exposure context in which one, or another, addiction-like behavior is formed leading to development of a second or multiple (Sussman, 2017). In these instances, developing interventions and treatments that draw from addiction science and that recognize the specific patterns of multiple and concurrent addictions may be more effective in treating tanning addiction than ones that simply target indoor tanning as the risk behavior of focus.

Given the potential neurobiological pathways of tanning addiction as extensively described in this chapter, pharmacological therapies may also have a role in treating tanning addiction. As the study by Kaur and colleagues demonstrated, the use of an opioid antagonist eliminated the subjective reinforcing effects of indoor tanning in excessive tanners, suggesting that such therapies may help to combat the reinforcing properties of UV light exposure and aid in cessation of tanning behavior (Kaur et al., 2006). In the case of SAD, as well, there are psychopharmacological treatment implications given the potential biological basis driving frequent tanning in individuals with seasonal depression. However, much more clinical research is needed regarding the neurobiological basis of tanning as an addiction and its interplay with psychosocial factors and other mental health conditions before such therapies might be clinically indicated.

Legislative change may also impact the initiation of indoor tanning at younger ages, thus curbing the development of tanning addiction. At the state level in the USA, as of 2015 more than forty states and the District of Columbia had in place policies aimed at restricting youth access to indoor tanning through minimum age and parental permission requirements (Guy et al., 2016). Despite population-level evidence that such policies can reduce the prevalence of indoor tanning among youth (Guy et al., 2014), a proposed national minimum age requirement by the Food and Drug Administration appears to have been abandoned (FDA, 2015). However, recent federal regulations to reclassify indoor tanning devices from class I to class II medical devices created additional premarket review requirements for manufacturers seeking to introduce new devices to the market, and require a black box warning stating they should not be used by consumers under the age of eighteen (FDA, 2014). Other population-based interventions such as mass media campaigns that have been effective for preventing and reducing addictive behaviors such as tobacco use are also strategies that could be implemented for tanning behavior (including indoor and outdoor tanning), particularly mass media messaging aimed at youth to prevent and reduce tanning exposure before it progresses to habitual, addictive use (Seidenberg et al., 2015). Such population-based strategies, coupled with clinical interventions delivered at the individual level to identify, prevent, and treat tanning addiction can form a comprehensive approach to reducing the associated morbidity and mortality and costs to society.

Conclusions

In conclusion, an empirical body of evidence has emerged over more than ten years that has identified tanning as an addiction. The importance of recognizing and addressing tanning addiction is an essential aspect of the overall issue of skin cancer as a significant public health crisis (US Department of Health and Human Services, 2014). While indoor tanning and sunbathing both increase the risk of skin cancer, excessive, addictive tanning substantially increases the risk of dermatological sequelae and may result in additional negative consequences such as financial, emotional, and other health (e.g., problem substance use) problems.

Despite clear evidence for the addiction-like properties of tanning for a subset of individuals, the specific behavioral and biological pathways warrant further research, particularly prospective research that enables a clearer understanding of the initiation and progression of tanning addiction. Future transdisciplinary work in this field, conducted with methodologic rigor, is required to effectively prevent, reduce, and mitigate this high-risk addiction.

REFERENCES

American Psychiatric Association [APA] (2000). *Diagnostic and Statistical Manual of Mental Disorders* (4th edition). Washington, DC: American Psychiatric Association.

American Psychiatric Association [APA] (2013). *Diagnostic and Statistical Manual of Mental Disorders* (5th edition). Washington, DC: American Psychiatric Association.

Ashrafioun, L. & Bonar, E. E. (2014a). Development of a brief scale to assess frequency of symptoms and problems associated with tanning. *Journal of the American Academy of Dermatology*, **70**(3), 588-589. doi:10.1016/j.jaad.2013.11.041

Ashrafioun, L. & Bonar, E. E. (2014b). Tanning addiction and psychopathology: Further evaluation of anxiety disorders and substance abuse. *Journal of the American Academy of Dermatology*, **70**(3), 473-480. doi:10.1016/j.jaad.2013.10.057

Ashrafioun, L. & Bonar, E. E. (2015). Psychometric assessment of the craving to tan questionnaire. *American Journal of Drug and Alcohol Abuse*, **41**(1), 74-81. doi:10.3109/00952990.2014.939754

Aubert, P. M., Seibyl, J. P., Price, J. L., et al. (2016). Dopamine efflux in response to ultraviolet radiation in addicted sunbed users. *Psychiatry Research*, **251**, 7-14. doi:10.1016/j.pscychresns.2016.04.001

Aumann, T. D., Raabus, M., Tomas, D., et al. (2016). Differences in number of midbrain dopamine neurons associated with summer and winter photoperiods in humans. *PLoS ONE*, **11**(7), e0158847. doi:10.1371/journal.pone.0158847

Baler, R. D. & Volkow, N. D. (2006). Drug addiction: the neurobiology of disrupted self-control. *Trends in Molecular Medicine*, **12**(12), 559-566. doi:10.1016/j.molmed.2006.10.005

Banerjee, S. C., Hay, J. L. & Greene, K. (2013). Cognitive rationalizations for tanning-bed use: a preliminary exploration. *American Journal of Health Behavior*, **37**(5), 577-586. doi:10.5993/ajhb.37.5.1

Berridge, K. C. & Robinson, T. E. (2016). Liking, wanting, and the incentive-sensitization theory of addiction. *American Psychologist*, **71** (8), 670-679. doi:10.1037/amp0000059

Blum, K. et al. (2020). Precision Behavioral Management (PBM): a novel genetically guided therapy to combat Reward Deficiency Syndrome (RDS) relevant to the opiate crisis. In S. Sussman (Ed.) *The Cambridge Handbook of Substance and Behavioral Addictions*. Cambridge, UK: Cambridge University Press, pp. 297-306

Boniol, M., Autier, P., Boyle, P. & Gandini, S. (2012). Cutaneous melanoma attributable to sunbed use: systematic review and meta-analysis. *BMJ*, **345**, e4757. doi:10.1136/bmj.e4757

Cartmel, B., Dewan, A., Ferrucci, L. M., et al. (2014). Novel gene identified in an exome-wide association study of tanning dependence. *Experimental Dermatology*, **23** (10), 757-759. doi:10.1111/exd.12503

Chait, S. R., Thompson, J. K. & Jacobsen, P. B. (2015). Preliminary development and evaluation of an appearance-based dissonance induction intervention for reducing UV exposure. *Body Image*, **12**, 68-72. doi:10.1016/j.bodyim.2014.09.004

Dulcis, D., Jamshidi, P., Leutgeb, S. & Spitzer, N. C. (2013). Neurotransmitter switching in the adult brain regulates behavior. *Science*, **340**(6131), 449-453. doi:10.1126/science.1234152

Earleywine, M., LaBrie, J. W. & Pedersen, E. R. (2008). A brief Rutgers Alcohol Problem Index with less potential for bias. *Addictive*

Behaviors, **33**(9), 1249–1253. doi:10.1016/j.addbeh.2008.05.006

FDA (2014). General and plastic surgery devices: reclassification of ultraviolet lamps for tanning, henceforth to be known as sunlamp products and ultraviolet lamps intended for use in sunlamp products. Final order. *Federal Registister*, **79**(105), 31205–31214.

FDA (2015). General and plastic surgery devices: restricted sale, distribution, and use of sunlamp products. Retrieved from www.federalregister.gov/documents/2015/12/22/2015-32024/general-and-plastic-surgery-devices-restricted-sale-distribution-and-use-of-sunlamp-products

Feldman, S. R., Liguori, A., Kucenic, M., et al. (2004). Ultraviolet exposure is a reinforcing stimulus in frequent indoor tanners. *Journal of the American Academy of Dermatology*, **51** (1), 45–51. doi:10.1016/j.jaad.2004.01.053

Fell, G. L., Robinson, K. C., Mao, J., Woolf, C. J. & Fisher, D. E. (2014). Skin beta-endorphin mediates addiction to UV light. *Cell*, **157**(7), 1527–1534. doi:10.1016/j.cell.2014.04.032

Feng, J., Frisard, C., Nahar, V. K., et al. (2017). Gender differences in indoor tanning habits and location. *Journal of the American Academy of Dermatology*. doi:10.1016/j.jaad.2017.10.015

First, M., Spitzer, R., Gibbon, M. & Williams, J. (1995). *Structured Clinical Interview for DSM-IV Axis I Disorders (SCID)*. New York: New York State Psychiatric Institute Biometrics Research Department.

Fisher, D. E. & James, W. D. (2010). Indoor tanning – science, behavior, and policy. *New England Journal of Medicine*, **363**(10), 901–903. doi:10.1056/NEJMp1005999

Flannery, B. A., Volpicelli, J. R. & Pettinati, H. M. (1999). Psychometric properties of the Penn Alcohol Craving Scale. *Alcoholism: Clinical and Experimental Research*, **23**(8), 1289–1295.

Flight, M. H. (2013). Synaptic transmission: summer blues. *Nature Reviews Neuroscience*, **14**(6), 378. doi:10.1038/nrn3517

Flores, K. G., Erdei, E., Luo, L., et al. (2013). A pilot study of genetic variants in dopamine regulators with indoor tanning and melanoma. *Experimental Dermatology*, **22**(9), 576–581. doi:10.1111/exd.12200

Gambichler, T., Bader, A., Vojvodic, M., et al. (2002). Plasma levels of opioid peptides after sunbed exposures. *British Journal of Dermatology*, **147**(6), 1207–1211.

Gibbons, F. X., Gerrard, M., Lane, D. J., Mahler, H. I. & Kulik, J. A. (2005). Using UV photography to reduce use of tanning booths: a test of cognitive mediation. *Health Psychology*, **24**(4), 358–363. doi:10.1037/0278-6133.24.4.358

Gillen, M. M. & Markey, C. N. (2012). The role of body image and depression in tanning behaviors and attitudes. *Journal of Behavioral Medicine*, **38**(3), 74–82. doi:10.1080/08964289.2012.685499

Guy, G. P., Jr., Berkowitz, Z., Everett Jones, S., et al. (2015). Trends in indoor tanning among US high school students, 2009–2013. *JAMA Dermatology*, **151**(4), 448–450. doi:10.1001/jamadermatol.2014.4677

Guy, G. P., Jr., Berkowitz, Z., Everett Jones, S., Watson, M. & Richardson, L. C. (2017). Prevalence of indoor tanning and association with sunburn among youth in the United States. *JAMA Dermatology*, **153**(5), 387–390. doi:10.1001/jamadermatol.2016.6273

Guy, G. P., Jr., Berkowitz, Z., Jones, S. E., et al. (2014). State indoor tanning laws and adolescent indoor tanning. *American Journal of Public Health*, **104**(4), e69–74. doi:10.2105/ajph.2013.301850

Guy, G. P., Jr., Berkowitz, Z., Watson, M., Holman, D. M. & Richardson, L. C. (2013). Indoor tanning among young non-Hispanic white females. *JAMA Internal Medicine*, **173** (20), 1920–1922. doi:10.1001/jamainternmed.2013.10013

Guy, G. P., Jr., Watson, M., Richardson, L. C. & Lushniak, B. D. (2016). Reducing indoor tanning – an opportunity for melanoma prevention. *JAMA Dermatology*, **152**(3), 257–259. doi:10.1001/jamadermatol.2015.3007

Harrington, C. R., Beswick, T. C., Graves, M., et al. (2012). Activation of the mesostriatal reward pathway with exposure to ultraviolet radiation (UVR) vs. sham UVR in frequent tanners: a pilot study. *Addiction Biology*, **17**(3), 680–686. doi:10.1111/j.1369-1600.2010.00312.x

Harrington, C. R., Beswick, T. C., Leitenberger, J., et al. (2011). Addictive-like behaviours to ultraviolet light among frequent indoor tanners. *Clinical and Experimental Dermatology*, **36**(1), 33–38. doi:10.1111/j.1365-2230.2010.03882.x

Heckman, C. J. & Manne, S. L. (2012). *Shedding Light on Indoor Tanning*. Dordrecht; New York: Springer.

Heckman, C. J., Cohen-Filipic, J., Darlow, S., et al. (2014a). Psychiatric and addictive symptoms of young adult female indoor tanners. *American Journal of Health Promotion*, **28**(3), 168–174. doi:10.4278/ajhp.120912-QUAN-442

Heckman, C., Darlow, S., Cohen-Filipic, J. & Kloss, J. (2016). Mood changes after indoor tanning among college women: associations with psychiatric/addictive symptoms. *Health Psychol Res*, **4**(1), 5453. doi:10.4081/hpr.2016.5453

Heckman, C. J., Darlow, S., Kloss, J. D., et al. (2014b). Measurement of tanning dependence. *Journal of the European Academy of Dermatology and Venereology*, **28** (9), 1179–1185. doi:10.1111/jdv.12243

Heckman, C. J., Darlow, S. D., Kloss, J. D., Munshi, T. & Manne, S. L. (2015). Contextual factors, indoor tanning, and tanning dependence in young women. *American Journal of Health Behavior*, **39**(3), 372–379. doi:10.5993/ajhb.39.3.10

Heckman, C. J., Egleston, B. L., Wilson, D. B. & Ingersoll, K. S. (2008). A preliminary investigation of the predictors of tanning dependence. *American Journal of Health Behavior*, **32**(5), 451–464. doi:10.5555/ajhb.2008.32.5.451

Hillhouse, J. J. & Turrisi, R. (2002). Examination of the efficacy of an appearance-focused intervention to reduce UV exposure. *Journal of Behavioral Medicine*, **25**(4), 395–409.

Hillhouse, J. J., Baker, M. K., Turrisi, R., et al. (2012). Evaluating a measure of tanning abuse and dependence. *Archives of Dermatology*, **148**(7), 815–819. doi:10.1001/archdermatol.2011.2929

Hillhouse, J., Stapleton, J. & Turrisi, R. (2005). Association of frequent indoor UV tanning with seasonal affective disorder. *Archives of Dermatology*, **141**(11), 1465. doi:10.1001/archderm.141.11.1465

Hillhouse, J., Turrisi, R. & Shields, A. L. (2007). Patterns of indoor tanning use: implications for clinical interventions. *Archives of Dermatology*, **143**(12), 1530–1535. doi:10.1001/archderm.143.12.1530

Hillhouse, J., Turrisi, R., Stapleton, J. & Robinson, J. (2008). A randomized controlled trial of an appearance-focused intervention to prevent skin cancer. *Cancer*, **113**(11), 3257–3266. doi:10.1002/cncr.23922

Hillhouse, J., Turrisi, R., Stapleton, J. & Robinson, J. (2010). Effect of seasonal affective disorder and pathological tanning motives on efficacy of an appearance-focused intervention to prevent skin cancer. *Archives of Dermatology*, **146**(5), 485–491. doi:10.1001/archdermatol.2010.85

Holman, D. M., Fox, K. A., Glenn, J. D., et al. (2013). Strategies to reduce indoor tanning: current research gaps and future opportunities for prevention. *American Journal of Preventative Medicine*, **44**(6), 672–681. doi:10.1016/j.amepre.2013.02.014

Jussila, A., Huotari-Orava, R., Ylianttila, L., Partonen, T. & Snellman, E. (2016). Narrow-band ultraviolet B radiation induces the expression of beta-endorphin in human skin in vivo. *Journal of Photochemistry and Photobiology B*, **155**, 104–108. doi:10.1016/j.jphotobiol.2016.01.007

Kaur, M., Liguori, A., Lang, W., et al. (2006). Induction of withdrawal-like symptoms in a small randomized, controlled trial of opioid blockade in frequent tanners. *Journal of the

American Academy of Dermatology, **54**(4), 709–711. doi:10.1016/j.jaad.2005.11.1059

Kourosh, A. S., Harrington, C. R. & Adinoff, B. (2010). Tanning as a behavioral addiction. *American Journal of Drug and Alcohol Abuse*, **36**(5), 284–290. doi:10.3109/00952990.2010.491883

Le Foll, B., Gallo, A., Le Strat, Y., Lu, L. & Gorwood, P. (2009). Genetics of dopamine receptors and drug addiction: a comprehensive review. *Behavioral Pharmacology*, **20**(1), 1–17. doi:10.1097/FBP.0b013e3283242f05

Leary, M. R., Saltzman, J. L. & Georgeson, J. C. (1997). Appearance motivation, obsessive-compulsive tendencies and excessive suntanning in a community sample. *Journal of Health Psychology*, **2**(4), 493–499. doi:10.1177/135910539700200406

Levins, P. C., Carr, D. B., Fisher, J. E., Momtaz, K. & Parrish, J. A. (1983). Plasma beta-endorphin and beta-lipoprotein response to ultraviolet radiation. *The Lancet*, **2**(8342), 166.

Levran, O., Yuferov, V. & Kreek, M. J. (2012). The genetics of the opioid system and specific drug addictions. *Human Genetics*, **131**(6), 823–842. doi:10.1007/s00439-012-1172-4

Lim, H. W., James, W. D., Rigel, D. S., et al. (2011). Adverse effects of ultraviolet radiation from the use of indoor tanning equipment: time to ban the tan. *Journal of the American Academy of Dermatology*, **64**(5), 893–902. doi:10.1016/j.jaad.2011.03.007

Mays, D., Atkins, M. B., Ahn, J. & Tercyak, K. P. (2017). Indoor tanning dependence in young adult women. *Cancer Epidemiology, Biomarkers & Preention*, **26**(11), 1636–1643. doi:10.1158/1055-9965.EPI-17-0403

Miller, K. A., Piombo, S. E., Cho, J., et al. (2018). Prevalence of tanning addiction and behavioral health conditions among ethnically and racially diverse adolescents. *Journal of Investigative Dermatology*, **138**(7), 1511–1517. doi:10.1016/j.jid.2018.02.018

Mosher, C. E. & Danoff-Burg, S. (2010a). Addiction to indoor tanning: relation to anxiety, depression, and substance use. *Archives of Dermatology*, **146**(4), 412–417. doi:10.1001/archdermatol.2009.385

Mosher, C. E. & Danoff-Burg, S. (2010b). Indoor tanning, mental health, and substance use among college students: the significance of gender. *Journal of Health Psychology*, **15**(6), 819–827. doi:10.1177/1359105309357091

Nilsen, L. T., Hannevik, M. & Veierod, M. B. (2016). Ultraviolet exposure from indoor tanning devices: a systematic review. *British Journal of Dermatology*, **174**(4), 730–740. doi:10.1111/bjd.14388

NIMH (2018). Seasonal Affective Disorder. Retrieved from www.nimh.nih.gov/health/topics/seasonal-affective-disorder/index.shtml

Petit, A., Lejoyeux, M., Reynaud, M. & Karila, L. (2014). Excessive indoor tanning as a behavioral addiction: a literature review. *Current Pharmaceutical Design*, **20**(25), 4070–4075.

Poorsattar, S. P. & Hornung, R. L. (2007). UV light abuse and high-risk tanning behavior among undergraduate college students. *Journal of the American Academy of Dermatology*, **56**(3), 375–379. doi:10.1016/j.jaad.2006.08.064

Poorsattar, S. P. & Hornung, R. L. (2010). Tanning addiction: current trends and future treatment. *Expert Review of Dermatology*, **5**(2), 123–125. doi:10.1586/edm.10.14

Rozin, P. & Stoess, C. (1993). Is there a general tendency to become addicted? *Addictive Behavior*, **18**(1), 81–87.

Schneider, S., Schirmbeck, F., Bock, C., et al. (2015). Casting shadows on the prevalence of tanning dependence: an assessment of mCAGE criteria. *Acta Dermato-Venereologica*, **95**(2), 162–168. doi:10.2340/00015555-1907

Seidenberg, A. B., Mahalingam-Dhingra, A., Weinstock, M. A., Sinclair, C. & Geller, A. C. (2015). Youth indoor tanning and skin cancer prevention: lessons from tobacco control. *American Journal of Preventative Medicine*, **48**(2), 188–194. doi:10.1016/j.amepre.2014.08.034

Skobowiat, C., Dowdy, J. C., Sayre, R. M., Tuckey, R. C. & Slominski, A. (2011). Cutaneous hypothalamic-pituitary-adrenal axis homolog: regulation by ultraviolet radiation. *American Journal of Physiology Endocrinology and Metabolism*, **301**(3), E484–493. doi:10.1152/ajpendo.00217.2011.10.1152/ajpendo.00217.2011

Spiro, J., Parker, S., Oliver, I., et al. (1987). Effect of PUVA on plasma and skin immunoreactive alpha-melanocyte stimulating hormone concentrations. *British Journal of Dermatology*, **117**(6), 703–707.

Stapleton, J. L., Hillhouse, J., Levonyan-Radloff, K. & Manne, S. L. (2017). Review of interventions to reduce ultraviolet tanning: need for treatments targeting excessive tanning, an emerging addictive behavior. *Psychology of Addictive Behaviors*, **31**(8), 962–978. doi:10.1037/adb0000289

Stapleton, J. L., Hillhouse, J. J., Turrisi, R., et al. (2016). The Behavioral Addiction Indoor Tanning Screener (BAITS): an evaluation of a brief measure of behavioral addictive symptoms. *Acta Dermato-Venereologica*, **96**(4), 552–553. doi:10.2340/00015555-2290

Sussman, S. (2017). *Substance and Behavioral Addictions: Concepts, Causes, and Cures*. Cambridge, UK; New York, NY: Cambridge University Press.

Sussman, S. & Sussman, A. N. (2011). Considering the definition of addiction. *International Journal of Environmental Research and Public Health*, **8**(10), 4025–4038. doi:10.3390/ijerph8104025

Turrisi, R., Mastroleo, N. R., Stapleton, J. & Mallett, K. (2008). A comparison of 2 brief intervention approaches to reduce indoor tanning behavior in young women who indoor tan very frequently. *Archives of Dermatology*, **144**(11), 1521–1524. doi:10.1001/archderm.144.11.1521

US Congress, t. C., 2nd Session (2010). Compilation of patient protection and affordable care act, as amended through May 1, 2010. Chapter 49, Section 5000B. Imposition of tax on indoor tanning services. Retrieved from http://housedocs.house.gov/energycommerce/ppacacon.pdf

US Department of Health and Human Services (2014). *The Surgeon General's Call to Action to Prevent Skin Cancer*. Washington, DC.

Volkow, N. D., Fowler, J. S., Wang, G. J. & Swanson, J. M. (2004). Dopamine in drug abuse and addiction: results from imaging studies and treatment implications. *Molecular Psychiatry*, **9**(6), 557–569. doi:10.1038/sj.mp.4001507

Warlow, S. M. et al. (2020). Sensitization of incentive salience and the transition to addiction. In S. Sussman (Ed.) *The Cambridge Handbook of Substance and Behavioral Addictions*. Cambridge, UK: Cambridge University Press, pp. 23–37.

Warthan, M. M., Uchida, T. & Wagner, R. F., Jr. (2005). UV light tanning as a type of substance-related disorder. *Archives of Dermatology*, **141**(8), 963–966. doi:10.1001/archderm.141.8.963

Wintzen, M., de Winter, S., Out-Luiting, J. J., van Duinen, S. G. & Vermeer, B. J. (2001a). Presence of immunoreactive beta-endorphin in human skin. *Experimental Dermatology*, **10**(5), 305–311.

Wintzen, M., Ostijn, D. M., Polderman, M. C., et al. (2001b). Total body exposure to ultraviolet radiation does not influence plasma levels of immunoreactive beta-endorphin in man. *Photodermatology, Photoimmunology & Photomedicine*, **17**(6), 256–260.

World Health Organization (2018). Ultraviolet Radiation (UV). Retrieved from www.who.int/uv/en/

31 Considering the Overlap and Nonoverlap of Compulsivity, Impulsivity, and Addiction

Austin W. Blum, MD, JD, and Jon E. Grant, JD, MD, MPH

Introduction

As reflected by the National Institutes of Health (NIH) Research Domain Criteria (RDoC) framework, various forms of mental illness are increasingly understood as disorders of neural circuitry involved in specific cognitive, affective, motivational, or social processes (Cuthbert & Insel, 2013; Insel et al., 2010). Within this research context, the concept of self-control has emerged as an important dimensional construct in psychiatry. In normal human behavior, the exercise of self-control – itself comprised of an array of distinct capacities – allows people to deliberate between conflicting goals and anticipate the possible consequences of their actions. By contrast, across a broad constellation of psychiatric disorders, the inability to exert self-control over a behavior contributes to significant distress or impairment. Therefore, the factors contributing to self-control and the biological processes that underpin them have emerged as the subject of intense scientific interest.

Three leading nosological frameworks for understanding self-control problems are impulsivity, compulsivity, and addiction. Impulsivity refers to behaviors or actions in a broad range of domains that are premature or unduly risky and that often result in negative consequences (Daruna & Barnes, 1993; Evenden, 1999). Compulsivity refers to a tendency toward repetitive or habitual behaviors, which are frequently maladaptive (Gillan et al., 2016; van den Heuvel et al., 2016). Addiction, finally, refers to persistent engagement in behavior that produces short-term reward in the face of adverse consequences (Potenza, 2006).

In addition to serving as useful clinical heuristics, these frameworks are also promising scientific tools in the search for biological markers of mental illness. Some early studies had suggested that impulsivity (also characterized by reward-seeking behavior) and compulsivity (motivated by harm avoidance or tension/anxiety reduction) represent opposite ends of a single dimension (Hollander & Wong, 1995; Stein et al., 1994). Impulsive and compulsive features, however, may be present concurrently in the same disorder or at different times within the same disorder, suggesting that they may share common neurobiological mechanisms (such as impaired "top-down" control of behavior; Fineberg et al., 2014). Adding to the conceptual boundary confusion, addiction is commonly associated with both impulsivity and compulsivity, providing additional evidence that these three concepts may intersect in complex, nonmutually-exclusive ways (Clark, 2014; Grant et al., 2010c). The concept of addiction has also faced fundamental challenges related to whether nonsubstance or "behavioral" addictions should be included under the same umbrella as substance use disorders (Grant & Chamberlain, 2016). These conceptual questions may have far-reaching implications for the diagnostic classification and treatment of psychiatric disorders characterized by diminished control.

In this chapter, we explore the roles that addiction and pathological impulsivity and compulsivity play in contemporary psychiatry. We begin by defining these concepts and providing a basic neurobiological framework for understanding them. After establishing these definitions, we discuss a classical example of each concept: attention-deficit/hyperactivity disorder (ADHD) (impulsivity), obsessive-compulsive disorder (OCD) (compulsivity), and gambling disorder (addiction). The chapter concludes by considering the overlapping features of impulsivity, compulsivity, and addiction, complicating any easy understanding of their contribution to mental illness.

Definitions and Descriptions of Transdiagnostic Concepts

Impulsivity

The ability to act on impulse carries a range of potential advantages as well as the possibility of deleterious consequences. On the one hand, making fast or intuitive decisions may be essential in life-or-death situations; socially, it can bring reputational rewards as these actions may be regarded by others as enterprising or bold (Daruna & Barnes, 1993). On the other hand, the inability to deliberate before acting is associated with a number of maladaptive behaviors and disorders (Moeller et al., 2001), including antisocial personality disorder (Swann et al., 2009), ADHD (Winstanley, Eagle & Robbins, 2006), and suicidality (Oquendo & Mann, 2000).

Measurement of Impulsivity. According to behavioral and neurocognitive data, impulsivity is a multidimensional (i.e., dissociable) construct (Dalley et al., 2008). Two major domains of impulsivity are impulsive action – evidenced by an inability to inhibit motor responses – and impulsive choice, referring to a tendency to make risky decisions (Dalley, Everitt & Robbins, 2011; Grant & Chamberlain, 2014; MacKillop et al., 2016). More specifically, impulsive action reflects an inability to inhibit a prepotent (habitual or dominant) behavioral response, whereas impulsive choice reflects a preference for immediate rewards to the detriment of long-term goals. These dissociable domains have been investigated using an array of personality- and laboratory-based measures.

Two common measures of motor impulsivity (an example of deficient response inhibition which characterizes impulsive action) are go/no-go

Declaration of interest Dr. Grant has received research grant support from the American Foundation for Suicide Prevention, Takeda Pharmaceuticals, and the TLC Foundation for Body-Focused Repetitive Behaviors; he receives yearly compensation from Springer Publishing for acting as Editor-in-Chief of the *Journal of Gambling Studies*; and he has received royalties from American Psychiatric Publishing, McGraw Hill, Norton Press, Johns Hopkins University Press, and Oxford University Press. Dr. Blum has nothing to disclose.

and stop-signal tasks (Band & van Boxtel, 1999). On go/no-go tasks, participants are required to suppress prepotent motor activity in response to a target stimulus. Participants are asked to make a rapid motor response whenever a "go" stimulus appears (e.g., horizontal lines appearing onscreen) but to withhold their responses when a different stimulus appears (e.g., vertical lines). Because go-trials are more frequent than no-go trials, participants develop a prepotent tendency to respond that requires effort to suppress. Motor impulsivity is assessed by the number of times participants incorrectly respond to a no-go trial. By contrast, stop-signal tasks measure a participant's ability to inhibit (or cancel) a motor response that has already been initiated (Aron & Poldrack, 2005; Logan, Cowan & Davis, 1984). In one version of the task, participants are instructed to press a button corresponding to directional arrows appearing onscreen. On a subset of trials ("stop" trials), an auditory tone follows presentation of the "go" stimulus, indicating that participants should attempt to suppress their motor response for the given trial. By varying the time between presentation of the "go" stimulus and the stop signal, the task provides an estimate of the time taken by the brain to inhibit a prepotent response. Participants who take longer to inhibit the response are said to be more impulsive.

As measured by performance on neuroscientific tasks, impulsive choice (i.e., deficient deferment of gratification) refers to either the discounting of a larger reward with increasing delay (time) or to irrational risk-taking. The ability to delay gratification is typically measured using temporal discounting tasks, in which participants are required to choose between an immediate reward (for example, $100) and a larger reward in the future (for example, $150 in six months) (Berns, Laibson & Loewenstein, 2007; Laibson, 1997; also see Reed et al., 2020). The more quickly the subjective value of a reward decreases over time, the more impulsive the participant is said to be (Peters & Büchel, 2011). Similarly, decision-making can be measured using the Iowa Gambling Task (Bechara et al., 1994, 1998) or the Cambridge Gambling Task (Rogers et al., 1999).

Finally, impulsivity can also be conceptualized as an aspect of personality. An extensive literature discusses the use of self-report questionnaires to measure trait impulsivity, including the Barratt Impulsiveness Scale (BIS-11; Patton, Stanford & Barratt, 1995; Stanford et al., 2009) and Eysenck Impulsiveness Questionnaire (I_7; Eysenck et al., 1985). Subscales of the BIS-11 include attentional, motor, and non-planning impulsiveness. The BIS-11 is well suited for use in the population at large and is also sensitive to the more extreme levels of impulsivity that characterize ADHD (Malloy-Diniz et al., 2007).

Neural Substrates of Impulsivity. Individual differences in impulsivity have been experimentally explained by variation in cortical and subcortical mechanisms. One key component underlying impulsive choice is aberrancy in reward-related decision-making, which is consistently associated with activity of the striatum and ventromedial prefrontal cortex (vmPFC; Kable & Glimcher, 2009). In tasks of intertemporal choice, more impulsive participants show sharply decreased neural activity in the medial prefrontal cortex and ventral striatum as delay increases, a pattern not seen in participants with a greater capacity to defer gratification (Kable & Glimcher, 2007). These and other findings suggest that the vmPFC and ventral striatum track the subjective value of both immediate and delayed rewards, taking into account the time at which the reward is received (Kable & Glimcher, 2010; Monterosso & Luo, 2010). In addition, the ability to suppress a motor response appears to be accomplished by distributed circuitry including the right inferior frontal gyrus (rIFG; Aron, Robbins & Poldrack, 2014), evidenced by studies showing that damage to this region is associated with impulsive motor behavior (Aron et al., 2003b; Dodds, Morein-Zamir & Robbins, 2011). A causal role of the rIFG in response inhibition has also been demonstrated using transcranial magnetic stimulation (Chambers et al., 2006).

In sum, different forms of impulsivity are likely driven by distinct but interrelated neural circuits. One such circuit – involved in making trade-offs between risk and reward – includes the vmPFC and the nucleus accumbens/ventral striatum (Robbins et al., 2012). A separate neural circuit underlying response inhibition may include the rIFG, anterior cingulate cortex, and presupplementary motor area (Bari & Robbins, 2013). According to pharmacological manipulations, response inhibition is mediated by the norepinephrine system (Robbins, 2017).

Compulsivity

Like impulsivity, compulsivity may be either adaptive or maladaptive under different circumstances. On the one hand, the ability to act on strong habit – a type of adaptive compulsive behavior – allows one to allocate scarce cognitive resources to more complex tasks (Neal, Wood & Quinn, 2006; Wood, Quinn & Kashy, 2002). Compulsivity has also been linked with the five-factor trait of conscientiousness, describing an orientation toward dependability, organization, and achievement (Samuel & Widiger, 2011). On the other hand, in a maladaptive sense, compulsivity may refer to the performance of repetitive or stereotyped behaviors that are inappropriate to the situation or have no relationship to an overall goal (Dalley et al., 2011). Compulsivity also relates to a sensation of imperfection, described as an unsettling feeling that a situation or act is not "just right" (Sica et al., 2015).

In the *Diagnostic and Statistical Manual of Mental Disorders,* fifth edition (DSM-5), disorders defined by the presence of obsessions and/or compulsions are grouped in a new class of Obsessive-Compulsive and Related Disorders (American Psychiatric Association, 2013). These disorders include OCD, body dysmorphic disorder, hoarding disorder, trichotillomania (hair-pulling disorder), and excoriation (skin-picking) disorder. Compulsivity is also crucial to addiction (Everitt & Robbins, 2013; Koob & Le Moal, 2005).

Measurement of Compulsivity. The domain of self-control most relevant to compulsivity is arguably cognitive flexibility, which indexes a participant's ability to change a behavior when exposed to new information. One common test of cognitive flexibility is the Intra-Extra Dimensional Set Shift (IED) task (Fineberg et al., 2015), a computerized analogue of the Wisconsin Card Sorting Test. In the IED, participants are presented with a screen showing boxes containing two artificial stimulus dimensions: white lines and pink shapes. Through trial and error, participants attempt to learn an underlying rule governing which of the pink shapes is correct. After a fixed number of correct responses, the stimuli and/or rules are changed, and participants must adapt accordingly – they must make a shift either within the shape dimension (the intradimensional shift) or from the shape dimension to the line dimension (the extradimensional shift). Impaired cognitive flexibility is indicated by a greater total number of errors on the task (Owen et al., 1991).

Compulsivity has also been examined as a personality trait and assessed using self-report questionnaires. Obsessive-compulsive thoughts and behaviors, for example, have been assessed with the Padua Inventory (Burns et al., 1996; Sanavio, 1988) and a tendency toward repetitive habitual behaviors has been indexed using the Cambridge–Chicago

Compulsivity Trait Scale (CHI-T; Chamberlain & Grant, 2018). The Padua Inventory has been validated in OCD and gambling disorder (Anholt et al., 2009; Grant & Potenza, 2006a; van den Heuvel et al., 2009), whereas the CHI-T was designed to capture aspects of compulsivity at the population level.

Neural Substrates of Compulsivity. Problematic forms of compulsivity (at least in the setting of OCD) are thought to result from aberrant functioning of cortico-striatal-thalamic-cortical (CSTC) networks, or "loops" (reviewed in Reghunandanan, Fineberg & Stein, 2015). Within these loops, abnormalities have been consistently documented in several structures known to be important in goal-directed behavior, including the prefrontal cortex, thalamus, caudate/putamen (dorsal striatum), and the neurocircuitry associated with these structures. More specifically, functional neuroimaging studies of OCD patients have shown decreased neural activation in brain regions implicated in goal-directed behavioral control (ventromedial prefrontal cortex, caudate) with concomitant over-activation of regions involved in habit learning (presupplementary motor area, putamen; Fineberg et al., 2018). Taken together, these and other studies suggest that the direct pathway of the basal ganglia may become hyperactive in OCD, thereby disrupting the delicate balance between habit-based striatal circuitry and top-down control. In fact, abnormal habit formation may be a common thread across a number of compulsive disorders, including binge eating (and associated obesity) and substance abuse (Voon et al., 2015). Multiple neurotransmitter systems (e.g., serotonin [5-HT], dopamine, and glutamate) have been implicated in compulsivity (see following discussion on the treatment of OCD).

Addiction

The framework of addiction has expanded to encompass a broad range of potentially harmful behaviors. In its historical sense, "addiction" referred to the state of being especially enthusiastic about or devoted to a particular activity (Alexander & Schweighofer, 1988). By the nineteenth century, addiction had acquired its modern signification of a harmful, uncontrolled involvement with drugs – at the time, especially alcohol or opium (Alexander & Schweighofer, 1988). The idea of compulsive drug use remained central to definitions of addiction through the second half of the twentieth century (Jaffe, 1990; O'Brien, Volkow & Li, 2006). In recent years, however, the understanding of addiction has undergone rapid changes. In 2001, Constance Holden wrote an article for *Science* discussing the emerging field of "behavioral" addictions (Holden, 2001), and since that time the question of which disorders should be evaluated under an addiction framework has remained controversial (Billieux et al., 2015; Fong, Reid & Parhami, 2012; Martin & Petry, 2005; Ziauddeen & Fletcher, 2013). Notably, DSM-5 placed gambling disorder within a new category of "substance-related and addictive disorders" in recognition of its similarities with substance use disorders (SUDs) (American Psychiatric Association, 2013; Grant et al., 2010c; Petry, 2006; Potenza, 2014). Although gambling disorder is currently the only nonsubstance-related disorder grouped with SUDs in DSM-5, Internet Gaming Disorder was included in the research appendix as a condition requiring further study (Petry & O'Brien, 2013). (Of note, a similar condition – gaming disorder – is provisionally recognized as an addiction by the 11th revision of the *International Classification of Diseases* [ICD-11]; see www.who.int/features/qa/gaming-disorder/en/; accessed December 10th, 2018.) Potential addictions related to sex (Kor et al., 2013; Reid, 2013; Reid et al., 2012), food (Avena et al., 2012; Ziauddeen, Farooqi & Fletcher, 2012a, 2012b), and shopping are not recognized as independent mental health disorders in DSM-5.

While consensus remains elusive about specific disorders, there is general agreement about some aspects of addiction. Core components of addiction, it seems clear, include: (1) continued engagement in a behavior despite adverse consequences; (2) an appetitive urge or craving state prior to engagement in the behavior; (3) compulsive engagement in the behavior; and (4) impaired control over the behavior (Potenza, 2006; Shaffer, 1999). Under these criteria, behaviors such as gambling could be considered potentially addictive. Recent research also shows that gambling disorder and SUDs share neurobiological features that support their inclusion in a single diagnostic class (Brewer & Potenza, 2008; Grant, Brewer & Potenza, 2006; Potenza, 2008).

Impulsive/Compulsive Features in Addiction. At least initially, drug seeking and using are motivated by the experience of satisfaction or pleasure (a "high"). Drug use and other reward-related behaviors are governed primarily by the mesolimbic dopamine pathway, which links the ventral tegmental area to the nucleus accumbens (NAc)/ventral striatum (Chambers, Taylor & Potenza, 2003; Everitt & Robbins, 2005; Jentsch & Taylor, 1999; Koob & Volkow, 2010). All known drugs of abuse – as well as natural rewards such as food – promote the release of dopamine in the NAc (Kenny, 2011; Sulzer, 2011). Although dopamine was initially associated with the sensation of pleasure, growing evidence suggests that dopaminergic transmission in the NAc plays a more complex role related to reward-based learning, reward processing (e.g., anticipation and outcome evaluation), and incentive salience (i.e., desire or motivation for reward) (Schultz, 2011; Volkow & Li, 2004).

As addiction progresses, control over drug use (or gambling) becomes increasingly habitual and ultimately compulsive. This transition from goal-directed to habitual behavior is underpinned by a shift in processing from the ventral to the dorsal striatum, a region involved in stimulus–response (S-R) habit learning (Everitt & Robbins, 2013; Koob & Volkow, 2010). This shift toward maladaptive S-R learning may represent a trait/vulnerability marker for the development of addiction (Hogarth & Chase, 2011; Hogarth, Chase & Baess, 2012), a consequence of recurrent engagement in the behavior (Belin et al., 2008; Corbit, Nie & Janak, 2012; Nelson & Killcross, 2006), or both.

In summary, the development of addiction may reflect an overall shift from goal-directed ("impulsive") to habitual ("compulsive") behavior (Belin-Rauscent, Everitt & Belin, 2012; Everitt, Dickinson & Robbins, 2001). The complex role of impulsivity and compulsivity in addiction is discussed in greater detail below.

Clinical Characteristics and Treatment

Attention-Deficit/Hyperactivity Disorder

ADHD is the prototypical disorder of impulsivity (Barkley, 1997). It is the most commonly diagnosed psychiatric condition in children, and symptoms persist into adulthood in approximately 60 percent of cases (Kessler et al., 2005). In adults, the consequences of ADHD may include impairment in occupational functioning, interpersonal problems, and increased risk of motor vehicle accidents (Kessler et al., 2005, 2006; Nigg, 2013). The worldwide prevalence of adult ADHD is estimated to be 3.4 percent (range 1.2 percent to 7.3 percent; Fayyad et al., 2007), but the disorder may be more common in young adults. In one study of university students, 8.3 percent met diagnostic criteria for ADHD (Mortier et al., 2015).

Clinical Presentation. In DSM-5, ADHD is defined by a behavioral pattern of impulsivity, hyperactivity, and/or inattention (American Psychiatric Association, 2013). Impulsivity may manifest as social intrusiveness (interrupting others, for example), or a tendency to make important decisions without considering the long-term consequences. Adults with ADHD also frequently have difficulties regulating their emotions (Corbisiero et al., 2013), contributing to functional impairment above and beyond the core ADHD symptoms of inattention and hyperactivity-impulsivity (Barkley & Fischer, 2010).

Psychiatric Comorbidity. ADHD cooccurs with a wide range of other disorders characterized by impulsivity (Kooij et al., 2012). Adolescents screening positive for ADHD have higher rates of gambling behavior and problem gambling than non-ADHD adolescents (Faregh & Derevensky, 2011), a finding that has also been reported in longitudinal studies of young adults (Breyer et al., 2009). In a sample of adult pathological and at-risk gamblers, 25 percent also had ADHD (Grall-Bronnec et al., 2011). Problematic use of the internet (Bernardi & Pallanti, 2009; Carli et al., 2013), substance use disorders (van Emmerik-van Oortmerssen et al., 2012), and compulsive sexual behavior (Odlaug et al., 2013) are also strongly associated with ADHD. Finally, ADHD is closely associated with eating disorders. In a large epidemiologic survey, 5.7 percent of respondents had a lifetime diagnosis of bulimia nervosa and 9.3 percent had been diagnosed with binge-eating disorder (Kessler et al., 2013).

Response to Treatment. Impulsivity in ADHD represents a key target for pharmacological intervention (Arnsten, 2006a). Given that the symptoms of ADHD are thought to be caused by dysregulation of fronto-striatal circuitry and norepinephrine/dopamine neurotransmission (Arnsten, 2006a, 2006b; Biederman, 2005), medications used to treat ADHD likely exert their beneficial effects by acting on these systems (Wilens, 2006).

The first-line treatments for ADHD are psychostimulant medications, such as *d*-amphetamine and methylphenidate. Methylphenidate treatment is linked with improvement in response inhibition, a core cognitive domain implicated in the pathophysiology of ADHD (Aron et al., 2003a; Boonstra et al., 2005). Even so, up to 30 percent of patients do not respond to stimulants or are unable to tolerate them (Madaan et al., 2006). As an alternative to stimulant medications, atomoxetine, a selective norepinephrine reuptake inhibitor, is effective in treating ADHD (Adler et al., 2005; Faraone et al., 2005; Michelson et al., 2003). Venlafaxine (a serotonin–norepinephrine reuptake inhibitor) has shown mixed results (Amiri et al., 2012; Ghanizadeh, Freeman & Berk, 2013). Finally, ADHD has been treated using the wakefulness-promoting agent modafinil (Greenhill et al., 2006). There is little evidence to support the use of serotonin reuptake inhibitors such as citalopram in ADHD (Biederman, Spencer & Wilens, 2004), consistent with neurochemical manipulations showing that the serotonin system is not involved in response inhibition (Chamberlain et al., 2006).

Obsessive–Compulsive Disorder

Obsessive–compulsive disorder (OCD) is a neuropsychiatric disorder characterized by obsessions (recurrent, intrusive thoughts), compulsions (repetitive and ritualistic actions), or both (American Psychiatric Association, 2013). OCD has a lifetime prevalence of 1 percent to 3 percent (Grant, 2014; Ruscio et al., 2010) and is associated with a significant global health burden (Hollander et al., 2016). It is considered the archetypal disorder of compulsivity (Fineberg et al., 2010, 2014).

Clinical Presentation. Based on factor analysis, the symptoms of OCD have been grouped into four distinct subtypes: (1) contamination obsessions with cleaning compulsions; (2) aggressive, sexual, somatic, or religious obsessions with checking compulsions; (3) symmetry obsessions with ordering compulsions; and (4) hoarding (Leckman et al., 1997; Mataix-Cols et al., 2004, 2005). These symptom dimensions have been associated with distinct patterns of psychiatric comorbidity (Hasler et al., 2005), specific genetic polymorphisms (Hasler, Kazuba & Murphy, 2006), and distinct but overlapping patterns of neural activation (Mataix-Cols et al., 2004), as well as differential response to treatment (Mataix-Cols et al., 1999, 2002). OCD usually emerges during childhood or early adulthood (Geller, 2006), with male patients tending to start at an earlier age (Narayanaswamy et al., 2012). If untreated, OCD is usually chronic, with symptoms following a waxing and waning course (Skoog & Skoog, 1999).

Psychiatric Comorbidity. OCD shows considerable overlap with other disorders on the obsessive–compulsive spectrum (Phillips et al., 2010). Patients with OCD have high lifetime rates of tic disorders (up to 30 percent; Leckman et al., 2010) and are at increased risk for developing body dysmorphic disorder (BDD), trichotillomania, and excoriation disorder (Bienvenu et al., 2012; Lochner & Stein, 2010). In studies of participants with BDD, 32 percent to 33 percent had a lifetime diagnosis of OCD (Gunstad & Phillips, 2003; Phillips et al., 2005). OCD also shows significant co-occurrence with obsessive–compulsive personality disorder (roughly 23 percent to 45 percent; Eisen et al., 2010; Starcevic et al., 2013).

Response to Treatment. Evidence-based treatments for OCD include cognitive-behavioral therapy involving exposure and response prevention (Foa, 2010; Simpson et al., 2011) and pharmacotherapy with selective serotonin reuptake inhibitors (SSRIs) or the tricyclic antidepressant clomipramine (Bandelow et al., 2008; Grant, 2014). SSRIs are used as the first-line pharmacologic treatment for OCD (over clomipramine) due to their relatively low adverse-effect profile (Fineberg et al., 2012). In treatment-resistant OCD, treatment options include switching to another SSRI or augmentation with a low-dose antipsychotic agent (Abudy, Juven-Wetzler & Zohar, 2011), especially in patients with tics (Fineberg et al., 2006).

Many patients (40 percent to 65 percent) respond to adequate trials of SSRIs or clomipramine (Mancebo et al., 2006; Reddy et al., 2010). The generally positive response of OCD to these drugs (collectively, serotonin reuptake inhibitors [SRIs]) supports a key role for serotonin dysregulation in the pathophysiology of the disorder (Chamberlain & Fineberg, 2013). Antidepressants which lack serotonergic action, such as desipramine (a relatively selective norepinephrine reuptake inhibitor), are typically ineffective in the treatment of OCD (Zohar & Insel, 1987).

Because up to 60 percent of OCD patients receive little or no benefit from SRIs, however, some new pharmacological approaches have targeted neurotransmitters other than serotonin. One of these targets is glutamate, the primary excitatory neurotransmitter in the cortico-striatal-thalamic-cortical (CSTC) circuit. Both neuroimaging and genetics studies have found that glutamatergic dysregulation may contribute to the pathophysiology of OCD (Pittenger, Bloch & Williams, 2011; Simpson et al., 2012; Wu et al., 2012). Glutamate-modulating agents have demonstrated therapeutic benefit in OCD as monotherapy (as in the case of the NMDA receptor antagonist ketamine; Rodriguez et al., 2013) or as augmentation to SRI treatment (Leppink & Grant, 2017).

For patients with severe, treatment-refractory OCD, neurosurgery provides a potential option. In 2009, the US Food and Drug Administration (FDA) approved deep brain stimulation (DBS) targeting the ventral capsule/ventral striatum for intractable OCD (Greenberg, Rauch & Haber, 2010). A recent meta-analysis determined that 60 percent of patients respond to DBS, as measured by a $\geq$35 percent reduction in symptom severity (Alonso et al., 2015). Although the mechanism of DBS remains unclear, it appears to exert complex and widespread changes in CSTC loops (Makris et al., 2016). Gamma knife ventral capsulotomy (a type of stereotactic radiosurgery) has also been used successfully in intractable OCD (Greenberg et al., 2003; Lopes et al., 2009).

Gambling Disorder

Gambling Disorder (GD, previously known as pathological gambling) is a psychiatric disorder characterized by persistent and recurrent maladaptive patterns of gambling behavior (American Psychiatric Association, 2013). Although most people who gamble do so without adverse consequences, those with GD continue to gamble despite significant personal, financial, and social costs (Hodgins, Stea & Grant, 2011). Disordered gambling is associated with a poor quality of life (Black, Moyer & Schlosser, 2003; Grant & Kim, 2005) and greater overall health problems (Hong, Sacco & Cunningham-Williams, 2009; Morasco & Petry, 2006). Suicide attempts are also relatively common (17 percent prevalence among treatment-seeking gamblers; Petry & Kiluk, 2002).

Clinical Presentation. Like substance addictions, GD is characterized by symptoms of craving, tolerance, and withdrawal. Disordered gambling usually begins in adolescence or early adulthood, with male gamblers tending to start at a younger age than females (Chambers & Potenza, 2003; Grant & Kim, 2001). Women, however, appear to progress from recreational to disordered gambling more quickly than men (Grant, Odlaug & Mooney, 2012) – a phenomenon called *telescoping* that has also been documented in some (but not all) studies of SUDs (Brady & Randall, 1999; Keyes et al., 2010). As in SUDs, up to one-third of people with GD recover without formal treatment (Slutske, 2006).

Psychiatric Comorbidity. Gambling Disorder frequently cooccurs with other psychiatric disorders. In clinical samples, 35 percent to 63 percent of disordered gamblers have screened positive for a lifetime SUD (Argo & Black, 2004; Grall-Bronnec et al., 2011; Wareham & Potenza, 2010), a rate substantially higher than that reported in the general population (26.6 percent; Kessler et al., 1994). Other studies have reported high rates of cooccurring mood, anxiety, and personality disorders among disordered gamblers (Grant, 2008; Kessler et al., 2008; Petry, Stinson & Grant, 2005). GD has also shown overlap with other putative behavioral addictions (compulsive sexual behavior and compulsive buying; Black & Moyer, 1998).

Response to Treatment. Multiple neurotransmitter systems (e.g., glutamatergic, opioidergic, serotonergic, dopaminergic) have been implicated in the pathophysiology of GD and other addictions (Clark & Limbrick-Oldfield, 2013; Leeman & Potenza, 2012, 2013; Limbrick-Oldfield, van Holst & Clark, 2013). The diversity of these systems and variety of pharmacologic agents used to treat GD (glutamate modulators, opioid antagonists, SRIs) reflect the considerable heterogeneity of GD. Although there are no FDA-approved treatments for GD, a meta-analysis of sixteen outcome studies found that pharmacological treatments were more effective for disordered gambling than placebo (overall effect size = 0.78; Pallesen et al., 2007).

The glutamate system plays a key role in drug reward, reinforcement, and relapse (Bowers, Chen & Bonci, 2010; Kalivas et al. 2009) and also appears to be dysfunctional in GD (Nordin, Gupta & Sjödin, 2007). Therefore, glutamate-modulating agents have been used to reduce reward-seeking behavior in a variety of substance and behavioral addictions (Olive et al., 2012). In one study, treatment with *N*-acetylcysteine – an amino acid that appears to normalize glutamatergic signaling in the nucleus accumbens – significantly decreased core symptoms of problem gambling (Grant, Kim & Odlaug, 2007). Memantine has also shown positive results in GD and may operate by improving cognitive measures related to compulsivity (Grant et al., 2010a). Taken together, these results suggest a role for glutamate in the pathophysiology of disordered gambling.

Opioid antagonists have also produced generally positive results. Opioid antagonists decrease dopamine release in the mesolimbic pathway and have been used successfully to dampen gambling-related excitement and cravings (Kim, 1998). The mu (μ)-opioid antagonist naltrexone has shown superiority to placebo in reducing gambling urges and behavior and may preferentially benefit participants with a positive family history of alcohol dependence (Grant, Kim & Odlaug, 2009; Kim et al., 2001). The opioid antagonist nalmefene has also demonstrated efficacy in treating GD (Grant et al., 2006, 2010b). These findings suggest that opioid pathways may play an important role in behavioral addictions (as in substance use disorders).

Although serotonergic dysfunction appears to be implicated in GD (Potenza, 2008), most placebo-controlled studies of SRIs (including paroxetine [Grant et al., 2003; Kim et al., 2002], fluvoxamine [Blanco et al., 2002; Hollander et al., 2000], and sertraline [Saiz-Ruiz et al., 2005]) have shown mixed results, with both positive and negative findings reported. Escitalopram, however, may be effective for gamblers with cooccurring anxiety disorders (Grant & Potenza, 2006b). Thus, individual differences among disordered gamblers may be relevant to treatment outcomes.

Our relatively limited understanding of the neurobiology of disordered gambling has hindered the development of targeted treatments for GD (Potenza et al., 2013). Future research should therefore continue to investigate whether intermediate phenotypes or endophenotypes relevant to addiction – such as compulsivity and impulsivity – represent viable therapeutic targets in GD.

Impulsivity/Compulsivity/Addiction: Overlapping Constructs

As discussed, impulsivity, compulsivity, and addiction seem to be governed by relatively dissociable neural and neurochemical systems. Impulsivity implicates a brain circuit including the ventral striatum, ventromedial prefrontal cortex, and anterior cingulate cortex. Compulsivity, by contrast, centers on a different neural circuit involving the dorsal striatum and orbitofrontal cortex. Despite their differences, however, impulsivity and compulsivity also share a key common factor: dysregulated function of prefrontal cortex/striatal circuitry. Furthermore, reflecting their hypothetical shared neurobiology, impulsive and compulsive behaviors may be seen either at different time points or simultaneously within the same disorder.

Most notably, impulsive and compulsive behaviors are both prominent in addiction, in which impulsive behaviors (such as gambling or drug use) may become compulsive due to neuroplastic changes within the ventral/dorsal striatum. Conversely, compulsive behaviors (such as handwashing rituals in OCD) may eventually become automatic or "impulsive." By better understanding the conceptual overlap among addiction, impulsivity, and compulsivity, new and more effective treatments may be devised.

Compulsivity/Impulsivity in Gambling Disorder

Like substance use disorders, gambling disorder is associated with behavioral and cognitive measures of impulsivity. According to one meta-analysis, the primary impulsive personality traits identified in problem gamblers included negative urgency and low premeditation, as measured by the UPPS Impulsive Behavior Scale (Maclaren et al., 2011). Moreover, impulsivity in these gamblers is evidenced by impaired risk/reward decision-making (measured by the Iowa Gambling Task) and steep discounting of delayed rewards (Conversano et al., 2012; Leeman & Potenza, 2012; van Holst et al., 2010a, 2010b).

In addition to impulsivity, problem gambling is associated with multiple features of compulsivity. Similar to disorders on the obsessive-compulsive spectrum, gambling disorder is characterized by repetitive or compulsive engagement in a behavior (gambling) and ritualistic behavior – for example, gambling on particular slot machines or performing gambling tasks in a specific order (Grant & Potenza, 2006a). In other studies examining aspects of compulsivity, disordered gamblers have shown higher scores than healthy controls on the Padua Inventory (a measure of compulsivity; Bottesi et al., 2015), greater response perseveration on reversal learning tasks (de Ruiter et al., 2009), and more total errors on the Intra-Extra Dimensional Set Shift (IED) task (Grant et al., 2010a). Problem gamblers are also relatively slow to adapt to new reward contingencies, indicating impaired flexibility in reward learning (Vanes et al., 2014). Further complicating matters, recent research has suggested a genetic link between gambling disorder and OCD (Scherrer et al., 2015).

Impulsive Features of OCD

Although OCD is commonly regarded as the prototypical disorder of compulsive behavior, it also exhibits impulsive features (Ettelt et al., 2007; Potenza, 2007). In one study, participants with OCD showed significantly higher scores of cognitive impulsiveness on the Barratt Impulsiveness Scale than matched controls (Ettelt et al., 2007). In the same study, cognitive–attentional impulsiveness was linked with aggressive obsessions and checking compulsions, but not washing (Ettelt et al., 2007). These findings suggest that certain subtypes of OCD may have more impulsive features than others. In addition, a subset of people with OCD has been noted to show increased positive affect (rather than distress) in anticipation of performing OCD-related compulsions (Kashyap et al., 2012).

From a neuroanatomical perspective, some have postulated that OCD-related behaviors may become increasingly driven by the ventral striatum over time, resulting in these behaviors taking on an "impulsive" or hedonic quality (Fontenelle et al., 2011). Further supporting this hypothesis, the nucleus accumbens/ventral striatum has demonstrated efficacy as a treatment target for deep brain stimulation in severe OCD (Denys et al., 2010). Thus, "impulsive compulsions" in OCD may be linked with ventral cortico-striatal circuits previously implicated in other impulsive behaviors.

Conclusions

Impulsivity and compulsivity are key transdiagnostic constructs in psychiatry. As top-level symptoms, impulsive and compulsive behaviors are listed explicitly in the diagnostic criteria for ADHD, OCD, gambling disorder, and several other conditions characterized by diminished control. From this perspective, particular impulsive or compulsive behaviors – such as acting out of turn, handwashing rituals, or repeated gambling – are seen as core elements of their respective disorders. Alternatively, from a neurobiological perspective, impulsivity and compulsivity have been viewed as separate neurocognitive constructs mediated by specific neural circuits and neurochemical systems. Under either frame of reference, however, impulsivity and compulsivity show substantial overlap. These constructs often have similar clinical presentations, arise from parallel brain circuits, and sometimes respond to the same classes of pharmacological agents. It is hoped that a better understanding of the complex relationship between impulsivity and compulsivity will promote the development of more effective therapies for impulsive, compulsive and addictive disorders.

REFERENCES

Abudy, A., Juven-Wetzler, A. & Zohar, J. (2011). Pharmacological management of treatment-resistant obsessive-compulsive disorder. *CNS Drugs*, **25**(7), 585–596. https://doi.org/10.2165/11587860-000000000-00000

Adler, L. A., Spencer, T. J., Milton, D. R., Moore, R. J. & Michelson, D. (2005). Long-term, open-label study of the safety and efficacy of atomoxetine in adults with attention-deficit/hyperactivity disorder: an interim analysis. *The Journal of Clinical Psychiatry*, **66**(3), 294–299.

Alexander, B. K. & Schweighofer, A. R. F. (1988). Defining "addiction." *Canadian Psychology/Psychologie Canadienne*, **29**(2), 151–162. https://doi.org/10.1037/h0084530

Alonso, P., Cuadras, D., Gabriëls, L., et al. (2015). Deep brain stimulation for obsessive-compulsive disorder: a meta-analysis of treatment outcome and predictors of response. *PLoS ONE*, **10**(7), e0133591. https://doi.org/10.1371/journal.pone.0133591

American Psychiatric Association (2013). *Diagnostic and Statistical Manual of Mental Disorders* (5th edition). Washington, DC: American Psychiatric Publishing.

Amiri, S., Farhang, S., Ghoreishizadeh, M. A., Malek, A. & Mohammadzadeh, S. (2012). Double-blind controlled trial of venlafaxine for treatment of adults with attention deficit/hyperactivity disorder. *Human Psychopharmacology*, **27**(1), 76–81. https://doi.org/10.1002/hup.1274

Anholt, G. E., van Oppen, P., Emmelkamp, P. M. G., et al. (2009). Measuring obsessive-compulsive symptoms: Padua Inventory-Revised vs. Yale-Brown Obsessive Compulsive Scale. *Journal of Anxiety Disorders*, **23**(6), 830–835. https://doi.org/10.1016/j.janxdis.2009.04.004

Argo, T. R. & Black, D. W. (2004). Clinical characteristics. In *Pathological Gambling: A Clinical Guide to Treatment*. Arlington, VA, US: American Psychiatric Publishing, Inc., pp. 39–53.

Arnsten, A. F. T. (2006a). Fundamentals of attention-deficit/hyperactivity disorder: circuits and pathways. *The Journal of Clinical Psychiatry*, **67** (Supplement 8), 7–12.

Arnsten, A. F. T. (2006b). Stimulants: therapeutic actions in ADHD. *Neuropsychopharmacology*, **31**(11), 2376–2383. https://doi.org/10.1038/sj.npp.1301164

Aron, A. R. & Poldrack, R. A. (2005). The cognitive neuroscience of response inhibition: relevance for genetic research in attention-deficit/hyperactivity disorder. *Biological Psychiatry*, **57**(11), 1285–1292. https://doi.org/10.1016/j.biopsych.2004.10.026

Aron, A. R., Dowson, J. H., Sahakian, B. J. & Robbins, T. W. (2003a). Methylphenidate improves response inhibition in adults with attention-deficit/hyperactivity disorder. *Biological Psychiatry*, **54**(12), 1465–1468.

Aron, A. R., Fletcher, P. C., Bullmore, E. T., Sahakian, B. J. & Robbins, T. W. (2003b). Stop-signal inhibition disrupted by damage to right inferior frontal gyrus in humans. *Nature Neuroscience*, **6**(2), 115–116. https://doi.org/10.1038/nn1003

Aron, A. R., Robbins, T. W. & Poldrack, R. A. (2014). Inhibition and the right inferior frontal cortex: one decade on. *Trends in Cognitive Sciences*, **18**(4), 177–185. https://doi.org/10.1016/j.tics.2013.12.003

Avena, N. M., Gearhardt, A. N., Gold, M. S., Wang, G.-J. & Potenza, M. N. (2012). Tossing the baby out with the bathwater after a brief rinse? The potential downside of dismissing food addiction based on limited data. *Nature Reviews Neuroscience*, **13**(7), 514; author reply 514. https://doi.org/10.1038/nrn3212-c1

Band, G. P. & van Boxtel, G. J. (1999). Inhibitory motor control in stop paradigms: review and reinterpretation of neural mechanisms. *Acta Psychologica*, **101**(2–3), 179–211.

Bandelow, B., Zohar, J., Hollander, E. & WFSBP Task Force on Treatment Guidelines for Anxiety, Obsessive-Compulsive and Post-Traumatic Stress Disoders (2008). World Federation of Societies of Biological Psychiatry (WFSBP) guidelines for the pharmacological treatment of anxiety, obsessive-compulsive and post-traumatic stress disorders – first revision. *The World Journal of Biological Psychiatry*, **9**(4), 248–312. https://doi.org/10.1080/15622970802465807

Bari, A. & Robbins, T. W. (2013). Inhibition and impulsivity: behavioral and neural basis of response control. *Progress in Neurobiology*, **108**, 44–79. https://doi.org/10.1016/j.pneurobio.2013.06.005

Barkley, R. A. (1997). Behavioral inhibition, sustained attention, and executive functions: constructing a unifying theory of ADHD. *Psychological Bulletin*, **121**(1), 65–94. https://doi.org/10.1037/0033-2909.121.1.65

Barkley, R. A. & Fischer, M. (2010). The unique contribution of emotional impulsiveness to impairment in major life activities in hyperactive children as adults. *Journal of the American Academy of Child and Adolescent Psychiatry*, **49**(5), 503–513.

Bechara, A., Damasio, A. R., Damasio, H. & Anderson, S. W. (1994). Insensitivity to future consequences following damage to human prefrontal cortex. *Cognition*, **50**(1–3), 7–15.

Bechara, A., Damasio, H., Tranel, D. & Anderson, S. W. (1998). Dissociation of working memory from decision making within the human prefrontal cortex. *Journal of Neuroscience*, **18**(1), 428–437. https://doi.org/10.1523/JNEUROSCI.18-01-00428.1998

Belin, D., Mar, A. C., Dalley, J. W., Robbins, T. W. & Everitt, B. J. (2008). High impulsivity predicts the switch to compulsive cocaine-taking. *Science*, **320**(5881), 1352–1355. https://doi.org/10.1126/science.1158136

Belin-Rauscent, A., Everitt, B. J. & Belin, D. (2012). Intrastriatal shifts mediate the transition from drug-seeking actions to habits. *Biological Psychiatry*, **72**(5), 343–345. https://doi.org/10.1016/j.biopsych.2012.07.001

Bernardi, S. & Pallanti, S. (2009). Internet addiction: a descriptive clinical study focusing on comorbidities and dissociative symptoms. *Comprehensive Psychiatry*, **50**(6), 510–516. https://doi.org/10.1016/j.comppsych.2008.11.011

Berns, G. S., Laibson, D. & Loewenstein, G. (2007). Intertemporal choice – toward an integrative framework. *Trends in Cognitive Sciences*, **11**(11), 482–488. doi.org/10.1016/j.tics.2007.08.011

Biederman, J. (2005). Attention-deficit/hyperactivity disorder: a selective overview. *Biological Psychiatry*, **57**(11), 1215–1220. https://doi.org/10.1016/j.biopsych.2004.10.020

Biederman, J., Spencer, T. & Wilens, T. (2004). Evidence-based pharmacotherapy for attention-deficit hyperactivity disorder. *The International Journal of Neuropsychopharmacology*, **7**(1), 77–97. https://doi.org/10.1017/S1461145703003973

Bienvenu, O. J., Samuels, J. F., Wuyek, L. A., et al. (2012). Is obsessive-compulsive disorder an anxiety disorder, and what, if any, are spectrum conditions? A family study perspective. *Psychological Medicine*, **42**(1), 1–13. https://doi.org/10.1017/S0033291711000742

Billieux, J., Schimmenti, A., Khazaal, Y., Maurage, P. & Heeren, A. (2015). Are we overpathologizing everyday life? A tenable blueprint for behavioral addiction research. *Journal of Behavioral Addictions*, **4**(3), 119–123. https://doi.org/10.1556/2006.4.2015.009

Black, D. W. & Moyer, T. (1998). Clinical features and psychiatric comorbidity of subjects with pathological gambling behavior. *Psychiatric Services*, **49**(11), 1434–1439. https://doi.org/10.1176/ps.49.11.1434

Black, D. W., Moyer, T. & Schlosser, S. (2003). Quality of life and family history in pathological gambling. *The Journal of Nervous and Mental Disease*, **191**(2), 124–126. https://doi.org/10.1097/01.NMD.0000050942.86352.47

Blanco, C., Petkova, E., Ibáñez, A. & Sáiz-Ruiz, J. (2002). A pilot placebo-controlled study of fluvoxamine for pathological gambling. *Annals of Clinical Psychiatry*, **14**(1), 9–15.

Boonstra, A. M., Kooij, J. J. S., Oosterlaan, J., Sergeant, J. A. & Buitelaar, J. K. (2005). Does methylphenidate improve inhibition and other cognitive abilities in adults with childhood-onset ADHD? *Journal of Clinical and Experimental Neuropsychology*, **27**(3), 278–298. https://doi.org/10.1080/13803390490515757

Bottesi, G., Ghisi, M., Ouimet, A. J., Tira, M. D. & Sanavio, E. (2015). Compulsivity and impulsivity in pathological gambling: does a dimensional-transdiagnostic approach add clinical utility to DSM-5 classification? *Journal of Gambling Studies*, **31**(3), 825–847. https://doi.org/10.1007/s10899-014-9470-5

Bowers, M. S., Chen, B. T. & Bonci, A. (2010). AMPA receptor synaptic plasticity induced by psychostimulants: the past, present, and therapeutic future. *Neuron*, **67**(1), 11–24. https://doi.org/10.1016/j.neuron.2010.06.004

Brady, K. T. & Randall, C. L. (1999). Gender differences in substance use disorders. *The Psychiatric Clinics of North America*, **22**(2), 241–252.

Brewer, J. A. & Potenza, M. N. (2008). The neurobiology and genetics of impulse control disorders: relationships to drug addictions. *Biochemical Pharmacology*, **75**(1), 63–75. https://doi.org/10.1016/j.bcp.2007.06.043

Breyer, J. L., Botzet, A. M., Winters, K. C., et al. (2009). Young adult gambling behaviors and their relationship with the persistence of ADHD. *Journal of Gambling Studies*, **25**(2), 227–238. https://doi.org/10.1007/s10899-009-9126-z

Burns, G. L., Keortge, S. G., Formea, G. M. & Sternberger, L. G. (1996). Revision of the Padua Inventory of obsessive compulsive disorder symptoms: distinctions between worry, obsessions, and compulsions. *Behaviour Research and Therapy*, **34**(2), 163–173.

Carli, V., Durkee, T., Wasserman, D., et al. (2013). The association between pathological internet use and comorbid psychopathology: a systematic review. *Psychopathology*, **46**(1), 1–13. https://doi.org/10.1159/000337971

Chamberlain, S. & Fineberg, N. A. (2013). The neurobiology of obsessive-compulsive disorder. In K. N. Ochsner & S. Kosslyn (Eds.), *The Oxford Handbook of Cognitive*

Neuroscience: Volume 2: The Cutting Edges. New York, NY: Oxford University Press. https://doi.org/10.1093/oxfordhb/9780199988709.013.0029

Chamberlain, S. R. & Grant, J. E. (2018). Initial validation of a transdiagnostic compulsivity questionnaire: the Cambridge–Chicago Compulsivity Trait Scale. *CNS Spectrums*, 1–7. https://doi.org/10.1017/S1092852918000810

Chamberlain, S. R., Müller, U., Blackwell, A. D., et al. (2006). Neurochemical modulation of response inhibition and probabilistic learning in humans. *Science*, **311**(5762), 861–863. https://doi.org/10.1126/science.1121218

Chambers, C. D., Bellgrove, M. A., Stokes, M. G., et al. (2006). Executive "brake failure" following deactivation of human frontal lobe. *Journal of Cognitive Neuroscience*, **18**(3), 444–455. https://doi.org/10.1162/089892906775990606

Chambers, R. A. & Potenza, M. N. (2003). Neurodevelopment, impulsivity, and adolescent gambling. *Journal of Gambling Studies*, **19**(1), 53–84.

Chambers, R. A., Taylor, J. R. & Potenza, M. N. (2003). Developmental neurocircuitry of motivation in adolescence: a critical period of addiction vulnerability. *The American Journal of Psychiatry*, **160**(6), 1041–1052. https://doi.org/10.1176/appi.ajp.160.6.1041

Clark, L. (2014). Disordered gambling: the evolving concept of behavioral addiction. *Annals of the New York Academy of Sciences*, **1327**, 46–61. https://doi.org/10.1111/nyas.12558

Clark, L. & Limbrick-Oldfield, E. H. (2013). Disordered gambling: a behavioral addiction. *Current Opinion in Neurobiology*, **23**(4), 655–659. https://doi.org/10.1016/j.conb.2013.01.004

Conversano, C., Marazziti, D., Carmassi, C., et al. (2012). Pathological gambling: a systematic review of biochemical, neuroimaging, and neuropsychological findings. *Harvard Review of Psychiatry*, **20**(3), 130–148. https://doi.org/10.3109/10673229.2012.694318

Corbisiero, S., Stieglitz, R.-D., Retz, W. & Rösler, M. (2013). Is emotional dysregulation part of the psychopathology of ADHD in adults? *Attention Deficit and Hyperactivity Disorders*, **5**(2), 83–92. https://doi.org/10.1007/s12402-012-0097-z

Corbit, L. H., Nie, H. & Janak, P. H. (2012). Habitual alcohol seeking: time course and the contribution of subregions of the dorsal striatum. *Biological Psychiatry*, **72**(5), 389–395. https://doi.org/10.1016/j.biopsych.2012.02.024

Cuthbert, B. N. & Insel, T. R. (2013). Toward the future of psychiatric diagnosis: the seven pillars of RDoC. *BMC Medicine*, **11**, 126. https://doi.org/10.1186/1741-7015-11-126

Dalley, J. W., Everitt, B. J. & Robbins, T. W. (2011). Impulsivity, compulsivity, and top-down cognitive control. *Neuron*, **69**(4), 680–694. https://doi.org/10.1016/j.neuron.2011.01.020

Dalley, J. W., Mar, A. C., Economidou, D. & Robbins, T. W. (2008). Neurobehavioral mechanisms of impulsivity: fronto-striatal systems and functional neurochemistry. *Pharmacology, Biochemistry, and Behavior*, **90**(2), 250–260. https://doi.org/10.1016/j.pbb.2007.12.021

Daruna, J. H. & Barnes, P. A. (1993). A neurodevelopmental view of impulsivity. In *The Impulsive Client: Theory, Research, and Treatment*. Washington, DC: American Psychological Association, pp. 23–37. https://doi.org/10.1037/10500-002

de Ruiter, M. B., Veltman, D. J., Goudriaan, A. E., et al. (2009). Response perseveration and ventral prefrontal sensitivity to reward and punishment in male problem gamblers and smokers. *Neuropsychopharmacology*, **34**(4), 1027–1038. https://doi.org/10.1038/npp.2008.175

Denys, D., Mantione, M., Figee, M., et al. (2010). Deep brain stimulation of the nucleus accumbens for treatment-refractory obsessive-compulsive disorder. *Archives of General Psychiatry*, **67**(10), 1061–1068. https://doi.org/10.1001/archgenpsychiatry.2010.122

Dodds, C. M., Morein-Zamir, S. & Robbins, T. W. (2011). Dissociating inhibition, attention, and response control in the frontoparietal network using functional magnetic resonance imaging. *Cerebral Cortex*, **21**(5), 1155–1165. https://doi.org/10.1093/cercor/bhq187

Eisen, J. L., Pinto, A., Mancebo, M. C., et al. (2010). A 2-year prospective follow-up study of the course of obsessive-compulsive disorder. *The Journal of Clinical Psychiatry*, **71**(8), 1033–1039. https://doi.org/10.4088/JCP.08m04806blu

Ettelt, S., Ruhrmann, S., Barnow, S., et al. (2007). Impulsiveness in obsessive-compulsive disorder: results from a family study. *Acta Psychiatrica Scandinavica*, **115**(1), 41–47. https://doi.org/10.1111/j.1600-0447.2006.00835.x

Evenden, J. L. (1999). Varieties of impulsivity. *Psychopharmacology*, **146**(4), 348–361.

Everitt, B. J., Dickinson, A. & Robbins, T. W. (2001). The neuropsychological basis of addictive behaviour. *Brain Research. Brain Research Reviews*, **36**(2–3), 129–138.

Everitt, B. J. & Robbins, T. W. (2005). Neural systems of reinforcement for drug addiction: from actions to habits to compulsion. *Nature Neuroscience*, **8**(11), 1481–1489. https://doi.org/10.1038/nn1579

Everitt, B. J. & Robbins, T. W. (2013). From the ventral to the dorsal striatum: devolving views of their roles in drug addiction. *Neuroscience & Biobehavioral Reviews*, **37**(9, Part A), 1946–1954. https://doi.org/10.1016/j.neubiorev.2013.02.010

Eysenck, S. B. G., Pearson, P. R., Easting, G. & Allsopp, J. F. (1985). Age norms for impulsiveness, venturesomeness and empathy in adults. *Personality and Individual Differences*, **6**(5), 613–619. https://doi.org/10.1016/0191-8869(85)90011-X

Faraone, S. V., Biederman, J., Spencer, T., et al. (2005). Efficacy of atomoxetine in adult attention-deficit/hyperactivity disorder: a drug-placebo response curve analysis. *Behavioral and Brain Functions*, **1**, 16. https://doi.org/10.1186/1744-9081-1-16

Faregh, N. & Derevensky, J. (2011). Gambling behavior among adolescents with attention deficit/hyperactivity disorder. *Journal of Gambling Studies*, **27**(2), 243–256. https://doi.org/10.1007/s10899-010-9211-3

Fayyad, J., De Graaf, R., Kessler, R., et al. (2007). Cross-national prevalence and correlates of adult attention-deficit hyperactivity disorder. *The British Journal of Psychiatry*, **190**, 402–409. https://doi.org/10.1192/bjp.bp.106.034389

Fineberg, N. A., Apergis-Schoute, A. M., Vaghi, M. M., et al. (2018). Mapping compulsivity in the DSM-5 obsessive compulsive and related disorders: cognitive domains, neural circuitry, and treatment. *The International Journal of Neuropsychopharmacology*, **21**(1), 42–58. https://doi.org/10.1093/ijnp/pyx088

Fineberg, N. A., Brown, A., Reghunandanan, S. & Pampaloni, I. (2012). Evidence-based pharmacotherapy of obsessive-compulsive disorder. *The International Journal of Neuropsychopharmacology*, **15**(8), 1173–1191. https://doi.org/10.1017/S1461145711001829

Fineberg, N. A., Chamberlain, S. R., Goudriaan, A. E., et al. (2014). New developments in human neurocognition: clinical, genetic, and brain imaging correlates of impulsivity and compulsivity. *CNS Spectrums*, **19**(1), 69–89. https://doi.org/10.1017/S1092852913000801

Fineberg, N. A., Day, G. A., de Koenigswarter, N., et al. (2015). The neuropsychology of obsessive-compulsive personality disorder: a new analysis. *CNS Spectrums*, **20**(5), 490–499. https://doi.org/10.1017/S1092852914000662

Fineberg, N. A., Potenza, M. N., Chamberlain, S. R., et al.B (2010). Probing compulsive and impulsive behaviors, from animal models to endophenotypes: a narrative review. *Neuropsychopharmacology*, **35**(3), 591–604. https://doi.org/10.1038/npp.2009.185

Fineberg, N. A., **Stein, D. J.**, **Premkumar, P.**, et al. (2006). Adjunctive quetiapine for serotonin reuptake inhibitor-resistant obsessive-compulsive disorder: a meta-analysis of randomized controlled treatment trials. *International Clinical Psychopharmacology*, **21**(6), 337–343. https://doi.org/10.1097/01.yic.0000215083.57801.11

Foa, E. B. (2010). Cognitive behavioral therapy of obsessive-compulsive disorder. *Dialogues in Clinical Neuroscience*, **12**(2), 199–207.

Fong, T. W., **Reid, R. C.** & **Parhami, I.** (2012). Behavioral addictions: where to draw the lines? *The Psychiatric Clinics of North America*, **35**(2), 279–296. https://doi.org/10.1016/j.psc.2012.03.001

Fontenelle, L. F., **Oostermeijer, S.**, **Harrison, B. J.**, **Pantelis, C.** & **Yücel, M.** (2011). Obsessive-compulsive disorder, impulse control disorders and drug addiction: common features and potential treatments. *Drugs*, **71**(7), 827–840. https://doi.org/10.2165/11591790-000000000-00000

Geller, D. A. (2006). Obsessive-compulsive and spectrum disorders in children and adolescents. *The Psychiatric Clinics of North America*, **29**(2), 353–370. https://doi.org/10.1016/j.psc.2006.02.012

Ghanizadeh, A., **Freeman, R. D.** & **Berk, M.** (2013). Efficacy and adverse effects of venlafaxine in children and adolescents with ADHD: a systematic review of non-controlled and controlled trials. *Reviews on Recent Clinical Trials*, **8**(1), 2–8.

Gillan, C. M., **Robbins, T. W.**, **Sahakian, B. J.**, **van den Heuvel, O. A.** & **van Wingen, G.** (2016). The role of habit in compulsivity. *European Neuropsychopharmacology*, **26**(5), 828–840. https://doi.org/10.1016/j.euroneuro.2015.12.033

Grall-Bronnec, M., **Wainstein, L.**, **Augy, J.**, et al. (2011). Attention deficit hyperactivity disorder among pathological and at-risk gamblers seeking treatment: a hidden disorder. *European Addiction Research*, **17**(5), 231–240. https://doi.org/10.1159/000328628

Grant, J. E. (2008). *Impulse Control Disorders: A Clinician's Guide to Understanding and Treating Behavioral Addictions*. New York: W. W. Norton.

Grant, J. E. (2014). Clinical practice: obsessive-compulsive disorder. *The New England Journal of Medicine*, **371**(7), 646–653. https://doi.org/10.1056/NEJMcp1402176

Grant, J. E. & **Chamberlain, S. R.** (2014). Impulsive action and impulsive choice across substance and behavioral addictions: cause or consequence? *Addictive Behaviors*, **39**(11), 1632–1639. https://doi.org/10.1016/j.addbeh.2014.04.022

Grant, J. E. & **Chamberlain, S. R.** (2016). Expanding the definition of addiction: DSM-5 vs. ICD-11. *CNS Spectrums*, **21**(4), 300–303. https://doi.org/10.1017/S1092852916000183

Grant, J. E. & **Kim, S. W.** (2001). Demographic and clinical features of 131 adult pathological gamblers. *The Journal of Clinical Psychiatry*, **62**(12), 957–962.

Grant, J. E. & **Kim, S. W.** (2005). Quality of life in kleptomania and pathological gambling. *Comprehensive Psychiatry*, **46**(1), 34–37. https://doi.org/10.1016/j.comppsych.2004.07.022

Grant, J. E. & **Potenza, M. N.** (2006a). Compulsive aspects of impulse-control disorders. *The Psychiatric Clinics of North America*, **29**(2), 539–551. https://doi.org/10.1016/j.psc.2006.02.002

Grant, J. E. & **Potenza, M. N.** (2006b). Escitalopram treatment of pathological gambling with co-occurring anxiety: an open-label pilot study with double-blind discontinuation. *International Clinical Psychopharmacology*, **21**(4), 203–209.

Grant, J. E., **Brewer, J. A.** & **Potenza, M. N.** (2006). The neurobiology of substance and behavioral addictions. *CNS Spectrums*, **11**(12), 924–930.

Grant, J. E., **Chamberlain, S. R.**, **Odlaug, B. L.**, **Potenza, M. N.** & **Kim, S. W.** (2010a). Memantine shows promise in reducing gambling severity and cognitive inflexibility in pathological gambling: a pilot study. *Psychopharmacology*, **212**(4), 603–612. https://doi.org/10.1007/s00213-010-1994-5

Grant, J. E., **Kim, S. W.** & **Odlaug, B. L.** (2007). N-acetyl cysteine, a glutamate-modulating agent, in the treatment of pathological gambling: a pilot study. *Biological Psychiatry*, **62**(6), 652–657. https://doi.org/10.1016/j.biopsych.2006.11.021

Grant, J. E., **Kim, S. W.** & **Odlaug, B. L.** (2009). A double-blind, placebo-controlled study of the opiate antagonist, naltrexone, in the treatment of kleptomania. *Biological Psychiatry*, **65**(7), 600–606. https://doi.org/10.1016/j.biopsych.2008.11.022

Grant, J. E., **Kim, S. W.**, **Potenza, M. N.**, et al. (2003). Paroxetine treatment of pathological gambling: a multi-centre randomized controlled trial. *International Clinical Psychopharmacology*, **18**(4), 243–249. https://doi.org/10.1097/01.yic.0000073881.93678.21

Grant, J. E., **Odlaug, B. L.** & **Mooney, M. E.** (2012). Telescoping phenomenon in pathological gambling: association with gender and comorbidities. *The Journal of Nervous and Mental Disease*, **200**(11), 996–998. https://doi.org/10.1097/NMD.0b013e3182718a4d

Grant, J. E., **Odlaug, B. L.**, **Potenza, M. N.**, **Hollander, E.** & **Kim, S. W.** (2010b). Nalmefene in the treatment of pathological gambling: multicentre, double-blind, placebo-controlled study. *The British Journal of Psychiatry*, **197**(4), 330–331. https://doi.org/10.1192/bjp.bp.110.078105

Grant, J. E., **Potenza, M. N.**, **Hollander, E.**, et al. (2006). Multicenter investigation of the opioid antagonist nalmefene in the treatment of pathological gambling. *The American Journal of Psychiatry*, **163**(2), 303–312. https://doi.org/10.1176/appi.ajp.163.2.303

Grant, J. E., **Potenza, M. N.**, **Weinstein, A.** & **Gorelick, D. A.** (2010c). Introduction to behavioral addictions. *The American Journal of Drug and Alcohol Abuse*, **36**(5), 233–241. https://doi.org/10.3109/00952990.2010.491884

Greenberg, B. D., **Price, L. H.**, **Rauch, S. L.**, et al. (2003). Neurosurgery for intractable obsessive-compulsive disorder and depression: critical issues. *Neurosurgery Clinics of North America*, **14**(2), 199–212.

Greenberg, B. D., **Rauch, S. L.** & **Haber, S. N.** (2010). Invasive circuitry-based neurotherapeutics: stereotactic ablation and deep brain stimulation for OCD. *Neuropsychopharmacology*, **35**(1), 317–336. https://doi.org/10.1038/npp.2009.128

Greenhill, L. L., **Biederman, J.**, **Boellner, S. W.**, et al. (2006). A randomized, double-blind, placebo-controlled study of modafinil film-coated tablets in children and adolescents with attention-deficit/hyperactivity disorder. *Journal of the American Academy of Child and Adolescent Psychiatry*, **45**(5), 503–511. https://doi.org/10.1097/01.chi.0000205709.63571.c9

Gunstad, J. & **Phillips, K. A.** (2003). Axis I comorbidity in body dysmorphic disorder. *Comprehensive Psychiatry*, **44**(4), 270–276. https://doi.org/10.1016/S0010-440X(03)00088-9

Hasler, G., **Kazuba, D.** & **Murphy, D. L.** (2006). Factor analysis of obsessive-compulsive disorder YBOCS-SC symptoms and association with 5-HTTLPR SERT polymorphism. *American Journal of Medical Genetics. Part B, Neuropsychiatric Genetics*, **141B**(4), 403–408. https://doi.org/10.1002/ajmg.b.30309

Hasler, G., **LaSalle-Ricci, V. H.**, **Ronquillo, J. G.**, et al. (2005). Obsessive-compulsive disorder symptom dimensions show specific relationships to psychiatric comorbidity. *Psychiatry Research*, **135**(2), 121–132. https://doi.org/10.1016/j.psychres.2005.03.003

Hodgins, D. C., **Stea, J. N.** & **Grant, J. E.** (2011). Gambling disorders. *The Lancet*, **378**(9806),

1874–1884. https://doi.org/10.1016/S0140-6736(10)62185-X

Hogarth, L. & Chase, H. W. (2011). Parallel goal-directed and habitual control of human drug-seeking: implications for dependence vulnerability. *Journal of Experimental Psychology: Animal Behavior Processes*, **37**(3), 261–276. https://doi.org/10.1037/a0022913

Hogarth, L., Chase, H. W. & Baess, K. (2012). Impaired goal-directed behavioural control in human impulsivity. *Quarterly Journal of Experimental Psychology*, **65**(2), 305–316. https://doi.org/10.1080/17470218.2010.518242

Holden, C. (2001). "Behavioral" addictions: do they exist? *Science*, **294**(5544), 980–982. https://doi.org/10.1126/science.294.5544.980

Hollander, E. & Wong, C. M. (1995). Body dysmorphic disorder, pathological gambling, and sexual compulsions. *The Journal of Clinical Psychiatry*, **56** (Supplement 4), 7–12; discussion 13.

Hollander, E., DeCaria, C. M., Finkell, J. N., et al. (2000). A randomized double-blind fluvoxamine/placebo crossover trial in pathologic gambling. *Biological Psychiatry*, **47** (9), 813–817.

Hollander, E., Doernberg, E., Shavitt, R., et al. **W** (2016). The cost and impact of compulsivity: a research perspective. *European Neuropsychopharmacology*, **26**(5), 800–809. https://doi.org/10.1016/j.euroneuro.2016.02.006

Hong, S.-I., Sacco, P. & Cunningham-Williams, R. M. (2009). An empirical typology of lifetime and current gambling behaviors: association with health status of older adults. *Aging & Mental Health*, **13**(2), 265–273. https://doi.org/10.1080/13607860802459849

Insel, T., Cuthbert, B., Garvey, M., et al. (2010). Research domain criteria (RDoC): toward a new classification framework for research on mental disorders. *The American Journal of Psychiatry*, **167**(7), 748–751. https://doi.org/10.1176/appi.ajp.2010.09091379

Jaffe, J. (1990). Drug addiction and drug abuse. In A. G. Gilman, L. Goodman & A. Gilman (Eds.), *Goodman & Gilman's The Pharmacological Basis of Therapeutics* (6th edition). New York: Macmillan.

Jentsch, J. D. & Taylor, J. R. (1999). Impulsivity resulting from frontostriatal dysfunction in drug abuse: implications for the control of behavior by reward-related stimuli. *Psychopharmacology*, **146**(4), 373–390.

Kable, J. W. & Glimcher, P. W. (2007). The neural correlates of subjective value during intertemporal choice. *Nature Neuroscience*, **10** (12), 1625–1633. https://doi.org/10.1038/nn2007

Kable, J. W. & Glimcher, P. W. (2009). The neurobiology of decision: consensus and controversy. *Neuron*, **63**(6), 733–745. https://doi.org/10.1016/j.neuron.2009.09.003

Kable, J. W. & Glimcher, P. W. (2010). An "as soon as possible" effect in human intertemporal decision making: behavioral evidence and neural mechanisms. *Journal of Neurophysiology*, **103**(5), 2513–2531. https://doi.org/10.1152/jn.00177.2009

Kalivas, P. W., Lalumiere, R. T., Knackstedt, L. & Shen, H. (2009). Glutamate transmission in addiction. *Neuropharmacology*, **56** (Supplement 1), 169–173. https://doi.org/10.1016/j.neuropharm.2008.07.011

Kashyap, H., Fontenelle, L. F., Miguel, E. C., et al. (2012). "Impulsive compulsivity" in obsessive-compulsive disorder: a phenotypic marker of patients with poor clinical outcome. *Journal of Psychiatric Research*, **46**(9), 1146–1152. https://doi.org/10.1016/j.jpsychires.2012.04.022

Kenny, P. J. (2011). Reward mechanisms in obesity: new insights and future directions. *Neuron*, **69**(4), 664–679. https://doi.org/10.1016/j.neuron.2011.02.016

Kessler, R. C., Adler, L., Ames, M., et al. (2005). The World Health Organization Adult ADHD Self-Report Scale (ASRS): a short screening scale for use in the general population. *Psychological Medicine*, **35**(2), 245–256.

Kessler, R. C., Adler, L., Barkley, R., et al. (2006). The prevalence and correlates of adult ADHD in the United States: results from the National Comorbidity Survey Replication. *The American Journal of Psychiatry*, **163**(4), 716–723. https://doi.org/10.1176/ajp.2006.163.4.716

Kessler, R. C., Berglund, P. A., Chiu, W. T., et al. (2013). The prevalence and correlates of binge eating disorder in the World Health Organization World Mental Health Surveys. *Biological Psychiatry*, **73**(9), 904–914. https://doi.org/10.1016/j.biopsych.2012.11.020

Kessler, R. C., Hwang, I., LaBrie, R., et al. (2008). DSM-IV pathological gambling in the National Comorbidity Survey Replication. *Psychological Medicine*, **38**(9), 1351–1360. https://doi.org/10.1017/S0033291708002900

Kessler, R. C., McGonagle, K. A., Zhao, S., et al. (1994). Lifetime and 12-month prevalence of DSM-III-R psychiatric disorders in the United States: Results from the National Comorbidity Survey. *Archives of General Psychiatry*, **51**(1), 8–19.

Keyes, K. M., Martins, S. S., Blanco, C. & Hasin, D. S. (2010). Telescoping and gender differences in alcohol dependence: new evidence from two national surveys. *The American Journal of Psychiatry*, **167**(8), 969–976. https://doi.org/10.1176/appi.ajp.2009.09081161

Kim, S. W. (1998). Opioid antagonists in the treatment of impulse-control disorders. *The Journal of Clinical Psychiatry*, **59**(4), 159–164. https://doi.org/10.4088/JCP.v59n0403

Kim, S. W., Grant, J. E., Adson, D. E. & Shin, Y. C. (2001). Double-blind naltrexone and placebo comparison study in the treatment of pathological gambling. *Biological Psychiatry*, **49**(11), 914–921. https://doi.org/10.1016/S0006-3223(01)01079-4

Kim, S. W., Grant, J. E., Adson, D. E., Shin, Y. C. & Zaninelli, R. (2002). A double-blind placebo-controlled study of the efficacy and safety of paroxetine in the treatment of pathological gambling. *The Journal of Clinical Psychiatry*, **63**(6), 501–507.

Koob, G. F. & Le Moal, M. (2005). Plasticity of reward neurocircuitry and the "dark side" of drug addiction. *Nature Neuroscience*, **8**(11), 1442–1444. https://doi.org/10.1038/nn1105-1442

Koob, G. F. & Volkow, N. D. (2010). Neurocircuitry of addiction. *Neuropsychopharmacology*, **35**(1), 217–238. https://doi.org/10.1038/npp.2009.110

Kooij, J. J. S., Huss, M., Asherson, P., et al. (2012). Distinguishing comorbidity and successful management of adult ADHD. *Journal of Attention Disorders*, **16**(5 Supplement), 3S–19S. https://doi.org/10.1177/1087054711435361

Kor, A., Fogel, Y., Reid, R. C. & Potenza, M. N. (2013). Should hypersexual disorder be classified as an addiction? *Sexual Addiction & Compulsivity*, **20**(1–2). https://doi.org/10.1080/10720162.2013.768132

Laibson, D. (1997). Golden eggs and hyperbolic discounting. *The Quarterly Journal of Economics*, **112**(2), 443–478. https://doi.org/10.1162/003355397555253

Leckman, J. F., Denys, D., Simpson, H. B., et al. (2010). Obsessive-compulsive disorder: a review of the diagnostic criteria and possible subtypes and dimensional specifiers for DSM-V. *Depression and Anxiety*, **27**(6), 507–527. https://doi.org/10.1002/da.20669

Leckman, J. F., Grice, D. E., Boardman, J., et al. (1997). Symptoms of obsessive-compulsive disorder. *The American Journal of Psychiatry*, **154**(7), 911–917. https://doi.org/10.1176/ajp.154.7.911

Leeman, R. F. & Potenza, M. N. (2012). Similarities and differences between pathological gambling and substance use disorders: a focus on impulsivity and compulsivity. *Psychopharmacology*, **219**(2), 469–490. https://doi.org/10.1007/s00213-011-2550-7

Leeman, R. F. & Potenza, M. N. (2013). A targeted review of the neurobiology and genetics of behavioural addictions: an emerging area of research. *Canadian Journal of Psychiatry*, **58**(5), 260–273. https://doi.org/10.1177/070674371305800503

Leppink, E. W. & Grant, J. E. (2017). Pharmacological augmentations of SRIs for obsessive compulsive disorder. In *The Wiley Handbook of Obsessive Compulsive Disorders*. Wiley-Blackwell, pp. 311–340. https://doi.org/10.1002/9781118890233.ch16

Limbrick-Oldfield, E. H., van Holst, R. J. & Clark, L. (2013). Fronto-striatal dysregulation in drug addiction and pathological gambling: consistent inconsistencies? *NeuroImage Clinical*, **2**, 385–393. https://doi.org/10.1016/j.nicl.2013.02.005

Lochner, C. & Stein, D. J. (2010). Obsessive-compulsive spectrum disorders in obsessive-compulsive disorder and other anxiety disorders. *Psychopathology*, **43**(6), 389–396. https://doi.org/10.1159/000321070

Logan, G. D., Cowan, W. B. & Davis, K. A. (1984). On the ability to inhibit simple and choice reaction time responses: a model and a method. *Journal of Experimental Psychology: Human Perception and Performance*, **10**(2), 276–291.

Lopes, A. C., Greenberg, B. D., Norén, G., et al. (2009). Treatment of resistant obsessive-compulsive disorder with ventral capsular/ventral striatal gamma capsulotomy: a pilot prospective study. *The Journal of Neuropsychiatry and Clinical Neurosciences*, **21**(4), 381–392. https://doi.org/10.1176/jnp.2009.21.4.381

MacKillop, J., Weafer, J., Gray, J. C., et al. (2016). The latent structure of impulsivity: impulsive choice, impulsive action, and impulsive personality traits. *Psychopharmacology*, **233**(18), 3361–3370. https://doi.org/10.1007/s00213-016-4372-0

Maclaren, V. V., Fugelsang, J. A., Harrigan, K. A. & Dixon, M. J. (2011). The personality of pathological gamblers: a meta-analysis. *Clinical Psychology Review*, **31**(6), 1057–1067. https://doi.org/10.1016/j.cpr.2011.02.002

Madaan, V., Kinnan, S., Daughton, J. & Kratochvil, C. J. (2006). Innovations and recent trends in the treatment of ADHD. *Expert Review of Neurotherapeutics*, **6**(9), 1375–1385. https://doi.org/10.1586/14737175.6.9.1375

Makris, N., Rathi, Y., Mouradian, P., et al. (2016). Variability and anatomical specificity of the orbitofrontothalamic fibers of passage in the ventral capsule/ventral striatum (VC/VS): precision care for patient-specific tractography-guided targeting of deep brain stimulation (DBS) in obsessive compulsive disorder (OCD). *Brain Imaging and Behavior*, **10**(4), 1054–1067. https://doi.org/10.1007/s11682-015-9462-9

Malloy-Diniz, L., Fuentes, D., Leite, W. B., Correa, H. & Bechara, A. (2007). Impulsive behavior in adults with attention deficit/hyperactivity disorder: characterization of attentional, motor and cognitive impulsiveness. *Journal of the International Neuropsychological Society*, **13**(4), 693–698. https://doi.org/10.1017/S1355617707070889

Mancebo, M. C., Eisen, J. L., Pinto, A., et al. (2006). The Brown Longitudinal Obsessive Compulsive Study: treatments received and patient impressions of improvement. *The Journal of Clinical Psychiatry*, **67**(11), 1713–1720.

Martin, P. R. & Petry, N. M. (2005). Are non-substance-related addictions really addictions? *The American Journal on Addictions*, **14**(1), 1–7. https://doi.org/10.1080/10550490590899808

Mataix-Cols, D., Marks, I. M., Greist, J. H., Kobak, K. A. & Baer, L. (2002). Obsessive-compulsive symptom dimensions as predictors of compliance with and response to behaviour therapy: results from a controlled trial. *Psychotherapy and Psychosomatics*, **71**(5), 255–262. https://doi.org/10.1159/000064812

Mataix-Cols, D., Rauch, S. L., Manzo, P. A., Jenike, M. A. & Baer, L. (1999). Use of factor-analyzed symptom dimensions to predict outcome with serotonin reuptake inhibitors and placebo in the treatment of obsessive-compulsive disorder. *The American Journal of Psychiatry*, **156**(9), 1409–1416. https://doi.org/10.1176/ajp.156.9.1409

Mataix-Cols, D., Rosario-Campos, M. C. do & Leckman, J. F. (2005). A multidimensional model of obsessive-compulsive disorder. *The American Journal of Psychiatry*, **162**(2), 228–238. https://doi.org/10.1176/appi.ajp.162.2.228

Mataix-Cols, D., Wooderson, S., Lawrence, N., et al. (2004). Distinct neural correlates of washing, checking, and hoarding symptom dimensions in obsessive-compulsive disorder. *Archives of General Psychiatry*, **61**(6), 564–576. https://doi.org/10.1001/archpsyc.61.6.564

Michelson, D., Adler, L., Spencer, T., et al. (2003). Atomoxetine in adults with ADHD: two randomized, placebo-controlled studies. *Biological Psychiatry*, **53**(2), 112–120. https://doi.org/10.1016/S0006-3223(02)01671-2

Moeller, F. G., Barratt, E. S., Dougherty, D. M., Schmitz, J. M. & Swann, A. C. (2001). Psychiatric aspects of impulsivity. *The American Journal of Psychiatry*, **158**(11), 1783–1793. https://doi.org/10.1176/appi.ajp.158.11.1783

Monterosso, J. R. & Luo, S. (2010). An argument against dual valuation system competition: cognitive capacities supporting future orientation mediate rather than compete with visceral motivations. *Journal of Neuroscience, Psychology, and Economics*, **3**(1), 1–14. https://doi.org/10.1037/a0016827

Morasco, B. J. & Petry, N. M. (2006). Gambling problems and health functioning in individuals receiving disability. *Disability and Rehabilitation*, 28(10), 619–623. https://doi.org/10.1080/09638280500242507

Mortier, P., Demyttenaere, K., Nock, M. K., et al. (2015). [The epidemiology of ADHD in first-year university students]. *Tijdschrift Voor Psychiatrie*, **57**(9), 635–644.

Narayanaswamy, J. C., Viswanath, B., Veshnal Cherian, A., et al. (2012). Impact of age of onset of illness on clinical phenotype in OCD. *Psychiatry Research*, **200**(2–3), 554–559. https://doi.org/10.1016/j.psychres.2012.03.037

Neal, D. T., Wood, W. & Quinn, J. M. (2006). Habits – a repeat performance. *Current Directions in Psychological Science*, **15**(4), 198–202. https://doi.org/10.1111/j.1467-8721.2006.00435.x

Nelson, A. & Killcross, S. (2006). Amphetamine exposure enhances habit formation. *The Journal of Neuroscience*, **26**(14), 3805–3812. https://doi.org/10.1523/JNEUROSCI.4305-05.2006

Nigg, J. T. (2013). Attention-deficit/hyperactivity disorder and adverse health outcomes. *Clinical Psychology Review*, **33**(2), 215–228. https://doi.org/10.1016/j.cpr.2012.11.005

Nordin, C., Gupta, R. C. & Sjödin, I. (2007). Cerebrospinal fluid amino acids in pathological gamblers and healthy controls. *Neuropsychobiology*, **56**(2–3), 152–158. https://doi.org/10.1159/000115782

O'Brien, C. P., Volkow, N. & Li, T.-K. (2006). What's in a word? Addiction versus dependence in DSM-V. *The American Journal of Psychiatry*, **163**(5), 764–765. https://doi.org/10.1176/ajp.2006.163.5.764

Odlaug, B. L., Lust, K., Schreiber, L. R. N., et al. (2013). Compulsive sexual behavior in young adults. *Annals of Clinical Psychiatry*, **25**(3), 193–200.

Olive, M. F., Cleva, R. M., Kalivas, P. W. & Malcolm, R. J. (2012). Glutamatergic medications for the treatment of drug and behavioral addictions. *Pharmacology, Biochemistry, and Behavior*, **100**(4), 801–810. https://doi.org/10.1016/j.pbb.2011.04.015

Oquendo, M. A. & Mann, J. J. (2000). The biology of impulsivity and suicidality. *The Psychiatric Clinics of North America*, **23**(1), 11–25.

Owen, A. M., Roberts, A. C., Polkey, C. E., Sahakian, B. J. & Robbins, T. W. (1991). Extra-dimensional versus intra-dimensional set shifting performance following frontal lobe excisions, temporal lobe excisions or amygdalo-hippocampectomy in man. *Neuropsychologia*, **29**(10), 993–1006.

Pallesen, S., Molde, H., Arnestad, H. M., et al. (2007). Outcome of pharmacological treatments of pathological gambling: a review and meta-analysis. *Journal of Clinical Psychopharmacology*, **27**(4), 357–364. https://doi.org/10.1097/jcp.013e3180dcc304d

Patton, J. H., Stanford, M. S. & Barratt, E. S. (1995). Factor structure of the Barratt Impulsiveness Scale. *Journal of Clinical Psychology*, **51**(6), 768–774.

Peters, J. & Büchel, C. (2011). The neural mechanisms of inter-temporal decision-making: understanding variability. *Trends in Cognitive Sciences*, **15**(5), 227–239. https://doi.org/10.1016/j.tics.2011.03.002

Petry, N. M. (2006). Should the scope of addictive behaviors be broadened to include pathological gambling? *Addiction*, **101** (Supplement 1), 152–160. https://doi.org/10.1111/j.1360-0443.2006.01593.x

Petry, N. M. & Kiluk, B. D. (2002). Suicidal ideation and suicide attempts in treatment-seeking pathological gamblers. *The Journal of Nervous and Mental Disease*, **190**(7), 462–469. https://doi.org/10.1097/01.NMD.0000022447.27689.96

Petry, N. M. & O'Brien, C. P. (2013). Internet gaming disorder and the DSM-5. *Addiction*, **108**(7), 1186–1187. https://doi.org/10.1111/add.12162

Petry, N. M., Stinson, F. S. & Grant, B. F. (2005). Comorbidity of DSM-IV pathological gambling and other psychiatric disorders: results from the National Epidemiologic Survey on Alcohol and Related Conditions. *The Journal of Clinical Psychiatry*, **66**(5), 564–574.

Phillips, K. A., Menard, W., Fay, C. & Weisberg, R. (2005). Demographic characteristics, phenomenology, comorbidity, and family history in 200 individuals with body dysmorphic disorder. *Psychosomatics*, **46**(4), 317–325. https://doi.org/10.1176/appi.psy.46.4.317

Phillips, K. A., Stein, D. J., Rauch, S., et al. (2010). Should an obsessive-compulsive spectrum grouping of disorders be included in DSM-V? *Depression and Anxiety*, **27**(6), 528–555. https://doi.org/10.1002/da.20705

Pittenger, C., Bloch, M. H. & Williams, K. (2011). Glutamate abnormalities in obsessive compulsive disorder: neurobiology, pathophysiology, and treatment. *Pharmacology & Therapeutics*, **132**(3), 314–332. https://doi.org/10.1016/j.pharmthera.2011.09.006

Potenza, M. N. (2006). Should addictive disorders include non-substance-related conditions? *Addiction*, **101** (Supplement 1), 142–151. https://doi.org/10.1111/j.1360-0443.2006.01591.x

Potenza, M. N. (2007). Impulsivity and compulsivity in pathological gambling and obsessive-compulsive disorder. *Revista Brasileira De Psiquiatria*, **29**(2), 105–106.

Potenza, M. N. (2008). Review. The neurobiology of pathological gambling and drug addiction: an overview and new findings. *Philosophical Transactions of the Royal Society of London, Series B, Biological Sciences*, **363** (1507), 3181–3189. https://doi.org/10.1098/rstb.2008.0100

Potenza, M. N. (2014). Non-substance addictive behaviors in the context of DSM-5. *Addictive Behaviors*, **39**(1), 1–2. https://doi.org/10.1016/j.addbeh.2013.09.004

Potenza, M. N., Balodis, I. M., Franco, C. A., et al. (2013). Neurobiological considerations in understanding behavioral treatments for pathological gambling. *Psychology of Addictive Behaviors*, **27**(2), 380–392. https://doi.org/10.1037/a0032389

Reddy, Y. C. J., Alur, A. M., Manjunath, S., Kandavel, T. & Math, S. B. (2010). Long-term follow-up study of patients with serotonin reuptake inhibitor-nonresponsive obsessive-compulsive disorder. *Journal of Clinical Psychopharmacology*, **30**(3), 267–272. https://doi.org/10.1097/JCP.0b013e3181dbfb53

Reed, D. D. et al. (2020). Behavioral economic considerations of novel addictions and nonaddictive behavior: research and analytic methods. In S. Sussman (Ed.) *The Cambridge Handbook of Substance and Behavioral Addictions*. Cambridge, UK: Cambridge University Press, pp. 73–86.

Reghunandanan, S., Fineberg, N. A. & Stein, D. J. (2015). Pathogenesis. In S. Reghunandanan, N. A. Fineberg & D. J. Stein (Eds.), *Obsessive-Compulsive and Related Disorders*. New York, NY: Oxford University Press, pp. 13–35.

Reid, R. C. (2013). Personal perspectives on hypersexual disorder. *Sexual Addiction & Compulsivity*, **20**(1–2), 4–18. https://doi.org/10.1080/10720162.2013.772876

Reid, R. C., Carpenter, B. N., Hook, J. N., et al. (2012). Report of findings in a DSM-5 field trial for hypersexual disorder. *The Journal of Sexual Medicine*, **9**(11), 2868–2877. https://doi.org/10.1111/j.1743-6109.2012.02936.x

Robbins, T. W. (2017). Cross-species studies of cognition relevant to drug discovery: a translational approach. *British Journal of Pharmacology*, **174**(19), 3191–3199. https://doi.org/10.1111/bph.13826

Robbins, T. W., Gillan, C. M., Smith, D. G., de Wit, S. & Ersche, K. D. (2012). Neurocognitive endophenotypes of impulsivity and compulsivity: towards dimensional psychiatry. *Trends in Cognitive Sciences*, **16**(1), 81–91. https://doi.org/10.1016/j.tics.2011.11.009

Rodriguez, C. I., Kegeles, L. S., Levinson, A., et al. (2013). Randomized controlled crossover trial of ketamine in obsessive-compulsive disorder: proof-of-concept. *Neuropsychopharmacology*, **38**(12), 2475–2483. https://doi.org/10.1038/npp.2013.150

Rogers, R. D., Everitt, B. J., Baldacchino, A., et al. (1999). Dissociable deficits in the decision-making cognition of chronic amphetamine abusers, opiate abusers, patients with focal damage to prefrontal cortex, and tryptophan-depleted normal volunteers: evidence for monoaminergic mechanisms. *Neuropsychopharmacology*, **20** (4), 322–339. https://doi.org/10.1016/S0893-133X(98)00091-8

Ruscio, A. M., Stein, D. J., Chiu, W. T. & Kessler, R. C. (2010). The epidemiology of obsessive-compulsive disorder in the National Comorbidity Survey Replication. *Molecular Psychiatry*, **15**(1), 53–63. https://doi.org/10.1038/mp.2008.94

Saiz-Ruiz, J., Blanco, C., Ibáñez, A., et al. (2005). Sertraline treatment of pathological gambling: a pilot study. *The Journal of Clinical Psychiatry*, **66**(1), 28–33.

Samuel, D. B. & Widiger, T. A. (2011). Conscientiousness and obsessive-compulsive personality disorder. *Personality Disorders*, **2** (3), 161–174. https://doi.org/10.1037/a0021216

Sanavio, E. (1988). Obsessions and compulsions: the Padua Inventory. *Behaviour Research and Therapy*, **26**(2), 169–177.

Scherrer, J. F., Xian, H., Slutske, W. S., Eisen, S. A. & Potenza, M. N. (2015). Associations between obsessive-compulsive classes and pathological gambling in a national cohort of male twins. *JAMA Psychiatry*, **72**(4), 342–349. https://doi.org/10.1001/jamapsychiatry.2014.2497

Schultz, W. (2011). Potential vulnerabilities of neuronal reward, risk, and decision mechanisms to addictive drugs. *Neuron*, **69** (4), 603–617. https://doi.org/10.1016/j.neuron.2011.02.014

Shaffer, H. J. (1999). On the nature and meaning of addiction. *National Forum*, **79**(4), 9–14.

Sica, C., Bottesi, G., Orsucci, A., et al. (2015). "Not Just Right Experiences" are specific to obsessive-compulsive disorder: further evidence from Italian clinical samples. *Journal of Anxiety Disorders*, **31**, 73–83. https://doi.org/10.1016/j.janxdis.2015.02.002

Simpson, H. B., **Maher, M. J.**, **Wang, Y.**, et al. (2011). Patient adherence predicts outcome from cognitive behavioral therapy in obsessive-compulsive disorder. *Journal of Consulting and Clinical Psychology*, **79**(2), 247–252. https://doi.org/10.1037/a0022659

Simpson, H. B., **Shungu, D. C.**, **Bender, J.**, et al. (2012). Investigation of cortical glutamate-glutamine and γ-aminobutyric acid in obsessive-compulsive disorder by proton magnetic resonance spectroscopy. *Neuro-psychopharmacology*, **37**(12), 2684–2692. https://doi.org/10.1038/npp.2012.132

Skoog, G. & Skoog, I. (1999). A 40-year follow-up of patients with obsessive-compulsive disorder. *Archives of General Psychiatry*, **56**(2), 121–127.

Slutske, W. S. (2006). Natural recovery and treatment-seeking in pathological gambling: results of two U.S. national surveys. *The American Journal of Psychiatry*, **163**(2), 297–302. https://doi.org/10.1176/appi.ajp.163.2.297

Stanford, M. S., **Mathias, C. W.**, **Dougherty, D. M.**, et al. (2009). Fifty years of the Barratt Impulsiveness Scale: an update and review. *Personality and Individual Differences*, **47**(5), 385–395. https://doi.org/10.1016/j.paid.2009.04.008

Starcevic, V., **Berle, D.**, **Brakoulias, V.**, et al. (2013). Obsessive-compulsive personality disorder co-occurring with obsessive-compulsive disorder: conceptual and clinical implications. *The Australian and New Zealand Journal of Psychiatry*, **47**(1), 65–73. https://doi.org/10.1177/0004867412450645

Stein, D. J., **Hollander, E.**, **Simeon, D. & Cohen, L.** (1994). Impulsivity scores in patients with obsessive-compulsive disorder. *The Journal of Nervous and Mental Disease*, **182**(4), 240–241.

Sulzer, D. (2011). How addictive drugs disrupt presynaptic dopamine neurotransmission. *Neuron*, **69**(4), 628–649. https://doi.org/10.1016/j.neuron.2011.02.010

Swann, A. C., **Lijffijt, M.**, **Lane, S. D.**, **Steinberg, J. L. & Moeller, F. G.** (2009). Trait impulsivity and response inhibition in antisocial personality disorder. *Journal of Psychiatric Research*, **43**(12), 1057–1063. https://doi.org/10.1016/j.jpsychires.2009.03.003

van den Heuvel, O. A., **Remijnse, P. L.**, **Mataix-Cols, D.**, et al. (2009). The major symptom dimensions of obsessive-compulsive disorder are mediated by partially distinct neural systems. *Brain*, **132**(4), 853–868. https://doi.org/10.1093/brain/awn267

van den Heuvel, O. A., **van Wingen, G.**, **Soriano-Mas, C.**, et al. (2016). Brain circuitry of compulsivity. *European Neuro-psychopharmacology*, **26**(5), 810–827. https://doi.org/10.1016/j.euroneuro.2015.12.005

van Emmerik-van Oortmerssen, K., **van de Glind, G.**, **van den Brink, W.**, et al. (2012). Prevalence of attention-deficit hyperactivity disorder in substance use disorder patients: a meta-analysis and meta-regression analysis. *Drug and Alcohol Dependence*, **122**(1–2), 11–19. https://doi.org/10.1016/j.drugalcdep.2011.12.007

van Holst, R. J., **van den Brink, W.**, **Veltman, D. J. & Goudriaan, A. E.** (2010a). Brain imaging studies in pathological gambling. *Current Psychiatry Reports*, **12**(5), 418–425. https://doi.org/10.1007/s11920-010-0141-7

van Holst, R. J., **van den Brink, W.**, **Veltman, D. J. & Goudriaan, A. E.** (2010b). Why gamblers fail to win: a review of cognitive and neuroimaging findings in pathological gambling. *Neuroscience & Biobehavioral Reviews*, **34**(1), 87–107. https://doi.org/10.1016/j.neubiorev.2009.07.007

Vanes, L. D., **van Holst, R. J.**, **Jansen, J. M.**, et al. (2014). Contingency learning in alcohol dependence and pathological gambling: learning and unlearning reward contingencies. *Alcoholism, Clinical and Experimental Research*, **38**(6), 1602–1610. https://doi.org/10.1111/acer.12393

Volkow, N. D. & Li, T.-K. (2004). Drug addiction: the neurobiology of behaviour gone awry. *Nature Reviews Neuroscience*, **5** (12), 963–970. https://doi.org/10.1038/nrn1539

Voon, V., **Derbyshire, K.**, **Rück, C.**, et al. (2015). Disorders of compulsivity: a common bias towards learning habits. *Molecular Psychiatry*, **20**(3), 345–352. https://doi.org/10.1038/mp.2014.44

Wareham, J. D. & Potenza, M. N. (2010). Pathological gambling and substance use disorders. *The American Journal of Drug and Alcohol Abuse*, **36**(5), 242–247. https://doi.org/10.3109/00952991003721118

Wilens, T. E. (2006). Mechanism of action of agents used in attention-deficit/hyperactivity disorder. *The Journal of Clinical Psychiatry*, **67** (Supplement 8), 32–38.

Winstanley, C. A., **Eagle, D. M. & Robbins, T. W.** (2006). Behavioral models of impulsivity in relation to ADHD: translation between clinical and preclinical studies. *Clinical Psychology Review*, **26**(4), 379–395. https://doi.org/10.1016/j.cpr.2006.01.001

Wood, W., **Quinn, J. M. & Kashy, D. A.** (2002). Habits in everyday life: thought, emotion, and action. *Journal of Personality and Social Psychology*, **83**(6), 1281–1297.

Wu, K., **Hanna, G. L.**, **Rosenberg, D. R. & Arnold, P. D.** (2012). The role of glutamate signaling in the pathogenesis and treatment of obsessive-compulsive disorder. *Pharmacology, Biochemistry, and Behavior*, **100**(4), 726–735. https://doi.org/10.1016/j.pbb.2011.10.007

Ziauddeen, H. & Fletcher, P. C. (2013). Is food addiction a valid and useful concept? *Obesity Reviews*, **14**(1), 19–28. https://doi.org/10.1111/j.1467-789X.2012.01046.x

Ziauddeen, H., **Farooqi, I. S. & Fletcher, P. C.** (2012a). Food addiction: is there a baby in the bathwater? *Nature Reviews Neuroscience*, **13**(7), 514. https://doi.org/10.1038/nrn3212-c2

Ziauddeen, H., **Farooqi, I. S. & Fletcher, P. C.** (2012b). Obesity and the brain: how convincing is the addiction model? *Nature Reviews Neuroscience*, **13**(4), 279–286. https://doi.org/10.1038/nrn3212

Zohar, J. & Insel, T. R. (1987). Obsessive-compulsive disorder: psychobiological approaches to diagnosis, treatment, and pathophysiology. *Biological Psychiatry*, **22**(6), 667–687.

32 Anhedonia in Addictive Behaviors

Walter G. Dyer, BS, BA, Adam M. Leventhal, PhD,
Nicholas I. Goldenson, PhD, and Mariel S. Bello, MA

Introduction

Addiction can be conceptualized as the pathological and paradoxical pursuit of and engagement in certain behaviors that are immediately reinforcing in nature, despite often causing long-term adverse consequences (Bickel et al., 2011). Initial engagement in addictive behaviors nearly always generates an appetitive, *positively* reinforcing (or rewarding) effect, often subjectively experienced in the form of pleasure (Kelley & Berridge, 2002). It is therefore intuitive that investigation of etiological mechanisms underlying addiction consider dysfunction in how organisms process and respond to positive reinforcers more broadly (both addictive and nonaddictive pleasurable acts) as a plausible driver of addictive behavior.

Anhedonia – a diminished interest in or ability to experience pleasure from rewards commonly encountered in the general population – has garnered increasing scientific attention as a putative etiological influence on addiction. There have been two emphases of study in anhedonia in addiction: (1) a trait-like tendency implicated in psychiatric disorders (transdiagnostic) that increases propensity toward the onset, escalation, and persistence of addictive behaviors and may be a mechanism of comorbidity between addiction and certain psychopathologies (Leventhal & Zvolensky, 2015); and (2) a temporary state or enduring trait caused by psychobiological dysregulation resulting from constant and chronic engagement in hyper-rewarding addictive behaviors (e.g., Koob & Le Moal, 2001). In either sense, anhedonia may motivate pursuit of addictive behaviors as a means for satisfying the inherent drive for positive reinforcement that is not otherwise met due an inherent lack of pleasure garnered from common (nonaddictive) behaviors that are enjoyable for most individuals under most conditions.

A handful of extant publications reviewing the empirical literature on anhedonia in addiction have been useful for identifying trends in results, and informing models to guide theory and treatment addressing anhedonia in addiction (D'Souza & Markou, 2010; Garfield, Lubman & Yücel, 2014; Hatzigiakoumis et al., 2011; Leventhal & Zvolensky, 2015). While of value, each are at least five years old, with dozens of published studies addressing anhedonia in addiction appearing since 2014. Additionally, the addiction landscape has changed recently, including the proliferation of novel tobacco products like e-cigarettes that were virtually unstudied several years back (Cobb et al., 2010), increasing normalization and legalization of cannabis use (Hall & Lynskey, 2016), and a rapidly evolving opioid crisis, resulting in unprecedented increases in opioid-related overdoses in many regions (Seth et al., 2018). Further advancement of the science of nonsubstance behavioral addictions has promoted an increased attention to and understanding of a broader range of addictions – illustrated in many chapters in this volume. With the constant evolution of technology to generate higher-performing and highly accessible addictive consumer products (e.g., smartphones and tablet applications) with high reinforcing value (Sussman & Dejong, 2018), the identification of anhedonia and other etiological underpinnings of behavioral addictions are of importance; however, no extant review has addressed anhedonia in nonsubstance addictions.

Overall Scope of the Chapter

This chapter reviews the published literature on anhedonia in substance-related and nonsubstance addictive behaviors. To provide a scientific context, the chapter first describes the anhedonia construct and two complimentary conceptual models of anhedonia's role in addiction etiology. Then, the methods and results of a systematic exhaustive review is presented that addresses all published empirical studies on anhedonia in addiction among humans, with the exception of those covered in our previous review of anhedonia in cigarette smoking research as of 2014 (Leventhal & Zvolensky, 2015). Finally, the chapter concludes by describing clinical implications of the review, remaining gaps in the literature, and areas that warrant future research.

Overview of the Construct of Anhedonia and Its Putative Role in Addiction

Anhedonia Construct Conceptualization and Measurement

Anhedonia has been studied under numerous perspectives, spanning psychopathology, personality and individual differences science, behavior analysis, social cognition, and neuroscience (Cohen et al.,, 2011; Harvey et al., 2007; Huys et al., 2013; Snaith, 1993; Treadway & Zald, 2011). A common theme across perspectives is the notion that anhedonia is a manifestation of deficient reward functioning. The subjective expression of anhedonia involves reduced frequency and intensity of experiential enjoyment as well as diminished pleasure from, and interest in, commonly rewarding stimuli. By commonly rewarding, we mean stimuli and behaviors commonly encountered in the general population that are experienced as reinforcing by most, and are unlikely to acquire addictive properties. Such commonly rewarding stimuli include natural reinforcers and do not include exogenous psychoactive substances or other artificially engineered, nondrug rewards designed to be hyperstimulating and potentially addictive (e.g., high-performance digital media). These include face-to-face social interactions, natural sensory experiences (e.g., a beautiful view), and traditional hobbies.

Anhedonia can be conceptualized as a higher-order, multidimensional construct that is composed of related, but distinct lower-order dimensions such as: (1) global anhedonia (reduced happiness and enjoyment derived in one's life; Carleton et al., 2013); (2) anticipatory anhedonia (diminished subjective interest in, and anticipation of, pleasant events; Gard et al., 2006); and (3) consummatory anhedonia (diminished ability to experience pleasure in response to rewarding stimuli; Gard et al., 2006). Based on prior work, anhedonia can be considered conceptually and empirically distinct from other emotional constructs, such as overall level depressive symptoms, alexithymia, affective flattening (i.e., dampened experience of both positive and negative emotions), extraversion, and negative affect (Fiorito & Simons, 1994; Franken, Zijlstra & Muris, 2006; Leventhal et al., 2006). Anhedonia can also be conceptualized as a continuous dimension with a broad distribution in the general population (Fawcett et al., 1983). The lower end of the anhedonia spectrum is characterized by a tendency to affectively and motivationally respond strongly to most rewards, whereas the upper end of this continuum is manifested as difficulty developing interest or pleasure in most rewards (Fawcett et al., 1983; Meehl, 1975). People with elevated anhedonia (deflated hedonia) typically do not unequivocally lack pleasure in all circumstances, and instead require a higher level of reward stimulation and more potent reinforcers to feel enjoyment (Schlaepfer et al., 2008; Wise, 2008). Low to moderate potency reinforcers that are pleasurable or interesting to most (e.g., smell of freshly baked bread) may have limited affective consequences in anhedonia, whereas hyper-rewarding experiences that are uncommon occurrences (e.g., a job offer for a desirable position) may produce pleasure despite anhedonia (Franken et al., 2006).

Subjective anhedonia is commonly measured in surveys in which respondents rate imagined affective responses to experiences that are commonly encountered and enjoyable to most (e.g., "I would be able to enjoy my favorite meal" from Snaith-Hamilton Pleasure Scale [SHAPS]; Snaith et al., 1995), or their interest, desire, and anticipation of such activities (e.g., "When something exciting is coming up in my life, I really look forward to it." from Temporal Experience of Pleasure Scale [TEPS]; Gard et al., 2006). Indirect (nonsubjective) measures of anhedonia using methods from psychophysiology, behavioral economics, or neuroscience typically involve experimental exposure to a commonly rewarding stimulus (e.g., picture depicting a beautiful nature scene) and measurement of a biological or behavioral response (Rømer Thomsen, 2015).

Conceptual Models of Anhedonia's Role in the Etiology of Addiction

Two distinct (yet complimentary) classes of conceptual models have been proposed. One identifies anhedonia as a neuroadaptation and consequence of chronic exposure to hyperrewarding addictive stimuli, generalizable to most individuals with addiction and across species (Koob & Le Moal, 2001). Another considers anhedonia to be an individual difference factor that increases risk of initiation, escalation, and maintenance of addictive behavior. This model proposes that anhedonia-mediated addiction vulnerability represents one characteristic etiologic pathway prominent in a subsample of the overall population of people with addiction, some of whom are vulnerable to addiction by alternate pathways (e.g., sensation seeking, distress intolerant, anxiety prone; Leventhal & Zvolensky, 2015).

Reward Allostasis Model (Koob & Le Moal, 2001). This model hypothesizes that acute exposure to addictive behaviors initially results in robust activation of brain reward pathways, raising the reward stimulation level far above baseline, resulting in a strong motivational effect, often including subjective euphoria. With repeated experiences, the level of stimulation produced by each acute exposure to the addictive behavior diminishes over time (i.e., habituation/desensitization, counteradaptation). Neuroadaptations caused by chronic hyperstimulation to the brain's reward system (mesolimbic dopamine) results in a compensatory response (innervation of the hypothalamic-pituitary-adrenal axis) whereby the "hedonic set point" lowers, such that postexposure states of anhedonic withdrawal ensue. During such withdrawal states, the reward system's activity level is temporarily diminished below the "baseline" premorbid level (prior to first exposure to the addictive behavior). In humans, the anhedonic withdrawal state can be manifested as reduced levels of interest in, pursuit of, and enjoyment from common nonaddictive rewards. Consequently, the organism is motivated to reinstate engagement of the addictive behavior to preserve a homeostatic level of pleasure and reward activity. That is, to maintain a level of reward functioning that is similar to the baseline (preaddictive behavior exposure) level, constant engagement in the addictive behavior is required without extended periods of abstinence.

Emotional Vulnerability Model (Leventhal & Zvolensky, 2015). This model (and other similar models) propose that individual differences in a person's tendency toward anhedonia may increase vulnerability to the onset, escalation, maintenance, and persistence of addictive behavior. It is hypothesized that, prior to addiction onset, people with anhedonia may (learn that they) feel pleasure only in response to high-potency rewards and may, therefore, develop beliefs that they are likely to enjoy any type of hyper-rewarding (potentially addictive) stimulus to a much greater extent than other common reinforcers. Therefore, they may be more likely to initiate engagement in an addictive behavior with the intent that this behavior may increase the capacity to experience enjoyment that they may otherwise be unable to derive.

Because exposure to commonly rewarding stimuli is unlikely to activate dopamine release in reward circuitry for anhedonic individuals, chronic reward hypoactivity may cause upregulation resulting in greater availability of postsynaptic dopamine receptors (Tremblay et al., 2005). When a high-potency reinforcer with addiction potential is encountered that generates robust neural activation and dopamine release, the level of ensuing receptor occupancy may be high, which may in turn result in a particularly robust reward response to the addictive agent. The strong reward may propel conversion from initial experimentation with an addictive behavior to escalation and frequent engagement in the behavior.

People with higher premorbid trait anhedonia may be more vulnerable to the neuroadaptive sequelae of postexposure hedonic dysregulation, anhedonia, and motivation to reinstate the active behavior described above in Koob et al.'s model. Thus, when they are deprived from the addictive behavior or attempt to quit engaging in the behavior, their preaddiction anhedonic temperament may be unmasked and potentially exacerbated due to the psychobiological dysregulation induced by chronic exposure to the addictive behaviors, taking them back to a hedonic state that is worse than before their addictive behavior began. As such, trait anhedonic individuals may be more liable to reinstate the behavior (or relapse back to the behavior) to counteract the pronounced deficient reward activity experienced.

A Systematic Review of the Empirical Literature on Anhedonia in Addictive Behaviors

Scope and Methodology of the Review

Articles were identified through searches of PubMed, PsycInfo, and Medline as of August 1, 2018. Searches used the *AND* function to identify articles that crossed both an anhedonia-related term (*anhedonia* OR hedonia OR *anhedonic, reduced pleasure, reduced interest*) and an addictive behavior (nicotine/tobacco products: *smoking, cigarette, nicotine, tobacco*; alcohol: *alcohol, ethanol, drink, binge drinking, alcohol consumption*; cannabis: *cannabis, marijuana, marihuana, tetrahydrocannabinol [THC]*; stimulants: *dextroamphetamine [Dexedrine], dextroamphetamine/amphetamine combination product [Adderall], methylphenidate [Ritalin, Concerta], Desoxyn, Ephedrine, cocaine, crack, methamphetamine*; opioids: *opioids, painkillers, hydrocodone [Vicodin], oxycodone [OxyContin, Percocet], oxymorphone [Opana], morphine, codeine, fentanyl, heroin, smack, china white, black tar*; nonsubstance behavioral addictions: *behavioral addiction, gambling disorder, food addiction, binge-eating disorder, sex addiction, hypersexuality disorder, internet addiction, Internet Gaming Disorder, compulsive buying disorder, and exercise addiction*). Studies were eligible for inclusion if they: (a) contained human subjects; and (b) were published in English. We excluded studies that examined anhedonia's role in nicotine/tobacco use that were published before May 2014, as a comprehensive review on this topic was published previously (Leventhal & Zvolensky, 2015).

The search yielded 4,187 total abstracts, of which 3,809 papers were evaluated for inclusion. After excluding 198 articles that lacked empirical data and 3,543 empirical papers that did not meet criteria, sixty-eight publications were included in the final review. Decisions for article inclusion in this review were based on a consensus across the study authors; no articles were identified that resulted in irreconcilable differing opinions across the authors regarding suitability for inclusion. The sixty-eight studies included were first categorized based by addictive agent and further subgrouped by study design or other qualitative similarities (e.g., sample characteristics, findings, addictive behavior outcome variable operationalization). Table 32.1 summarizes the methodology and results of each of the 68 studies included in the review.

Nicotine/Tobacco Product Use

As our previous publication (Leventhal & Zvolensky, 2015) systematically reviewed all research on cigarette smoking and anhedonia occurring on or prior to May 1, 2014, only studies of anhedonia in nicotine/tobacco product use published afterwards are reviewed below. The section summary integrates the post-2014 review with the conclusions of the Leventhal and Zvolenksy 2015 review.

Self-Report Studies in Adolescents and Young Adults. Three recent studies have examined anhedonia in noncigarette tobacco product use in youth and young adults. In a cross-sectional study of ninth-grade students aged fourteen years, on average, Stone et al. (2017) demonstrated that, for every one standard deviation (SD) unit greater in anhedonia level, there were 27 percent to 42 percent higher odds of smoking initiation, and 9 percent to 19 percent increase in susceptibility to smoke combustible cigarettes among never-smokers. Within an overlapping sample of ninth-grade adolescents, Leventhal et al. (2016) found that adolescents who ever used electronic (e-) cigarettes exclusively had higher levels of anhedonia compared to nonusers, but lower levels of anhedonia compared to adolescents who used combustible cigarettes exclusively or used both combustible cigarettes and e-cigarettes. In the only study of anhedonia in hookah use identified in this exhaustive review, Brikmanis et al. (2017) found that young adults with higher levels of anhedonia at a baseline survey reported higher frequency of hookah use across three-, six-, and nine-month follow-ups; however, anhedonia was not associated with frequency of e-cigarette, cigar, smokeless tobacco, or snus use.

Self-Report Studies in Adults. Several recent studies identified in this review explored the intersection of anhedonia with affective psychopathology or personality traits in cigarette smoking. A cross-sectional study in adult cigarette smokers found positive associations of anhedonia symptoms with trait levels of urgency (i.e., a subconstruct of impulsivity defined as the tendency to respond rashly within the context of high-intensity affect) and cigarette dependence severity (Roys et al., 2016). In the same study, anhedonia symptoms moderated the relation between urgency and severity of cigarette dependence, such that trait urgency was only related to nicotine dependence at average and high levels (one standard deviation [SD] above the mean) of anhedonia, but not low levels of anhedonia (one SD below the mean; Roys et al., 2016). In a separate cross-sectional study of military veterans with current major depression, depressed smokers reported significantly greater levels of anhedonia than depressed nonsmokers, suggesting that smoking may be linked with anhedonic subtypes of depression (Liverant et al., 2014). In a study of fifty-five healthy participants (thirty adults with nicotine dependence and twenty-five nonsmokers), smokers scored significantly higher on anhedonia measures than nonsmokers (Peechatka et al., 2015).

Studies of the intersection between anhedonia and certain smoking-related motivational variables fail to show a consistent pattern of association. A cross-sectional study of adult nontreatment-seeking cigarette smokers found that anhedonia was associated with a greater number of cigarettes smoked per day, higher cigarette dependence levels, and PTSD symptom severity (Mathew et al., 2015). This study also found that anhedonia was not significantly associated with either negative reinforcement (i.e., desire to smoke to alleviate cravings and/or nicotine withdrawal symptoms) or positive reinforcement (i.e., desire to smoke due to novelty seeking, reward dependence, and/or pleasurable sensations when smoking) smoking motives, and was not a significant mediator of the relation between PTSD symptom severity and smoking motives (Mathew et al., 2015). In a separate investigation of the intersection of anhedonia and smoking motives in adult regular smokers, Pang and colleagues (2014) found that anhedonia did not moderate relations between either negative reinforcement or positive reinforcement smoking expectancies and cigarette dependence severity, suggesting that the extent to which beliefs that smoking alters affect translates into cigarette dependence vulnerability is not amplified amongst those with anhedonia.

Studies of Smoking Cessation and Withdrawal. In a longitudinal cohort study of Spanish-speaking Mexican-Americans, participants with higher mean levels of anhedonia during a quit attempt were less likely to be abstinent; however, this association was no longer significant after statistically controlling for nonanhedonic symptoms of depression (Haslam et al., 2018). A recent study utilized ecological momentary assessment to determine whether specific variables related to tobacco withdrawal (i.e., cravings to smoke, negative affect) exerted time-varying associations with anhedonia during the first ten days following a quit attempt (Cook et al., 2017). In this study, researchers found that smokers with baseline high nicotine dependence (versus those with lower levels of nicotine dependence) reported significantly greater levels of postquit anhedonia through approximately Day 9 (Cook et al., 2017). This study also investigated mean postquit anhedonia levels over time by treatment group (placebo, nicotine replacement therapy [NRT], and bupropion) and found that anhedonia levels were significantly higher in the placebo group relative to the NRT group during the first two days of the quit attempt, whereas there were no significant differences in postquit anhedonia between bupropion and placebo at any point in time (Cook et al., 2017).

Table 32.1 Overview of articles included in the review

Study	Sample	Design	Anhedonia measure	Main finding
Nicotine/tobacco product use				
Brikmanis et al. (2017)	N = 518 young adults (*mean age* [SD] = 20.5 [1.8]	Observational longitudinal	SHAPS	Anhedonia (Anh) predicted hookah use frequency (days smoked at three months, six months, and nine months) ($p < 0.001$, IRR = 1.04 [1.02, 1.06]), but not e-cigarette, cigars, smokeless tobacco, or snus use frequency
Cook et al. (2015)	N = 1,175 current smokers (*mean age* [SD] = 44.80 [11.05]	Observational analysis in clinical trial	Selected SHAPS items	Postquit Anh was associated with a decreased latency to relapse (*HR* = 1.09, 95%CI [1.02, 1.17]) and with lower eight-week point prevalence abstinence (*OR* = 0.91, 95% CI[0.86, 0.97]) Abstinence-induced increase in Anh was near fully suppressed by nicotine replacement therapy relative to the placebo (*beta* = −0.66, $p < 0.001$)
Cook et al. (2017)	Smokers N = 1,122 (*mean age* [*SD*] = 45.1 [11.0])	Observational analysis in clinical trial	Selected SHAPS items	Anh was significantly greater among those high in dependence relative to lower dependent smokers starting from the day of cessation out to day nine postquit Anh was higher immediately post-quit in placebo (vs. both Bupropion and NRT treatment groups), which fell to levels similar to groups receiving NRT by day seven Anh and its time-varying association with craving early in quit attempt was reduced by nicotine replacement therapy
Guillot et al. (2017)	N = 125 nontreatment seeking smokers (*mean age* [SD] = 43.74 [11.34]	Quasi-experimental	SHAPS	Greater trait Anh predicted greater pleasantness of smoking, lower perceived pleasantness of positive pictures, and less unpleasantness of negative pictures (*betas* = 0.18 to 0.35, *ps* = 0.007 to 0.07)
Haslam et al. (2018)	Spanish-speaking Mexican-Americans N = 199 (*mean age* [*SD*] = 38.7 [10.42]	Observational longitudinal	CESD-D-A	Mean scores on the low positive affect / Anh subscale (range 0–3) from CESD was not related to later smoking cessation at quit day (OR 1.06, 95% CI [0.67, 1.67]), week 3 (OR 0.92, 95% CI [0.57, 1.45]), or week 26 (OR 0.63, 95% CI [0.32, 1.18])
Hughes et al. (2017)	Current smokers N = 211 (*mean age* [*SD*] = 40 [15])	Observational longitudinal	TEPS	Anh scores were significantly higher after four weeks of abstinence than at baseline (*mean scores* = 43.5 vs. 41.7, $p < 0.05$)
Leventhal et al. (2016)	Ninth-grade students N = 189 electronic and conventional cigarette smokers, N = 152 conventional cigarette only users, N = 412 electronic cigarette only users, and N = 2,557 nonusers (*mean age* = 14)	Observational cross-sectional	SHAPS	Anh was higher in e-cigarette only ever users than nonusers (*mean scores* [SD] = 1.79 [0.49] vs.1.65 [0.47]; $p < 0.05$) E-cigarette only ever users had lower levels of Anh compared to combustible cigarette ever users or dual users (*mean scores* [SD] = 1.79 [0.49] vs. 1.86 [0.60] vs. 1.94 [0.61])
Liverant et al. (2014)	N = 36 depressed smokers and N = 44 depressed nonsmokers	Observational cross-sectional	MASQ-AD	Depressed smokers reported greater Anh than depressed nonsmokers (t [77] = 2.01, p = 0.048)
Mathew et al. (2015)	N = 342 smokers (*mean age* [SD] = 43.7 [10.8])	Observational cross-sectional	SHAPS	Anh was positively associated with nicotine dependence (r = 0.14; $p < 0.05$)

Table 32.1 (*cont.*)

Study	Sample	Design	Anhedonia measure	Main finding
				Anh was positively associated with cigarettes per day ($r = 0.14$; $p < 0.05$) Anh was not associated with positive reinforcement smoking motives ($r = -0.02$) Anh was not associated with negative reinforcement smoking motives ($r = 0.03$) Anh was not a significant mediator of the relation between PTSD symptoms and smoking motives
Pang et al. (2014)	*N* = 317 daily cigarette smokers (*mean age* [SD] = 43.89 [10.71])	Observational cross-sectional	MASQ-S	Anh did not moderate relations between either negative reinforcement or positive reinforcement smoking expectancies and cigarette dependence severity (*beta* = 0.11, $p = 0.06$)
Peechatka et al. (2015)	*N* = 30 nicotine dependent smokers and *N* = 25 nonsmokers	Observational cross-sectional	BDI-Anh	Anh was higher in nicotine dependent group than in the group of nonsmokers (*mean scores [SD]* = 0.37 [0.67] vs. 0.00 [0.00]; $p = 0.001$)
Piper et al. (2017)	Adult smokers *N* = 1,236	Observational longitudinal	Author-constructed EMA	Smokers who reported notably high levels of craving and anhedonia (high craving-Anh group determined by latent class analysis model; 8% of overall sample) were more dependent on nicotine products and relapsed sooner than those in the Moderate Withdrawal group (64% of sample) (*mean scores* [SD] = 6.2 [1.9] vs. 5.3 [2.1]; $p < 0.01$) and relapsed sooner (*mean days to relapse* = 105.89 vs. 153.19; $p < 0.05$)
Powers et al. (2016)	Adult smokers *N* = 525 (*mean age* = 46; 48.2% Black/African American)	Observational longitudinal	SHAPS	Rate of Anh was higher among men (16.6%) than among women (10.2%) ([$\chi^2$1] = 4.72, $p = 0.03$) Participants classified as Anh at baseline were significantly more likely to be abstinent at week 8 (*OR* = 3.23, 95% CI = 1.40–7.5, $p = 0.006$); however, gender did not significantly moderate this association
Roys et al. (2016)	Adult smokers *N* = 1125 (*mean age* [SD] = 31.56 [12.61])	Observational cross-sectional	MASQ-S	Anh was positively related to nicotine dependence (*beta* = 0.05, $p = 0.02$) Urgency was related to nicotine dependence at average (*beta* = 0.05, $p < 0.05$) and high (*beta* = 0.08, $p < 0.01$) levels of Anh, but not when Anh was low (*beta* = 0.02, $p = 0.43$)
Stone et al. (2017)	Ninth grade students *N* = 3299 (*mean age* [*SD*] = 14.1 [0.42])	Observational cross-sectional	SHAPS	Increasing levels of Anh was associated with a 27%–42% increase in odds of smoking initiation in overall sample (OR [95% CI] = 1.42 [1.30–1.56]; $p < 0.0001$) Increasing levels of Anh was associated with a 9%–19% increase in odds of smoking initiation susceptibility in the subsample never-smokers (*beta* = 0.10–0.19; $p \leq 0.002$)

Table 32.1 (*cont.*)

Study	Sample	Design	Anhedonia measure	Main finding
Alcohol use				
Cano et al. (2017)	N = 181 Hispanic adults aged 18–25 years old	Observational cross-sectional	CES-D	Higher levels of Anh were associated with higher alcohol use severity (*beta* = 0.20) Gender did not moderate associations between Anh and alcohol use severity
Carton et al. (2018)	N = 38, 694 French adults	Observational cross-sectional	MINI	Anh was associated with alcohol abuse (OR = 1.66), but not alcohol dependence (OR = 1.27) in participants with major depression and comorbid nonalcohol, substance use disorder In samples that excluded participants with comorbid substance use disorders, Anh was no longer associated with alcohol abuse (OR = 1.46)
Chuang et al. (2016)	N = 807 ninth-grade adolescents	Observational cross-sectional	SHAPS	Lifetime alcohol/drug use, without comorbid nicotine product use, had higher symptoms of Anh (d = 0.28)
Erwin et al. (2017)	N = 1,484 US military veterans	Observational cross-sectional	Trauma history screen and PTSD Checklist for DSM-5	Anh symptom cluster was strongly associated with past-year alcohol consequences (r = 0.29)
Dervaux et al. (2010)	N = 34 patients with schizophrenia and lifetime alcohol abuse or dependence and N = 66 patients with schizophrenia without lifetime substance abuse or dependence	Observational cross-sectional	SSS; PAS	There were no significant group differences between patients with schizophrenia with (vs. without) comorbid alcohol use disorder on PAS score (F = 0.00; p = 0.99)
Janiri et al. (2005)	N = 70 participants who met DSM-IV criteria for alcohol, opioid, or multiple drug dependence	Observational cross-sectional	SHAPS; SANS; BRMES	SANS and SHAPS total scores assessed during early days of abstinence were significantly correlated with alcohol use craving during treatment (rs = 0.32 and 0.37; $p < 0.01$), but not duration of alcohol use abstinence or severity of alcohol withdrawal
Leibenluft et al. (1993)	N = 26 healthy volunteers and N = 35 patients with major depression and N = 117 patients with seasonal affective disorder and N = 16 patients with alcohol dependence and N = 24 patients with comorbid depression and alcohol dependence	Observational cross-sectional	HRS	Patients with alcohol dependence were more likely than patient without alcohol dependence to report drinking to alleviate Anh symptoms (F = 222.81; $p < 0.001$)
Luby et al. (2018)	N = 305 children aged three to six years old at baseline, oversampled for symptoms of depression	Observational longitudinal	PASA; CDI-Anh	Children with higher Anh scores had higher orbitofrontal cortical volumes prior to 11.25 years old relative to those with lower Anh scores Greater volume and thickness of the orbitofrontal cortex was associated with higher alcohol use frequency at age twelve (*beta* = -0.21)
Marra et al. (1998)	N = 44 hospitalized patients with alcoholism recruited one to two weeks after detoxification	Observational longitudinal	PAS; SA; PDS	Anh symptoms following two weeks of detoxification did not predict relapse at six months after treatment
Martinotti et al. (2008b)	N = 102 detoxified participants meeting criteria for alcohol dependence in remission	Observational longitudinal	SHAPS; SANS-Anh	In patients who were ultimately abstinent between fifteen days to one month over a twelve-month follow-up period, SHAPS at fifteen to thirty days of abstinence was positively correlated with nausea

Table 32.1 (*cont.*)

Study	Sample	Design	Anhedonia measure	Main finding
				and vomiting withdrawal symptoms ($r = 0.41$) and SANS-Anh was positively correlated to overall alcohol withdrawal symptoms ($r = 0.34$), "paroxysmal sweats" ($r = 0.34$), and "headache, fullness in head" ($r = 0.49$) alcohol withdrawal symptoms during treatment In patients abstinent between one month to three months, SHAPS was positively correlated to overall alcohol withdrawal symptoms ($r = 0.47$), anxiety ($r = 0.78$), agitation ($r = 0.60$), auditory disturbances ($r = 0.78$), visual disturbances ($r = 0.78$), and orientation ($r = 0.78$), whereas SANS-Anh was positively correlated to overall alcohol withdrawal symptoms ($r = 0.69$) and anxiety ($r = 0.64$) during treatment In patients abstinent between three months to six months, SHAPS was positively correlated to overall alcohol withdrawal symptoms ($r = 0.70$), tremors ($r = 0.59$), and orientation ($r = 0.67$), while SANS-Anh to overall alcohol withdrawal ($r = 0.53$), tremors ($r = 0.75$), tactile disturbances ($r = 0.59$), visual disturbances ($r = 0.54$), headache, fullness in head ($r = 0.54$), and orientation ($r = 0.55$) during treatment In patients abstinent between six months to one year, SANS-Anh was associated with overall withdrawal ($r = 0.56$), nausea and vomiting ($r = 0.78$), tremors ($r = 0.78$), paroxysmal sweats ($r = 0.78$), anxiety ($r = 0.78$), agitation ($r = 0.78$), headaches ($r = 0.78$), and orientation ($r = 0.78$) alcohol withdrawal symptoms during treatment Alcohol craving was positively correlated to SHAPS ($r = 0.30$) and SANS-Anh ($r = 0.26$) measure in the total sample
Martinotti et al. (2011)	$N = 64$ Anh alcohol dependent patients randomized to one of three conditions: 23 received Acetyl-I-Carnitine (ALC) at a dosage of 3 g/day, 21 received ALC at a dosage of 1 g/day, and 20 were given placebo	Observational analysis in clinical trial	SHAPS; VASa	Anh symptoms in the placebo group showed a decline until day thirty and remains stable for the rest of the study Levels of Anh significantly reduced in both ALC 3 g ($\Delta = -3.3$) and ALC 1 g ($\Delta = -2$) groups relative to placebo Intravenous ALC accelerated the improvement of Anh symptoms reaching constant low levels earlier by the tenth day
Noordsy et al. (1991)	$N = 75$ DSM-III-R outpatients with schizophrenia	Observational cross-sectional	AUI	Over half of the sample reported that drinking alcohol had positive effects on symptoms of Anh (57.6%)
Nunn et al. (2001)	$N = 196$ undergraduates from University College, London and Goldsmiths College, London	Observational cross-sectional	O-LIFE; PDI; HADS	Alcohol users had significantly lower introvertive Anh scores relative to cannabis and alcohol users and no drink/drug users ($F = 9.30$)

Table 32.1 (*cont.*)

Study	Sample	Design	Anhedonia measure	Main finding
Parrish et al. (2016)	N = 674 Mexican-origin youth	Observational longitudinal	MASQ	Frequent alcohol use at fourteen years old led to subsequent increases in Anh depression from age fourteen to sixteen years old, and higher levels of Anh depression at age fourteen would contribute to subsequent increases in alcohol use from age fourteen to sixteen years old (*betas* = 0.05–0.08)
Pozzi et al. (2008)	N = 70 participants who met DSM-IV criteria for alcohol, opioid, or multiple drug dependence	Observational cross-sectional	SHAPS; SANS	Mean levels of Anh (SHAPS; SANS) did not significantly differ between subgroups (alcohol, opioid, or drug dependent participants) Alcohol or drug use demonstrated a weak predictive capacity on Anh scales (R^2 = 0.10–0.22)
Cannabis use				
Albertella et al. (2018)	N = 114 occasional cannabis users (mean age = 20.5) and N = 41 frequent cannabis users (mean age = 20.3)	Observational longitudinal	OLIFE	Among frequent cannabis users, younger age was associated with increasing levels of introvertive Anh over time, whereas among occasional cannabis users, younger age was associated with decreasing levels of introvertive Anh over time
Bersani et al. (2002)	Males with schizophrenia N = 25 cannabis users (mean age = 29.3) and N = 25 nonusers (mean age = 30.0)	Observational cross-sectional	SANS-Anh	Anh was higher in nonusers than in cannabis users (*mean scores* = 14.88 vs. 12.2; p = 0.005)
Bovasso (2001)	N = 849 community members reporting no depressive symptoms at baseline and N = 1,837 community members no diagnosis of cannabis use at baseline	Observational longitudinal	DISa	Incidence of Anh was approximately four times greater odds in cannabis users than in nonusers (Odds Ratio [OR] = 4.32, 95% Confidence Interval [CI] = 1.32–14.16; Wald χ^2 = 5.8, df = 1, $p < 0.05$) Baseline cannabis use predicted likelihood for experiencing Anh in follow-up period (χ^2 = 12.1, df = 1, $p < 0.01$)
Dorard et al. (2008)	N = 32 adolescent / young adult cannabis abusers (mean age 17.2) and N = 30 adolescent / young adult nonusers control (mean age 16.7)	Observational cross-sectional	SA; PAS	Physical Anh was significantly associated with cannabis use (*betas* = 2.961; p = 0.04) but not social Anh (*betas* = 1.392; p = 0.101)
Dumas et al. (2002)	Healthy university students (mean age 21.17) N = 126 never cannabis users; N = 65 cannabis past or occasional users; N = 41 cannabis regular users	Observational cross-sectional	PhA; SA	No significant difference between levels of Anh in cannabis regular users and cannabis never users
Feingold et al. (2017)	Individuals with Major Depressive Disorder N = 2,283 noncannabis users, N = 173 cannabis users without cannabis use disorder, N = 77 individuals with cannabis use disorder	Observational longitudinal	AUDADIS-IV	Individuals with a cannabis use disorder had significantly greater odds of reporting Anh relative to nonusers (adjusted OR = 2.62; 95% CI = 1.36 – 5.08; p = 0.0048)
Johnson et al. (2009)	N = 154 young adult past thirty-days cannabis users	Observational cross-sectional	MASQ-AD	Anh was not significantly/uniquely associated with frequency of cannabis use (t = 0.19, *beta* = 0.02, $p > 0.05$)
Lawn et al. (2016)	N = 20 cannabis-dependent participants and N = nondependent, drug-using controls	Quasi-experimental	SHAPS; TEPS	Anh did not differ between those who received placebo, 8 mg THC (Cann – CBD), and 8 mg THC + 10 mg CBD (Cann + CBD; F 2,32 = 0.248, p = 0.782)
Leventhal et al. (2017)	N = 3394 high school students	Observational longitudinal	SHAPS	Baseline Anh level was positively associated with rate of increase in cannabis use frequency across

Table 32.1 (*cont.*)

Study	Sample	Design	Anhedonia measure	Main finding
				follow-ups (beta, [95% CI] = 0.115 [0.022, 0.252], $p = 0.03$) Association of baseline Anh with faster cannabis use escalation was amplified among adolescents with (versus without) friends who used cannabis at baseline (beta, [95% CI] = 0.179 [0.043, 0.334] versus 0.064 [−0.071, 0.187], interaction $p = 0.04$)
Nunn et al. (2001)	$N = 49$ undergraduate cannabis users (mean age = 21.4) and $N = 49$ undergraduate noncannabis or alcohol users (mean age = 22.0)	Observational cross-sectional	OLIFE	Cannabis users had lower levels of Anh than nonusers ($F[1,192] = 7.12, p < 0.01$)
Stimulant drug use				
Crits-Christoph et al. (2018)	$N = 79$ adults with current diagnosis of cocaine dependence	Observational longitudinal	Three-item Anh scale from BDI-I	Greater severity of self-reported Anh significantly predicted nonabstinence from cocaine in month three (*OR* = 5.40) and month six (*OR* = 5.60), even when controlling for overall depression
Kirkpatrick et al. (2016)	$N = 97$ healthy stimulant-naïve volunteers	Quasi-experimental	SHAPS and TEPS	Greater anticipatory pleasure (TEPS) at baseline predicted greater amphetamine-induced increases in positive mood (*betas* = 0.46) Nonsignificant trend indicating that higher baseline Anh (SHAPS) predicted greater amphetamine-related increases in positive mood ($p = 0.09$)
Leventhal et al. (2008)	$N = 204$ psychiatric outpatients with past stimulant use disorder in full remission for $\geq$ two months (STIM+) and $N = 2070$ psychiatric outpatients with no history of stimulant use disorder (STIM−)	Observational cross-sectional	SCID-IV	Relative to those without a history of stimulant use disorder, STIM+ participants reported greater prevalence of current Anh (*OR* = 1.58)
Leventhal et al. (2010)	$N = 43{,}093$ American adults (NESARC-I)	Observational cross-sectional	Alcohol Use Disorder and Associated Disabilities Interview Schedule-IV	Anh was significantly associated with lifetime amphetamine use (*OR* = 1.56) and cocaine use (*OR* = 1.24) in adjusted combined models controlling for depression In participants without a lifetime stimulant-dependent diagnosis, Anh also predicted lifetime use of cocaine in adjusted combined models (*OR* = 1.27) Among a subsample of lifetime cocaine users, Anh, but not depressed mood, was also significantly associated with cocaine dependence (*OR* = 2.22) Among lifetime amphetamine users, Anh was significantly associated with lifetime amphetamine dependence (*OR* = 1.85)
Lichlyter et al. (2011)	$N = 37$ adults with stimulant dependence abstinent for 31–1,533 days	Observational cross-sectional	SAS	Preferred method of drug administration, duration of abstinence, latency from first use to regular use, and prior solicitation of treatment were not related to SAS scores

Table 32.1 (*cont.*)

Study	Sample	Design	Anhedonia measure	Main finding
McGregor et al. (2005)	N = 21 inpatients with methamphetamine dependence and N = 9 sex- and age-matched controls	Observational cross-sectional	AWQ	For inpatients undergoing methamphetamine withdrawal, Anh and other depression-related symptoms declined from a high initial peak within twenty-four hours of the last use of amphetamines, resolving to near comparison group levels by the first week of abstinence (*mean score* = 0.65, SEM = 0.05)
Morie et al. (2014)	N = 27 healthy controls with no drug use history and N = 23 current cocaine abusers	Quasi-experimental	SHAPS (State Anh) and Chapman Physical and Social Anh Scales (trait Anh)	Cocaine users (vs. controls) had significantly higher trait levels of physical (t =5.4) and social Anh (t = 10.2) and state Anh (t = 2.6) Physical Anh was significantly associated with addiction severity (r = 0.58) State Anh was correlated with cocaine withdrawal severity (r = 0.44), but not trait Anh measures
Newton et al. (2004)	N = 19 nontreatment-seeking methamphetamine-dependent participants	Observational longitudinal	BDI	Individuals in the early study entry group (abstinent for one to three days) reported greater levels of Anh than late study entry group participants (abstinent for twelve to fourteen days) (*mean score* [SD] = 14.5 [8.1] vs. 7.2 [5.4])
Tremblay et al. (2002)	N = 36 healthy controls with no reported history of mood disorders or other psychiatric illnesses and N = 50 patients with DSM-IV major depressive disorder	Observational analysis in clinical trial	SHAPS	Anh (as measured by the Snaith-Hamilton Pleasure Scale [SHAPS]) was not predictive of the level of dextroamphetamine-induced rewarding effects (F = 1.54); however, a single item related to Anh on the Hamilton Rating Scale for Depression (HAM-D; "loss of interest in activities") showed a positive correlation with dextroamphetamine reward
Tremblay et al. (2005)	N = 12 healthy controls with no reported history of mood disorders or other psychiatric illnesses and N = 12 patients with DSM-IV major depressive disorder	Quasi-experimental	SHAPS	Patients with major depression (vs. healthy controls) had a hypersensitive response to the rewarding effects of dextroamphetamine, and the degree of the dextroamphetamine's rewarding effects was associated with severity of Anh symptoms (r = 0.58)
Voce et al. (2018)	N = 636 adults who had used amphetamine within their lifetime and had an ICD-10 diagnosis of schizophrenia or affective psychotic disorder	Observational cross-sectional	DIP-Anh	Past year users of amphetamine with schizophrenia had significantly higher prevalence of Anh symptoms (*OR* = 2.01) relative to former amphetamine users with schizophrenia
Wardle et al. (2017)	N = 85 treatment-seeking adults with cocaine use disorder	Observational analysis in clinical trial	SHAPS and Progressive Ratio Task	Greater Anh was associated with poorer treatment outcomes involving contingency management (Bayesian = 92.6% probability that negative relationship between SHAPS and treatment outcomes exists) Baseline Anh levels did not moderate the effect of L-DOPA treatment ($\chi^2[1]$ = 0.01)

Table 32.1 (*cont.*)

Study	Sample	Design	Anhedonia measure	Main finding
Opioid use				
Garfield et al. (2017)	N = 90 participants who were prescribed opioid maintenance pharmacotherapy and N = 31 opioid-dependent participants and N = 33 control participants	Observational analysis in clinical trial	SHAPS and TEPS	Opioid-dependent participants had significantly higher scores for Anh than healthy controls (F = 8.84) Healthy controls' mean TEPS scores were significantly higher than those of both pharmacotherapy (p = 0.01) and abstinent (p = 0.01) groups, which did not significantly differ from each other
Huhn et al. (2016)	N = 36 prescription opioid dependent patients and N = 10 healthy controls	Experimental	SHAPS and Affect-Modulated Acoustic Startle Response	Prescription opioid dependent patients (PODP) reported higher Anh scores (mean score = 1.6, SD = 2.1) relative to controls (*mean score* = 0.2, *SD* = 0.4) PODP showed less startle suppression when viewing positive stimuli relative to controls (t = –2.87)
Janiri et al. (2005)	N = 24 participants who met DSM-IV criteria for opioid dependence	Observational cross-sectional	SHAPS and VAS Craving	Among opioid dependent participants, greater levels of Anh were significantly associated with increased opioid drug cravings (r = 0.32), duration of abstinence (r = –0.28), and opioid withdrawal symptoms (r = 0.44)
Krupitsky et al. (2002)	N = 73 patients with heroin addiction who voluntarily admitted to an inpatient substance abuse program for opioid dependency treatment	Observational analysis in clinical trial	Zung Depression Scale, Spielberger Anxiety Scale, and Visual Scale for Craving of Heroin	Anh symptoms were significantly reduced in patients who were treated with citalopram during the first few weeks of treatment, such that patients treated with active medication showed marked reduction in Anh on the fourteenth and twenty-first days of treatment relative to baseline
Krupitsky et al. (2016)	N = 306 participants meeting criteria for DSM-IV opioid dependence	Observational analysis in clinical trial	Ferguson Anh Scale and Chapman Scale of Physical and Social Anh	Anh levels were moderately elevated at baseline and gradually decreased to levels that were at or near normal within first one to two months of biweekly drug counseling and oral or implantable naltrexone treatment Oral or implantable naltrexone did not increase Anh levels among patients who continued in treatment and did not relapse
Lubman et al. (2018)	N = 121 participants who met criteria for current or past-year opioid dependence	Observational longitudinal	TEPS	Participants TEPS scores significantly dropped (i.e., Anh increased) following a month with above-average opioid use TEPS scores rose following a month with below-average opioid use Between-subject and within-subject TEPS scores did not significantly predict opioid use in the subsequent month (*beta* = –0.24)
Martinotti et al. (2008a)	N = 25 participants who met DSM-IV criteria for opioid dependence and N = 25 participants who met DSM-IV criteria for alcohol dependence	Observational longitudinal	SHAPS and Tubingen Anh Questionnaire (TAF)	There were significant group differences in levels of Anh symptoms (F = 5.969), such that patients with prescription opioid dependence reported higher levels of Anh after three to twelve months of detoxification treatment relative to patients with alcohol dependence

Table 32.1 (*cont.*)

Study	Sample	Design	Anhedonia measure	Main finding
Meshesha et al. (2017)	N = 35 undergraduate students who reported past year nonprescription opioid use and N = 36 healthy controls with no past year drug use	Quasi-experimental	SHAPS and Affective Picture Task	Participants who reported past year nonprescription opioid use rated pleasant images as less pleasant compared to controls (F = 4.84) Participants who reported past year nonprescription opioid use reported greater levels of Anh compared to controls (F = 4.78)
Miotto et al. (2001)	N = 5 patients who were diagnosed with heroin dependence and schizophrenia	Observational analysis in clinical trial	Clinical Interview	Patients with schizophrenia and comorbid heroin dependence undergoing methadone treatment reported an improvement in Anh levels after receiving therapeutic dosages (50–80 mg/day)
Stevens et al. (2007)	N = 25 male poly-drug abusers with opioid dependence and N = 26 poly-drug abusers abstinent from opioids for more than 3 months and N = 26 nondrug healthy males	Observational cross-sectional	SHAPS and TAF	Group differences in frequency and intensity of hedonic activities (TAF) were found, such that poly-drug abusers with opioid dependence had lower scores than healthy controls (F = 7.82), while there were no differences between poly-drug users who were abstinent for more than three months and poly-drug abusers with opioid dependence Group differences in levels of Anh (SHAPS) were found, such that both poly-drug abusers with opioid dependence and poly-drug users who were abstinent for more than three months had greater levels of Anh than healthy controls (F = 5.97)
Nonsubstance behavioral addictions				
Davis and Woodside (2002)	Female patients with eating disorders (mean age, standard deviation = 27.0, 8.4) N = 78 with restrictive anorexia (AN) and N =76 with bulimia nervosa (BN) and N = 32 not otherwise specified	Observational cross-sectional	PAS	Higher mean physical Anh scores for women with anorexia nervosa relative to age-matched population values, while women with bulimia nervosa had slightly lower physical Anh scores relative to age-matched scores (mean scores, *SD* = 17.8, 7.2; 17.8, 9.6 vs. 13.3, 7.2; 14.5, 8.0) Group differences in physical Anh were associated with differences in physical activity level, such that women with bulimia nervosa who did not exercise excessively had significantly lower Anh scores (*mean score* [SD] = 13.3 [7.2]) than those with bulimia nervosa who exercised excessively (*mean score* [SD] = 17.8 [7.2])and women with anorexia nervosa who either exercised excessively (*mean score* [SD] = 20.7 [9.3]) or did not (*mean score* [SD] = 20.9 [7.5])
Eiber et al. (2002)	Women N = 20 with restrictive anorexia and N = 20 with anorectic-bulimia and N = 20 with bulimia and N = 20 healthy controls	Observational cross-sectional	SPSH	Social and physical Anh did not differ between disorderd eating groups, however, scores on physical Anh approximately 20 points higher in those with eating disorders versus healthy controls Social Anh but not physical Anh correlated positively with "Drive for Thinness" and "fear of swallowing sucrose solution" in overall sample ([*beta*, *ps*] 0.328, < 0.05; 0.268, < 0.05 respectively)

Table 32.1 (*cont.*)

Study	Sample	Design	Anhedonia measure	Main finding
Franken et al. (2006)	$N = 37$ high risk (skydivers) (mean age = 27.8 [SD = 8.3]) and $N = 34$ low risk (rowers) (mean age = 27.0 [SD = 6.1])	Observational cross-sectional	R-PAS; SHAPS	High-risk group (skydivers) showed higher levels of Anh than the low-risk group (rowers) on R-PAS (mean scores [SD], *ps* = 18.5 [8.1] vs. 14.9 [7.0], <0.05) and SHAPS (mean scores [SD], *ps* = 24.6 [6.9] vs. 19.9 [4.3], <0.005)
Guillot et al. (2017)	$N = 503$ at-risk emerging adults	Observational longitudinal	SHAPS	Trait Anh prospectively predicted greater levels of compulsive internet use and internet addiction ([*betas*, *ps*] 0.08, <0.021; 0.09, <0.041 respectively) as well as a greater likelihood of video game addiction (*OR* [95% CI], p = 1.33 [1.11–1.60] 0.003)
Heirene et al. (2016)	Male rock climbers $N = 4$ high ability (mean age = 24.75 [SD = 3.3]) and $N = 4$ average ability (mean age = 23.75 [SD = 6.2]	Observational cross-sectional	S-SI	Climbers of both ability levels reported experiencing Anh during periods of abstinence from their sport (e.g., "I compare everything I do to climbing, and nothing compares", "Other things don't excite me as much") All participants reported engaging in fewer other recreational activities (e.g., weight lifting) that they viewed may hinder their climbing performance Climbers of both ability levels reported that they felt their enjoyment threshold had increased since they started climbing, resulting in the need for more stimulating activities to achieve enjoyment (e.g., "It changes your expectations of enjoyment")
Pettorruso et al. (2014)	Individuals with Parkinson's disease (PD) $N = 11$ with Pathological Gambling (PG) and $N = 23$ with nongambling other impulse control disorders (ICDs) and $N = 120$ PD only controls	Observational cross-sectional	SHAPS	PG group reported significantly higher incidence of Anh than the ICDs group and PD controls (45%, 9%, 14% respectively) PG group reported significantly higher Anh scores than the ICDs group and PD controls (2.0 ± 1.3, 1.0 ± 1.1, 1.0 ± 1.2 respectively)

Note: CESD-D-A = Center for Epidemiologic Studies-Depression Scale- items loading on the low positive affect/ anhedonia subscale; SHAPS = Snaith-Hamilton Pleasure Scale; TEPS = Temporal Experience of Pleasure; MASQ-S = Mood and Anxiety Symptoms Questionnaire-Short Form; BDI-Anh = Beck Depression Inventory-II - Anhedonia subscale; SHS = Subjective Happiness Scale; TEPS = Temporal Experience of Pleasure Scale; MASQ-AD = Mood and Anxiety Symptom Questionnaire – anhedonia subscale; DIS[a] = The National Institute of Mental Health Diagnostic Interview Schedule – Anhedonia screener; Anh = Anhedonia;; MASQ-AD = Mood and Anxiety Symptom Questionnaire – Anhedonic Depression Scale; OLIFE = Oxford-Liverpool Inventory of Feelings and Experiences- Introvertive Anhedonia Scale; PhA = Revised Physical Anhedonia Scale; SA = Revised Social Anhedonia Scale; PAS = Physical Anhedonia Scale; SANS-Anh = Scale for Assessment for Negative Symptoms- Anhedonia Subscale; NESARC = National Epidemiologic Survey on Alcohol and Related Conditions; AUDADIS-IV = Alcohol Use Disorder and Associated Disabilities Interview Schedule – DSM-IV Version; SPSH = Scale for Physical and Social Anhedonia; PAS = Physical Anhedonia Scale; S-SI = Semi-structured Interview; R-PAS = Revised-Physical Anhedonia Scale; DIP-Anh = Diagnostic Interview for Psychosis – Anhedonia Scale; PRT = Progressive Ratio Task (a task measuring the amount of effort participants are willing to give to receive a consistent monetary reward); AWQ = Amphetamine Withdrawal Questionnaire; APT = Affective Picture Task; TAF = Tubingen Anhedonia Questionnaire; POMS = Profile of Mood States; BAES = Biphasic Alcohol Effects Scale; VASa = Visual Analogue Scale for Anhedonia; SSS = Zuckerman Sensation Seeking Scale; CDI = Children Depression Inventory – Anhedonia Subscale; PASA = Preschool Age Psychiatric Assessment; ASR = Acoustic Startle Response; BRMS = Bech-Rafaelsen Melancholia Scale; ZDS = Zung Depression Scale; SAS = Social Anhedonia Scale; VSCH = Visual Scale for Craving Heroin; THS = Trauma History Screen; PDS = Pleasure-Displeasure Scale; HRS = Hamilton Rating Scale for Depression; HADS = Hospital Anxiety and Depression Scale; MINI = Mini International Neuropsychiatric Interview

Moreover, this study demonstrated significant time-varying associations between craving and anhedonia early in the quit attempt (Days 1 through 4) and negative affect and anhedonia immediately upon quitting through the tenth day (Cook et al., 2017); post-quit anhedonia and its time-varying association with cigarette craving early in a quit attempt was reduced by NRT (Cook et al., 2017).

Other studies examining postquit anhedonia outcomes have found that adult smokers report significantly greater levels of anhedonia after four weeks of abstinence (Hughes et al., 2017), and post-quit levels of anhedonia were associated with relapsing more quickly and a significantly higher likelihood of having smoked within eight weeks postquit (Cook et al., 2015, 2017; Piper et al., 2017). In contrast, a recent study showed that participants classified as anhedonic at pretreatment were three times more likely than hedonic participants to have successfully quit smoking at Week 8, but gender did not significantly moderate this association (Powers et al., 2016).

Laboratory Studies. We identified one laboratory study of nontreatment seeking adult smokers (Guillot et al., 2017), which found suggestive evidence that trait anhedonia was associated with greater ratings of pleasantness of smoking-related pictures at both nicotine-deprived and nicotine-sated conditions. There was no evidence that the association between anhedonia and affective reactivity to pleasant, aversive, or smoking pictures was significantly moderated by smoking deprivation.

Summary. The findings of this review (that includes research published after May 2014) largely concord with a 2014 review of the anhedonia-tobacco literature (Leventhal & Zvolensky, 2015), and presents new evidence that largely corroborates past work identifying anhedonia as a risk factor for smoking cessation failure, cessation-related withdrawal, and heavier smoking in adulthood; though some exceptions were noted. New evidence in youth and young adult samples reviewed here implicates anhedonia in susceptibility to smoking initiation as well as use of non-cigarette tobacco products.

Alcohol Use

Self-Report Studies in Adolescents and Young Adults. Among 305 children aged three to six years old at baseline, children with higher (versus lower) anhedonia had higher orbitofrontal cortical volumes in a follow-up assessment occurring prior to eleven years old, and greater volume and thickness of the orbitofrontal cortex was positively associated with subsequent frequency of alcohol use at age twelve years old (Luby et al., 2018). In a study of 807 teens, youth who had ever used alcohol or drugs, but did not use nicotine/tobacco products, had higher symptoms of anhedonia compared to nonusers of any substances (Chuang, Chan & Leventhal, 2016). Furthermore, a longitudinal study of 674 Mexican-origin youth found that frequent alcohol use at fourteen years old was associated with subsequent increases in anhedonic depression symptoms from age fourteen to sixteen years old, and higher levels of anhedonic depression at age fourteen was associated with subsequent increases in alcohol use from age fourteen to sixteen years old (Parrish et al., 2016), indicating a bidirectional association between anhedonia and alcohol use in mid-adolescence.

Cross-sectional studies in emerging adults have shown that greater levels of anhedonia symptoms are associated with higher severity of alcohol use disorder symptomatology (Cano et al., 2017) and past-year alcohol use consequences, such as blackouts (Erwin et al., 2017) but are not higher in drinkers versus non-drinkers (Nunn, Rizza & Peters, 2001).

Studies of Alcohol Abstinence and Withdrawal During or After Alcohol and Other Substance Use Treatment. Three studies have examined associations of anhedonia with alcohol relapse or withdrawal symptomatology in patients with alcohol use disorder undergoing detoxification and other forms of alcohol use treatment. Marra and colleagues (1998) collected data on *physical anhedonia* – diminished ability to feel rewarded by physical sensations such as touch movement, eating, smell, and sound – and *social anhedonia* – reduced desire for social affiliation and reduced pleasure from interpersonal interactions – following two weeks of detoxification since last alcohol use. In this study, both physical and social anhedonia during treatment did not significantly predict relapse at 6 months after treatment (Marra et al., 1998). A separate study though demonstrated that severity of anhedonia assessed during the early days of abstinence was positively correlated with greater alcohol use craving during treatment, but – similar with the other study – not with duration of abstinence or severity of alcohol withdrawal symptoms (Janiri et al., 2005). One study that explored associations of alcohol withdrawal symptoms with anhedonia levels during the first twelve months of alcohol use abstinence recruited 102 detoxified subjects at various times during remission and subdivided the overall sample into four groups according to length of abstinence (Group 1: 15–30 days; Group 2: 30–90 days; Group 3: 90–180 days; Group 4: 180–360 days; Martinotti et al., 2008b). Results of this study showed significant relations between greater anhedonia levels and elevated alcohol withdrawal symptoms across the four time-points: 15–30 days (e.g., nausea and vomiting, paroxysmal sweats), 30–90 days (e.g., anxiety, agitation, visual disturbances), 90–180 days (e.g., headaches, tactile disturbances), and 180–360 days (e.g., tremors) during observation (Martinotti et al., 2008b).

Studies in Populations with Cooccurring Behavioral Health Disorders. Some studies provide evidence of an intersection between psychiatric disorders, alcohol use, and anhedonia. One survey study found that over half of patients with schizophrenia self-reported that drinking alcohol had positive effects on alleviating symptoms of anhedonia (Noordsy et al., 1991). A cross-sectional study comparing anhedonia across groups with different diagnoses illustrated that patients with alcohol dependence and comorbid major depression were more likely than patients with seasonal affective disorder or major depression and without cooccurring alcohol dependence to report drinking to alleviate anhedonia symptoms (Leibenluft et al., 1993). A cross-sectional study of patients with schizophrenia showed that those with (versus without) comorbid alcohol use disorder did not differ in physical anhedonia (Dervaux et al., 2010), failing to provide additional corroborating evidence of an additive effect of schizophrenia and alcohol use disorder on likelihood of anhedonia. The results of Dervaux and colleagues should be interpreted in context – this study focused on a subgroup of only thirty-four patients with lifetime history of alcohol use disorder, who were heterogenous with regards to severity and remission length of alcohol use by combining those with alcohol abuse and dependence into a single group. Whether more reliable (or robust) associations with anhedonia are evident in larger schizophrenia patient samples with more severe current alcohol use disorders warrants inquiry.

Some studies have examined anhedonia–alcohol use relations in the context of poly-substance use. A recent investigation conducted in a nationally representative sample of 38,694 French adults (Carton et al., 2018) found that anhedonia was positively associated with alcohol abuse amongst those with major depression and a nonalcohol substance use disorder, but anhedonia was not associated with alcohol abuse among participants without nonalcohol substance use disorders (Carton et al., 2018), suggesting possible interplay of poly-substance use in the alcohol–anhedonia connection. However, Pozzi et al. (2008) found that mean values of anhedonia symptoms did not significantly differ among patients with alcohol dependence, patients with opioid dependence, and patients with multiple drug dependence undergoing substance use treatment, and anhedonia was weakly associated with frequency of alcohol or drug use in the past thirty days. This study included a small sample of patients with alcohol dependence ($N = 20$), raising question as to whether statistical power was sufficient to identify clinically meaningful associations.

Summary. Anhedonia may be a risk factor for alcohol use initiation and escalation of use, particularly for youth and young adults. Amongst those in alcohol use treatment or recovery, anhedonia may be linked with more severe alcohol withdrawal symptoms and frequent use in certain contexts. Evidence suggests an additive association of alcohol use with other behavioral disorders in the prediction of anhedonia and a potential functional relationship between anhedonia and other behavioral health conditions – drinking could alleviate anhedonia for patients with serious mental illness.

Cannabis Use

Self-Report Studies in Adolescents and Young Adults. In a longitudinal study of 3,396 high-school students, Leventhal et al. (2017) found associations of greater levels of anhedonia at age fourteen with increased risk of cannabis use escalation across a two-year follow-up period, and that association was amplified among adolescents with (versus without) friends who also used cannabis. This study did not find evidence that cannabis use at age fourteen predicted changes in anhedonia over two-year follow-up (Leventhal et al., 2017). Similarly, a separate study found that adolescents with cannabis dependence had significantly higher levels of *physical anhedonia* – diminished ability to feel rewarded by physical sensations such as touch movement, eating, smell, and sound – relative to healthy adolescents who reported not regularly using cannabis; nonsignificant relations were found for social anhedonia ($p = 0.13$; Dorard et al., 2008). Albertella et al. (2018) found that, for youth aged fifteen to twenty (versus twenty-one to twenty-four) changes in anhedonia over a twelve-month follow up was positively associated with frequency of cannabis use, suggesting a potential vulnerable period for anhedonia-cannabis use linkages at younger ages. Cross-sectional studies of young adults using smaller samples have not found positive associations between cannabis use status and anhedonia (Dumas et al., 2002; Nunn et al., 2001).

Self-Report Studies in General Adult Samples. Johnson et al. (2009) demonstrated that anhedonic depression was not a significant predictor of frequency of cannabis use above and beyond controlling for other covariates (daily nicotine product use, alcohol consumption, and gender) in a cross-sectional analysis of young adult current cannabis users (those who reported using cannabis in the past thirty days). This study found a positive association between anhedonia and cannabis use coping motives (using cannabis to regulate affect).

Raising the possibility that different facets of anhedonia may be important to differentiating a cannabis–anhedonia connection, another cross-sectional study including behavioral measures of reward processing found that twenty cannabis-dependent (versus twenty drug-using noncannabis-dependent control) participants exhibited greater anhedonia in the form of impaired reward learning but did not differ on motivation to obtain rewards (Lawn et al., 2016).

In the sole longitudinal study of cannabis use in a general adult sample, Bovasso (2001) reported that individuals with (versus without) cannabis abuse and no depressive symptoms at baseline had a four times greater incidence of anhedonia at a follow up fourteen to sixteen years later, after controlling for sociodemographic factors and psychiatric characteristics in the Baltimore Epidemiologic Catchment Area Study ($N = 849$).

Studies in Populations with Cooccurring Psychiatric Disorders. In a small cross-sectional study including individuals at an inpatient psychiatric facility, Bersani et al. (2002) observed significantly higher anhedonia scores among cannabis nonusers ($N = 25$) and users ($N = 25$) with schizophrenia. By contrast, in a study of a nationally representative sample of US adults with major depressive disorder, researchers found that individuals with cannabis use disorder (versus cannabis nonusers) had significantly greater odds of reporting anhedonia symptoms two years later (Feingold, Rehm & Lev-Ran, 2017). Possibly, anhedonia is predictive of cannabis use among mood disorders but not thought disorders.

Summary. Large-scale studies of adolescent and general adult samples suggest a fairly consistent association between cannabis use and use disorder with anhedonia, which aligns with the notion that anhedonia may increase risk of cannabis use escalation. In adults, cannabis use may increase subsequent risk of anhedonia in those with or without a prior history of significant depression symptoms. The young adult literature on this topic is small, restricted to studies published nearly two decades ago, and has not corroborated these findings; the reasons for this discrepancy are unclear. Whether anhedonia affects maintenance of cannabis use, relapse, and withdrawal symptomatology, use of other types of cannabis products (e.g., cannabis edibles, cannabis vaping, blunts), and generalizes to psychiatric populations has yet to be fully determined, as these data are scarce and seem to be inconclusive.

Stimulant Drug Use

Self-Report Studies in Adults. One study of individuals seeking outpatient psychiatric treatment used diagnostic data to demonstrate that patients with past stimulant use disorder in full remission for two months or longer (versus those with no history of stimulant use disorder) reported greater prevalence of current anhedonia at the outset of treatment (Leventhal et al., 2008). Stimulant use disorder was a combined category that amalgamated several psychostimulant drugs (i.e., cocaine, amphetamine, methamphetamine, dextroamphetamine). This finding suggests that anhedonia may be a protracted consequence of stimulant use or perhaps a preexisting risk factor that precedes and follows stimulant use disorder onset and offset, respectively; however, the correlational nature also leaves open the possibility of unmeasured confounds, though a host of psychiatric and demographic covariates were adjusted for in that study, increasing confidence that there may be a specific link between anhedonia and stimulant use disorder. Consistent with this result, patients with schizophrenia who were past-year users of amphetamine reported significantly higher prevalence of anhedonia symptoms relative to former amphetamine users with schizophrenia (Voce et al., 2018), further suggesting that recent use is linked with anhedonia amongst patients with psychiatric conditions.

Leventhal et al. (2010) found that anhedonia was incrementally associated with lifetime cocaine or amphetamine use in a representative population-based sample of American adults, after accounting for depressed mood in the same model (Leventhal et al., 2010). The association with lifetime stimulant use generalized across those who did versus did not ultimately progress to stimulant dependence. Among the subsample of lifetime cocaine or amphetamine users, anhedonia, but not depressed mood, was also significantly associated with progression to dependence (Leventhal et al., 2010). Thus, these results suggest that anhedonia may be associated with amphetamine and cocaine use initiation as well as risk of transition from initiation to dependence.

Studies of Stimulant Use Abstinence and Withdrawal. Generally, behavioral interventions such as contingency management – a reward-based approach where individuals receive monetary incentives for objectively verified abstinence (Higgins, Silverman & Heil, 2007) – have been shown to be efficacious for stimulant dependence treatment (Dutra et al., 2008). However, analyses of subgroups who respond best to contingency management found that patients with cocaine use disorder with greater anhedonia levels exhibited poorer treatment outcomes involving contingency management (Wardle et al., 2017), and greater severity of self-reported anhedonia at the beginning of contingency management treatment was significantly associated with relapse after three and six months of abstinence, even when controlling for overall depression (Crits-Christoph et al., 2018). A collective interpretation of or speculation from this set of findings is that because anhedonic individuals are less sensitive to nondrug reinforcers, contingency management incentives may be insufficiently motivating enough to promote choosing reinforced abstinence over cocaine.

In a separate smaller study, twenty-three participants with current cocaine abuse who were abstinent from cocaine for twenty-four hours completed surveys assessing both trait (i.e., physical and social anhedonia) and state anhedonia (as measured by the Snaith–Hamilton Pleasure Scale [SHAPS]) as well as cocaine addiction severity and cocaine withdrawal symptoms during a single session (Morie et al., 2014). Results showed that, compared to twenty-seven healthy controls with no drug use history, participants with current cocaine abuse had significantly higher scores on trait measures of physical and social anhedonia and state measures of anhedonia (Morie et al., 2014). Furthermore, Morie and colleagues found that greater levels of trait physical anhedonia, but not trait social anhedonia, was significantly associated with higher addiction severity of cocaine dependence, and state anhedonia, but not trait anhedonia measures, was significantly related to cocaine withdrawal severity (Morie et al., 2014). In a retrospective cross-sectional investigation of abstinent (more than thirty days from past usage) stimulant using adults, preferred method of drug administration (i.e., injecting, smoking, swallowing, or snorting), duration of abstinence, latency from first use to regular use, and prior solicitation of treatment were not related to social anhedonia scores (Lichlyter, Purdon & Tibbo, 2011), thus aligning with other studies that found nonsignificant associations between substance use behavior and social anhedonia scores (Dorard et al., 2008; Marra et al., 1998; Morie et al., 2014).

Research observing the time course of methamphetamine withdrawal during the first three weeks of abstinence, as measured by self-report, interviews, and observer ratings, generally show that anhedonia is a reliable withdrawal symptom with an initial peak within twenty-four hours of the last use of amphetamines and then ultimately resolves to near comparison group levels within one week of abstinence (McGregor et al., 2005; Newton et al., 2004).

Laboratory Studies. To date, there are three laboratory studies that have examined whether levels of anhedonia predict the magnitude of acute subjective effects of drug administration using dextroamphetamine in placebo-controlled experimental designs. One such study demonstrated that anhedonia (as measured by the SHAPS) was not predictive of the level of subjective rewarding effects produced by 30 mg of *d*-amphetamine (versus placebo) in the overall sample; however, a single item related to anhedonia on the Hamilton Rating Scale for Depression (HAM-D; "loss of interest in activities") was positively with dextroamphetamine rewarding effects in patients with major depression (Tremblay et al., 2002). A separate laboratory study conducted in healthy stimulant-naïve volunteers demonstrated that greater trait anticipatory pleasure at the baseline session predicted greater amphetamine-induced increases in positive mood, whereas, there was a marginal association between higher consummatory anhedonia at baseline and greater amphetamine-related increases in positive mood ($p = 0.09$; Kirkpatrick et al., 2016). Another laboratory study revealed that patients with major depression (versus healthy controls) had a hypersensitive response to the rewarding effects of dextroamphetamine, and the degree of the dextroamphetamine's rewarding effects was associated with severity of anhedonia symptoms prior to drug administration (Tremblay et al., 2005).

Summary. While some of the results are equivocal, in general, stimulant drug dependence is associated with a greater prevalence of anhedonia, and anhedonia is associated with an increased risk of progression along the entire stimulant use disorder developmental continuum (e.g., initiation, progression, maintenance, and relapse) and severity of stimulant dependence and withdrawal symptomatology. Anhedonia may increase sensitivity to the rewarding subjective effects of amphetamine, which could explain why anhedonic individuals are more likely to progress from initiation to dependence. Anhedonia is also a manifestation of stimulant withdrawal that is linked with poorer treatment outcomes and may hinder efforts to remain abstinent in patients undergoing treatment, particularly among individuals treated with contingency management.

Opioid Use

Self-Report Studies in Adults. A recent longitudinal investigation found that adult participants who reported past year nonmedical prescription opioid use (versus healthy controls) report greater anhedonia at baseline and at six- and twelve-month follow-up assessment (Meshesha et al., 2017). A separate study of patients who met criteria for current or past-year opioid dependence found anhedonia symptoms significantly increased following a month of above-average opioid use while anhedonia symptoms decreased with below average opioid use levels (Lubman et al., 2018). Furthermore, one cross-sectional study compared anhedonia in twenty-five male adults with poly-drug abuse and concurrent opioid dependence, twenty-six poly-drug abusers abstinent from opioids for more than three months, and twenty-six nondrug healthy males (Stevens et al., 2007). Results showed that participants with poly-drug abuse and opioid dependence and participants with poly-drug abuse who were abstinent for three months or longer had greater levels of anhedonia compared to healthy controls.

Studies of Opioid Abstinence and Withdrawal During or After Treatment. In twenty-four opioid-dependent participants during treatment, Janiri and colleagues (2005) found that greater levels of anhedonia during the early days of abstinence were significantly associated with increased opioid drug cravings, a shorter duration of abstinence, and greater severity of opioid withdrawal symptoms during treatment. Similarly, Martinotti, Cloninger & Janiri (2008a) demonstrated that patients with prescription opioid dependence reported higher levels of anhedonia after three to twelve months of detoxification treatment relative to patients with alcohol dependence measured at the same time point, suggesting that anhedonia may be a preexisting risk factor for or protracted consequence of opioid dependence that may be more robust than alcohol use, at least in the context of the treatment seeking population.

Regarding the role of anhedonia in response to different opioid use disorder pharmacotherapies, Krupitsky et al. (2016) found that anhedonia levels were moderately elevated during pretreatment, but significantly decreased within the first one to two months of biweekly drug counseling and oral or implantable naltrexone treatment (Krupitsky et al., 2016). This study also showed that oral or implantable naltrexone treatment (versus placebo) did not significantly increase levels of anhedonia among patients who continued in treatment and who relapsed during treatment (Krupitsky et al., 2016). A prior study of heroin-dependent patients in treatment found that patients who were treated with citalopram during the first few weeks of treatment showed marked reduction in anhedonia on fourteenth and twenty-first day of treatment relative to pretreatment anhedonia levels (Krupitsky et al., 2002). Similarly, an observational study also found that patients with schizophrenia and comorbid heroin dependence undergoing methadone treatment reported an improvement in anhedonia levels after receiving therapeutic dosages of methadone (50–80 mg/day; Miotto, Preti & Frezza, 2001). Garfield et al. (2017) demonstrated that opioid dependent participants who were prescribed opioid maintenance pharmacotherapy (i.e., methadone or buprenorphine) had significantly higher anhedonia symptoms during treatment relative to healthy controls, but anhedonia during treatment did not associate with duration of abstinence (Garfield et al., 2017). Taken together, these findings implicate that specific opioid use disorder pharmacotherapies (i.e., oral or implantable naltrexone treatment, citalopram, methadone) may significantly impact levels of anhedonia during treatment, but only for certain populations (e.g., patients with heroin dependence, patients with schizophrenia and comorbid heroin dependence).

Laboratory Studies. Huhn et al. (2016) utilized an affect-modulated acoustic startle response task to assess hedonic responses to standardized reward-related stimuli and found that patients with prescription opioid dependence (versus healthy controls) exhibited less startle suppression when viewing positive stimuli (Huhn et al., 2016), indicative of a less positive hedonic evaluation of putatively positive images relative to controls. Meshesha et al. (2017) showed that standardized images commonly perceived as pleasant were perceived as less pleasant among participants who reported past year nonmedical prescription opioid use than healthy controls (Meshesha et al., 2017).

Summary. The literature is fairly consistent that opioid use and dependence are associated with anhedonia in several populations. Among opioid-dependent patients, pretreatment levels of anhedonia may also increase the risk of opioid use relapse and opioid-related withdrawal symptoms during abstinence, and various pharmacotherapies either alleviate anhedonia or do not exacerbate anhedonia.

Nonsubstance Behavioral Addictions

Studies of Internet Use and Addiction. In a study of at-risk emerging adults who formerly attended alternative remediation high schools, Guillot et al. (2017) found that trait levels of anhedonia prospectively predicted greater levels of compulsive internet use and addiction to online activities (i.e., internet browsing, social media, or online shopping), as well as a higher likelihood of addiction to online/offline video games at a follow up nine to eighteen months later.

Studies of Participation in Extreme Sports. Two studies examined the role of anhedonia in thrill-seeking extreme sports – a class of behaviors that promote intense stimulation and addictiveness. One cross-sectional study found higher levels of anhedonia among thirty-seven adults who regularly engaged in skydiving and other thrill-seeking sports activities as compared to a control group of rowers who did not partake in high-risk activities (Franken et al., 2006). Another study utilized detailed semistructured interviews to explore the anhedonic experiences of high-ability and average-ability male rock climbers (Heirene et al., 2016). This study found climbers of both ability levels reported experiencing anhedonia during periods of abstinence from their sport (e.g., "I compare everything I do to climbing, and nothing compares," "Other things don't excite me as much") and that they felt their enjoyment threshold had increased since they started climbing, resulting in the need for more stimulating activities to achieve enjoyment (e.g., "It changes your expectations of enjoyment"; Heirene et al., 2016).

Studies of Eating and Other Addictive Behaviors. Recent research conducted in 154 patients with Parkinson's disease determined that thirty-four out of the 154 patients with Parkinson's disease also met diagnostic criteria for cooccurrence of impulse control disorders (eleven with pathological gambling, twenty with hypersexuality, nine with binge-eating problems, and five with compulsive shopping; Pettorruso et al., 2014). Findings of this study showed that patients with pathological gambling had a greater incidence of anhedonia and reported greater state levels of anhedonia relative to patients with nongambling impulse control disorders and patients with Parkinson's disease only (Pettorruso et al., 2014).

Summary. Collectively, these results suggest that anhedonia my increase risk in engagement in nonsubstance addictive behaviors, and that repeated execution of such behaviors may be followed by "withdrawal"-like states involving anhedonia. The association of anhedonia with behavioral conditions involving impulsive/compulsive eating, such as bulimia, suggests a hypersensitivity to the rewarding effects of foods that may be addictive and are involved in binge eating episodes in concert with a hyposensitivity to other rewards.

Targeting Anhedonia in Treatment of Addictive Behaviors

Pharmacological Treatments

Prior preclinical work suggests that the dopamine and norepinephrine reuptake inhibitor antidepressant medication bupropion, which is an FDA approved smoking cessation treatment, may improve anhedonia (Bruijnzeel & Markou, 2003; Cryan et al., 2001, 2004). However, one study demonstrated that the standard dose of bupropion did not significantly moderate the relation of pre-quit lifetime anhedonia to poor smoking cessation outcome (Leventhal et al., 2014). In a depression treatment trial, Tomarken et al. (2004) found that maximal clinical benefit from bupropion-related alleviation of anhedonia was found for a high dose (400 mg/day) that is larger than the standard dose for smoking cessation (300 mg/day). It is possible that higher doses of bupropion are required to provide sufficiently robust dopamine reuptake inhibition to improve reward processing and alleviate anhedonia (to the extent that in has downstream effects on anhedonia-related risk of smoking relapse). A randomized controlled trial testing the efficacy of the high dose of bupropion for anhedonic smokers could be a promising avenue for pharmacotherapy research options for anhedonia in addictive behaviors.

Recently, a laboratory study of acutely abstinent smokers found that the varenicline – a partial agonist of the α4β2 nicotinic acetylcholine receptor – versus placebo significantly reduced improved the relative reward value of a nondrug reinforcer (i.e., money) relative to smoking in a behavioral economics task (McClure et al., 2012). To the extent to which these findings indicate varenicline-mediated improvement of processing of nondrug rewards, further exploration of the effectiveness of varenicline for treatment of anhedonia among smokers and perhaps other addictive behaviors may warrant consideration.

Acetyl-L-carnitine (ALC), an endogenous compound that has been shown to significantly increase dopamine outflow in the nucleus accumbens, has been proposed as a method of addressing anhedonic indivdiuals alcohol use disorder (Martinotti et al., 2011). Martinotti et al. (2011) found that anhedonia was significantly reduced among patients with alcohol use disorder receiving a ten-day intravenous treatment of ALC at 1 g/day and 3 g/day relative to placebo in a detoxication program (Martinotti et al., 2011). ALC may be a potentially beneficial pharmacological treatment for targeting anhedonia in anhedonic patients with alcohol dependence or other addictive behaviors.

Levodopa – a dopamine precursor that is typically used in treatment of Parkinson's disease – has shown some promise as a candidate medication in treatment of cocaine dependence (Schmitz et al., 2008). Results from a study conducted in a sample of 161 treatment-seeking cocaine dependent participants receiving sustained release levodopa/carbidopa (400/100 mg) or placebo in combination with clinical management + cognitive behavioral therapy or clinical management + cognitive behavioral therapy + voucher-based reinforcement therapy found that levodopa treatment with vouchers demonstrated higher proportions of cocaine-negative urine tests, longer periods of continuous cocaine use abstinence, and less craving for cocaine versus other treatment combinations (Schmitz et al., 2008). One possible explanation is that levodopa-related increases in dopaminergic tone may heighten reward processing, which may in turn improve the saliency and reinforcing effects of contingent nondrug rewards (Schmitz et al., 2008). Future study of levadopa and other dopaminergic agonists with low abuse liability for the treatment of anhedonic individuals with addictive behaviors may be fruitful.

There may be an intersection between treatment with naltrexone, a mu (μ)-opioid receptor antagonist that blocks opioid effects, and anhedonia in opioid use disorder. In one trial, anhedonia levels decreased in patients with opioid dependence within one to two months of oral or implantable naltrexone treatment relative to the placebo (Krupitsky et al., 2016). A recent randomized controlled opioid use disorder treatment trial of voucher-based contingency management and support from a significant other to enhance retention on oral naltrexone discovered that participants who dropped out of treatment consistently reported higher rates of anhedonia and other affective symptoms relative to those who remained in treatment (Carroll et al., 2018). Thus, future studies examining the role of anhedonia on treatment adherence and relapse risk in opioid use disorder treatment is necessary to increase response to pharmacological treatment in anhedonic individuals.

There are no studies regarding behavioral addictions, modification of anhedonia and pharmacologic treatments. This is research that may be needed in due course.

Psychotherapy

Specific psychotherapeutic techniques such as behavioral activation – a behavior-based treatment approach that is designed to improve an individual's ability to engage in healthy, substance-free activities to increase exposure to positively rewarding experiences (Lejuez, Hopko & Hopko, 2001) – may be one therapeutic strategy for enhancing the reward and hedonic effects of alternative nonaddictive reinforcers in anhedonic individuals. A tailored version of this treatment approach was recently developed (Behavioral Activation Treatment for Smoking [BATS]) to address smoking cessation in smokers with elevated depressive symptoms, which incorporated behavioral activation strategies (e.g., activity monitoring, identifying and planning of pleasurable activities) to improve positive affect via increased engagement in rewarding experiences and enjoyment of nonsmoking, daily activities (MacPherson et al., 2010). In a pilot study that compared the effects of BATS (n = 35) with standard smoking cessation counseling (n = 33) among underserved smokers from diverse backgrounds, results had shown that an eight-session BATS generated significantly higher rates of smoking abstinence and greater reductions in depressive symptoms over the course of twenty-six weeks relative to standard cessation counseling alone (14.3 percent versus 0 percent at six-months follow-up; MacPherson et al., 2010). While this study did not present data specifically on anhedonia outcomes, future researchers should consider anhedonia's prevalence as a depression phenotype as support for BATS as a treatment strategy for individuals with cooccurring addictive behaviors and anhedonia. A recently published pilot study testing the effects of another modified behavioral activation treatment called LETS ACT (life enhancement treatment for substance use), which teaches participants to increase positively reinforcing value-driven activities to counter depression and relapse, found that those receiving LETS ACT had significantly higher abstinence rates at three months, six months, and twelve months post-treatment relative to those receiving supportive counseling (Daughters et al., 2018). Behavioral activation may be a promising therapeutic strategy for treatment of anhedonia among individuals with addictive behaviors.

Mindfulness-based therapy, which involve increasing awareness and acceptance of present-moment experiences as well as cultivating adaptive coping strategies to address triggers, cravings, and relapse of addictive behaviors (Witkiewitz et al., 2014) could be useful for reducing anhedonia in addictive behaviors. Mindfulness-based interventions may increase hedonic capacity and responsiveness to natural reward in patients with a history of depression (Geschwind, Peeters, Drukker, van Os & Wichers, 2011) and among samples of opioid using chronic pain patients (Garland, Froeliger & Howard, 2014, 2015). Furthermore, a recent cross-sectional study demonstrated that trait levels of mindfulness were associated with heightened hedonic capacity in a sample of chronic pain patients on extended opioid pharmacotherapy (Thomas & Garland, 2017). Future investigation of the effects of mindfulness-based addiction treatments on anhedonia would be of value.

Positive psychotherapy, which aims to cultivate positive emotions and traits (Seligman, Rashid & Parks, 2006), could presumably address anhedonia in addictive behaviors. Recent adaptations to address smoking cessation (i.e., Positive Psychotherapy for Smoking Cessation; PPT-S; Kahler et al., 2014) incorporated several exercises designed to teach anhedonic smokers on how to obtain pleasure, satisfaction, and meaning without smoking (e.g., focusing on positive life experiences and writing down three good things that happened each day, savoring experiences [e.g., morning coffee, the sun on their face] each day for one week, for at least two to three minutes per experience). Results of a preliminary study for PPT-S that was conducted in a sample of highly anhedonic smokers demonstrated significantly higher rates of smoking abstinence at eight weeks (47.4 percent), sixteen weeks (36.9 percent), and twenty-six weeks (31.6 percent; Kahler et al., 2014), which was substantially greater than abstinence benchmarks reported in prior meta-analyses (Fiore et al., 2008).

However, a subsequent larger pilot trial found that the effects of PPT-S were weaker for smokers with lower baseline levels of positive affect (i.e., higher CESD-anhedonia scores) relative to smokers with higher baseline positive affect (Kahler et al., 2015). Thus, despite a conceptual premise that PPT-S could be useful for anhedonic smokers by counteracting their hedonic deficits, the data was not supportive of this hypothesis. As PPT-S aims to cultivate existing psychological resources, it may be that anhedonic smokers may inherently lack such resources to cultivate and therefore may have a hard time experiencing pleasure enhancement from the intervention. Since the evidence base is small, more work is needed before definitively ruling out PPT-S as a candidate psychotherapy for anhedonia in addictive behaviors.

Remaining Gaps in Literature and Future Directions for Research

Cross-Population Differences in the Role of Anhedonia in Addictive Behaviors

There is limited work that has assessed the degree to which *gender* moderates associations between anhedonia and addictive behaviors (cf., Powers et al., 2016). Yet, a large body of evidence has shown relatively greater prevalence rates of mood disorders among women (Seney & Sibille, 2014) and some research supports gender differences in expression and experience of emotion as well as pleasurable events (Deng et al., 2016; van Roekel et al., 2016). Such data could inform whether sex-specific treatments that address anhedonia in addictive behaviors should be considered.

Examining risk factors associated with *adolescent and young adult substance users* is an emerging field of research that has largely focused on nicotine, cannabis, and alcohol use. Some of the first increases in opioid-related overdose deaths in adolescents and young adults were observed recently in the USA following years of decline (Curtin, Tejada-Vera & Warmer, 2017). Extending existing research on anhedonia in opioid use disorder to youths is warranted.

There is almost no literature on *ethnicity*, anhedonia, and addiction. A previous study of 2,423 postpartum women found that Asians and Pacific Islander women reported higher rates of anhedonia followed by African American women, Hispanic women, and white women (Liu & Tronick, 2014). It is plausible that certain racial/ethnic groups, particularly those from minority or underrepresented populations, may be differentially at risk for substance use, given varying prevalence rates of anhedonia across race/ethnic groups. Data addressing this question is absent.

Alternative Nicotine and Cannabis Products

With recent changes in technology, policy, and cultural trends, a highly diverse commercialized marketplace for alternative nicotine and cannabis products has emerged (e.g., e-cigarettes, heat-not-burn products, high-potency cannabis concentrates, cannabis edibles). Outside of a few studies of anhedonia in e-cigarette and hookah use (e.g., Leventhal et al. 2016; Brikmanis et al. 2017), very little is known regarding whether anhedonia may be a risk factor for use of alternative nicotine and cannabis products. Different methods of nicotine and cannabis administration may result in different pharmacokinetic profiles of drug absorption and, in turn, unique drug effects (e.g., edible versus smoked cannabis). Also, some products are available in flavored variants (e.g., edibles, cannabis vaporizer e-liquids), whereas traditional products are available in unflavored or tradition flavors (e.g., menthols). Given anhedonic individuals respond differently to the subjective perception-altering effects of sensory stimuli, studying whether anhedonia may be a relatively more robust risk factor for flavored products warrants consideration. Finally, high concentrations of nicotine and THC are available in certain products (e.g., Pod-mod e-cigarettes, dabs), which may alter their abuse liability and potential reinforcing effects, particularly in anhedonic individuals who are more sensitive to the subjective rewarding effects of certain drugs of abuse (e.g., Tremblay et al., 2005).

Poly-Drug Use and Poly-Product Use

In light of the proliferation of alternative nicotine, cannabis, and other substance use products, substance use has begun to take on an increasingly more complex form, as prevalence of poly-drug use – the concurrent utilization of two or more drugs – has substantially increased in youth and young adults (Creamer et al., 2015; Lee et al., 2015; Peters et al., 2018). To date, there have only been a small number of studies described above that have examined anhedonia-substance use associations within the context of poly-drug use (Carton et al., 2018; Pozzi et al., 2008; Stevens et al., 2007). These studies have been conducted in mixed populations and yielded relatively mixed results. A recent investigation illuminated that anhedonia may be an underlying mechanism of associations between family history of substance use and poly-drug use patterns across mid-adolescence (Cho, Stone & Leventhal, 2019), suggesting that trait levels of anhedonia that may arise in adolescence may increase susceptibility to engagement in poly-drug use and familial transmission of substance use. Whether the use of two or more drugs (versus use of a single drug) or different combinations of poly-product drug use (e.g., consumption of cigarettes, cannabis edibles, and prescription drugs) additively or synergistically increase anhedonia symptoms is currently unknown. Further exploration of the impact of availability and use of different types of opioids (e.g., prescription or illicit opioids, different synthetic compounds [i.e., Fentanyl versus Oxycontine]) on anhedonia symptoms would also be a critical research avenue, given the increasing prevalence of opioids misuse and addiction and rising opioid overdose deaths within the United States (Vivolo-Kantor et al., 2018).

Novel Nondrug Addictive Products

Considering rapidly evolving trends in digital communication and technology device use patterns, digital media platforms are becoming increasingly stimulating and addictive. Only one study has addressed anhedonia in digital media use. This study found anhedonia confers risk for problematic internet use in data collected more than a decade ago (Guillot et al., 2017). Whether anhedonia may be a risk factor (and a potential consequence) of excessive use of new media products (e.g., social media platforms, mobile gaming, media streaming) should be investigated.

Conclusions

Anhedonia may be a manifestation of psychobiological dysregulation generated by the chronic exposure to addictive behaviors as well as a premorbid trait, which, in either case, increase motivation to engage in addictive behaviors to offset deficient pleasure. Anhedonia may also play a unique role in the transitions across multiple stages of the addiction trajectory (i.e., initiation, escalation/progression, maintenance, cessation/relapse) across various substance and nonsubstance addictions. Some treatment and prevention interventions have shown promise in reducing anhedonia-related risk of addictive behaviors. Future work is needed to further clarify whether these associations generalize to diverse populations or engagement in certain addictive behaviors or use/couse of certain products. Further work evaluating the efficacy of prevention and intervention programs targeting anhedonia in mitigating risk for and treatment of addictive behaviors in individuals facing anhedonia may contribute to advances in clinical and scientific efforts that reduce the public health burden of anhedonia-addiction comorbidity.

REFERENCES

Albertella, L., Le Pelley, M. E., Yücel, M. & Copeland, J. (2018). Age moderates the association between frequent cannabis use and negative schizotypy over time. *Addictive Behaviors*, **87**, 183–189.

Bersani, G., Orlandi, V., Gherardelli, S. & Pancheri, P. (2002). Cannabis and neurological soft signs in schizophrenia: absence of relationship and influence on psychopathology. *Psychopathology*, **35**(5), 289–295.

Bickel, W. K., Jarmolowicz, D. P., Mueller, E. T. & Gatchalian, K. M. (2011). The behavioral economics and neuroeconomics of reinforcer pathologies: implications for etiology and treatment of addiction. *Current Psychiatry Reports*, **13**(5), 406.

Bovasso, G. B. (2001). Cannabis abuse as a risk factor for depressive symptoms. *American Journal of Psychiatry*, **158**(12), 2033–2037.

Brikmanis, K., Petersen, A. & Doran, N. (2017). Do personality traits related to affect regulation predict other tobacco product use among young adult non-daily smokers? *Addictive Behaviors*, **75**, 79–84.

Bruijnzeel, A. W. & Markou, A. (2003). Characterization of the effects of bupropion on the reinforcing properties of nicotine and food in rats. *Synapse*, **50**(1), 20–28.

Cano, M. Á., de Dios, M. A., Correa-Fernández, V., et al. (2017). Depressive symptom domains and alcohol use severity among Hispanic emerging adults: examining moderating effects of gender. *Addictive Behaviors*, **72**, 72–78.

Carleton, R. N., Thibodeau, M. A., Teale, M. J., et al. (2013). The center for epidemiologic studies depression scale: a review with a theoretical and empirical examination of item content and factor structure. *PLoS ONE*, **8**(3), e58067.

Carroll, K. M., Nich, C., Frankforter, T. L., et al. (2018). Accounting for the uncounted: physical and affective distress in individuals dropping out of oral naltrexone treatment for opioid use disorder. *Drug and Alcohol Dependence*, **192**, 264–270.

Carton, L., Pignon, B., Baguet, A., et al. (2018). Influence of comorbid alcohol use disorders on the clinical patterns of major depressive disorder: a general population-based study. *Drug and Alcohol Dependence*, **187**, 40–47.

Chuang, C. W. I., Chan, C. & Leventhal, A. M. (2016). Adolescent emotional pathology and lifetime history of alcohol or drug use with and without comorbid tobacco use. *Journal of Dual Diagnosis*, **12**(1), 27–35.

Cho, J., Stone, M. D. & Leventhal, A. M. (2019). Anhedonia as a phenotypic marker of familial transmission of polysubstance use trajectories across midadolescence. *Psychology of Addictive Behaviors*, **33**(1), 15–25.

Cobb, N. K., Byron, M. J., Abrams, D. B. & Shields, P. G. (2010). Novel nicotine delivery systems and public health: the rise of the "e-cigarette". *American Journal of Public Health*, **100**(12), 2340–2342.

Cohen, A. S., Najolia, G. M., Brown, L. A. & Minor, K. S. (2011). The state-trait disjunction of anhedonia in schizophrenia: potential affective, cognitive and social-based mechanisms. *Clinical Psychology Review*, **31** (3), 440–448.

Cook, J. W., Lanza, S. T., Chu, W., Baker, T. B. & Piper, M. E. (2017). Anhedonia: its dynamic relations with craving, negative affect, and treatment during a quit smoking attempt. *Nicotine & Tobacco Research*, **19**(6), 703–709.

Cook, J. W., Piper, M. E., Leventhal, A. M., et al. (2015). Anhedonia as a component of the tobacco withdrawal syndrome. *Journal of Abnormal Psychology*, **124**(1), 215.

Creamer, M. R., Perry, C. L., Harrell, M. B. & Diamond, P. M. (2015). Trends in multiple tobacco product use among high school students. *Tobacco Regulatory Science*, **1**(3), 204–214.

Crits-Christoph, P., Wadden, S., Gaines, A., et al. (2018). Symptoms of anhedonia, not depression, predict the outcome of treatment of cocaine dependence. *Journal of Substance Abuse Treatment*, **92**, 46–50.

Cryan, J. F., Dalvi, A., Jin, et al. (2001). Use of dopamine-β-hydroxylase-deficient mice to determine the role of norepinephrine in the mechanism of action of antidepressant drugs. *Journal of Pharmacology and Experimental Therapeutics*, **298**(2), 651–657.

Cryan, J. F., O'Leary, O. F., Jin, S. H., et al. (2004). Norepinephrine-deficient mice lack responses to antidepressant drugs, including selective serotonin reuptake inhibitors. *Proceedings of the National Academy of Sciences*, **101**(21), 8186–8191.

Curtin, S. C., Tejada-Vera, B. & Warmer, M. (2017). Drug overdose deaths among adolescents aged 15-19 in the United States: 1999-2015. *NCHS Data Brief*, **282**, 1–8.

Daughters, S. B., Magidson, J. F., Anand, D., et al. (2018). The effect of a behavioral activation treatment for substance use on post-treatment abstinence: a randomized controlled trial. *Addiction*, **113**(3), 535–544.

D'Souza, M. S. & Markou, A. (2010). Neural substrates of psychostimulant withdrawal-induced anhedonia. In *Behavioral Neuroscience of Drug Addiction*. Berlin, Heidelberg: Springer, pp. 119–178.

Davis, C. & Woodside, D. B. (2002). Sensitivity to the rewarding effects of food and exercise in the eating disorders. *Comprehensive Psychiatry*, **43**(3), 189–194.

Deng, Y., Chang, L., Yang, M., Huo, M. & Zhou, R. (2016). Gender differences in emotional response: inconsistency between experience and expressivity. *PLoS ONE*, **11**(6), e0158666.

Dervaux, A., Laqueille, X., Bourdel, M. C., Olié, J. P. & Krebs, M. O. (2010). Impulsivity and sensation seeking in alcohol abusing patients with schizophrenia. *Frontiers in Psychiatry*, **1**, 135.

Dorard, G., Berthoz, S., Phan, O., Corcos, M. & Bungener, C. (2008). Affect dysregulation in cannabis abusers. *European Child & Adolescent Psychiatry*, **17**(5), 274–282.

Dumas, P., Saoud, M., Bouafia, S., et al. (2002). Cannabis use correlates with schizotypal personality traits in healthy students. *Psychiatry Research*, **109**(1), 27–35.

Dutra, L., Stathopoulou, G., Basden, S. L., et al. (2008). A meta-analytic review of psychosocial interventions for substance use disorders. *American Journal of Psychiatry*, **165** (2), 179–187.

Eiber, R., Berlin, I., de Brettes, B., Foulon, C. & Guelfi, J. D. (2002). Hedonic response to sucrose solutions and the fear of weight gain in patients with eating disorders. *Psychiatry Research*, **113**(1-2), 173–180.

Erwin, M. C., Charak, R., Durham, T. A., et al. (2017). The 7-factor hybrid model of DSM-5 PTSD symptoms and alcohol consumption and consequences in a national sample of trauma-exposed veterans. *Journal of Anxiety Disorders*, **51**, 14–21.

Fawcett, J., Clark, D. C., Scheftner, W. A. & Gibbons, R. D. (1983). Assessing anhedonia in psychiatric patients: the pleasure scale. *Archives of General Psychiatry*, **40**(1), 79–84.

Feingold, D., Rehm, J. & Lev-Ran, S. (2017). Cannabis use and the course and outcome of major depressive disorder: a population based longitudinal study. *Psychiatry Research*, **251**, 225–234.

Fiore, M. C., Jaen, C. R., Baker, T. B., et al. (2008). *Treating Tobacco Use and Dependence: 2008 Update*. Rockville, MD: US Department of Health and Human Services.

Fiorito, E. R. & Simons, R. F. (1994). Emotional imagery and physical anhedonia. *Psychophysiology*, **31**(5), 513–521.

Franken, I. H., Zijlstra, C. & Muris, P. (2006). Are nonpharmacological induced rewards related to anhedonia? A study among skydivers. *Progress in Neuro-psychopharmacology and Biological Psychiatry*, **30**(2), 297–300.

Gard, D. E., Gard, M. G., Kring, A. M. & John, O. P. (2006). Anticipatory and consummatory components of the experience of pleasure: a scale development study. *Journal of Research in Personality*, **40**(6), 1086–1102.

Garfield, J. B., Cotton, S. M., Allen, N. B., et al. (2017). Evidence that anhedonia is a symptom of opioid dependence associated with recent use. *Drug and Alcohol Dependence*, **177**, 29–38.

Garfield, J. B., Lubman, D. I. & Yücel, M. (2014). Anhedonia in substance use disorders: a systematic review of its nature, course and clinical correlates. *Australian & New Zealand Journal of Psychiatry*, *48*(1), 36–51.

Garland, E. L., Froeliger, B. & Howard, M. O. (2014). Effects of Mindfulness-Oriented Recovery Enhancement on reward responsiveness and opioid cue-reactivity. *Psychopharmacology*, **231**(16), 3229–3238.

Garland, E. L., Froeliger, B. & Howard, M. O. (2015). Neurophysiological evidence for remediation of reward processing deficits in chronic pain and opioid misuse following treatment with Mindfulness-Oriented Recovery Enhancement: exploratory ERP findings from a pilot RCT. *Journal of Behavioral Medicine*, **38**(2), 327–336.

Geschwind, N., Peeters, F., Drukker, M., van Os, J. & Wichers, M. (2011). Mindfulness training increases momentary positive emotions and reward experience in adults vulnerable to depression: a randomized controlled trial. *Journal of Consulting and Clinical Psychology*, **79**(5), 618.

Guillot, C. R., Halliday, T. M., Kirkpatrick, M. G., Pang, R. D. & Leventhal, A. M. (2017). Anhedonia and abstinence as predictors of the subjective pleasantness of positive, negative, and smoking-related pictures. *Nicotine & Tobacco Research*, 19(6), 743–749.

Hall, W. & Lynskey, M. (2016). Evaluating the public health impacts of legalizing recreational cannabis use in the United States. *Addiction*, **111**(10), 1764–1773.

Harvey, P. O., Pruessner, J., Czechowska, Y. & Lepage, M. (2007). Individual differences in trait anhedonia: a structural and functional magnetic resonance imaging study in non-clinical subjects. *Molecular Psychiatry*, **12**(8), 767.

Haslam, A. K., Correa-Fernández, V., Hoover, D. S., et al. (2018). Anhedonia and smoking cessation among Spanish-speaking Mexican-Americans. *Health Psychology*, **37**(9), 814.

Hatzigiakoumis, D. S., Martinotti, G., Di Giannantonio, M. & Janiri, L. (2011). Anhedonia and substance dependence: clinical correlates and treatment options. *Frontiers in Psychiatry*, **2**, 10.

Heirene, R. M., Shearer, D., Roderique-Davies, G. & Mellalieu, S. D. (2016). Addiction in extreme sports: an exploration of withdrawal states in rock climbers. *Journal of Behavioral Addictions*, **5**(2), 332–341.

Higgins, S. T., Silverman, K. & Heil, S. H. (Eds.) (2007). *Contingency Management in Substance Abuse Treatment*. Guilford Press.

Hughes, J. R., Budney, A. J., Muellers, S. R., et al. (2017). Does tobacco abstinence decrease reward sensitivity? A human laboratory test. *Nicotine & Tobacco Research*, **19**(6), 677–685.

Huhn, A. S., Meyer, R. E., Harris, J. D., et al. (2016). Evidence of anhedonia and differential reward processing in prefrontal cortex among post-withdrawal patients with prescription opiate dependence. *Brain Research Bulletin*, **123**, 102–109.

Huys, Q. J., Pizzagalli, D. A., Bogdan, R. & Dayan, P. (2013). Mapping anhedonia onto reinforcement learning: a behavioural meta-analysis. *Biology of Mood & Anxiety Disorders*, **3**(1), 12.

Janiri, L., Martinotti, G., Dario, T., et al. (2005). Anhedonia and substance-related symptoms in detoxified substance-dependent subjects: a correlation study. *Neuropsychobiology*, **52**(1), 37–44.

Johnson, K. A., Bonn-Miller, M. O., Leyro, T. M. & Zvolensky, M. J. (2009). Anxious arousal and anhedonic depression symptoms and the frequency of current marijuana use: testing the mediating role of marijuana-use coping motives among active users. *Journal of Studies on Alcohol and Drugs*, **70**(4), 543–550.

Kahler, C. W., Spillane, N. S., Day, A., et al. (2014). Positive psychotherapy for smoking cessation: treatment development, feasibility, and preliminary results. *The Journal of Positive Psychology*, **9**(1), 19–29.

Kahler, C. W., Spillane, N. S., Day, A. M., et al. (2015). Positive psychotherapy for smoking cessation: a pilot randomized controlled trial. *Nicotine & Tobacco Research*, **17**(11), 1385–1392.

Kelley, A. E. & Berridge, K. C. (2002). The neuroscience of natural rewards: relevance to addictive drugs. *Journal of Neuroscience*, **22** (9), 3306–3311.

Kirkpatrick, M. G., Goldenson, N. I., Kapadia, N., et al. (2016). Emotional traits predict individual differences in amphetamine-induced positive mood in healthy volunteers. *Psychopharmacology*, **233**(1), 89–97.

Koob, G. F. & Le Moal, M. (2001). Drug addiction, dysregulation of reward, and allostasis. *Neuropsychopharmacology*, **24** (2), 97.

Krupitsky, E. M., Burakov, A. M., Didenko, T. Y., et al. (2002). Effects of citalopram treatment of protracted withdrawal (syndrome of anhedonia) in patients with heroin addiction. *Addictive Disorders & Their Treatment*, **1**(1), 29–33.

Krupitsky, E., Zvartau, E., Blokhina, E., et al. (2016). Anhedonia, depression, anxiety, and craving in opiate dependent patients stabilized on oral naltrexone or an extended release naltrexone implant. *The American Journal of Drug and Alcohol Abuse*, **42**(5), 614–620.

Lawn, W., Freeman, T. P., Pope, R. A., et al. (2016). Acute and chronic effects of cannabinoids on effort-related decision-making and reward learning: an evaluation of the cannabis 'amotivational' hypotheses. *Psychopharmacology*, **233**(19–20), 3537–3552.

Lee, Y. O., Hebert, C. J., Nonnemaker, J. M. & Kim, A. E. (2015). Youth tobacco product use in the United States. *Pediatrics*, **135**(3), 409–415.

Leibenluft, E., Fiero, P. L., Bartko, J. J., Moul, D. E. & Rosenthal, N. E. (1993). Depressive symptoms and the self-reported use of alcohol, caffeine, and carbohydrates in normal volunteers and four groups of psychiatric outpatients. *American Journal of Psychiatry*, **150**, 294–294.

Lejuez, C. W., Hopko, D. R. & Hopko, S. D. (2001). A brief behavioral activation treatment for depression: treatment manual. *Behavior Modification*, **25**(2), 255–286.

Leventhal, A. M. & Zvolensky, M. J. (2015). Anxiety, depression, and cigarette smoking: a transdiagnostic vulnerability framework to understanding emotion–smoking comorbidity. *Psychological Bulletin*, **141**(1), 176.

Leventhal, A. M., Brightman, M., Ameringer, K. J., et al. (2010). Anhedonia associated with stimulant use and dependence in a population-based sample of American adults. *Experimental and Clinical Psychopharmacology*, **18**(6), 562.

Leventhal, A. M., Chasson, G. S., Tapia, E., Miller, E. K. & Pettit, J. W. (2006). Measuring hedonic capacity in depression: a psychometric analysis of three anhedonia scales. *Journal of Clinical Psychology*, **62**(12), 1545–1558.

Leventhal, A. M., Cho, J., Stone, M. D., et al. (2017). Associations between anhedonia and marijuana use escalation across mid-adolescence. *Addiction*, **112**(12), 2182–2190.

Leventhal, A. M., Piper, M. E., Japuntich, S. J., Baker, T. B. & Cook, J. W. (2014). Anhedonia, depressed mood, and smoking cessation outcome. *Journal of Consulting and Clinical Psychology*, **82**(1), 122.

Leventhal, A. M., Ramsey, S. E., Brown, R. A., LaChance, H. R. & Kahler, C. W. (2008). Dimensions of depressive symptoms and smoking cessation. *Nicotine & Tobacco Research*, **10**(3), 507–517.

Leventhal, A. M., Strong, D. R., Sussman, S., et al. (2016). Psychiatric comorbidity in adolescent electronic and conventional cigarette use. *Journal of Psychiatric Research*, **73**, 71–78.

Lichlyter, B., Purdon, S. & Tibbo, P. (2011). Predictors of psychosis severity in individuals with primary stimulant addictions. *Addictive Behaviors*, **36**(1–2), 137–139.

Liverant, G. I., Sloan, D. M., Pizzagalli, D. A., et al. (2014). Associations among smoking, anhedonia, and reward learning in depression. *Behavior Therapy*, **45**(5), 651–663.

Liu, C. H. & Tronick, E. (2014). Prevalence and predictors of maternal postpartum depressed mood and anhedonia by race and ethnicity. *Epidemiology and Psychiatric Sciences*, **23**(2), 201–209.

Lubman, D. I., Garfield, J. B., Gwini, S. M., et al. (2018). Dynamic associations between opioid use and anhedonia: a longitudinal study in opioid dependence. *Journal of Psychopharmacology*, **32**(9), 957–964.

Luby, J. L., Agrawal, A., Belden, A., et al. (2018). Developmental trajectories of the orbitofrontal cortex and anhedonia in middle childhood and risk for substance use in adolescence in a longitudinal sample of depressed and healthy preschoolers. *American Journal of Psychiatry*, **175**(10), 1010–1021.

MacPherson, L., Tull, M. T., Matusiewicz, A. K., et al. (2010). Randomized controlled trial of behavioral activation smoking cessation treatment for smokers with elevated depressive symptoms. *Journal of Consulting and Clinical Psychology*, **78**(1), 55.

Marra, D., Warot, D., Payan, C., et al. (1998). Anhedonia and relapse in alcoholism. *Psychiatry Research*, **80**(2), 187–196.

Martinotti, G., Cloninger, C. R. & Janiri, L. (2008a). Temperament and character inventory dimensions and anhedonia in detoxified substance-dependent subjects. *American Journal of Drug and Alcohol Abuse*, **34**(2), 177–183. doi:10.1080/00952990701877078

Martinotti, G., Di Nicola, M., Reina, D., et al. (2008b). Alcohol protracted withdrawal syndrome: the role of anhedonia. *Substance Use & Misuse*, **43**(3–4), 271–284.

Martinotti, G., Andreoli, S., Reina, D., et al. (2011). Acetyl-l-carnitine in the treatment of anhedonia, melancholic and negative symptoms in alcohol dependent subjects. *Progress in Neuro-Psychopharmacology and Biological Psychiatry*, **35**(4), 953–958.

Mathew, A. R., Cook, J. W., Japuntich, S. J. & Leventhal, A. M. (2015). Post-traumatic stress disorder symptoms, underlying affective vulnerabilities, and smoking for affect regulation. *The American Journal on Addictions*, **24**(1), 39–46.

McClure, E. A., Vandrey, R. G., Johnson, M. W. & Stitzer, M. L. (2012). Effects of varenicline on abstinence and smoking reward following a programmed lapse. *Nicotine & Tobacco Research*, **15**(1), 139–148.

McGregor, C., Srisurapanont, M., Jittiwutikarn, J., et al. (2005). The nature, time course and severity of methamphetamine withdrawal. *Addiction*, **100**(9), 1320–1329.

Meehl, P. E. (1975). Hedonic capacity: some conjectures. *Bulletin of the Menninger Clinic*, **39**(4), 295–307.

Meshesha, L. Z., Pickover, A. M., Teeters, J. B. & Murphy, J. G. (2017). A longitudinal behavioral economic analysis of non-medical prescription opioid use among college students. *The Psychological Record*, **67**(2), 241–251.

Miotto, P., Preti, A. & Frezza, M. (2001). Heroin and schizophrenia: subjective responses to abused drugs in dually diagnosed patients. *Journal of Clinical Psychopharmacology*, **21**(1), 111–113.

Morie, K. P., De **Sanctis, P., Garavan, H. & Foxe, J. J.** (2014). Executive dysfunction and reward dysregulation: a high-density electrical mapping study in cocaine abusers. *Neuropharmacology*, **85**, 397–407.

Newton, T. F., Kalechstein, A. D., Duran, S., Vansluis, N. & Ling, W. (2004). Methamphetamine abstinence syndrome: preliminary findings. *The American Journal on Addictions*, **13**(3), 248–255.

Noordsy, D. L., Drake, R. E., Teague, G. B., et al. (1991). Subjective experiences related to alcohol use among schizophrenics. *Journal of Nervous and Mental Disease*, **179**(7), 410–414.

Nunn, J. A., Rizza, F. & Peters, E. R. (2001). The incidence of schizotypy among cannabis and alcohol users. *The Journal of Nervous and Mental Disease*, **189**(11), 741–748.

Pang, R. D., Khoddam, R., Guillot, C. R. & Leventhal, A. M. (2014). Depression and anxiety symptoms moderate the relation between negative reinforcement smoking outcome expectancies and nicotine dependence. *Journal of Studies on Alcohol and Drugs*, **75**(5), 775–780.

Parrish, K. H., Atherton, O. E., Quintana, A., Conger, R. D. & Robins, R. W. (2016). Reciprocal relations between internalizing symptoms and frequency of alcohol use: findings from a longitudinal study of Mexican-origin youth. *Psychology of Addictive Behaviors*, **30**(2), 203.

Peechatka, A. L., Whitton, A. E., Farmer, S. L., Pizzagalli, D. A. & Janes, A. C. (2015). Cigarette craving is associated with blunted reward processing in nicotine-dependent smokers. *Drug and Alcohol Dependence*, **155**, 202–207.

Peters, E. N., Bae, D., Barrington-Trimis, J. L., Jarvis, B. P. & Leventhal, A. M. (2018). Prevalence and sociodemographic correlates of adolescent use and polyuse of combustible, vaporized, and edible cannabis products. *JAMA Network Open*, **1**(5), e182765.

Pettorruso, M., Martinotti, G., Fasano, A., et al. (2014). Anhedonia in Parkinson's disease patients with and without pathological gambling: a case-control study. *Psychiatry Research*, **215**(2), 448–452.

Piper, M. E., Vasilenko, S. A., Cook, J. W. & Lanza, S. T. (2017). What a difference a day makes: differences in initial abstinence response during a smoking cessation attempt. *Addiction*, **112**(2), 330–339.

Powers, J. M., Carroll, A. J., Veluz-Wilkins, A. K., et al. (2016). Is the effect of anhedonia on smoking cessation greater for women versus men? *Nicotine & Tobacco Research*, **19**(1), 119–123.

Pozzi, G., Martinotti, G., Reina, D., et al. (2008). The assessment of post-detoxification anhedonia: influence of clinical and psychosocial variables. *Substance Use & Misuse*, **43**(5), 722–732.

Rømer Thomsen, K. (2015). Measuring anhedonia: impaired ability to pursue, experience, and learn about reward. *Frontiers in Psychology*, *6*, 1409.

Roys, M., Weed, K., Carrigan, M. & MacKillop, J. (2016). Associations between nicotine dependence, anhedonia, urgency and smoking motives. *Addictive Behaviors*, **62**, 145–151.

Schlaepfer, T. E., Cohen, M. X., Frick, C., et al.**K** (2008). Deep brain stimulation to reward circuitry alleviates anhedonia in refractory major depression. *Neuropsychopharmacology*, **33**(2), 368.

Schmitz, J. M., Mooney, M. E., Moeller, F. G., et al. (2008). Levodopa pharmacotherapy for cocaine dependence: choosing the optimal behavioral therapy platform. *Drug and Alcohol Dependence*, **94**(1–3), 142–150.

Seligman, M. E., Rashid, T. & Parks, A. C. (2006). Positive psychotherapy. *American Psychologist*, **61**(8), 774.

Seney, M. L. & Sibille, E. (2014). Sex differences in mood disorders: perspectives from humans and rodent models. *Biology of Sex Differences*, **5**(1), 17.

Seth, P., Rudd, R. A., Noonan, R. K. & Haegerich, T. M. (2018). Quantifying the epidemic of prescription opioid overdose deaths. *American Journal of Public Health*, **108**(4), 500–502.

Snaith, P. (1993). Anhedonia: a neglected symptom of psychopathology. *Psychological Medicine*, **23**(4), 957–966.

Snaith, R. P., Hamilton, M., Morley, S., et al. (1995). A scale for the assessment of hedonic tone the Snaith–Hamilton Pleasure Scale. *The British Journal of Psychiatry*, **167**(1), 99–103.

Stevens, A., Peschk, I. & Schwarz, J. (2007). Implicit learning, executive function and hedonic activity in chronic polydrug abusers, currently abstinent polydrug abusers and controls. *Addiction*, **102**(6), 937–946.

Stone, M. D., Audrain-McGovern, J. & Leventhal, A. M. (2017). Association of anhedonia with adolescent smoking susceptibility and initiation. *Nicotine & Tobacco Research*, **19**(6), 738–742.

Sussman, N. & DeJong, S. M. (2018). Ethical considerations for mental health clinicians working with adolescents in the digital age. *Current Psychiatry Reports*, **20**(12), 113.

Thomas, E. A. & Garland, E. L. (2017). Mindfulness is associated with increased hedonic capacity among chronic pain patients receiving extended opioid pharmacotherapy. *The Clinical Journal of Pain*, **33**(2), 166.

Tomarken, A. J., Dichter, G. S., Freid, C., Addington, S. & Shelton, R. C. (2004). Assessing the effects of bupropion SR on mood dimensions of depression. *Journal of Affective Disorders*, **78**(3), 235–241.

Treadway, M. T. & Zald, D. H. (2011). Reconsidering anhedonia in depression: lessons from translational neuroscience. *Neuroscience & Biobehavioral Reviews*, **35**(3), 537–555.

Tremblay, L. K., Naranjo, C. A., Cardenas, L., Herrmann, N. & Busto, U. E. (2002). Probing brain reward system function in major depressive disorder: altered response to dextroamphetamine. *Archives of General Psychiatry*, **59**(5), 409–416.

Tremblay, L. K., Naranjo, C. A., Graham, S. J., et al. (2005). Functional neuroanatomical substrates of altered reward processing in major depressive disorder revealed by a dopaminergic probe. *Archives of General Psychiatry*, **62**(11), 1228–1236.

van Roekel, E., Bennik, E. C., Bastiaansen, J. A., et al. (2016). Depressive symptoms and the experience of pleasure in daily life: an exploration of associations in early and late adolescence. *Journal of Abnormal Child Psychology*, **44**(5), 999–1009.

Vivolo-Kantor, A. M., Seth, P., Gladden, R. M., et al. (2018). Vital signs: trends in emergency department visits for suspected opioid overdoses – United States, July 2016–September 2017. *Morbidity and Mortality Weekly Report*, **67**(9), 279.

Voce, A., McKetin, R., Burns, R., Castle, D. & Calabria, B. (2018). The relationship between illicit amphetamine use and psychiatric symptom profiles in schizophrenia and affective psychoses. *Psychiatry Research*, **265**, 19–24.

Wardle, M. C., Vincent, J. N., Suchting, R., et al. (2017). Anhedonia is associated with poorer outcomes in contingency management for cocaine use disorder. *Journal of Substance Abuse Treatment*, **72**, 32–39.

Wise, R. A. (2008). Dopamine and reward: the anhedonia hypothesis 30 years on. *Neurotoxicity Research*, *14*(2–3), 169–183.

Witkiewitz, K., Bowen, S., Harrop, E. N., et al. (2014). Mindfulness-based treatment to prevent addictive behavior relapse: theoretical models and hypothesized mechanisms of change. *Substance Use & Misuse*, **49**(5), 513–524.

33 Mindfulness-Based Interventions Applied to Addiction Treatments

Afton Kechter, PhD, and David S. Black, PhD, MPH

> Mindfulness allows us to see more clearly into the nature of our pain, and the stories we construct about it.
>
> -Jon Kabat-Zinn (2013, p. 414)

Introduction

Treatments for substance and behavioral addictions are often comprehensive and tailored to fit the specific needs and preferences of the individual client. The path to recovery may range from generalized supportive services where the individual engages in anonymous groups to intensive inpatient or residential treatment where they engage in evidence-based psychotherapy groups (SAMHSA, 2017). One of the leading, second-wave, evidence-based treatments for addictions is cognitive-behavioral therapy (CBT). CBT is a short-term, problem-focused, and action-oriented treatment that teaches participants to understand how their cognitive processes relate to their behavioral processes in order to change their behaviors (Bass, 2014). While most leading addiction treatment programs are effective in the short term, the majority of recipients will relapse within a year of treatment (Criscitelli & Avena, 2016).

Understanding the limitations of current addiction treatments will allow researchers and clinicians to appropriately tailor and deliver longer-lasting, efficacious treatments for addictive behaviors. One notion is that leading treatment programs, such as CBT, may fail to connect individuals with developing awareness of triggers in order to relearn how to accept and respond to cravings in an adaptive way. Mindfulness-based interventions (MBIs) have emerged as a set of programs that shift from CBT, which teaches participants to modify thoughts, feelings, and behaviors, to teaching participants to be mindfully aware and accept those same thoughts, feelings, and behaviors without effort to modify the content. For a clinical example, the CBT therapist may invite participants to evaluate, or judge, the usefulness of cognitions and challenge them in order to inhibit the maladaptive behavior it is connected to. Conversely, the MBI therapist may invite participants to notice cognitions and behavioral urges without judgment and allow them to be fully experienced and then pass, without reactivity or behavioral response.

MBIs represent a family of third-wave psychotherapeutic programs developed with the goal of helping people cultivate an ongoing daily practice of mindfulness. Mindfulness is commonly operationalized as the awareness that emerges through paying attention on purpose, in the present moment, and nonjudgmentally to the unfolding of experience moment by moment (Black, 2012, 2014; Kabat-Zinn, 2003). The lineage of MBIs stem from the Mindfulness-Based Stress Reduction (MBSR) program, which was originally developed to help people with chronic pain symptoms (Kabat-Zinn, 1982) and improve their mental health by increasing their ability to self-regulate and actively participate in their own healing process. There are now several MBIs adapted from the original MBSR program to meet the unique needs of different patient populations. These programs include Mindfulness Based Cognitive Therapy (MBCT), Mindfulness Based Relapse Prevention (MBRP), Mindfulness Oriented Recovery Enhancement (MORE), and Mindfulness Based Eating Awareness Training (MB-EAT).

MBCT was developed by Segal et al. for people suffering from recurrent major depressive episodes to prevent relapse (Segal, Williams & Teasdale, 2018). MBRP was developed by Bowen et al. for people in aftercare substance use disorder treatment (Bowen et al., 2009). MORE was developed by Garland et al. for people with chronic pain and opioid use disorder to target common underlying mechanisms (Garland et al., 2014b). Less commonly tested is MB-EAT, which was developed by Kristeller and Wolever for treatment of binge-eating disorder (BED) and related issues to develop a balanced relationship with food and regulated intake (Kristeller & Wolever, 2011). These programs range in delivery from six weekly ninety-minute sessions to ten weekly two-hour sessions, with the most common format being the original eight weekly two-hour sessions (Kechter, Amaro & Black, 2018). Central to all MBIs is teaching participants the principles and practices of mindfulness and how to apply these practices in daily life to prevent the onset of symptoms and to stymie the suffering caused by symptoms.

Altogether, MBIs have emerged with promise as a distinct treatment in reducing relapse and other maladaptive behaviors. Through mindfulness meditation practice, MBIs aim to raise an individual's metacognitive awareness and adaptive coping skills to modify risk mechanisms underlying triggers and cravings that often lead to relapse (Garland, Froeliger & Howard, 2014a; Witkiewitz et al., 2014). This metacognitive awareness gained from MBIs allows the participant to self-monitor their cognitive and emotional processes and then develop skills to modify maladaptive coping and habitual behaviors underlying addiction (Garland et al., 2014a; Garland, Gaylord & Park, 2009). Next, we discuss commonalities in maladaptive coping behaviors (i.e., substance use and binge eating disorders) in order to further explain how MBIs target similar mechanisms across addictions.

Similarities between Substance Use Disorder and Binge-Eating Disorder

Before we discuss similarities between substance use disorder (SUD) and binge-eating disorder (BED) as maladaptive coping behaviors and summarize literature on MBI efficacy in treating these disorders, we explain our rationale for focusing on these two specific disorders. First, we focus on BED rather than the broader category of eating disorders (ED) given the current conceptualizations of other eating disorders like anorexia nervosa (AN), which is considered to resemble anxiety disorders such as obsessive-compulsive disorder rather than as an addiction disorder (Sussman, 2017). Furthermore, little research exists on MBI for AN, despite research suggesting a similar activation and dysregulation of endogenous opioids in animal models (Avena & Bocarsly, 2012). Second, while food addiction has been postulated as one potential cause of the obesity epidemic, conceptualizing food as a drug of abuse remains controversial given the survival properties of food. Not all people who are obese have BED or people with BED are obese; only 25 percent to 30 percent of people with food addiction are obese (Criscitelli & Avena, 2016). However, a growing body of literature indicates excess sugar intake leads to signs of tolerance, drug-like withdrawal when sugar is unavailable, craving-like behaviors, and changes in dopamine and opioid systems in reward-related brain regions; which is nearly identical to animals using substances such as alcohol or nicotine (Avena, 2011; Avena & Bocarsly, 2012; Avena & Gold, 2011; Avena et al., 2012; Criscitelli & Avena, 2016; Murray et al., 2014; Murray, Kroll & Avena, 2015). Given the obesity epidemic and prediction that 60 percent of people will be obese by 2030 (Kelly et al., 2008), examining treatments and mechanisms to target and prevent such weight gain is crucial. Third, both SUD and ED have many disorder-specific diagnoses in the DSM-5 (i.e., alcohol use disorder vs. opioid use disorder and binge-eating disorder vs. anorexia nervosa). Furthermore, there is overlap in the DSM-5 diagnostic criteria for **SUD** and **BED** (American Psychiatric Association, 2013), such that both are characterized by overconsumption (of food and alcohol/drugs, respectively) and loss of control (see Table 33.1). However, MBIs for SUD treatment is often not alcohol and drug specific, but rather collapsed into the same addiction treatment (i.e., MBRP, described in following section). The MBI for ED reviewed here were all developed specifically for BED (i.e., MB-EAT, described in previous section). We discuss implications and limitations of disorder-specific versus nonspecific MBIs at the end of the chapter.

The first main commonality between SUD and BED are the psychosocial triggers and cravings/urges to alleviate negative emotionality. It is well established that acute and chronic stress leads to increased addiction vulnerability (Sinha, 2008). Research has shown high levels of emotional and psychological stress or negative affect decrease behavioral control, which increases impulsivity and distress (Sinha, 2008). Persistent stress leads to greater risk of maladaptive behaviors (Sinha, 2008). When maladaptive behaviors become habitual reactions to pleasant and unpleasant experiences, craving and attachment are established (Brewer, Elwafi & Davis, 2013). These cravings are often triggered by an internal or external cue, that leads to the desire for a substance of abuse, and heightened risk of relapse, or recurrence of a substance or food binge after a period of remission (Kristeller & Wolever, 2010; Witkiewitz & Marlatt, 2005). This reward-based learning can be applied to all addictive or maladaptive behaviors including gambling, internet/electronic addictions, shopping, exercise, work, sex, and love (Sussman, 2017; Sussman & Black, 2008; Sussman et al., 2011) – we expand on this toward the end of the chapter.

Neurobiological research lends additional insight into stress and addiction vulnerability common in SUD and BED. Neuroimaging research has shown high levels of stress are associated with decreased prefrontal functioning and increased limbic-striatal level responding,

Table 33.1 Key DSM-5 diagnostic criteria that characterize alcohol use disorder versus binge-eating disorder (APA, 2013)

Alcohol use disorder (AUD)	Binge-eating disorder (BED)
A. A problematic pattern of alcohol use leading to clinically significant impairment or distress, as manifested by at least two of the following, occurring within a twelve-month period. 1. Alcohol is often taken in larger amounts or over a longer period than was intended. 2. There is a persistent desire or unsuccessful effort to cut down or control alcohol use. 3. A great deal of time is spent in activities necessary to obtain alcohol, use alcohol, or recover from its effects. 4. Craving, or a strong desire or urge to use alcohol. 5. Recurrent alcohol use resulting in a failure to fulfill major role obligations at work, school, or home. 6. Continued alcohol use despite having persistent or recurrent social or interpersonal problems causes or exacerbated by the effects of alcohol. 7. Important social, occupational, or recreational activities are given up or reduced because of alcohol use. 8. Recurrent alcohol use in situations in which it is physically hazardous. 9. Alcohol use is continued despite knowledge of having a persistent or recurrent physical or psychological problem that is likely to have been caused or exacerbated by alcohol. 10. Tolerance, as define by either of the following: a. A need for markedly increased amounts of alcohol to achieve intoxication or desired effect. b. A markedly diminished effect with continued use of the same amount of alcohol. 11. Withdrawal, as manifested by either of the following: a. The characteristic withdrawal syndrome for alcohol. b. Alcohol (or closely related substance, such as benzodiazepine) is taken to relieve or avoid withdrawal symptoms.	A. Recurrent episodes of binge eating. An episode of binge eating is characterized by both of the following: 1. Eating, in a discrete period of time (e.g., within any two-hour period), and amount of food that is definitely larger than what most people would eat in a similar period of time under similar circumstances. 2. A sense of lack of control over eating during the episode (e.g., a feeling that one cannot stop eating or control what or how much one is eating). B. The binge-eating episodes are associated with three (or more) of the following: 1. Eating much more rapidly than normal. 2. Eating until feeling uncomfortably full. 3. Eating large amounts of food when not feeling physically hungry. 4. Eating alone because of feeling embarrassed by how much one is eating. 5. Feeling disgusted with oneself, depressed, or very guilty afterward. C. Marked distress regarding binge eating is present. D. The binge eating occurs, on average at least once a week for three months. E. The binge eating is not associated with the recurrent use of inappropriate compensatory behavior as in bulimia nervosa and does not occur exclusively during the course of bulimia nervosa or anorexia nervosa.

Note. AUD is used as an example here and other drug-specific disorders have similar criteria. Specifications under each diagnosis regard remission and severity. Under AUD, severity is classified from "mild=presence of 2–3 symptoms" to "severe=presence of 6 or more symptoms." Contrarily, under BED, severity is classified from "mild=1–3 binge eating episodes per week" to "extreme=14 or more binge-eating episodes per week."

which results in low behavioral and cognitive control (Sinha, 2008). Low inhibitory control has been associated with people diagnosed with SUDs and BEDs (Volkow, Wang & Baler, 2011). Several regions of the brain and neurotransmitter systems are involved in reward pathways associated with drugs and highly palatable foods (i.e., sugar; Volkow et al., 2011), including release of dopamine, endorphins, and opioids when exposed to substances in the form of drugs and food. For a full review on these complex pathways see Yau et al. (2014).

It is well known that reinforcing properties of drugs involve activation of the brain's reward center and leads to a decreased production of dopamine without the drug (Sinha, 2008), essentially hijacking the naturally occurring reward system (Brewer, 2017). Volkow et al. describe four main circuits – i.e., (1) reward-saliency, (2) motivation-drive, (3) learning-conditioning, and (4) inhibitory control-emotion regulation-executive function – in addictive pathways, where food high in sugars and fats are potent rewards and notably similar to drug addiction (Volkow et al., 2011). Consumption of highly palatable food (or drug in addiction) can hijack balanced reward pathways similar to nicotine and cocaine (increased dopamine), resulting in enhanced reinforcing value of food (or drugs) and weakening inhibitory control (Criscitelli & Avena, 2016; Murray et al., 2014). Using drugs or eating highly palatable foods all activate the opioid system in reward-related brain areas and creates a sense of elatedness (Avena & Bocarsly, 2012). When prolonged and repeated use creates symptoms of tolerance and withdrawal, the drug and food is now required for maintenance, rather than elated effects, the addiction becomes neuro-biologically based (more on dopamine "wanting" than opioid-based "liking"; Warlow et al., 2020). In summary, current evidence suggests individuals with SUD and BED may be self-medicating in an effort to compensate for a disrupted dopaminergic system.

Transdiagnostic Application of MBIs

A number of theoretical models of mindfulness-based treatments for SUDs exist. Overall, these treatments aim to liberate the root issue that limit the person within the addiction loop (Brewer et al., 2013) by targeting three key paths. The first path is the risk from lack of awareness and being on auto-pilot; leading to the second path of craving, negative affect, stress reactivity; finally leading to the third path of substance use (Witkiewitz et al., 2014). Mindfulness training targets each of these paths and enhances mindfulness skills so that the habitual reaction is decoupled and blocked.

SUD and BED involve disorder-specific MBIs with overlapping mechanisms of therapeutic action. These target mechanisms include self regulation, self-exploration, and self-liberation by cultivating awareness of internal experience, interrupting conditioned patterns, developing higher-level cognitive processes, decreasing stress reactivity, and empowering a sense of self-control and acceptance (Black, 2012, 2014; Kabat-Zinn, 2003; Kristeller & Wolever, 2011). Multiple addiction scholars have proposed a transdiagnostic framework for mechanisms underlying maladaptive disorders and reasoned for a paradigm shift that examines and addresses the commonalities of multiple disorders (Greeson, Garland & Black, 2014; Leventhal & Zvolensky, 2015).

While MBIs for BED are less examined in the scientific literature, these programs target similar pathways and mechanisms as MBIs for SUDs. Mindfulness training for EDs trains participants in mindfulness meditation, self-awareness, and self-acceptance (Kristeller & Wolever, 2011). Given the survival properties of food (versus drugs), mindfulness training for BED focuses on developing adaptive eating behaviors by developing insight into triggers and cravings that lead to binge eating episodes. Altogether, through mindfulness training, people learn to cultivate awareness of cravings and skills to allow triggers to pass thereby preventing binge relapses.

Mindfulness is used as a training paradigm or transdiagnostic tool across illnesses to target underlying mental processes of rumination, inflexibility, and distress (i.e., anxiety, depression, posttraumatic stress, substance use, eating disorders, sleep disturbance, and chronic pain; Greeson et al., 2014). The following six mechanisms all underlie maladaptive behaviors and are counteracted through transtherapeutic qualities of mindfulness: (1) negative affectivity and emotional reactivity, (2) repetitive negative thoughts, (3) experiential avoidance, (4) attentional bias, (5) reappraisal, and (6) suppression (Greeson et al., 2014). Altogether, mindfulness training offers a transtherapeutic approach for treatment of addictions and common comorbid symptomology such as stress and psychopathology.

One theory posits that two mindfulness components may be most critical in participant improvement and common factors across MBIs. Specifically, Monitor and Acceptance Theory (MAT) proposes that the two key mechanisms across MBIs that participants develop from mindfulness training are (1) attention and (2) acceptance (Lindsay & Creswell, 2017). This theory suggests attention monitoring and acceptance interact to improve stress, affect and health outcomes; such that high monitoring skills combined with high acceptance correlate with more adaptive responses (i.e., less rumination, higher reappraisal, and lower symptoms of anxiety and depression). Interestingly, this interaction has predicted that people with greater emotional and body awareness in the absence of acceptance report with greater psychological distress and maladaptive behaviors. While authors discuss limitations of their theory and review of the literature, such as exclusion of considering therapeutic effects from group-based intervention, the evidence is convincing that awareness and acceptance are two active components in the multifaceted effects of MBIs. Further exploration is warranted to clarify the active components of mindfulness training in order to appropriately tailor the intervention for a variety of populations and outcomes. See Table 33.2 for techniques used across MBIs to target awareness and acceptance.

The Efficacy of MBIs for Treating SUD and BED

We synthesize key findings from four of the most recent reviews of the literature examining effects of MBIs on people with SUD and BED (Godfrey, Gallo & Afari, 2015; Grant et al., 2017; Katterman et al., 2014; Li et al., 2017; O'Reilly et al., 2014), two reviews for each disorder. Grant et al. set strict study eligibility criteria by only including RCTs for MBRP among adult patients with diagnosed SUD. Median age of participants was thirty-nine years old and median proportion of male participants was 72 percent. Comparison conditions included relapse prevention, CBT and treatment as usual (TAU).

Li et al. set more inclusive study eligibility criteria by including quasi-experimental trials of SUD with repeated measures and RCT. Programs included MBRP, MORE, MBSR, Vipassana Meditation, Mindfulness Meditation, Motivational interviewing plus mindfulness meditation, mind-body training, etc. Participants ranged from adolescents to adults and comparison conditions included TAU, alternative psychotherapeutic treatment, and inactive control.

Table 33.2 Core mindfulness constructs and common practices across interventions

Mindfulness concepts	Mindfulness practices	Example instructions
Awareness and attention		
Defined as attention monitoring to momentary body sensations, thoughts, and emotional experiences Improves selective and executive attention ability and working memory	• Body scan • Sitting/walking breath awareness meditation • Noticing triggers • Raisin exercise • Gentle mindful yoga	Sitting awareness meditation: "Find a comfortable seated position where your feet are grounded on the floor and your hands rest in your lap. Allow eyes to gently close and body to be still and relaxed. First notice your breath without trying to change it. Then begin to lengthen your inhale to full capacity; exhale tension or stress. Repeat. Notice the natural rise and fall of your diaphragm with each breath. Continue to bring your awareness back to the breath, noticing when it drifts. You may get distracted from body sensations and focus on emotions and thoughts that arise and are connected to the past or future. Simply observe this shift and imagine it floating away on a passing cloud, returning to riding with the flow of your breath. Letting go of whatever tries to capture your attention and allowing yourself to be fully present moment to moment. When you are ready, gently flutter your eyes open and notice any shifts in thoughts, feelings, and body sensations."
Acceptance		
Defined as recognizing one's experience without trying to change it Improves affective, stress, and physical health outcomes	• Loving kindness meditation • Compassion meditation • Noticing and observing without reactivity and judgment	Noticing and observing without reactivity and judgment: "When we relate to experiences as right or wrong, good or bad, like or don't like, want or don't want we limit ourselves in that judgment. This can become a habit we do automatically, which often leads to an less adaptive reaction. However, developing the ability to recognize and understand our experiences unfold without judgment liberates us. For example, welcoming and not trying to change experiences such as cravings allows them to pass quicker. In fact, cravings only last 90 seconds and it's one's reaction to the craving that may determine our behavior regarding whether one uses a drug or binge eats. Next time you notice a craving, try to observe it in stillness – simply watch it come and go without judgment."

Note. These mindfulness constructs and practices are core to MBIs (i.e., MBSR, MBCT, MBRP, MB-EAT). Quotations in the example column represent what the mindfulness instructor may say to guide that respective practice. See Linsday and Creswell (2017).

Similar to Grant et al., Katterman et al. set strict inclusion criteria by only including MBSR and MBCT with a binge eating, emotional eating, or weight related outcome. Participants were mostly women ranging from eighteen to seventy-five years old, with most being between forty and sixty years old. Comparison conditions included CBT and dosage of treatment-control.

Similar to Li et al., O'Reilly et al. expanded study eligibility criteria to include MBIs and mindful exercise program with an outcome of obesity-related eating behavior. Thirty-eight percent of these studies were RCTs and 62 percent were pre-post design. Age range and intensity of comparison groups varied due to the loosened exclusion criteria.

The reviews for both SUD and BED found mixed results regarding decreased frequency and quantity of addiction-related behaviors. Among thirty-four RCTs evaluating MBIs for substance misuse, meta-analytic results revealed superior effects of mindfulness treatment versus comparison conditions in reducing frequency and amount of substance use (medium effect size, d = -0.33, 95% CI [-0.88, -0.14]; Li et al., 2017). The other systematic review and meta-analysis of SUD identified nine RCTs evaluating MBRP-only for samples with SUD, but failed to find a significant difference between MBRP and comparison groups on relapse (OR = 0.72, 95% CI [0.46–1.13]), frequency of use (Standardized Mean Difference [SMD] = 0.02, 95% CI [-0.40–0.44]), and a number of other relevant mechanisms (Grant et al., 2017).

In one of the BED reviews, over 90 percent of studies using a MBI to treat binge eating (n = 11) reported a significant reduction in binge eating frequency and/or severity (d = 1.39); (O'Reilly et al., 2014). Sixty-three percent of studies targeting emotional eating (n = 8) reported improvement in emotional eating occurrence and/or urge to emotionally overeat (d = 0.67). Sixty-seven percent of studies targeting emotional eating (n = 6) reported improvements in external eating frequency (d = 0.65; O'Reilly et al., 2014). The majority of intervention studies that showed null effects involved participants who did not have emotional eating concerns and reported low levels of emotional eating at baseline (see Katterman et al., 2014).

Outcomes Targeted by MBIs

Although not all reviews found common effects, we identified three key outcomes that improved across MBIs: decreased craving/withdrawal, improved mental health, and effects on weight and dietary intake. Both reviews on SUD identified a decreased craving and withdrawal and improvement in mental health. Among thirty-four RCTs evaluating mindfulness treatments for substance misuse, meta-analytic results revealed a large effect on intensity of craving for psychoactive substances (d = -0.63, 95% CI [-1.17,-0.08]; Li et al., 2017). The systematic review and meta-analysis which identified nine RCTs evaluating MBRP only also for substance use disorder and found small clinical effects in favor of MBRP for craving/withdrawal (SMD = 0.13, 95% CI = 0.19–0.08; Grant et al., 2017). Furthermore, indirect evidence suggests MBRP may lead to greater reductions in withdrawal/craving among alcohol use disorders rather than any subtype of SUDs (SMD = 0.09, 95% CI = 0.18–0.01; Grant et al., 2017). Among thirty-four RCTs evaluating mindfulness treatments for substance misuse, meta-analytic results revealed a large effect on severity of stress for psychoactive substances (d = -1.12, 95% CI [-2.72, -0.01]; Li et al., 2017). Furthermore, MBRP may lead to greater reductions in depressive symptoms among those with stimulant use disorders compared to other SUD categories of use (SMD = 0.46, 95% CI = 0.81–0.11; Grant et al., 2017).

While results suggest mindfulness training effectively reduces binge eating and emotional eating in populations engaging in these behaviors, evidence for effect on weight and dietary intake are mixed. O'Reilly et al. identified 90 percent (n = 10) that reported weight loss or maintenance (Cohen's d = 0.19; O'Reilly et al., 2014). Katterman et al. identified 60 percent of studies evaluated (n = 10) that provided nutrition education and/or exercise-related components, however results seem biased because those that focused on weight loss as primary outcome found significant decreases in weight (Katterman et al., 2014). Furthermore, there was lack of support for ability of MBIs to improve dietary intake (O'Reilly et al., 2014).

Rigor and Reproducibility of MBIs

Delivering MBI curriculum is a dynamic process. MBI facilitators transition between didactic teachings, guided experiential activities in mindfulness meditation, and discussion of personal experiences of the practice often shared in a group-based setting. This multifaceted role may mean that no two facilitators or sessions are alike and therefore inferring concrete intervention effects per study becomes challenging (Borrelli, 2011; Breitenstein et al., 2010; Gould et al., 2016). Utilizing strategies to enhance the rigor and reproducibility of MBIs is important for reliably and validly interpreting participant outcomes. Treatment fidelity is a methodology used to monitor and enhance the delivery of a behavioral intervention (Bellg et al., 2004; Resnick et al., 2005). More rigorous treatment fidelity methods not only offers more confidence in specifying the underlying mechanisms of change but has also been associated with stronger treatment outcomes (Carroll et al., 2007). There are a number of treatment fidelity frameworks that have evolved over time to help researchers implement strategies.

The Treatment Fidelity Workgroup of the National Institutes of Health Behavior Change Consortium (BCC) synthesized existing frameworks for treatment fidelity in behavioral interventions and put forth recommendations into an all-encompassing framework. This framework covers five components of fidelity: design, training, delivery, receipt, and enactment (Bellg et al., 2004; Borrelli, 2011; Resnick et al., 2005). Design encompasses strategies used to ensure same dose within and across conditions and planning for implementation setbacks. Training encompasses strategies used to standardize training using curriculum manuals, ensuring provider skills acquisition, minimizing drift in provider skills, and accommodating for provider differences. Delivery encompasses strategies used to control for provider differences, reducing differences in treatment delivery, ensuring adherence to treatment protocol, and minimizing contamination between conditions. Receipt encompasses strategies used to ensure participant comprehension including cognitive capacity and behavioral performance. Enactment encompasses strategies used ensure participants' use of behavioral and cognitive skills. Strategies from these components are flexible and should vary based on MBI phase and stage.

Our recent review of the literature identified reporting of treatment fidelity in MBI leading trials using this framework. We identified low and inconsistent reporting of these five treatment fidelity components across 25 MBI RCTs, which limits the interpretability and transparency of the MBI evidence base (Kechter et al., 2019). Specifically, varying methods and measures may contribute to discrepant findings and a more standardized practice is warranted to reliably and validly interpret MBI trials. In the following section, we expand on this work using the same framework and definitions in order to highlight gaps and future directions given that it is unclear if and how variation in implementation is related to outcomes across trials. This is a particularly critical field limitation since extensive research is being conducted to identify underlying mechanisms of change (i.e., which techniques work for whom and why) in order to enhance the dissemination in clinical settings and close the research-to-practice gap.

An Assessment of Treatment Fidelity in MBI Efficacy Studies

Two of the four reviews we discussed reported on treatment fidelity. Grant et al. acknowledged all five elements of design (i.e., control conditions included TAU, relapse prevention, health education, or CBT), training (i.e., providers ranged from trained graduate level therapists with experience in CBT and mindfulness meditation [MM] to certified mindfulness instructors), delivery (i.e., MBRP adaptations and implementation), receipt (i.e., dosage or contact time, homework), and enactment (i.e., daily logs) across studies evaluating MBRP. Katterman et al. focused on receipt and enactment across the fourteen studies reviewed. Authors reported "average time spent practicing mindfulness" was available for 43 percent of studies and ranged from eight to thirty minutes per day. Furthermore, 21 percent of studies reported collecting measures of mindfulness and/or acceptability, both of which increased from pre-post. Attendance was reported in 36 percent of studies and ranged from 70 percent to 100 percent. Only one of the fourteen studies excluded participants if they missed a set number of sessions (i.e., four out of sixteen sessions consecutively). Retention at postintervention was reported for all studies and ranged from 60 percent to 100 percent. Katterman et al. found nonsignificantly different attrition rates across study conditions with the exception of the investigation of Kristeller, Wolever and Sheets (2014), which showed higher retention in the mindfulness condition versus CBT control at one of two study sites.

Among MBI trials targeting SUD, the following limitations should be considered when interpreting findings. First, less than half of studies reviewed by Li et al. reported an objective verification of SUD outcome variables such as a urine test, only 16.7 percent followed participants for more than six months, and 40.5 percent did not have adequate power for statistical analyses. All of these methodological omissions limit interpretation of findings, and there is a need for objective verification, longer follow-up, and adequately powered samples in future studies. Additionally, in lieu of Li et al.'s meta-analytic findings of significant improvements among the MBI participants versus control participants, Grant et al. found contradicting findings of nonsignificant difference between comparisons for relapse, frequency use, dropout, depressive and anxiety symptoms, or mindfulness. It is important to note Li et al. reviewed RCT and quasi-experimental MBIs while Grant et al. only reviewed RCTs of MBRP. That is, MBRP is one intervention program where the curriculum has been specifically tailored for substance use disorders, while MBIs include MBRP as well as MBSR, MBCT and others. Inclusion criteria for MBI versus MBRP likely differed in substance use disorder severity, which may explain the difference in findings. Nonetheless, meta-results suggest MBRP is on par with certain current gold standard treatments that were used as comparison conditions (Relapse Prevention and CBT). Findings from individual MBRP trials reporting superior effects to control conditions may be a result of (1) combined data from MBRP and RP +TAU, (2) focus on select positive results, or (3) differences in treatment fidelity (e.g., participant attrition; Grant et al., 2017). Therefore, while all of these interventions stem from the same theory and practice, it is hard to draw conclusions based on these findings and more research is needed to identify which program elements are efficacious and for whom.

Among MBI trials targeting BED, the following limitations should be considered when interpreting findings. First, samples were small and nondiverse (i.e., mostly white and female participants), which inhibits our ability to generalize to other populations and have confidence in findings based on limited power. Second, half of studies did not measure mindfulness pre- to post-intervention so it is unclear whether improved mindfulness was a mechanism functioning on observed outcomes in some of the studies (O'Reilly et al., 2014). Lastly, only a few researchers are doing this work so larger-scale RCT of MBIs for different or combined eating disorders (i.e., anorexia nervosa, bulimia nervosa, binge-eating disorder) and heterogenous samples is warranted for improving theoretical and clinical implications.

We identified areas for improvement in measurement that can be addressed across fields. There is a longstanding need for mental and behavioral intervention research to incorporate eating behavior and nutrition measures; as well as eating and nutrition interventions to incorporate mental and behavioral health measures (Kiecolt-Glaser, 2010). Additionally, the majority of studies reviewed in this chapter did not report adequately on treatment fidelity. The interaction of including more comprehensive (1) mind-body assessments (e.g., Five-Facet Mindfulness Questionnaire using ecological momentary assessment of mindfulness to behaviors in real time) and (2) treatment fidelity measures may offer insights into transdisciplinary mechanisms of MBI treatment.

MBIs Applied to Behavioral Addictions

While food and drug addictions have a physical agent that effects the neurochemistry of the brain (or phenotypic parallels), the same reward-based learning process applies across substances and behaviors. That is, an individual learns that when they engage in an addictive behavior they experience a reward. Behavioral addictions may include gambling, shopping, exercise, work, sex, or love (Sussman & Black, 2008; Sussman et al., 2011). Given that MBIs target the avoidance of unpleasant experiences by training one to develop adaptive (versus maladaptive) responses, MBI techniques may translate across all substance and behavioral addictions. Due to the recent popularization the recent popularization of MBIs, the majority of peer-reviewed research exists on MBIs for gambling.

A recent systematic review and meta-analysis assessed the effects of MBIs for treatment of *disordered gambling* among adults (Maynard et al., 2018). Thirteen studies were included in the review, of which seven were RCTs and were the ones included in the meta-analysis. Findings suggest MBIs have a moderate treatment effect on gambling behaviors, symptoms, and urges (g = 0.68–0.69, $p \leq 0.01$) and large treatment effect on financial outcomes (g = 0.75, $p < 0.01$). While these statistical pooled effects are promising, it is important to note the common limitations specific to treatment fidelity. The intervention curriculum delivered varied drastically, such that some studies used "MBCT for problem gambling" (de Lisle, Dowling & Allen, 2011) while others used "imaginal desensitization" (Blaszcynski, Maccallum & Joukhador, 2005) or "brief DBT" (Christensen et al., 2013), which include mindfulness techniques but would not be considered derivatives of MBSR. Furthermore, the settings and dosage were also inconsistent, such that the intervention was delivered individually (vs. group) for most studies and ranged from one to twenty sessions over one to twenty-four weeks. Altogether, these findings suffer from methodological shortcomings and future research should first aim to standardize the MBI curriculum for disordered gambling (and other addictive behaviors) and then deliver that protocol in a standardized group format across large, diverse samples.

Next, we briefly report on findings from single research studies of MBIs for behavioral addictions. Li et al. used data from a RCT of MORE for *internet gambling disorder* (IGD) to examine therapeutic mechanisms (Li, Garland & Howard, 2018). This study reported, among a sample of thirty adults, changes from preintervention to postintervention cognitive process- mediated reductions in IGD and cravings. Van Gordon et al. looked at *sex addiction* in a case study (Van Gordon, Shonin & Griffiths, 2016) and *workaholism* in a single controlled trial (Van Gordon et al., 2017) following a second-generation mindfulness-based intervention known as Meditation Awareness Training (MAT). In both of these reports, the MAT intervention led to significant improvements in each respective behavior of addiction as well as other measures of well-being suggesting transtherapeutic effects of mindfulness training on addictions. However, more studies are needed to replicate findings and add to the evidence base before we can draw conclusions on MBI effect sizes and/or mechanisms of change for these behavioral addictions.

Conclusions

In this chapter we discussed MBIs as a transtherapeutic treatment in reducing craving and relapse across substance and behavioral addictions. Specifically, we highlighted commonalities between SUD and BED and summarized the evidence base of treatment outcomes for MBIs applied to both. We also touched on the emerging literature for MBIs being applied to internet gambling, sex, and work addictions. Our review of the literature aligns with previous work that suggests MBIs are on par with other gold standard treatments such as CBT – and in some instances superior (Garland & Howard, 2018). While findings across all MBIs applied to addiction studies are promising for reducing addictions through decreased craving/withdrawal and improved mental/physical health, much more research is needed to replicate findings across diverse samples and identify mechanisms of action. Maintaining high treatment fidelity will be essential for confident interpretations of MBI outcomes and mechanisms of action.

Identifying change mechanisms is warranted in order to pragmatically tailor and deliver the intervention for a variety of populations and settings. We found that MBI literature for SUD treatment incorporated change mechanisms while MBI literature for BED did not. This is likely because of the quantity of research on MBIs for SUDs versus BEDs, which raises the concern that by focusing too narrowly on separate conditions we may overlook transtherapeutic mechanisms that could be applied across conditions. Research identifying mechanisms of maladaptive intake behaviors underlying stress and addiction processes that MBIs target is an important gap to address across fields in order to produce the most robust transtherapeutic effects. To conclude, we discuss emerging theories and research needed to answer questions such as: Which techniques work for which person or addiction type? How does someone know if they are practicing in the "right" way? How do MBIs improve addiction-related behaviors? For whom do MBIs work most optimally to improve addiction-related behaviors?

Many models of stress, addiction, and mindfulness exist (see Avena, 2011; Brewer et al., 2013; Greeson et al., 2014; Lazarus & Folkman, 1984;

Sinha, 2008; Volkow et al., 2011; Witkiewitz et al., 2014). Many of them also share overlapping concepts and ideas across addictive intake behaviors (food and drug) and how mindfulness training cuts across disorder-specific treatments to decouple and liberate people from addiction loops. As discussed previously, one theory posits that two key mindfulness mechanisms of action are acceptance and awareness such that together they produce synergistic and protective effects (Lindsay & Creswell, 2017). Future research should aim to test this theory alongside individual differences to shed light on which skills and for whom are MBIs optimal for improving addiction-related behaviors.

There are a number of pragmatic considerations for enhancing MBI implementation and dissemination. As we discussed throughout this chapter, treatment fidelity includes methods and measures used across the intervention to enhance implementation and testability of the active program ingredients. Standardizing and reporting treatment fidelity methods and measures is an area of needed improvement to enhance confidence in MBI interpretability. The enhancement of this practice will help researchers draw stronger conclusions on concepts such as: How many sessions do participants need to attend to reap optimal benefits? How much and what kinds of daily practice do participants need to engage in to reap optimal benefits? How does one's acceptability of the MBI or quality of home practice impact their outcomes? Utilization of the *Treatment Fidelity Tool for MBIs* (Kechter et al., 2018) may offer a potential solution to the field's inconsistent methods and measures used and reported in MBI research literature.

Additional pragmatic issues relate to treatment sequencing and mindfulness instructors. First, treatment sequencing refers to the assessment of MBI within complex treatments. For example, some participants are receiving a MBI embedded in medication regimen, individual therapy, and other group-based therapy. This examination would allow MBIs to be more prescriptive in the sense that we could individually tailor based on decision rules that dictate how the type or dosing of treatment should change based on the specific clinical needs of the patient. Tools for quality of practice versus quantity of practice may also be developed to provide insight into whether there is a right way or level of requirement in mindfulness practices for better outcomes. Second, mindfulness instructors are often required to be MBSR certified, which can cost more than $10,000 and take approximately three years to complete (Garland & Howard, 2018). While we acknowledge the complexity that goes into proper delivery of a MBI and maintaining a threshold of treatment integrity, this criterion limits the in-clinic treatment fidelity and dissemination. Identifying more efficient ways to train therapists and interventionists is essential to avoid the research-to-practice gap.

The research-to-practice implementation gap refers to when treatments transition from research staff and resources for fidelity procedures to clinical settings without any of this protocol. Often, without knowing the key ingredients and active change mechanisms that need to be delivered, nonresearch clinicians may not deliver the intervention with the same adherence and competence leading to less robust results and/or mixed findings across studies. Research is needed to address the following research questions in order to avoid this implementation cliff. First, identify which techniques for which people/conditions are most robust. Second, identify what degree of training and fidelity is required to produce clinically relevant outcomes while sparing time and resources. Third, examine treatment sequence in clinical settings to determine whether the order in which participants receive an MBI impacts outcomes. And finally, research is needed to examine mindfulness as a long-term, regular, health behavior practice that sustains addiction recovery.

REFERENCES

American Psychiatric Association [APA] (2013). *Diagnostic and Statistical Manual of Mental Disorders* (5th edition). Arlington, VA: American Psychiatric Association.

Avena, N. M. (2011). Food and addiction: implications and relevance to eating disorders and obesity. *Current Drug Abuse Reviews*, **4** (3), 131–132.

Avena, N. M. & Bocarsly, M. E. (2012). Dysregulation of brain reward systems in eating disorders: Neurochemical information from animal models of binge eating, bulimia nervosa, and anorexia nervosa. *Neuropharmacology*, **63**(1), 87–96.

Avena, N. M. & Gold, M. S. (2011). Food and addiction – sugars, fats and hedonic overeating. *Addiction*, **106**(7), 1214–1215. doi:10.1111/j.1360-0443.2011.03373.x

Avena, N. M., Gold, J. A., Kroll, C. & Gold, M. S. (2012). Further developments in the neurobiology of food and addiction: update on the state of the science. *Nutrition*, **28**(4), 341–343. doi:10.1016/j.nut.2011.11.002

Bass, C., Van Nevel, J. & Swart, J. (2014). A comparison between dialectical behavior therapy, mode deactivation therapy, cognitive behavioral therapy, and acceptance and commitment therapy in the treatment of adolescents. *The International Journal of Behavioral Consultation and Therapy*, **9**(2), 4.

Bellg, A. J., Borrelli, B., Resnick, B., et al. (2004). Enhancing treatment fidelity in health behavior change studies: best practices and recommendations from the NIH Behavior Change Consortium. *Health Psychology*, **23**(5), 443–451. doi:10.1037/0278-6133.23.5.443

Black, D. S. (2012). Mindfulness and substance use intervention. *Substance Use & Misuse*, **47** (3), 199–201. doi:10.3109/10826084.2011.635461

Black, D. S. (2014). Mindfulness-based interventions: an antidote to suffering in the context of substance use, misuse, and addiction. *Substance Use & Misuse*, **49**(5), 487–491. doi:10.3109/10826084.2014.860749

Blaszczynski, A., Maccallum, F. & Joukhador, J. (2001). A comparative evaluation of imaginal desensitisation and group cognitive therapy in the treatment of pathological gambling. In G. Coman (Ed.), *Lessons of the Past: Proceedings of the 10th Conference of the National Association for Gambling Studies.* Victoria, Australia: National Association for Gambling Studies, pp. 40–49.

Borrelli, B. (2011). The assessment, monitoring, and enhancement of treatment fidelity in public health clinical trials. *Journal of Public Health Dentistry*, **71**, S52–S63.

Bowen, S., Chawla, N., Collins, S. E., et al. (2009). Mindfulness-based relapse prevention for substance use disorders: a pilot efficacy trial. *Substance Abuse*, **30**(4), 295–305. doi:10.1080/08897070903250084

Breitenstein, S. M., Gross, D., Garvey, C. A., et al. (2010). Implementation fidelity in community-based interventions. *Research in Nursing & Health*, **33**(2), 164–173. doi:10.1002/nur.20373

Brewer, J. A. (2017). *The Craving Mind : From Cigarettes to Smartphones to Love – Why We Get Hooked and How We Can Break Bad Habits*. New Haven: Yale University Press.

Brewer, J. A., Elwafi, H. M. & Davis, J. H. (2013). Craving to quit: psychological models and neurobiological mechanisms of mindfulness training as treatment for addictions. *Psychology of Addictive Behaviors*, **27**(2), 366–379. doi:10.1037/a0028490

Carroll, C., Patterson, M., Wood, S., et al. (2007). A conceptual framework for implementation fidelity. *Implementation Science*, **2**, 40. doi:10.1186/1748-5908-2-40

Christensen, D. R., Dowling, N. A., Jackson, A. C., et al. (2013). A proof of concept for using brief dialectical behavior therapy as a treatment for problem gambling. *Behaviour Change*, **30**, 117–137.

Criscitelli, K. & Avena, N. M. (2016). The neurobiological and behavioral overlaps of nicotine and food addiction. *Preventive Medicine*, **92**, 82–89. doi:10.1016/j.ypmed.2016.08.009

de Lisle, S. M., Dowling, N. A. & Allen, J. S. (2011). Mindfulness-based cognitive therapy for problem gambling. *Clinical Case Studies*, **10**, 210–228.

Garland, E. L. & Howard, M. O. (2018). Mindfulness-based treatment of addiction: current state of the field and envisioning the next wave of research. *Addiction Science & Clinical Practice*, **13**(1), 14. doi:10.1186/s13722-018-0115-3

Garland, E. L., Froeliger, B. & Howard, M. O. (2014a). Mindfulness training targets neurocognitive mechanisms of addiction at the attention-appraisal-emotion interface. *Front Psychiatry*, **4**, 173. doi:10.3389/fpsyt.2013.00173

Garland, E., Gaylord, S. & Park, J. (2009). The role of mindfulness in positive reappraisal. *Explore (NY)*, **5**(1), 37–44. doi:10.1016/j.explore.2008.10.001

Garland, E. L., Manusov, E. G., Froeliger, B., et al. (2014b). Mindfulness-oriented recovery enhancement for chronic pain and prescription opioid misuse: results from an early-stage randomized controlled trial. *Journal of Consulting and Clinical Psychology*, **82**(3), 448–459. doi:10.1037/a0035798

Godfrey, K., Gallo, M. & Afari, L. . (2015). Mindfulness-based interventions for binge eating: A systematic review and meta-analysis. *Journal of Behavioral Medicine*, **38**(2), 348–362.

Gould, L. F., Dariotis, J. K., Greenberg, M. T. & Mendelson, T. (2016). Assessing fidelity of implementation (FOI) for school-based mindfulness and yoga interventions: A systematic review. *Mindfulness (NY)*, **7**(1), 5–33. doi:10.1007/s12671-015-0395-6

Grant, S., Colaiaco, B., Motala, A., et al. (2017). Mindfulness-based relapse prevention for substance use disorders: A systematic review and meta-analysis. *Journal of Addiction Medicine*, **11**(5), 386–396.

Greeson, J., Garland, E. L. & Black, D. S. (2014). Mindfulness: A transtherapeutic approach for transdiagnostic mental processes. In C. T. N. Amanda Ie & E. J. Langer (Eds.), *The Wiley Blackwell Handbook of Mindfulness* (1st edition). John Wiley & Sons, Ltd.

Kabat-Zinn, J. (1982). An outpatient program in behavioral medicine for chronic pain patients based on the practice of mindfulness meditation: Theoretical considerations and preliminary results. *General Hospital Psychiatry*, **4**(1), 33–47. https://doi.org/10.1016/0163-8343(82)90026-3

Kabat-Zinn, J. (2003). Mindfulness-based interventions in context: Past, present, and future. *Clinical Psychology: Science and Practice*, **10**, 144–156.

Kabat-Zinn, J. (2013). *Full Catastrophe Living : Using the Wisdom of Your Body and Mind to Face Stress, Pain, and Illness – Revised and Updated Edition*. New York: Bantam Books.

Katterman, S. N., Kleinman, B. M., Hood, M. M., Nackers, L. M. & Corsica, J. A. (2014). Mindfulness meditation as an intervention for binge eating, emotional eating, and weight loss: A systematic review. *Eating Behaviors*, **15** (2), 197–204.

Kechter, A., Amaro, H. & Black, D. S. (2019). Reporting of treatment fidelity in mindfulness-based intervention trials: A review and new tool using NIH behavior change consortium guidelines. *Mindfulness*, **10**(2), 215–233.

Kelly, T., Yang, W., Chen, C. S., Reynolds, K. & He, J. (2008). Global burden of obesity in 2005 and projections to 2030. *International Journal of Obesity*, **32**(9), 1431–1437. doi:10.1038/ijo.2008.102

Kiecolt-Glaser, J. K. (2010). Stress, food, and inflammation: Psychoneuroimmunology and nutrition at the cutting edge. *Psychosomatic Medicine*, **72**(4), 365–369. doi:10.1097/PSY.0b013e3181dbf489

Kristeller, J. L. & Wolever, R. Q. (2011). Mindfulness-based eating awareness training for treating binge eating disorder: The conceptual foundation. *Eating Disorders*, **19** (1), 49–61. doi:10.1080/10640266.2011.533605

Kristeller, J., Wolever, R. Q. & Sheets, V. (2014). Mindfulness-based eating awareness training (MB-EAT) for binge eating: A randomized clinical trial. *Mindfulness*. http://dx.doi.org/10.1007/s12671-012-0179-1

Lazarus, R. S. & Folkman, S. . (1984). *Stress, Appraisal, and Coping*. New York: Springer.

Leventhal, A. M. & Zvolensky, M. J. (2015). Anxiety, depression, and cigarette smoking: A transdiagnostic vulnerability framework to understanding emotion-smoking comorbidity. *Psychological Bulletin*, **141**(1), 176–212. doi:10.1037/bul0000003

Li, W., Garland, E. L. & Howard, M. O. (2018). Therapeutic mechanisms of Mindfulness-Oriented Recovery Enhancement for internet gaming disorder: Reducing craving and addictive behavior by targeting cognitive processes. *Journal of Addictive Diseases*, **37**, 5–13. doi:10.1080/10550887.2018.1442617

Li, W., Howard, M. O., Garland, E. L., McGovern, P. & Lazar, M. (2017). Mindfulness treatment for substance misuse: A systematic review and meta-analysis. *Journal of Substance Abuse Treatment*, **75**, 62–96.

Lindsay, E. K. & Creswell, J. D. (2017). Mechanisms of mindfulness training: Monitor and Acceptance Theory (MAT). *Clinical Psychology Review*, **51**, 48–59. doi:10.1016/j.cpr.2016.10.011

Maynard, B. R., Wilson, A. N., Labuzienski, E. & Whiting, S. W. (2018). Mindfulness-based approaches in the treatment of disordered gambling: A systematic review and meta-analysis. *Research on Social Work Practice*, **28** (3), 348–362.

Murray, S., Kroll, C. & Avena, N. M. (2015). Food and addiction among the ageing population. *Ageing Research Reviews*, **20**, 79–85. doi:10.1016/j.arr.2014.10.002

Murray, S., Tulloch, A., Gold, M. S. & Avena, N. M. (2014). Hormonal and neural mechanisms of food reward, eating behaviour and obesity. *Nature Reviews Endocrinology*, **10**(9), 540–552. doi:10.1038/nrendo.2014.91

O'Reilly, G., Cook, L., Spruijt-Metz, D. & Black, D. (2014). Mindfulness-based interventions for obesity-related eating behaviours: A literature review. *Obesity Reviews*, **15**(6), 453–461.

Resnick, B., Bellg, A. J., Borrelli, B., et al. (2005). Examples of implementation and evaluation of treatment fidelity in the BCC studies: Where we are and where we need to go. *Annals of Behavioral Medicine*, **29** (Supplement), 46–54. doi:10.1207/s15324796abm2902s_8

SAMHSA (2017). *Behavioral Health Treatments and Services*. Retrieved from https://www.samhsa.gov/treatment

Segal, Z. V., Williams, M. & Teasdale, J. (2018). *Mindfulness-Based Cognitive Therapy for Depression*. Guilford Publications.

Sinha, R. (2008). Chronic stress, drug use, and vulnerability to addiction. *Annals of the New York Academy of Sciences*, **1141**, 105–130.

Sussman, S. (2017). *Substance and Behavioral Addictions: Concepts, Causes, and Cures*. Cambridge, Great Britain: Cambridge University Press.

Sussman, S. & Black, D. S. (2008). Substitute addiction: A concern for researchers and practitioners. *Journal of Drug Education*, **38** (2), 167–180. doi:10.2190/DE.38.2.e

Sussman, S., Reynaud, M., Aubin, H. J. & Leventhal, A. M. (2011). Drug addiction, love, and the higher power. *Evaluation & the Health Professions*, **34**(3), 362–370. doi:10.1177/0163278711401002

Van Gordon, W., Shonin, E., Dunn, T. J., et al. (2017). Meditation awareness training for the treatment of workaholism: A controlled trial. *Journal of Behavioral Addictions*, **6**(2), 212–220. doi:10.1556/2006.6.2017.021

Van Gordon, W., Shonin, E. & Griffiths, M. D. (2016). Meditation awareness training for the treatment of sex addiction: A case study. *Journal of Behavioral Addictions*, **5**(2), 363–372. doi:10.1556/2006.5.2016.034

Volkow, N. D., Wang, G. & Baler, R. D. (2011). Reward, dopamine, and the control of food intake: Implications for obesity. *Trends in Cognitive Sciences*, **15**(1), 37–46.

Warlow, S. M., et al. (2020). Sensitization of incentive salience and the transition to addiction. In S. Sussman (Ed.) *The Cambridge Handbook of Substance and Behavioral Addictions*. Cambridge, UK: Cambridge University Press, pp. 23–37.

Witkiewitz, K. Bowen, S., Harrop, E. N., et al. (2014). Mindfulness-based treatment to prevent addictive behavior relapse: Theoretical models and hypothesized mechanisms of change. *Substance Use & Misuse*, **49**(5), 513–524.

Witkiewitz, K. & Marlatt, G. A. (2005). Emphasis on interpersonal factors in a dynamic model of relapse. *American Psychologist*, **60**(4), 341–342. doi:10.1037/0003-066X.60.4.341

Yau, Y. H. C., Gottlieb, C. D., Krasna, L. C. & Potenza, M. N. (2014). Food addiction – Chapter 7: Evidence, evaluation, and treatment. In *Behavioral Addictions*, pp. 143–184.

34 American Legal Issues in Addiction Treatment and Research

Daniel H. Willick, PhD, JD

Introduction

This chapter addresses legal issues faced by healthcare professionals in the United States who treat addicts or conduct addiction research. It explores the law's competing goals of encouraging treatment and research while also seeking to apprehend addicts engaged in the possession or use of illegal substances, persons who enable such possession or use, and persons engaged in illegal conduct as a result of their addiction.

Legally Relevant Addictions

Before focusing on the competing goals of addiction treatment and apprehension of addicts, it is appropriate to identify three types of addiction which are legally relevant. They are addiction to controlled substances or illegal drugs, alcoholism, and behavioral addictions. Each of these addictions is treated differently by the criminal law and by civil rights law.

The law has long recognized and regulated addiction to illegal drugs and controlled substances by the outright prohibition of the use of illegal drugs and of controlled substances which are procured without a proper prescription. It has also penalized actions, such as driving a vehicle while impaired by drugs. In the case of alcoholism, the law prohibits being drunk in public and operating vehicles while impaired by alcohol. Behavioral addictions were only recognized as a new diagnostic category in 2013 in the American Psychiatric Association *Diagnostic and Statistical Manual of Mental Disorders*, fifth edition (2013) ("DSM-5"). So far, while criminal and civil punishments may be imposed for acts caused by certain behavioral addictions, such as criminal conviction for viewing or possessing pornography due to sexual addiction (*U.S. v. Lighthall*, 2004); loss of a professional license due to the professional's misappropriation of client funds to support a gambling addiction (*In Re: Menna*, 1995); or a mother's loss of child custody due to an internet addiction which resulted in multiple liaisons with men (*Bower v. Bower*, 2000), most behavioral addictions have only achieved limited recognition by the law.

Each of the three types of addiction has received different treatment in the criminal law. In the landmark United States Supreme Court case of *Robinson v. California* (1962), the Court held that the prohibition against cruel and unusual punishment found in the Eighth Amendment of the United States Constitution bars criminal conviction for the diseases or status of drug addiction. This contrasts with the later ruling of the United States Supreme Court in *Powell v. Texas* (1968) that it is permissible under the Eighth Amendment to impose criminal punishment upon a person for being an alcoholic because alcoholism involves the act of drinking rather than the status of addiction. However, there are legal scholars who argue that, in light of modern knowledge of addiction, *Powell* was wrongly decided (M. Slater, 2018). To date, behavioral addiction has not received much legal recognition.

Gambling addiction and sexual addiction have had limited success in mitigating punishment for federal criminal convictions although Federal sentencing guidelines (United States Sentencing Guidelines, Section 5K2.13) permit sentence reduction if "the defendant committed the offense while suffering from a significantly reduced mental capacity... [which] contributed substantially to the commission of the offense." However, such mitigation is not available if the reduced mental capacity was caused by voluntary use of drugs or other intoxicants, if there is a need to protect the public from the defendant's violence, serious threat of violence, or criminal history or if the defendant was convicted of obscenity, sexual abuse, sexual exploitation, or certain other sex crimes. (*Id.*) Gambling addiction justified reduced sentences for criminal convictions for fraud or theft in *U.S. v. Liu* (2003) and *U.S. v. Sadolsky* (2000). However, it was rejected as grounds to reduce criminal sentences in *U.S. v. Carucci* (1999), *U.S. v. Miller* (2006), and *Venezia v. U.S.* (1995). Sexual addiction has achieved limited success in lessening the sentence for a federal crime (*U.S. v. Lighthall*, 2004) and usually is rejected as a basis for sentence mitigation (*U.S. v. Brooks*, 2011; *U.S. v. Caro*, 2002; *U.S. v. Davis*, 2006, *U.S. v. Long*, 2001; and *U.S. v. Romualdi*, 1996).

Drug addiction and alcoholism are granted limited protection under the Americans With Disabilities Act ("ADA") (42 U.S.C. sections 12101, *et seq.*) which protects the civil rights to employment and public accommodations and services to persons suffering from certain disabilities, including mental impairment (42 U.S.C. section 12102(1)(A)). To date, behavioral addictions have not been granted similar protection. State laws, such as California's Unruh Act (California Civil Code sections 51, 51.5) often contain protections like those granted by the ADA.

Under the ADA, a person suffering from drug addiction (42 U.S.C. sections 12210, 12214) may not be discriminated against so long as he or she is no longer engaged in the illegal use of drugs. The ADA also recognizes alcoholism as a protected disability, so long as the alcoholic is not using or under the influence of alcohol while on the job (42 U.S.C. section 12114).

Behavioral addictions appear to be excluded from protection as a disability under the ADA by its exclusion of disability protection for "sexual behavior disorders; ...compulsive gambling, kleptomania, or pyromania" (42 U.S.C. section 12211). It is important to point out that persons diagnosed with a legally relevant addiction, which qualifies for little or no legal protection, may also qualify for more robust protection because they suffer from a cooccurring mental disorder, such as depression, which has protection as a disability under the ADA.

The Competing Goals of Apprehension versus Treatment and Research

The law and government policy, including legislation, regulations, precedential court decisions, and government agency documents, express the competing goals of diagnosis and treatment versus apprehension. For example:

> The laws and regulations governing the confidentiality of substance use disorder records were written out of a great concern about the potential use of substance use disorder information against individuals, causing individuals with substance use disorders not to seek needed treatment.
>
> (82 Federal Register 6053, Confidentiality of Substance Use Disorder Patient Records, 2017).

> Effective psychotherapy. . .depends upon an atmosphere of confidence and trust in which the patient is willing to make a frank and complete disclosure of facts, emotions, memories and fears.
>
> (*Jaffee v. Redmond*, 1996).

> This disclosure of records authorized herein is required for official use including investigation and possible administrative and/or criminal proceedings regarding any violation of the laws of the State of California.
>
> (2018 Authorization For Release Of Alcohol And Drug Abuse Information routinely used by Medical Board of California to obtain patient substance abuse treatment records).

Treatment and research rest on laws protecting confidentiality, privilege, and informed consent, while the apprehension of addicts and others for violation of civil and criminal laws relies on laws mandating or permitting disclosure of otherwise protected addiction treatment and research information. This clash of laws, which is a focus of this chapter, plays out in a legal system where American federal law may conflict with the law of a particular state. Additionally, there often are multiple and sometimes conflicting laws within a state or within federal law. This complexity is intensifying as the political system enacts new laws in reaction to the public's recognition of a drug abuse and addiction crisis with a growing number of drug overdose deaths. The annual totals of drug overdose deaths in the United States were 52,404 in 2015, 63,632 in 2016, and 70,237 in 2017 (Hedegaard, Minino & Warner, 2018; Seth et al., 2018). Each of these numbers easily exceeds the total number of American deaths between 2000 and 2018 due to terrorism and to military combat.

This chapter focuses on the recurrent clash of confidentiality of treatment and apprehension of addicts and their enablers. An awareness of these legal themes is essential to alert a healthcare professional when to seek expert legal advice. The following discussion of laws distills multiple, sometimes conflicting, and often complex legal requirements which are subject to change. It should not be relied on as legal advice.

Relevant Statuses

The law consists of governmentally sanctioned rules for the purpose of regulating human conduct to achieve various goals. Legal rules apply to persons who occupy particular legally recognized statuses. These rules endow each status with certain prerogatives (e.g., rights or privileges), on the one hand, and certain obligations or duties, on the other hand. Two statuses are the focus of the present discussion (i.e., patient and healthcare professional) and are central to confidentiality and disclosure in addiction law.

Patient

A patient, in the context of addiction law, is an individual who is diagnosed or treated for addiction or substance abuse by a licensed healthcare professional. A patient possesses certain legal prerogatives (e.g., rights or privileges), such as the right to confidentiality, established to further the goals of effective diagnosis and treatment. However, those prerogatives are not unlimited and may be overridden when the patient acts or is accused of acting in violation of legal duties or obligations, such as the obligation to refrain from possessing or using an addictive substance which is illegal or illegally obtained. Ironically, a patient's confidentiality may also be breached when the healthcare professional providing care is under investigation for illegal or unprofessional acts or the treatment is not provided by a licensed healthcare professional.[1]

Patient Rights to Confidentiality

The most basic right possessed by a patient, who is treated for addiction, is the right to confidentiality of information about his or her diagnosis, treatment, and communications with each healthcare professional rendering treatment. This right derives from multiple federal laws and multiple state laws. It rests on the proposition, which is supported by empirical research, that a patient is more likely to seek and to remain in treatment when assured of the confidentiality of that treatment (Surgeon General of the United States, 1999).

The basic federal statute protecting the confidentiality of substance disorder diagnosis and treatment is 42 U.S.C. section 290dd-2, subsection (a) which states: "(a) Requirement. Records of the identity, diagnosis, prognosis, or treatment of any patient which are maintained in connection with the performance of any program or activity relating to substance abuse education, prevention, training, treatment, rehabilitation, or research, which is conducted, regulated, or directly or indirectly assisted by any department or agency of the United States shall, except as provided in subsection (e), be confidential and be disclosed only for the purposes and under the circumstances expressly authorized under subsection (b)." Subsection (e) exempts the exchange of information within or between the armed services or the Department of Veterans Affairs from confidentiality protection. Subsection (b) permits disclosure with patient written consent for a medical emergency, for research or program evaluation or by court order to avert a substantial risk of death or serious bodily harm. There are detailed federal regulations implementing the requirement of confidentiality (42 C.F.R. Part 2).

The federal law provides for confidentiality of substance disorder diagnosis and treatment records for most addiction treatment. There are two requirements for the obligation of confidentiality to apply to such records maintained by a healthcare professional. First, the healthcare professional must be considered a "program" covered by the law. Second, the professional must be "directly or indirectly" federally assisted.

A healthcare professional meets the definition of a covered program "if it is an individual or entity that holds itself out as providing, and provides, alcohol or drug abuse diagnosis, treatment, or referral for treatment" (SAMHSA, 2017). A professional is federally assisted if he or she prescribes controlled substances to treat substance abuse disorders pursuant to a Drug Enforcement Administration ("DEA") license (SAMHSA, 2017).

Exceptions to confidentiality are quite limited (42 U.S.C. section 290dd-2, subsection (b)). Disclosure may be authorized by the patient; may be authorized by a court upon a showing of good cause to avert "a substantial risk of death or serious bodily harm" (42 U.S.C. section

[1] The law does <u>not</u> protect information shared in Alcoholics Anonymous sessions from disclosure in court because the treatment provided is not from a licensed healthcare professional (*Cox v. Miller*, 2002).

290dd-2, subsection (b)(2)(C)); and otherwise may not occur in criminal proceedings (42 U.S.C. section 290dd-2, subsection (c)). Furthermore, "no State law may authorize any disclosure prohibited" by federal law (42 C.F.R. section 2.20). However, state laws which are more protective of confidentiality than federal law will be enforced (*Id.*).

Unfortunately, multiple laws may come into play as to confidential treatment information regarding substance abuse, addiction, and related healthcare. For example, the following federal laws and regulations may apply in addition to the federal law identified above:

(1) Privacy regulations (45 C.F.R. Parts 160 and 164) promulgated under the authority of the Health Insurance Portability and Accountability Act (42 U.S.C. sections 1320d, et seq.), commonly referred to as "HIPAA."
(2) The psychotherapist-patient privilege which protects confidential psychotherapist-patient communications and records from disclosure in judicial proceedings (*Jaffee v. Redmond*, 1996).
(3) The federal Constitutional right to privacy (*Roe v. Wade*, 1973, *Whalen v. Roe*, 1977).

California provides an illustration of the myriad of state laws which may impact healthcare records of the diagnosis or treatment of addiction. Like federal law, California has laws which provide special protections for the confidentiality of records of alcohol or drug abuse diagnosis or treatment (California Health and Safety Code sections 11812, 11845.5). If the care involves the expenditure of County funds, disclosure requires authorization by the patient plus the consent of the attending healthcare professional (California Health and Safety Code section 11812(c), California Welfare and Institutions Code section 5328(a)(2)). Records of care which are regulated by the State may only be released if there is a Court order after an application showing probable cause (California Health and Safety Code section 11845.5(c)(5),(d)). As of 2018, there is scant or no Court guidance on the interpretation of these laws.

In addition to the California state laws protecting the confidentiality of alcohol and drug abuse records, there are a number of other California laws concerning the confidentiality of diagnosis and treatment records which may come into play, including:

(1) Confidentiality of Medical Information Act (California Civil Code sections 56.10, 56.104).
(2) Insurance Information and Privacy Protective Act (California Insurance Code sections 791.01-791.22).
(3) Patient Access To Health Records (California Health and Safety Code sections 123100-123149.5).
(4) Lanterman, Petris, Short Act confidentiality provisions (California Welfare and Institutions Code sections 5328-5330).
(5) Physician-patient privilege (California Evidence Code sections 990-1007).
(6) Psychotherapist--patient privilege (California Evidence Code sections 1010-1027).
(7) Constitutional Right to Privacy (California Constitution, Article I, section 1).

Healthcare Professional

A healthcare professional is a person licensed by state law to provide care or to conduct research regarding addiction within the scope of that license. The license is a prerogative, which is a privilege, granted by state law and regulated by state agencies. The privilege to prescribe controlled substances is subject to federal regulation.

Treatment or research concerning addiction or substance abuse may involve many different categories of healthcare professionals licensed by the state, such as physician, psychologist, marriage and family therapist, social worker, professional counselor, addiction counselor, nurse, nurse practitioner, or physician's assistant. These professionals are authorized by their state-issued license to render certain types of treatment and are restricted from providing care in excess what their license or other legal rules authorize. For example, therapies to treat addiction which rely on the use of medication (e.g., treatment of opioid addiction through the prescription of methadone or Suboxone) require that the treating healthcare professional possesses a state-issued license authorizing the prescription of the treatment medications and, if those medications are controlled substances, possesses an appropriate federal Drug Enforcement Administration (DEA) registration (21 U.S.C. sections 822, 823, 824).

A central principle of treatment is that the healthcare professional providing treatment must obtain the patient's informed consent to the care proposed to be rendered. Not only does this involve a discussion with the patient of risks and benefits, but it should also involve disclosure of when confidentiality of treatment may or may not occur.

Healthcare professionals are obligated by state and federal law to maintain the confidentiality of information about persons who are diagnosed or treated for a disease or medical condition, such as addiction. The laws cited above, which establish a patient's right to confidentiality, and which make patient-provider communications privileged and confidential, necessarily create an obligation on the part of the healthcare professional to protect that confidentiality and privilege. Sometimes penalties may accrue to professionals who breach confidentiality. For example, HIPAA permits the federal government or state government to take legal action, including the imposition of fines, against healthcare professionals who breach HIPAA's privacy regulations by the unauthorized disclosure of a patient's protected health information (42 U.S.C. section 300gg-22). However, a patient does not have the right to bring a lawsuit or to seek damages for a breach of HIPAA confidentiality (*Webb v. Smart Document Solutions, LLC*, 2007). Nevertheless, state law may authorize a lawsuit by a patient for damages based on a breach of the patient's right to medical privacy. (See, e.g., California Civil Code section 56.35.)

Recent Legal Reforms to Address the Addiction Crisis

First, a brief review of legal reforms which address America's crisis of addiction to prescription drugs is presented. Next, the conflict between laws encouraging treatment of addiction by protecting confidentiality and laws which breach confidentiality to assist in the apprehension of addicts and their enablers is discussed.

The SUPPORT Act

In 2018, in a rare instance of bipartisanship, Congress passed the "Substance Use Disorder Prevention That Promotes Opioid Recovery And Treatment For Patients And Communities Act" ("the SUPPORT Act"). The SUPPORT Act was promptly signed by the President as Public Law No. 115-271. It nationalizes and coordinates federal and State efforts to fight opioid addiction. Provisions of the SUPPORT Act (PL No. 115-271):

(1) Initiate changes in the Medicare and Medicaid programs to expand prevention and treatment of opioid addiction through measures, such as innovative use of telemedicine and expanded use of

medication assisted treatment using buprenorphine (PL No. 115-271, sections 6031-6032).

(2) Prohibit kickbacks for referrals of patients in addiction treatment to recovery homes, clinical treatment facilities, and laboratories (*id.*, section 8122).
(3) Encourage the testing of treatment models for behavioral health care (*id.*, section 6001).
(4) Support and coordinate effective prescription drug monitoring programs (PDMP) in all fifty states (*id.*, sections 5041-5042).

Prescription Drug Monitoring Programs

With federal encouragement and support (42 U.S.C. section 280g-3), every state in the United States has adopted a prescription drug monitoring program (PDMP). A PDMP is an electronic database which collects information on all prescription of addictive medication without the consent of patients or prescribing physicians (Unger, 2014).

All programs monitor at least [DEA rated] Schedule II drugs [which are the most dangerous and addictive drugs that may be prescribed]. . .. Almost all programs authorize both prescribers (doctors) and dispensers (pharmacists) to use and access the information. Almost all programs also authorize law enforcement to use the program to obtain evidence in criminal [and civil licensing] investigations, but states vary with regard to the scope of access afforded to law enforcement.

(*Id.*, p. 350.)

A good description of the various PDMPs has been published by the National Alliance for Model State Drug Laws (2014). Recent reforms have expanded PDMPs to include prescribing by veterinarians, optometrists, and other providers who prescribe addictive medications (Petersen et al., 2018). The SUPPORT Act provides federal funding of state-operated PDMPs and encourages data-sharing among PDMPs. (PL No. 115-271, sections 5041-5042.)

Mandatory and Advisory Practice Guidelines

In 2016, the federal Centers for Disease Control and Prevention (CDC) issued guidelines for the prescribing of opioids to treat pain (CDC, 2016). The CDC Guidelines recommended lower doses of opioids to treat chronic pain and a detailed risk-benefit analysis before prescribing opioids for chronic pain. Such prescribing is to be followed by ongoing monitoring. Various states, such as Oregon and Virginia, have adopted versions of the CDC Guidelines as mandatory treatment requirements (Petersen et al., 2018).

Among the mandatory requirements adopted in some states is a requirement for healthcare professionals to check the PDMP before and after prescribing controlled substances to a patient (*id.*, California Health and Safety Code section 11165.4). This is for the purpose of determining if the patient is "doctor shopping" to obtain excessive addictive medications.

Another treatment directive which may be adopted by a state is the requirement that a healthcare professional who prescribes an opioid or treats a patient at risk of opioid overdose must offer to prescribe naloxone or another FDA-approved drug for reversal of opioid overdose (California Business and Professions Code sections 740-742).

These new governmental guidelines restricting prescriptions of opioids stand in marked contrast to governmental guidelines and law enacted in the 1990s and early 2000s. The earlier guidelines and law encouraged use of opioids to treat intractable pain (California Business and Professions Code section 2241.5; Medical Board of California 2010).

Conflicting Legal Goals

Effective Treatment Based on Confidentiality and Informed Consent. Protection of confidentiality in the treatment of addiction stems from the legal recognition of the use of psychotherapeutic techniques and psychotherapists in rendering that treatment. Confidentiality is necessary and legally protected because of the belief that effective treatment is:

dependent upon the fullest revelation of the most intimate and embarrassing details of the patient's life. . .. Unless a patient. . .is assured that such information can and will be held in utmost confidence, he will be reluctant to make the full disclosure upon which diagnosis and treatment. . .depends. . .. Although it is recognized that the granting of the [psychotherapist-patient] privilege may operate in particular cases to withheld relevant information, the interests of society will be better served if psychiatrists [and other psychotherapists] are able to assure patients that their confidences are protected.

(*People v. Gonzales*, 2013.)

The purest expression of the principle is that effective treatment of addiction must rest on the "absolute right of confidentiality." Bollas and Sundelson (1995), in their book *The New Informants: The Betrayal of Confidentiality in Psychoanalysis and Psychotherapy*, clearly articulate this principle in lamenting and opposing any exceptions to confidentiality which the law has permitted. For example, they argue (Bollas & Sundelson, 1995, p. 176) that mandatory reporting to the authorities of child abuse or the required reporting of a patient's serious threat of violence against a third party compromises the confidentiality and hence the effectiveness of treatment:

It is more effective to get an abusing parent into treatment and to have the other members of the family seen immediately by fellow practitioners than to call in the police. A patient who is intending to harm another person is not by any means beyond his psychoanalyst's remedial action. A psychoanalyst can, if in his view it is warranted, have a patient committed or sectioned in the hospital if the person is a threat to himself or others. . .. By exercising his judgment he [the psychotherapist] can act with a greater range of options than he can under the current reporting laws, which mandate reporting to the police and lead only to incarceration.

Reporting of possible addiction and addiction treatment has become pervasive in the mandatory disclosure through PDMPs to law enforcement of the use of addictive medications and of many medications used to treat addiction. Furthermore, the healthcare professional providing addiction treatment may be required or permitted to breach confidentiality to protect third persons or the patient, if the patient is a danger to others or a danger to self (*Tarasoff v. Regents of the University of California*, 1976, California Civil Code sections 43.92, 56.10(c)(19)). These disclosures call into question the assurance of confidentiality which, as explained above, presumably underlies treatment of addiction. Indeed, these disclosures raise the issue of whether a proper balance of disclosure and confidentiality may ever be achieved.

Effective Apprehension of Lawbreakers: The Government's Right to Confidential Information. An obvious question is how to reconcile mandatory monitoring by PDMPs with the requirement of confidentiality which is deemed to be crucial for effective treatment of addiction and substance abuse. While the Courts have not yet definitively addressed this issue, they have upheld PDMPs as not violating the federal constitutional right to privacy (*Whalen v. Roe*, 1977) and have permitted state agencies to use PDMPs to monitor the prescription of addictive medications without notice to or the consent of the involved patients or the prescribing physician (*Lewis v. Superior Court*, 2017).

Lewis v. Superior Court (2017) is particularly instructive in revealing the logic a court might use to justify use of a PDMP by government to apprehend addicts and healthcare professionals who improperly prescribe addictive drugs. In *Lewis v. Superior Court* (2017), the California Supreme Court ruled that, notwithstanding California's Constitutional Right To Privacy, the Medical Board of California, the state agency which licenses physicians, was empowered to access California's PDMP to monitor, collect, and use over 200 pages of a physician's prescribing records to prosecute the physician in an administrative proceeding for his alleged unsafe prescribing. This access was permitted although neither the physician nor his patients knew of, or authorized, disclosure of their prescriptions or treatment records. The Court ruled this was proper based upon the complaint of one patient about a matter unrelated to the physician's prescribing practices. The investigation of the physician's prescribing was initiated because a patient complained that the physician had rudely encouraged her to undertake a particular weight-loss program. The Medical Board of California used the PDMP to identify five patients where it questioned the safety of the physician's prescribing. It then obtained authorizations from three of the five patients for release of the physician's full medical records and enforced subpoenas to obtain the records of the two other patients who did not authorize disclosure. Although the Medical Board of California failed to obtain a finding in the administrative proceeding that the physician had engaged in unsafe prescribing for any patient, it sustained disciplinary actions against the physician for negligent patient care and failure to maintain adequate records.

The California Supreme Court ruled that the Medical Board of California's use of the PDMP to review a physician's prescribing, without the knowledge of the involved patients, and successfully to subpoena other treatment records, without the authorization of involved patients, was an invasion of privacy "justified by the state's dual interest in protecting the public from the unlawful use and diversion of a particularly dangerous class of prescription drugs and protecting patients from negligent or incompetent physicians" (*Lewis v. Superior Court*, 2017, p. 572).

Since *Lewis v. Superior Court* (2017) did not involve the treatment of addiction, the open question is whether the law permits addiction treatment records to be disclosed without the patient's authorization, notwithstanding the patient's Constitutional right to privacy, as well as the federal and state statutes providing for the confidentiality of substance abuse diagnosis and treatment (e.g., 42 U.S.C. section 290dd-2; California Health and Safety Code sections 11812, 11845.5). However, regardless of the answer to this question, it is undisputed that PDMPs presently can and are being used by law enforcement to identify patients being treated for addiction with opioids (i.e., methadone, buprenorphine) and to identify the physicians prescribing that treatment. The open question is whether such PDMP data may be used to investigate and prosecute the addicts receiving this treatment, notwithstanding the Fourth Amendment of the US Constitution, which limits unreasonable search and seizure, or under similar state constitutional restrictions of search and seizure, such as Article I, Section 13 of the California Constitution. A related issue is whether patients will be less likely to seek treatment for addiction using therapeutic opioids, such as methadone and buprenorphine, because the government will learn of their addiction and treatment through mandatory reports to a PDMP.

What Is the Proper Legal Balance of Treatment and Apprehension of Addicts? The law continues to grapple with the issue of how to resolve the competing values of patient confidentiality to encourage treatment of addiction and disclosure of addiction treatment information to the government to assist in apprehension of addicts and healthcare professionals who facilitate addiction. Relevant considerations in resolving this clash of values include:

(1) Whether fear of disclosure of treatment for addiction discourages addicts from seeking treatment.
(2) Whether disclosure of addiction treatment will result in criminal prosecution of the addict who is receiving treatment or result in encouragement of diversion to a treatment program, successful completion of which will avoid criminal prosecution.
(3) The resolution of these issues ultimately depends on the balance struck between criminal law, with its incarceration, other punishments, and stigmatization, and civil law, with its use of diversion without the stigma of criminal conviction. Which type of law will be used as the predominant means to deter and to treat addiction?

As the costs of mass incarceration for drug crimes and the spread of addiction to all social strata have become more apparent, there is a movement to rely less on criminal punishment to deal with the epidemic of addiction. However, the increase of effective and immediate identification of addicts, including those in treatment, due to the use of computers and electronic data processing using PDMPs, means there is increased detection, with the possibility of criminal prosecution, of addicts in treatment. How these conflicting issues and trends will be resolved is far from clear.

Conflicting Roles for Healthcare Professionals

Treatment or Apprehension?

The tension between the conflicting legal goals of treatment or apprehension creates difficult choices for a healthcare professional in obtaining informed consent to addiction treatment or in choosing to provide such treatment. Given the lack of certainty over whether, or to what extent, the government is entitled to obtain addiction treatment records, by means other than information available on a PDMP, healthcare professionals rendering addiction treatment face difficult and often unresolved issues.

First, there is the question of what to disclose to a patient entering addiction treatment about the confidentiality of his or her treatment records. Given that there is a significant probability that a patient entering addiction treatment has engaged in behavior which might be characterized as criminal (e.g., use of illegal substances; obtaining prescription medications through questionable means; driving while under the influence), the treating healthcare professional has an ethical obligation to disclose the risk that the government will breach the patient's confidentiality and obtain treatment records. Such a disclosure should include a warning that treatment by methadone or buprenorphine will be reported to a PDMP along with the patient's identity. If possible, the custom and practice of government agencies to prosecute patients in treatment for addiction using treatment records or to use treatment records to trigger other investigational techniques should be disclosed. Another situation to be discussed as part of informed consent is that a treating healthcare professional may disclose otherwise confidential information about addiction treatment to other persons, including the government, if the patient is a danger to self or to others as a result of his addiction (*Tarasoff v. Regents of the University of California*, 1976, California Civil Code sections 43.92, 56.10(c)(19)). In other words, there is a strong basis to conclude medical ethics requires such disclosure when obtaining a patient's informed consent to addiction treatment.

Second, given the risk of treatment records being obtained by prosecutors, the treating healthcare professional must decide whether to include any admissions of illegal criminal behavior in the patient's treatment records. Although in virtually all jurisdictions there is an obligation to keep adequate treatment records, an argument can be made that it is not prudent to include a patient's admission of criminal behavior in those records, unless there is a requirement of mandatory reporting of the risk of behaviors that are dangerous to self or others, and are the result of addictive drugs. Competent care may also require a healthcare professional to include evidence of a patient's illegal acts in the medical record, such as when a pregnant patient is addicted to heroin, and it is important to document this in the medical record to alert other healthcare professionals treating the patient, the fetus or the infant.

Third, there is the question of how a treating healthcare professional should respond to a government subpoena for a patient's addiction treatment records. Sometimes, such subpoenas are issued as part of a licensing investigation of the treating healthcare professional. In any event, ethics and the law in many jurisdictions may require the healthcare professional to object to the subpoena based on privilege or confidentiality of substance abuse treatment records. (See, e.g., California Evidence Code sections 995, 1015.)

Fourth, addiction treatment may be imposed as part of a diversion program, such as diversion in lieu of criminal prosecution or diversion at the direction of a licensing board. If so, the diversion program itself may be conditioned on disclosure of otherwise confidential treatment information as a condition of the diversion.

Fifth, addiction treatment provided to persons convicted of crimes by government employed or approved healthcare professionals frequently involves disclosure to the government of treatment records. Is there any confidentiality in such treatment? For example, in California, certain classes of convicted sex offenders are required to participate in psychotherapy as a condition of probation with their psychotherapists required to share therapy information with the parole officer and to assist polygraph examiners with the administration of periodic lie detector tests of the patient (*People v. Ignacio Garcia*, 2017; California Penal Code section 1203.067, subd.(b)(3)).

Finally, there should be concern that the considerations described above will dissuade many healthcare professionals from choosing to provide addiction treatment. For those who choose to provide such treatment, a careful weighing out of costs and benefits may be made on a case-by-case basis due to legal considerations.

Healthcare Professionals in Treatment

Healthcare professionals who have been treated for addiction or substance abuse present an interesting problem. Title II of the American With Disabilities Act (42 U.S.C. section 12132) prohibits state healthcare licensing boards from discriminating against persons, including healthcare professionals, with a past diagnosis and successful treatment for substance abuse and for a mental health disorder (*Hason v. Medical Board of California*, 2002). This is because a history of mental health diagnosis or treatment does not mean that a healthcare professional is presently impaired such that he or she is or will be unable to practice the healthcare profession competently. While it may be appropriate to inquire into whether the healthcare professional's present use of addictive drugs or mental illness impairs present or future ability to practice their profession, it is not proper to inquire into past diagnosis, addiction, or treatment (*id.*, American Psychiatric Association, 2018). An American Psychiatric Association (APA) position statement (2018) makes the point as follows:

> [T]he APA believes that prior diagnosis and treatment of a mental disorder are, *per se*, not relevant to the question of current impairment and that oversight entities should not include questions about past diagnosis and treatment of a mental disorder as a component of a general screening inquiry.

Nevertheless, licensing boards and other entities which screen healthcare professionals, such as insurers and hospital medical staffs, may continue to make such general inquiries. So long as such practices continue, there will be an incentive for healthcare professionals who have addiction issues to avoid treatment. The issue stated bluntly is whether it is appropriate or legally permissible for the adage "once an addict, always an addict" to be relevant in licensing and credentialing decisions.

A more difficult situation is presented where the addiction treatment is being rendered to a healthcare professional who is continuing to practice and is so impaired that he is a danger to his patients. In such a situation, the healthcare professional who is providing addiction treatment is arguably compelled to breach confidentiality to seek government assistance to protect the patients of the addicted healthcare professional (*Tarasoff v. Regents of the University of California*, 1976, California Civil Code section 56.10(c)(19)). Similarly, a breach of confidentiality could be required if the addicted healthcare professional is a danger to himself, including if he is suicidal.

Addiction Research

The laws governing human research, including addiction research, rest on three fundamental ethical principles identified in the Belmont Report (1979):

> Respect for persons acknowledges human subjects' autonomy and requires consent as a prerequisite to research. Beneficence obliges researchers to maximize benefits to society while minimizing risks of harm to human subjects. Justice demands fairness in balancing the benefits conferred and burdens imposed through research. Even with modern advances in research and technology, these ethical principles remain valid
>
> (Azim, 2018, p. 1708, footnotes omitted).

Operationalization of these three fundamental principles has proven to be a challenge. Unfortunately, the laws governing addiction research are as complex as, or more complex than, the laws governing the confidentiality of addiction treatment. There are at least three sets of federal laws regarding research (the new Common Rule of the federal Department of Health and Human Services and at least sixteen other federal agencies, the Food and Drug Administration's research rules, and the research provisions of HIPAA Privacy Rule). Additionally, many states have laws governing research. On top of the laws governing research are the laws, discussed earlier in this chapter, providing for privacy and confidentiality of treatment, which may impact addiction research, which involves treatment of research subjects.

The following federal laws govern research:

(1) The new Common Rule (45 C.F.R. Part 46) is a "Federal Policy for the Protection of Human Subjects" which is being implemented by no less than seventeen federal agencies, each of which has promulgated its own regulations adopting the rule's provisions.
(2) The federal Food and Drug Administration has its own longstanding regulations (21 C.F.R. Parts 50 and 56) which differ in limited but significant respects from the new Common Rule.
(3) The federal HIPAA privacy regulations (45 C.F.R. Parts 160 and 164) have specific provisions applicable to research privacy protections (45 C.F.R. sections 164.508, 164.512).

States may have enacted laws dealing with research. For example, California has the following laws related to research. Some of these laws have particular applicability to addiction research:

(1) California Health and Safety Code sections 11480-11481 concern the process for approval of research concerning cannabis or hallucinogenic drugs.
(2) California Health and Safety Code sections 24170-24179.5 concern human experimentation and set forth requirements to protect the rights of human subjects in medical experiments, including requiring informed consent.
(3) California Health and Safety Code sections 111515-111545 concern research involving the experimental use of drugs, including the need for approval by an Institutional Review Board and obtaining informed consent of research subjects.
(4) California Penal Code sections 3500 and 3521-3523 concern research with prisoners as research subjects and require that they have rights comparable to other research subjects.

Uncertainty over the phased implementation of the new Common Rule, the interaction between the various federal laws, the interaction between state law and federal law and which law preempts when there is a conflict between laws, has created a complex legal landscape.

A taste of the myriad of complexities involved in navigating the various laws governing human research is found in the following discussion by a federal Secretary of Health and Human Services committee of the new Common Rule's loosening of HIPAA privacy protections for "secondary research":

> The application of this new exemption – like the application of HIPAA itself – is complex, and without sufficient guidance, research institutions, IRBs [Institutional Review Boards], and the general public may have difficulty understanding the circumstances under which the HIPAA Exemption may and may not be relied upon as an exemption from Common Rule requirements. Understanding the contours of the HIPAA Exemption will be significant for researchers involved in secondary research activities, particularly records research, as investigators conducting research activities that qualify for the exemption will be permitted to forego the requirement of securing IRB approval and informed consent (traditional informed consent, or 'broad consent') or waiver of consent for such secondary research
>
> (Secretary's Advisory Committee On Human Research Protections, 2017).

The Committee goes on to justify the new "complex" exemption as "predicated on an understanding that when both HIPAA and the Common Rule apply to specific human subjects research activities, the overlapping regulatory requirements can lead to confusion, duplicative review, and extra burden on the researcher and his or her institution." (*Id.*) Given the complicated and changing rules governing addiction research, the best advice for a healthcare professional conducting addiction research is to conduct that research in a setting, such as a research university, where there are institutional supports to assist with compliance with the rules.

Conclusions

The addiction crisis has resulted in significant and ongoing changes in the law. This chapter identifies significant legal issues which are at the center of these changes with the hope that this will assist healthcare professionals and other interested persons involved in addiction treatment or research in navigating the complex and shifting legal currents by identifying areas of legal concern and knowing when to seek expert advice.

REFERENCES

American Psychiatric Association (2013). *Diagnostic and Statistical Manual of Mental Disorders* (5th edition). Arlington: American Psychiatric Association.

American Psychiatric Association (2018). *Position Statement on Inquiries about Diagnosis and Treatment of Mental Disorders in Connection with Professional Credentialing and Licensing.*

Americans with Disabilities Act, 42 U.S.C. sections 12101, *et seq.*, 12102(1)(A), 12114, 12210, 12211, 12214.

Azim, A. (2018). Note: Common sense; Rethinking the new Common Rule's weak protections for human subjects. *Vanderbilt Law Review*, **71**, 1704–1736.

Belmont Report (1979). National Commission for the Protection of Human Subjects of Biomedical and Behavioral Research. *The Belmont Report: Ethical Principles and Guidelines for the Protection of Human Subjects of Research.* www.hhs.gov/ohrp/sites/default/files/the-belmont-report-508c_Final.pdf.

Bollas, C. & Sundelson, D. (1995) *The New Informants: The Betrayal of Confidentiality in Psychoanalysis and Psychotherapy.* Northvale, N.J.: Jason Aronson, Inc.

Bower v. Bower, 758 So.2d 405 (Miss. 2000).

California Business and Professions Code sections 740-742, 2241.5.

California Civil Code sections 43.92, 51, 51.5, 56.10(c)(19), 56.104, 56.35.

California Confidentiality of Medical Information Act, Civil Code sections 56.10(c)(19), 56.104, 56.35.

California Constitution, Article I, sections 1 and 13.

California Evidence Code sections 990-1007. Physician-patient privilege.

California Evidence Code sections 995, 1015.

California Evidence Code sections 1010-1027. Psychotherapist-patient privilege.

California Health and Safety Code sections 11165.4, 11480-11481, 11812, 11845.5, 24170-24179.5, 111515-111545, 123100-123149.5.

California Insurance Code sections 791.01-791.22. California Insurance Information And Privacy Protection Act.

California Penal Code sections 1203.067(b)(3), 3500, 3521-3523.

California Welfare and Institutions Code section 5328-5330. Lanterman, Petris, Short Act confidentiality provisions.

Centers for Disease Control and Prevention (2016), *Guideline for Prescribing Opioids for Chronic Pain.* www.cdc.gov/drugoverdose/pdf/Guidelines_Factsheet-a.pdf.

Cox v. Miller, 296 F.3d 89 (2d Cir. 2002).

Hason v. Medical Board of California, 279 F.3d 1167 (9th Cir. 2002).

Hedegaard, H., Minino, A. & Warner, M. (2018). *Drug Overdose Deaths in the United States, 1999–2017. National Center for Health Statistics Data Brief* No. 329, Nov. 2018. www.cdc.gov/nchs/products/databriefs/db329.htm.

In Re: Menna, 11 Cal.4th 975 (1995).

Jaffee v. Redmond, 116 S.Ct. 1923 (1996).

Lewis v. Superior Court, 3 Cal.5th 561 (2017).

Medical Board of California (2010). *Guidelines for Prescribing Controlled Substances for Pain.*

Medical Board of California (2018). *Authorization for Release of Alcohol and Drug Abuse Information.*

National Alliance for Model State Drug Laws (2014) *Prescription Drug Abuse, Addiction and Diversion, Part 1.* www.namsdl.org/library/884CB2C5-1372-636C-DD54DCC00FD31313/.

People v. Ignacio Garcia, 2 Cal.5th 792 (2017).

People v. Gonzales, 56 Cal.4th 353, 371-372 (2013).

Petersen, A., Peters, S. C., Richard, M. H. & Whites, A. (2018). State legislative responses to the opioid crisis: Leading examples. *Journal of Health & Life Sciences Law*, Feb. 2018, **11**, 30.

Powell v. Texas, 392 U.S. 514 (1968).

Robinson v. California, 370 U.S. 660 (1962).

Roe v. Wade, 410 U.S. 113, 93 S.Ct. 705 (1973).

SAMHSA (2017). *Substance Abuse Confidentiality Regulations, Frequently Asked Questions (FAQs regarding the Substance Abuse Confidentiality Regulations).* September 15, 2017. www.samhsa.gov/about-us/who-we-are/laws-regulations/confidentiality-regulations.htm.

Secretary's Advisory Committee on Human Research Protection (SACHRP) (2017). Attachment B to December 12, 2017, *SACHRP Letter to the HHS Secretary Recommendations on the Interpretation and Application of Exemption §_.104(d)(4), the "HIPAA Exemption".* www.hhs.gov/ohrp/sachrp-committee/recommendations/attachment-b-december-12-2017/index.html.

Seth, P., Scholl, L., Rudd, R. & Bacon, S. (2018). Overdose deaths involving opioids, cocaine, and psychostimulants in United States, 2015–2016. *Centers for Disease Control and Prevention, Morbidity, Mortality Weekly Report*, March 30, 2018, **67**(12), 349–358. www.cdc.gov/mmur/volume/67/wr/mm6712al.htm.

Slater, M. (2018) Note: Is *Powell* still valid? The Supreme Court's changing stance on cruel and unusual punishment. *Virginia Law Review*, **104**, 547–588.

SUPPORT ACT (Public Law No. 115-271).

Surgeon General of the United States (1999). *Mental Health – A Report of the Surgeon General*, Chapter 7, pp. 440–441. https://profiles.nlm.nih.gov/ps/access/NNBBHS.pdf.

Tarasoff v. Regents of the University of California, 17 Cal.3d 425 (1976).

Unger, D. (2014). Student note: Minding your meds: Balancing the needs for patient privacy and law enforcement in prescription drug monitoring programs. *West Virginia Law Review*, **117**, 345–388.

United States Constitution, Fourth Amendment, Eighth Amendment.

United States Sentencing Guidelines (2004) Section 5K2.13.

U.S. v. Brooks, 628 F.3d 79 (6th Cir. 2011).

U.S. v. Caro, 309 F.3d 1348 (11th Cir. 2002).

U.S. v. Carucci, 33 F.Supp.2d 302 (S.D.N.Y. 1999).

U.S. v. Davis, 182 Fed.Appx. 741 (9th Cir. 2006).

U.S. v. Lighthall, 389 F.3d 791 (8th Cir. 2004).

U.S. v. Liu, 267 F.Supp.2d 371 (E.D.N.Y. 2003).

U.S. v. Miller, 178 Fed.Appx. 70 (2d Cir. 2006).

U.S. v. Long, 185 F.Supp.2d 30 (D.D.C. 2001).

U.S. v. Romualdi, 101 F.3d 971 (3d Cir. 1996).

U.S. v. Sadolsky, 234 F.3d 938 (6th Cir. 2000).

Venezia v. U.S., 884 F.Supp. 919 (D.N.J. 1995) affd. without opin., 77 F.3d 465 (3d Cir. 1995).

Webb v. Smart Document Solutions, LLC, 499 F.3d 1078, 1081 (9th Cir. 2007).

Whalen v. Roe, 429 U.S. 589, 97 S.Ct. 869 (1977).

21 C.F.R. Parts 50 and 56.

21 U.S.C. sections 822-824.

42 C.F.R. Part 2.

42 U.S.C. section 280g-3.

42 U.S.C. section 290dd-2.

42 U.S.C. section 300gg-22.

42 U.S.C. sections 1320d, et seq.

42 U.S.C section 12132.

45 C.F.R. Part 46.

45 C.F.R. Parts 160 and 164.

45 C.F.R. sections 164.508 and 164.512.

82 Federal Register 6053, Confidentiality of Substance Use Disorder Patient Records (2017).

Index